Scott-Brown's Otolaryngology

Sixth edition

Paediatric Otolaryngology

Scott-Brown's Otolaryngology

Sixth edition

General Editor

Alan G. Kerr FRCS

Consultant Otolaryngologist, Royal Victoria Hospital, Belfast and Belfast City Hospital;
Formerly Professor of Otorhinolaryngology, The Queen's University, Belfast

Other volumes

1 **Basic Sciences** *edited by* Michael Gleeson

2 **Adult Audiology** *edited by* Dafydd Stephens

3 **Otology** *edited by* John B. Booth

4 **Rhinology** *edited by* Ian S. Mackay and T. R. Bull

5 **Laryngology and Head and Neck Surgery** *edited by* John Hibbert

Paediatric Otolaryngology

Editors

David A. Adams BSc, MSc, FRCS(Ed)

Senior Lecturer, Department of Otorhinolaryngology, Queen's University, Belfast

Michael J. Cinnamond FRCS(Ed), FRCSI

Professor, Department of Otorhinolaryngology, Queens University, Belfast

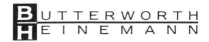

BUTTERWORTH
HEINEMANN

Butterworth-Heinemann
Linacre House, Jordan Hill, Oxford OX2 8DP
A division of Reed Educational and Professional Publishing Ltd

 A member of the Reed Elsevier plc group

OXFORD   BOSTON   JOHANNESBURG
MELBOURNE   NEW DELHI   SINGAPORE

First published 1952
Second edition 1965
Third edition 1971
Fourth edition 1979
Fifth edition 1987
Sixth edition 1997

British Library Cataloguing in Publication Data
A catalogue record for this book is
available from the British Library

Library of Congress Cataloguing in Publication Data
A catalogue record for this book is
available from the Library of Congress

ISBN 0 7506 0595 2 (Volume 1)
     0 7506 0596 0 (Volume 2)
     0 7506 0597 9 (Volume 3)
     0 7506 0598 7 (Volume 4)
     0 7506 0599 5 (Volume 5)
     0 7506 0600 2 (Volume 6)
     0 7506 1935 X (set of six volumes)
     0 7506 2368 3 (Butterworth-Heinemann International Edition, set of six volumes)

Printed and bound in Great Britain by Bath Press, Bath

Contents

vi   *Contents*

Colour plates in this volume

Between pages 6/19/30 and 6/19/31 (continued)

Plate 6/19/II Photographs of 'before and after' lip repair using the Millard technique. (*a*) Unilateral cleft of lip and palate at birth; (*b*) cleft lip repaired at 3 months old. The lip scar is quite red and raised; (*c*) unilateral cleft lip and palate at birth; (*d*) at 2 years and 6 months the old lip scar has flattened and paled becoming less obvious

Plate 6/23/I Microlaryngoscopy showing (*a*) mucosal ulceration of the vocal cords and right false cord 24 hours after intubation for ventilatory support for respiratory distress; (*b*) granulation tissue filling the glottis in front of the endotracheal tube; (*c*) a fibrous subglottic stenosis; (*d*) mild congenital subglottic stenosis; (*e*) severe congenital subglottic stenosis; (*f*) mucus retention cysts after intubation; (*g*) post-mortem specimen showing an abnormally thick cricoid and hyperplasia of the submucosa (courtesy of Mr R. Pracy); (*h*) interarytenoid fixation

Contributors to this volume

David A. Adams BSc, MSc, FRCS(Ed)
Senior Lecturer, Department of
Otorhinolaryngology, Queen's University, Belfast

David Albert FRCS
Consultant Otolaryngologist, The Hospitals for Sick
Children, Great Ormond Street, London

C. M. Bailey BSc, FRCS
Consultant Otolaryngologist, The Hospitals for Sick
Children, Great Ormond Street, London and Royal
National Throat, Nose and Ear Hospital, London

E. F. Battersby MB ChB, DA, FFARCS
Formerly Consultant Anaesthetist, The Hospitals for
Sick Children, Great Ormond Street, London

S. Bellman FRCSI
Consultant Audiological Physician, The Hospitals
for Sick Children, Great Ormond Street, London

Alexander W. Blayney MCh, FRCS(Lond), FRCSI
Consultant Otolaryngologist, University College
Dublin, The Mater and The Children's Hospitals,
Dublin

P. J. Bradley MB, BCh, BAO, DCH, FRCS(Ir), FRCS(Ed)
Consultant Otolaryngologist/Head and Neck
Oncologist, University Hospital, Queen's Medical
Centre, Nottingham

Michael J. Cinnamond FRCS(Ed), FRCSI
Professor, Department of Otorhinolaryngology, The
Queen's University, Belfast

R. Corbett MRCP
Consultant Paediatric Oncologist, Christchurch
Hospital, Christchurch, New Zealand

David L. Cowan MB, ChB, FRCS(Ed)
Consultant Otolaryngologist and Honorary Senior
Lecturer, City Hospital and Royal Hospital for Sick
Children, Edinburgh

C. B. Croft MB, FRCS, FRCS(Ed)
Consultant Otolaryngologist, Royal National
Throat, Nose and Ear Hospital, London

R. Dinwiddie MB, FRCP, DCH
Consultant Paediatrician, The Hospitals for Sick
Children, Great Ormond Street, London

P. D. M. Ellis MA, FRCS
Consultant ENT Surgeon, Addenbrooke's Hospital,
Cambridge

J. N. G. Evans MB, BS, DLO, FRCS
Consultant Ear, Nose and Throat Surgeon, The
Hospitals for Sick Children, Great Ormond Street,
London

Andrew P. Freeland MB, BS, FRCS
Consultant Otolaryngologist, Radcliffe Infirmary,
Oxford

Kevin P. Gibbin MA, MB, BChir, FRCS
Consultant Otolaryngologist, University Hospital,
Queen's Medical Centre, Nottingham

Roger F. Gray FRCS
Consultant ENT Surgeon, Department of
Otolaryngology, Addenbrooke's Hospital, Cambridge

Terry Gregg FDS
Consultant Paediatric Dental Surgeon, School of
Dentistry, Royal Victoria Hospital, Belfast

John Hibbert MA, ChM, FRCS
Consultant ENT Surgeon, Guy's Hospital, London

David R. James FRCS(Ed), FDSRCS(Eng)
Consultant Oral and Maxillofacial Surgeon, Centre
for Craniofacial Anomalies, The Hospitals for Sick
Children, Great Ormond Street, London

Barry McCormick PhD
Consultant Audiological Scientist, Professor and
Director, Children's Hearing Assessment Centre,
Nottingham

A. Richard Maw MB, BS(Lond), FRCS, MS
Consultant Otolaryngologist, Bristol Royal
Infirmary and Royal Hospital for Sick Children,
Bristol; Clinical Lecturer and Head of Department of
Otolaryngology, University of Bristol

P. D. Phelps MD, FRCS, FFR, FRCR, DMRD
Consultant Radiologist, Royal National Throat, Nose
and Ear Hospital, London

P. N. Plowman MA, MD, MRCP, FRCP
Consultant Oncologist, The Hospitals for Sick
Children, Great Ormond Street, London

J. Pritchard FRCP
Consultant Oncologist, The Hospitals for Sick
Children, Great Ormond Street, London

David W. Proops BDS, MB, ChB, FRCS
Consultant ENT Surgeon, The University Hospital
and The Children's Hospital, Birmingham; Honorary
Senior Lecturer, University of Birmingham

Peter Ramsay-Baggs BDS, MB, BCh, BAO, FDSRCS(Eng),
FFDRCSI, FRCS(Ed)
Consultant Oral and Maxillofacial Surgeon, The
Ulster Hospital, Dundonald and The Royal Victoria
Hospital, Belfast

William Reardon MD, MRCPI, DCH
Honorary Senior Registrar in Medical Genetics,
Institute of Child Health, London

Andrew Richardson MSc, BDS, DPD, DOrth, FFD
Professor, Orthodontic Division, School of Clinical
Dentistry, Royal Victoria Hospital, Belfast

J. H. Rogers MA, BM, BCh, FRCS, DLO
Consultant Ear, Nose and Throat Surgeon, Royal
Liverpool Hospital and The Royal Liverpool
Children's NHS Trust, Liverpool

Lewis Spitz MB, CHB, PhD, FRCS(Edin), FRCS(Eng), FAAP
Nuffield Professor of Paediatric Surgery, The
Hospitals for Sick Children, Great Ormond Street,
London

Sylvia Thompson RegMCSLT, MSc, MSc(Clin.Aud)
Senior Speech and Language Therapist, Christie
Brown Centre, Tralee, Eire

I. Vanniasegaram MSc, FRCS
Consultant Audiological Physician, Barking
Havering and Brentwood Community Health Care
NHS Trust; Honorary Consultant Audiological
Physician, The Hospitals for Sick Children, Great
Ormond Street, London

A. P. Walby FRCS(Ed)
Consultant Otolaryngologist, Royal Victoria
Hospital, Belfast

Rosalind Wilson RGN, RSCN
Ward Sister, Royal National Throat, Nose and Ear
Hospital, London

Introduction

When I started work on this Sixth Edition I did so in the belief that my experience with the Fifth Edition would make it straightforward. I was wrong. The production of the Fifth Edition was hectic and the available time short. The contributors and volume editors were very productive and in under two and a half years we produced what we, and happily most reviewers, considered to be a worthwhile academic work. On this occasion, with a similar team, we allowed ourselves more time and yet have struggled to produce in four years. One is tempted to blame the health service reforms but that would be unfair. They may have contributed but the problems were certainly much wider than these.

The volume editors, already fully committed clinically, have again been outstanding both in their work and in their understanding of the difficulties we have encountered. Once again there was an excellent social spirit among the editors. They have been very tolerant of the innumerable telephone calls and it has always been a pleasure to work with them. The contributors have also been consistently pleasant to deal with, even those who kept us waiting.

There have been technical problems in the production of this work and I want to pay tribute to the patience of all those who suffered under these, not least the publishing staff at Butterworth-Heinemann. One of the solutions to the problems has been the use of a system of pagination that I consider to be ugly and inefficient for the user and I wish to apologize in advance for this. Unfortunately anything else would have resulted in undue delay in the publication date.

Medicine is a conservative profession and many of us dislike change. Some will feel that we have moved forward in that most Latin plurals have been replaced by English, for example we now have polyps rather than polypi. We have also buried acoustic neuromata, with an appropriate headstone, and now talk about vestibular schwannomas. It has taken about two decades for this to become established in otological circles and may take even longer again, to gain everyday usage in the world of general medicine.

I am pleased with what has been produced. Some chapters have altered very little because there have been few advances in those subjects and we have resisted the temptation of change for change's sake. There have been big strides forward in other areas and these have been reflected in the appropriate chapters.

Despite, and because of, the problems in the production of these volumes, the staff at Butterworth-Heinemann have worked hard and have always been pleasant to deal with. I wish to acknowledge the co-operation from Geoff Smaldon, Deena Burgess, Anne Powell, Mary Seager and Chris Jarvis.

It would be impossible to name all those others who have helped, especially my colleagues in Belfast, but I want to pay tribute to the forbearance of my wife Paddy who graciously accepted the long hours that were needed for this work.

As I stated in my introduction to the Fifth Edition, I was very impressed by the goodwill and generosity of spirit among my Otolaryngological colleagues and am pleased that there has been no evidence of any diminution of this during the nine years between the editions. I remain pleased and proud to be a British Otolaryngologist and to have been entrusted with the production of this latest edition of our standard textbook.

Alan G. Kerr

Preface

In his preface to the Fifth Edition John Evans pointed out that Paediatric Otolaryngology is now an established branch of the specialty, so justifying a separate volume in this standard text. In this edition we have, out of necessity, changed about half the contributors, but not the overall style of the book. We would, therefore, wish to acknowledge John Evans' role in laying the strong foundations which have made our task much easier.

We are grateful to all those who have written chapters in this book, especially those who did so at relatively short notice. We were encouraged by the willingness of all to contribute their expertise and time in doing so.

Several authors did express concern that, of necessity, a book such as this is dated by the time of publication. No blame for this, however, can be attached to Alan Kerr who has gently bullied us since 'honouring' us with the editorship of this volume. We are grateful to Alan for his support, guidance and patience.

Our secretary, Deirdre McGrath, has provided invaluable help on many occasions.

We are pleased to pay tribute to our wives and families for their tolerance and understanding during the preparation of this book. We are grateful to two registrars, Robin Adair and Peter Leyden, for undertaking the difficult task of proofreading in the final stages.

Finally, this volume could not have been finished without considerable help and support from Butterworth–Heinemann, the publishers. It has been reassuring always to be able to pick up the telephone and get immediate advice.

David A. Adams
Michael J. Cinnamond

1

Improving the paediatric otolaryngological consultation

David Albert

Imagine an adult otolaryngological consultation in which the patient arrived with four relatives, of whom two were in wheelchairs, one was screaming and the other announced she wanted to go to the toilet just as you were about to look at the patient. Next, the patient had to be cajoled into an examination but just as you were finishing, pulled all your instruments on the floor. While this may seem extreme, paediatric otolaryngological clinics can easily turn into this kind of nightmare with stressed parents and doctors and precious little time or peace for any discussion about treatment options. To be controversial I could suggest that the percentage of paediatric patients being offered surgery might vary inversely with the time available to the surgeon and the overall tranquillity of the clinic. As an important part of routine paediatric otolaryngology is to reassure parents that surgery is often not necessary, it is clearly vital that clinics are planned so that this is possible.

Making life easy for yourself even before you see the patient

If one is working in a resource-constrained environment, the most that may be achievable is to conduct a paediatric otolaryngological clinic in a paediatric, rather than otolaryngological setting as this is much more likely to have been designed with the child in mind. Few are likely to have the opportunity to design a paediatric otolaryngological clinic from scratch, but the following points about the physical layout of the clinic area should be useful in any discussions about upgrading existing space to provide a more child-friendly environment. The aim is to make the visit a pleasant experience for child and parent alike, with a more rewarding and efficient consultation for both sides.

Special facilities required for paediatric clinics

Inexperienced hospital planners often forget that children's clinics need *more* rather than *less* space to accommodate the various buggies, siblings, nannies and grandparents that often accompany the patient. Space needs also to be put aside for baby feeding and changing rooms and this is now included in most hospital quality standards. While it is important to design the clinic time-table to avoid delay *as much as possible*, some waiting is inevitable. A play room or play area is essential for the smaller children with television, video or computers for the older children. Toys should be available for children of all ages. This does not have to be anything elaborate and, indeed, merely providing paper, pencils and/or colouring books is a huge step forward from expecting children to sit quietly in the waiting room. Some system of informing parents of the length of delay is also useful so that they can plan trips to the toilet and drinks machine (or the other way around).

Clinic room layout

Ideally the doctor should be able to greet the family as they enter the consultation room and should therefore be seated facing the door. A traditional arrangement across a desk is rather confrontational and it is often better therefore to have the desk along the side of the room so that the doctor can move freely from the desk area to the examination area. Right-handed surgeons would have the desk on the right as they look at the parents and child. If the surgeon uses a wheeled chair this allows for easy movement from examination to hospital notes. The child should not be hemmed into one corner of the room. It is important to consider space for buggies and also a small play area both to observe the patient and to occupy siblings. The play area should be close to the mother so that the child feels secure but not too distant from the doctor so that the child becomes accustomed to the doctor's presence prior to examination. Similarly when the child moves to the examination area, the mother as well as the doctor needs to be close. The nurse, if present, should be able to switch roles between occupying the patient and siblings to helping with the examination.

Equipment

As vast arrays of complex equipment and daunting instruments can be off putting to children, a compact examination trolley that combines suction, examination lamp, fibreoptic light source and otoscope with drawers for instruments is a useful starting point in designing a paediatric otolaryngological consultation room. Only a small proportion of available instruments should be on view such as the otoscope tips and tongue depressors which will be used for every patient. It is safer and less threatening to use an electric mirror warmer rather than a spirit lamp and while it is rather bulky, the immediate access to correctly warmed mirrors that it provides does encourage examination of the postnasal space in children. Similarly, while it is easier in some children to use a microscope with them lying down, the convenience of having a microscope immediately available with the child sitting in the normal examination chair, does allow microscopic examination of the tympanic membrane in more children. Surprisingly, children tolerate microscopic suction clearance remarkably well sitting on the examination chair and supported from behind by a nurse or parent.

Optimizing the consultation

History taking

Younger children and siblings should be settled into distractive play by the clinic nurse, so that the parents can give their attention to telling their story. Airway obstruction in small children, suspected hearing loss, speech delay and repeated infections are all scenarios that are understandably accompanied by parental anxiety. The golden rule is to believe the parents unless and until you can legitimately reassure them that all is well. Parents are usually the best witnesses to the child's problem, but also ask the child if appropriate.

Examination

While taking the history from the parent, assess the child's airway, play and general alertness. If the child is uneasy proceed slowly because once the child's confidence is lost it may take a long time to recover.

Smaller children should be examined on a parent's lap for reassurance and this will also allow gentle positioning if needed. Let the child touch the instruments and avoid sudden movements. Explain what is about to happen, especially if it may be uncomfortable.

Ear examination

Small children should sit sideways on the parent's lap with one arm cuddling the child and controlling the arms while supporting the child's head against the chest with the other hand. The position is reversed for examination of the other ear. Older children can be encouraged to put the contralateral ear on their shoulder affording the surgeon an excellent head position for otoscopy. The pinna is pulled posteriorly to straighten the external canal in both infants and children, the otoscope tip is then gently inserted and steadied by the little finger against the child's face. In neonates the membrane lies obliquely, distorting the normal appearances. Otoscopy in this age group should thus be interpreted carefully so as not to diagnose wrongly otitis media in a sick neonate. Children of all ages will accept gentle removal of wax and foreign bodies, though will need to be reassured about the strange looking headmirror.

Pneumatic otoscopy produces a rather unexpected and strange sensation in children; explanation is essential if you want to test both ears! For pneumatic otoscopy to be reliable an airtight seal needs to made with the ear canal using special ear speculae. If these are not available, tympanic mobility is better assessed with tympanometry. Accurate diagrams of the tympanic membrane are not only essential for good serial records but are also helpful to explain disease to the parents.

The gold standard for paediatric otoscopy is a video-camera attached to a short Hopkins rod or to a purpose-designed otoscope and speculum combined. The view with a video-otoscope (Figure 1.1) (Jedmed

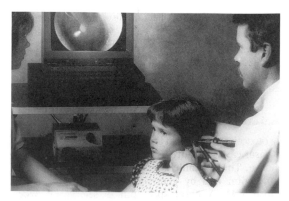

Figure 1.1 Video-otoscope

Instrument Company, England) is comparable to conventional otoscopy but allows accurate records to be kept as video-prints. The view on the monitor encourages children to participate in examination and makes explanations to parents quicker and more convincing.

Testing for mastoid tenderness does require the good ear to be examined first as otherwise the reliability can be poor. Mastoiditis has often been treated with broad-spectrum antibiotics masking the clinical signs, though if a laterally displaced ear (Figure 1.2) is present the diagnosis is seldom in doubt. Look for evidence of skin disease if otitis externa or histiocytosis is suspected. If bat ears are found as an incidental finding, it is probably best not to ask if these are a concern, or at least discuss this finding with the parent out of earshot of the child.

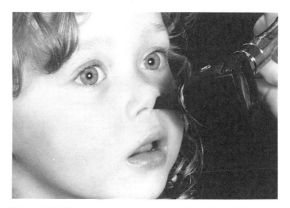

Figure 1.3 The otoscope gives an excellent view of the paediatric nasal cavity

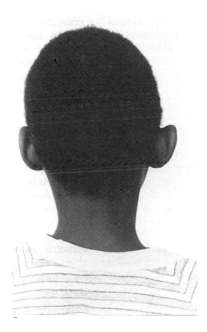

Figure 1.2 Mastoiditis with laterally displaced pinna

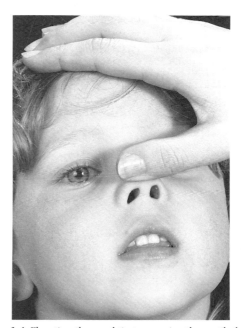

Figure 1.4 Elevating the nasal tip to examine the vestibule without the need for a speculum

Informal clinic testing of hearing and tuning fork tests are notoriously unreliable in younger children and are no substitute for experienced paediatric audiological assessment.

Nasal examination

The otoscope provides an excellent view of the paediatric nasal cavity (Figure 1.3) and is well tolerated by children. The vestibule is examined with headmirror illumination and by gently elevating the nasal tip (Figure 1.4). A nasal speculum is seldom, if ever required and is poorly tolerated. It is important to

remember that what may seem like a cosmetically unattractive nose may grow into a well proportioned nose in time.

If topical anaesthesia is required for cautery or nasendoscopy, a cotton wool pledget sparingly soaked in 10% cocaine provides excellent vasoconstriction and anaesthesia in 5–10 minutes, though it is easy to exceed recommended doses. A spray delivers a smaller dose but is less well tolerated and achieves less vasoconstriction. Topical cocaine makes foreign body removal from the nose much easier and eliminates the need for general anaesthesia in almost all cases.

Throat examination

This should be kept till last as it is the least well tolerated. A wooden tongue depressor is much less threatening than a cold metal spatula. Be gentle, once the child has gagged, even the thought of an approaching spatula will produce further gagging. As in much of paediatric examination the first time is always the best. It takes no time to lose a child's confidence but forever to regain that lost trust.

Postnasal examination with a 12–14 mm mirror is possible in two-thirds of 5 year olds, though merely visualizing the adenoids does not necessarily help assess obstruction. Most 5 year olds will cooperate with indirect laryngoscopy but the view obtained is often inadequate because of the posteriorly placed epiglottis.

Neck examination

Remember to palpate the neck but remember also that cervical adenopathy (Figure 1.5) is a common incidental finding in children. Cystic hygroma (Figure 1.6) in the neck often extends into the floor of mouth

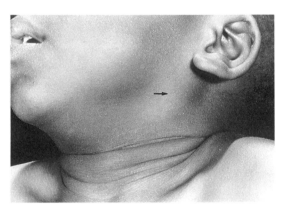

Figure 1.5 Cervical adenopathy; the history may be more important than the clinical findings

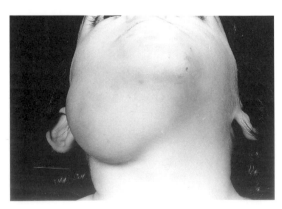

Figure 1.6 Cystic hygroma

so palpate this area bimanually. The classic position for a branchial cyst (Figure 1.7) is one-third of the way down the anterior border of sternomastoid. Thyroglossal cysts (Figure 1.8) typically lie just to the left of the midline in the anterior neck. In children it is often difficult to demonstrate elevation on tongue protrusion.

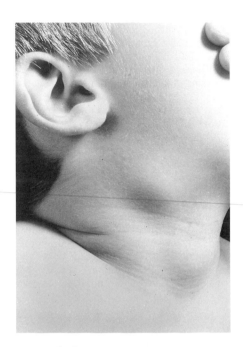

Figure 1.7 Branchial cyst

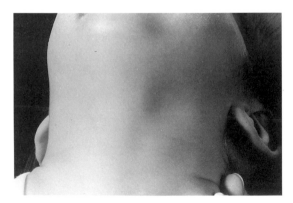

Figure 1.8 Thyroglossal cyst

General examination

By assessing the child as a whole, important diagnostic pointers will not be missed such as syndromic features, general skin disease, cavernous haemangiomas or a pectus excavatum. Particular conditions will be suggested by the history and an extended examination will then be necessary. The cranial nerves can be tested in older children who can also perform most tests of balance.

Discussing the findings

It comes as something of a surprise to some surgeons that parents are actually interested in your findings in their child. A moment's explanation as you examine the child will help later when discussing treatment. Diagrams are useful as well as printed notes or booklets on common conditions.

Investigation

Investigations are generally unnecessary in the common childhood otolaryngological conditions such as adenotonsillar hypertrophy, allergic rhinitis and recurrent tonsillitis. One notable exception is the need for accurate audiometric assessment for the multitude of young patients attending otolaryngological clinics with otitis media with effusion. Particularly in children, invasive investigations should be used only if they will alter the management for the child. Rare but important conditions however must not be missed, even if the presentation may seem unremark-able. Lymphoma may present as unexceptional cervical lymphadenopathy and an angiofibroma usually presents as nasal obstruction and epistaxis.

In a more specialist paediatric otolaryngological practice, careful audit of investigations should determine a cost-benefit analysis for investigations which have become 'routine' without accurate appraisal.

Discussing management

This is what the parents have come to hear – your opinion. Some parents will come merely expecting confirmation that surgery is required and have little interest in complex explanations. Others will favour a more conservative approach and will need every detail explained and every therapeutic option explored.

The surgeon's views may not coincide with the parents', but it is better to be forewarned and then to offer a number of options with the advantages outlined for each. Surgeons should remember that it is rare for there to be only one option available and the indications for surgery are seldom absolute. The public perception of otolaryngological surgeons has been marred by criticism of decision making for routine paediatric operations. It is up to us to put our house in order and ensure that this decision making is beyond reproach.

2

Radiology in paediatric otolaryngology

P. D. Phelps

The principles of technique which apply to imaging in adults apply equally to the demonstration of head and neck lesions in infants and children. Optimum spatial and density resolution with the lowest possible level of patient irradiation and freedom from movement artefacts must be achieved. Limitation of radiation dose is particularly important in this age group, and minimal patient movement is hard to obtain. Consequently, many of the more sophisticated modes of imaging such as xerography, conventional tomography and computerized tomography (CT) are used less in the younger age group and most imaging assessments rely on plain films. However, the role of CT continues to increase and, with scan times of a few seconds possible on the latest machines, these examinations can now usually be performed without sedation.

Upper respiratory tract

Air within the structures of the upper respiratory tract provides a natural contrast medium for the accurate delineation and evaluation of the adjacent soft tissues of the neck. Most of these assessments are made on the lateral neck film obtained during inspiration with the neck partially extended. Additional views can be employed as the need arises and radiology can often provide information as to the specific cause of airway obstruction and to its site. Well-coned frontal and lateral films are obtained; inspiratory and expiratory films may be needed in each projection to reveal the abnormality fully.

The prevertebral soft tissues and the airway in general are extremely pliable in infants and with expiration and flexion of the neck a wide variety of

distortions and bizarre appearances can result; these are discussed in Chapter 24. High kilovoltage techniques with special filters in the X-ray beam can give detailed radiographs of the upper airway with reduced radiation dose. Such techniques obviate the need for xerography. Although xerography can give an enhanced demonstration of the air-soft tissue interface (Figure 2.1), the radiation dose is higher, and the technique is no longer used.

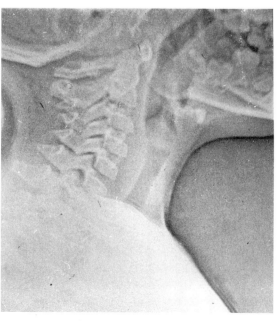

Figure 2.1 Lateral neck xerogram in a child. Note the high position of the larynx

Inflammatory disease of the pharynx, larynx and epiglottis are common causes of upper respiratory obstruction and potentially very serious. Radiological examination is rarely necessary to demonstrate these conditions directly but is needed to exclude pulmonary disease. A soft tissue lateral view of the neck may show soft tissue swelling of the larynx and can reveal the extent of a retropharyngeal abscess (see Figure 24.6).

Conventional tomography is particularly useful in the frontal projection for showing subglottic stenosis and webs (Figure 2.2). It can be combined with CT to assess congenital abnormalities such as vascular rings or developmental cysts which cause stridor by distortion of the trachea at a lower level (Figure 2.3).

Magnetic resonance imaging is replacing CT for the investigation of the upper aerodigestive tract in the paediatric age group. It has two distinct advantages: no ionizing radiation is involved and imaging can be carried out in any plane. Sagittal views are particularly useful especially in congenital

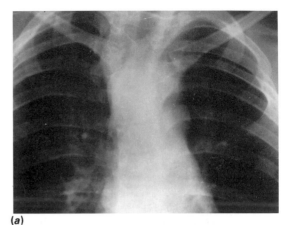

(a)

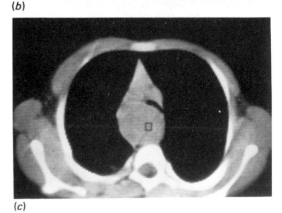

(b)

(c)

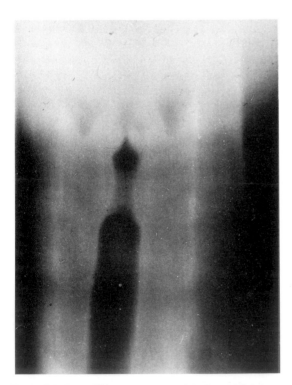

Figure 2.2 Frontal linear tomogram of the larynx showing subglottic stenosis. Note the vocal cords in full adduction

Figure 2.3 A child with stridor due to a mediastinal tracheal duplication cyst. (*a*) Chest radiograph shows an ill-defined midline soft tissue mass and a vertebral anomaly at the same level. The presence of such a congenital osseous abnormality suggests that the soft tissue lesion may also be of congenital origin; (*b*) lateral tomogram shows the cyst indenting and narrowing the trachea from behind; (*c*) axial CT shows the round cyst at the level of the right main bronchus which is slightly compressed. Attenuation values in the area depicted by the square confirmed a cyst

abnormalities causing stridor (Figure 2.4). Some of these, which may be difficult to assess clinically or by other imaging methods, are often well shown (Figure 2.5).

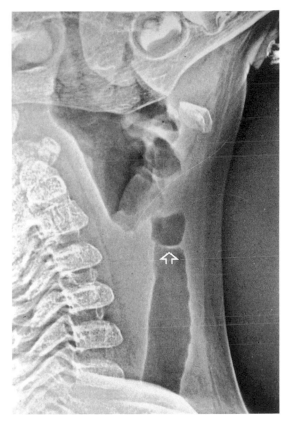

Figure 2.4 Sagittal magnetic resonance view showing a subglottic web (arrow)

Barium studies

Barium swallow and meal are little used for pharyngeal abnormalities but have an important application for various well-known adult disorders which can occur in children. Achalasia of the cardia is usually diagnosed by imaging as is hiatus hernia or oesophageal stricture and ulceration which may result from it (Figure 2.6).

Face and sinuses

The sinuses are present in the infant and can become infected. At birth small antra and ethmoids can be demonstrated radiologically. The frontal and sphe-

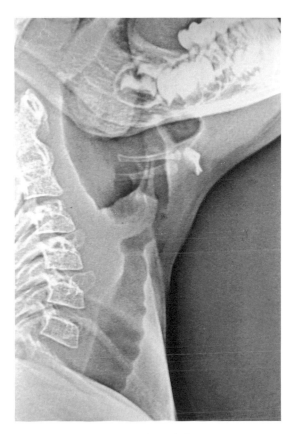

Figure 2.5 Sagittal MRI reveals a subglottic stenosis

noid sinuses develop later. The lateral view does not present any problem, but proper positioning is essential to show infant sinuses. The most important plain film sinus view in the adult is the occipitomental with the baseline at 45° to the plane of the film (see Volume 4). In the older child this angle must be decreased to about 28° or the projection will be too steep for proper evaluation of the maxillary antra. In the infant the angle must be even less so that the view is almost a posteroanterior view. Radiographically the findings of sinusitis vary according to age but, as in the adult, loss of the normal radiolucency usually indicates disease. As well as the loss of normal aeration, more specific features such as mucosal thickening and fluid levels may be recognized (Figure 2.7). A mucocoele from obstruction of the sinus ostium is rare in children, and is best demonstrated by sectional imaging (Figure 2.8).

Choanal atresia

Choanal atresia is the commonest congenital abnormality of the nose but it cannot be demonstrated by

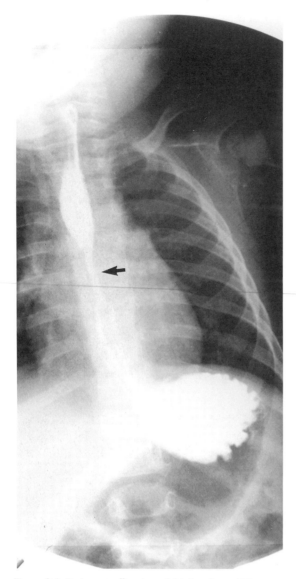

Figure 2.6 Barium swallow in a child showing a sliding type of hiatus hernia with a stricture above it (arrow)

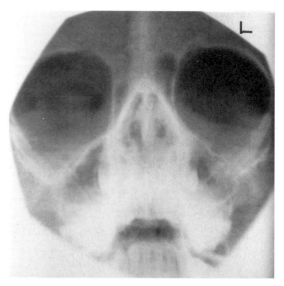

Figure 2.7 Occipitomental view of the sinuses. There is mucosal thickening in the left antrum. The frontal sinuses are unformed

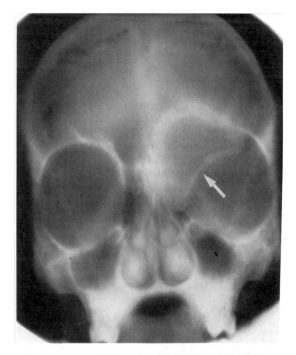

Figure 2.8 Expansile lesion depressing the roof of the orbit (arrow). Hypocycloidal coronal section tomogram

plain film views. Formerly contrast medium was instilled into the nose and a plain lateral view obtained to show the site of obstruction. Now, however, axial CT is the investigation of choice and will show bony or membranous atresia (Figure 2.9). Bilateral atresias are usually diagnosed soon after birth. It is most important that adequate preparation by suction of the nasal cavities is undertaken immediately prior to scanning. Choanal atresia is often combined with other congenital anomalies as in the CHARGE (**c**oloboma, **h**eart disease, **a**tresia of choanae, **r**etarded growth, **g**enital hypoplasia, **e**ar abnormalities) association.

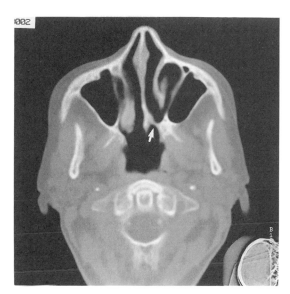

Figure 2.9 Axial CT scan showing unilateral choanal atresia (arrow)

Developmental mass lesions

Developmental mass lesions affecting the upper respiratory tract include meningoencephalocoeles and arachnoid or dermoid cysts. Encephalocoeles occur in the midline in the nasofrontal and nasoethmoidal regions (Figure 2.10). Although they may be demonstrated by conventional imaging techniques, CT scanning is the investigation of choice. This is particularly so for the much rarer lateral protrusions through the base of the skull. They may present as masses in the infratemporal fossa which subsequently expand and bulge into the aerodigestive tract (Figure 2.11). Dehiscences in the skull base occur with neurofibromatosis and defects in the back of the orbit may result in proptosis (Figure 2.12).

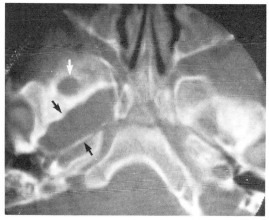

(*a*)

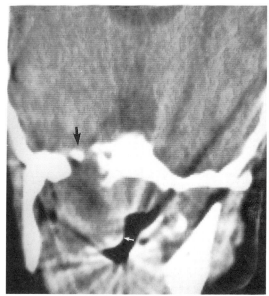

(*b*)

Figure 2.11 (*a*) Axial, (*b*) coronal CT scans showing a large meningocoele protruding through a grossly widened sphenopetrosal suture (black arrows) and bulging into the nasopharynx (small white arrow). Note the enlargement of the ipsilateral foramen ovale and the low attenuation within the mass

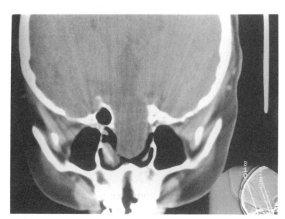

Figure 2.10 Coronal CT showing a large midline meningoencephalocoele

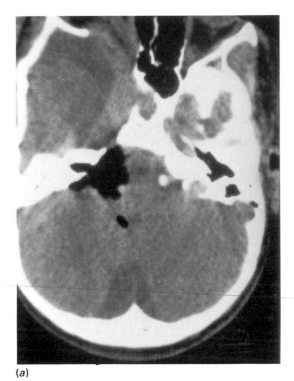

(a)

Magnetic resonance has few advantages over CT but can differentiate meningocoele from encephalocoele by showing that the mass contains either CSF or brain (Figure 2.13). Other midline masses are nasal gliomas which probably have a common origin with meningoencephalocoeles and nasal dermoids. Although these are demonstrated best by MRI, there are some potential diagnostic pitfalls (Barkovich *et al.*, 1991), in particular the normal fat deposition that occurs in the developing skull base structures (Figure 2.14).

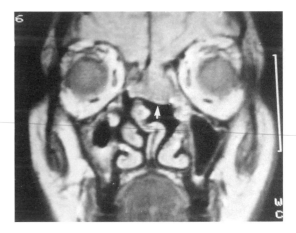

Figure 2.13 Coronal MR section shows a midline encephalocoele (arrow)

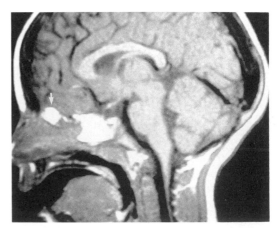

Figure 2.14 A normal T1-weighted sagittal MR section showing high signal from fat in the basisphenoid and crista galli (arrow)

(b)

Figure 2.12 (*a*) Axial CT section on a patient with neurofibromatosis and deficient floor of the middle cranial fossa and back of the orbit. The patient was deaf, and the air meatogram examination was performed to exclude an acoustic neuroma. (*b*) The encephalocoele (asterisk) appears as a soft tissue mass in the infratemporal fossa

Inflammatory disease of the sinuses

Acute inflammation of the sinuses is uncommon in children but can lead to serious intraorbital and intracranial complications. Young people still lose vision in an eye from orbital cellulitis and, although most cases recover after antibiotic therapy, adequate drainage of the infected sinuses may be necessary. Thus orbital cellulitis with proptosis constitutes, along with the intracranial complications of suppurative otitis media, one of the few indications for emergency CT within 24 hours (Figure 2.15). Fluid levels within the sinus or orbit which can be seen on plain films are an indication of a collection of pus

(Figure 2.16). Mucosal thickening of the sinuses is uncommon in children and should raise the suspicion of fibrocystic disease (Figure 2.17).

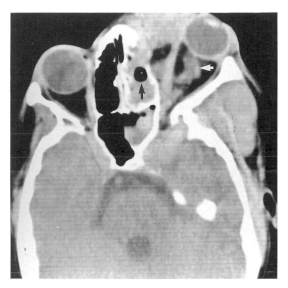

Figure 2.16 Axial CT scan shows an inflammatory mass which has extended from the ethmoids. There is a fluid level (black arrow). The patient also has an haemangioma in the orbit (white arrow)

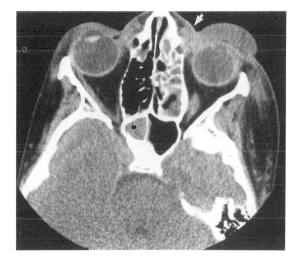

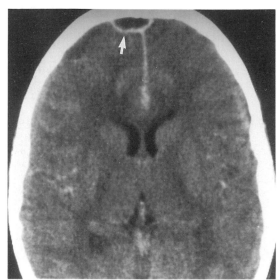

Figure 2.15 (*a*) Axial CT scan with contrast shows a soft tissue mass at the inner canthus of the left eye (arrow) as well as oedema of the eyelid and a collection in the opposite sphenoid sinus. (*b*) A section at a higher level shows an extradural abscess (arrow)

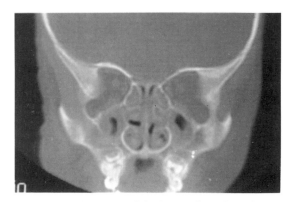

Figure 2.17 Diffuse mucosal thickening throughout the sinuses

Juvenile angiofibroma

Although the pathogenesis of so-called juvenile nasopharyngeal angiofibroma is uncertain and it occurs in an older age group, this vascular tumour also appears to be of developmental origin. Lloyd and Phelps (1986) in a study of 30 cases have shown that the angiofibroma takes origin at the sphenopalatine foramen. It enlarges the foramen and erodes bone locally at the base of the medial pterygoid plate, the floor of the sphenoid sinus and the posterior wall of the maxillary antrum. Further extension leads to invasion of the infratemporal fossa, orbit and middle cranial fossa (Figure 2.18). Severe bleeding may accompany biopsy and for this reason most surgeons are reluctant to undertake biopsy of a nasopharyngeal mass in an adolescent male patient, preferring to rely upon clinical and radiological features to decide whether the mass is likely to be an angiofibroma or a non-vascular lesion such as an antrochoanal polyp. Traditionally this involved angiography to show the characteristic vascular blush, supported by the 'antral sign' or indentation of the posterior wall of the maxillary antrum shown on lateral plain films or tomography.

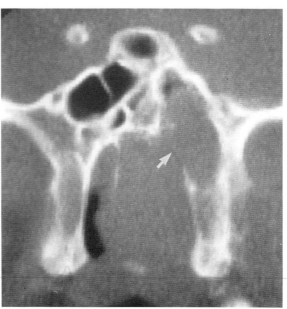

Figure 2.19 Coronal CT section at the level of the choana. A juvenile angiofibroma has eroded the base of the medial pterygoid plate (arrow) and extended into the sphenoid sinus

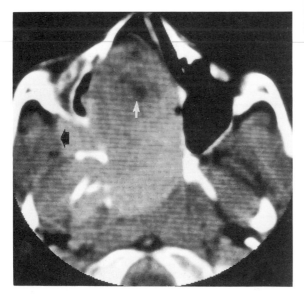

Figure 2.18 A large juvenile angiofibroma fills the nasal cavity and extends through the pterygomaxillary fissure into the infratemporal fossa (black arrow). The white arrow indicates an area of necrosis. Axial enhanced CT section

The 'antral sign' however is not specific for angiofibromas. It can occur with any slow-growing mass in the infratemporal fossa and was only positive in 81% of the author's patients with angiofibroma.

A more reliable sign is erosion of the base of the medial pterygoid plate, associated with enlargement of the sphenopalatine foramen which was demonstrated in 100% of 28 patients examined by conventional or computerized tomography (Figure 2.19). Once the diagnosis is established then the role of the radiologist is to define the limits of the tumour prior to surgery since this may influence the surgical approach. Three-plane magnetic resonance tomography is the method of choice (Figure 2.20). It best

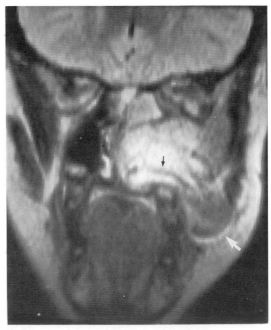

Figure 2.20 Coronal MR section showing an angiofibroma which has extended into the soft tissues of the cheek (white arrow). The black arrow points to a large vessel on the surface of the tumour. Demonstration of these vessels by MR can be diagnostic. (From Lloyd and Phelps, 1986, *Clinical Otolaryngology*, with permission)

demonstrates the extent of the tumour, it uses non-ionizing radiation and it will show the vascular nature of the angiofibroma and confirm the diagnosis. Angiography need only be performed if embolization is deemed necessary prior to surgery (Figure 2.21).

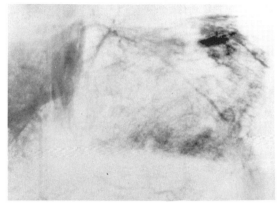

(a)

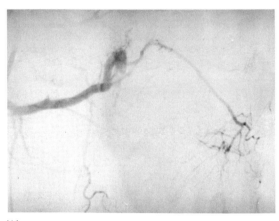

(b)

Figure 2.21 External carotid angiogram with subtraction to show the blood supply to a large juvenile angiofibroma (*a*) before and (*b*) after therapeutic embolization. (Courtesy of Dr Brian Kendall, The National Hospital London)

The natural history of angiofibroma, treated or untreated, is highly variable. It has long been known that there is a tendency to involute with age. These clinical observations have been supported by histological evidence that individual tumours show an increase in fibrous elements with time. However, at least partly because of the difficulty of assessment of the area of origin, and because of the reluctance of clinicians to intervene in the absence of symptoms, there seems to be no firm evidence in the literature that spontaneous involution of untreated lesions occurs (Chandler *et al.,* 1984). Complete regression of a small tumour that persisted after surgical removal of the original mass has been described (Stansbie and Phelps, 1986). Involution of this tumour was fully documented by serial CT scans over a period of 4 years (Figure 2.22).

Lesions of the jaws

Congenital deformities of the face and jaws usually present to plastic surgeons or to oral surgeons and orthodontists because of bite problems. The two most important of the first arch syndromes are:

1 *Hemifacial microsomia* in which there is under-development of one half of the face (Figure 2.23). In the 20% of cases where the deformity is bilateral there is always dissymmetry between the two sides.
2 *Mandibulofacial dysostosis* or the *Treacher Collins syndrome,* where there is characteristic bilateral and symmetrical hypoplasia of jaw and ear structures. The pathogenesis of both conditions has been discussed by Poswillo (1974).

Underdevelopment of the ascending ramus and condyle of the mandible appears to be the hallmark of hemifacial microsomia, and these abnormalities can be well shown by lateral and frontal radiographs and especially by orthopantomography (Figure 2.24). It has long been recognized that this hypoplasia affects not only bony structures but also the soft tissues, and in particular the muscles and the parotid gland. Only recently has the use of CT enabled this

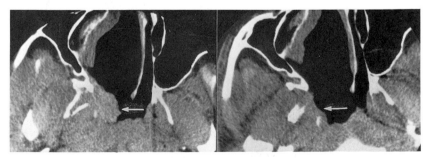

Figure 2.22 Axial CT sections 4 years apart, showing regression of a small angiofibroma which had reappeared after surgical removal. (From Stansbie and Phelps, 1986, *Journal of Laryngology and Otology*, with permission)

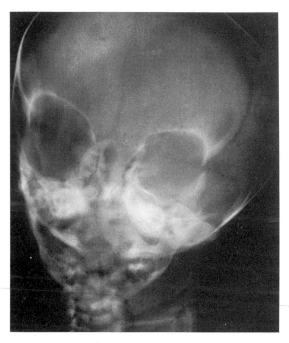

Figure 2.23 Underdevelopment of one half of the face, including the orbit, in a child with oculo-auricular-vertebral dysplasia

soft tissue hypoplasia to be adequately demonstrated (Figure 2.25). Characteristically there is most under-development of the masseter muscle and the parotid gland, a feature often apparent on clinical examination, although the pterygoid muscles are also commonly affected.

Symmetrical hypoplasia of jaws and muscles is a feature of the Treacher Collins syndrome, but this is more uniform and less pronounced than in hemifacial microsomia and the salivary glands are not affected. Antegonal notching of the body of the mandible is a feature of the condition and crowding of teeth causes orthodontic problems.

Trauma

Plain films are the standard initial investigation for facial trauma and can reveal much useful informa-tion besides showing the fracture lines (Figure 2.26), but CT is now the investigation needed in most severe cases (Figure 2.27).

Fibrous dysplasia

Tumours and tumour-like lesions of the jaws are uncommon in children, and fibro-osseous abnormali-ties such as fibrous dysplasia predominate (Figure 2.28). They cause a painless and slowly developing expansion of the jaws and may have characteristic appearances on plain films or CT, but are more often cystic with non-specific features, although a well corticated margin confirms the benign nature of the lesion. A giant cell reparative granuloma of

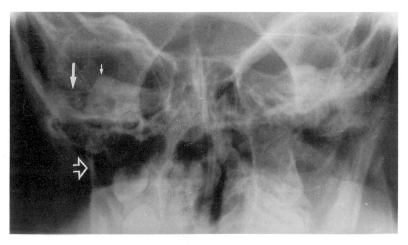

Figure 2.24 Another case of oculo-auricular-vertebral dysplasia. The Towne's view shows a large foramen magnum which was associated with an occipital meningocoele. The open arrow points to the hypoplastic mandibular ramus; the small arrow points to the arcuate eminence; the large arrow points to the depressed tegmen, so typical of hemifacial microsomia

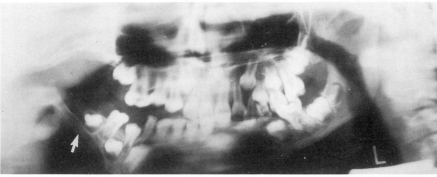

(a)

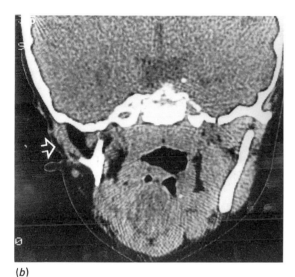

(b)

Figure 2.25 Hemifacial microsomia. (*a*) Orthopantomograph showing gross underdevelopment of part of the body of the mandible on the right (arrow); (*b*) coronal CT section shows the hypoplastic musculature and can be compared to the normal muscles shown on the left. The open arrow points to temporalis, which inserts into a horizontal shelf of bone, presumably representing a deformed coronoid process

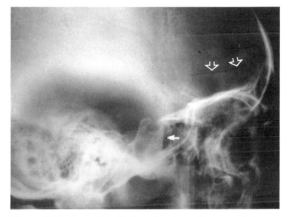

Figure 2.26 Lateral skull view showing a fracture of the skull vault (open arrows) as well as a fluid level in the sphenoid sinus (white arrow)

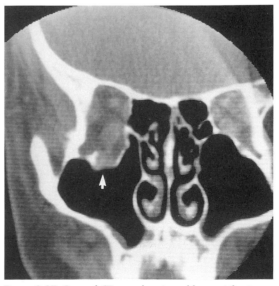

Figure 2.27 Coronal CT scan showing a blow-out fracture through the orbital floor (arrow)

the upper alveolus is shown in Volume 4 (Figure 2.30).

Rare malignant neoplasms cause extensive ragged destruction of the jaws. Sometimes calcification or even new bone formation within the tumour may be diagnostic, especially in osteogenic sarcoma (Figure 2.29).

Bone marrow tumours

Bone marrow tumours in children not infrequently involve the mandible. Leukaemia, lymphoma and

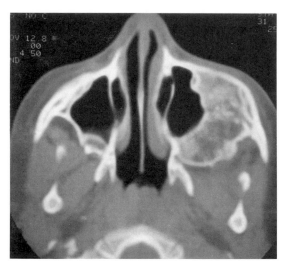

Figure 2.28 Fibrous dysplasia of the maxilla in a 4-year-old child. This axial CT scan shows the lesion to be of the mixed type with islands of bone in a largely fibrous bed

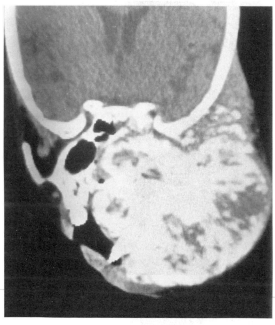

Figure 2.29 Coronal CT scan showing a massive osteogenic sarcoma arising from the maxilla

metastatic neuroblastoma can produce mottled destruction of the mandible and destruction or disruption of the teeth. Lytic destructive lesions are a common feature of histiocytosis and the mandible is often involved (Figure 2.30).

Chordomas

Chordomas are slow-growing destructive tumours that arise in the skull base usually in the midline. There is a wide age range at presentation and therefore chordomas can occur in children. MRI is the

investigation of choice. The tumours usually have a non-homogeneous appearance on T1-weighted images and show some degree of contrast enhancement (Figure 2.31).

Carcinoma of the nasopharynx

This also affects a wide age range and may occur

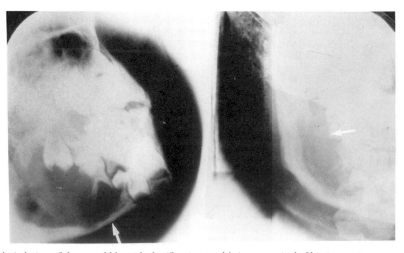

Figure 2.30 Large lytic lesion of the mandible with the 'floating teeth' sign so typical of histiocytosis

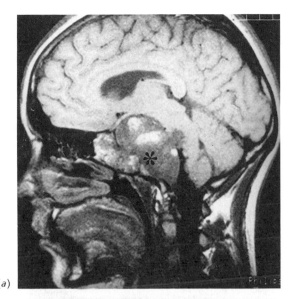

(a)

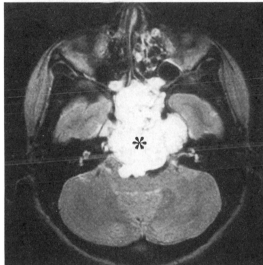

(b)

Figure 2.31 A large midline chordoma of the basisphenoid shows a non-homogeneous appearance on the sagittal T1-weighted MR section (*a*) and high signal on the T2-weighted axial section (*b*) (asterisk)

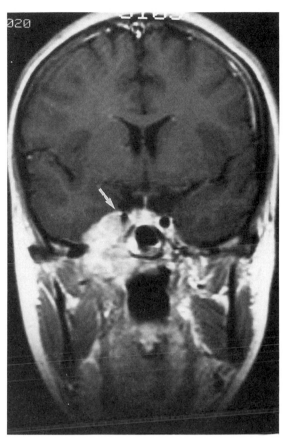

Figure 2.32 A nasopharyngeal carcinoma in a teenage girl shows a mass extending through the skull base into the parasellar region on this coronal gadolinium-enhanced MR scan. The tumour surrounds the internal carotid artery in the cavernous sinus (arrow)

in young people. Coronal section MRI is again the investigation of choice, especially for showing intracranial extension (Figure 2.32).

The petrous temporal bone

The middle and inner ears are fully developed at birth, but the temporomandibular joint and mastoid process are not. Postnatal changes in the temporal bone consist of growth and pneumatization of the mastoid process and alteration in the shape of the tympanic ring. Prior to full ossification of the petrous pyramid, the dense bone of the labyrinthine capsule can be clearly identified on plain mastoid views, enabling gross developmental abnormalities to be identified without the need for sectional imaging (Figure 2.33). In the middle ear the ossicles can be shown and, in the neonate, even marrow spaces.

Congenital ear deformities

Many congenital abnormalities of the hearing organ do not involve bony structures and therefore cannot be shown by radiological methods. Nevertheless, structural abnormalities of the inner, middle and external ear can be shown in considerable detail by *imaging*. Unfortunately, affected children are usually

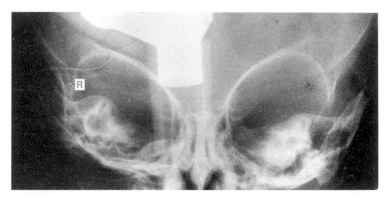

Figure 2.33 Perorbital view. Normal appearances on the left. On the right there is no labyrinth, but just a primitive otocyst with endolymphatic appendage

referred between the ages of 2 and 4 years, when the deafness is first confirmed, and sedation or a general anaesthetic is required for the examination. If, after careful consideration, it is felt that the results of the investigation would be unlikely to affect patient management it may be reasonable to defer the examination until the child can cooperate. In the neonatal period a few CT sections can usually be obtained for those relevant external deformities or syndromes in which temporal bone abnormalities are a feature. These syndromes with recognized structural abnormalities of the temporal bone are reviewed in Chapter 4 of *Diagnostic Imaging of the Ear* (Phelps and Lloyd, 1990).

The purpose of the radiological examination is first to demonstrate any bony abnormality of the inner ear, and particularly of the cochlea. This is complementary to the audiological assessment and ideally electrophysiological studies (either auditory brain stem response or electrocochleography) should be undertaken at the same time. Deformities associated with an actual or potential cerebrospinal fluid fistula may be demonstrated.

Congenital abnormalities of the middle and external ears are shown much more often than deformities of the inner ear, although combined deformities occur in about 20% of cases. The study of the outer ear relates to the prospects for surgical intervention to improve the sound conducting mechanisms and is mandatory before any exploration of congenital atresia. Surgery is now, however, rarely performed for unilateral lesions, but in bilateral atresias the radiological examination is crucial to indicate the best side for exploration, especially the all-important assessment of the presence, state and size of the middle ear cavity.

Inner ear deformities

Congenital malformations of the bony labyrinth, internal auditory meatus and vestibular aqueduct, which

vary widely in severity from minor anomalies with normal cochlear function to severe deformities which preclude any level of hearing whatever, may be suggested by audiological assessment. Traditionally two eponyms are enshrined in accounts of congenital deafness and so need to be defined:

1 *Michel defect* (Michel, 1863) – complete lack of development of any inner ear structures.
2 *Mondini defect* (Mondini, 1791) – a cochlea with one and a half turns and the apical coil replaced by a distal sac. Although the subject of Mondini's dissection had been completely deaf, the normal basal turn of the true Mondini defect means that some hearing is possible. Mondini's case also had very dilated vestibular aqueducts (Phelps, 1986).

Line drawings of some examples of labyrinthine deformities are shown in Figure 2.34. A primitive sac

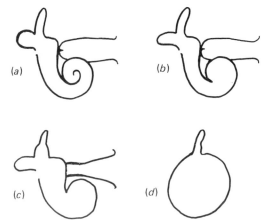

Figure 2.34 Line drawings of some important abnormalities of the inner ear, based on coronal section imaging. (*a*) Solitary dysplastic semicircular canal; (*b*) Mondini deformity with a deficient bony spiral in the cochlea; (*c*) dilated dysplastic labyrinth with tapering internal auditory meatus; (*d*) primitive otocyst

with one or more appendages (Figures 2.33 and 2.34) is more common than a Michel deformity.

The semicircular canals may be missing or dilated in varying degree, but the commonest labyrinthine anomaly, namely a solitary dilated dysplastic lateral semicircular canal (see Figure 2.34) is often associated with normal cochlear function. Dilatation of the vestibular aqueduct often accompanies minor abnormalities of the bony cochlea and vestibule and congenital hearing loss (Figure 2.35) (Valvassori, 1983). The deafness may be fluctuant and/or progressive giving rise to speculation that endolymphatic hydrops is also a feature.

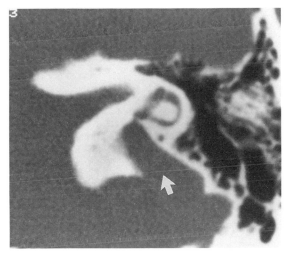

Figure 2.35 Axial CT scan showing a widely dilated vestibular aqueduct in a child with progressive sensorineural deafness. Note the normal vestibule and lateral semicircular canal ('signet ring' sign, see Volume 3, Chapter 2)

Anomalies of the internal auditory meatus include the bulbous type which is usually of no significance; unusual direction which is the result of skull base aberrations; and very narrow or double internal auditory meatus which usually indicate severe or total deafness (Phelps and Lloyd, 1983).

Inner ear lesions associated with cerebrospinal fluid fistula

Congenital cerebrospinal fluid fistula into the middle ear cavity is a rare but potentially fatal condition which is frequently misdiagnosed. When the fistula occurs spontaneously it usually presents in the first 5 or 10 years of life as:

1 Cerebrospinal fluid rhinorrhoea if the eardrum is intact. Cerebrospinal fluid passes down the eustachian tube causing a nasal discharge

2 Cerebrospinal fluid otorrhoea if there is a perforation in the eardrum, or if myringotomy has been performed for presumed serous otitis media
3 Attacks of meningitis which are usually recurrent. At times meningitis is the sole presenting manifestation of a cerebrospinal fluid fistula.

Deafness is usually severe or complete, but it is difficult to diagnose and assess, especially in a young child. It is frequently unrecognized if unilateral. The conductive and sensorineural components of the deafness are also hard to define.

Spontaneous cerebrospinal fluid fistulae from the subarachnoid space into the middle ear cavity may be classified as perilabyrinthine or translabyrinthine. The very rare perilabyrinthine group, through bony defects close to but not involving the labyrinth, usually have normal hearing initially. The commoner translabyrinthine group is nearly always associated with anacusis, severe labyrinthine dysplasia and a route via the internal auditory meatus. The labyrinthine deformity is more severe than the type classically described by Mondini, and evidence of a dilated cochlear aqueduct in these cases is also unconvincing.

The perilabyrinthine and translabyrinthine routes are discussed in a paper by Phelps (1986). The most important route is via an abnormally-shaped internal auditory meatus that usually tapers at its lateral end (Figure 2.36). The cochlea is an amorphous sac which lacks a modiolus or central bony spiral. The cochlear sac may be bigger or smaller than a normal cochlea. No proper basal turn can be recognized as in a true Mondini deformity, and there is a wide communication between the cochlear sac and the vestibule which is itself abnormal and enlarged, especially in the horizontal plane (Figure 2.37). The semicircular canals may be dilated to a varying degree, especially the lateral.

The labyrinthine malformation is often accompanied by a defective stapes, usually a hole in the footplate, and the exit route of cerebrospinal fluid into the middle ear is via the oval or, less commonly, the round window. It should be stressed that the fistula is usually spontaneous or the result of a minor head injury.

Congenital fixation of the stapes footplate is likely to be associated with a profuse perilymph or cerebrospinal fluid leak following stapedectomy. The surgical results of stapedectomy for congenital stapedial fixation are not very satisfactory, but there is little radiological evidence of structural abnormalities of the labyrinth in these 'gushers'.

The management of cerebrospinal fluid fistulae into the middle ear depends on a high degree of clinical suspicion. Perilabyrinthine fistulae are extremely rare and usually associated with normal hearing. Bony defects around the labyrinth may be shown by sophisticated bone imaging, but tracer cerebrospinal fluid

Translabyrinthine

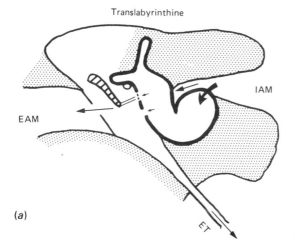

(a)

Perilabyrinthine

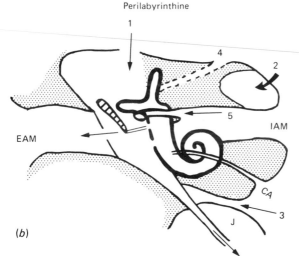

(b)

Figure 2.36 (*a*) Diagram to show the commonest inner ear anomaly associated with cerebrospinal fluid fistula. Note the wide communication between the vestibule and cochlear sac. This diagram is based on coronal section tomograms. (*b*) Diagram based on coronal section tomograms to show the various routes of perilabyrinthine fistulae around a labyrinth of normal configuration: (1) through the tegmen tympani; (2) through large apical air cells; (3) via Hyrtl's fissure; (4) via petromastoid canal (not a proven route); (5) via the facial nerve canal. EAM = external auditory meatus; ET = eustachian tube; CA = cochlear aqueduct; J = jugular fossa. (From Phelps, P.D., 1986, *Clinical Otolaryngology*, with permission)

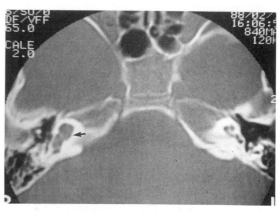

Figure 2.37 A dilated dysplastic cochlea incompletely separated from a dilated vestibule is shown on this axial CT scan (arrow). Compare with the normal side. The child presented with otogenic meningitis

mandatory. When a basal turn of normal calibre is associated with a distal sac, i.e. a true Mondini deformity, then some hearing is possible and there is no risk of meningitis or a fistula (Figure 2.38).

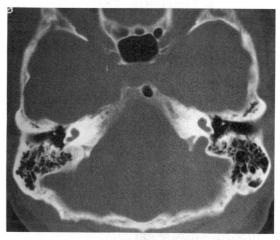

Figure 2.38 Bilateral Mondini deformities with some hearing present

Middle ear deformities

Radiology of congenital deformities of the middle and external ear relates almost exclusively to the prospects of improvement of conductive deafness by surgical intervention. The size and shape of the middle ear cavity is the most important assessment to be made, especially where there is atresia of the external auditory meatus.

contrast studies may be necessary to confirm the aural route. The commoner translabyrinthine type is almost always associated with labyrinthine dysplasia. Sensorineural deafness or two unexplained attacks of meningitis make CT study of the temporal bones

In the majority of unilateral atresias with associated deformity of the pinna but no other congenital abnormality, there is a normally formed mastoid with good pneumatization and the middle ear cavity is of relatively normal shape. Even in the most severe deformities there is rarely complete absence of the middle ear and usually at least a slit-like hypotympanum can be shown lateral to the basal turn of the cochlea. The middle ear cavity may be reduced in size by encroachment of the atretic plate laterally, by a high jugular bulb inferiorly or by descent of the tegmen superiorly. In craniofacial microsomia and mandibulofacial dysostosis, the attic and antrum are typically absent or slit-like, being replaced in varying degrees by solid bone or by descent of the tegmen (Figure 2.39).

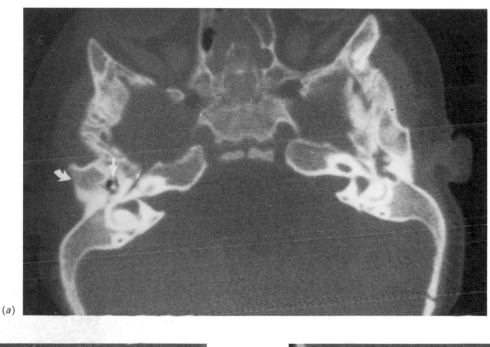

(a)

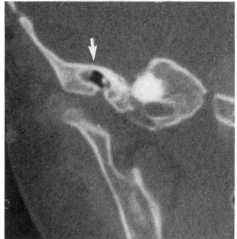

(b)

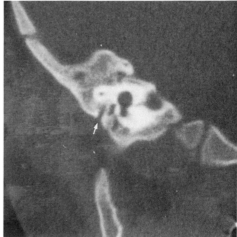

(c)

Figure 2.39 Severe congenital deformity of the middle and external ears in a case of Treacher Collins syndrome. The inner ears are normal. (a) Axial section at the level of the lateral semicircular canals. On both sides the antrum is replaced by solid bone. On the right a very small air-containing attic encloses a diminutive ossicle (large arrow). The curved arrow indicates the uncannulated tympanic bone and the small arrow the second part of the facial nerve canal which is in a relatively normal position; (b) coronal section anteriorly shows the small attic; (c) more posterior coronal section through the vestibule shows the short descending facial canal. (Courtesy of Dr E. A. Burrows)

If the middle ear cavity is air-containing, its shape and contents are relatively easy to assess. Frequently, however, the middle ear in congenital abnormalities contains undifferentiated mesenchyme, a thick glue-like substance which is radiologically indistinguishable from soft tissue or retained mucus. Thin bony septa may divide the middle ear cavity into two or more compartments.

Facial nerve

The next most important structure from a surgical point of view is the facial nerve. The nerve is very rarely absent, although it might be hypoplastic. The main problem is aberration in the course of the nerve.

In early embryonic life, the developing VIIth cranial nerve lies anterior to the otocyst, so if development is arrested at this stage, a tract for the facial nerve is found anterior to a primitive otic sac. If development is arrested at a later stage, after the cochlea has formed to some extent, then the first part of the facial nerve is found in its usual situation above and lateral to the cochlea. The facial nerve is, therefore, relatively unaffected by developmental abnormalities of the labyrinth, and aberrations of the first part of the facial nerve canal are most unusual.

The course of the second and third parts is, however, dependent on normal development of the branchial arches, the facial nerve being the nerve of the second arch. During its development and migration, the facial nerve curves behind the branchial cartilage to reach the anterior aspect of the same cartilage. At the same time, part of the cartilage adheres to the otic capsule to form the fallopian canal. If, during development, the external pharyngeal groove of the first branchial arch is active and atresia is due only to maldevelopment of the tympanic ring, then the second and third parts of the facial canal follow a relatively normal course (Figure 2.40).

The greater the deformity the more marked is the tendency for the facial nerve to follow a more direct route out into the soft tissues of the face. Exposed

facial nerves in the middle ear cavity are the most common abnormalities recorded at surgery for congenital malformations. Usually the fallopian canal is dehiscent but the descending segment may also be exposed, and overhang of the facial ridge with absence of the second genu is a usual finding in the Treacher Collins syndrome, making access to the oval window difficult for the surgeon. A short vertical segment of the facial canal and high stylomastoid foramen mean that the nerve turns forwards into the cheek in a high position (see Figure 2.40).

In the preoperative radiological assessment, the descending facial canal and its relationship to other structures must be demonstrated, preferably in both lateral (Figure 2.41) and coronal sections (Figure 2.42). Axial CT sections will show the descending canal in cross-section and identification is less certain. Grossly displaced nerves crossing the middle ear cavity are more difficult to identify even by CT, but two useful signs of aberrant pathways through the middle ear cavity are:

1 An exit foramen through the floor of the middle ear cavity or lateral atretic plate may be identified
2 Absence of the pyramidal eminence at the back of the middle ear cavity which normally contains the stapedius muscle and tendon (see Volume 3, Chapter 2).

The pyramid was identified in only two of the cases noted at operation to have anomalies of the facial canal in the middle ear and, in these, the dehiscence was in the second part. Absence of the

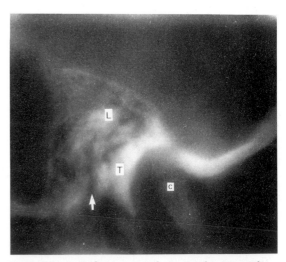

Figure 2.41 Lateral tomogram of congenital atresia with a well-pneumatized mastoid. T = the uncannulated tympanic bone; L = lateral semicircular canal; c = condyle of the mandible. The arrow points to the descending facial canal which is in a normal position

FACIAL NERVE

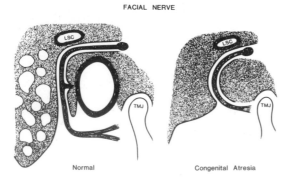

Normal   Congenital Atresia

Figure 2.40 Facial nerve. LSC = Lateral semicircular canal; TMJ = temporomandibular joint

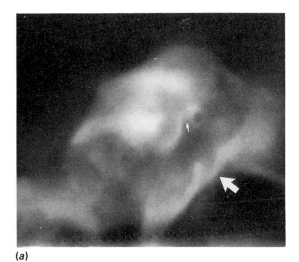

(a)

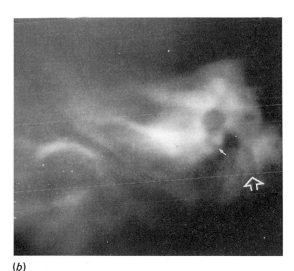

(b)

Figure 2.42 Congenital bony atresia with a normal-sized air-containing middle ear cavity. (*a*) Semiaxial section shows the oval window (small arrow) obscured by an overhanging fallopian canal. This feature would make it difficult or impossible to insert any form of strut during attempts at reconstructive surgery. (*b*) Coronal section slightly more posterior at the level of the short descending facial canal (open arrow). The small arrow points to the round window niche. Note the absence of the normal pyramidal eminence, suggesting that there is dehiscence of the facial nerve at the second genu

pyramid is, therefore, good presumptive evidence of an exposed facial nerve. Bifurcation of the descending portion is far more common with congenital malformations than in normal patients. The descending facial canal is often short (Figure 2.43).

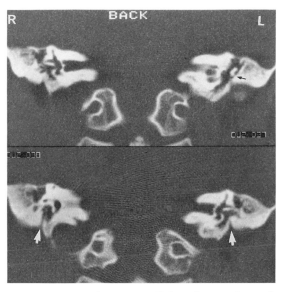

Figure 2.43 Coronal CT section of bilateral external meatal atresia with air-containing middle ears. Note the ossicular mass on the left (black arrow) and the anterior position of the descending facial nerves (white arrows)

Ossicles

A normal ossicular chain is rarely found where there is atresia of the external ear, but complete absence of the ossicles is also unusual. In most cases at least some vestige of the ossicular chain is evident. The ossicles are often thicker and heavier than normal (Figure 2.44) or, less frequently, thin and spidery. They may be fixed to the walls of the middle ear cavity by bosses of bone, but the more usual deformity

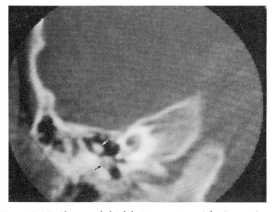

Figure 2.44 Abnormal thick but separate ossicles in an air-containing middle ear behind a pneumatized atretic plate. This axial CT section was made at the level of the round window niche

discovered at surgery is a fusion of the bodies of malleus and incus. The ankylosis varies in degree and may be bony or fibrous. The radiological recognition of this ossicular union is difficult but is, in any case, not of great practical importance and an irregular lump of bone in the middle ear cavity usually represents an ossicular mass.

Because of the partial or complete replacement of the tympanic membrane by a bony plate, the handle of the malleus is not surprisingly that part of the chain which is most often abnormal and most easily recognized on the tomograms. If the handle is absent the molar tooth appearance of the ossicles will no longer be evident in the lateral projection and a triangular appearance of the ossicular mass will be seen. Often the handle of the malleus is bent towards the atretic plate to which it may be fixed and this gives the typical L-shaped appearance to the ossicular mass. A slit-like attic so typical of Treacher Collins syndrome or an overhanging facial ridge may obstruct the free movement of the ossicular chain.

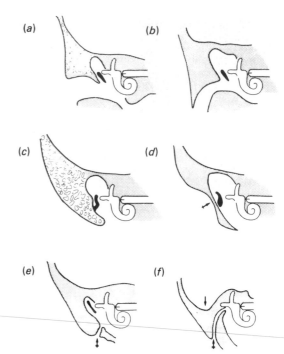

Figure 2.45 A diagrammatic representation of congenital deformities of the middle and external ears based on coronal section tomograms. (*a*) Normal appearances; (*b*)–(*f*) various types of atretic plate, reduced middle ear cavity, ossicular deformity and anterior facial nerve ⇥. → = thin atretic plates; → = depression of the tegmen. (From Phelps, Lloyd and Shelton, 1977, *British Journal of Radiology*, with permission)

External auditory meatus

In congenital deformities of the external ear, the external auditory meatus may be narrow, short, completely or partially atretic or it may run in an abnormal direction. It often slopes up towards the middle ear and in such cases it may be curved in two planes, becoming more horizontal at its medial end. The obstruction in atresia may be due to soft tissue or bone but usually both are involved. The tympanic bone may be hyperplastic (rarely), deformed or absent.

The so-called atretic plate may, therefore, be composed partly of a deformed tympanic bone and partly of downwards and forward extension of squamous temporal and mastoid bones, in which case it may be pneumatized.

A diagrammatic representation of some of the congenital structural abnormalities of the middle and external ears, as shown by coronal section imaging, is given in Figure 2.45.

Syndromes

It is not intended to discuss the radiological features of syndromic ear deformities except for the two commonest and most important.

Hemifacial microsomia

The ear lesions are usualy bizarre and severe. The pinna is often represented by a small tag. Meatal atresia and middle ear abnormalities are almost constant findings and there may be gross descent of the tegmen to, or even below, the level of the lateral semicircular canal (see Figure 2.24). Occasionally, some degree of hyperplasia of the external ear structures, particularly the tympanic bone, occurs but the mastoid is hypoplastic and unpneumatized. The middle ear cavity is usually small, being encroached upon by the low tegmen and thick atretic plate. The ossicles in such cases are absent or hypoplastic and malformed (Figure 2.46). Three of the author's patients had an ossicular mass displaced laterally far from the oval window. This anomaly is only seen in cases of facial microsomia. The condition is not exclusively unilateral and often involves the bones of the skull base. Though bilateral, there is always considerable dissymmetry between the two sides. This dissymmetry distinguishes the syndrome from Treacher Collins syndrome, with which it has often been confused in the past. There is no hereditary factor in craniofacial microsomia. It is the most common of the otocraniofacial syndromes (Phelps, Lloyd and Poswillo, 1983).

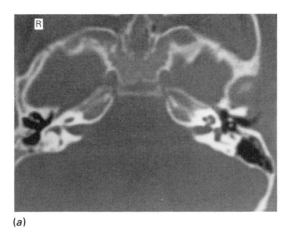

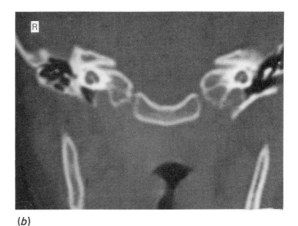

(a)   (b)

Figure 2.46 Hemifacial microsomia. (a) Axial, (b) coronal sections. Normal appearances on the left. On the right there is some depression of the tegmen and thin bony atresia, but there is a large air containing middle ear cavity. Note, however, that the small hypoplastic ossicles lie medial and lateral instead of anterior and posterior as on the normal side

Treacher Collins syndrome

The middle ear abnormalities in Treacher Collins syndrome are symmetrical and characteristic, although they may vary in severity (Phelps, Poswillo and Lloyd, 1981). The mastoid is unpneumatized and the attic and antrum are often reduced to slit-like proportions (Figure 2.47). Atresia of the external auditory meatus is a less constant feature and in 50% of patients the meatus may be patent, although

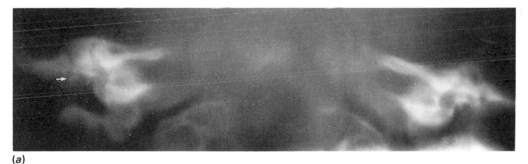

(a)

Figure 2.47 Treacher Collins syndrome. (a) Coronal section tomogram showing normal external auditory meatus and relatively normal lower middle ear cavities. There are, however, virtually no attics present and some hypoplastic ossicles (arrow). (b) Axial CT section at the level of the lateral semicircular canals showing solid bone replacing the antrum on each side. Note the typical symmetry of these lesions

(b)

it tends to be curved, running upwards in its lateral part. Ossicular abnormalities are common and, in nearly all the operated ears in the author's series, the facial nerve followed a more direct path with opening out of the bends. It usually appeared at surgery as an overhanging facial ridge.

Bone dysplasias

Deafness is a common childhood feature of rare congenital generalized bony dysplasias. Only a brief account of the radiological features of osteogenesis imperfecta and of the dysplasias with increased bone density is given here. For more extensive descriptions other works need to be consulted (Booth, 1982; Phelps and Lloyd, 1983).

Deafness in osteogenesis imperfecta tarda may be conductive, sensorineural or mixed. The radiological appearances consist of demineralization of the labyrinthine capsule indistinguishable from otospongiosis but, in contrast to otospongiosis which only affects the capsule, dehiscent ossification occurs in other sites in the petrous pyramid (Figure 2.48).

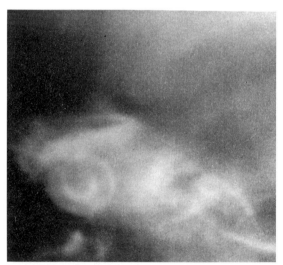

Figure 2.48 Demineralization of bone surrounding the cochlea in a case of osteogenesis imperfecta, shown on this coronal tomogram

The osteopetroses are a group of uncommon genetic disorders characterized by increased skeletal density and abnormalities of bone modelling. Common to all of these disorders is a proclivity for involvement of the calvarium and skull base. An associated constellation of neurotological symptoms may result, presumably secondary to bony encroach-

ment on the cranial foraminae. Sectional imaging of the petrous temporal bone shows generalized sclerosis and narrowing of the internal auditory meatus. Encroachment by bosses of bone in the attic may also be revealed (Figure 2.49).

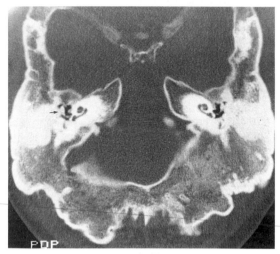

Figure 2.49 Craniometaphyseal dysplasia; a congenital bone dysplasia causing narrowing of the attic and encroaching upon the ossicles (arrow) shown on this axial CT scan

Otitis media

Radiology has little part to play in conditions such as otitis media, which is essentially a clinical diagnosis. Loss of aeration of the middle ear cleft and mastoid may suggest infection, but cell wall breakdown (coalescent mastoiditis) and abscess formation in mastoiditis are hard to demonstrate on plain films, and are better shown by CT (Figure 2.50).

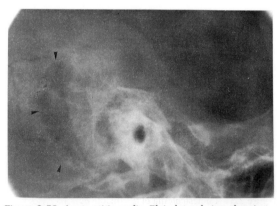

Figure 2.50 Acute otitis media. Plain lateral view showing mastoid cell wall breakdown (coalescent mastoiditis)

Cholesteatoma in children

Cholesteatoma in childhood is less common than in adults but is more aggressive and dangerous and shows some special features. Often large cholesteatomas are associated with small perforations of the eardrum and well pneumatized mastoids (Jahnke, 1982). The cholesteatomas in the author's patients appeared to be primary attic lesions and were considered to be 'acquired' even when the eardrum was intact. There was usually no bony erosion seen on radiological examination.

While not wishing to discuss the aetiology of cholesteatoma, it does seem that a high proportion of childhood cholesteatomas affecting the middle ear have a congenital origin with an intact, unscarred eardrum and no bone erosion (Figure 2.51). Characteristically they are localized in the mesotympanum and later extend to the attic. Any discussion of congenital childhood cholesteatoma is complicated by two phenomena which are difficult to explain:

1 Cholesteatoma of the base of the skull not affecting the middle ear cavity, and therefore undoubtedly of congenital origin, is predominantly a disease of later life. These lesions which are thought to arise from squamous cell rests are therefore considered in Volume 3, Chapter 2.
2 The external auditory meatus develops by recannulation of a solid plug of ectodermal cells of the first branchial arch. This process begins at the medial end, with the membrane separating the primitive meatus from the tubotympanic recess developing into the eardrum. Failure of recannulation will result in congenital atresia of the external auditory meatus, potentially with the epidermis trapped medial to the atretic plate. This situation would seem to have all the potential for develop-

ment of a cholesteatoma, especially if, as is often found at operation, there is a vestigial eardrum present.

Congenital atresia of the external auditory meatus is not rare but, surprisingly, cholesteatoma beyond the atresia is most unusual. It is probable that in such cases lack of a stimulus, such as infection, means that any squamous cell rests remain dormant. In theory, MR should be able to distinguish cholesteatoma from surrounding soft tissues but, in practice, this is difficult.

Labyrinthitis ossificans and cochlear implants

Now that multi-electrode implants are being used in children the recognition of labyrinthitis ossificans has assumed considerable importance in the preoperative assessment. The ossification comes about as a result of suppurative otitis interna, usually bacterial, of meningitic or otogenic origin and is a relative contraindication to electrode insertion (Figure 2.52).

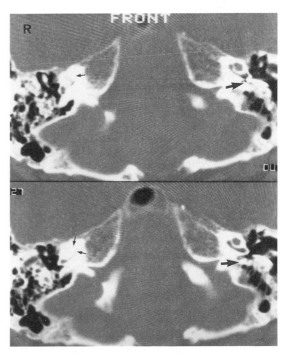

Figure 2.52 Two axial CT sections of the ears of a child deafened by labyrinthitis. The coils of the right cochlea are almost completely obliterated by labyrinthitis ossificans (small arrows). There is a single channel cochlear implant in the round window niche on the other side (large arrows)

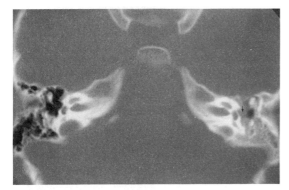

Figure 2.51 Cholesteatoma of the middle ear in a child. Note the typical erosion of the incudo-stapedial region (arrow) and compare to the other normal side

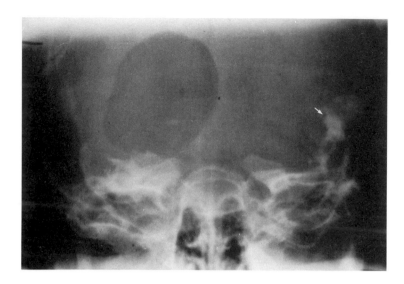

Figure 2.53 Gross disruption of the base of the skull by Hand-Schüller-Christian disease. Only a part of the labyrinth remains on the left (arrow). More typical of this condition is the punched out erosion in the skull vault. Plain Towne's view

Neoplasms

Occasionally tumours such as rhabdomyosarcoma or tumour-like conditions such as Hand-Schüller-Christian disease (histiocytosis X) may affect the temporal bone or mastoid (Figure 2.53). Massive destruction of bone is the usual feature.

References

BARKOVICH, A. J., VENDERMARCK, P., EDWARDS, M. S. and COGEN, P. H. (1991) Congenital nasal masses: CT and MR imaging features in 16 cases. *American Journal of Neuroradiology*, **12**, 105–116

BOOTH, J. B. (1982) Medical management of sensorineural hearing loss. *Journal of Laryngology and Otology*, **96**, 673–684

CHANDLER, J. R., GOULDING, G. R., MOSKOWITZ, L. and QUENCER, R. M. (1984) Nasopharyngeal angiofibromas, staging and management. *Annals of Otology, Rhinology and Laryngology*, **93**, 322–329

JAHNKE, V. (1982) Clinical, pathological and therapeutic aspects of cholesteatoma in children. In: *Cholesteatoma and Mastoid Surgery*, edited by J. Sade. Amsterdam: Kugler Publications. p. 25

LLOYD, G. A. S. and PHELPS, P. D. (1986) Juvenile angiofibroma: imaging by magnetic resonance, CT and conventional techniques. *Clinical Otolaryngology*, **11**, 247–259

MICHEL, E. M. (1863) Memoire sur les anomalies congenitals de o'oreille interne. *Gazette Medicale de Strasbourg*, **4**, 55–58

MONDINI, C. (1791) Anatomica surdi nati sectio. Bononiensi scientarium et artium instituto atque academia commentarii. *Bononiae*, **VII**, 419–428

PHELPS, P. D. (1986) Congenital cerebrospinal fluid fistulae of the petrous temporal bone. *Clinical Otolaryngology*, **11**, 79–92

PHELPS, P. D. and LLOYD, G. A. S. (1983) Syndromes with congenital hearing loss. In: *Radiology of the Ear*. Oxford: Blackwell Scientific Publications. p. 121

PHELPS, P. D. and LLOYD, G. A. S. (1990) *Diagnostic Imaging of the Ear*. Berlin: Springer-Verlag

PHELPS, P. D., LLOYD, G. A. S. and SHELDON, P. W. E. (1977) Congenital deformity of the middle and external ear. *British Journal of Radiology*, **50**, 714–727

PHELPS, P. D., LLOYD, G. A. S. and POSWILLO, D. (1983) The ear deformities in craniofacial microsomia and oculo-auriculo-vertebral dysplasia. *Journal of Laryngology and Otology*, **97**, 995–1005

PHELPS, P. D., POSWILLO, D. and LLOYD, G. A. S. (1981) The ear deformities in mandibulofacial dysostosis (Treacher Collins syndrome). *Clinical Otolaryngology*, **6**, 15–18

POSWILLO, D. (1974) Otomandibular deformity: pathogenesis as a guide to reconstruction. *Journal of Maxillofacial Surgery*, **2**, 64–72

STANSBIE, J. M. and PHELPS, P. D. (1986) Involution of juvenile nasopharyngeal angiofibroma (a case report). *Journal of Laryngology and Otology*, **100**, 599–603

VALVASSORI, G. E. (1983) The vestibular aqueduct and associated anomalies of the inner ear. *Otolaryngologic Clinics of North America*, **16**, 95–101

3

Genetic factors and deafness

William Reardon

Mendelian, mitochondrial and multifactorial genetics

There are five main types of genetically determined disease – chromosomal, single gene disorders, mitochondrial disorders, multifactorial conditions, and somatic cell genetic disorders. Somatic cell disorders have not been shown to be of importance in the genetics of deafness and will not be considered further. All genetic disease stems from aberrations in the coding function or the processing of human DNA. DNA totalling approximately 3×10^9 base pairs exists within every nucleated cell. Although DNA has a complex structure, involving the sugar, deoxyribose, phosphate and the four bases, adenine, thymine, guanine and cytosine, its arrangement under the light microscope is as discrete chromosomes. The functions of DNA are twofold: first to encode an estimated 100 000 genes and, secondly to transmit genetic information from generation to generation. Virtually every protein, be it structural, regulatory or otherwise in function, results from a gene in the nucleus encoding the amino acid sequence. The particular amino acid sequence is a function of the combination of the DNA base sequence, each *triplet* of bases encoding a single amino acid. As a result, each of the 20 amino acids has its own triplet code(s) in DNA. Considering the complexity of this system, errors are surprisingly infrequent, but may occur at several levels.

Most grossly, *chromosomal abnormalities* may be identified. The normal human chromosome number of 46 has been known since 1956 and the first human chromosomal disease, Down's syndrome, since 1959. Modern techniques of chromosome banding have improved resolution to such a degree that by 1990 over 600 chromosomal abnormalities had been identified in addition to several normal variants

(Connor and Ferguson-Smith, 1990). To the clinician a possible chromosomal abnormality will be suggested by the identification of several single gene disorders in the same patient or, more commonly, by unexplained developmental delay and a recognized single gene disorder not usually associated with developmental delay in the same patient.

Although Mendel's observations in peas had been known since 1865, it was not until 1902 that the first *single gene disorder* in humans, alkaptonuria, was identified as such by Garrod at the suggestion of Bateson. Over 5700 single gene disorders and traits are now recognized (McKusick, 1992). Improved molecular techniques in recent years have facilitated the chromosomal localization of over 2500 of these conditions. The actual DNA sequence responsible for encoding a designated protein (i.e. the gene) has been identified for several single gene disorders and the nature of the underlying mutations elucidated in affected individuals at DNA level (Collins, 1992). Mendel's experiments described the independent segregation of single traits in peas, each trait being governed by a discrete gene. Essentially then, mendelian genetics pertains to single genes and disorders thereof. Several different patterns of inheritance may underlie single gene disorders, but essentially these depend on whether the gene in question is autosomal (chromosome pairs 1–22) or sex chromosomal (X and Y) in its location and whether the gene is dominant or recessive. These patterns of inheritance are usually easily identifiable from the family tree.

The 44 autosomes comprise 22 chromosome pairs, one of maternal and one of paternal origin. Within a chromosome pair the order of the genes is exactly alike. Alternative forms of the gene are known as alleles and may or may not interfere with the function of the gene. If both alleles of the pair are the same, then the individual is homozygous at that gene locus and if two different allelic forms of the gene exist within the pair, then the individual is heterozygous. When a gene is expressed (i.e. apparent in the phenotype) in the heterozygous state, that allele is said to be dominant. Thus, if an allele undergoes a disease causing dominant mutation, the individual will manifest the disease even though there is a normal allele present at the same locus on the paired chromosome. The affected individual is heterozygous at the locus and at reproduction has a 50% chance of passing the normal allele to the offspring and a 50% chance of passing the disease-bearing allele to the offspring. This is the situation with autosomal dominant single gene disorders, an example of which is Marfan's syndrome. The family tree will show vertical transmission of the condition from one generation to the next.

In contrast, autosomal recessive disorders require that the individual must have disease causing mutations on both maternal and paternal alleles before the disease manifests itself clinically. Consequently the risk of transmitting the disease to the next generation is much smaller, requiring the reproductive partner also to be a carrier for the same disease. Once an affected child has been identified with a disease transmitted in this way, the recurrence risk in future pregnancies is 25% for these patients. It follows then that autosomal recessive disease is seen more frequently in populations where there is a high rate of consanguinity. This is the most common form of mendelian inheritance. In terms of the family tree, autosomal recessive disease is usually seen in a single generation, unless there is consanguinity in successive generations which would facilitate the emergence of the disorder in several generations of the same family, a phenomenon known as pseudodominance. Since autosomal recessive disease manifestation requires homozygosity, there will be far more people heterozygous for the disease-bearing allele – the carrier state – than there will be affected individuals. Many autosomal recessive conditions are rare and clinical investigations of the carrier state have not been performed. In some such conditions the carrier state may itself be pathological under certain circumstances, sickle cell disease carriers being an example. However, most carriers of autosomal recessive mutations are clinically asymptomatic and it is uncertain how reliable clinical investigations targetted at carrier identification are likely to prove in terms of sensitivity and specificity. The ultimate answer to accurate carrier detection for autosomal recessive conditions is molecular analysis of the gene in question in the patient. Tests of this nature will actually look at the DNA sequence of the gene and see if one of the alleles has a mutation present. This is the mode of carrier detection now used for cystic fibrosis, the gene for which was identified in 1989 (Kerem *et al.*, 1989; Rommens *et al.*, 1989; Riordan *et al.*, 1989), as abnormalities of the sweat test and other measures proved unsatisfactory in predicting the carrier state.

Some may find this heterozygote manifestation in autosomal recessive disease puzzling. After all, the hallmark of dominance is that the heterozygous state is phenotypically identifiable, so why are sickle cell disease and other conditions which similarly cause heterozygote manifestation not classified as dominants? It is important to appreciate that dominance and recessivity are not intrinsic properties of a gene or a mutant allele, but rather describe the relationship between the phenotypes of three genotypes – the mutant homozygote, the wildtype (normal allele) homozygote and the heterozygote. In theory, an allele may behave as a dominant or a recessive characteristic depending on its partner allele and several examples of this are recognized in animal genetics where, unlike human genetics, specific experimental crosses may be performed to verify a point. Essentially then dominance and recessivity are not as distinct as might first be assumed, although in clinical practice, they tend to be referred to as absolute phenomena.

Alternatively, if the gene involved in a mutation is on the X chromosome, then the condition will be apparent in males who are hemizygous for most loci on this chromosome. This is the basis of X-linked recessive inheritance. A mutation which is recessive and consequently rarely causes discernible clinical consequences in the carrier female who is heterozygous, has a 50% chance of being passed to male offspring, who consequently manifest the disease. Similarly the other 50% of males will be mutation free and clinically unaffected. Among female offspring 50% will be carriers and 50% non-carriers. The hallmarks of this pattern of transmission on the family tree are disease confined to males or, if affected, females will usually have a milder form of the condition. Classically the condition will be passed from the affected grandfather through his clinically normal carrier daughter to his grandson who is also affected. A common example of this type of inheritance are the haemophilias A and B. X-linked dominant mutations are generally lethal in the male as the normal allele is required in order for the patient to survive. Females with X-linked dominant conditions have dominant mutations on one of the X chromosomes which are fully expressed in the heterozygous state and are compatible with life due to the presence of the normal allele. An example of an X-linked dominant condition is focal dermal hypoplasia (Goltz syndrome).

Carrier characteristics of X-linked recessive disorders in females are likely to be much more variable than is the situation for autosomal recessive disorders. This is because of lyonization of one or other X chromosome in every cell, so that in any particular cell the female has only one active X chromosome. Which of the two X chromosomes is inactivated is a purely random event. Consequently, in any group of females who are known carriers for the same X-linked recessive condition there will be some in whom the mutant chromosome predominates, some in whom the active proportions of mutant and wildtype are comparable, and some in whom the wildtype predominates. In clinical terms this makes for very mixed findings ranging from those who manifest the disease as a reflection of their disproportionately active mutant X chromosome, to those who have almost no trace of the disorder on clinical testing due to their disproportionately active wildtype X chromosome. As with autosomal recessive disorders, the ultimate detection of mutation carriers rests with actual examination of the sequence of bases in the DNA. Since most genes for mendelian conditions have hardly been localized yet, this type of mutational analysis is available only for those few conditions in which the gene has actually been cloned and its mutations studied.

Almost all proteins are encoded by nuclear DNA. Several subunits of the mitochondrial respiratory chain are, however, coded by the *mitochondrial genome*, a single circular chromosome within the mitochondrion, several of which are present within each cell. Mitochondrial chromosomes are almost exclusively maternal in their transmission between generations. Mutations in the mitochondrial chromosomes have widespread effects throughout several tissue types, particularly those with a high energy requirement such as skeletal muscle, giving rise to a variable clinical picture which may be difficult to recognize. Clinical features, apart from myopathy and encephalopathy, may include external ophthalmoplegia, seizures, ataxia, dementia, stroke-like episodes, retinopathy, deafness, cardiac conduction defects, renal dysfunction and endocrine disorders such as diabetes mellitus (Harding, 1989). In consequence of maternal transmission of mitochondrial DNA the family tree will show a pattern of affected individuals of both sexes who are related through their mothers. Offspring of affected males are spared, unlike offspring of affected females who are prone to develop the condition, albeit in varying degrees and with variable clinical manifestations, depending on the tissues involved in the individual.

In direct contrast to mendelian genetics, the *multifactorial model* of inheritance attributes phenotypic variation between individuals to a large number of causes, each in itself having only a small effect, but when acting together, producing a disorder with the clinical phenotype. Clinically this is indistinguishable from other causes of the same phenotype. The increased risk to relatives of the patient reflects, not only their shared genes, but also their shared environment. Continuous variables in the population such as height and weight are examples of multifactorial characteristics. It is highly likely that several genetic loci, acting in an additive manner, and interacting with environmental factors determine the phenotype in these situations. Such a model takes account of continuous distribution but can also accommodate familial aggregation where the prevalence of a disorder

among relatives is less than expected by the single gene model of transmission, but more than expected by chance (Bishop, 1990).

Principles of genetic counselling in deafness

Harper (1988) defined genetic counselling as 'the process by which patients or relatives at risk of a disorder that may be hereditary are advised of the consequences of the disorder, the probability of developing and transmitting it and of the ways in which this may be prevented or ameliorated'. Implicit to this is the estimation of risk and it is important to appreciate that not all risk estimates are of similar type. Estimates of risk are based on the information available to the counsellor. This will include the family history, medical details of the patient and relatives, the clinical examination of the patient and any investigations arising therefrom. Mendelian disorders, once the condition in question has been recognized, lend themselves to *specific risks* of recurrence within a pedigree and of transmission to offspring. The crucial point is the recognition of the condition, since many single gene disorders are rare and only described in a small number of families. *Modified mendelian risks* are used where an individual is at a known 'prior' risk of having inherited a mutant gene, but some other information is available which changes the overall risk of having inherited the condition. An example is the use of creatine kinase enzyme levels in females thought to be at risk of carrying Duchenne muscular dystrophy mutations. *Empiric risks*, in contrast, are based on observed data of recurrence in sibships involving several families with the same clinical problem, but where a simple mendelian pattern of inheritance does not apply. The most common reason for giving empiric risks to a family is that a mendelian disorder cannot be recognized. This could be due to a chromosomal basis for the condition or, more commonly, because the condition in question has several aetiological causes which are not clinically identifiable. Genetic deafness is a good example. Although environmental and genetic aetiologies are well documented, it is impossible to infer aetiology in an isolated case with a negative family history and negative investigations. Consequently an empiric risk is appropriate and is calculated as follows (Baraitser and Winter, 1983):

$$7/10 \times 2/3 \times 1/4 = 1/9 \text{ approximately.}$$

Although 50% of congenital deafness is thought to be environmental, if all investigations for such causes are negative, approximately 70% of the remainder would be estimated to be genetic. Of these, most studies suggest that approximately two-thirds are of autosomal recessive inheritance, which have a one in four recurrence risk. Hence the risk of recurrence in a subsequent pregnancy to the normal parents of a single deaf child is approximately one in nine. Empiric risks are unsatisfactory, because their calculation implicitly recognizes that some families have a higher risk of recurrence and some a lower risk. Of course there is a need for ongoing review of families counselled empirically, since the birth of a second affected child will confirm that the deafness in the family is almost definitely autosomal recessive, with a one in four chance of recurrence.

It is evident from the foregoing that much of the work of a geneticist is focused on securing a specific diagnosis to provide a basis for satisfactory counselling. Moreover several factors have been documented in regard to genetic deafness which may have a bearing on counselling. Marriage between deaf individuals is commonplace, thus introducing the possibility of several independent genetic causes of deafness arising in the one pedigree. Likewise this assortive mating may mean that genetic counselling for deafness is appropriate for deaf people with a definite environmental aetiology. Frequently a diagnosis of acquired deafness may have been made in childhood, which does not withstand rigorous investigation, thus changing the basis for risk estimation in the next generation. Finally, it is important to be aware of cultural factors within the deaf community, as many affected individuals are deeply hostile to any suggestion that the aim of counselling is to minimize the risk of transmitting deafness (Arnos, Israel and Cunningham, 1991; Christiansen, 1991; King, 1991).

Prevalence of genetic deafness

It should be emphasized that 'deafness' in genetic terms usually refers to sensorineural deafness. Few genetically determined conditions cause a pure conductive deafness or a mixed deafness picture. Several studies have independently indicated that approximately 50% of all childhood deafness is 'genetic' in aetiology and a suggested incidence of 1/2000 livebirths is appropriate to genetic deafness, although it must be emphasized that the cohorts studied in each of the many such surveys are not strictly comparable (Beighton 1990; Reardon, 1992). In these circumstances 'genetic' usually refers to single gene disorders which give rise to deafness and other possible sources of genetic deafness have not been specifically sought.

The clinical spectrum of inherited deafness is broad and ranges from simple deafness without other clinical abnormalities to genetically-determined syndromes affecting several different body systems in which deafness is only one of many signs which together comprise the syndrome. The diagnosis of syndromic deafness may appear uncomplicated but the variability in phenotype from one affected individual to the next, as a reflection of clinical expressivity of the gene, can often be quite confusing. Consequently, it is often useful, even where the diagnosis seems relatively clearcut, to seek the advice of an expert dysmorphologist.

Malformations, deformations, disruptions and syndromes

Based on a comprehensive review of the world literature Kennedy (1974) found a prevalence for congenital malformation of 1.08% to 4.5%, depending on the method of ascertainment. Major malformations are present in 2% of all liveborn children and account for over 20% of neonatal deaths. The form or structure of tissues and organs may be altered in three basic ways:

1 Malformations, in which the developmental process was always abnormal, e.g. polydactyly
2 Deformations, in which developmentally normal processes are modified by mechanical forces to produce an abnormal outcome, e.g. plagiocephaly
3 Disruption, in which an extrinsic breakdown or interference with an originally normal developmental process leads to altered morphology, e.g. the phocomelia of thalidomide embryopathy.

The term 'syndrome', meaning 'running together' is used to describe one of the relationships which may exist between observed abnormalities of morphology in a patient. By definition a syndrome consists of multiple abnormalities thought to be causally related, e.g. in Down's syndrome the trisomy 21 accounts for the congenital heart disease and characteristic dysmorphology seen in affected patients.

It is worth recalling the natural history of syndrome delineation. All syndromes began as clinical descriptions, frequently in unrelated patients. Subsequent expansion of the syndrome may have involved the reporting of other clinical stigmata in patients with apparently the same condition. This delineated the syndrome into various subtypes on the basis of distinctive clinical characteristics. Perhaps the recognition of the syndrome in related individuals, sometimes in a manner suggestive of a mendelian inheritance pattern, indicated a single genetic mutation as the basis for the multiple abnormalities observed in patients with the syndrome and, finally, the identification of the cause of the syndrome, be it a single gene event, a chromosomal event, or an environmentally induced event. Some of the syndromes to be considered later in this chapter have reached this endpoint and their cause is known thereby allowing a consideration of the clinical signs as a reflection of the underlying cause. Most syndromes are at the clinical description or pedigree level and their exact aetiologies remain to be defined (Cohen, 1982).

Syndrome recognition is valuable, not only for the assistance it offers to the geneticist in estimating recurrence risks, but because if the phenotypic spectrum of a syndrome is well delineated, the identification of that syndrome in a given patient facilitates the search for cryptic defects which might lead to clinical problems at a later stage in the disease process. Examples of this are radiological examination of the vertebrae in Goldenhar syndrome to look for hemivertebrae, and ophthalmological examination in Stickler syndrome to detect early signs of retinal detachment. Finally, it is worth remembering that syndromes due to single gene disorders are a reflection, not just of the mutant gene, but of the interaction of that gene and its protein product with several other genes and with environmental influences. Hence the pattern of clinical signs attributable to a given syndrome is in no way stereotyped and can sometimes overlap with clinical phenomena described in aetiologically distinct syndromes. This range of clinical variability can mask the correct syndromic diagnosis and suggest an alternative, incorrect, diagnosis with obvious detrimental consequences for management, genetic counselling and risk estimation.

The identification of genetic loci

The clinician who identifies a large family, several of whom are affected by the same single gene disorder, may feel that the identification of the locus and cloning the gene is only a short step away. Unfortunately this is not the case and several years may separate the family identification and sample collection stage from the ultimate cloning of the responsible gene. Good clinical data are an essential prerequisite of any genetic study. For an autosomal dominant or X-linked disorder a single pedigree may be large enough to be used as the basis for a linkage study. More frequently, and always in the case of autosomal recessively transmitted disease, several families sharing the same condition are studied to see if chromosomal localization of the locus can be achieved. This is the strategy known as family linkage studies. The major pitfall of this strategy is that by including several families there is a risk that not all problems are due to mutation at the same genetic locus and statistically significant results about gene localization may be obscured. To a degree, careful selection of families for entry to the study and well-defined clinical criteria help overcome this hurdle and this is particularly true of syndromic conditions.

The genetic localization of a disorder is investigated by looking for cosegregation of the gene, as defined by affected and unaffected family members, with markers of known chromosomal location. Any two loci have a 50% chance of being coinherited, but if enough marker loci are tested, then cosegregation between marker loci from a specific chromosomal region and the disease locus may be observed. Special statistical methods are applied to the analysis of such studies, the outcome being expressed in terms of LOD ($\log_{10}$ of the odds) scores. A score of $+3$ or greater is taken as significant at the 5% level. Such a result in a

linkage study will be followed by detailed mapping studies of the disease locus and a much wider range of marker loci from the chromosomal region of interest to confirm the linkage and to refine the disease localization. Several complex strategies for gene identification may then be adopted, although in any particular case the decision as to which is most appropriate may be governed by factors such as whether a specific candidate gene has already been identified in this chromosome region whose malfunction might conceivably lead to the disease phenotype, whether clinical material from patients with chromosomal anomalies of this region is available etc. Further discussion of these strategies is beyond the scope of this text but an excellent short review is given by Davies and Read (1992).

These steps are designed to identify the disease locus. Identification of a specific mutation within that DNA sequence may require significant further effort and time. While mutations lead to disease by virtue of the abnormal gene product, the precise biological reason as to why mutation at a specific locus may cause deafness is likely to be different for most of the deafness causing loci. The disturbance of cellular biology resulting in deafness may be unique to each genetically distinct cause of deafness.

Classification of genetic deafness

There are as many classifications as there are textbooks and none is perfect. However if genetic deafness is considered in relation to underlying aetiology, four broad categories need to be discussed:

1 Monogenic (i.e single gene disorders)
  a undifferentiated deafness
    autosomal dominant
    autosomal recessive
    X-linked recessive
  b syndromic
    autosomal dominant
    autosomal recessive
    X-linked
  c miscellaneous single gene disorders, which may be associated with deafness
2 Mitochondrial mutations causing deafness
3 Chromosomal disorders associated with deafness
4 Deafness due to aetiologically heterogeneous disorders of development.

Monogenic

Undifferentiated deafness (i.e. non-syndromic deafness)

Approximately 70% of monogenic deafness is said to be undifferentiated. The only clinical finding is deafness and the only clue to aetiology is the pattern of inheritance in the pedigree. Autosomal dominant, autosomal recessive and X-linked forms are described and it is likely that there are several loci responsible for each, the phenomenon known as genetic heterogeneity. Clearly, recognition of the genetic basis is impossible in the sporadic case, underlining the role of empiric counselling for such situations. It is estimated that more than 75% are autosomal recessive in aetiology, with a further 10–20% being autosomal dominant and 2–3% being X-linked recessive. Konigsmark and Gorlin (1976) have attempted to document undifferentiated deafness in terms of inheritance pattern, audiogram characteristics, vestibular function profile and histopathological observations. It seems very likely however that these parameters are insufficient to discriminate accurately between forms of undifferentiated deafness due to different underlying mutations. It is a measure of the resistance of genetic deafness to molecular advances that the Konigsmark and Gorlin classification remains in common use despite well recognized limitations and the distorted genetic picture it creates.

Autosomal dominant undifferentiated deafness

Konigsmark and Gorlin (1976) suggested six different types, according to age of onset and audiogram characteristics of the deafness, but McKusick (1992), on reviewing the published pedigree data accepts only three types with certainty – progressive low tone, mid tone and progressive high tone. All are of sensorineural deafness, but as emphasized by Beighton (1990) the precise recognition of these types in practice is not always so clearcut. Fraser (1976) reiterated the observation that gene penetrance is known to be quite variable in this group of disorders and several examples have been documented in which the gene has appeared to skip a generation only to reappear among the offspring.

The number of genetic loci which cause autosomal dominant undifferentiated deafness remains unknown. To date only one such locus has been localized on the basis of linkage studies in a large inbred Costa Rican family (Leon *et al.*, 1992). There has been no further report of this gene being more closely defined and the molecular pathology of this form of autosomal dominant deafness remains undetermined at the time of writing.

Autosomal recessive undifferentiated deafness

Quite how many forms of this exist has been widely debated with estimates ranging from three (Konigsmark and Gorlin, 1976) on the basis of audiogram characteristics and age of onset, to six (Stevenson and Cheeseman, 1956), based on mathematical calculations of a population survey of hereditary deaf with hereditary deaf matings, to 35 (Morton, 1960), based on complex mathematical analysis. Furthermore, Morton suggested that the carrier rate for autosomal

recessive deafness genes may be as high as 16%, although the usually quoted heterozygote figure for autosomal recessive deafness is 10% (Fraser, 1976). The variability of these estimates emphasizes the current deficiencies in our knowledge about this group of conditions. Genetically distinct forms are not recognizable at the clinical level nor is there evidence that modern techniques of cochlear function assessment can help overcome this problem. Unlike the situation with a clearcut autosomal dominant pedigree, the distinction between genetic and environmental causes of the deafness is obscured, unless consanguinity in the family tilts the balance of suspicion towards this aetiology. The recognition of a second affected child is usually confirmatory. Several subpopulations have been described with a higher prevalence of this form of deafness (Beighton, 1990). In such communities the empiric risk calculations which form the basis of counselling to the family of the sporadic case will need to be modified to take account of these local factors. Clinical and audiological evaluations of obligate gene carriers have not been helpful in identifying the carrier state.

X-linked recessive undifferentiated deafness

A male-to-female disproportion among deaf patients with a preponderance of males was first alluded to by Wilde (1853) and subsequent studies have suggested that 2–3% of genetic deafness is due to this form of inheritance (Fraser, 1976; Reardon, 1990). While it seems likely on the basis of genetic linkage studies that there are at least two distinct forms (Reardon *et al.*, 1991), the more common of these, characterized by stapes fixation and perilymphatic 'gusher' at surgery, is characterized by a distinctive radiological profile which almost certainly underlies the observation of a 'gusher' in some of the pedigrees published (Phelps *et al.*, 1991). Although many of these families have a mixed pattern of deafness, thought to reflect the stapes fixation, this is by no means exclusively true and a range of disturbance of other otoneurological parameters has also been defined in such subjects (Glasscock, 1973; Reardon *et al.*, 1993a). Family linkage studies have suggested a localization for this form of deafness at Xq13–q21 (Brunner *et al.*, 1988; Wallis *et al.*, 1988; Reardon *et al.*, 1991), but the gene has not been cloned at the time of writing.

Several obligate carrier females may show disturbed auditory function and if present this may be a useful aid to counselling (Reardon *et al.*, 1992a) and a smaller number have anatomical abnormalities on CT scan of the cochlea (Phelps *et al.*, 1991). However, the nature and extent of such changes are very variable and the absence of such abnormalities cannot be taken as synonymous with the non-carrier state in females from pedigrees with this form of deafness (Reardon *et al.*, 1993a).

Syndromic deafness

Autosomal dominant syndromic forms of deafness

Under this category are considered syndromes primarily associated with deafness. Only a few of the commoner syndromes encountered in clinical practice will be described. Comprehensive details are provided by Winter and Baraitser (1993).

Waardenburg syndrome

Probably the single most recognized form of syndromic deafness, this condition is characterized by pigmentary disturbance, lateral displacement of the inner canthi of the eye and deafness. The pigmentary abnormalities range from the classical white forelock to iris heterochromia to depigmented skin patches. Sometimes it is more subtle, affecting only the eyelash (Figure 3.1). It is important to recognize that the clinical features of this condition are highly variable and the classical stigmata may be present in any combination and to varying degrees. Based on the clinical features and their segregation within families, heterogeneity has been proposed and the syndrome has been subdivided into types 1 and 2 on the basis of the presence of dystophia canthorum (lateral displacement of the inner punctum of the eye) in type 1 and its absence in type 2. Deafness is observed in approximately 25% of all cases of Waardenburg syndrome but is said to occur in a higher proportion of those with type 2 (Arias, 1971). Vestibular hypofunction is an often overlooked feature, estimated to have a prevalence of 75% in the condition (Konigsmark and Gorlin, 1976).

A single case report in 1989 (Ishikiriyama *et al.*, 1989) of a boy with dystophia canthorum, sensorineural deafness, heterochromia iridis, partially albinotic fundi and skin depigmentation was seminal to the identification of the gene for Waardenburg syndrome type 1. This patient was reported to have a *de novo* chromosome rearrangement involving the long arm of chromosome 2, confirmed by the normal karyotypes in both his parents. This fortuitous observation of the disease phenotype in a patient with a *de novo* chromosomal rearrangement has been valuable in the gene localization of several other conditions. Subsequently family linkage studies strengthened the likely localization on chromosome 2q when significant cosegregation of gene markers from this area and Waardenburg syndrome was found (Foy *et al.*, 1990). More recently mutations in the DNA of the HuP2 gene have been identified in several families with Waardenburg syndrome type 1 and also in a single family with Waardenburg syndrome type 2 (Tassabehji *et al.*, 1993).

Overall about 56% families with Waardenburg syndrome are thought to be linked to chromosome 2q and these appear to be mainly of the type 1 group. However, it appears likely that some more type 2 families will also be due to mutations at the HuP2 locus, and likewise that some type 1 families will be due to mutations involving another locus or loci. It remains to be defined at the time of writing how many other loci exist, mutations at which may underlie the Waardenburg phenotype. It is already clear however that the strict delineation of the Waardenburg syndrome into distinct types on the basis of clinical characteristics is not altogether valid at a genetic level.

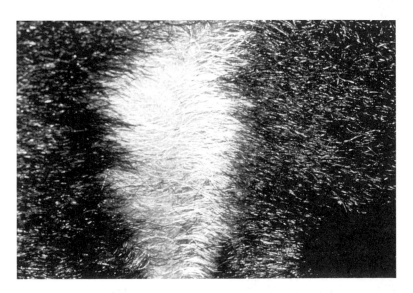

Figure 3.1 Waardenburg syndrome: note the pigmentary disturbance of the hair characteristic of this autosomal dominant condition

LEOPARD syndrome

The acronym LEOPARD signifies *l*entigines, *e*lectrocardiograph abnormalities, *o*cular hypertelorism, *p*ulmonary stenosis, *a*bnormalities of genitalia, *r*etardation of growth and sensorineural *d*eafness. Typically affected patients have numerous small dark brown spots on the skin over the arms and trunk, and may involve the face. These are usually present from birth or the early neonatal period and spare mucosal surfaces (Figure 3.2). Valvular pulmonary stenosis is the single most common structural heart lesion but a wide variety of other heart abnormalities have been described, including atrial septal defects, infundibular or supravalvular pulmonary stenosis, subaortic stenosis and hypertrophic cardiomyopathy. Although not present in all patients with the syndrome, the ECG abnormality is said to be unique and is characterized by a superiorly oriented mean QRS axis in the frontal plane, generally between $-60°$ and $-120°$. Even in the absence of skin pigmentary signs and structural heart lesions this ECG observation is said to be diagnostic of the syndrome. Heart block has been reported in several patients. Mental retardation, usually in the mild range, has been noted in up to 25% of cases. Male patients frequently have cryptorchidism and in some female patients ovarian hypoplasia is a feature of the syndrome. Stature tends to be short and the face is characterized by a triangular shape, hypertelorism, ptosis, epicanthic folds and the lentigenes, if present. Sensorineural deafness is a feature in about 25% of cases, although the degree can be variable (Pickering *et al.*, 1971).

Branchio-oto-renal syndrome

This is a highly variable condition characterized by the presence of auricular or preauricular pits in association with ear malformations, branchial sinuses and renal abnormalities in the full blown phenotype. However preauricular pits are a frequent non-specific minor malformation in neonates and are generally not associated with any other anomalies. In families where the syndrome is segregating the diagnosis may be made in the absence of auricular pitting or branchial sinuses (Figure 3.3). In the sporadic case, however, where the possibility of a new mutation has to be considered, the diagnosis may be much more difficult to confirm. Allied to these considerations is the fact that a degree of confusion exists in the literature with some authors separating 'earpits-deafness' syndrome from branchio-oto-renal syndrome and the use of term branchio-oto-urethral syndrome. Essentially it is thought that these clinical entities all refer to the same condition (Cremers and Fikkers-van Noord, 1980), although whether these are genetically homogeneous or not remains to be elucidated. In light of the confusion surrounding this entity it is not surprising that accurate data as to prevalence of the different features in patients with the condition are deficient. Current estimates suggest that the branchial signs are present in approximately 60% of patients, otological signs apparent in 80%, deafness in 66% and renal anomalies in 10%. This latter figure may represent an underestimate as renal investigations have frequently been omitted in reported families. Indeed, it is noteworthy in this respect that Konigsmark and Gorlin (1976) did not refer to the renal system in their summary of clinical and investigative data about the condition, signifying the relative neglect that has characterized the renal manifestations of this syndrome. However, structural anomalies of the kidney and ureteric system have been documented ranging from renal agenesis and hypoplasia to glomerular lesions. While Konigsmark and Gorlin (1976) referred to sensorineural deafness of variable degree in several members of a large pedigree, more recent authors have indicated that the deafness is more characteristically mixed in type (Slack and Phelps, 1985; Beighton, 1990).

As with Waardenburg syndrome, a chromosomal clue to the possible locus for this syndrome has been published. Haan *et al.* (1989) described eight patients

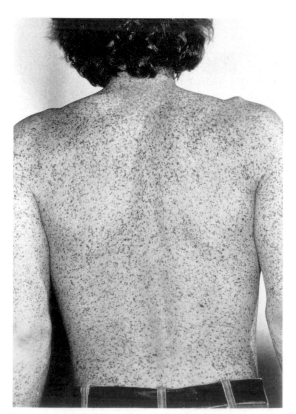

Figure 3.2 LEOPARD syndrome: Note the typical pigmentary lentigines of this condition.

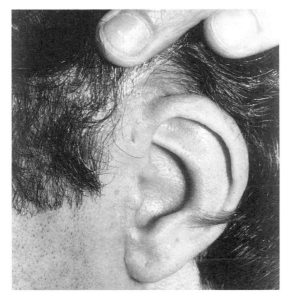

(*a*)

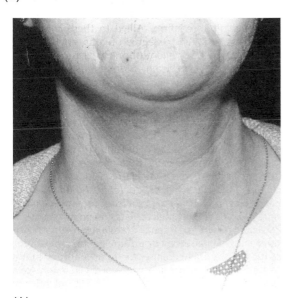

(*b*)

Figure 3.3 Branchio-oto-renal syndrome: note the preauricular pit in the classical branchio-oto-renal position in this male patient (*a*). His mother shows the neck scar of previous surgery for her branchial sinus (*b*).

in the same pedigree with branchio-oto-renal syndrome and tricho-rhino-phalangeal syndrome in association with a rearrangement of chromosome 8q. Linkage studies of pedigrees with the syndrome has since shown significant linkage to this region (Smith *et al.*, 1992a) and it is likely that mutations in most,

if not all, families will be documented at this locus in the future.

Treacher Collins syndrome

Mandibulofacial dysostosis, also known eponymously after Treacher Collins, is characterized by a recognizable facial appearance. The palpebral fissures are downslanting and there is marked malar hypoplasia. The mandible is small causing a receding chin appearance. Frequently there is a lower eyelid coloboma. The pinna is frequently deformed or misplaced and the external auditory canal atretic or narrow (Figure 3.4). Deafness may be conductive, mixed or sensorineural, depending on the nature of the structural malformations in a given patient.

Although several chromosomal abnormalities have been described in patients with Treacher Collins syndrome, the report of a single patient with a *de novo* translocation between the long arm of chromosome 5 and the short arm of chromosome 13 has been most helpful in terms of gene localization (Baelestrazzi *et al.*, 1983). Both Jabs *et al.* (1991) and Dixon *et al.* (1991) independently reported significant linkage results between the Treacher Collins locus and chromosome 5q markers. To date the precise nature of the locus and its underlying mutations has not been reported.

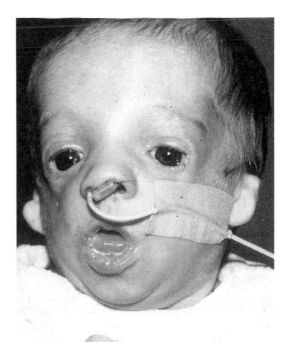

Figure 3.4 Treacher Collins syndrome: note the down slanting palpebral fissures and abnormal ears. Frequently there will be colobomata of the lower eyelid.

Neurofibromatosis type II

Also known as central neurofibromatosis or bilateral acoustic neurofibromatosis, this autosomal dominant condition is quite distinct from von Recklinghausen's disease (neurofibromatosis type I or peripheral neurofibromatosis). The cardinal feature of the condition is bilateral acoustic neuroma. This results in pressure on the VIIIth cranial nerve leading to deafness in many affected cases. The age of onset of the deafness is variable, most commonly in the second or third decade, although instances of onset in the eighth decade have been recorded. Other tumours involving the central nervous system are common in affected patients and their families. Although glial tumours and meningiomas have been recorded in this condition many times, schwannomas are a more characteristic occurrence.

Café-au-lait patches are a feature of the condition but are fewer in number than required for the diagnosis of neurofibromatosis type I. In one large series the authors did not document any patient with more than six such patches in association with neurofibromatosis type II (Kanter *et al.*, 1980). Between one and five patches were found in approximately half of affected patients. Similarly, the occasional observation of neurofibromas or plexiform neuromas may suggest a diagnosis of neurofibromatosis type I in which these clinical features are more characteristic (Baraitser, 1990). The gene was localized to chromosome 22 in 1988 (Wertelecki *et al.*) following the observation that chromosome 22 abnormality is common in meningiomatous tissue and the demonstration by Seizinger, Martiza and Gusella (1986) that part of chromosome 22 was lost in acoustic neuroma tissue.

Stickler syndrome

The clinical limits of this autosomal dominantly transmitted condition are still uncertain, some clinicians believing that the disorder of hearing loss, cleft palate and retinal degenerative changes described by Stickler is the same as the vitreoretinal degenerative condition described by Wagner and probably represents the same entity also as the familial radiological abnormalities known as Weissenbacher–Zweymuller syndrome (Gorlin, Cohen and Levin, 1990). It is certain however, that many patients with Pierre-Robin sequence are affected by one of the conditions grouped under the Stickler syndrome flag. Other features in infancy include flattening of the midface, prominence of the eyes and early onset of high myopia (Figure 3.5). High tone sensorineural deafness of a progressive nature is common (approximately 70–80% of cases). Retinal degenerative changes are a fundamental part of the syndrome, often leading to frank detachment and the assessment of a suspected case is not complete without expert ophthalmological exami-

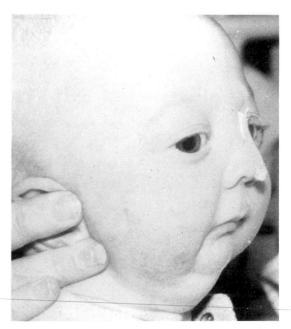

Figure 3.5 Stickler syndrome: lateral view of the face emphasizing the micrognathia which is characteristic of the condition in the neonatal period.

nation. Approximately half of patients will also have a cataract. Early radiological changes of rhizomelic shortening and metaphyseal widening are the forerunners of osteoarthritic changes which tends to be earlier in onset than usual (Temple, 1989).

Stickler syndrome and clinically overlapping disorders are most likely to represent mutations of collagen genes, of which there are several. Consequently it is not surprising that this group of disorders is genetically heterogeneous. Several families with Stickler syndrome do map to the COL2A1 locus on chromosome 12q (Francomano *et al.*, 1987) and mutation in the COL2A1 gene has been identified in one family (Ahmad *et al.*, 1991). However there have been enough instances of families with Stickler syndrome showing recombinations with this locus to demonstrate that other genetic loci for Stickler syndrome-like conditions remain to be identified. The biological basis of the deafness is not understood at present.

Autosomal recessive syndromic deafness

As with the autosomal dominant forms, only a small selection of the more commonly encountered syndromes will be considered.

Usher's syndrome

As many as four different types of Usher's syndrome have been postulated on the basis of the degree of clinical involvement and postulated mode of inheritance. However, McKusick (1992) lists only two types and there is little evidence to support clinical classification beyond this. Both forms are characterized by deafness and retinitis pigmentosa (Figure 3.6). Type I is characterized by severe to profound deafness, absent vestibular responses and prepubertal onset of retinitis pigmentosa. In contrast, type II tends towards a less severe form of deafness, has normal vestibular responses and a later onset of retinal changes (Davenport and Ommen, 1977). Posterior subcapsular cataracts are a frequent late complication. Mental retardation has been described in up to 25% of cases in one series (Hallgren, 1959), though these figures have not been replicated and are generally felt to be a substantial overestimation.

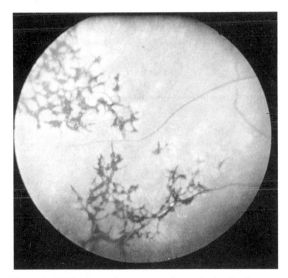

Figure 3.6 Usher's syndrome: note the typical retinal appearance of retinitis pigmentosa in an adult patient with Usher syndrome Type 1.

Using a family linkage study approach and without the guidance of fortuitous chromosomal rearrangements, two research groups mapped a gene for Usher's syndrome type II to chromosome 1q (Lewis *et al.*, 1990; Kimberling *et al.*, 1990). Subsequent work has shown that most Usher II pedigrees are consistent with this gene localization, but at least one family with this diagnosis maps elsewhere, although a precise localization has not been reported.

Families consistent with the Usher I phenotype do not show linkage to 1q, confirming that Usher's syndrome is a genetically heterogeneous condition. Three distinct chromosomal regions have been shown to have significant linkage with Usher's syndrome type I. These are 14q in a French study, which possibly represents a genetically isolated subpopulation in Western France (Kaplan *et al.*, 1992), 11q in French-Acadian and some British families (Smith *et al.*, 1992b) and 11q in families of British, Irish, American non-Acadian and South African origin (Kimberling *et al.*, 1992).

Essentially, at present there is evidence to support at least five distinct gene loci responsible for the two closely related phenotypes of Usher I and II. Three of these loci appear consistent with the type I phenotype in different populations and the chromosome 1q localization appears consistent with the type II phenotype. The fifth locus, responsible for families with type II which do not map to 1q has yet to be identified.

Jervell and Lange-Nielsen syndrome

Although only recognized since 1957, this is one of the most dramatic of syndromes involving deafness in view of the life-threatening consequences of failure to detect the condition. Clinically there is usually a history of fainting in otherwise well deaf children. Approximately 50% of all cases reported died before adolescence during a fainting attack (Fraser, 1976). The fainting is due to cardiac conduction disturbance, manifest as prolonged QT interval on the ECG. This predisposes to arrhythmia of the 'torsade de pointe' type. No localization for the gene has been reported.

Pendred's syndrome

This condition is comprised of deafness and goitre, although it is by no means certain that all patients with this diagnosis share the same underlying gene defect. The deafness is usually sensorineural and abnormal vestibular responses have been recorded in some cases (Konigsmark and Gorlin, 1976). Dyshormonogenesis in the thyroid gland leads to goitre, usually present in childhood. However, goitre is not invariable and definitive diagnosis may require a perchlorate test, although interpretation of the latter as a diagnostic tool may be fraught with difficulty (Fraser, 1976). Theoretically, if perchlorate is given after a tracer dose of ^{131}I, there is an abnormal fall in activity in the gland. Notwithstanding the block in the enzyme pathway in the thyroid, compensatory hyperplasia of the gland is usually adequate to avoid overt hypothyroidism and most cases are euthyroid. Radiological examination of the cochlea has been reported to show a Mondini type malformation, but this has not been a feature of all cases examined (Phelps and Lloyd, 1983). The underlying gene defect(s) have not been identified, although a possible gene localization has been suggested on the basis of the coincidental observation of an unbalanced chromosomal complement involving deletion of 8q in a mentally retarded, deaf girl with thyroid hormone dysgenesis (van Wouwe *et al.*, 1986). As yet this localization is unconfirmed.

X-linked syndromic deafness

Alport's syndrome

Many of the early classic family studies in families with nephritis with or without deafness appeared to support an autosomal dominant form of inheritance for this condition. It is likely that several different genetic conditions were represented in these studies, each sharing the common feature of an inherited nephritis. An extensive review of the genetics of 'classic' Alport's syndrome was performed by Flinter *et al.* (1988). Crucially these authors defined strict diagnostic criteria for the condition, and so avoided the type of diagnostic confusion which bedevilled previous studies. The genetics of 'classic' Alport's syndrome are compatible with X-linked recessive inheritance, with males being affected more severely and with no male-to-male transmission being recorded. The clinical course in males progresses from haematuria in early childhood, with progressive sensorineural deafness developing during school years, to chronic renal failure by the early 20s and characteristic ophthalmic signs of anterior lenticonus and macular flecks manifesting in late teenage years. The course in females is much milder and more variable. A minority of 15% progress to chronic renal failure by 40 years, but almost all others remain asymptomatic throughout life, although microscopic haematuria is an almost constant finding among carrier females.

The subsequent course of developments represents a series of triumphs for molecular genetics. Initial linkage to markers on Xq (Flinter, Abbs and Bobrow, 1989) indicated an approximate localization of the gene. The subsequent recognition that one of the genes for type IV collagen (the COL4A5 gene), known to be a major structural component of basement membrane, mapped to this same region of the X chromosome (Myers *et al.*, 1990) sparked intense investigation of this gene in Alport families to see if actual mutations at DNA level could be identified. This proved to be the case, Barker *et al.* (1990) confirming the X-linkage of 'classic' Alport's syndrome by demonstrating COL4A5 abnormalities in individuals with this condition. It is important to realize that this finding does not preclude other mutations in different components of the type IV collagen gene, such as COL4A1 and COL4A2, both of which are located on chromosome 13, as causes of autosomally transmitted forms of basement membrane disease which may present clinically with nephritis with or without deafness. These mimic the Alport picture and provide the likely reason for the controversy which surrounded the genetics of Alport's syndrome prior to Flinter's study.

In summary, genetically determined abnormalities of type IV collagen may present with a nephritis and deafness profile. Since type IV collagen is composed of several units, some autosomally encoded, and at least one (COL4A5) encoded on the long arm of the X chromosome, the pattern of inheritance in an individual family will depend upon the site of mutation in that family. 'Classic' Alport's syndrome, as defined by Flinter *et al.* (1988), relates to the clinical phenotype consequent on X-linked mutations. However, several pedigrees exist which are almost certainly examples of autosomal dominant transmission which have been well reviewed elsewhere (McKusick, 1992) and which may ultimately prove to be due to mutations of the autosomally encoded units of type IV collagen.

Otopalatodigital syndrome

This is a rare condition memorable for the cleft palate, distinctive facies, widely separated toes, short stature and conductive deafness in several of the affected cases reported (Figure 3.7). Most have had a mild degree of mental retardation and abnormal ossicular development has been documented in a few instances (Gorlin, Cohen and Levin, 1990).

Miscellaneous single gene disorders which may be associated with deafness

These are so many that any selection is bound to be idiosyncratic. Particularly noteworthy are osteogenesis imperfecta and the syndromes of craniosynostosis, of which there are over 100. Only the commonly recognized phenotypes will be discussed here.

Osteogenesis imperfecta

This comprises a complex and heterogeneous group of genetic disorders involving abnormalities of type I collagen for the most part. The classification of Sillence, Senn and Danks (1979) incorporating clinical, genetic and radiological data is the almost universal choice. Many of the underlying mutations have now been characterized at DNA level and their phenotypic correlations clarified. Essentially there are two classes of collagen mutation. In the first the quantity of type I collagen produced is reduced but that which is produced is of normal quality, whereas in the second class of mutation, the structure of the collagen produced is abnormal. The latter has more deleterious consequences (Byers, Wallis and Willing, 1991). The pattern of inheritance may be autosomal dominant or autosomal recessive, varying from mutation to mutation.

Deafness is most common in osteogenesis imperfecta types I and III. Type I patients are characteristically of normal stature, with little or no bony deformity and blue sclerae. Type III, in contrast, is characterized by progressive skeletal deformity, short stature and, usually, dentinogenesis imperfecta. Scleral colour is not as characteristic in this form. Both tend

been documented which may give rise to either phenotype and indeed deafness has also been recorded in association with some mutations which give an osteogenesis imperfecta type IV phenotype, which is clinically milder. Consequently, osteogenesis imperfecta is not a single diagnosis but each family represents clinical manifestations of a particular mutation involving collagen, usually collagen type I.

Saethre-Chotzen syndrome

This is a very variable autosomal dominant condition, essentially comprising craniosynostosis, facial asymmetry, ptosis, brachydactyly with or without syndactyly, and several skeletal anomalies (Gorlin, Cohen and Levin, 1990) (Figure 3.8). Although mild to moderate hearing loss is commonly described in this disorder, thought to be the result of compression of the VIIIth nerve, the exact prevalence of deafness as part of the syndrome remains ill defined. Several cases have been identified with cytogenetic abnormalities of 7p21. The most convincing in terms of suggesting this area as the site of the causative locus being the report of a classical Saethre-Chotzen phenotype in association with a *de novo* translocation (Reardon *et al.*, 1993b). Linkage to this area has been documented in several large pedigrees (Brueton *et al.*, 1992), but the gene has yet to be defined.

Crouzon's syndrome

The phenotype of Crouzon's syndrome is more consistently recognizable than that of Saethre-Chotzen syndrome, largely due to the characteristic maxillary hypoplasia, shallow orbits and proptosis (Figure 3.9). It is also an autosomal dominant condition, with a high incidence of new mutation, perhaps accounting for greater than 50% of cases (Gorlin, Cohen and Levin, 1990). Deafness of an unspecified nature has been documented in 55%, and external auditory canal atresia in 13% (Kreiborg, 1981). The gene for the condition remains unknown, but it has been established that it is not an allelic form of any of the mapped craniosynostosis genes (Reardon *et al.*, 1994).

Apert's syndrome

This autosomal dominant condition is characterized by craniosynostosis with midfacial flattening and syndactyly, often giving the typical 'mitten' hands and feet (Figure 3.10). Many patients with this condition are mentally retarded, thus reducing the likelihood of reproducing, hence most cases represent new mutations. No consistent chromosomal abnormality has been reported and no linkage clues for gene localization have emerged. Otitis media is common, perhaps related to the high prevalence of cleft palate. Likewise

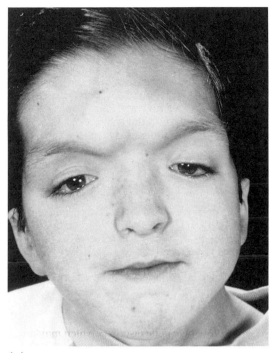

(a)

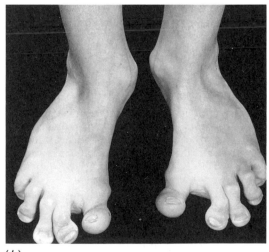

(b)

Figure 3.7 Otopalatodigital syndrome: (a) Face–note the prominent supra-orbital ridges and down slanting palpebral fissures. There is also hypertelorism and a broad nasal root. (b) Feet–there is exaggerated clefting between the hallux and the other toes. Note the typical tree frogging appearance.

to be inherited as autosomal dominant conditions although there are exceptions to this (Byers, Wallis and Willing, 1991). Several different mutations have

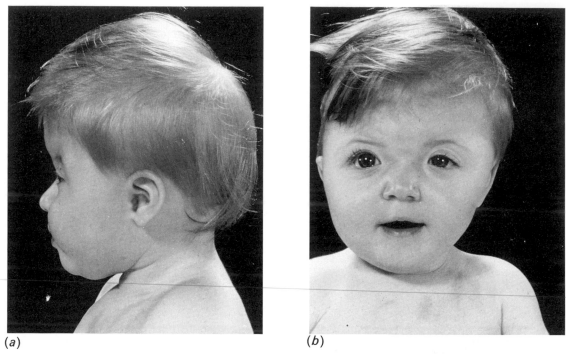

(*a*)   (*b*)

Figure 3.8 Saethre-Chotzen syndrome: AP (*a*) and lateral (*b*) views of the face to emphasize the facial asymmetry, ptosis, brachy-cephaly and prominence of the crus helicisis which are the major featuress of this variable condition in the patient shown.

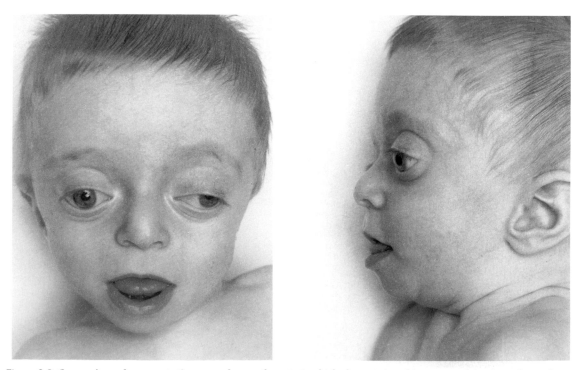

Figure 3.9 Crouzon's syndrome: note the severe degree of proptosis which characterizes this autosomal dominant form of craniosynostosis

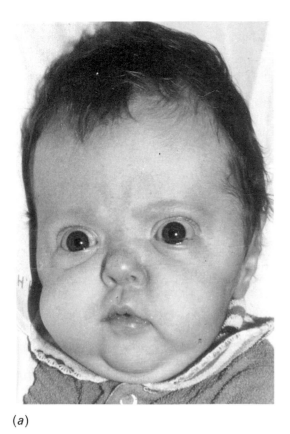

(a)

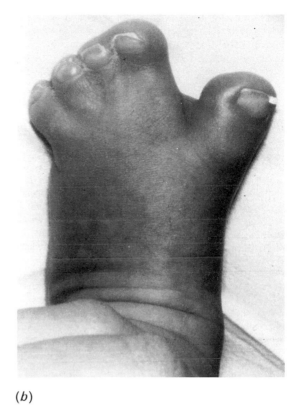

(b)

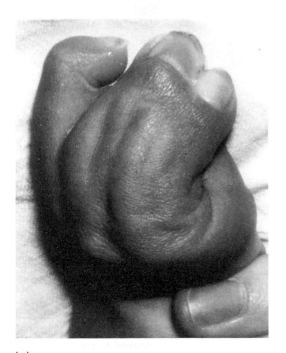

(c)

Figure 3.10 Apert's syndrome: there is marked
craniosynostosis with midface hypoplasia and depression of
the nasal bridge (a). The hands and feet show skin and
bony syndactyly (b and c).

a congenitally fixed stapes footplate is a frequent observation. An exact figure for prevalence of deafness in this patient group remains unclear (Gorlin, Cohen and Levin, 1990).

Mitochondrial mutations causing deafness

Although mitochondrially-mediated genetic disease has been perceived to be primarily a disorder with clinical neuromuscular presentation, this is not exclusively true. Historically this group of disorders has been recognized on the basis of an abnormal muscle biopsy showing ragged red fibres when stained by the Gomori trichrome method. Given this ascertainment bias, it seems likely that the full spectrum of mitochondrially-mediated genetic disease remains unappreciated. Nonetheless, several different types of mitochondrial mutations have been shown to be associated with deafness. Careful documentation of the clinical findings in four separate studies, using different populations of mitochondrially-mediated disease has consistently uncovered deafness as a feature in all cohorts studied (Petty, Harding and Morgan-Hughes, 1986; Holt *et al.*, 1989; Poulton, Deadman and Gardiner, 1989; Reardon *et al.*, 1992b). The striking feature is the variability of clinical presentation and the extent of disease, irrespective of whether the method of ascertainment was clinical and histological (Petty, Harding and Morgan-Hughes, 1986) or clinical and molecular (Holt *et al.*, 1989; Poulton, Deadman and Gardiner, 1989; Reardon *et al.*, 1992b).

This phenomenon is readily understandable in the context of mitochondrial genetics, where a proportion of cells have normal DNA and a proportion have mutant DNA. While the fine cellular and molecular mechanisms remain obscure, current thinking suggests that the higher the proportion of mutant-DNA-containing-cells in any given tissue or organ, the more likely that tissue or organ is to show pathology. Obviously some tissues are more prone to mitochondrially-mediated damage than others, in particular those tissues with a high metabolic turnover would seem to be most vulnerable. Although all affected members within a family will have inherited the same mutation from the mother's mitochondrial genome, the proportion of abnormal DNA present in each individual is purely a random event. This is the genetic basis of the clinical variability. Consequently, a consistent clinical profile for mitochondrially-determined deafness is most unlikely to emerge. The best approach is to combine family history taking with an integrated view of the patient's symptoms as a whole rather than a series of unrelated diseases in the same patient.

Finally, three particular reports deserve special mention, because they specifically correlated deafness with mitochondrial mutations. Higashi (1989) noted that familial streptomycin-induced deafness appeared to be transmitted predominantly through females, compatible with mitochondrial inheritance. Secondly in a large Arab–Israeli pedigree maternally inherited sensorineural deafness was described in which formal segregation analysis suggested that the deafness represented a two-locus model due to simultaneous inheritance of the mitochondrial mutation and an autosomal recessive gene (Jaber *et al.*, 1992). A mitochondrial DNA point mutation has now been identified in both these conditions which is thought to underlie the deafness (Prezant *et al.*, 1993). This mutation leads to an amino acid substitution in the ribosomal RNA, thought to enhance aminoglycoside binding. Finally Ballinger *et al.* (1992) observed deafness of an unspecified nature in association with diabetes mellitus in a family shown to have a deletion of the mitochondrial DNA. As with the other two reports the clue to the true nature of the condition lay with the recognition that the condition was maternally transmitted.

Chromosomal disorders associated with deafness

Specific chromosomal disorders and, in particular, Down's syndrome (trisomy 21) may be significantly associated with deafness. However, deafness is a highly non-specific finding among patients with chromosomal problems. There are over 150 discrete chromosomal abnormalities documented which have been associated with deafness in reported cases and it is likely that there may be many others unreported. The chromosomal anomalies reported in these patients have covered virtually every chromosome and the nature of the chromosomal irregularity has included deletions, duplications, ring chromosomes, trisomy, triploidy and mosaicism. The reason for this diversity both in chromosome region and in the nature of abnormality in patients with abnormal karyotype and deafness is that a chromosomal anomaly reflects problems due to a deficiency or an excess of several genetic loci. Consequently deafness will only be part of the clinical picture in such patients.

The observation of deafness associated with a specific chromosomal abnormality may be enormously important to researchers attempting to identify a deafness locus in that particular chromosomal region. X-linked recessive undifferentiated deafness is a case in point. Although a possible locus at Xq21 had been identified in linkage studies and several patients with deletions of this and surrounding regions of the chromosome were found to be deaf, it was unclear whether these observations were due to involvement of the same locus or two discrete loci in the same cytogenetic region. The report of a patient with a cytogenetic deletion, whose CT scan showed the typical abnormality seen in the cytogenetically normal members of the families used in the linkage study, confirmed that the two data sets related to the same disease locus (Reardon *et al.*, 1992c). Similarly the important contributions of the coincidental observation of syndromic deafness and cytogenetic abnormalities have already been highlighted.

Deafness due to aetiologically heterogeneous disorders of development

Many of the conditions which clinicians associate with deafness are not strictly 'genetic' in that they are not related to a chromosomal disorder nor is an identifiable pattern of inheritance always apparent. Nonetheless familial examples or a skewed sex distribution may suggest a genetic input to the aetiology in a proportion of cases at least. Examples are oculoauriculovertebral phenotype (Goldenhar's syndrome) and Klippel-Feil syndrome.

The Goldenhar phenotype is characterized by hemifacial microsomia, associated with vertebral anomalies and epibulbar dermoids (Figure 3.11). Aetiological heterogeneity is not in question, the condition having been observed in association with several chromosomal abnormalities, teratogenic agents, as an autosomal dominant trait, and as a possible autosomal recessive trait in different affected individuals and their families (Cohen, Rollnick and Kaye, 1989). Deafness is common, perhaps a feature of 50% of cases, and not associated with any particular aetiology. The ear pathology may be extensive, involving the external auditory canal, ossicular development in the middle ear and, occasionally, sensorineural deafness. Clearly there is a genetic contribution to this phenotype in some cases but most cases are not genetic in that mendelian forms of the condition are rare and this is reflected in the small recurrence risk given to clinically normal parents of an affected child (Harper, 1988).

Klippel-Feil anomaly is clinically identified by the fusion of two or more cervical vertebrae, which may extend to involve the lower spine. The condition is due to a failure of normal segmentation in embryonic life. Classification is based on the degree and extent of fusion and mendelian forms have been recognized, autosomal dominant inheritance being the most commonly suggested mode of inheritance (McKusick, 1992). However, there have been several instances of affected siblings born to unaffected parents, suggesting that a proportion of the genetically determined cases may be autosomal recessive in transmission. Most cases are sporadic events with no evidence of cervical malformation in the parents and a low risk of recurrence (Harper, 1988) reflecting the aetiologi-

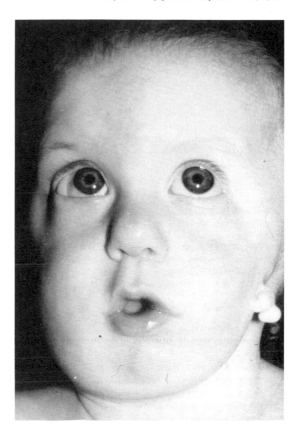

Figure 3.11 Goldenhar's syndrome: this patient has a marked degree of facial asymmetry with a malformed, lowset pinna.

cal heterogeneity which is thought to underlie the condition.

Klippel-Feil malformation may be seen as an isolated finding or in association with more extensive abnormalities. The association of Klippel-Feil malformation, congenital deafness and Duane syndrome (abducens palsy with retraction bulbi) comprises the Wildervanck syndrome, also known as cervico-oculoacusticus syndrome. Several patients also have malformation of the bony cochlea (Phelps and Lloyd, 1983). The inheritance pattern is not established, the condition having been observed almost exclusively in females. Although models proposing polygenic, autosomal dominant with incomplete penetrance and multifactorial inheritance have been postulated the reason for the female preponderance in prevalence is unknown.

Acknowledgements

Drs Michael Baraitser and Robin Winter generously agreed to allow publication of pictures of several patients featured on the London Dysmorphology Database. I should also like to acknowledge Dr Caroline Berry for the picture of LEOPARD syndrome.

References

AHMAD, N. N., ALA-KOKKO, L., KNOWLTON, R. G., JIMINEZ, S. A., WEAVER, E. J., MAGUIRE, J. I. *et al.* (1991) Stop codon in the procollagen II gene (COL2A1) in a family with the Stickler syndrome (arthro-ophthalmopathy). *Proceedings of the National Academy of Sciences*, **88**, 6624–6627

ARIAS, S. (1971) Genetic heterogeneity in the Waardenburg syndrome. *Birth Defects Original Article Series*, **VII**, 87–101

ARNOS, K. S., ISRAEL, J. and CUNNINGHAM, M. (1991) Genetic counselling of the deaf. Medical and cultural considerations. *Annals of the New York Academy of Science*, **630**, 236–239

BAELESTRAZZI, P., BAETEMAN, M. A., MATTEI, M. G. and MATTEI, J. (1983) Franceschetti syndrome in a child with a de novo balanced translocation (5; 13) (q11; p11) and significant decrease of hexosaminidase B. *Human Genetics*, **64**, 305–308

BALLINGER, S. W., SHOFFNER, J. M., HEDAYA, E. V., TROUNCE, I., POLAK, M. A., KOONTZ, D. A. *et al.* (1992) Maternally transmitted diabetes and deafness associated with a 10.4kb mitochondrial DNA deletion. *Nature Genetics*, **1**, 11–15

BARAITSER, M. (1990) *The Genetics of Neurological Disorders*, 2nd edn. Oxford: Oxford University Press

BARAITSER, M. and WINTER, R. M. (1983) *A Colour Atlas of Clinical Genetics*. London: Wolfe Medical Publications

BARKER, D. F., HOSTIKKA, S. L., ZHOU, J., CHOW, L. T., OLIPHANT, A. R., GERKEN, S. C. *et al.* (1990) Identification of mutations in the COL4A5 collagen gene in Alport syndrome. *Science*, **248**, 1224–1227

BEIGHTON, P. (1990) Hereditary deafness. In: *Principles and Practice of Medical Genetics* 2nd edn, edited by A. E. Emery and D. L. Rimoin. Edinburgh: Churchill Livingstone

BISHOP, D. T. (1990) Multifactorial inheritance. In: *Principles and Practice of Medical Genetics*, 2nd edn, edited by A. E. Emery and D. L. Rimoin. Edinburgh: Churchill Livingstone

BRUETON, L. A., VAN HERWERDEN, L., CHOTAI, K. and WINTER, R. M. (1992) The mapping of a gene for craniosynostosis: evidence for linkage of the Saethra–Chotzen syndrome to distal chromosome 7p. *Journal of Medical Genetics*, **29**, 681–685

BRUNNER, H. G., VAN BENNEKOM, C. A., LAMBERMON, E. M. M., LIAN OEI, T., CREMERS, C. W. R. J., WIERINGA, B. *et al.* (1988) The gene for X-linked progressive mixed deafness with perilymphatic gusher during stapes surgery is linked to PGK. *Human Genetics*, **80**, 337–340

BYERS, P. H., WALLIS, G. A. and WILLING, M. C. (1991) Osteogenesis imperfecta: translation of mutation to phenotype. *Journal of Medical Genetics*, **28**, 433–442

CHRISTIANSEN, J. B. (1991) Sociological implications of hearing loss. *Annals of the New York Academy of Science*, **630**, 230–235

COHEN, M. M. JR (1982) *The Child with Multiple Birth Defects*. New York: Raven Press

COHEN, M. M, JR, ROLLNICK, B. R. and KAYE, CL. (1989) Oculoauriculovertebral spectrum: an updated critique. *Cleft Palate Journal*, **26**, 276–286

COLLINS, F. S. (1992) Positional cloning: let's not call it reverse anymore. *Nature Genetics*, **1**, 3–6

CONNOR, J. M. and FERGUSON-SMITH, M. A. (1990) *Essential Medical Genetics*, 3rd edn. Oxford: Blackwell Scientific Publications

CREMERS, C. W. R. J. and FIKKERS-VAN NOORD, M. (1980) The earpits-deafness syndrome: clinical and genetic aspects. *International Journal of Pediatric Otorhinolaryngology*, **2**, 309–322

DAVENPORT, S. L. H. and OMMEN, G. S. (1977). The heterogeneity of Usher syndrome. *Vth International Conference on Birth Defects*, Montreal

DAVIES, K. E. and READ, A. P. (1992) *Molecular Basis of Inherited Disease*, 2nd edn. Oxford: IRL Press at Oxford University Press

DIXON, M. J., READ, A. P., DONNAI, D., COLLEY, A., DIXON, J. and WILLIAMSON R., (1991) The gene for Treacher Collins syndrome maps to the long arm of chromosome 5. *American Journal of Human Genetics*, **49**, 17–22

FLINTER, F. A., ABBS, S. and BOBROW, M. (1989) Localization of the gene for classic Alport syndrome. *Genomics*, **4**, 335–338

FLINTER, F. A., CAMERON, J. S., CHANTLER, C., HOUSTON, I. and BOBROW, M. (1988) The genetics of 'classic' Alport syndrome. *Lancet*, ii, 1005–1007

FOY, C., NEWTON, V., WELLESLEY, D., HARRIS, R. and READ, A. (1990) Assignment of the locus for Waardenburg syndrome type I to human chromosome 2q37 and possible homology to the splotch mouse. *American Journal of Human Genetics*, **46**, 1017–1023

FRANCOMANO, C. A., LIBERFARB, R., HIROSE, T., MAUNEMEE, I. H., STREETEN, E. A., MEYERS, D. A. *et al.* (1987) The Stickler syndrome: evidence for close linkage to the structural gene for Type II collagen. *Genomica*, **1**, 293–296

FRASER, G. R. (1976) *The Causes of Profound Childhood Deafness*. Baltimore: Johns Hopkins University Press

GARROD, A. E. (1902) The incidence of alkaptonuria: a study in chemical individuality. *Lancet*, ii, 1616–1620

GLASSCOCK, M. E. (1973) The stapes gusher. *Archives of Otolaryngology*, **98**, 82–91

GORLIN, R. J., COHEN, M. M. JR and LEVIN, L. S. (1990) *Syndromes of the Head and Neck*, 3rd edn. New York: Oxford University Press

HAAN, E. A., HULL, Y. J., WHITE, S., COCKINGTON, R., CHARLTON, P. and CALLEN, D. F. (1989) Trichorhino-phalangeal and branchio-oto syndromes in a family with an inherited rearrangement of chromosome 8q. *American Journal of Medical Genetics*, **32**, 490–494

HALLGREN, B. (1959) Retinitis pigmentosa combined with congenital deafness: with vestibulo-cerebellar ataxia and mental subnormality in a proportion of cases. *Acta Psychiatrica Neurologica Scandinavica*, **34** (suppl. 138), 9–101

HARDING, A. E. (1989) The mitochondrial genome – breaking the magic circle. *New England Journal of Medicine*, **320**, 1341–1343

HARPER, P. S. (1988) *Practical Genetic Counselling*, 3rd edn. London: Wright

HIGASHI, K. (1989) Unique inheritance of streptomycin-induced deafness. *Clinical Genetics*, **35**, 433–436

HOLT, I. J., HARDING, A. E., COOPER, J. M., SCHAPIR, A. H., TOSCANO, A., CLARK, J. B. *et al.* (1989) Mitochondrial myopathies: clinical and biochemical features of 30 patients with major deletions of muscle mitochondrial DNA. *Annals of Neurology*, **26**, 699–708

ISHIKIRIYAMA, S., TONOKI, H., SHIBUYA, Y., CHIP, S., HARADA, N., ABE, K. *et al.* (1989) Waardenburg syndrome type 1 in a child with *de novo* inversion (2) (q35q37.3). *American Journal of Medical Genetics*, 33, 505–507

JABER, L., SHOHAT, M., BU, X., FISCHEL-GHODSIAN, N., YANG, H.-Y. Y., WANG, S.-J. *et al.* (1992) Sensorineural deafness inherited as a tissue specific mitochondrial disorder. *Journal of Medical Genetics*, 29, 86–90

JABS, E. W., LI, X., COSS, C., TAYLOR, E. W., MEYERS, D. A. and WEBER, J. L. (1991) Mapping the Treacher Collins locus to 5q31.3-q33.3. *Genomics*, 11, 193–198

KANTER, W. R., ELDRIDGE, R., FABRICANT, R., ALLEN, J. C. and KOERBER, T. (1980) Central neurofibromatosis with bilateral acoustic neuroma: genetic, clinical and biochemical distinctions from peripheral neurofibromatosis. *Neurology*, 30, 851–859

KAPLAN, J., GERBER, S., BONNEAU, D., ROZET, J. M., DELRIEU, O., BRIARD, M. L. *et al.* (1992) A gene for Usher syndrome type 1 (USH1A) maps to chromosome 14q. *Genomics*, 14, 979–987

KENNEDY, W. P. (1974) Epidemiologic aspects of the problem of congenital malformation. *Birth Defects Original Article Series*, 3, 1–18

KEREM, B. -S., ROMMENS, J. M., BUCHANAN, J. A., MARKIEWICZ, D., COX, T. K., CHAKRAVARTI, A. *et al.* (1989) Identification of the CF gene: genetic analysis. *Science*, 245, 1073–1080

KIMBERLING, W. J., WESTON, M. D., MOLLER, C. G., DAVENPORT, S. L. H., SHUGART, Y. Y., PRILUCK, I. A. *et al.* (1990) Localisation of Usher syndrome type II to chromosome 1q. *Genomics*, 7, 245–249

KIMBERLING, W. J., MOLLER, C. G., DAVENPORT, S., PRILUCK, I. A., GREENBERG, J., REARDON, W. *et al.* (1992) Linkage of Usher syndrome type 1 gene (USH1B) to the long arm of chromosome 11. *Genomics*, 14, 988–994

KING, J. I. (1991) Ethical issues in the genetic study of deafness. *Annals of the New York Academy of Science*, 630, 236–239

KONIGSMARK, B. W. and GORLIN, R. J. (1976) *Genetic and Metabolic Deafness*. Philadelphia: W. B. Saunders Co

KREIBORG, S. (1981) Crouzon syndrome. *Scandinavian Journal of Plastic and Reconstructive Surgery*, Suppl. 18, 1–198

LEON, P. E., RAVENTOS, H., LYNCH, E., MORROW, J. and KING, M. -C. (1992) The gene for an inherited form of deafness maps to chromosome 5q31. *Proceedings of the National Academy of Sciences*, 89, 5181–5184

LEWIS, R. A., OTTERUD, B., STAUFFER, D., LALOUEL, J. M. and LEPPERT, M. (1990) Mapping recessive ophthalmic diseases: linkage of the locus for Usher syndrome type II to a DNA marker on chromosome 1q. *Genomics*, 7, 250–256

MCKUSICK, V. A. (1992) *Mendelian Inheritance in Man*, 10th edn. Baltimore: Johns Hopkins University Press

MORTON, N. E. (1960) The mutational load due to detrimental genes in man. *American Journal of Human Genetics*, 12, 348–364

MYERS, J. C., JONES, T. A., POHJOLAINEN, E. -R., KADRI, A. S., GODDARD, A. D., SHEER, D. *et al.* (1990) Molecular cloning of alpha 5(IV) collagen and assignment of the gene to the region of the X chromosome containing the Alport syndrome locus. *American Journal of Human Genetics*, 46, 1024–1033

PETTY, R. K. H., HARDING, A. E. and MORGAN-HUGHES, J. A. (1986) The clinical features of mitochondrial myopathy. *Brain*, 109, 915–938

PHELPS, P. D. and LLOYD, G. S. (1983) *Radiology of the Ear*. Oxford: Blackwell Scientific Publications

PHELPS, P. D., REARDON, W., PEMBREY, M., BELLMAN, S. and LUXON, L. M. (1991) X-linked deafness, stapes fixation and a distinctive defect of the inner ear. *Neuroradiology*, 33, 326–330

PICKERING, D., LASKI, B., MACMILLAN, D. and ROSE, V. (1971) 'Little LEOPARD' syndrome. *Archives of Disease in Childhood*, 46, 85–90

POULTON, J., DEADMAN, M. E. and GARDINER, R. M. (1989) Duplications of mitochondrial DNA in mitochondrial myopathy. *Lancet*, i, 236–240

PREZANT, T. R., AGAPIAN, J. V., BOHLMAN, C., BU, X., OZTAS, S., QIU, W.-Q. *et al.* (1993) Mitochondrial ribosomal RNA mutation associated with both antibiotic-induced and non-syndrome deafness. *Nature Genetics*, 4, 289–294

REARDON, W. (1990) Sex-linked deafness – Wilde revisited. *Journal of Medical Genetics*, 27, 376–379

REARDON, W. (1992) Genetic deafness. *Journal of Medical Genetics*, 29, 521–526

REARDON, W., MIDDLETON-PRICE, H., SANDKUIJL, L., PHELPS, P., BELLMAN, S., LUXON, L. *et al.* (1991) A multipedigree linkage study of X-linked deafness: linkage to Xq13-q21 and evidence for genetic heterogeneity. *Genomics*, 11, 885–894

REARDON, W., MIDDLETON-PRICE, H. R., MALCOLM, S., PHELPS, P., BELLMAN, S., LUXON, L. M. *et al.* (1992a) Clinical and genetic heterogeneity in X-linked deafness. *British Journal of Audiology*, 26, 109–114

REARDON, W., ROSS, R. J. M., SWEENEY, M. G., LUXON, L. M., PEMBREY, M. E., HARDING, A. E. *et al.* (1992b) Diabetes mellitus associated with a pathogenic point mutation in mitochondrial DNA. *Lancet*, ii, 1376–1379

REARDON, W., ROBERTS, S., PHELPS, P. D., THOMAS, N. S., BECK, L., ISSAC, R. *et al.* (1992c) Phenotypic evidence for a common pathogenesis in X-linked deafness pedigrees and in Xq13-q21 deletion related deafness. *American Journal of Medical Genetics*, 44, 513–517

REARDON, W., BELLMAN, S., PHELPS, P. D., PEMBREY, M. E. and LUXON, L. M. (1993a) Neuro-otological function in X-linked deafness: a multipedigree assessment and correlation with other parameters. *Acta Otolaryngologica*, 113, 706–714

REARDON, W., MCMANUS, S. P., SUMMERS, D. and WINTER, R. M. (1993b) Cytogenetic evidence that the Saethre-Chotzen gene maps to 7p21.2. *American Journal of Medical Genetics*, 47, 633–636

REARDON, W., VAN HERWERDEN, L., ROSE, C., JONES, B., MALCOLM, S. and WINTER, R. M. (1994) Crouzon syndrome is not linked to craniosynostosis loci at 7p and 5qter. *Journal of Medical Genetics*, 31, 219–221

RIORDAN, J. R., ROMMENS, J. M., KEREM, B. -S., ALAN, N., ROZMAHEL, R., GRZELCZAK, Z. *et al.* (1989) Identification of the cystic fibrosis gene: cloning and characterisation of complementary DNA. *Science*, 245, 1066–1073

ROMMENS, J. M., IANUZZI, M. C., KEREM, B.-S., DRUMM, M. L., KELMER, G., DEAN, M. *et al.* (1989) Identification of the cystic fibrosis gene: chromosome walking and jumping. *Science*, 245, 1059–1065

SEIZINGER, B. R., MARTUZA, R. L. and GUSELLA, J. F. (1986) Loss of genes on chromosome 22 in tumorigenesis of human acoustic neuroma. *Nature*, 322, 644–647

SILLENCE, D. O., SENN, A. and DANKS, D. M. (1979) Genetic heterogeneity in osteogenesis imperfecta. *Journal of Medical Genetics*, 16, 101–116

SLACK, R. W. T. and PHELPS, P. D. (1985) Familial mixed deafness with branchial arch defects (earpits-deafness syndrome). *Clinical Otolaryngology*, 10, 271–277

SMITH, R. J. H., COPPAGE, K. B., ANKERSTJERNE, J. K. B., CAPPER, D. T., KUMAR, S., KENYON, J. *et al.* (1992a) Localization of the gene for branchiootorenal syndrome to chromosome 8q. *Genomics*, **14**, 841–844

SMITH, R. J. H., LEE, E. C., KIMBERLING, W. J., DAIGER, S. P., PELIAS, M. Z., KEATS, B. J. B. *et al.* (1992b) Localisation of two genes for Usher syndrome type 1 to chromosome 11. *Genomics*, **14**, 995–1002

STEVENSON, A. C. and CHEESEMAN, E. A. (1956) Hereditary deaf mutism with particular reference to Northern Ireland. *Annals of Human Genetics*, **20**, 177–231

TASSABEHJI, M., READ, A. P., NEWTON, V. E., PATTON, M., GRUSS, P., HARRIS, R. *et al.* (1993) Mutations in the PAX3 gene causing Waardenburg syndrome type 1 and type 2. *Nature Genetics*, **3**, 26–30

TEMPLE, I. K. (1989) Stickler's syndrome. *Journal of Medical Genetics*, **26**, 119–126

WALLIS, C., BALLO, R., WALLIS, G., BEIGHTON, P. and GOLDBLATT, J. (1988) X-linked mixed deafness with stapes fixation in a Mauritian kindred: linkage to Xq probe pDP34. *Genomics*, **3**, 299–301

WERTELECKI, W., ROULEAU, G. A., SUPERNEAU, D. W., FOREHAND, L. W., WILLIAMS, J. P., HAINES, J. L. *et al.* (1988) Neurofibromatosis 2: clinical and DNA linkage studies of a large kindred. *New England Journal of Medicine*, **319**, 278–283

VAN WOUWE, J. P., WIJNANDS, M. C., MOURAD-BAARS, P. E., GERAEDTS, J. P. M., BEVERSTOCK, G. C. and VAN DE KAMP, J. J. P. (1986) A patient with dup(10p) del(8q) and Pendred syndrome. *American Journal of Medical Genetics*, **24**, 211–217

WILDE, W. R. (1853) *Practical Observations on Aural Surgery and the Nature and Diagnosis of Diseases of the Ear*. London: Churchill

WINTER, R. M. and BARAITSER, M. (1993) *The London Dysmorphology Database*. Oxford: Oxford University Press

4

The causes of deafness

David A. Adams

Newton (1985) described the problems associated with assigning a cause to the hearing loss for many children. An example of this is provided by a child diagnosed as having sensorineural hearing loss at the age of 2 years who has viruria and specific IgG antibody to cytomegalovirus. In this situation the infection may be congenital but it is possible that it is postnatal and coincidental. Newton also emphasized that the earlier the hearing loss is diagnosed and investigations commenced, the greater the likelihood of concluding that the hearing loss is due to congenital infection. Fraser (1976) pointed out that the search is not of purely academic interest, but does have considerable practical implications. Parents want to know the cause of deafness in the child and often this is one of the first questions they ask. Awareness of the causes of deafness helps to identify high-risk groups and is therefore useful in assisting early detection. It also helps in the planning of programmes for prevention or reduction in the size of the problem.

Classification

The causes of deafness in children can be classified in a number of ways, e.g. incidence or prevalence, congenital or postnatal and genetic or non-genetic.

A good history, examination, and full audiological investigation will usually permit classification of the deafness. Confusion may occur when attempts are made to classify deafness according to whether it is congenital or acquired. In this chapter deafness is considered under the main headings of conductive, sensorineural, mixed and non-organic, and where appropriate, subdivided in the following way.

Congenital disorders causing or predisposing to deafness

1 Genetic, with anatomical abnormalities of the external or middle ear
   a deafness present at birth
   b hearing probably normal at birth, deafness begins in childhood
2 Non-genetic, due to disease affecting the developing embryo or fetus
3 Other congenital disorders predisposing to development of deafness during childhood.

Perinatal causes of deafness

Acquired disorders causing deafness

Conductive deafness

The conditions in which the hearing loss is mainly conductive are summarized in Table 4.1. Many other syndromes present with external and middle ear deformity, although the hearing loss is usually mixed or predominantly sensorineural. These are discussed later.

Congenital disorders causing conductive deafness

Down's syndrome (trisomy 21)

Down's syndrome is a common disorder occurring in 1 in 600 of all live births. The incidence has been

Table 4.1 Causes of conductive deafness

1   *Congenital disorders*
a   Genetic, with abnormality of external or middle ear
    i   Deafness present at birth
        Down's syndrome
        Crouzon's disease
        Marfan's syndrome
        Treacher Collins syndrome
        Pierre Robin syndrome
        achondroplasia
        Duane syndrome
        Apert's syndrome
        otopalatodigital syndrome
    ii   Deafness appearing in childhood
        osteogenesis imperfecta
        otosclerosis
b   Congenital disorders predisposing to otitis media with
    effusion or infection (see Table 4.2)
c   Miscellaneous disorders (see Table 4.3)

2   *Acquired disorders* (see Table 4.4)

estimated at 1 in 1000 births in mothers under the age of 25 years and 1 in 100 births in mothers aged 40 or older. The affected individual usually has an extra number 21 chromosome. The characteristic facies makes the disorder easily recognizable.

Children with Down's syndrome present multiple problems to the otologist. Cunningham and McArthur (1981) estimated that as many as 50% of Down's syndrome children with hearing loss passed the normal childhood screening tests as carried out by local authorities. Maurizi *et al.* (1985) concluded that middle ear pathology is more common than might be expected on a purely clinical basis and that objective tests including evoked response audiometry are essential for reliable evaluation. The present author has found this technique to be of limited value if there is only a slight conductive loss, since it is often difficult to determine if there is a response present at near normal threshold levels.

These children are very susceptible to repeated upper respiratory tract infections, including sinusitis and otitis media, both suppurative and with effusion. In one series, 60% of children with Down's syndrome, examined during the summer months, were found to have otitis media with effusion (Schwartz and Schwartz, 1978). Down's syndrome is associated with narrow external auditory canals, making it difficult to insert ventilation tubes.

In addition, there may be ossicular chain abnormalities, usually of the stapes. Balkany *et al.* (1979) found that 40% of a group of Down's syndrome children had a conductive deafness not due to infection or otitis media with effusion. Exploratory surgery in 17 of these children revealed congenital ossicular malformations or destruction, probably as a consequence of previous chronic infection.

There may also be an underlying sensorineural deafness, a short cochlea being the commonest reported finding.

It is therefore important to re-assess hearing thresholds after insertion of ventilation tubes as residual hearing loss is a major additional handicap in these children (Cunningham and McArthur, 1981).

Pappas (1985) stated that early detection and treatment of otological problems in patients with Down's syndrome would undoubtedly result in them developing better communication skills and possibly a higher level of academic achievement.

Crouzon's disease (craniofacial dysostosis)

As with most of the hereditary causes of conductive deafness this is inherited as an autosomal dominant trait. Affected children have hypoplasia of the mandible and maxilla with a parrot-beak nose. There is usually skull deformity (craniostenosis) and exophthalmos.

Associated with the syndrome may be stenosis or atresia of the external auditory canal. The tympanic membrane may be absent and the malleus fused to the bony wall of the epitympanum. Other features include a deformed stapes, often fused to the promontory and a narrow round window niche. A conductive hearing loss is present in one-third of children with Crouzon's disease.

Marfan's syndrome

This is inherited as an autosomal dominant trait. Affected children are tall, often with scoliosis and have long fingers and toes. Other features include hypotonic muscles, a tendency for lens dislocation and cardiac problems, especially aortic aneurysm. Deafness is a rare finding (Konigsmark and Gorlin, 1976).

Treacher Collins syndrome (mandibulofacial dysostosis)

The features of this autosomal dominant trait are confined to the head. The commonest feature of the syndrome is hypoplasia of the malar bones and maxilla. There is an antimongoloid slant to the palpebral fissures. The mandible is usually hypoplastic.

There may be deformities of the pinna, usually microtia, with stenosis or atresia of the external auditory canal. The tympanic membrane may be replaced by a bony plate. The ossicular chain can have a variety of malformations and, in some cases, the middle ear cleft is absent. Tensor tympani and stapedius muscles are often absent. Inner ear abnormalities, if present, would appear to be confined to the vestibular labyrinth (Schuknecht, 1993).

Taylor and Phelps (1993) used CT to demonstrate

a number of abnormalities in 13 patients with Treacher-Collins syndrome (Figure 4.1). These included absence of mastoid pneumatization, hypoplastic middle ear, ossicular chain abnormality and occlusion or stenosis of the external auditory meatus. They found inner ear abnormalities in only one patient.

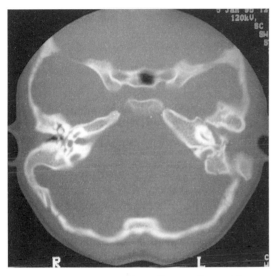

Figure 4.1 CT scan – Treacher Collins syndrome. (Courtesy of Peter Phelps)

The results of corrective surgery are poor (Jahrsdoerfer *et al.*, 1989). These children may be suitable for a bone-anchored hearing aid when the skull bones are sufficiently thick to accept an osseointegrated screw.

In spite of their appearance the distribution of intelligence in these children would appear to be similar to that in the normal population (Fisch, 1981).

Pierre Robin syndrome

This is considered to be an autosomal dominant trait although, in some cases, it may be due to intrauterine disease during the first trimester. The features of this syndrome include cleft palate, hypoplasia of the mandible, glossoptosis, congenital dislocation of the hip and club foot. There may be mental retardation associated with either microcephaly or hydrocephalus.

The external ears may be cup-shaped and appear to be low set because of the hypoplastic mandible (Figure 4.2). The middle ear cleft may be absent, or there may be thickening of the stapes footplate and crura. Inner ear deformities include abnormal commu-

nications between the middle and apical turns of the cochlea, a poorly developed modiolus or a narrow internal auditory canal.

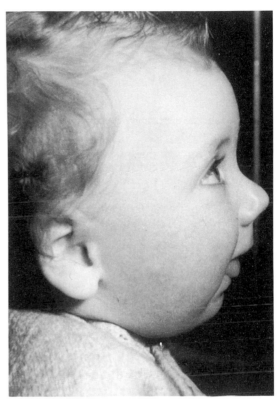

Figure 4.2 Pierre Robin syndrome

The audiogram shows a conductive deafness, but in cases with inner ear abnormalities the hearing loss is mixed.

Achondroplasia (dwarfism)

Although this is inherited as an autosomal dominant trait, about three-quarters of cases may be due to fresh mutation. The incidence rises with increasing parental age.

The main effects are on the skeletal system. There is slow growth of cartilage and delayed endochondral ossification. The result is stunted growth, with disproportionately short limbs and a large head with prominent forehead and depressed nasal bridge.

In the middle ear, the ossicles may be fused to the bony margins of the middle ear cleft. The cochlea may be deformed. The hearing loss, if present, is usually conductive as a result of the middle ear abnormality and also of a predisposition to otitis media with effusion.

Duane syndrome (cervical oculoacoustic dysplasia)

The affected children with this autosomal dominant syndrome have a very short neck, congenital paralysis of the VIth cranial nerve and enophthalmos with conductive deafness.

Abnormalities of the external ear include microtia and atresia of the external auditory canal. In the middle ear, the ossicles may be fused and not connected to the oval window. The oval window may be closed by a membrane. Some children have a mixed hearing loss.

Apert's syndrome (acrocephalosyndactyly)

This is inherited as an autosomal dominant trait, although it is thought that some of the cases are the result of fresh mutation with a high mutation rate related to advancing parental age. These children have a high, tower skull and a flat forehead (acrocephaly). There is maxillary hypoplasia with a high-arched usually cleft palate and saddle nose. The fingers and toes are fused (syndactyly).

The audiogram shows a flat conductive loss of varying degrees. Surgical exploration has demonstrated congenital fixation of the stapes footplate. There is also a high incidence of otitis media perhaps due to the associated cleft palate.

Otopalatodigital syndrome

This X-linked trait is characterized by bossing of the frontal and occipital bones. There is hypertelorism, hypoplasia of the mandible and cleft palate. The fingers are short and clubbed. Most cases show mild mental retardation.

The pinnae are low set and small. There is a conductive deafness due to abnormalities of the ossicular chain (Gorlin, Cohen and Levin, 1990).

Osteogenesis imperfecta

The complexity of this group of genetic disorders is described in Chapter 3. The basic defect of osteogenesis imperfecta seems to be that collagen does not mature properly giving a faulty framework for the hydroxyapatite crystals deposited during ossification.

Morrison (1979) reported a series in which the onset of deafness started as early as 6 years and as late as 51 years, with a peak in the third decade. The deafness is conductive initially, although some cases develop a mixed loss. Schuknecht (1993) summarized the findings of several authors, noting that the disease was characterized by the presence of new soft vascular bone in the region of the oval window, resembling that found in otosclerosis. Bergstrom (1977) reported deformity of the stapes.

Stewart and O'Reilly (1990) described the findings of a group of patients suffering from this disorder and stated that the hearing loss first appeared in the first and second decades as a conductive deafness which then progressed to a mixed loss.

It has been argued that otosclerosis is a localized form of osteogenesis imperfecta as they share many common featuers. Shea and Postma (1982), however, reported that the results of surgery in a group of patients with osteogenesis imperfecta were not as good as those obtained in otosclerotic ears. This, with the earlier age of onset of deafness in osteogenesis imperfecta, would suggest that the two conditions are at least clinically distinct.

Otosclerosis

This is a disease of uncertain aetiology. In many cases it is inherited as an autosomal dominant trait with variable penetrance (Sando, Suehira and Wood, 1983).

Deafness does not usually begin until puberty and is, on average, later than that in osteogenesis imperfecta. Cawthorne (1955) reported that 70% of patients with clinical otosclerosis first noticed their hearing loss between the ages of 11 and 30 years. In another large series of 610 patients, in whom the deafness began before 18 years of age, the average age of onset of deafness was surprisingly low at 11.5 years (Robinson, 1983). One-half of the patients in this series had a family history of otosclerosis.

There is general agreement that the deafness in children is conductive, with normal or good inner ear function. The results of stapedectomy in children are good, but it should be remembered that middle ear infection is common in this age group. The additional risk to the cochlea which this might present may be avoided by fitting a hearing aid until the child is older.

Congenital disorders predisposing to otitis media with effusion or infection
(Table 4.2)

Children with congenital infections, who have been exposed to adverse perinatal factors or have chromosomal abnormalities do seem to have a higher prevalence of middle ear infection or otitis media with effusion than other children (Das, 1990).

Table 4.2 **Congenital disorders predisposing to otitis media with effusion or infection**

Cystic fibrosis
Immotile cilia syndrome
Cleft palate
Immune deficiency disease

Cystic fibrosis (mucoviscidosis)

Cystic fibrosis is the commonest autosomal recessive disease in the UK, occurring in approximately 1 in 2000 births. The precise nature of the defect is unknown. It affects both mucus and non-mucus secreting glands. The nasal airway, sinus ostia, eustachian tube and middle ear are blocked by viscid mucus. There is also involvement of the salivary glands, bile duct and intestine with fat malabsorption and impaired digestion.

Children with this disease are probably not more susceptible to otitis media with effusion and middle ear infection. These children are often treated with potentially ototoxic antibiotics in high dosage and are therefore at risk of developing a sensorineural deafness.

The diagnosis is established by the finding of an increased concentration of sodium in the sweat to above 60 mmol/l.

Immotile cilia syndrome

In this rare disease there is impairment of the normal ciliary mechanism of respiratory tract mucosa. The clinical spectrum of disease varies from children with a chronic cough to the sinusitis, bronchiectasis and situs inversus of Kartagener's syndrome. These children are very susceptible to otitis media with effusion. The diagnosis is confirmed by electron microscopy of biopsies of upper respiratory tract mucosa.

Cleft palate

The incidence of cleft lip-palate is 1 in 500–750 live births (Rood and Stool, 1981). Otitis media, especially with effusion is common. Paradise, Bluestone and Felder (1969) found that virtually all children with cleft palates under the age of 20 months had otitis media usually with effusion.

Two factors may be responsible for this. Regurgitation of irritant food and fluids around the eustachian tube orifice will cause oedema and obstruction. Second, there is usually some degree of eustachian tube dysfunction associated with failure of the tube to open properly on swallowing. There is no midline anchorage in the unrepaired cleft palate and this prevents the tensor palati muscle exerting sufficient force on the eustachian tube orifice to open it.

Rood and Stool (1981) found that the incidence of otitis media with effusion reduced after palatal repair and also with advancing age. Repair of the cleft palate does not, however, always solve the eustachian tube problem. Scarring may inhibit movement of the tensor palati. Furthermore, infracture of the pterygoid hamulus is sometimes used to relieve tension on the palatal repair. This in itself disturbs the functional opening of the eustachian tube.

Robson *et al.* (1992) suggested that, although otitis media with effusion is common in children with cleft palate, ventilators or grommets should only be inserted when clinically indicated rather than routinely at the time of the cleft palate repair.

Immune deficiency disease

Disorders of the immune system predispose to infection of various body systems, including the middle ear.

Miscellaneous congenital causes of conductive deafness (Table 4.3)

Isolated malformations of the external and middle ears

These and their management are discussed in Chapter 5.

Table 4.3 Congenital disorders with conductive deafness – miscellaneous conditions

Isolated malformations
Congenital cholesteatoma
Rhabdomyosarcoma
Fibrous dysplasia
Goldenhar's syndrome

Congenital cholesteatoma

True congenital (primary) cholesteatoma may be due to an epithelial rest left behind as the otic cyst sinks in from the surface of the developing embryo. Aimi (1983) postulated that most congenital cholesteatomas occurred near the tympanic isthmus of the middle ear, at the junction of first and second branchial arches. This would suggest that the origin of the cholesteatoma was related to migration of external canal ectoderm into the middle ear at an early stage of development, perhaps because of the failure of the inhibitory function of the tympanic ring.

Derlacki and Clemis (1965) outlined three criteria for diagnosis:

1 Development behind an intact tympanic membrane
2 No history of ear infections
3 The lesion must arise from inclusion of squamous epithelium during embryonic development.

It must not be forgotten, however, that cholesteatoma, limited to the middle ear and mastoid behind an intact tympanic membrane, may be due to epidermal ingrowth followed by healing of a perforation of the tympanic membrane (Schuknecht, 1993).

Congenital cholesteatoma may be classified according to the site of origin (Schuknecht, 1993):

1 The petrous apex
2 The cerebellopontine angle
3 The mastoid
4 The middle ear
5 The external auditory canal.

The lesion behaves in the same way as acquired
cholesteatoma with enlargement of the cyst and bony
erosion. The spectrum of symptoms ranges from conductive deafness to facial paralysis and the intracranial complications of the disease. In some cases the
hearing may be normal because sound is conducted
from the tympanic membrane through the cyst to
the stapes footplate.

McDonald, Cody and Ryan (1984) reported a series
of 21 patients considered to have congenital cholesteatoma. This group represented 2% of all the cholesteatomas considered by the authors, suggesting that
congenital cholesteatoma may not be as rare as previously supposed. Conductive deafness was the commonest presenting symptom in 18 patients and in 13
of those the tympanic membrane was described as
opaque, white or had a cyst visible through it. The
disease was confined to the middle ear and mastoid
in 20 patients, in the other patient there was extension to the petrous apex.

Brooker and Smyth (1991) described a series of
nine congenital cholesteatomas developing within the
middle ear behind an intact tympanic membrane.
They felt that these middle ear cholesteatomas were
distinct from primary cholesteatomas originating in
the apical petrous temporal bone. These authors also
felt that there was still a place for combined approach
tympanoplasty in the management of congenital
middle ear cholesteatoma.

Rhabdomyosarcoma

Rhabdomyosarcoma, although rare, is the commonest
type of malignant neoplasm arising in the soft tissues
of the head and neck in children (Chasin, 1984).

The tumour probably originates from a primitive
skeletal muscle cell (the myoblast) or from a mesenchymal stem cell. Those related to the ear present
with a friable mass in the external auditory canal.
There is discharge, bleeding, conductive deafness and
occasionally facial paralysis.

The prognosis is poor, although treatment with a
combination of radiotherapy, chemotherapy and surgery may give some benefit.

Fibrous dysplasia of bone

A comprehensive review of this disorder was provided
by Nager, Kennedy and Kopstein (1982). It is a
disease of unknown aetiology. There are two types –
monostotic and polyostotic. In monostotic disease, a

single bone is involved with the skull or face being
the site in about 10% of cases. If the lesion involves
the temporal bone, it may present as a slowly progressive, hard, painless swelling in the mastoid or squamous portion. Temporal bone disease usually becomes
evident during childhood with progressive conductive
deafness, increase in size or change in shape of the
temporal bone, and progressive obliteration of the
external auditory canal (Nager and Holliday, 1984).

Polyostotic fibrous dysplasia, if associated with
café-au-lait spots and precocious sexual development,
is known as McCune Albright syndrome. In polyostotic disease both temporal bones may be affected.

The radiological features vary with the amount of
fibrosis and calcification, with areas of radiotranslu-
cency adjacent to areas of increased bony density.

The complications include exposure of dura, predisposition to acquired cholesteatoma and cranial nerve
involvement.

Hereditary fibrous dysplasia is very rare. Adams *et
al.* (1991) described a unique family, many members
of which have polyostotic fibrous dysplasia of bone.
In this family the disorder would appear to be inherited as an autosomal dominant trait with variable
penetrance. Deafness is an early symptom in affected
children and is purely conductive. The tympanogram
shows a very high compliance in most cases. The
hearing loss is progressive and eventually becomes
mixed. Seven of the patients have had exploratory
middle ear surgery with the commonest finding being
the replacement of the long process of the incus by
fibrous tissue. There is at present considerable debate
as to the nature of the disease in this family. The
histology has some features in keeping with the diagnosis of Paget's disease, although the clinical and
biochemical findings are quite different.

Goldenhar's syndrome (oculoauriculovertebral dysplasia)

The aetiology of this condition is unknown, although
in some cases there would appear to be a hereditary
trait (Chapter 3). Lesions of the eye include a cleft
upper lid, dermoids and defects of the extraocular
muscles. There may be auricular appendages, microtia and atresia of the external auditory canal (Figure
4.3). There is often unilateral hypoplasia of the mandible with hemivertebrae and club foot.

Approximately 50% of cases have a conductive
deafness due to the external ear abnormalities.

Acquired disorders causing conductive deafness

The conditions acquired during childhood which
cause hearing loss are summarized in Table 4.4.
Otitis media, whether suppurative or with effusion, is
the commonest cause of deafness in childhood. These

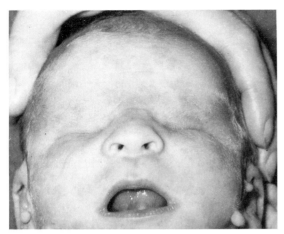

Figure 4.3 Goldenhar's syndrome

Table 4.4 Acquired causes of conductive deafness

Inflammation
   otitis externa
   acute (suppurative) otitis media
   chronic (suppurative) otitis media
   acute otitis media with effusion
   chronic otitis media with effusion
Trauma
Foreign body
Wax

disorders are discussed in Chapters 8 and 7 respectively.

Otitis externa

In children acute (infected) otitis externa and eczematous otitis externa are the commonest forms of this disorder.

Swimming in chlorinated pools predisposes to the condition. The irritation of the skin of the external canal makes the child scratch and the subsequent trauma allows the skin to become infected.

Some children develop an allergy to acrylic or silicone earmoulds. This can be successfully overcome by using non-allergic moulds made from vulcanite, although these are expensive.

Conductive deafness is not a feature of otitis externa unless the external canal is blocked by debris or oedematous skin.

Trauma

Conductive deafness can be caused by direct or indirect trauma to the ear. Direct trauma is from a foreign body perforating the tympanic membrane or a fracture of the petrous temporal bone.

Many parents are obsessed with the need to remove wax manually from a child's ear using cotton buds. The child's head may jerk during this manoeuvre and the object may be driven through the tympanic membrane. There may be damage to the ossicular chain and on occasions to the cochlea. Perforation of the tympanic membrane also occurs during clumsy attempts to syringe an ear.

Head injuries, as the result of accidents involving traffic or falls at home, are common in the young. The child's skull is more deformable than that of an adult and will often dent without fracture (Pond fracture). The sutures have not united and fissure fractures may persist as separated sutures. As in adults, fractures of the temporal bone are classified relative to the axis of the petrous portion (Schuknecht, 1993). Longitudinal fractures are commonest (80% of cases) and are associated with a blow to the side of the head. The fracture line usually spares the cochlea and the deafness tends to be conductive in nature but may be sensorineural or mixed. There is often bleeding from the ear if the skin of the external canal is lacerated and the tympanic membrane torn. In other cases there may be a haemotympanum or cerebrospinal fluid behind an intact tympanic membrane. The ossicular chain may be damaged by dislocation or fracture.

The hearing loss in a child may not be noticed until some time after the injury. The child may be unconscious, or admitted to a paediatric unit and not complain of deafness.

Williams, Ghorayeb and Yeakley (1992) carried out a retrospective study of temporal bone fractures in children over a 6-year period. Most of these were caused either by motor vehicles or by falling from heights. In this group of children the fracture line was commonly oblique. Facial palsy and sensorineural hearing loss were less common in children than adults.

Radiology is difficult in children as they tend to be restless and uncooperative. In some cases, fractures of the temporal bone are not visible on X-ray.

Most cases will settle spontaneously with healing of the perforation and the hearing will return to normal assuming there is no damage to the ossicular chain or cochlea. Cholesteatoma, as a result of entrapment of squamous cells in the fracture line, is a rare complication (Freeman, 1983).

Indirect trauma occurs as the result of a slap on the ear, an explosion or barotrauma. Children are more likely than adults to have eustachian tube dysfunction and may experience problems when flying, usually during descent.

Foreign body

Children often present with a foreign body in the external auditory canal and in many cases it is an incidental finding.

Foreign bodies may be of two types: those which

are hygroscopic (peas, beans, paper) and those which are not (beads, gravel). A foreign body will only cause deafness if it completely occludes the ear canal or is pushed through the tympanic membrane during attempts to remove it.

Most are easily removed by syringing, although this must be avoided if the foreign body is hygroscopic. If the object is in the outer one-third of the ear canal it can often be removed using a hooked probe. This is not always easy since children are much more likely to move about with subsequent risk of damage to the tympanic membrane. It is best to try once only and if unsuccessful to arrange removal of the foreign body under general anaesthesia.

Wax

The ear's self-cleansing mechanism will usually keep the external ear free of wax. The use of cotton buds may cause impaction of wax deep in the external canal.

Children who use hearing aids often have excessive wax in the ear canal. This must be removed on each visit to the clinic as it may block the earmould. In a profoundly deaf child, with high-powered aids, accumulation of wax in the ear canal can cause feedback and limit the useful output of the aid.

Sensorineural deafness

Sensorineural deafness in children may result from the various known congenital or acquired disorders summarized in Table 4.5. In published series the incidence of deafness with an unknown cause may be as high as 50%.

Table 4.5 Causes of sensorineural deafness

1 *Congenital disorders*
a Genetic
  i Deafness present at birth
    deafness alone
    syndromes associated with deafness
  ii Deafness appearing in childhood
    deafness alone
    syndromes associated with deafness
b Non-genetic, due to intrauterine disease
    infections
    ototoxic drugs
    metabolic disorders

2 *Perinatal disorders* (see Table 4.6)

3 *Acquired disorders* (see Table 4.7)

Four patterns of pathological abnormality of the cochlea have been described in patients with sensorineural deafness.

Michel dysplasia is the most severe, with total ab-

sence of the labyrinth, perhaps as a result of failure of the otic vesicle to separate from the neural ridge.

Mondini dysplasia affects the cochlea and semicircular canals. The cochlear duct is reduced to the basal coil only. The organ of Corti may be absent or reduced to a mound of undifferentiated cells. This type of dysplasia is seen in the Klippel-Feil and Pendrel's syndromes. It may be visible on polytomography. Alexander (1904) described this dysplasia in association with auditory nerve involvement.

In *Bing-Siebenmann dysplasia*, the bony labyrinth is normal with underdevelopment of the membranous part.

Scheibe (cochleosaccular) dysplasia is the least severe and is thought to be present in about 70% of cases of congenital deafness. The stria vascularis has alternating areas of aplasia and hyperplasia. The organ of Corti is rudimentary and the hair cells sparse or absent. The saccule is collapsed. The utricle and semicircular canals are normal. It has been identified in Waardenburg's, Usher's and Refsum's syndromes and also in rubella deafness.

Genetic disorders with deafness present at birth

A full discussion of the genetics of deafness is given in Chapter 3.

Klippel-Feil syndrome (brevicollis)

The aetiology of this condition is uncertain (Chapter 3). In some cases it would appear to be the result of an autosomal recessive trait although the majority would appear to be inherited as an autosomal dominant.

The external ear may have microtia with preauricular appendages and atresia of the external auditory canal. Middle ear manifestations include deformity of the incudostapedial joint or stapes and fusion of the short process of incus to the floor of the attic. The cochlea is short and there may be distortion of the internal auditory meatus. Most have a sensorineural loss, although it may be mixed or occasionally conductive (Dubey and Ghosh, 1993). These authors presented a literature review of children with Klippel-Feil syndrome who had conductive hearing loss. The complications of corrective surgery include perilymph 'gusher', total deafness and meningitis (Stewart and O'Reilly, 1989). The success rate of surgery to correct conductive loss would appear to be only 50%.

Turner's syndrome (gonadal aplasia)

These patients have an abnormal genetic constitution, with an XO pattern. It is present in 1 in 5000 live births. The external ears are low set, with large lobes. The mastoid air cell system is poorly developed and there may be abnormalities of the stapes. There is some debate as to whether or not the disorder is associated with sensorineural deafness, although cases have been reported. Anderson *et al.* (1969) stated that, in their series, 64% of patients had a sensorineural deafness with a bilaterally symmetrical loss in the mid-frequency range. A conductive or mixed loss, was present in 22%; perhaps, in some cases, as a consequence of repeated attacks of otitis media.

Fanconi's syndrome

This autosomal recessive condition presents with congenital anaemia, skin pigmentation, skeletal deformities and mental retardation. The hearing loss appears to affect the high frequencies first and is slowly progressive.

Pili torti

In this autosomal recessive disease dry, brittle hair is associated with sensorineural deafness.

Usher's syndrome

Usher's syndrome is inherited as an autosomal recessive trait (Chapter 3). It is an association of retinitis pigmentosa with progressive sensorineural deafness. These children may also have vertigo and epilepsy. Chan (1994) estimated that Usher's syndrome accounts for 3–6% of children with congenital deafness. One of the difficulties with the disorder is that the retinal changes do not usually appear until the child is 5 or 6 years of age. In younger children a retinogram may be necessary to establish a diagnosis because the changes are not visible by fundoscopy (Chan, 1994).

Pendred's syndrome

This is inherited as an autosomal recessive trait. A congenital defect in thyroxine synthesis eventually cause goitre, which usually becomes obvious between the age of 5 and 10 years. The sensorineural deafness is severe to profound, is said to be present at birth, and is certainly present by 6 months. This condition may not be diagnosed in the first child until 8–10 years of age when the goitre appears. The diagnosis will then be made much earlier in subsequent siblings.

Congenital hypothyroidism (cretinism)

The cause of the hearing loss in this condition is different from that in Pendred's syndrome (Fisch, 1981). The detection of partial deafness, sensorineural or mixed, is often made difficult by associated mental or physical abnormalities. Objective assessment is usually necessary. Fisch pointed out that this cause of deafness might be prevented by effective screening of neonates for hypothyroidism.

Waardenburg's syndrome

This is inherited as an autosomal dominant trait. Chan (1994) estimated that it accounts for about 2% of children with congenital deafness. There are two types. In type 1 the medial canthi of the eyes are displaced laterally and in type 2 the medial canthi are not displaced laterally. Twenty per cent have a white forelock, 45% have irides of different colours or have different colours in one iris (heterochromia iridis). Chan estimated that type 2 was 20 times more common than type 1 and that 20% of those with type 1 Waardenburg's syndrome had a sensorineural hearing loss whereas 55% of those with type 2 were affected. Newton, Liu and Read (1994) found that a profound sensorineural hearing loss and hypoplastic blue irides appeared more frequently in those with type 1 Waardenburg's syndrome, whereas partial iris heterochromia and asymmetrical audiograms seemed more frequent in those with the type 2 syndrome. The hearing loss may be moderate or profound, unilateral or bilateral. If the hearing loss is partial it may affect the low rather than the high frequencies.

Jervell and Lange-Nielsen syndrome

One-half of affected children with this autosomal recessive disorder die before the age of 20 years. The deafness is bilateral and severe to profound. It is associated with abnormalities of the electrocardiograph, in particular a prolongation of the Q–T interval.

Genetic disorders with deafness developing after birth

The diseases associated with progressive sensorineural hearing loss are described later in this chapter. Various authors have reported examples of hereditary sensorineural deafness with no other abnormality, in which the hearing appears to be normal at birth with a gradual onset of deafness, which may progress, occurring during childhood (Konigsmark and Gorlin, 1976; Holmes, 1977; Cremers, 1979).

Alport's syndrome

There is debate as to the aetiology of this disorder. This is discussed in detail in Chapter 3. Children present with haematuria and albuminuria within the first decade. Males are much more seriously affected than females and often die before 30 years of age.

In approximately 50% of patients a high frequency

sensorineural deafness begins around the age of 10 years. This loss usually progresses to become severe. Ruben (1985) suggested that a renal lesion must be excluded in all adolescents with a newly found progressive sensorineural deafness.

Renal tubular acidosis

This is a rare autosomal recessive disorder with only 23 cases reported in the world literature (Takanobu *et al.*, 1984). The author has seen one child, thought to be the first in Ireland (McShane *et al.*, 1987). His deafness was first noticed at 3 years of age and was found at that time to be a flat, moderate to severe sensorineural hearing loss. His most recent audiogram shows a profound loss, worse for the high frequencies.

Refsum's disease

Retinitis pigmentosa with peripheral neuropathy and cerebellar ataxia are the features of this autosomal recessive disorder. Sensorineural deafness usually starts between the ages of 10 and 20 years and is asymmetrical in some cases.

Cogan's syndrome

The aetiology of this is unknown, although it has been suggested that it is an autoimmune disease and, as such, is a localized manifestation of polyarteritis nodosa (Stephens, Luxon and Hinchcliffe, 1982). There is non-syphilitic interstitial keratitis with sensorineural deafness and vertigo. It usually first manifests in adolescence with sudden onset of vertigo, tinnitus and rapidly progressive deafness. Treatment with high doses of steroids may halt the deterioration in hearing.

Norrie's syndrome

In this X-linked recessive disorder there is progressive blindness with, in some cases, mental retardation. Progressive sensorineural deafness is present in about one-third of patients.

Non-genetic disorders: deafness due to intrauterine disease

These conditions, sometimes referred to as the embryopathies, are common and often preventable causes of congenital sensorineural deafness. The best known of these are the maternal infections which may be transmitted to the fetus across the placenta, through the cervix or at the time of birth.

Rubella

Martin (1982) described rubella as being the commonest identifiable cause of congenital sensorineural hearing loss in children. Newton (1985) described a

cohort of children in Manchester. She found that, although congenital rubella was relatively common, the number of children affected by it had declined compared to a previous study of a similar population. The other significant finding in Newton's series was that 75% of the children with rubella deafness were born to mothers who had not been immunized. Davis (1993) also found that the part played by rubella as a cause of deafness in the UK had decreased. He noted however a large increase in the number of preterm babies surviving with hearing impairment. Similar findings were reported by Parving and Hauch (1994) in a study of the causes of profound hearing impairment in a school for the deaf.

Deafness occurs in about one-third of rubella children. Affected children may also have microcephaly with mental retardation, eye lesions including cataracts and retinitis, abnormalities of the cardiovascular system and lower limb deformities.

There is a mistaken belief that deafness only occurs if infection is within the first trimester. Hardy (1973) pointed out that infection with rubella at any stage in the pregnancy can cause deafness; infection at 0–8 weeks – 86% of children born with deafness, 9–12 weeks – 85%, 13–20 weeks 53%, 21–35 weeks – 20%.

The virus enters the mother either through the nose or mouth and is transmitted through the placenta to the fetus. The maternal infection may be subclinical in about 40% of cases. Deafness is sometimes the only abnormality.

There is seasonal variation in the incidence of rubella (Martin, 1982). The numbers of children with rubella deafness born in December and January are much greater than those born in the summer months (Figure 4.4). This is not due to a seasonal

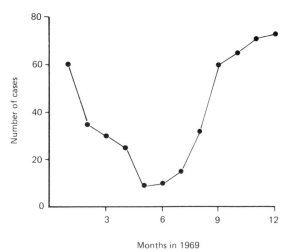

Figure 4.4 Distribution by month of birth for all cases of perceptive deafness due to rubella (EC 469 cases). (From Martin, J. A. M., 1982, *Audiology*, **21**, by courtesy of the author and publisher)

variation in birth rate. It would appear that children conceived in March and April are more at risk of rubella than at any other time of the year.

Hemenway, Sando and McChesney (1969) described the abnormal findings in the ear. There may be abnormalities of the stapes or cartilaginous fixation of the stapes footplate. The child's middle ear may contain fetal mesenchyme. The cochlea and saccule have Scheibe-type dysplasia.

The sensorineural hearing loss is usually severe to profound. Fisch (1981) described the typical loss as flat, affecting all frequencies more or less evenly, although it may be trough-shaped with a maximum loss for the middle frequencies. Wild *et al.* (1989) found the hearing loss to be flat with an average of 93 dB. Only one child in their series of 57 had a progressive hearing loss.

The diagnosis of rubella is often made on clinical grounds. It is possible to culture the virus from throat swabs or samples of stool or urine up to the age of 6 months. Persistence of IgG antibody after the disappearance of maternal IgG indicates congenital infection. Rubella specific IgM is present in the infected child for about the first 6 months after birth. Newton (1985) pointed out that the earlier the hearing loss is diagnosed and investigations commenced, the greater the likelihood of concluding that the hearing loss is due to a congenital infection such as rubella.

Martin (1982) pointed out that eradication of rubella would abolish one-fifth of all congenital sensorineural deafness. The policy in the UK at present is to offer vaccination to all girls between 10 and 14 years of age and also to screen all women at antenatal clinics. There are several problems with this policy. For it to be successful in abolishing congenital rubella there would have to be almost a 100% uptake in the target population. This is known not to be the case. In addition, the vaccine would need to be 100% effective (Begg and Noah, 1985). At present no check is made on girls after vaccination. Around 40% of babies damaged by rubella are first born. Antenatal screening for rubella is therefore too late since the fetus may already be infected (Kudesia *et al.*, 1985). These authors advocated a change in policy with testing before and after vaccination to ensure a primary response. This technique would also distinguish women who were protected by the vaccine from those with antibodies to the natural virus.

Cytomegalovirus

There is controversy as to the importance of cytomegalovirus in the aetiology of congenital sensorineural deafness. Fraser (1976) thought that it was a relatively minor cause of hearing loss. More recently, several authors have suggested that the importance of cytomegalovirus as a cause of congenital deafness has been underestimated. Pappas (1983), in a review of children with subclinical infection, found that cytomegalovirus was the most common viral agent causing sensorineural deafness in children. It may well be that many cases of congenital sensorineural deafness in the 'cause unknown' group are due to cytomegalovirus.

Cytomegalovirus infection can be either congenital, occur during the perinatal period or be acquired. Newton (1985) felt that the perinatal group were commoner than congenital but caused less auditory damage.

There are two clinical types of infection. The systemic infection (10% of patients) is obvious at birth or in the neonatal period. This has a much worse prognosis with the child often being severely handicapped. Children with focal infection (90% of patients) appear to be normal at birth and, in other words, have subclinical disease.

Pappas (1983) summarized the pathological findings. Cells with intranuclear inclusion bodies were found in Reissner's membrane and the stria vascularis. Immunofluorescent techniques demonstrate viral antigens among the inner ear cells including the organ of Corti and neurons of the spiral ganglion. Cytomegalovirus infection can cause destruction of both cochlear and labyrinthine structures.

The hearing loss is usually severe to profound and bilateral, but may, in a few cases, be unilateral (Saigal *et al.*, 1982; Pappas, 1983). Strauss (1990) reported a significant hearing loss in 33–48% of children with symptoms and in 6.9% of those without symptoms. Some of the children had a progressive hearing loss. Strauss also stated that acquired cytomegalovirus infection could be associated with sudden deafness and acute labyrinthitis. Hickson and Alcock (1991) found that, in all five children in their series with congenital cytomegalovirus, a significant deterioration of hearing was noted within the first 4 years of life. These authors felt that it was essential that neonates with cytomegalovirus be referred for hearing assessment and that the child's hearing be monitored on a long-term basis. Asymptomatic children, with apparently normal hearing thresholds, may have impairment of higher centre function (Connolly *et al.*, 1992). The important clinical application of this finding relates to auditory processing of children in noisy classroom situations.

If the disorder is suspected at birth the virus can be cultured from urine samples. This is only useful during the first few weeks of life. Serological tests which show either a rising titre of IgG antibody or the presence of cytomegalovirus-specific IgM will confirm the diagnosis.

Toxoplasmosis

The causative organism of this infection is *Toxoplasma gondii*. The disease is much less common than either rubella or cytomegalovirus infection. The condition is usually subclinical at birth but may eventually manifest itself with progressive blindness because of chorioretinitis. Some children present with hepatosplenomegaly and jaundice. In some, cerebral calcification may result in epilepsy or hydrocephalus.

Kelemen (1958) reported the pathological findings in two children. Both had calcium deposits in the stria vascularis and spiral ligament.

The diagnosis may be made by injecting material from a lymph node or cerebrospinal fluid into mice and examining the brain for calcification 4–6 weeks later. The Sabin–Feldman dye test and the indirect fluorescent antibody test will confirm the presence of infection. Radiology of the skull can be useful if there is focal calcification of the brain.

McGee *et al.* (1992) presented the findings of a cohort of 30 children with congenital toxoplasmosis. Twenty eight had had treatment and two had not. There was no evidence of significant sensorineural hearing loss in any of the children in this group, although the study was of younger children only and there was no information as to whether or not a loss had developed later in life. They also presented a literature survey which suggested 10–15% of children with congenital toxoplasmosis have a significant hearing loss. The literature, however, does confirm that the symptoms develop in later years and not in young children.

Congenital syphilis

Deafness caused by congenital syphilis may begin in childhood, although in most cases the onset occurs between the ages of 25–35 years (Karmody and Schuknecht, 1966). In early onset disease the infection is severe and often fatal. The ear symptoms are overshadowed by systemic disease. In the later onset or tardive form, deafness with vertigo and tinnitus may be present. There may be profound unilateral deafness.

In the middle ear there may be thickening of the malleus with fusion of the malleus head and incus. There is osteitis of the temporal bone with mononuclear leucocytic infiltration. Obliterative endarteritis and hydrops are found, resulting in degeneration of the cochlear and vestibular end organs.

Herpes simplex

Congenital deafness has been attributed to infection with herpes simplex virus (Veltri *et al.*, 1981). These authors demonstrated, histopathologically, infection of the labyrinthine sensory cells. Herpes may be transmitted during the passage through the birth canal and the consequent risk of direct infection is about 40% (Gerber, 1990).

Dahle and McCollister (1988) described only two children with sensorineural hearing loss in a group of 20 with symptomatic neonatal infection.

Ototoxic drugs

The effect of these drugs on the fetal cochlea will be discussed in the section dealing with acquired causes of deafness.

Irradiation

Irradiation can cause deafness in adults. It is sometimes quoted as a potential cause of congenital sensorineural deafness. The present author cannot find any reports in the literature in which this relationship has been established.

Ultrasound

Pye, Knight and Arnett (1984) described cochlear hair cell damage in guinea-pigs due to ultrasound of 12.5 kHz. Ultrasonic scanning, using frequencies of 3.5 or 5 MHz, is a commonly employed technique in obstetric practice. At present, there is no evidence that this is harmful to the fetal ear (Hepper and Shahidullah, 1994).

Maternal diabetes

Fraser (1976) stated that the role of maternal diabetes as a cause of congenital deafness had not been established. Gratz, Pollack and Zimmerman (1981) described the radiological findings in two children of unrelated, insulin-dependent mothers. In each case there was hypoplasia of the internal auditory meatus. The cochlea, vestibule and semicircular canals were radiologically normal.

Fetal alcohol syndrome

The author has seen two children with fetal alcohol syndrome both of whom have moderate, bilateral sensorineural hearing loss. Church and Gerkin (1988) found that in a group of children with fetal alcohol syndrome, about one-third had bilateral sensorineural hearing loss.

Perinatal disorders causing sensorineural deafness

There is general agreement that because of the decrease in perinatal mortality over the last two decades, more children are surviving with handicaps such as deafness (Newton, 1985; Davis, 1993; Razi and Das, 1994). The main risk factors in the perinatal period are summarized in Table 4.6. One of the difficulties with this group is that more than one risk factor is usually present and this makes the contribution of each difficult to ascertain.

Table 4.6 Perinatal causes of sensorineural deafness

Hypoxia
Hyperbilirubinaemia
Preterm delivery and low birthweight

Hypoxia

Hall (1964) described the otopathological findings in neonatal asphyxia, including a decrease in cell numbers in the cochlear nuclei. The cochlea appeared histologically normal. A review of the other literature would suggest that perinatal asphyxia only rarely causes a hearing loss (D'Souza *et al.*, 1981). Karjalainen *et al.* (1982) found no evidence of sensorineural deafness in a group of 20 children in which there was known severe placental insufficiency and intrauterine hypoxia. More recently, however, other authors have suggested that periods of neonatal apnoea and hypoxia strongly predispose to subsequent hearing loss (Duara *et al.*, 1986; Salamay, Eldredge and Tooley, 1989).

Hyperbilirubinaemia

Rhesus disease is now uncommon in the UK, although hyperbilirubinaemia may also be found with other blood group incompatibilities, hereditary spherocytosis and liver immaturity. Gerber (1990) questioned the definition of hyperbilirubinaemia and how frequently hyperbilirubinaemia is associated with with congenital deafness. It would appear that with modern methods of management and prevention, neonatal jaundice has virtually disappeared as the cause of congenital deafness.

Low birthweight and preterm children

Preterm delivery (before the end of the thirty-seventh week) and low birthweight (weighing less than 2500 g) are usually concomitant conditions and are therefore best considered together.

These infants have a higher incidence of hearing loss than normal (Bergman *et al.*, 1985). There are several reasons for this. They are more likely to have suffered episodes of hypoxia or acidosis. In addition, these children have immature metabolic functions and kernicterus can result from smaller increases in serum bilirubin levels than in mature neonates. There is also the possibility that the deafness and low birthweight are concomitantly caused by the same factor, e.g. rubella.

In the immediate postnatal period these children spend a variable amount of time in intensive care units in noisy incubators. This is discussed later in this chapter. They are very prone to life-threatening infections and are given antibiotics which are potentially ototoxic.

Some experimental animals seem to have a 'critical period' during which structural and functional development of hearing occurs (Uziel, 1985). Deafness is likely to result from exposure to noxious agents at different times during this critical period. There is no evidence at present that there is a similar critical period in humans.

In summary, it is often difficult to ascertain the causative agent in these children because of the number of potential risk factors. It is possible that these factors exert a synergistic effect on the auditory system.

Acquired disorders causing sensorineural deafness

These conditions are summarized in Table 4.7. The extension of middle ear infection to cause cochlear damage is discussed in Chapter 8.

Table 4.7 Acquired conditions causing sensorineural deafness

Infections
    complications of otitis media
    viral labyrinthitis
Immunization
Autoimmune deafness
Meningitis
Ototoxic drugs
Trauma
Metabolic disease
Neoplastic disease

Various different viral agents, in addition to those already discussed, have been identified as pathogenic in the ear. These include mumps, measles, herpes simplex, varicella-zoster and influenza viruses.

Davis (1982) provided the first experimental evidence for viraemic spread to the ear and it seems likely that this is the common route by which the viruses reach the auditory system. Labyrinthitis may also be caused by extension of infection from the meninges.

It is obviously difficult to be certain that any viral illness is a cause of subsequent sensorineural hearing loss.

Mumps

Mumps is considered to be the commonest cause of unilateral sensorineural hearing loss in children (Baloh, 1982; Kirk, 1987).

Measles

Schuknecht (1993) reported the incidence of deafness with measles as the suspected cause to be about 4–

10% in populations of deaf children. The hearing loss tends to be bilateral and moderate to severe.

The pathological findings include degeneration of the organ of Corti, spiral ganglion and vestibular sensory cells.

Reye's syndrome

This acute, and sometimes fatal, illness usually starts during recovery from a viral illness especially influenza and varicella. More recently it has been linked to the use of aspirin in children. Clinically the child's condition deteriorates with vomiting, lethargy or irritability. In severe cases cerebral oedema will progress to coma and death. Rarey *et al.* (1983) described the pathological features in a 2-month old child with Reye's syndrome. The inner hair cells of the organ of Corti were damaged more severely than the outer cells with various degrees of degeneration of non-sensory epithelial cells lining the cochlear duct. Similar lesions were found in the vestibular end organs.

The present author is not aware of any published reports of auditory function in children who have recovered from Reye's syndrome; those seen in Belfast to the present have normal hearing.

Immunization

Tetanus immunization and antitoxin are known to cause peripheral neuropathies in some patients. In a review of the literature, Mair and Elverland (1977) identified nine cases in which deafness occurred 2–10 days after tetanus immunization or tetanus antitoxin. These authors pointed out that it is extremely difficult to be certain that the two events are related, although in the absence of other aetiological factors, a cause–effect relationship may be assumed. The present author has seen one child in which triple vaccination was followed 2 days later by a 'flu-like illness and severe bilateral sensorineural loss.

There are no reports in the literature of deafness after diphtheria or polio immunization.

Measles, mumps and rubella immunization (MMR) is now widely available. Stewart and Prabhu (1993) reported nine cases of an alleged sensorineural hearing loss after immunization with MMR vaccine as reported by the yellow cards surveillance scheme. Three of the nine cases were not caused by the vaccine, of the other six, two were bilateral and four had unilateral sensorineural hearing loss. There was no other obvious cause for the hearing loss in these six children. The authors concluded that the risk of deafness after MMR is small and must be weighed against the risks of deafness due to the natural disease.

Autoimmune sensorineural hearing loss

Immunological destruction of the auditory and vestibular systems is a recognized feature of many dis-

eases (Stephens, Luxon and Hinchliffe, 1982; Brookes, 1985; Naclerio, 1985).

Damage may be caused in several ways. Immune complexes lodge in the microcirculation of the ear causing obstruction and hypoxia in the distal tissues. Complement fixation may cause a vasculitis with subsequent inflammatory response. It is also possible that there is an inappropriate direct immune reaction against cells derived from the neural crest.

Brookes and Newland (1986) presented eight cases, one a child of 11 years, with deafness and evidence of circulating immune complexes. Plasma exchange, thought to remove the immune complexes, was of marginal benefit in restoring hearing in about one-half of the cases, although in some, relief was only temporary.

Meningitis

The most frequent cause of acquired sensorineural deafness in childhood is meningitis (Martin, 1982; Davis and Wood, 1992). The latter estimated that about 90% of acquired deafness was due to this cause. Fortnum (1992) reviewed the literature. The incidence of post-meningitic hearing impairment is reported as varying from 3.5% to as high as 37.2%. This large range reflects the sampling errors associated with small samples, the type and severity of the hearing impairment included, the timing of the assessment after the onset of the illness, the age range of the children, the profile of the infecting organisms, the sophistication of the tests used and the reliability of the referral system. In Belfast it was found that only about 50% of children with bacterial meningitis were referred for hearing assessment. Subsequently a protocol has been devised to ensure that all children have their hearing assessed within 1 month of discharge from hospital. It would appear that the true incidence of sensorineural hearing loss after meningitis lies between 8 and 12% with about one-quarter of these having profound sensorineural deafness.

Fortnum and Davis (1993) considered the risk factors for sensorineural hearing loss in children with meningitis. These included the following: the presence of associated hydrocephalus, children aged less than 1 month or greater than 5 years, children whose length of stay was greater than 16 days in the hospital, admission during the winter months (October–March), and a cerebrospinal fluid (CSF) glucose concentration of less than 2.2 mmol/l. It would appear that there is no differential risk for the infecting organisms.

The ear may be affected in different ways by meningitis. Bacterial labyrinthitis due to direct spread of the infection from the subarachnoid space through the cochlear aqueduct, internal acoustic meatus or endolymphatic duct is associated with profound sensorineural hearing loss. In children who have partial or reversible hearing loss there may be toxic or serous labyrinthitis.

The deafness is usually bilateral and profound although may be less severe and even unilateral (Rasmussen, Johnsen and Bohr, 1991). There have been reports of improvements in the hearing after meningitis even in children with profound bilateral sensorineural hearing loss, although improvements are more often reported in cases with less severe problems. Fortnum considered that some of these may have been due to improvements in the reliability and accuracy of hearing tests as the child got older, or to resolution of a simultaneously present conductive hearing loss due to fluid in the middle ear.

The common organisms associated with sensorineural hearing loss after meningitis are *Streptococcus pneumoniae*, *Haemophilus influenzae* and *Neisseria meningitidis*. In spite of previous publications suggesting that *Neisseria meningitidis* is the most dangerous organism with respect to hearing loss, it would appear that bacterial meningitis of any type can result in sensorineural hearing loss of any degree in a child of any age and that meningitic sensorineural hearing loss is not truely organism specific (Fortnum, 1992).

Parving and Hauch (1994) noted a small reduction in recent years of the number of children deaf due to meningitis. Fortnum (1992) described recent advances in both prevention and treatment of bacterial meningitis. Immunization against *Haemophilus influenzae* infections (Hib) is now available. Bent and Beck (1994) considered the implications of this treatment. There is also considerable interest in the use of dexamethasone in meningitis (Meningitis Working Party of the British Paediatric Association Immunology and Infectious Disease Group, 1992). American studies suggested that dexamethasone probably reduces the likelihood of deafness after *Haemophilus influenzae* meningitis but its usefulness in pneumococcal and meningococcal meningitis has not yet been proven. The authors of this report argued that it is too early to say if steroids are of benefit and suggested the need for multicentre placebo-controlled trials.

Nadol (1978) considered the findings in 304 patients thought to have viral meningitis. The causative virus was identified in only one-sixth of the group and included mumps, measles, herpes simplex and varicella-zoster viruses. None of these patients had a sensorineural hearing loss. Fortnum (1992) in a review of the literature, found only a few documented cases of hearing impairment after viral meningitis.

Ototoxic drugs

The potential ototoxicity of many drugs is well recognized, the two most important groups being the 'loop' diuretics and the aminoglycoside antibiotics. A comprehensive summary of the pharmacology of these drugs and pathological lesions produced was provided by Harper (1982).

Animal research has demonstrated that aminoglycosides will cause intrauterine cochlear damage (Uziel, 1985). There also appears to be interspecies and interstrain variability. In humans, there are surprisingly few reports of deafness due to the administration of aminoglycosides either during pregnancy or childhood (Crifo *et al.*, 1980; Scott and Griffiths, 1994). It would appear that neonates and older children have reduced risks from the ototoxic effects of these drugs. Children with cystic fibrosis often receive prolonged treatment with high doses of these drugs. Crifo *et al.* (1980) found only one such child, in a group of 30, with a bilateral slight high frequency loss assumed to be due to gentamicin.

Similar findings were reported in 53 children with cystic fibrosis who were given tobramycin. Only one developed a transient high frequency loss (Thomsen and Friis, 1979).

Erythromycin is commonly used in children with a history of penicillin allergy. Schweitzer and Olson (1984) presented a case report in which pharmacological doses were used. The patient developed a hearing loss 5 days after erythromycin was first given. On stopping the drug the hearing improved, although the high frequency loss persisted. A survey of the literature revealed a further 32 cases with a reversible high frequency loss. Similar findings were reported by Haydon, Thielin and Davis (1984).

This apparent lack of ototoxicity in children must not be allowed to induce a feeling of complacency. Bernard (1981) demonstrated alterations in the brain stem evoked potentials of preterm babies due to conventional doses of aminoglycosides. Colding *et al.* (1989) carried out audiometry at the age of 4 years in 69 out of 105 surviving children who had continuous intravenous gentimicin in a neonatal intensive care unit. Two of these had a hearing loss of 20 dB. Kastanioudakis *et al.* (1993) found a significant number of children with hearing loss and vestibular dysfunction due to the administration of streptomycin sulphate in Albanian children. Gray (1989) described a similar problem in India. As with adults, the serum peak and trough levels must be carefully monitored, especially in children with renal disease.

Chemotherapy for childhood malignancy has also been reported as a cause of sensorineural hearing loss (Schell, McHaney and Green, 1989). These authors found that the probability of the hearing loss was related to the accumulative dose of cisplatin given and that the hearing loss was more likely if the patient had had previous irradiation. They noted that irradiation alone did not affect the child's hearing.

Trauma

The effects of trauma on the cochlea are fully discussed in Volumes 2 and 3.

A blow to the head, sufficient to render a child unconscious can cause cochlear concussion with a fracture of the temporal bone (Schuknecht, 1993). Transverse fractures of the petrous temporal bone are associated with damage to the cochlea or auditory nerve. In children, the deafness may not be noticed for some time after the injury. Rupture of the round or oval window may be caused by sudden violent exercise and is predisposed to by anatomical abnormalities (Pashley, 1982). Surgical trauma, even after minor procedures such as myringotomy may damage the cochlea.

Perilymph fistulae have been described in paediatric patients after trauma (Myer *et al.*, 1989; Pappas and Schneiderman, 1989). The children had sudden, fluctuating or progressive sensorineural hearing loss.

The effects of noise exposure on the adult ear are well known. The effects on fetal and neonatal ears are not. Most women continue to work for the first few months of their pregnancy. The mother's abdominal and uterine walls will provide protection from noise. Smeja *et al.* (1979) found that when the mother was exposed to 100 dB noise, there was a change in fetal heart rhythm and also fetal movements. These may reflect distress. The effects of excessive environmental noise on the ears of the fetus are unknown (Hepper and Shahidullah, 1994).

Many neonates spend their first few days or weeks of life in incubators in constant noise levels of 60–80 dB. Added to this is the 5–25 dB generated by other life-support equipment such as ventilators, humidifiers and monitors. Medical and nursing staff will often stimulate apnoeic babies by striking the side of the incubator. This can cause impulse signals up to 140 dB SPL (Bess, Peek and Chapman, 1979).

Animal experiments have demonstrated outer hair cell loss in neonatal guinea-pigs and rats exposed to noise (Douek *et al.*, 1976; Uziel, 1985). In human neonates, however, the noise levels currently found in incubators do not seem to cause a hearing loss (Schulte and Stennert, 1978). It would seem possible that the affects of incubator noise and ototoxic antibiotics might summate and this has been shown in animals (Scott and Griffiths, 1994).

Children and adolescents live in a self-induced noisy environment. The MRC Institute of Hearing Research (1985) published a report which examined the potential damage to hearing arising from leisure noise. The major source of auditory hazard to the population from non-occupational noise is from amplified music. Portable stereo radiocassette players with headphones can generate noise intensity levels potentially hazardous to human ears (Catalano and Levin, 1985). Much has been written about the potential dangers of rock concert music and there are many reports of temporary threshold shifts in both musicians and the audience. West and Evans (1990) used sweep frequency Bekesy tracking audiometry to investigate hearing loss after noise exposure in 60 young subjects. They concluded that exposure to amplified music is harmful, the earliest sign being a decrease in frequency resolution. Ruben (1985) pointed out that an adolescent with a seemingly insignificant high frequency loss may become severely handicapped in middle age due to the additive effects of industrial noise exposure and other causes of sensorineural deafness.

Concern has been expressed about the potential additional hearing loss caused by high powered hearing aids. Markides (1971) could not find sufficient evidence at that time to support this. More recently Fradis and Feiglin (1984) and Newton and Rowson (1988) could find no evidence of hearing aids causing deterioration in hearing.

Menière's disease

This is an extremely rare cause of deafness in children and presents a similar clinical picture to that found in adults.

Metabolic disease

Disorders of the microcirculation are common in diabetes mellitus and it is quoted as a cause of deafness. Seiger *et al.* (1983), in a survey of the literature, found conflicting views. One explanation of this was the heterogenicity of the different groups studied. These authors presented the findings in a group of 51 insulin-dependent diabetic children. None had evidence of deafness. This may have been due to many factors including short duration of the illness and lack of sensitivity in the auditory tests used.

Neoplastic disease

Acoustic neuroma (schwannoma) may be present at birth, but only become clinically obvious in later life. There are very few reported cases of acoustic neuroma in children. Allcutt *et al.* (1991) reported three acoustic neuromas in children all of which were detected late and only when they were large and vascular.

Leukaemia may affect the temporal bone in two ways (Schuknecht, 1993). Leukaemic infiltrates may be found in middle ear mucosa and perilymph spaces, or haemorrhage may cause sudden deafness, usually with dizziness.

Sudden deafness

Children rarely complain of sudden loss of hearing. Tierei *et al.* (1984) suggested the following as possible causes:

1 Infection – mumps, measles, meningitis, varicella
2 Trauma – concussion, fractures of temporal bone, perilymph fistula
3 Idiopathic – the mechanism may be vascular with spasm, thrombosis, embolism or haemorrhage causing cell anoxia and death.

Progressive sensorineural hearing loss in children

Newton and Rowson (1988) found that 9% of a cohort of children assessed had a progressive sensorineural hearing loss. These authors felt that this was an underestimate of the size of the problem. Progressive deafness has been found with infection such as rubella, cytomegalovirus and meningitis. It may also occur in association with a perilymph fistula (Mayer *et al.*, 1989; Pappas and Schneiderman, 1989).

There have been several descriptions of dilatation of the vestibular aqueduct (Jackler and De la Cruz, 1989; Arcand *et al.*, 1991). The latter authors performed routine CT of the mastoids of 130 deaf children. Eighteen were found to have an enlarged vestibular aqueduct. Phelps (1994) suggested that the investigation of choice was a CT scan using axial sections (Figure 4.5).

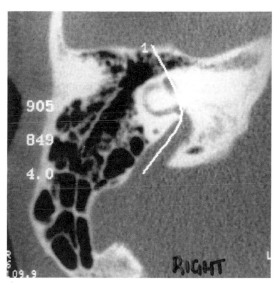

Figure 4.5 Dilated vestibular aqueduct. (Courtesy of Peter Phelps)

Mixed deafness

The conditions which cause a mixed deafness are summarized in Table 4.8. Otosclerosis in children is usually associated with conductive deafness only.

Earpits-deafness syndrome

Slack and Phelps (1985) presented a description of four families and a review of the literature. The condition is characterized by unilateral or bilateral auricular deformities in 75% of cases. These are preauricular pits or appendages with unilateral or bilateral branchial fistulae or cysts in 50% of affected children. The ossicular chain may be abnormal and

Table 4.8 Causes of mixed deafness

1 Congenital abnormalities, deafness present at birth
    earpits-deafness syndrome
2 Congenital abnormalities, deafness occurring in childhood
    osteopetrosis (Albers-Schönberg disease)
    Langerhans cell histiocytosis
    mucopolysaccharidosis
3 Acquired disease
    infection

there is distortion of the basal turn of the cochlea. Two of the patients in this series had ossiculoplasties with no improvement in hearing. This confirmed the findings of other otologists dealing with this condition.

Osteopetrosis (Albers-Schönberg disease)

This may be inherited in a dominant form (benign) or as a recessive trait (clinically malignant). There is abnormal bone growth with failure of reabsorption of calcified cartilage and persistence of primitive bone. The bony labyrinths and ossicles consist of dense calcified cartilage. The mastoid is usually not pneumatized. These patients present to otologists with mixed deafness and recurrent facial nerve palsy.

Langerhans cell histiocytosis

The 1985 Philadelphia workshop adopted the term Langerhans cell histiocytosis to cover histiocytosis X, eosinophilic granuloma, Hand-Schuller-Christian disease and Letterer-Siwe disease (D'Angio, Favara and Ladisch, 1986).

The symptoms in this disorder in children include otorrhoea, temporal bone lesions including swelling and polyps in the external auditory canal (Irving, Broadbent and Jones, 1994; Quraishi, Blayney and Breatnach, 1993). The latter authors pointed out that this disorder can mimic otitis externa, otitis media and even acute mastoiditis. It is important to remember the possibility of this disorder in a child with persistent symptoms. Treatment is usually a combination of curettage, chemotherapy and radiotherapy.

Mucopolysaccharidoses

The best known of these are Hurler's (type 1) and Hunter's (type 2) syndromes. There is abnormal metabolism of intracellular high molecular weight carbohydrates. Most of the mucopolysaccharidoses are autosomal recessive traits except for Hunter's syndrome which is X-linked.

Fisch (1981) noted that all affected children examined by him had a hearing loss. In many of the children the hearing loss was conductive, although it was sometimes superimposed on a moderate high frequency sensorineural deafness to give a mixed loss. Schuknecht (1993) indicated that deafness is not always present in these children but, if present, is of the mixed type.

Schachern, Shea and Paparella (1984) presented the findings from the temporal bones of three patients with Hurler's syndrome. They included otitis media, residual mesenchyme in the round window niche, partial occlusion of the middle ear and basophilic concretions in the stria vascularis. Other reports note the absence of the incudostapedial joint and obliteration of both oval and round windows with fibrous tissue invading the otic capsule.

Infection

This is the commonest cause of mixed deafness in children and is discussed in Chapter 8.

Non-organic deafness (psychogenic deafness)

There are three types of this condition.

Functional (hysterical) deafness

This is apparent deafness in the absence of a pathological process affecting the auditory pathway. The deafness is a product of the subconscious. It is estimated that functional deafness is responsible for about 5% of all audiological clinic attendances. It would appear to be very uncommon under the age of 5 years.

It may be a reaction to stress, especially if the child is not doing well at school and the parents' expectations are unrealistically high. In some cases it is a means of identifying with another member of the family who has a hearing problem.

The deafness may be moderate to severe with evidence of other psychological disturbances such as mutism, tremors, aggressive or withdrawn behaviour. The child's voice is usually unaltered with no deterioration in the quality of speech. These children often give different serial audiograms with better speech discrimination scores than would be expected from the pure-tone readings. Clinically the child's hearing is usually much better than the audiogram would suggest. This group must be differentiated from those children who seem to have difficulty in understanding what is involved in pure-tone audiometry.

Malingering

In this type there is intention on the part of the child to deceive. This is rare in children as most are not sophisticated enough to maintain the pretence for long and there is rarely the motivation for financial gain as sometimes seen in adults.

Organic deafness with psychogenic overlay

Children with true ear disease occasionally appear to be much deafer than can be explained by the pathology.

In all three types of non-organic deafness, objective tests, including evoked response audiometry, will reveal the true hearing thresholds (Yoshida, Noguchi and Uemura, 1989). The author has found otoacoustic emission testing useful in these children.

These children present difficult management problems. It is important to stress to parents the need to avoid accusing the child of feigning a hearing loss. Attempts should be made to look for areas of conflict at home or school. This may mean referral to a child psychologist or psychiatrist. These children must not be issued with hearing aids for fear of reinforcing their 'deafness'. Brooks and Geoghegan (1992) presented the findings of a retrospective follow up 6–27 years after first presentation. They found that a small number still had non-organic hearing loss, one of whom was a self-confessed malingerer. They concluded that although non-organic hearing loss appears to resolve in the short-term, there are some children who have persistent problems.

Conclusions

This chapter attempts to cover the major causes of deafness in children. The space given to each is not a reflection of its importance or prevalence. Taylor (1979) discussed the reasons for the differences in prevalence rates between various studies (Table 4.9). In retrospective studies serological data are not available, access to accurate hospital records is not always possible and sample groups differ. True comparisons are therefore difficult to make.

A more recent multicentre study of EEC children with a hearing loss of 50 dB or worse was reported by Martin (1982). In this study rubella was responsible for 20% of deafness in children in the UK. Deafness was identified as having a genetic basis in about 12% of cases, caused by perinatal anoxia or jaundice in 10% and in 40% of cases the cause was unknown.

Davis and Parving (1993) demonstrated differences in causes of deafness in populations of children in

Table 4.9 **Different prevalence rates of deafness between various studies**

Causes	Percentage of cases
Genetic	24–39
Embryopathies (mainly rubella)	6–24
Perinatal	6–23
Unknown	25–45

Denmark and England, although they pointed out that the scarcity of prevalence data for childhood hearing impairment worldwide is exacerbated by the difficulty of interpretating existing data. Vanniasegaram, Tungland and Bellman (1993) found higher prevalence rates of mendelian deafness and rubella in a Bengali community compared to nationally expected rates. Prevalence rates also change with time (Newton, 1985; Parving and Hauch, 1994). In general there would appear to be a reduction in the number of children born with deafness due to prenatal infection and an increase in those born with hereditary hearing loss or exposure to perinatal factors, such as preterm delivery and low birthweight.

The large size of the 'cause unknown' group is a feature of all reported series. Much discussion has ensued as to possible aetiologies in this group. At present, it is generally assumed that most of these are the result of recessive genes or to gene mutations. Many of the others are caused by undiagnosed intrauterine infection or to the effects of other unrecognized cochlear pathogens. Barr (1982) underlined the marked interspecies differences in response to thalidomide. This suggests an interaction between genetic factors and exogenous pathogens in the causation of deafness. It would seem that a genetically deficient auditory pathway is more susceptible to external agents. A better understanding of the processes causing deafness, together with appropriate and early investigation of the deaf child, should reduce the size of the 'cause unknown' group.

References

ADAMS, D. A., GORMLEY, P. K., KERR, A. G., SMYTH, G. D. L., OSTERBERG, P. and SLOAN, J. (1991) Otological manifestations of a new familial polyostotic bone disorder. *Journal of Laryngology and Otology*, **105**, 80–84

AIMI, K. (1983) Role of the tympanic ring in the pathogenesis of congenital cholesteatoma. *Laryngoscope*, **93**, 1140–1146

ALEXANDER, G. (1904) Zur Pathologie und pathologishen Anatomie der kongenitalen Taubheit. *Archiv für klinische und experimentelle Ohren-, Nasen-und Kehlkopfheilkunde*, **61**, 183–219

ALLCUTT, D. A., HOFFMAN, H. J., ISLA, A., BECKER, L. E. and HUMPHREYS, R. P. (1991) Acoustic schwannomas in children. *Neurosurgery*, **21**, 14–18

ANDERSON, H., FILIPSSON, R., FLUUR, E., KOCH, B., LINDSTEN, J. and WEDENBERG, E. (1969) Hearing impairment in Turner's syndrome. *Acta Otolaryngologica Supplementum*, **247**, 1–26

ARCAND, R., DESSOSIERS, M., DUBE, J. and ABELA, A. (1991) The large vestibular aqueduct syndrome and sensorineural hearing loss in the pediatric population. *Journal of Otolaryngology*, **20**, 247–250

BALKANY, T. J., MISCHKE, R. E., DOWNS, M. P. and JAFEK, O. W. (1979) Ossicular abnormalities in Down's syndrome. *Otolaryngology and Head and Neck Surgery*, **87**, 372–384

BALOH, R. W. (1982) Hearing loss. In: *Cecil Textbook of Medicine*, edited by J. B. Wyngaarden and L. H. Smith. Philadephia: W. B. Saunders. pp. 1958–1961

BARR, B. (1982) Teratogenic hearing loss. *Audiology*, **21**, 111–127

BEGG, N. T. and NOAH, N. D. (1985) Immunisation targets in Europe and Britain. *British Medical Journal*, **291**, 1370–1371

BENT, J. P. and BECK, R. A. (1994) Bacterial meningitis in the pediatric population: paradigm shifts and ramifications for otolaryngology – head and neck surgery. *International Journal of Pediatric Otorhinolaryngology*, **31**, 41–49

BERGMAN, I., HIRSCH, R. P., FRIA, T. J., SHAPIRO, S. M., HOLZMAN, I. and PAINTER, M. J. (1985) Cause of hearing loss in the high-risk premature infant. *Journal of Pediatrics*, **106**, 95–101

BERGSTROM, L. (1977) Osteogenesis imperfecta. Otologic and maxillofacial aspects. *Laryngoscope*, **87** (suppl. 6), 1–42

BERNARD, P. A. (1981) Freedom from ototoxicity in aminoglycoside treated neonates: a mistaken notion. *Laryngoscope*, **91**, 1985–1994

BESS, F. H., PEEK, B. E. and CHAPMAN, J. J (1979) Further observation on noise levels in infant incubators. *Pediatrics*, **63**, 100–106

BROOKER, D. S. and SMYTH, G. D. L. (1991) Treatment of congenital cholesteatoma of the middle ear. *Australian Journal of Otolaryngology*, **1**, 9–11

BROOKES, G. B. (1985) Immune complex associated deafness. *Journal of the Royal Society of Medicine*, **78**, 47–55

BROOKES, G. B. and NEWLAND, A. C. (1986) Plasma exchange in the treatment of immune complex associated sensorineural deafness. *Journal of Laryngology and Otology*, **100**, 25–33

BROOKS, D. N. and GEOGHEGAN, P. M. (1992) Non-organic hearing loss in young persons: transient episode or indication of deep seated difficulty. *British Journal of Audiology*, **26**, 347–350

CATALANO, P. J. and LEVIN, S. M. (1985) Noise induced hearing loss and portable radios with headphones. *International Journal of Pediatric Otorhinolaryngology*, **9**, 59–67

CAWTHORNE, T. (1955) Otosclerosis. *Journal of Laryngology and Otology*, **69**, 437–456

CHAN, K. H. (1994) Sensorineural hearing loss in children – classification and evaluation. Paediatric otology. *Otolaryngologic Clinics of North America*, **27**, 473–486

CHASIN, W. D. (1984) Rhabdomyosarcoma of the temporal bone. *Annals of Otology, Rhinology and Laryngology*, **93** (suppl. 112), 71–73

CHURCH, M. W. and GERKIN, K. P. (1988) Hearing disorders in children with fetal alcohol syndrome: findings from case reports. *Pediatrics*, **82**, 147–154

COLDING, H., ANDERSON, E. A., PRYTZ, S. and WULFFSBERG, H. (1989) Auditory function after continuous infusion of gentamycin to high risk neonates. *Acta Paediatrica Scandinavica*, **78**, 840–843

CONNOLLY, P. K., JERGER, S., WILLIAMSON, W. D., SMITH, R. J. H. and DENMLER, G. (1992) Evaluation of higher level auditory function in children with asymptomatic congenital cytomegalovirus infection. *American Journal of Otology*, **13**, 185–192

CREMERS, C. W. R. J. (1979) Autosomal recessive non-syndromal progressive sensorineural deafness in childhood: a separate clinical and genetic entity. *International Journal of Pediatric Otorhinolaryngology*, **1**, 193–199

CRIFO, S., ANTONELLI, M., GAGLIARDI, M., LUCARELLI, N. and MAROLINI, P. (1980) Ototoxicity aminoglycoside antibiotics in long-term treatment for cystic fibrosis. *International Journal of Pediatric Otorhinolaryngology*, **1**, 193–199

CUNNINGHAM, C. C. and MCARTHUR, K. (1981) Hearing loss and treatment in young Down's syndrome children. *Child: Care, Health and Development*, **7**, 357–374

DAHLE, A. J. and MCCOLLISTER, F. P. (1988) Audiological findings in children with neonatal herpes. *Ear and Hearing*, **9**, 256–258

D'ANGIO, G. J., FAVARA, B. E. and LADISCH, S. (1986) Workshop on the childhood histiocytosis: concepts and controversies. *Medical and Pediatric Oncology*, **14**, 104–117

DAS, V. K. (1990) Prevalence of otitis media with effusion in children with bilateral sensorineural hearing loss. *Archives of Disease in Childhood*, **65**, 757–759

DAVIS, A. (1993) The prevalence of deafness. In: *Deafness*, 5th edn, edited by J. Ballantyne, M. C. Martin and A. Martin. London: Whurr. pp. 1–11

DAVIS, A. and PARVING, A. (1993) Towards appropriate epidemiological data in childhood hearing disability: a comparative European study of birth cohorts. *Journal of Audiological Medicine*, **3**, 35–47

DAVIS, A. and WOOD, S. (1992) The epidemiology of childhood hearing impairment: factors relevant to planning of services. *British Journal of Audiology*, **26**, 77–90

DAVIS, L. E. (1982) Experimental viral infections of the inner ear. III. Viraemic spread of reovirus to hamster eighth nerve ganglion cells. *Annals of Otology, Rhinology and Laryngology*, **91**, 90–93

DERLACKI, E. and CLEMIS, J. (1965) Congenital cholesteatoma of the middle ear and mastoid. *Annals of Otology, Rhinology and Laryngology*, **74**, 706–727

DOUEK, E., DODSON, H. C., BANNISTER, L. H., ASHCROFT, P. and HUMPHRIES, K. N. (1976) Effects of incubator noise on the cochlea of the newborn. *Lancet*, ii, 1110–1113

D'SOUZA, S., MCCARTNEY, E., NOLAN, M. and TAYLOR, I. G. (1981) Hearing, speech and language in survivors of severe perinatal asphyxia. *Archives of Disease in Childhood*, **56**, 245–252

DUARA, S., SUTER, C. M., BESSARD, K. K. and GUTBERLET, R. L. (1986) Neonatal screening with auditory brainstem responses: results of follow-up audiometry and risk factor evaluation. *Journal of Pediatrics*, **108**, 276–281

DUBEY, S. P. and GHOSH, L. M. (1993) Klippel-Feil syndrome with congenital conductive deafness: report of a case and review of the literature. *International Journal of Pediatric Otorhinolaryngology*, **25**, 201–208

FISCH, L. (1981) Syndromes associated with hearing loss. In: *Audiology and Audiological Medicine*, vol. II, edited by H. A. Beagley. Oxford: Oxford University Press. pp. 559–639

FORTNUM, H. M. (1992) Hearing impairment after bacterial meningitis. *Archives of Disease in Childhood*, **67**, 1128–1133

FORTNUM, H. and DAVIS, A. (1993) Hearing impairment in children after bacterial meningitis: incidence and resource implications. *British Journal of Audiology*, **27**, 43–52

FRADIS, M. and FEIGLIN, H. (1984) Effects of hearing aids on hearing. *Laryngoscope*, **94**, 113–117

FRASER, G. R. (1976) *The Causes of Profound Deafness in Childhood*. London: Bailliere Tindall

FREEMAN, J. (1983) Temporal bone fractures and cholesteatoma. *Annals of Otology, Rhinology and Laryngology*, **92**, 558–560

GERBER, S. E. (1990) Review of a high risk register for congenital or early-onset deafness. *British Journal of Audiology*, **24**, 347–356

GORLIN, R. J., COHEN, M. M. JR and LEVIN, L. S. (1990) *Syndromes of the Head and Neck*, 4th edn. New York: Oxford University Press

GRATZ, E. S., POLLACK, M. A. and ZIMMERMAN, R. D. (1981) Congenital facial palsy and ipsilateral deafness: association with maternal diabetes mellitus. *International Journal of Pediatric Otorhinolaryngology*, **3**, 335–341

GRAY, R. J. (1989) Causes of deafness in schools for the deaf in Madras. *International Journal of Pediatric Otorhinolaryngology*, **18**, 97–106

HALL, J. G. (1964) The cochlea and cochlear nuclei in neonatal asphyxia. *Acta Otolaryngologica Supplementum*, **194**, 1–93

HARDY, J. B. (1973) Foetal consequences of maternal viral infections in pregnancy. *Archives of Otolaryngology*, **98**, 218–227

HARPER, E. S. (1982) The pharmacology of ototoxic drugs. *British Journal of Audiology*, **16**, 81–93

HAYDON, R. C., THIELIN, J. W. and DAVIS, W. E. (1984) Erythromycin ototoxicity: analysis and conclusions based on 22 case reports. *Otolaryngology and Head and Neck Surgery*, **92**, 678–684

HEMENWAY, W., SANDO, I. and MCCHESNEY, D. (1969) Temporal bone pathology following maternal rubella. *Archiv für klinische und experimentelle Ohren- Nasen- und Kehlkopfheilkunde*, **193**, 287–300

HEPPER, P. G. and SHAHIDULLAH, S. (1994) Noise and the foetus: a critical review of the literature. *Health and Safety Executive Research Report no 63*. London: HMSO

HICKSON, L. M. and ALCOCK, D. (1991) Progressive hearing loss in children with congenital cytomegalovirus. *Journal of Paediatrics and Child Health*, **27**, 105–107

HOLMES, L. B. (1977) Medical genetics. In: *Hearing Loss in Children*, edited by B. J. Jaffe. Baltimore: University Park Press. pp. 253–265

IRVING, R. M., BROADBENT, V. and JONES, N. S. (1994) Langerhans cell histiocytosis of childhood. Management of head and neck manifestations. *Laryngoscope*, **104**, 64–70

JACKLER, R. K. and DE LA CRUZ, A. (1989) The large vestibular aqueduct. *Laryngoscope*, **99**, 1238–1242

JAHRSDOERFER, R. A., AGUILAR, E. A., YEAKLEY, J. W. and COLE, R. R. (1989) Treacher-Collins syndrome: an otologic challenge. *Annals of Otology, Rhinology and Laryngology*, **98**, 807–812

KARJALAINEN, S., KARJA, J., SUMONIO, S. and YLISKOSKI, M. (1982) Intrauterine hypoxia as a cause of hearing impairment in children. *International Journal of Pediatric Otorhinolaryngology*, **4**, 233, 243

KARMODY, C. S. and SCHUKNECHT, H. F. (1966) Deafness in congenital syphilis. *Archives of Otolaryngology*, **83**, 18–27

KASTANIOUDAKIS, J., SKEVAS, A., ASSIMAKOPOULOUS, D. and ANASTASOPOULOS, D. (1993) Hearing loss and vestibular dysfunction in childhood from the use of streptomycin in Albania. *International Journal of Pediatric Otorhinolaryngology*, **26**, 109–115

KELEMEN, G. (1958) Toxoplasmosis and congenital deafness. *Archives of Otolaryngology*, **68**, 547–561

KIRK, M. (1987) Sensorineural hearing loss and mumps. *British Journal of Audiology*, **21**, 227–228

KONIGSMARK, B. W. and GORLIN, R. J. (1976) *Genetic and Metabolic Deafness*. Philadelphia: W. B. Saunders

KUDESIA, G., ROBINSON, E. T., WILSON, W. D., WILSON, T. S., STEWART, I. M., CAMPBELL, A.T. *et al.* (1985) Rubella: immunity and vaccination in schoolgirls. *British Medical Journal*, **290**, 1406–1408

MCDONALD, T. J., CODY, D. T. R. and RYAN, R. E. J. (1984) Congenital cholesteatoma of the ear. *Annals of Otology, Rhinology and Laryngology*, **93**, 637–640

MCGEE, T., WOLTERS, C., STEIN, L., KRAUS, N., JOHNSON, D., BOYER, K. *et al.* (1992) Absence of sensorineural hearing loss in treated infants and children with congenital toxoplasmosis. *Otolaryngology, Head and Neck Surgery*, **106**, 75–80

MCSHANE, M. A., CARSON, D., REDMOND, A. and ADAMS, D. A. (1987) Renal tubular acidosis with nerve deafness. *Ulster Medical Journal*, **56**, 137–141

MAIR, I. W. S. and ELVERLAND, H. H. (1977) Sudden deafness and vaccination. *Journal of Laryngology and Otology*, **91**, 323–329

MARKIDES, A. (1971) Do hearing aids damage the user's residual hearing? *Sound*, **5**, 99–105

MARTIN, J. A. M. (1982) Aetiological factors relating to childhood deafness in the European community. *Audiology*, **21**, 149–158

MAURIZI, M., OTTAVIANI, F., PALUDETTI, G. and LUNGAROTTI, S. (1985) Audiological findings in Down's children. *International Journal of Pediatric Otorhinolaryngology*, **9**, 227–232

MENINGITIS WORKING PARTY OF THE BRITISH PAEDIATRIC ASSOCIATION IMMUNOLOGY AND INFECTIOUS DISEASE GROUP (1992) Should we use dexamethasone in meningitis? *Archives of Disease in Childhood*, **68**, 1398–1401

MORRISON, A. W. (1979) Diseases of the otic capsule II. Other diseases. In: *Scott Brown's Disesases of the Ear, Nose and Throat*, vol. 2. 4th edn. edited by J. Ballantyne and J. Groves. London: Butterworths. pp. 465–496

MRC INSTITUTE OF HEARING RESEARCH (1985) *Damage to the Hearing Arising from Leisure Noise: a Review of the Literature*. Health and Safety Executive. London: HMSO

MYER, C. M., FARRER, S. M., DRAKE, A. F. and COTTON, R. T. (1989) Perilymph fistulas in children: rationale for therapy. *Ear and Hearing*, **10**, 112–116

NACLERIO, R. (1985) Recent advances in immunology with reference to otolaryngology. *Otolaryngologic Clinics of North America*, **18**, 821–832

NADOL, J. B. (1978) Hearing loss as a sequela of meningitis. *Laryngoscope*, **88**, 739–750

NAGER, G. T. and HOLLIDAY, M. J. (1984) Fibrous dysplasia of the temporal bone. Update with case reports. *Annals of Otology, Rhinology and Laryngology*, **93**, 630–633

NAGER, G. T., KENNEDY, D. W. and KOPSTEIN, E. (1982) Fibrous dysplasia. A review of the disease and its manifestations in the temporal bone. *Annals of Otology, Rhinology and Laryngology*, **91** (suppl. 92), 1–52

NEWTON, V. E. (1985) Aetiology of bilateral sensorineural hearing loss in young children. *Journal of Laryngology and Otology*, Suppl. 10, 1–57

NEWTON, V. E. and ROWSON, V. J. (1988) Progressive sensorineural hearing loss in childhood. *British Journal of Audiology*, **22**, 287–295

NEWTON, V. E., LIU, X.-Z. and READ, A. (1994) The association of sensorineural hearing loss and pigmentation abnormalities in Waardenburg syndrome. *Journal of Audiological Medicine*, **3**, 69–78

PAPPAS, D. G. (1983) Hearing impairment and vestibular abnormalities among children with subclinical cytomegalovirus. *Annals of Otology, Rhinology and Laryngology*, **92**, 552–557

PAPPAS, D. G. (1985) *Diagnosis and Treatment of Hearing Impairment in Children*. London: Taylor and Francis

PAPPAS, D. G. and SCHNEIDERMAN, T. S. (1989) Perilymph fistula in pediatric patients with a pre-exisiting sensorineural loss. *American Journal of Otology*, **10**, 499–501

PARADISE, J. L., BLUESTONE, C. D. and FELDER, H. (1969) The universality of otitis media in 50 infants with cleft palate. *Pediatrics*, **44**, 35–42

PARVING, A. and HAUCH, A. M. (1994) The causes of profound hearing impairment in a school for the deaf – a longitudinal study. *British Journal of Audiology*, **28**, 63–69

PASHLEY, N. R. T. (1982) Simultaneous round and oval window fistulae in a child. *Annals of Otology, Rhinology and Laryngology*, **91**, 332–335

PHELPS, P. D. (1994) Dilatation of the vestibular aqueduct, the association with congenital deafness. *Clinical Otolaryngology*, **19**, 93–94

PYE, A., KNIGHT, J. J. and ARNETT, J. M. (1984) Sensory hair cell damage from high frequency noise exposure. *British Journal of Audiology*, **18**, 231–236

QURAISHI, M. S., BLAYNEY, A. W. and BREATNACH, F. (1993) Aural symptoms as primary presentation of Langerhans cell histiocytosis. *Clinical Otolaryngology*, **18**, 317–323

RAREY, K. E., DAVIS, J. A., DAVIS, L. E. and HAWKINS, J. E. JR (1983) Inner ear pathology associated with Reye's syndrome. *International Journal of Pediatric Otorhinolaryngology*, **6**, 255–263

RASMUSSEN, N., JOHNSEN, N. J. and BOHR, V. A. (1991) Otologic sequelae after pneumococcal meningitis: a survey of 164 consecutive cases with a follow-up of 94 survivors. *Laryngoscope*, **101**, 876–882

RAZI, M. S. and DAS, V. K. (1994) Effects of adverse perinatal events on hearing. *International Journal of Pediatric Otorhinolaryngology*, **30**, 29–40

ROBINSON, M. (1983) Juvenile otosclerosis – a 20 year study. *Annals of Otology, Rhinology and Laryngology*, **92**, 561–565

ROBSON, A. K., BLANSHARD, J. D., JONES, K., ABERY, E. H., SMITH, M. G. and MAW, A. R. (1992) A conservative approach to the management of otitis media with effusion in cleft palate children. *Journal of Laryngoloty and Otology*, **106**, 788–792

ROOD, S. R. and STOOL, S. E. (1981) Current concepts of aetiology, diagnosis and management of cleft palate related otopathologic disease. *Otolaryngologic Clinics of North America*, **14**, 865–884

RUBEN, R. J. (1985) Otolaryngologic disorders of adolescents: a review. *International Journal of Pediatric Otorhinolaryngology*, **9**, 1–30

SAIGAL, S., LUNYK, O., LARKE, R. P. B. and CHERVESKY, M. A. (1982) Outcome in children with congenital cytomegalovirus infection: a longitudinal follow-up study. *American Journal of Diseases of Children*, **136**, 896–901

SALAMAY, A., ELDREDGE, L. and TOOLEY, W. H. (1989) Neonatal status and hearing loss in high risk infants. *Journal of Pediatrics*, **114**, 847–852

SANDO, I., SUEHIRA, S. and WOOD, R. P. (1983) Congenital anomalies of the external and middle ear. In: *Pediatric Otolaryngology*, edited by C. D. Bluestone and S. E. Stool. Philadelphia: W. B. Saunders. pp. 309–346

SCHACHERN, P. A., SHEA, D. A. and PAPARELLA, M. M. (1984) Mucopolysaccharidosis I-H (Hurler's syndrome) and human temporal bone histopathology. *Annals of Otology, Rhinology and Laryngology*, **93**, 65–69

SCHELL, M. J., MCHANEY, V. A. and GREEN, A. A. (1989) Hearing loss in children and young adults receiving cisplatin with or without prior cranial radiation. *Journal of Clinical Oncology*, **7**, 754–760

SCHUKNECHT, H. F. (1993) *Pathology of the Ear*, 2nd edn. Philadephia: Lea and Febiger

SCHULTE, F. J. and STENNERT, E. (1978) Hearing defects in pre-term infants. *Archives of Disease in Childhood*, **53**, 260–270

SCHWARTZ, D. M. and SCHWARTZ, R. M. (1978) Acoustic impedance and otoscopic findings in young children with Down's syndrome. *Archives of Otolaryngology*, **104**, 652–656

SCHWEITZER, V. G. and OLSON, N. R. (1984) Ototoxic effect of erythromycin therapy. *Archives of Otolaryngology*, **100**, 258–260

SCOTT, R. M. J. and GRIFFITHS, M. V. (1994) A clinical review of ototoxicity. *Clinical Otolaryngology*, **19**, 3–8

SEIGER, A., WHITE, N. H., SKINNER, M. W. and SPECTOR, G. J. (1983) Auditory function in children with diabetes mellitus. *Annals of Otology, Rhinology and Laryngology*, **92**, 237–241

SHEA, J. J. and POSTMA, D. S. (1982) Findings and long-term surgical results in the hearing loss of osteogenesis imperfecta. *Archives of Otolaryngology*, **108**, 467–470

SLACK, R. W. T. and PHELPS, P. D. (1985) Familial mixed deafness with branchial arch defects (earpits-deafness syndrome). *Clinical Otolaryngology*, **10**, 271–277

SMEJA, Z., SLOMKO, Z., SIKORSKI, K. and SOWINSKI, H. (1979) The risk of hearing impairment in children from mothers exposed to noise during pregnancy. *International Journal of Pediatric Otorhinolaryngology*, **1**, 221–229

STEPHENS, S. D. G., LUXON, L. and HINCHCLIFFE, R. (1982) Immunological disorders and auditory lesions, *Audiology*, **21**, 128–148

STEWART, B. J. A. and PRABHU, P. U. (1993) Reports of sensorineural deafness after measles, mumps and rubella immunisation. *Archives of Disease in Childhood*, **69**, 153–154

STEWART, E. J. and O'REILLY, B. F. (1989) Kleppel–Feil syndrome and conductive loss. *Journal of Laryngology and Otology*, **103**, 947–949

STEWART, E. J. and O'REILLY, B. F. (1990) A clinical and audiological investigation of osteogenesis imperfecta in Scottish patients. *Clinical Otolaryngology*, **15**, 93 (abstract)

STRAUSS, M. (1990) Human cytomegalovirus labyrinthitis. *American Journal of Otolaryngology*, **11**, 292–298

TAKANOBU, A., YAMAMOTO, J., MATSUDA, I., TANIGUCHI, N. and NAGAI, B. (1984) Siblings with renal tubular acidosis and nerve deafness. The first family in Japan. *Human Genetics*, **66**, 282–285

TAYLOR, D. J. and PHELPS, P. D. (1993) Imaging of ear deformitites in Treacher Collins syndrome. *Clinical Otolaryngology*, **18**, 263–267

TAYLOR, I. G. (1979) The deaf child. In: *Scott–Brown's Diseases of the Ear, Nose and Throat*, vol. 2, 4th edn, edited by J. Ballantyne and J. Groves. London: Butterworth pp. 499–532

THOMSEN, J. and FRIIS, B. (1979) High dose tobramycin treatment of children with cystic fibrosis. Bacteriological effect and clinical ototoxicity. *International Journal of Pediatric Otorhinolaryngology*, **1**, 33–40

TIERI, L., MASI, R., MARSELLA, P and PINELLI, V. (1984) Sudden deafness in children. *International Journal of Pediatric Otorhinolaryngology*, **7**, 257–264

UZIEL, A. (1985) Non-genetic factors affecting hearing development. *Acta Otolaryngologica*, Suppl. 421, 57–61

VANNIASEGARAM, I., TUNGLAND, O. P. and BELLMAN, S. (1993) A 5-year review of children with deafness in a multiethnic community. *Journal of Audiological Medicine*, **2**, 9–19

VELTRI, R. W., WILSON, W. R., SPRINKLE, P. M., RODMAN, S. M. and KAVESH, D. A. (1981) The implication of virus in idiopathic sudden hearing loss: primary infection or re-activation of latent virus. *Otolaryngology Head and Neck Surgery*, **89**, 137–141

WEST, P. D. B. and EVANS, E. F. (1990) Early detection of hearing damage in young listeners resulting from exposure to amplified music. *British Journal of Audiology*, **24**, 90–103

WILD, N. J., SHEPPARD, S., SMITHELLS, R. W., HOLZEL, H. and JONES, G. *et al.* (1989) Onset and severity of hearing loss due to congenital rubella infection. *Archives of Disease in Childhood*, **64**, 1280–1283

WILLIAMS, W. T., GHORAYEB, B. Y. and YEAKLEY, J. W. (1992) Pediatric temporal bone fractures. *Laryngoscope*, **102**, 600–603

YOSHIDA, M., NOGUCHI, A. and UEMURA, I. (1989) Functional hearing loss in children. *International Journal of Pediatric Otorhinolaryngology*, **17**, 287–295

5

Testing hearing in children

S. Bellman and I. Vanniasegaram

When assessing the hearing of young children different methods may be used from those employed with older children and adults, but the information sought is similar – to identify and quantify any hearing impairment, to localize the site of any pathological process and to assess any resulting hearing disability. Hearing thresholds are identified, wherever possible, by age appropriate behavioural techniques. If these are impossible because of the age or level of cooperation of the child, then objective measures of threshold measurement are used, in practice usually measuring auditory evoked potentials (AEP). There are now a number of techniques which may identify areas of abnormal pathology in the auditory system. Impedance audiometry (otoadmittance measurement) is a common procedure used to assess middle ear function. Otoacoustic emissions are measured to demonstrate normal outer hair cell function in the cochlea. Tympanic membrane displacement can indicate abnormal cochlear (and cerebrospinal fluid) pressures and cochlear blood flow. Electric response audiometry (ERA) can be used to measure auditory evoked potentials, in particular the auditory brain stem response (ABR), to assess not only auditory thresholds but also abnormalities of the auditory pathways. Any disability resulting from a hearing impairment can be assessed either by a questionnaire approach, or by speech audiometry in a quiet room and, if relevant, in noise.

Hearing assessment is only one aspect in the overall care of children with hearing problems. If a hearing problem is found investigations into the cause of the hearing loss will be needed, followed by appropriate management and rehabilitation. These topics are covered elsewhere.

Development of response to sound

The behavioural response to sound matures with the child's development in the same way as other skills. Before a tester can start to assess the hearing of children it is essential to have a good working knowledge of how these responses develop in a normal child. It is also necessary to understand the normal development of the child in other fields, as hearing responses and communication skills have to be viewed in the context of the child's overall level of maturation. The responses described below are related to the child's developmental, rather than chronological age.

Neonatal responses

During the first weeks of life a baby responds to loud sounds by a startle reflex. This response includes the aural-palpebral reflex, which remains one of the most consistent responses to sound, a change in heart rate and pattern of respiration and a backwards head jerk and body movement (the Moro reflex). These responses are not elicited by quiet sounds and the intensity of sound producing a reaction depends very much on the psychophysiological state of the child. For these reasons it is not possible to assess a neonate's hearing thresholds accurately by behavioural techniques.

Responses of infants under 4 months age

As the infant matures she begins to notice sounds and to respond by stilling and listening. By 4 months of age an infant stills and smiles to a parent's voice, even when the source is not within the visual field, and obviously vocalizes in response to voice in a communicative way. The response is mainly seen to louder sounds and there is no consistent response to quieter sounds that could reliably be used for threshold estimation.

Responses at 4–6 months

At this age an infant is beginning to turn the head to the source of a sound with increasing consistency. Not only is the response more reliable, but it also occurs to sounds of lower intensity, so that estimates of the hearing threshold using behavioural techniques are sometimes possible. However, because the localization of sound is still developing at this age, the response varies from the prompt localization of sound seen in an older infant.

The turn to an auditory stimulus is often delayed and a longer presentation of the stimulus is necessary, without raising the intensity of the sound. The sound may also need to presented nearer to the child than the usual 1m distance. A child of this age may learn to localize sound to the first side tested, but then only turn to this direction wherever the source of the sound. This could lead to a suspicion of a unilateral hearing loss if the child's developmental age is not taken into account. The child may also turn to the correct side, but with a half turn that does not visualize the sound source, or may assume the sound to come from the first object or person identified on turning, again not recognizing the actual source of sound. These are normal responses for many children of this age. Children of this developmental age also respond better to the more traditional test sounds and do not turn to warble tones at the same quiet levels, which could lead to a suspicion of hearing impairment if only the latter are used.

Responses at 7–9 months

By this age a child can localize quiet sounds accurately on a horizontal plane, although many children still have problems in identifying a source of sound below, and in particular above their heads on testing. A child will turn readily to a parent's voice across a room and search for the source of interesting sounds. The child should also be babbling tunefully and during this time may begin to copy sounds more noticeably.

Responses at 10–12 months

At this age a child can localize quiet sounds on any plane when not otherwise occupied. Verbal comprehension is developing for single words, such as her name, 'no' and well-known objects. The range of vocalizations increases and by their first birthday some children are attempting to say and repeat a few words.

Responses at 13–24 months

A child of this age localizes sounds readily but begins to anticipate and search for the sound source during behavioural testing, so that more active distraction may be necessary. Understanding of words increases so that by 18 months many children will identify some body parts. By the age of 2 years children will often pick out toys when requested, and simple speech discrimination tests can be introduced into the assessment. The child's vocabulary increases over the second year of life and children usually start joining two words together by 18–21 months. Even before speech is recognizable the vocalizations should show good intonation patterns with a speech-like rhythm.

Responses over 2 years of age

As the child gets older she becomes increasingly able to inhibit the earlier ready response to sound. Such a child will usually turn to a particular stimulus on first presentation only, and will subsequently ignore the sound. The ability consciously to avoid turning to an anticipated sound, e.g. during testing, also develops, although an eye-glide is often seen. However, as many parents will testify, an older child can appear to be completely unaware of unwelcome requests or demands. As this stage is reached simple distraction techniques of testing become more difficult and eventually impossible to carry out reliably, and conditioning or play audiometry in free field can be attempted. Many children will carry out pure-tone audiometry before 3 years of age given appropriate test conditions, the limiting factor being the acceptance of headphones.

Behavioural audiometry

Behavioural testing of infants and young children is usually carried out sound (free) field, using stimuli delivered either live or through loudspeakers. Various extra factors need to be considered in this situation, both because of the nature of sound field testing, as opposed to conventional audiometry using headphones, and also the difficulty of working with such young and often uncooperative children.

Environment

The environment in which the testing of a young child takes place is vitally important if the results are to be accurate. The room must be not only acoustically acceptable, but must also be a comfortable and inviting place, where a child can relax. An insecure and worried child will not cooperate fully in the necessary assessment. While older children and adults may perform hearing tests in small sound-treated booths, the testing of younger children should take place in an acoustically-treated normal-sized room. There needs to be space for the child and caregiver to sit comfortably in the room while testers can move freely around the child.

The room, as for a booth, should be extremely quiet, and such rooms are expensive to provide. A reasonable compromise for diagnostic audiometric testing is an overall sound level not exceeding 30 dB(A). However, because the testing of young children is carried out in free field, ideally even lower background sound levels are necessary. The design of audiometric rooms is a very specialized area, but certain features of a room used for young children are worthy of consideration. For example the sound absorbent lining to the walls is often acoustic tiling, but a fabric finish can give a more welcoming feel to a room.

In addition to reducing the acoustic interference, the visual aspects of such a room need consideration. The lighting is extremely important in sound field testing with live stimuli. There should be even illumination, with no possibility of shadows alerting a hearing impaired child to the tester's position. There should be no large windows overlooking interesting and, in particular, moving objects, that may distract a child and make testing unreliable. Within the room itself there should be no distracting features, such as pictures or attractive toys, which could be in the child's visual field while testing. When testing a child it is important to ensure that there are no reflective surfaces, particularly two way mirrors for observation, which are in a position to be used by a child to gain clues which would invalidate results. In this respect a window becomes a mirror in the dark, and suitable blinds and curtains may be needed.

Stimulus

Frequency

In the past a wide variety of uncalibrated sounds have been used 'live' to assess hearing. While some of these may still have a place during an asssessment, it is now recognized that sounds have to be far more frequency specific if accurate and meaningful hearing levels are to be obtained. The aim is to build up information about a child's hearing for different frequencies in the same way that one carries out an audiogram in an older child. During the test for threshold levels the minimum requirement should be an accurate assessment of hearing at low, middle and high frequencies in both ears.

One traditional screening sound which is cheap and readily available and still used in many centres is the cup/spoon combination. Rubbing of the back of a spoon around the rim of an unchipped cup gives a low intensity sound with a wide frequency spectrum. However, any roughness of the cup or clinking sound will alter this, affecting its reliability as a test sound (Figure 5.1). The human voice is also used in many centres as a stimulus, although more frequently for screening than testing. The sound 'oo' is usually around 500 Hz, the hummed 'mm' about 1 kHz and the 's' sound around 3 kHz. In addition high frequency rattles (Figure 5.2) are very practical for screening and assessing hearing at 3–4 kHz and above.

More recently instruments producing warble tones have been introduced. These give a reproducible, frequency specific stimulus which will not produce standing waves, with variation in intensity, when used for sound field testing. Some are small devices with a limited output, more suitable for screening, but others can deliver sound up to 120 dB(A)SPL for frequencies of 125 Hz to 8 kHz. This type of frequency specificity is essential to provide information for appropriate hearing aid fitting. In addition to hand held instruments, the sound can be delivered by loudspeaker with the same frequency specificity.

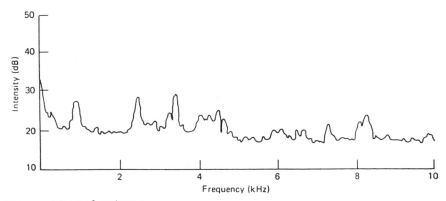

Figure 5.1 Frequency spectrum of cup/spoon

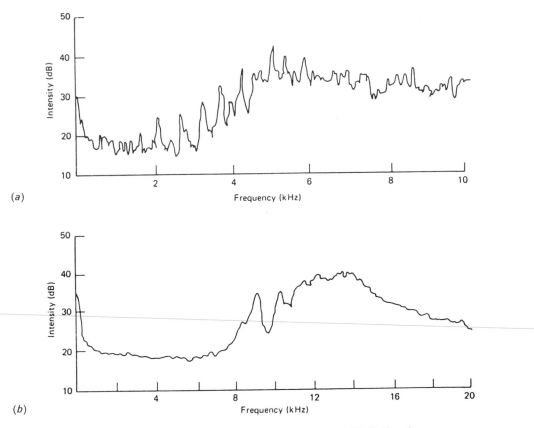

Figure 5.2   (a) Frequency spectrum of Manchester rattle. (b) Frequency spectrum of Nuffield rattle

Intensity

During an assessment of hearing it is essential to know not only the frequency of a sound to which the child responds, but also the intensity of the quietest sound responded to at each frequency. The only accurate way of monitoring the delivery of sounds is with a sound level meter, calibrated to measure at low enough intensities. Sounds measured in free field are usually measured in dB(A)SPL, and rooms can be individually calibrated so that these recordings can be compared with dB HTL measures. In practical terms a sound level meter that records sound pressure levels down to 20 dB(A)SPL is adequate for normal test purposes. When using live sound delivery each sound needs to be measured at the level of the child's ear. The distance from sound source to ear can have a marked effect on intensity, as sound diminution in intensity follows the inverse square law. When using sound delivered by loudspeaker the intensity levels need to be calibrated for the child's test position, and again a slight change in the child's position can alter the perceived sound levels.

Subject

As already described, a child's response to sound matures with age, and it is very important to use the appropriate test method for the child's overall developmental stage. Application of the wrong method will lead to lack of cooperation from the child and unreliable results. Some measure of a child's developmental age can be obtained by providing suitable toys for the child to play with while taking a history from the care-giver, and observing the use of the toys. For example, a child who understands the use of real objects but does not have any concept of the symbolic significance of miniature toys is likely to need testing by distraction techniques. A child who shows reasonable play with miniature objects is usually able to condition to sound in free field, and may accept headphones and proceed to an audiogram.

Distraction test of hearing

This technique which requires two trained testers, was originally described by Ewing (1957) and later

in greater detail by Sheridan (1968). One tester remains in front of the child and is responsible for
maintaining the child's attention in the correct state
for testing and able to observe the reactions of the
child. The other tester produces the test sounds
behind the child when the child's attention is appropriate. This requires good coordination between the
testers, best achieved when the two are used to
working as a pair.

The test layout is demonstrated in Figure 5.3, with
test sounds being produced 1 m from the child's ear
and on a horizontal plane. The sounds are produced
behind the child, and it is essential that the tester
and equipment do not come into the child's visual
range, and that the distractor does not look at the
tester at any time. There should be no chance of
tactile stimulation, as can occur if a tester is too close
to a child, particularly with shaken rattles which can
produce air currents. It is also important that the
distractor should be experienced in judging the attention levels of young children. The younger the child
the easier it is to attract and fix attention visually, so
overdistraction, which parents frequently quote as a
problem, should be avoided. As a child gets older,
and in particular over 12–15 months of age, continuous distraction, varying in degree, may become necessary, as these children start to look round when
there is nothing of interest in front. In addition,
children of this age quickly realize that there is someone behind them, and start to look round even if
unable to hear, which needs to be controlled by the
distractor. Occasional episodes when no sound is
produced should help identify this problem.

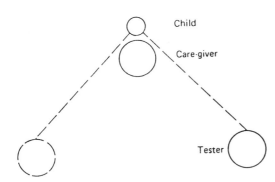

Figure 5.3 Lay-out of room for distraction testing

Visual reinforcement audiometry

This method of testing is used to supplement and
sometimes replace distraction audiometry. The sound
is presented through a loudspeaker at suprathreshold
levels to condition the child, and the response is
reinforced by a visual stimulus, such as a flashing
light or moving toy near the loudspeaker. This
method is said to reduce the habituation to sound
seen in children over 1 year of age, and to reinforce
localization of a sound stimulus. The distractor is still
essential during the test to control the child's pre-
stimulus activity and attention.

Thompson and Weber (1974) reported median
thresholds to sound through a loudspeaker of 45–55
dB SPL at 3–5 months, 35–45 dB SPL at 6–11
months and 35–40 dB SPL at 12–17 months when
testing by behavioural observation audiometry. However Moore and Wilson (1978) reported that, using a
complex sound at 70 dB SPL for conditioning, they
obtained thresholds of under 20 dB SPL at 500 Hz, 1
kHz and 4 kHz on testing the older infant. They felt
that this approach was reliable from 5 months of
age. They also commented that an animated toy
provided the best reinforcement.

Conditioning audiometry

This is also known as performance testing and play
audiometry, as the child is taught to join in a 'game'
with the tester. Although some children under 2
years of age can carry out this type of task, and
many 2 year olds are able to cooperate reasonably in
the test, it is most useful for children of 30 months
and over. Basically the child is taught to carry out
some simple task in response to a sound stimulus.
This may be, for example, putting a brick in a box, a
wooden man in a bus, or a peg in a board, the range
of activities being limited only by imagination. The
task is first taught with visual reinforcement, using
either the word 'go' with visible lip movements and
facial expressions, or a free field audiometer with the
stimulus button visible. For a hearing impaired child
a louder stimulus, such as a visible drum, may be
necessary to teach the task. The visual stimulus is
then withdrawn and the minimum intensity recorded
for response to a range of stimuli. Thompson and
Weber (1974) reported median thresholds to noise
on using play audiometry of 26 dB SPL at 24–29
months of age, and 13 dB SPL at 30–35 months of
age.

With the younger child various strategies may be
used during testing in order to complete the task.
Several different play activities may be used in succes-
sion, to keep attention, and occasional suprathreshold
stimuli may be interspersed as necessary to reinforce
conditioning. The crucial ability in the child is not
that of carrying out an action when there is a sound.

The important thing is that a child can wait and not respond when there is no stimulus. The younger child or those with attention problems may respond after a time, regardless of stimuli, and this activity has to be discouraged without losing the child's confidence. It is essential that a child should feel she is succeeding throughout testing if cooperation is to be maintained.

Once children are able to condition reliably to sound, the only factor preventing them from carrying out an unmasked pure tone audiogram is the acceptance of headphones. With modern technology many young children have seen or even used headphones for stereo radios and hi-fi units and will happily cooperate at 30 months of age. However, some children are more wary of strange instruments, and may be over 3 years of age before they will carry out an audiogram. Warren (personal communication, 1986) has suggested the use of an earphone mounted on a Flexarm to overcome the difficulty in accepting headphones. Some children will accept a bone vibrator more readily, and bone conduction thresholds may be obtained first. Many children can cope with masking from the age of 4–6 years, and from 7 years virtually all normal children can be tested for hearing thresholds in the same way as adults.

Testing the 'difficult' child

As already discussed, the appropriate test to measure hearing thresholds in a child depends on the overall developmental age of a child, and not the chronological age. Thus a child who is developmentaly at the 9-month level will be best tested by distraction methods or visual reinforcement audiometry, regardless of actual age. The validity of this approach was assessed by Flexner and Gans (1985) who tested children with different degrees of mental handicap finding comparable results with children of similar developmental levels.

When a child's developmental level is below 3–4 months, behavioural methods of testing are not appropriate for hearing assessment and one of the so-called 'objective' methods is necessary, in particular electric response audiometry using electrocochleography or auditory brain stem response. Although these tests have their limitations (see below) they may be the only way of gaining information on the hearing ability of a very young or handicapped child.

Children with visual problems may respond differently to sound from their normal hearing peers, and this must be taken into account on testing their hearing. A young child with very poor vision is unable to relate a sound to its source and will react to a sound by stilling and listening. If the sound is familiar he may reach out a hand for the object, while keeping his body and head still and continuing

to listen. Many visually impaired children respond reasonably well to a voice at minimal intensities, but do not respond to other test sounds, particularly warble tones, unless presented at suprathreshold levels. It can be difficult with some of these children to be sure that they can hear at minimal levels, and if any doubt remains an 'objective' test should be used, as optimal hearing is essential for a visually impaired child to receive maximum sensory input. Otoacoustic emission measurement may be sufficient to confirm adequate hearing in this group.

Once partially-sighted children are able to use their residual vision effectively, following either correction or training, they will attempt to localize a sound source and start to respond clearly at lower intensities. When distracting these children a large, bright coloured object is required, and sometimes a torch light may be helpful to attract attention. When a visually impaired child reaches the age where conditioning tests are more suitable, the task chosen must be suitable for the child's visual–motor skills. This includes the use of larger objects and simpler tasks, such as dropping a brick in a basket, rather than fitting games, e.g. using small pegs in a board.

Some children, particularly those with various forms of cerebral palsy, may be difficult to test because of limitations in carrying out voluntary movements. This may occur against a background of involuntary movement, making the presence or absence of a response difficult to assess with certainty. Even when a child can localize a sound by head or eye movements, the response may be slow and require prolonged presentation of the stimulus. The older child may understand the task during conditioning, but only be capable of one or two different movements in response. A familiar care-giver is essential to interpret the child's communications. Again 'objective' tests are needed when there remains any doubt about hearing levels. Some of these children may have been affected by perinatal problems, e.g. severe asphyxia or hyperbilirubinaemia, and are thus at high risk of hearing impairment.

Children with autistic features can be difficult to test, partly because of problems in gaining their attention. They may show only fleeting regard for a distractor and any objects used, and are sometimes very difficult to keep in one place for testing. These children frequently show little if any interest in voice, but will often respond promptly to warble tones and rattles. If there are persistent problems in obtaining results then 'objective' methods can be used, but experienced testers can usually obtain hearing levels in these children.

In a similar way a hyperactive child or one with attention problems may be difficult to test and may require a variety of different tests and techniques to complete a hearing assessment, however, 'objective' testing is not normally necessary.

Electric response audiometry

Objective audiometry is usually performed when the child will not give satisfactory responses to conventional behavioural tests (above), as these tests do not depend upon a voluntary behavioural response from the child. Although there are other 'objective' tests of hearing, including the use of acoustic stapedial reflex thresholds, in much of the literature objective audiometry is used synonymously with electric response audiometry. Electric response audiometry is the general term covering a whole class of procedures, and many different auditory evoked potentials can be used for objective audiometry. Details of these procedures are not considered in this chapter, but good overall reviews are given by Davis (1976), Beagley (1981) and Hyde (1987).

In electric response audiometry used in routine audiological assessments, the electric potentials are recorded from surface electrodes placed in the ear or on the scalp. The electrode position depends on the response to be measured, but for most audiological applications the response is measured between inverting mastoid and non-inverting vertex electrodes, with a further ground electrode placed either on the forehead or opposite mastoid to ensure correct preamplifier function.

The potentials generated are very small in comparison with the ongoing electrical activity of the brain (EEG), and would be swamped and uninterpretable were it not for specialized techniques to reduce the signal-to-noise ratio. First the response is filtered to pass unchanged as much as possible of the energy of the particular auditory evoked potential, with as little as possible of that of the noise. The second technique involves averaging a large number of sweeps of the response each time-locked to stimulus, to enhance the signal-to-noise ratio. The number of sweeps required depends on the auditory evoked potential and noise size, and varies for different auditory evoked potentials. The third technique used to enhance the recorded response is alternation of stimulus polarity. If the responses are then averaged, any components related to the stimulus waveform should be eliminated. In addition the responses are collected in two separate channels which can be compared to improve response recognition. In addition to enhancement of the signal-to-noise ratio, the recording conditions have to be optimal to ensure reliable results. This includes the minimizing of muscular activity which interferes with the signal. In adults this can be carried out by lying or seating the subject comfortably, but in children this normally means that the child has to be asleep, with sedation if necessary, or on occassion anaesthetized. Electrode impedance has to be reduced to 2 kΩ, (maximum of 5kΩ), if a good recording is to be obtained. All the conditions used during the test, including filter settings, state of the subject, number of sweeps and electrode impedance should be recorded to aid interpretation of the data.

Auditory evoked potentials are recorded along the auditory pathway but the origins of many auditory evoked potentials are still uncertain and open to debate. It is simplistic to expect a one-to-one correspondence between auditory evoked potentials and specific anatomical sites; however, there is reasonable evidence to suggest possible response sites (Davis 1976; Picton, Stapells and Campbell, 1981; Scherg, 1984; Moller and Jannetta, 1985). The imputed anatomical source depends on the latency of the response recorded. Latency is divided into five subclasses, from first to late. Electrocochleography records activity within the first few milliseconds (first) and includes the cochlear microphonic (from hair cells) and the action and summation potentials. The auditory brain stem response is recorded within the first 10 ms (fast) and includes the activity from the auditory nerve up to the inferior colliculus. Within the latency of 10–75 ms (middle) the middle latency responses occur, including the 40 Hz event-related potentials. These are thought to originate from the thalamus and primary auditory cortex. Myogenic auditory evoked potentials also occur within these latencies and may overlap with and obscure neurogenic responses. The responses between 75 and 300 ms (slow) include the slow vertex response, routinely used for threshold measurement in cooperative alert adults. The responses above 300 ms (late) include P_{300} and contingent negative variation, and are more usually administered for physiological psychology research purposes and as tests for disorders of higher cortical function.

Clinical applications

There is no single auditory evoked potential or procedure which is best for all circumstances and the clinician should appreciate the strengths and weaknesses of different techniques which may be employed. In children most testing is carried out for threshold estimation, and although electric response audiometry is extremely useful in this context, the limitations of the tests make it desirable to confirm objective testing by behaviourable methods as soon as the child is able to respond.

Ideally a test used in infants and young children should be non-invasive, robust during sleep and anaesthesia and should give accurate frequency specific thresholds. In practice such a procedure does not as yet exist. The auditory evoked potentials which yield good frequency specific thresholds are the middle and particularly the slow responses. However, they require a still, cooperative, alert subject and, if present, are very variable during sleep, as demonstrated by Osterhammel, Shallop and Terkildsen (1985) and, as shown by Proser and Arslan (1985), may be abolished by anaesthesia. This is a critical factor limiting the use of middle latency response and 40 Hz response in young children. Furthermore, postauricular myogenic responses also occur in the same latency interval and could cause interference. The fast latency responses are best elicited by a click stimulus and therefore their frequency specificity is low. However these responses are not affected by sleep or anaesthesia, and they are thus suitable for use in children. In practice the auditory evoked potentials normally used in children are the auditory brain stem response and rarely the cochlear nerve compound action potential, recorded by electrocochleography.

Electrocochleography

The cochlear nerve compound action potential is an exogenous transient response recorded in the first 10 ms interval, and comprising wave I of the auditory brain stem response. It can be recorded with small amplitudes from a number of sites in and around the ear. Intermediate amplitudes are found from recordings from the external auditory meatus, however the largest and most reliable recordings are yielded using a transtympanic needle electrode, because the signal-to-noise ratio is relatively high. Most adults can tolerate electrode insertion but a drawback to the transtympanic approach in children is the need for a general anaesthetic as the needle has to be inserted through the tympanic membrane on to the promontory. In addition, as the electrode has to be placed by a physician, the procedure cannot be carried out by a technician or scientist working alone. For these reasons electrocochleography is rarely performed in children for hearing threshold estimation alone. It may be justified however, as an alternative to auditory brain stem response, when combined with a necessary surgical procedure, e.g. insertion of ventilation tubes. Frequency specificity is suspect when using clicks or tone pip stimuli, but Bellman, Barnard and Beagley (1984) showed reasonable correlation between thresholds obtained and actual hearing thresholds for 2–4 kHz.

Auditory brain stem response

Jewett and Williston (1971) gave a description of auditory brain stem response and this was later reviewed by Jewett (1983). It is an exogenous transient response recorded in the 1–10 ms interval (fast) elicited best by very brief stimuli, such as clicks, at moderate to high levels. The waveform loses much of its structure when close to threshold and using tone pip stimuli. Though seven waves can be recorded the first five waves are commonly employed (Figure 5.4) and the most prominent feature, the wave V complex, is used for threshold estimation. A comprehensive description of the auditory brain stem response and its clinical applications is given by Jacobson (1985). As already noted, during auditory brain stem response recording the brain activity and the noise levels should be as low as possible. Young infants

will often fall asleep following a feed and on testing the stimulus intensity needs to start at around 50 dB in these babies, so that a normal hearing baby is not woken by the initial test sequence. Older and more disturbed children require sedation or anaesthesia for testing and auditory brain stem responses have been shown to be preserved during anaesthesia by Duncan, Sanders and McCullough (1979), and Cohen and Britt (1982). The robust nature of the auditory brain stem response has meant that in recent years it has achieved prominence in hearing assessment of infants and auditory brain stem response is the most commonly used objective test in children in the UK for hearing threshold estimation.

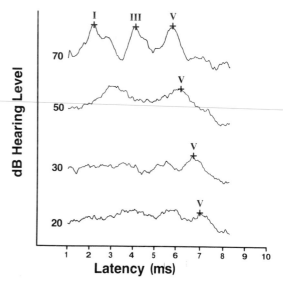

Figure 5.4 Auditory brain stem response tracing in an infant – hearing threshold 20 dB HL (within normal limits)

When testing infants and young children it is important to take into account the effects of maturation on the auditory brain stem response. Starr *et al.* (1977) have shown that the change in interwave latency (wave I to wave V) may be as much as 0.4 ms from 32 to 34 weeks' conceptional age. Gorga *et al.* (1989) reported normative data on 535 normal hearing children from 3 months to 3 years of age. There was no significant change in the latency of wave I, but wave V latency and I–V interval decreased until stable levels were reached by 18 months of age. Hyde *et al.* (1991) reported that the latency of wave V decreases 0.1 ms per month. Jiang *et al.* (1993) showed that the amplitude of all auditory brain stem response waves increases with age from birth, with wave I reaching adult size by 6 months and wave V by 2 years. In the newborn only wave I and wave V are clearly seen and wave III becomes prominent at about 2 weeks of age. Any team using auditory brain stem response measurements will need to collect its own normative data against which to compare test results.

The hearing threshold is determined by the lowest stimulus intensity at which the auditory evoked potential is detectable visually. As auditory brain stem response is usually evoked by click stimuli any information on hearing is mainly between frequencies 2 kHz and 4 kHz. In good conditions the click auditory brain stem response threshold can be within 10 dB of behavioural thresholds, but in the individual child the difference between the observed auditory brain stem response threshold and the behavioural threshold may be anywhere between 5 and 25 dB. A child with a low frequency hearing loss may pass the test and conversely a child who fails the test may have good hearing in the low frequencies. There have been attempts made to obtain information on mid and low frequency hearing using the auditory brain stem response, using either a 1 kHz tone pip stimulus or notch masking, but these results do not correspond as well to hearing levels, and may prolong the test too long for natural sleep.

In addition to hearing threshold estimation, auditory evoked responses provide useful information on the neurological status as described by Fria (1980). For example patients with multiple sclerosis may have neuronal desynchronization which abolishes the auditory brain stem response while the pure-tone audiogram remains normal, as reported by Paludetti *et al.* (1985). In infants a prolonged I–V latency with normal thresholds would suggest neurological damage to the auditory pathways. Marshall, Reichert and Kerley (1980) suggested that infants may also fail auditory brain stem response screening because of physiological immaturity. Auditory brain stem response thresholds may also be unreliable in infants with other conditions, e.g. kernicterus as confirmed by Kuriyama, Konishi and Mikawa (1986) and in the presence of high CSF pressure (author's observation). Patients with idiopathic auditory brain stem response depression have also been reported by Worthington and Peters (1980). The hearing threshold must thus be interpreted with caution in the presence of these conditions or, as noted by Kilney and Robertson (1985), in the presence of a neurological lesion. Conversely for ears with severe or profound hearing loss at 2 kHz or above absence of auditory brain stem response has no diagnostic significance neurologically.

Having detected a hearing loss and excluded confounding neurological disease, the differentiation between conductive, cochlear and mixed loses may not be easy using auditory brain stem response measures. Otomicroscopy can rule out only gross middle/external ear abnormalities, and tympanometry can be misleading in infancy. As noted earlier, wave I is present at birth and there is no significant change in latency from 3 months to 3 years. Definite prolongation of wave I latency would suggest a conductive hearing problem. Bone conduction auditory brain stem response testing has been reported with some success by Kramer (1992) and Yang *et al.* (1993), but has not found favour in most centres because of technical difficulties. This could further elucidate a conductive loss. The relationship between stimulus intensity and wave V latency is used to plot 'latency-intensity' function. In normal hearing, with increasing intensity of stimulation, the amplitude of the waves are enhanced and the latencies are reduced but the interwave latencies are relatively independent of click intensity. Conductive hearing losses, recruiting hearing losses and high frequency hearing losses are reported to give different 'latency-intensity' functions, but Eggermont (1983) felt the predictive value of the slope was questionable in distinguishing types of hearing losses in any individual.

Period evoked potential

This is a promising new technique based on the frequency following response. The frequency following response reflects auditory units predominantly in the brain stem and is recorded primarily to low frequency tone burst stimuli. The collection of sufficient sweeps takes as long as for the auditory brain stem response. However Parker and Matsebula (1992) reported that the phase-locked activity recorded at the vertex in response to a continuous pure tone stimulus can be acquired and averaged and the period evoked potential recorded in less than 5 s. They reported that this rapid test gives good low frequency information, below 1 kHz, and may develop into a useful supplement to the auditory brain stem response in audiological practice.

Impedance audiometry

The middle ear is an impedance matching device for optimizing the transfer of acoustic energy from air to the much denser fluid medium of the inner ear. Without the middle ear at least 97% of the incident energy would be reflected at the oval window. The efficiency of the middle ear system is highly dependent on the condition of the various component parts. As with any mechanical system the various structural components provide mass, friction and elasticity. In the middle ear the major components involving mass are the ossicles, in particular the malleus and incus. Friction occurs throughout the middle ear mechanism. Elasticity is mainly provided by the tympanic membrane and the volume of gases contained in the middle ear cleft. The three types of mechanical component react differently to an applied oscillating force such as sound and the efficiency of the middle ear system varies according to the frequency of the incoming sound. At low frequencies the effects of elasticity dominate, at high frequencies mass dominates. Changes in mass are rare, while changes in elasticity are common. Thus, though high frequency sound is available for testing, a low frequency sound (220 Hz) is most commonly employed in impedance audiometry, to maximize efficiency in detecting middle ear disorders.

Acoustic impedance refers to the inhibition of the flow of acoustic energy and was historically the first term to gain acceptance. Admittance is the reciprocal of this, and indicates the readiness of the middle ear to allow the flow of acoustic energy. In the past this term has been used almost interchangeably with impedance, and is now becoming the accepted term, thus the present terminology of otoadmittance measurement is replacing that of impedance audiometry.

The basic components of a device for measuring otoadmittance are shown in Figure 5.5. A small probe unit, sealed to the ear canal by a soft plastic cuff, is inserted in the ear. This probe contains a miniature earphone which delivers a 220 Hz probe tone, amplified after generation of a driving signal by an external oscillator. The probe also contains a microphone to measure the sound pressure level in the ear canal and an air line. The signal to the earphone is adjusted automatically to maintain a sound pressure level of around 85 dB. The admittance of the middle ear system is directly related to the changes in the driving signal required to maintain this constant sound pressure level in in the ear canal. If the elasticity of the tympanic membrane is low (increased stiffness), the admittance of the sound to the middle ear will be low and only a small amount of amplification will be needed to maintain the chosen sound pressure level of the probe tone. Conversely if the tympanic membrane is flaccid and absorbent the admittance of sound will be higher and more amplification of the probe tone will be needed.

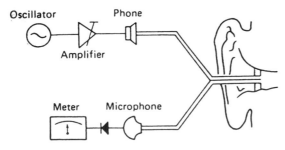

Figure 5.5 Electrostatic impedance instrument

Tympanometry

Tympanometry is the graphical representation of the admittance (or impedance, or compliance) of the middle ear. The mobility or compliance of the tympanic membrane is maximal when the air pressure in the middle ear is equal to that of the external auditory canal, and the membrane is thus free from stress and at its most efficient. Under normal conditions the pressure in the middle ear is maintained equal or close to atmospheric pressure by the functioning of the eustachian tube.

In tympanometry the otoadmittance measuring device changes the air pressure (measured in decapascals, daPa) in the external auditory canal, usually between +200 daPa and -400 daPa, while constantly monitoring the admittance of the system to sound. The compliance or admittance is highest when the pressures in the external and middle ears are equal, i.e. at pressures between +50 and -150 daPa in the normal ventilated middle ear. From a tympanogram one can calculate the ear canal volume, the middle ear pressure and the degree of admittance of the middle ear. Tympanometry uses the principle that sound pressure level is a function of closed cavity volume. Thus both the canal volume and compliance values are given in millilitres (ml).

Clinical applications

With an intact tympanic membrane the canal volume in a child may vary from 0.4 ml to 1.0 ml. This also depends on how far forward the probe tip is inserted. Values of 0.3 ml or lower usually indicate either cerumen or that the probe tip has been directed towards the canal wall. Rarely it could be due to very narrow external auditory canals, especially in infants. Children with Down's syndrome may also have very narrow ear canals, easily blocked with cerumen, which can create problems clinically as these children require regular monitoring of middle ear function because of the high incidence of abnormalities.

When there is a perforation or patent ventilation tube (grommet) it may not be possible to obtain a seal. If a seal is obtained the canal volume is usually greater than 2 ml, a measure of the combined volumes of the ear canal and middle ear and it may possible to record the pressure at which the eustachian tube opens. This is not a physiological test as the eustachian tube normally operates against a negative pressure gradient. A more realistic approach is to reduce the pressure in the external auditory canal to -200 daPa and then ask the subject to swallow. If tubal function is satisfactory then with each swallow the negativity of the pressure is reduced to normal atmospheric pressure.

There have been a number of attempts to categorize the shape of the tympanogram, and a classification scheme originally described by Jerger (1970) is commonly used. The tympanograms were divided into three basic shapes: a normal curve was type A, the flat curve typical of middle ear effusion was type B, and a normal shaped curve with reduced pressure was type C. This classification was found to be simplistic and further subdivisions were designated, but the classification remains imprecise. Figure 5.6 shows examples of various shapes of tympanogram in the presence of an intact tympanic membrane: (*a*) the normal middle ear produces a peaked curve that is almost symmetrical about the point of maximum admittance; (*b*) when the admittance is decreased in the presence of normal middle ear pressure as in otosclerosis or thickened tympanic membrane the peak becomes shallower; (*c*) if the tympanic membrane is thin or scarred, or the ossicular chain is disrupted in the presence of normal middle ear pressure then admittance is increased and the peak would be higher than normal; (*d*) when there is dysfunction of the eustachian tube the middle ear pressure becomes negative with shift of the peak to the left and frequently reduced admittance; (*e*) if there is fluid in the middle ear, damping the movement of the tympanic membrane, the tracing will become flat.

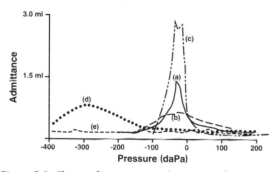

Figure 5.6 Shapes of tympanogram (a–e; see text)

Although tympanograms are extremely useful in children as a means of monitoring changes in middle ear pressure, the tympanogram has to be interpreted with caution in infants less than 7 months of age. Keith (1973) found 'W' shaped tympanograms in seven out of 40 newborn infants, a pattern associated with an abnormally compliant system. Paradise, Smith and Bluestone (1976) found normal tympanometry in 24 of 40 ears confirmed to have effusions. Wright *et al.* (1985) reported abnormal results in the presence of a normal middle ear in children up to 2 years of age. Caution also needs to be exercised in drawing conclusions from the shape of tympanograms as pathologies can coexist and there is considerable overlap in responses between abnormal and normal ears.

Tympanograms that vary over short periods of time may be of diagnostic significance. If the variation is synchronous with respiration, the most probable cause is a patent eustachian tube. A faster variation, synchronous with the pulse is sometimes seen where there is some acute inflammation of the middle ear

or tympanic membrane. More rarely it may indicate a glomus tumour (Black *et al.*, 1979).

Acoustic stapedial reflex

Tensor tympani muscle contraction in response to sound only occurs when the intensity is such as to cause a generalized startle reaction as shown by Djupesland (1965) and is inconsistent both between and within subjects. It is thus of no value when assessing children. In contrast the stapedial muscle reflex is commonly used both in adults and children. Contraction of the stapedius muscle produces a stiffening of the ossicular chain, observable as a decrease in admittance of sound. The lowest signal intensity at which the stapedius muscle contracts is defined as the acoustic reflex threshold (ART). For mid-frequency sounds it is normally elicitable at 85 dB (+/− 10 dB) above normal hearing threshold. It is a bilateral reflex and therefore its recording may be either ipsilateral or contralateral. The afferent limb includes the external ear, middle ear conducting system, the cochlea, the auditory nerve and the nucleus in the brain stem. The reflex travels bilaterally through the superior olivary complex to the facial nerve nucleus in the brain stem. The efferent arc is completed by the facial nerve supplying the stapedius muscle.

Acoustic reflex threshold testing should be carried out at frequencies of 0.5 kHz, 1 kHz, 2 kHz and 4 kHz. The reflex at 4 kHz may be absent in normal hearing subjects and in a small number of subjects the stapedius reflex may be absent altogether.

Clinical applications

Abnormalities of the acoustic reflex threshold can occur due to pathology affecting any part of the reflex system. In the presence of a conductive hearing loss of 10 dB, Jerger *et al.* (1974a) found the acoustic reflex threshold to be absent 80% of the time. Lutman (1984) demonstrated a 50% incidence of abnormal acoustic reflex thresholds in the presence of a 20 db air–bone gap and Brooks (1987) felt that a detectable stapedius reflex indicated, with a better than 95% probability, that the middle ear was within normal limits.

In the presence of a cochlear hearing loss, according to Jerger, Jerger and and Mauldin (1972), there is a 90% chance of observing a reflex if the hearing threshold is less than 60 dB. This was assumed to be related to the recruitment of loudness seen in cochlear hearing loss. They also felt that if the acoustic reflex was absent with a sensorineural hearing loss of less than 60 dB it was more likely to be a retrocochlear hearing loss. Although the simple association of recruitment with cochlear pathology and absence of recruitment with a neural pathology is now known to be invalid, measurement of recruitment remains one of a battery of tests which together help in localizing a lesion. A further adaptation of acoustic reflex threshold measurement involves that of acoustic reflex threshold decay. This is analogous to tone decay and Anderson, Barr and Wedenberg (1970) reported that a decay to half the initial magnitude of contraction in 4 s was strongly associated with retrocochlear pathology.

With brain-stem lesions both ipsilateral and contralateral reflexes can be abnormal. If both the contralaterals are abnormal and the ipsilaterals are normal it is very suggestive of brain-stem pathology. If facial nerve function is decreased the reflex on the affected side will be absent or elevated.

Early testing of acoustic reflex thresholds in young children suggested that there were problems in obtaining a response. For example Robertson, Peterson and Lamb (1968) found acoustic reflex thresholds in only 30% of children up to 1 year of age, and 70% in children of 18–36 months. Bennett and Weatherby (1979) reported that the percentage of observable reflexes increased to 100% when the probe tone was increased to 800 Hz. A probe tone of 660 Hz is helpful when testing young infants, but is not usually available on screening tympanometers which may limit their usefulness with this population.

Estimation of hearing threshold

The presence of an acoustic reflex may be useful in non-organic hearing loss and difficult-to-test children but it would be unwise to rely only on this measurement. As discussed above, in the presence of recruitment, it could be present with a 60 dB hearing loss. Attempts have been made to predict hearing levels by measuring reflex thresholds for pure tones and broad band noise. White noise elicits an acoustic reflex at about 65 dB, and Niemeyer and Sesterhenn (1974) observed that, as the severity of hearing loss increased, the difference between the pure tone and noise induced reflexes decreased. Jerger *et al.* (1974b) used this method to assign subjects to hearing categories of normal, mild/moderate, severe or profound and found that 60% were correctly assigned. However, this method is clearly not as accurate as the objective tests using electric response audiometry recordings. Other methods developed have not been clinically applicable.

One of the main limitations in very young children and infants is that vocalizing, speaking, crying, eating and swallowing can alter compliance and frequently render it impossible to obtain a record. The compliance can be altered by the acoustic reflex contraction and eustachian tube changes. An experienced audiologist should be able to manage most of these problems, but distraction techniques may be needed to calm these children.

New related techniques

Tympanic membrane diplacement measurement

This technique was first described by Marchbanks (1984). It relies on the fact that changes in hydrostatic pressure of the cochlear perilymph produce a small but measurable variation in the kinematics of the ossicles and tympanic membrane. Movement of the tympanic membrane is induced by acoustical stimulation of the stapedial reflex and the resulting tympanic membrane displacement measured over time. Although this technique is not of direct use in hearing testing, it may give information on implied pathology of hearing problems, e.g the fluctuations in hearing levels observed with changes in CSF pressure in some children.

Acoustic reflectometry

The tympanogram is the most useful test in children to confirm the presence or absence of middle ear fluid. Because of the difficulties in obtaining cooperation from young children the acoustic otoscope was developed by Teele and Teele (1984). This device does not require an air-tight seal and can also be used in a crying child. The speaker of the instrument emits a multifrequency (2–4 kHz) tone at 80 dBSPL and a microphone picks up any sound reflected from the tympanic membrane. In essence the greater the sound reflected by the middle ear, the greater the chance of there being a middle ear effusion. Although there are still problems standardizing the results of this device, Duoniadakis *et al.* (1993) found the sensitivity and specificity of the procedure to be 86% and 79% respectively in detection of otitis media. It may thus be a useful addition to the assessment of the difficult child.

Otoacoustic emissions

Otoacoustic emissions were first reported by Kemp (1978). They reflect a release of acoustic energy which can be recorded in the external ear canal. They are thought to originate from the outer hair cells of the cochlea. Otoacoustic emissions can occur spontaneously in 40–60% of healthy ears. However, the clinically useful responses are evoked otoacoustic emissions. These can be transient otoacoustic emissions in response to a click or tone burst, distortion product otoacoustic emissions occurring at intermodulation frequencies when two tones are presented simultaneously, or stimulus frequency otoacoustic emissions which occur at the same frequency as the stimulus. Most of the clinical research has been in respect of transient otoacoustic emissions.

Anderson and Kemp (1979) felt that the presence of evoked otoacoustic emissions was evidence of a normal functioning cochlea. Transient otoacoustic emissions are present with good low and middle frequency hearing to click stimuli and with development of computer software it is now possible to obtain higher frequency information. It is also possible to obtain thresholds at different frequencies with distortion product otoacoustic emissions as reported by workers such as Kimberley and Nelson (1989). Transient otoacoustic emissions have been reported by many workers to reflect a hearing threshold of 15–25 dB or better. For example Stevens (1988) found no emissions could be detected in subjects with a threshold of 18 dBnHL or higher. Transient otoacoustic emissions can be recorded from birth, with large amplitude emissions, making this an excellent tool for hearing screening in neonates. The level of the response is significantly higher than in adults but Bonfils, Uziel and Pujol (1988) reported that otoacoustic emissions were always absent with auditory brain stem response thresholds of greater than 40 dB HL. Similarly distortion product otoacoustic emissions have been found to be absent if the hearing threshold exceeds 15dB (Gaskill and Brown, 1993).

Clinical applications

The main use of evoked otoacoustic emissions is in screening for hearing impairment in neonates. They are also useful in screening cooperative children with a variety of handicaps where it is not possible to perform behavioural testing. This includes the monitoring of hearing in children on ototoxic agents. Most of these children are very ill and it may be difficult for them to perform any other form of audiometry. Unfortunately these drugs first affect hearing for the high frequencies and evoked otoacoustic emissions using clicks may not detect an early ototoxic hearing loss. However, they are certainly of value in identifying a problem before any marked hearing loss has occurred.

Apart from their use to identify reasonably normal hearing, otoacoustic emissions have a very limited place in the testing of children's hearing. They can be of value in identifying the site of a hearing impairment, as although absent in peripheral auditory disorders, they are present in central auditory disorders. Otoacoustic emissions may however be abnormal in VIIIth nerve lesions, the exact mechanism is not well understood. It may be due to interference with the blood supply to the cochlea. In addition, evoked otoacoustic emissions may be absent with conductive hearing losses. This may limit their clinical application in children.

Assessment of hearing disability

Hearing impairment can lead to a number of disabilities. These include a lack of awareness of sound, the inability to hear warning signals and environmental sounds clearly, difficulty in localizing sound and difficulties with communication. In adults there are a number of problem questionnaires which concentrate on different aspects of hearing disability, such as the Hearing Measurement Scale developed by Noble and Atherley (1970) and the Hearing Performance Inventory of Giolas (1982). These are not relevant on the whole to children, although they are helpful in putting hearing disability into a wider perspective. The most important effect of hearing impairment in children is on spoken language development. Most work around auditory disability in children concentrates on the measurement of their developing sound then speech recognition skills. There is now a very large number of tests applicable to hearing impaired children, mainly stimulated by the need to monitor and understand the use of cochlear implants.

Speech audiometry in routine clinical practice

In the older child speech detection and speech discrimination tests can be carried out in a similar way to tests in adults. This is by presentation of phonetically balanced word lists through headphones, with instruction to the child to repeat the word/sound heard, and scoring for correctly heard phonemes. The word lists for younger children may have to be simplified and suitable material would include the Manchester junior word lists, commonly used in the UK. However, such open-set tasks are not suitable for children under the age of 7–8 years, and even above this age some difficulties may be encountered. Young children frequently fail to give any response if they are unable to recognize a complete word thus giving an underestimate of their ability. In addition, some children have articulatory problems which can make it difficult to score a response accurately.

In younger children tests are normally closed-set, with the child picking out an item from a finite number of objects or pictures. The quickest and easiest parameters to measure are the optimal discrimination score and sound level at which this is achieved. The results are not directly comparable to open-set tests and need to be individually standardized for set size and number of test repetitions, to ensure accuracy. Test words can be delivered by live voice or loud speakers. The test is administered as a game in which the child must not feel he or she is failing as cooperation will quickly cease. The approach has to be appropriate to the child's developmental age and the vocabulary appropriate to the child's level of verbal comprehension. It is also important that the test is carried out first live with lipreading and facial expression visible to ensure that the child can reliably carry out the test in these conditions before using an auditory only mode.

From the age of 18 months a rough measure of

speech discrimination can be obtained by using a small number of items such as cup, shoe and spoon, and a small number of recipients, such as daddy, teddy and dolly. The child can then be asked to give, for example, the shoe to teddy and the quietest sound level at which this can be done recorded.

As children get older toys from an established toy test can be used, for example the Kendal toy test or its modification by McCormick (1977). This latter can be used live or in an automated form. Other suitable toy tests include the E2L toy test developed by Bellman and Marcuson (1991), which is particularly useful for young children with English as a second language. In a normal hearing child, in good listening conditions, 100% discrimination is found at 35 dB(SPL). A raised level is noted, as are any particular word confusions, which may give a clue to the type of hearing impairment. Picture tests can be used as the children get a little older and a combination of test materials may be neccesary to obtain results in children with a short attention span.

Again as children get older the range of vocabulary suitable for speech tests increases. A discussion on suitable word pairs for screening and testing English speaking 5 year olds was given by Haggard, Wood and Carroll (1984). At this stage it may be possible to extend a test session to measure the percentage of correct responses at different intensities so that speech reception or half peak elevation levels can be recorded.

Children may well have other problems that necessitate a modification to these test procedures. For example a child with a visual problem may need large objects or pictures, or those of a particular colour for ease of identification. This may mean that a smaller number of items can be presented, and the test protocol will need to be modified to take account of this. The child will also need time to become familiar with the test items so that they can be identified easily without prolonged scanning of the whole field for each individual item.

A child who has difficulty controlling voluntary movements accurately will need fewer objects with wide spacing to make the task physically possible, and the items will also need to be well spread out if a child can only eyepoint as a form of identification. Again the protocol for the test will need to take any smaller set size into account.

Speech perception in the hearing impaired

This is a very specialized subject and full coverage is not appropriate in this chapter. Hearing impaired children (and adults) gain their information on speech content from both visual and auditory inputs, and a full assessment should encompass both modes separately and in combination. Although some hear-ing impaired children may be able to carry out some form of speech discrimination task, many will have insufficient understanding of spoken language even to attempt such a test. There are also some children who can identify words using speech or lipreading, but cannot carry out the task with auditory input alone. Five speech perception categories have been defined by Geers and Moog (1987) on the basis of a child's auditory performance on a variety of cognitively and linguistically appropriate tests. The first level is that of detection of sound but inconsistent pattern perception. The next stage is consistent pattern recognition, e.g. discrimination of monosyllable and multisyllable words, including spondees and trochees. Many profoundly deaf individuals can only function at this level. The next level is that of inconsistent closed-set word identification, where some spectral information is perceived. There is a large number of tests appropriate for this, including those mentioned above. The next stage is that of consistent closed-set identification using the same tests. The final level is that of open-set word recognition, again using a wide range of test material. This stage is reached by most severely hearing impaired children with appropriate amplification, and increasingly by profoundly/totally deaf children using cochlear implants. Discourse tracking can then be tested, depending on the level of linguistic competence, to gain a functional idea of a child's auditory skills.

It is important to understand the general hierarchy of speech perception skills, but not to remember the enormous plethora of tests available. The choice of test material should be made on the basis of the population for which it is to be used.

Conclusion

Although the interpretation of individual tests may seem difficult in young children, a decision regarding a child's exact hearing status should be possible using a combination of the various tests outlined in this chapter. Even with neonates adequate information can be obtained for early hearing aid fitting and rehabilitation. In addition early confirmation of hearing impairment makes it easier to reach an aetiological diagnosis.

References

ANDERSON, H., BARR, B. and WEDENBERG, E. (1970) Early diagnosis of VIII nerve tumours by acoustic reflex tests. *Acta Otolaryngologica Supplementum*, **263**, 232–237

ANDERSON, S. D. and KEMP, D. T. (1979) The evoked cochlear mechanical response in laboratory primates. *Archives of Otolaryngology*, **224**, 47–54

BEAGLEY, H. A. (ed.) (1981) Electrophysiological tests of hearing. In: *Audiology and Audiological Medicine*, vol. 2. Oxford: Oxford University Press. pp. 781–808

BELLMAN, S. C., BARNARD, S. and BEAGLEY, H. A. (1984) An eight year follow-up of electrocochleography in children. *Journal of Laryngology and Otology*, **98**, 1–9

BELLMAN, S. C. and MARCUSON, M. (1991) A new toy test to investigate the hearing status of young children who have English as a second language. *British Journal of Audiology*, **25**, 317–322

BENNETT, M. J. and WEATHERBY, L. A. (1979) Multiple probe frequency acoustic reflex measurements. *Scandinavian Audiology*, **8**, 233–239

BLACK, M. J., BERGER, H., TRITT, R. A. and SCHLOSS, M. D. (1979) Impedance audiometry: its use in the diagnosis of glomus tympanicum tumors. *Journal of Otolaryngology*, **8**, 360–366

BONFILS, P., UZIEL, A. and PUJOL, R. (1988) Screening for auditory dysfunction in infants by evoked oto-acoustic emissions. *Archives of Otolaryngology*, **114**, 887–890

BROOKS, D. (1987) Impedance audiometry. In: *Scott-Brown's Otolaryngology*, 5th edn. volume 6. Paediatric Otolaryngology, edited by J. Evans. London: Butterworths. pp. 104–115

COHEN, M. S. and BRITT, R. H. (1982) Effects of sodium phenobarbitone, ketamine, halothane and chloralose on brainstem auditory evoked responses. *Anaesthesia and Analgesia*, **61**, 338–343

DAVIS, H. (1976) Principles of electric response audiometry. *Annals of Otology, Rhinology and Laryngology*, **85**, (suppl. 28), 1–96

DJUPESLAND, G. (1965) Electromyography of the tympanic muscles in man. *International Audiology*, **4**, 34–41

DUONIADAKIS, D. F., NIKOLOPOULOS, T. P., TSAKANIKOS, M. D., VASSILIADIS, S. V. and APOSTOLOPULOS, N. J. (1993) Evaluation of acoustic reflectometry in detecting otitis media in children. *British Journal of Audiology*, **27**, 409–414

DUNCAN, P. G., SANDERS, R. A. and MCCULLOUGH, D. W. (1979) Preservation of auditory-evoked brainstem responses in anaesthetised children. *Canadian Anaesthetists Society Journal*, **26**, 492–495

EGGERMONT, J. J. (1983) Audiologic disorders. In: *Bases of Auditory Brain-Stem Evoked Responses*, edited by E. J. Moore. New York: Grune & Stratton. pp. 287–316

EWING, I. R. (1957) Screening tests and guidance clinics for babies and young children. In: *Educational Guidance of the Deaf Child*, edited by A. W. G. Ewing. Manchester: Manchester University Press. p. 21

FLEXNER, C. and GANS, D. P. (1985) Comparative evaluation of the auditory responsiveness of normal and profoundly multihandicapped children. *Journal of Speech and Hearing Research*, **28**, 163–168

FRIA, T. J. (1980) The auditory brain stem responses: background and clinical applications. *Monographs in Contemporary Audiology*, **2**, 1–44

GASKILL, S. A. and BROWN, A. M. (1993) Comparing the level of the acoustic distortion product $2f_1-f_2$ with behavioural threshold audiograms from normal hearing and hearing-impaired ears. *British Journal of Audiology*, **27**, 397–408

GEERS, A. E. and MOOG, J. S. (1987) Predicting spoken language acquisition of profoundly hearing-impaired children. *Journal of Speech and Hearing Disorders*, **52**, 83–94

GIOLAS, T. G. (1982) *Hearing Handicapped Adults*. Englewood Cliffs: Prentice Hall

GORGA, M. P., KAMINSKI J. R., BEAUCHAINE, K. L. and NEELY, S. T. (1989) Auditory brainstem responses from children three months to three years of age: normal pattern of

response II. *Journal of Speech and Hearing Research*, **32**, 281–288

HAGGARD, M. P., WOOD, E. J. and CARROLL, S. (1984) Speech, admittance and tone-tests in school screening. Reconciling economics with pathology and disability perspectives. *British Journal of Audiology*, **18**, 133–154

HYDE, M. L. (1987) Evoked potential audiometry. In *Scott-Brown's Otolaryngology*, volume 6, Paediatric Otolaryngology, edited by J. Evans. London: Butterworths. pp. 80–103

HYDE, M. L., MALZIA, K., RIKO, K. and ALBERTI, P. W. (1991) Audiometric estimation error with the ABR in high risk infants. *Acta Otolaryngologica*, **111**, 212–219

JACOBSON, J. T. (ed.) (1985) *The Auditory Brainstem Response*. San Diego: College-Hill Press

JERGER, J. F. (1970) Clinical experience with impedance audiometry. *Archives of Otolaryngology*, **92**, 311–324

JERGER, J. T., JERGER, S. and MAULDIN, L. (1972) Studies impedance audiometry: I. Normal and sensorineural ears. *Archives in Otolaryngology*, **96**, 513–523

JERGER, J., ANTHONY, L., JERGER, S. and MAULDIN, L. (1974a) Studies in impedance audiometry. III. Middle ear disorders. *Archives of Otolaryngology*, **99**, 165–171

JERGER J., BURNEY, P., MAULDIN, L. and CRUMP, B. (1974b) Predicting hearing loss from the acoustic reflex. *Journal of Speech and Hearing Disorders*, **39**, 1–11

JEWETT, D. L. (1983) Introduction. In: *Bases of Auditory Brain-Stem Evoked Responses*, edited by E. J. Moore. New York: Grune & Stratton. pp. xxi–xxx

JEWETT, D. L. and WILLISTON, J. S. (1971) Auditory evoked far field average from the scalp of humans. *Brain*, **94**, 681–696

JIANG, Z. D., ZHANG, L., WU, Y. Y. and LIU, X. Y. (1993) Brainstem auditory evoked responses from birth to adulthood: development of wave amplitude. *Journal of Hearing Research*, **68**, 35–41

KEITH, R. W. (1973) Impedance audiometry with neonates. *Archives of Otolaryngology*, **97**, 465–467

KEMP, D. T. (1978) Stimulated acoustic emissions from within the human auditory system. *Journal of the Acoustical Society of America*, **64**, 1386–1391

KILNEY, P. and ROBERTSON, S. M. (1985) Neurological aspects of hearing assessment. *Journal of Otolaryngology*, **14** (suppl.), 34–39

KIMBERLEY, B. P. and NELSON, D. A. (1989) Distortion product emissions and sensorineural hearing loss. *Journal of Otolaryngology*, **18**, 365–369

KRAMER, S. J. (1992) Frequency-specific auditory brainstem responses to bone-conducted stimuli. *Audiology*, **31**, 61–71

KURIYAMA, M., KONISHI, Y. and MIKAWA, H. (1986) The effect of hyperbilirubinemia on the auditory brainstem response. *Brain Development*, **8**, 240–245

LUTMAN, M. E. (1984) The relationship between acoustic reflex threshold and air-bone gap. *British Journal of Audiology*, **18**, 223–229

MCCORMICK, B. (1977) The toy discrimination test: an aid to screening the hearing of children above a mental age of two years. *Public Health* (London), **91**, 67–73

MARCHBANKS, R. J. (1984) Measurement of tympanic membrane displacement arising from aural cardiovascular activity, swallowing and intra-aural muscle reflex. *Acta Otolaryngologica*, **98**, 119–129

MARSHALL, R., REICHERT, T. and KERLEY, S. M. (1980) Auditory function in newborn intensive care unit patients revealed by auditory brain-stem potentials. *Journal of Pediatrics,* **96**, 731–735

MOLLER, A. R. and JANNETTA, P. J. (1985) Neural generators of auditory brainstem response. In: *The Auditory Brainstem Response,* edited by J. T. Jacobson. San Diego: College-Hill Press. pp. 13–32

MOORE, J. M. and WILSON, W. R. (1978) Visual reinforcement audiometry (VRA) with infants. In: *Early Diagnosis of Hearing Loss,* edited by S. E. Gerber and G. T. Mencher New York: Grune and Stratton. pp. 177–213

NIEMEYER, W. and SESTERHENN, G. (1974) Calculating the hearing threshold from the stapedius reflex threshold for different sound stimuli. *Audiology,* **13**, 421–427

NOBLE, W. G. and ATHERLEY, G. R. C. (1970) The hearing measurement scale: a questionnaire for the assessment of auditory disability. *Journal of Auditory Research,* **10**, 229–250

OSTERHAMMEL, P. A., SHALLOP, J. K. and TERKILDSEN, K. (1985) The effect of sleep on the auditory brainstem response (ABR) and the middle latency response (MLR). *Scandinavian Audiology,* **14**, 47–50

PALUDETTI, G., OTTAVIANI, F., GALLAI, V., TASSON, A. and MAURIZI, M. (1985) Auditory brainstem responses (ABR) in multiple sclerosis. *Scandinavian Audiology,* **14**, 27–34

PARADISE, J. L., SMITH, C. G. and BLUESTONE, C. D. (1976) Tympanometric detection of middle ear effusion in infants and children. *Pediatrics,* **58**, 198–210

PARKER, D. J. and MATSEBULA, D. (1992) The period evoked potential: a rapid technique for acquisition of phase-locked responses to continuous pure-tone stimulation. *British Journal of Audiology,* **26**, 335–338

PICTON, T. W., STAPELLS, D. R. and CAMPBELL, K. B. (1981) Auditory evoked potentials from the human cochlea and brainstem. *Journal of Otolaryngology,* **10** (suppl. 9), 1–41

PROSER, S. and ARSLAN, E. (1985) Does anaesthesia affect child's auditory middle latency (MLR)? *Scandinavian Audiology,* **14**, 105–107

ROBERTSON, E. O., PETERSON, J. L. and LAMB, L. F. (1968) Relative impedance measurements in young children. *Archives of Otolaryngology,* **88**, 162–168

SCHERG, M. (1984) Spatio-temporal modelling of early auditory evoked potentials. *Revue de Laryngologie,* **105**, 163–170

SHERIDAN, M. D. (1968) *Manual for Stycar Tests of Vision and Hearing.* Windsor: National Foundation for Educational Research

STARR, A., AIMLIE, R. N., MARTIN, W. H. and SANDER, S. (1977) Development of auditory function in newborn infants revealed by auditory brainstem potentials. *Paediatrics,* **60**, 831–839

STEVENS, J. C. (1988) Click-evoked oto-acoustic emissions in normal and hearing impaired adults. *British Journal of Audiology,* **22**, 45–50

TEELE, D. W. and TEELE, J. (1984) Detection of middle -ear effusion by acoustic reflectometry. *Journal of Pediatrics,* **104**, 832–838

THOMPSON, G. and WEBER, B. A. (1974) Response of infants and young children to behavioural observation audiometry (BAO). *Journal of Speech and Hearing Disorders,* **39**, 140–147

WORTHINGTON, D. W. and PETERS, J. F. (1980) Quantifiable hearing and no ABR: paradox or error. *Ear and Hearing,* **1**, 281–285

WRIGHT, P., MCCONNEL, K., THOMPSON, J., VAUGHN, W. and SELLS, S. (1985) A longitudinal study of the detection of otitis media in the first two years of life. *International Journal of Pediatric Otorhinolaryngology,* **10**, 245–252

YANG, E. Y., STUART, A., STENSTROM, R. and GREEN, W. B. (1993) Test-retest variability of the auditory brainstem response to bone-conducted clicks in newborn infants. *Audiology,* **32**, 89–94

6

Screening and surveillance for hearing impairment in pre-school children

Barry McCormick

General issues in the UK

To bring screening/surveillance tests and systems into perspective it is useful to consider the child health setting in which they operate. In the UK, child health surveillance has been the focus of much discussion and debate in recent years. In 1989 a working party led by the British Paediatric Association published a report entitled 'Health for all children: A Programme for Child Health Surveillance' (The Hall Report, 1991).

In 1990 another working party was convened by the Royal College of General Practitioners. A report of their recommendations was published in 1992 by Oxford University Press.

These documents reiterate the need for district health authorities and family services authorities to review their joint policies on child health surveillance and stress the need for appropriate training and accreditation for those providing such services. They also stress the need for one person in each district to coordinate the screening programme. They define the aims of child health surveillance broadly to ensure that:

1 All children have the opportunity to realize their full potential in terms of good health, well being and development.
2 Remediable disorders are identified and acted upon as early as possible.

In addition to the reports from professional organizations there is now legislation in the UK which protects the rights of deaf children (and children with other special needs). Under the *Children Act* (1989) deaf children now fit into a legal framework and the authority has a statutory duty to serve them and their families. The authority has a responsibility to minimize the impact of the child's disability and

enable the child to lead as normal a life as possible. The Act highlights the dangers of delayed detection and reinforces the need for health authorities to have procedures and skills available so as not to hinder the assessment of a child who is deaf.

Although there is considerable agreement about the objectives, the means by which these can be achieved are subject to individual interpretation and variation between authorities. Important changes have been introduced in the *National Health Service and Community Care Act* (1990) which, for the first time, introduces a purchaser/provider split and internal market competition. This market system together with the introduction of fundholding general practitioner practices poses a challenge to screening and surveillance systems which, to be effective, need some sort of district coordination with central record keeping, clinical audit and epidemiological monitoring. Concerns have been expressed that the competitive market system might be driven by cost rather than quality and could inhibit service development and research.

The time has never been more opportune for professional and voluntary bodies to define acceptable quality standards to guide purchasers *and* providers and an example of a quality guideline document is included later in this chapter.

Example of a non-UK approach – The USA

The USA does not have the same community health structure and it is not surprising, therefore, that its early identification programmes have concentrated on neonatal screening. Despite this practice, which has only been a feature of the UK system over the past 5 years or so (and only in a few areas), the record of success in early detection is no better in the USA than in the UK and there is evidence that it may be worse. The average age of identification of deaf children in the USA is 3 years (National Institutes of Health Development Consensus Statement, 1993). The reasons why returns from neonatal screening programmes have been poor will be discussed later in this chapter but, having set the scene, it is important to discuss the philosophy of screening and surveillance programmes in some detail.

Screening

Definition and philosophy

The term screening needs definition. In the most extensive review to date on the subject of screening children's hearing, Haggard and Hughes (1991) defined screening as, 'A proactive centrally administered system to ensure testing of a high percentage of the members of a population or specified population stratum for a specified condition'. The test is not diagnostic in nature, that is, it does not establish the presence of the condition, or for example a level of hearing, but if well conducted it should highlight a subgroup of the population which is likely to exhibit the condition.

In an earlier publication (McCormick, 1988a), the author likened a screening test to the activity of fishing a flowing stream with a net the size and mesh of which can be adjusted to suit the intended catch. If the mesh is too fine a large quantity of unwanted catch will complicate the sorting stage. Conversely a large mesh will fail to catch all but the largest of the desired fish. A good hearing screening programme will filter out from the population a fairly small target group of cases likely to exhibit a hearing disorder with a high degree of sensitivity (i.e. it should catch affected cases efficiently and effectively) and with a high degree of specificity (i.e. it should correctly identify unaffected cases). A sensitive test rarely misses disease and a specific test causes few false alarms.

The formulae for quantifying these two descriptions of validity are:

$$\text{Sensitivity} = \frac{a}{a + c}$$

$$\text{Specificity} = \frac{d}{b + d}$$

Where   a = impairment present, test positive
        b = impairment absent, test positive
        c = impairment present, test negative
        d = impairment absent, test negative

Using the same notation:

$$\text{the false-negative proportion} = \frac{c}{a + c}$$

$$\text{and the false-positive proportion} = \frac{b}{b + d}$$

There is a trade off between sensitivity and specificity, just as with the fishing net mesh. It is not possible to achieve perfection for both simultaneously, but a target of 80–90% should be set for each and it must be accepted that false-positive and false-negative cases are unavoidable. The false-negative cases are much more serious in terms of the consequences to the individual and delayed development resulting from the late issuing of hearing aids, is one example. The false positives are likely to overload any follow-up system if they exist to any great extent and they might cause unnecessary parental anxiety.

Haggard (1992) rightly pointed out that it is not practicable in most service contexts to document the sensitivity of screening tests for rare conditions because the coverage is never perfect and there is no affordable gold standard for follow up to provide adequate numbers. Better descriptions of a screening system performance include the *positive predictive value* (PPV) of the test and the *incremental yield*.

The positive predictive value is the proportion of patients with a positive result who actually have the disease. In the previous notation we have

$$\text{PPV} = \frac{a}{a + b}$$

The concept of incremental yield takes account of the fact that various tests and procedures may contribute to the catch and each should be evaluated according to the potential catch still remaining. It would be misleading to conclude that a certain fishing net is useless because it did not catch fish of a certain size when, in fact, higher up stream a fishing net of the same or smaller mesh had already caught the majority of the fish. The net in question might be perfectly good if used at the correct place and time. It is a question of applying an effective strategy to maximize the efficiency and effectiveness of each procedure and being objective when evaluating the contribution of each test or procedure. An example of misguided interpretation of a test technique can be found in numerous papers in which the results of the health visitors' 7-month hearing screening test (the distraction test) is reported to contribute to detecting only 30% of cases when, in fact, there may be only 40–50% still left to find after successful neonatal screening. The successful find of 30% of total cases from the 50% still left to find is very commendable. It would be quite wrong to imply that the distraction test *missed* 70% of cases as is often implied from such analysis.

Benefits and disadvantages of screening

Chamberlain (1984) listed benefits and disadvantages of screening and these are listed below followed by the present author's comments.

Benefits

1 *Improved prognosis for cases detected by screening.* This is certainly considered to be the case for hearing impaired babies/children with severe or profound degrees of hearing loss. It seems logical that early detection and intervention will benefit the child by lessening the period of auditory deprivation and some evidence for this is presented by Markides (1986), White and White (1987) and Ramkalawan and Davis (1992).

2 *Less radical treatment which cures some early cases.* A convincing case cannot be made for 'curing' deafness. Avoidance of complications from cholesteatoma following early detection of this condition could be construed as one argument here but the strength of the screening system rests more with the considerations in (1) above.

3 *Resource savings.* The early detection of hearing problems requires prompt resource allocation which would not be available to cases of late detection for several months or years. It is considered, however, that such prompt support will lessen the need for more expensive special school needs or later special vocational requirements if the child is given a better chance to integrate in hearing society.

4 *Reassurance for those with negative test results.* This could be a major consideration for parents for whom a strong family history of deafness exists but, for the majority of parents, the question of hearing impairment is not even considered in the first year or so of life because of the lack of overt signs.

Disadvantages

1 *Longer morbidity for cases whose prognosis is unaltered.* This is probably not of any great significance for hearing impairment given that the prognosis is improved with the correct provision of remedial treatment and support.

2 *Overtreatment of questionable abnormalities.* This is of topical relevance given the continuing debate about grommet insertion and its long-term effects. For full cover of this topic and debate the reader is referred to Haggard and Hughes (1991) but for the sake of this chapter it must be appreciated that with persistent hearing losses lasting for more than 6 months with hearing levels in excess of 35 dB there are obvious and significant short-term effects and possible long-term consequences which are still not fully understood.

3 *Resource costs.* The cost of screening for a rare condition is considerable per case detected even though the cost per test may be small.

4 *False reassurance for those with false-negative results.* If the validity and reliability of the test are low the screening system will do more harm than good. This has been the case with badly administered health visitor distraction testing in some districts and with some neonatal screening techniques at the evaluation stage.

5 *Anxiety and sometimes morbidity for those with false-positive results.* The issuing of hearing aids to false-positive cases with normal hearing is a serious matter. The assessment of cases with self-remitting conductive hearing loss may introduce unnecessary anxiety for families. Although these are not true false-positive cases they are likely to be viewed as such by families who had no anxiety prior to the screen.

6 *Hazard of screening test.* Most hearing screening tests are completely non-invasive and safe given that sedation and general anaesthetics are not used at the screening stage. The risk of skin irritation from surface mounted electrodes or cross-infection from ear inserts might be considered to be minor hazards.

Chamberlain's checklist above is useful for any screening system. There is an additional consideration of significance with neonatal hearing screening and that is the influence of a negative result on parent–child bonding. Studies (e.g. Ramkalawan and Davis, 1992) have investigated this matter by retrospectively interviewing parents of deaf children. Most parents wished to know the diagnosis and prognosis as soon as possible after birth. Indeed late detection often instils guilt feelings in parents because they have lost time in treating the condition. Nevertheless parent–child bonding is important and must be respected. There is a need for very careful conveyance of results and sensitive handling of parents at all times, but most particularly at the time of confirmation of the hearing disorder.

Requirements for a screening programme

The tests used in screening should be quick, simple, inexpensive and safe to administer (Cochrane and Holland, 1971). Wilson and Junger (1968) have established the following criteria for screening:

1 The disease should be common and serious.
2 The natural history of the disease should be understood.
3 There should be a good screening test which is both simple and safe.
4 The screening programme should be acceptable to the public and authorities.

5 The screening programme should demonstrate that the benefits outweigh the costs.
6 The screening test should be able to identify and separate those at low risk from those at high risk with good sensitivity and specificity. There should be clearly defined and agreed cut-off points and intervention targets.

This framework is very useful in the context of hearing screening. Most of the requirements have been covered already but what information do we have on the incidence and prevalence of the condition in childhood? Davis and Wood (1992) studied a 3-year birth cohort in Nottingham and found that 1.8% (95% confidence interval 1.2–2.3) per thousand children were fitted with hearing aids by the age of 3 years (that is one child in 566). The prevalence decreased as the severity increased such that the rates were 0.74, 0.48, 0.29 for losses greater than 65 dBHL, 80 dBHL and 95 dBHL respectively (averaged across the frequencies 500 Hz, 1 kHz, 2 kHz and 4 kHz). Eighteen per cent of children in this study had acquired pathologies, predominantly meningitis. In another paper Davis (1993), reviewing nine UK studies, found one in 2000 children at about 5 years of age had a hearing loss greater than or equal to 80 dBHL. This estimate increases to 1 in 770 for hearing losses greater than or equal to 50 dBHL. European data give broadly similar estimates but those from Israel and Australia appear to be marginally different for unknown reasons. Reference should be made to Davis (1993) for more detailed discussion of prevalence and incidence data. These terms are often used incorrectly. *Prevalence* refers to the number or percentage of people with a stated characteristic at a particular time (e.g. the number of people who had a hearing problem in a stated year). *Incidence* is defined as the number of *new* cases in a defined population with a stated characteristic over a particular period (e.g. the number of people with a hearing problem arising between 1 January 1993 and 31 December 1993). Prevalence is a compound of incidence and duration. The age of detection of congenital hearing impairment and its prevalence are examples of performance indicators for preventive systems (e.g. the median age of detection of bilateral 50 dB or more congenital hearing impairment for 1983–1986 was 10 months for the Nottingham Health District according to Davis and Wood, 1992). It is this sort of performance indicator that should be used to monitor the success of screening and surveillance programmes.

Strategies for achieving success

In an ideal world all cases of congenital hearing disorder would be detected at the neonatal stage thus enabling the prompt provision of amplification to lessen the period of auditory deprivation. The favoured techniques for this purpose are the recordings of *auditory brain stem responses* (ABR), *otoacoustic emissions* (OAE) and automated recording of behavioural responses (*auditory response cradle*). It is debatable as to whether these tests should be applied universally or to a targetted high-risk group.

It is clearly more cost effective to concentrate on a high risk group for whom the yield should be relatively high. According to Davis (1994), a neonatal hearing screening programme targetted on the neonatal special care group using a highly sensitive test such as evoked otoacoustic emissions or abbreviated automated auditory brain stem responses might detect up to one-third of all hearing impaired children at a cost of about £30–£40 per child screened. This cost is very small compared with the cost of a child's stay in the neonatal special care unit (Haggard, 1992; Davis and Haggard, 1994). It has been reported in numerous studies that babies who require admission to special care units are ten times more likely to have hearing disorders than babies from normal maternity units (McCormick et al., 1984; Davis and Wood, 1992). If other risk factors are used as criteria for justifying neonatal screening the yield of the test can be improved. For example if all neonates with craniofacial abnormalities and family history of deafness (from childhood) are added to the special care group it should be possible, theoretically, to identify up to 50% of all cases with congenital or neonatally acquired hearing disorders by neonatal hearing screening.

The remaining 50% still require consideration within a screening/surveillance programme. Universal screening will be needed at some stage to identify this remaining group either at the neonatal stage or within the first months of life, accepting that only 50% of hearing impaired babies remain undetected and it will require the screening of 2000 babies to identify one with severe/profound hearing-impairment. The cost per child detected will be high even if the procedure costs only a modest amount per test. If, for example, it costs £5 to administer each test (or surveillance check) then it will cost £10 000 to detect one such case if the test is very sensitive. If lesser degrees of hearing loss are to be detected then the cost effectiveness improves dramatically. A well-administered distraction test will detect cases with mild and moderate hearing-impairment including those with high frequency losses and those with conductive disorders.

Haggard *et al.* (1992) undertook a retrospective study of the paediatric otological caseload resulting from improved screening in the first year of life and found that for every child with a permanent sensorineural hearing loss detected as a result of the screening system there were 34 children with very significant conductive disorders in excess of 47 dB(A). A screening system based on a good distraction test can detect these babies at a cost of approximately £300 per case but, if such cases are to be identified, it is necessary to have a policy for dealing with their needs. Very few require middle ear surgery in the first year of life and care should be directed more towards auditory compensation strategies, parental guidance, and continuing surveillance until the condition has resolved or until surgery or temporary hearing aid provision are indicated. It is necessary to have a coherent plan for service delivery with clearly stated targets and actions. In 1993 the author and a group of colleagues from throughout the UK were commissioned by the National Deaf Children's Society (NDCS) to produce a consensus document entitled 'Quality Standards in Paediatric Audiology: part 1, Guidelines on standards for early identification of hearing-impairment in children'. This report is very relevant to the present discussion and, as its compiler, the author has obtained permission from the NDCS to reproduce a substantial proportion of it (see Appendix 6.1).

The report provides important information for consideration by service providers and purchasers.

The screening tests

The report given in Appendix 6.1 provides a health care framework within which infant hearing screening tests can operate. The essential principles and requirements for each test are described below.

Auditory brain stem response tests (ABR)

It was the early work of Berger (1930) on the recording of the electroencephalogram (EEG) from the human scalp and the follow-up work by Davis *et al.* (1939) which led to subsequent refinements in recording specific changes in the EEG, and gave birth to ABR techniques as we now know them. Dawson's introduction of the average computer (Clark, 1958) provided the means by which responses could be detected and recorded with fine precision.

The electrical activity evoked in the auditory nerve and brain stem pathway is known collectively as the auditory brain stem response (ABR) and the recording of this, utilizing click stimuli and surface electrodes on the scalp, lends itself ideally to testing babies and difficult-to-test children. Babies can be tested without sedation though sedation, anaesthesia or sleep will not affect the recording. ABR recordings using click stimuli do not provide frequency specific information across the entire speech frequency range, but rather a general response in the mid- to high-frequency region centralized on 2.5–3 kHz. Caution must be exercised when interpreting the results be-

cause high or low frequency hearing losses might remain undetected by the technique.

The application of ABR measurements as a screen became a reality with the introduction of simplified instrumentation. Highly automated instruments have been introduced, some of which use machine scoring, thus removing the need for the operator to interpret waveforms. These automated packages have been reviewed by Mason (1993) and one example is the Nottingham ABR screener (Mason, 1984, 1985). This system provides a display of the on-line signal baseline and all the averaged waveforms as well as incorporating machine scoring. The device can be used by relatively inexperienced personnel. In a pilot study on 500 neonates, Mason (1993) reported that 7% of at-risk babies failed the screen at 50 dBHL of which 1.8% failed bilaterally; 44% of neonates referred by the screen were found to have normal hearing at follow up and it is likely that transient middle ear pathology was a factor in many of these cases. All eight babies (1.6% of the total at-risk population screened) with confirmed severe to profound hearing loss failed the screen. Further studies are needed to explore the technique in more detail, but the early signs are very encouraging and this method has already been shown to have good sensitivity and specificity.

Otoacoustic emissions (OAE)

Kemp (1978) discovered that low intensity sound energy, generated by the cochlea, could be recorded in the ear canal and he termed this phenomenon otoacoustic emissions. These measurements are now used routinely in audiology and they have found application in neonatal hearing screening programmes. There is general agreement that delayed otoacoustic emissions are generated only in a healthy or partially healthy cochlea and that their presence indicates mechanically active outer hair cells. The technique is ideal for neonatal screening because it is non-invasive, it can be undertaken during sleep, requiring only the insertion of an ear probe (rather like an impedance probe in appearance) and it is relatively quick to administer. Stevens *et al.* (1989) compared ABR and otoacoustic emission methods on at-risk neonates and found both measurements to be feasible. The sensitivity and specificity values for otoacoustic emissions were 93% and 84% respectively on a sample of 723 neonates.

ABR was used as the standard against which the sensitivity and specificity values were calculated because the ABR technique does permit threshold values to be determined. The intrinsic cut-off for recording of otoacoustic emissions appears to be about 25–35 dBHL and ears with a loss of this magnitude or greater will not produce emissions. The middle ear must be mobile and free from effusion.

Although lack of middle ear mobility does not appear to be a problem in well baby units (if the test is undertaken shortly after birth), it is known that special care neonates are more prone to effusion and this may affect the results in this group.

Broad band click stimuli are the stimuli of choice and responses are averaged in a similar way to ABR recordings.

Auditory response cradle (ARC)

The auditory response cradle is a microprocessor-controlled device designed to record behavioural responses to intense (85 dBSPL) high pass noise (2.6–4.4 kHz). The responses include head turn, body activity, startle response and respiration changes. The ARC has evolved through several models in the past decade and the latest version, the PARC comes in a portable brief-case-sized package.

Evaluation of early implementations on special care babies (McCormick, Curnock and Spavins, 1984) were only partially successful and improvements in the instrumentation and scoring algorithm were suggested by Davis (1984).

The ARC was, however, reported to be reliable when used on well babies and Tucker and Bhattacharya (1992) presented the results of trials on 6000 babies including follow-up data on these babies after 3 years. One hundred and two (1.7%) of the babies failed two ARC tests and 20 were found to have a hearing impairment of some degree. The reported false-positive rate was 1.3%.

The advantage of a behavioural technique is that it samples the entire auditory pathway, but there are uncertainties as to whether children with high tone hearing loss and/or loudness recruitment will be detected. The technique does not appear to be consistently reliable with special care babies and this is the priority group for testing.

Further independent studies are needed to satisfy the sceptics and it is regrettable that these have not appeared in the literature given all the hard work and effort that has been expended in the development of this equipment.

Utilizing parental suspicion

If parents are suspicious about their babies' hearing they are normally correct (Latham and Haggard, 1980; Lilholdt *et al.*, 1980; Hitchings and Haggard, 1983). Absence of suspicion does not, however, necessarily indicate normal hearing and typically only 20% of parents with severely/profoundly deaf children are responsible for initiating a referral for diagnostic testing (McCormick, 1988a; Watkins, Baldwin and Laoide, 1990).

The formalization of a referral system based on parental suspicion is justified even if the yield is only 20% because such a system can be applied from birth and can be based on long-term observation. Such a system is also very cheap to administer and many authorities now use the author's hints for parents handout leaflet entitled 'Can Your Baby Hear You?' shown in Figure 6.1. This may be given to the parents in the neonatal unit or at the health visitor's birth visit. Some authorities have incorporated the form in their parent-held record booklets. With proven validity of this simple health care system there is really no excuse for parental suspicions to be ignored by professionals.

The distraction test

The distraction test was first described by Ewing and Ewing (1944) and is based on the principle that babies turn to locate sounds in a reflex fashion. This response can be demonstrated easily by the age of 6 or 7 months when the baby has sufficient back, neck and head control to sit erect on a caregiver's knee and to turn to sounds located in the horizontal plane level with the ears. Two trained testers are required, one to present the stimulus sounds outside the baby's peripheral vision, and the other to control the baby's attention in the forward direction prior to each sound presentation (Figure 6.2). If frequency specific sounds are used and the basic principles described by the author (McCormick, 1988a) are adhered to the test can be extremely effective and efficient as a screening tool.

The distraction test is normally undertaken in the UK by two trained health visitors and a good record of success has been documented over a period of a decade in the Nottingham district (McCormick, 1983; McCormick *et al.*, 1984; Haggard *et al.*, 1992). Haggard *et al.* (1992) reported a median positive predictive value of 84% for the test from referrals from 14 different health centres and a sensitivity in the region of 90%. Unfortunately this record of success is rare and the reasons for poor performance are well known. Basically they result from lack of specification of standards at local levels and lack of commitment to national standards. In practice, to be successful with the distraction test or any other procedure in the community, it is necessary to have one person in each district with the responsibility for training and coordination. The standards have been set (McCormick, 1988a) and a training package exists and is available for immediate application ('Screening and Surveillance for Hearing Impairment in Young Children,' a video training package, Nottingham Community Health, Linden House, Beechdale Road, Bilborough, Nottingham). The finer points of detail are given full coverage in this training package and include:

erThe screening tests   6/6/7

Hints for Parents

"Can your baby hear you?"

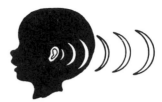

Here is a checklist of some of the general signs you can look for in your baby's first year:-

YES/NO

Shortly after birth
Your baby should be startled by a sudden loud noise such as a hand clap or a door slamming and should blink or open his eyes widely to such sounds.

By 1 Month
Your baby should be beginning to notice sudden prolonged sounds like the noise of a vacuum cleaner and he should pause and listen to them when they begin.

By 4 Months
He should quieten or smile to the sound of your voice even when he cannot see you. He may also turn his head or eyes toward you if you come up from behind and speak to him from the side.

By 7 Months
He should turn immediately to your voice across the room or to very quiet noises made on each side if he is not too occupied with other things.

By 9 Months
He should listen attentively to familiar everyday sounds and search for very quiet sounds made out of sight. He should also show pleasure in babbling loudly and tunefully.

By 12 Months
He should show some response to his own name and to other familiar words. He may also respond when you say 'no' and 'bye bye' even when he cannot see any accompanying gesture.

> Your health visitor will perform a routine hearing screening test on your baby between six and eight months of age. She will be able to help and advise you at any time before or after this test if you are concerned about your baby and his development. If you suspect that your baby is not hearing normally, either because you cannot answer yes to the items above or for some other reason, then seek advice from your health visitor.

©
Produced by Dr. Barry McCormick
Children's Hearing Assessment Centre, General Hospital, Nottingham NG1 6HA
Printed by The Sherwood Press (Nottingham) Limited

Figure 6.1 The Hints for Parents 'Can Your Baby Hear You?' form

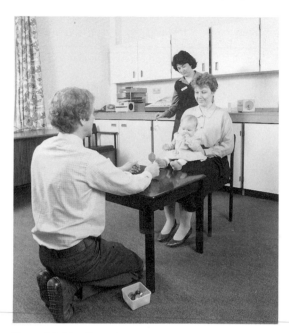

Figure 6.2   The distraction test situation

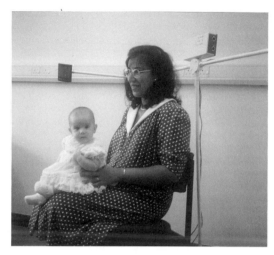

Figure 6.3   The behavioural screening test (BeST) prototype

1 The use of frequency specific stimuli.
2 The use of sound and no sound (control) trials.
3 The timing of stimulus presentation.
4 The method of attention control.
5 The scoring procedure.

When these techniques are correctly applied the test can function with a high degree of specificity and sensitivity as reported above, but considerable effort is required to maintain this record of success. Standards can soon deteriorate in the absence of regular appraisal, audit, training and refresher training.

The behavioural screening test (BeST) – a semi-automated distraction test

Numerous attempts have been made to develop equipment to automate features of the distraction test, but apart from hand held warblers no other technique has reached the manufacturing stage. A prototype of the BeST setup is shown in Figure 6.3 and this represents the first affordable alternative to the normal two person distraction test for screening application. The introduction of this method should have far reaching consequences because it requires only one tester and it removes many of the variables from the test situation by providing automated stimulus selection and a record of responses.

The timing of the stimulus presentation is controlled by the tester who is positioned at the front and controls the baby's attention in the normal way. A hand held transmitter/controller, concealed in the palm of one hand, enables the tester to present the next stimulus from one of the two speakers and to score the response. Correct responses are rewarded with a visual reinforcer on each speaker. An in-built algorithm selects the stimulus sound and side of presentation and aborts the test when it is complete. A visual display of the test results is then given for the tester to document in the child's notes. This test should bring added validity and precision to the test procedure at low cost.

Surveillance as an alternative to a screening test

A few districts in the UK have redirected resources from health visitor testing to neonatal screening and health visitor surveillance. In West Berkshire the distraction test has been suspended for a trial period during which time targetted neonatal screening and vigilant surveillance will be introduced. The surveillance method utilizes the author's 'Can Your Baby Hear You?' form (see Figure 6.1) and an additional questionnaire for parents. The results of the trial will be examined to assess any trends in the age of detection (Scanlon and Bamford, 1990).

An important point to note is that this district had documented improvements in the distraction test in recent years but did not emulate the level of success achieved within other districts, e.g. Nottingham. The distraction test they abandoned had a sensitivity rating of only 50% and this is far below that of 90% in Nottingham. The results so far appear to demonstrate that their success in early detection has not declined (Scanlon, personal communication), although it has not yet been established whether this can be attributed mostly to the introduction of the neonatal screening programme.

It is important to recognize that this is not a cost-cutting exercise and the initiators of the changes in West Berkshire are very careful to point this out. The resources are being redirected with equal demands on health visitor training, support, and commitment. The administration of the questionnaire and the recording of parents' responses in an interview setting may occupy as much time as a distraction test although only one health visitor will be needed.

It will take several years before valid conclusions can be drawn from the surveillance approach. Davis (1993) discussed the problems of evaluating data for a typical district when screening for a uncommon condition such as deafness. A long latency period is required to find any missed cases and the condition can fluctuate. Davis suggested that a statistically useful performance indicator for the age of identification of children (with a definite degree of bilateral impairment ≥ 50 dBHL) might be an unweighted running average, over a 5-year period, of the median and upper quartiles of the ages of referral, confirmation and hearing aid fitting. The start and end dates of the five cohorts would have to be arranged 6–10 years previously to ensure that any late detected cases are included and measures would have to be taken to chase the records of *all* children screened including the follow-up data for those who have moved out of the area.

Other performance indicators are needed such as the degree of coverage and the positive predictive value for screening, though these give no more than an indication of the present performance. There should be some value in data from a quality assurance perspective if these measures are combined with the yield of the current service and the trend over the previous 5 years or so in the detection of babies identified in, say, the first year of life. There will be limitations in this approach from an epidemiological (and therefore research) perspective but there will be value within the routine audit process.

The results of the West Berkshire trial are awaited with interest and will provide reference data to evaluate further studies. It is likely, however, that the newly developed BeST test will be quicker to administer than a surveillance interview and it does share the same benefit of only requiring one member of staff. The BeST test will also detect high tone deafness and sensorineural losses with marked loudness recruitment, neither of which could be detected by a surveillance approach in the first year or so of life.

Screening beyond the first year of life
The toy discrimination test

The techniques discussed so far in this chapter are used in the first year of life. Haggard and Hughes (1991) and Hall (1991) do not recommend a universal screen beyond the first year until school entry when the familiar pure tone sweep screening test can be applied. They indicate that all children with risk factors (including parental suspicion) should be referred to an audiology service and although this may appeal on theoretical grounds the practical application of this could overload any secondary or tertiary level clinic. There is a need for a 'sifting' procedure to isolate those who justifiably need onward referral and it is within this context that the *toy discrimination test* (McCormick, 1977) has found widespread application. Other techniques such as the *performance test* (McCormick, 1988a and later in this chapter) are sometimes used. Experience has shown that staff trained in both methods tend to use the toy discrimination test in preference unless a child does not understand the English language. The toy discrimination test is illustrated in Figure 6.4 and consists of a series of seven paired toy items chosen to have acoustically overlapping features and to be known by most children from a mental age of 2 years. A display of the paired items known to each particular child is presented and the child is conditioned to point to each toy upon request. The voice level is lowered to $\leq$ 40 dB(A) and the child passes the test if he or she responds to four items correctly within five requests (i.e. an 80% score) when not permitted to watch the speaker's face. It is desirable to measure the voice level with a sound level meter but, in the absence of this, a rule of thumb method to check the level is to ask an adult with normal hearing to stand at a distance of 3m and to listen to the words. They should be able to detect the level of voice (*not* whisper) but not be able to separate the items consistently if the voice level is at the target ≤ 40 dB(A) level.

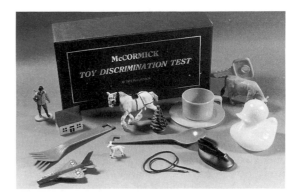

Figure 6.4 The McCormick toy discrimination test

This test can be applied in any routine clinic or home setting, if care is taken to exclude distracting noise, and it provides a more direct measure of hearing disability for speech and language than other procedures such as the distraction or performance test.

The automated IHR/McCormick toy discrimination test

This test (Ousey *et al.*, 1989; Palmer, Sheppard and Marshall, 1991) is illustrated in Figure 6.5 and is an example of a high technology approach to testing which lends itself to screening application because it reduces demands on the tester and proves a rapid test with high precision, but at a cost. The initial outlay on the equipment equates to about one-fifth of the salary of a clinic nurse or health visitor and, if a long-term pragmatic approach is adopted, it will be appreciated that this outlay will be recovered in a year or so by the saving of staff time.

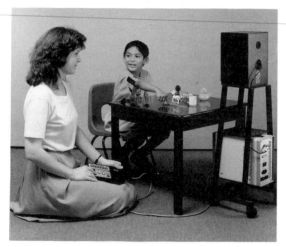

Figure 6.5 The automated IHR/McCormick toy discrimination test

The equipment consists of a speaker through which the toy discrimination test stimulus words are presented. The words are recorded on microchip memory thus giving the facility for random access to the words at any output level, and the test sequence and scoring are all automatic. The tester controls the timing of word presentation according to the child's state of attention and scores the response correct or incorrect. The level of presentation of the next word is automatically decreased or increased respectively. A scoring algorithm is used to establish the threshold. A hand-held keypad controls the operation of the test.

This test is used widely in tertiary level clinics and it should gradually find application in secondary level settings and perhaps even primary settings because

of its advantage in providing a direct and standardized measure of hearing disability with the requirement of only a modest level of staff training.

Added features for audiological service application include speech in noise and warble tone facilities.

The performance test

This test, first described by Ewing and Ewing (1944), provides pre-conditioning for pure tone audiometry. Full details of its application with up-to-date technology are given by the author in McCormick 1988a,b and 1994. It is a play technique suitable for children with developmental ages greater than 30 months and all that is required is a simple toy providing the facility for the repetition of a play sequence (e.g. placing a ball on a stick or a man in a boat). The test should be performed using *frequency specific sounds* to which the child is conditioned to respond. Skilled child handling is required to ensure that the child is conditioned correctly and is not responding impulsively. The timing of the stimulus presentation is crucial and long and short waits are required to check the consistency of the responses. It is also vital that the child does not gain any visual clue as to when the stimulus is presented.

In a screening context the sounds are presented at a set level of 35 dB(A) and the child passes the test if low and high frequencies are responded to at this level for each ear. The test does have the advantage of not being language dependent and it is ideal for use with non-English speaking children for whom the toy discrimination test cannot be used.

The author has been training health visitors to do this test, and the toy discrimination test, for many years and it is apparent that very few people use the performance test routinely because they find the toy disrimination test much more accessible. Both tests are used to assess whether 'at risk' cases should be referred onwards. The flaw in this process is that insufficient practice may be gained with normal straightforward children to develop and retain a good level of tester skill. In the ideal world both tests should be applied because both sample different aspects of auditory response, but this rarely happens in practice partly because of time shortage and partly because practice with each procedure is not maintained.

Conclusions

It is desirable to identify hearing problems as early as possible and methods for achieving this have been presented in this chapter. Recent health service changes in the UK challenge the very structure of services in which screening procedures can operate. To be effective the service requires district-wide coordination, monitoring and training commitment with a central figure taking ultimate responsibility for the outcome.

It is likely that only well proven, simple and reliable tests, which are quick to administer, will survive and medium to high technology will be needed. The questions to be addressed are:

1 Will the providers of health care be able to afford to equip themselves with appropriate test facilities?
2 Will they be motivated to do so?
3 Who will act as watchdogs to overview the efficiency and effectiveness of the screening service?

Challenges lie ahead as the process of decentralization of decision making and assigning of responsibility gradually shifts within the UK.

Appendix 6.1

Quality standards in paediatric audiology I

Guidelines on standards for early identification of hearing impairment in children

1. Introduction

Early detection and management of hearing impairment will help to lessen the impact of the condition on the child's social, emotional, intellectual and linguistic development. The child and family will benefit from such early detection and management. Tests and procedures are now available to achieve these objectives.

The situation in the UK is currently far from satisfactory (see for example the NDCS publication 'Audiological Services for Children'). Urgent action is required to raise standards to a satisfactory level and the introduction of a comprehensive system of quality control should enhance this process. The responsibility for securing good quality is shared by purchasers and providers. The targets listed below have all been achieved in centres within the UK and they are realistic.

2.0 Targets

2.1 To detect 80% of bilateral congenital hearing impairment in excess of 50 dBHL (averaged across the frequencies 500 Hz, 1 kHz, 2 kHz and 4 kHz) within the first year of life and 40% by the age of 6 months.
2.2 To fit hearing aids within 4 weeks of confirmation of hearing loss in appropriate cases.
2.3 To provide audiological assessment within 4 weeks of referral or fitness to test for children at high risk of acquired hearing loss (e.g. following meningitis).
2.4 To ensure that by 1 year of age all children

resident in the district will have benefited from either a formal screen or a specific surveillance procedure to see if they are at risk of hearing loss.

3. Audit and minimum requirements for a good quality service. Documenting the achievement of the above targets

Targetted neonatal screening and improved child health surveillance procedures need to be introduced as a matter of priority. The alternative approach of universal neonatal screening should be given careful thought and consideration for the future. Operation of the procedures recommended below should be subject to adequate data collection and audit utilizing a minimum data sheet approach for every child who comes under suspicion. This could be manual or, more ideally, computerized (for example the Paediatric Audiology Record System – PARS, a section of which is included in Appendix 6.2).

The results of the audit should be accessible to interested parties including parents and the voluntary bodies, e.g. NDCS, RNID, accepting, of course, the need for individual privacy and confidentiality. Monitoring birth cohorts over a 5-year period is essential to ensure that false-negative cases are not missed and acquired impairment is detected without delay.

4.0 Targetted neonatal hearing screening
(Approximately 7% of neonates)

Who should be tested?

4.1 Neonates at high risk including those:

i) admitted to special care baby units for a total of 48 hours or more,
ii) where there is a family history of deafness from birth,
iii) born with abnormalities of the head and neck,
iv) where there has been suspicion of significant intrauterine infection during pregnancy,
v) where there has been consanguineous marriage (e.g. cousin).

4.2 Coverage

To be effective the screening for risk factors should cover all babies resident in the district. Vigilance on the part of the primary health care team is essential to aid this process.

4.3 Parental information

Parents should be informed of the nature of the testing and have an explanation as to why it is undertaken. Written information should be available in an accessible style for parents with details of the screening and follow-up programme taking account of the sensitive needs of parents with newborn babies.

Good parental support is vital at all stages and they should have clear advice as to whom to contact for information or support.

4.4 Test methods and procedures

4.4.1 When and where should testing be undertaken?

High coverage is achieved by testing high risk neonates just before discharge from the maternity unit. Where this is not possible tests should be undertaken on an outpatient basis either at the maternity unit or at a paediatric audiology centre. For outpatients it is recommended that the initial screen is carried out as soon as possible and preferably within 6 weeks of the expected date of delivery.

Parents should be invited to be present during the test whenever possible and the testing must be undertaken in an appropriate environment.

4.4.2 Who should manage the service and who should test?

The service should be managed, and quality controlled, by a trained professional in audiology. Given the nature of the tests involved the most appropriate person would be an audiological scientist or a medical consultant trained in audiological science to at least Masters' degree level. The screen could be carried out by an appropriately trained person and the test should be carried out in a setting providing emergency resuscitation facilities and appropriate scientific monitoring and nursing care.

4.4.3 Method

Current preferred methods for screening use click evoked otoacoustic emissions or auditory brainstem response procedures.

The service needs to be planned carefully and advice taken before purchasing equipment or recruiting staff. Procedures for follow-up need to be considered and the diagnostic audiology service needs to be well developed, able to cope with the testing and management of the babies referred and sensitive to the needs of families.

4.4.4 Test results and follow-up procedure

Follow-up testing will be necessary for neonates who a) do not show a clearly defined acoustic emission or b) do not pass the auditory brainstem test at 50 dBnHL or c) are untestable.

4.4.5 Actions if first screen passed

The parents should be given an explanation of the test results (and a written record). They should also be given a handout such as the 'Can Your Baby Hear You?' form (see Figure 6.1). Professionals should be aware that this group remains at higher risk of hearing impairment of delayed onset. Parents should be advised that if they become concerned they should contact their health visitor, community doctor or general practitioner to arrange for an early appointment at the Paediatric Audiology Centre. Some centres accept direct referrals from parents.

The neonatal screening test results should be forwarded to the GP and Child Health Service.

4.4.6 Action if first screen failed

An auditory brainstem evoked response screen (without sedation) should be undertaken, or repeated if this was the first line screen, before discharge from the neonatal unit.

4.4.7 Action if second screen passed

The action in 4.4.5 should be taken.

4.4.8 Action if second screen failed

GP should be notified routinely and informed of follow-up actions.

Parents should receive sensitive counselling about the test results and be given clear information about the planned follow-up which should include:

a) Full ABR testing to estimate auditory thresholds. (This may include air and bone conduction.) This may be performed whilst still in the neonatal unit or as an outpatient appointment within 6 weeks from expected date of delivery. Beyond this age sedation might be needed. Tympanometry should be undertaken at the same time.

b) Shortly after the ABR testing full audiological assessment should be undertaken at the Paediatric Audiology Centre including:
   i) The taking of a full history.
   ii) Behavioural testing (according to level of maturity) to observe auditory sensitivity and tolerance levels.
   iii) Middle ear impedance and stapedial reflex testing.
   iv) Recording startle and auropalpebral reflex activity.
   v) Full otoacoustic emission testing (where indicated).

   This testing should be undertaken by appropriately trained staff with postgraduate qualifications in audiology (MSc minimum) and several years' experience in paediatric audiology.

c) The results of these investigations should be discussed with, and explained to, the parents and reports with interpretations of results should be sent to the GP, Child Health Service, paediatrician etc as appropriate.

d) Contact should be made with families who fail to attend for follow-up appointments. If they do not take advantage of the facilities offered it will be necessary to be particularly vigilant within the normal surveillance programme.

e) The clinical management and quality care issues highlighted in the Patient's Charter should be satisfied (see Appendix 6.3).

4.5 Audiological assessment indicates normal hearing

Action in 4.4.5 should be taken.

4.6 Audiological assessment confirms hearing impairment

4.6.1 Hearing aid required

The child should continue under the management of the Paediatric Audiology Service with hearing aid provision and follow-up where indicated. The levels of care expected at this stage include:

a) A prompt appointment (within a week) to see a consultant otolaryngologist or, if not already seen, an audiological physician, preferably at a Paediatric Audiology Centre. Genetic counselling should be offered to parents if indicated.
b) A prompt appointment for further audiological assessment and hearing aid fitting/assessment sessions. (The target here should be to fit the hearing aid within 4 weeks of confirmation of the hearing problem).
c) The allocation of a key person (clinician) with whom to relate for continuing information (visiting cards helpful here).
d) Information about voluntary sector to be offered to parents (e.g. NDCS).
e) Immediate contact and liaison to be made with local education support service, and social service department where indicated.
f) Contact to be made with a paediatrician (or delegated SCMO) for paediatric assessment unless already under a paediatrician.

4.6.2 Hearing aid not required

Where there is a mild hearing loss with evidence of otitis media with effusion it is reasonable to undertake further testing within 3–6 months to check for persistence and then to:

a) issue information leaflets about otitis media with effusions and compensation strategies,
b) arrange an ENT consultation if the problem persists,
c) discharge if the problem has cleared and the hearing levels are within normal limits,
d) undertake further assessment where indicated.

Where there is a mild sensorineural hearing loss of insufficient severity to require hearing aids at this early stage (typically less than 35 dB) the child should be kept under regular surveillance at 3-monthly intervals and brought forward for hearing aid fitting as appropriate. A key person (clinician) should be allocated to each family to be the direct contact point for information and advice (visiting cards desirable).

5.0 Non high-risk/normal birth neonates
(approximately 93% of neonates)

For the vast majority of neonates there will be no known risk factors associated with deafness and for these cases a surveillance approach should be adopted. This should include:

5.1 The questioning of parents at the antenatal stage about any family history of sensorineural deafness in childhood.
5.2 The issuing of a handout/checklist, along the lines of the 'Can Your Baby Hear You?' form (see Figure 6.1) on discharge from the maternity unit or during the Health Visitor's birth visit.
5.3 Treating parents' concern about their neonate/baby's hearing seriously with prompt referral to the Paediatric Audiology Centre where doubts are expressed. Such referrals should be accepted from the parents, the health visitors, GPs or any other professional. Open access audiology services have proved to be effective and desirable.

6.0 Babies from 0–6 months

No formal community screening of hearing should be undertaken. The procedures in 5.2 and 5.3 should be followed.

7.0 Babies 6–18 months

Unless there is an alternative surveillance method, of proven effectiveness from active monitoring, all babies should receive a hearing screening test at 6–7 months and this should be undertaken by two well-trained community health staff, at least one of whom is a health visitor and the second might be a trained nursing auxiliary. The testing should conform to a nationally recognised standard procedure (e.g. McCormick, *Screening for Hearing Impairment in Young Children*, London, Whurr Publishers (1994); and training package *Screening and Surveillance for Hearing Impairment in Young Children*, Nottingham Community Health, Linden House, Beechdale Road, Bilborough, Nottingham). There should be regular updating of the procedure and facilities for testing the hearing of the testers every 2 years or so. The coverage of this test should be in excess of 95% and the results should be subject to regular monitoring by the health visitor management and the audiological scientist/physician.

Where 95% true coverage is not achieved consideration should be given to other active methods, e.g. surveillance.

Results of the general audit on the distraction test should be reviewed at least annually and in retrospect taking account of the fact that the false-negatives (any missed cases) may take 2 or 3 years to surface in the system when delays in speech and language development have become apparent.

7.1 First distraction test passed

The parents should be reminded about the 'Can Your Baby Hear You?' document (see Figure 6.1) or be issued with another copy and be guided through this by the health visitor. They should be advised that although the baby has passed the screening test they should not hesitate to request another test or an appointment at the Paediatric Audiology Centre if they become concerned in the future. The procedure for routine developmental checks and further hearing tests should be explained.

7.2 First distraction test failed

The need for a second screening test and the timing of this should be explained in the light of the test results. The timing for the second test should be:

a) within 7–10 days if parents are concerned about their baby's hearing and the baby has not responded to sound.

b) between 6–8 weeks if the parents are not concerned and the baby shows some evidence of responding to sound, but not at the screening level.

7.3 Second distraction test passed

The action in 7.1 should be followed.

7.4 Second distraction test failed

An immediate referral should be made to the Paediatric Audiology Centre and this should be marked as urgent if the parents express particular concern. Such urgent referrals should be given an appointment to be seen within 2 weeks. All other cases should be seen within 6 weeks.

The actions from 4.4.8, 4.5 and 4.6 should be followed with exception of 4.4.8(a) which (if it is needed at all) should be deferred until after the diagnostic audiological investigation.

Conclusion and summary

This paper has covered the early identification area and encroached upon the initial diagnostic requirements within the Paediatric Audiology Centre. Clear guidelines have been offered for the operation and quality control for an effective service.

Appendix 6.2

Neonatal hearing screening data record

Biographical data

Name:_____   DOB_____   Sex_____

Serial Number_____   Hospital/Körner number_____

Consultant code_____   GP code_____   HV code_____

District code_____   Region code_____   NICU history_____

Family history_____   Birthweight_____gms _____lbs oz   Gestation_____wks

High risk factors_____   _____   _____   Syndrome_____

Test details   Test 1 – Date_____   Test 2 – Date_____

Reason/Tester   _____/_____   _____/_____

Left ear result   _____   _____

Right ear result   _____   _____

Method   _____   _____

Time taken   _____   _____

Screening level and scale   _____   _____

Onward referral to: Diagnostic ABR_____   Audiological Scientist_____   Genetic Counsellor

ENT_____   Paediatrician_____   Social worker_____   Other_____

(S)CMO_____   Ophthalmologist_____   GP_____

Follow up (to be completed for all children with abnormal ABR results)

At confirmation of hearing impairment: Severity   Left ear_____   Right ear_____   Date_____

Hearing aid fitted:_____   Type of Loss   Left ear_____   Right ear_____

Field choices

High risk factors:
1 None
2 Rubella
3 Meningitis
4 CMV
5 Jaundice
6 Respiratory problems
7 Asphyxia
8 Transfusion
9 Ototoxic drugs
10 Abnormal cranial scan
11 Cleft palate
12 Ear deformity
13 Cerebral palsy
14 Syndrome
15 Consanguinity
16 Other

Syndrome:
1 Wildervants syndrome
2 Downs syndrome
3 Mandibulo facial dysostosis (MFO)
4 Pierre-Robin syndrome (PRS)
5 Deafness earpits syndrome (DES)
6 Alports syndrome (deafness with neuritis DNS)
7 Deafness with optic atrophy (DOA)
8 Pendreds syndrome
9 Jervell and Lange Neilsen syndrome
10 Usher syndrome
11 X-linked
12 Waardenbergs syndrome
13 CHARGE
14 Other

Reason for test:
1 Not done
2 Universal
3 SCBU
4 HR screen
5 Concern

Result:
1 No result
2 Refer
3 Doubtful
4 Pass

Method:
1 ACR
2 POEMS
3 ILO 88/92
4 ILO screener
5 DP emissions
6 ALGO
7 ABR (SM)
8 ABR
9 Other

Scale:
1 dBA
2 dBSPL
3 dBHL
4 dBnHL

Severity:
0 < 20 dB HL
1 20–40 dB HL
2 41–70 dB HL
(2a 41–49 dB HL)
(2b 50–70 dB HL)
3 71–95 dB HL
4 96–120 dB HL
5 > 120 dB HL

Type:
1 No conductive element
2 Conductive element (abnormal tymp)

Appendix 6.3

The Patient's Charter
Clinical management and the Quality Care

The following specific requirements should be satisfied for each clinic appointment:

i) Appointment letters should include a map showing the location of the department relative to parking and public transport facilities together with contact names and a telephone number in case of difficulties with the appointment.

ii) Name badges and/or plaques should be displayed for all staff.

iii) 90% of cases should be seen within 15 minutes of the appointment time and if there are unavoidable delays such information should be given on arrival with updated information as the clinic progresses.

iv) Interpreters and the provision of other special communication needs must be arranged when indicated.

v) Appointments should be free from interruptions.

vi) Explanation of test procedures should be given and the results discussed with the parents with agreement of follow-up actions.

vii) Interested parties should receive copies of results with the GP and child health service and the referrer receiving these as a matter of routine.

The full range of other requirements within the Patient's Charter should also be satisfied.

References

BERGER, H. (1930) On the electroencephalogram of man. In: Hans Berger on the electroencephalogram of man. *Electroencephalography and Clinical Neurophysiology*, Suppl. 28, 37

CHAMBERLAIN, J. M. (1984) Screening programmes. *Journal of Epidemiology and Community Health*, **38**, 270–277

CLARK, W. A. JR. (1958) Average response computers (ARC-1). *Quarterly Progress Report No 49*, Research Laboratory of Electronics, Massachusetts Institute of Technology, Cambridge, Massachusetts, (MIT Press)

COCHRANE, A. and HOLLAND, W. W. (1971) Validation of screening procedures. *British Medical Bulletin*, **27**, 3–8

DAVIS, A. C. (1984) Detecting hearing-impairment in neonates – the statistical decision criterion for the auditory response cradle. *British Journal of Audiology*, **18**, 163–168

DAVIS, A. C. (1993) A public health perspective on childhood hearing impairment. In *Paediatric Audiology 0–5 years*, edited by B. McCormick, London: Whurr Publishers. Ch. 1, pp. 1–41

DAVIS, A. C. and HAGGARD, M. P. (1994) Costs involved in different screening for hearing impairment strategies: a Monte-Carlo simulation. Personal communication

DAVIS, A. C. and WOOD, S. (1992) The epidemiology of childhood hearing impairment: factors relevant to planning of services. *British Journal of Audiology*, **26**, 77–99

DAVIS, H., DAVIS, P. A., LOOMIS, A. L., HARVEY, E. N. and HOBART, G. (1939) Electrical reactions of the human brain to auditory stimulation during sleep. *Journal of Neurophysiology*, **2**, 500–514

EWING, I. R. and EWING, A. W. G. (1944) The ascertainment of deafness in infancy and early childhood. *Journal of Laryngology and Otology*, **59**, 309–338

HAGGARD, M. P. (1992) Screening children's hearing. *British Journal of Audiology*, **26**, 209–215

HAGGARD, M. P. and HUGHES, E. G. (1991) *Screening Children's Hearing – a Review of the Literature and the Impact of Otitis Media*. London: HMSO

HAGGARD, M. P., MCCORMICK, B., GANNON, M. M. and SPENCER, H. (1992) The paediatric otological caseload resulting from improved screening in the first year of life. *Clinical Otolaryngology*, **17**, 34–43

HALL, D. M. B. (ed) (1991) *Health for All Children* 2nd edn. Oxford: Oxford University Press

HITCHINGS, V. and HAGGARD, M. P. (1983) Incorporation of parental suspicions in screening infants' hearing. *British Journal of Audiology*, **17**, 71–75

KEMP, D. T. (1978) Stimulated acoustic emissions from within the human auditory system. *Journal of the Acoustical Society of America*, **64**, 1386–1391

LATHAM, A. M. and HAGGARD, M. P. (1980) A pilot study to detect hearing impairment in the young. *Midwife, Health Visitor and Community Nurse*, **9**, 370–374

LILDHOLDT, T., COURTOIS, J., KORTHOLM, B., SCHOU, J. W. and WARRER, H. (1980) The diagnosis of negative middle-ear pressure in children. The accuracy of symptoms and signs assessed by tympanometry. *Acta Otolaryngologica*, **89**, 459–464

MCCORMICK, B. (1977) The Toy Discrimination Test: an aid for screening the hearing of children above a mental age of two years. *Public Health (London)*, **91**, 67–73

MCCORMICK, B. (1983) Hearing screening by health visitors: a critical appraisal of the distraction test. *Health Visitor*, **56**, 449–451

MCCORMICK, B. (1988a) *Screening for Hearing Impairment in Young Children*. London: Chapman and Hall. (Republished 1994 by Whurr Publishers Ltd, London)

MCCORMICK, B. (ed.) (1988b) *Paediatric Audiology 0–5 years*. London: Whurr

MCCORMICK, B., CURNOCK, D. A. and SPAVINS, F. (1984) Auditory screening of special care neonates using the auditory response cradle. *Archives of Disease in Childhood*, **59**, 1168–1172

MCCORMICK, B., WOOD, S. A., COPE, Y., and SPAVINS, F. M. (1984) Analysis of records from an open access audiology service. *British Journal of Audiology*, **18**, 127–132

MARKIDES, A. (1986) Age at fitting hearing aids and speech intelligibility. *British Journal of Audiology*, **20**, 165–168

MASON, S. M. (1984) On line computer scoring of the auditory brainstem response for estimates of hearing threshold. *Audiology*, **23**, 277–296

MASON, S. M. (1985) Objective waveform detection in electric response audiometry. Unpublished *PhD Thesis*, University of Nottingham

MASON, S. M. (1993) Electric response audiometry. In: *Paediatric Audiology 0–5 years*, edited by B. McCormick London: Whurr Publishers. pp. 187–249

NIH CONSENSUS STATEMENT (1993) *Early Identification of*

Hearing Impairment of Infants and Young Children. Bethesda, Md: National Institutes of Health. Vol II, 1

OUSEY, J., SHEPPARD, S., TWOMEY, T. and PALMER, A. R. (1989) The IHR/McCormick automated toy discrimination test – description and initial evaluation. *British Journal of Audiology*, **23**, 245–251

PALMER, A. R., SHEPPARD, S. and MARSHALL, D. H. (1991) Prediction of hearing thresholds in children using an automated toy discrimination test. *British Journal of Audiology*, **25**, 351–356

RAMKALAWAN, T. W, and DAVIS, A. C. (1992) The effects of hearing loss and age of intervention on some language metrics in a population of young hearing impaired children. *British Journal of Audiology*, **27**, 97–107

ROYAL COLLEGE OF GENERAL PRACTITIONERS (1992) *Report of the Second Working Party on Child Health Surveillance.* Oxford: Oxford University Press

SCANLON, P. E. and BAMFORD, J. M. (1990) Early identification of hearing loss: screening and surveillance methods. *Archives of Disease in Childhood*, **65**, 479–485

STEVENS, J. C., WEBB, H. D., HUTCHINSON, J., CONNELL, J., SMITH, M. F. and BUFFIN, J. T. (1989) Click evoked otoacoustic emissions compared with brainstem electric response. *Archives of Disease in Childhood*, **64**, 1105–1111

TUCKER, S. M., and BHATTACHARYA, J. (1992) Screening of hearing-impairment in the newborn using the auditory response cradle. *Archives of Disease in Childhood*, **67**, 911–919

WATKINS, P. M., BALDWIN, M. and LAOIDE, S. (1990) Parental suspicion and identification of hearing impairment. *Archives of Disease in Childhood*, **65**, 846–850

WHITE, S. J. and WHITE, R. E. C. (1987) The effects of hearing status of the family and the age of intervention on receptive and expressive oral language skills in hearing-impaired infants. In: *Development of Language and Communication in Hearing-Impaired Children*, edited by H. Levitt, N. McGarr and D. Geffner. American Speech and Hearing Association, Monographs No 26. Rockville, Maryland. **26**, 9–24

WILSON, J. M. G. and JUNGER, G, (1968) Principles and practice of screening for disease. *Public Health Papers, number 34*, Geneva: World Health Organization

7

Otitis media with effusion

A. Richard Maw

Otitis media with effusion is the commonest cause of hearing difficulty and one of the most frequent reasons for elective admission to hospital for surgery during childhood. A variety of synonyms describes the condition. It has been termed catarrhal, exudative, seromucinous, serous, secretory and non-suppurative otitis media. Following sequential discussions at international symposia the terms middle ear effusion and otitis media with effusion are currently acceptable (Bluestone, 1984; Lim et al., 1993). To many clinicians and lay persons, however, it is known as 'glue ear'. Use of the term otitis media with effusion permits subdivision according to the nature of the effusion and its duration. A reasonable definition of the condition is the presence within the middle ear cleft of an effusion which may be serous or mucoid but not frankly purulent. Although not associated clinically with obvious signs or symptoms of infection, bacteria may be cultured from the effusion in approximately one-third to one-half of cases (Senturia et al., 1958). The condition results from an alteration of the mucociliary system within the middle ear and eustachian tube with accumulation of serous or mucoid fluid in the middle ear cleft, where there is usually a negative pressure. The changes result in part from infection to which is added an element of eustachian tube dysfunction. There is increasing evidence that the infection originates in the nasopharynx (Hemlin et al., 1991).

Middle ear effusions frequently persist for a short time following episodes of acute suppurative otitis media although 90% of such effusions have resolved within 3 months (Teele, Klein and Rosner, 1980).

Otitis media with effusion runs a relapsing and remitting course before ultimately resolving in later childhood. Fifty per cent of ears resolve spontaneously within 3 months and only 5% persist for more than 12 months (Zielhuis, Rach and Van den Broek, 1989). Certain risk factors have been identified in relation to the development of otitis media with effusion. It is very common in infants with cleft palate and is frequent in certain syndromes affecting the morphology of the nasopharynx and skull base. The relationship with the adenoid probably reflects the combined effects of nasopharyngeal disproportion, ascending eustachian tube infection and tubal dysfunction. Problems may also result from chronic infective and obstructive conditions of the nasal passages and sinuses. Any conditions which affect the proper function of the mucociliary system of the upper respiratory tract may predispose to development of middle ear effusion. There is a relationship between the presence of middle ear fluid and hearing impairment, though in younger children the hearing loss is not always obvious. When covert it may present as speech, language or learning delay and sometimes as behavioural and educational problems. Hearing loss may be first detected on routine screening examination at 7–9 months, 3 years of age or later at pre-school testing. There is still insufficient evidence to demonstrate a causal link between otitis media with effusion and clinically significant disablement in children (Haggard and Hughes, 1991), but a number of developmental disabilities may result from the persisting hearing loss which results from the condition (Chalmers et al., 1989). Episodes of acute suppurative otitis media are often superimposed on chronic effusions when the relatively symptomless condition may present with otalgia and sometimes otorrhoea.

Treatment varies widely and should depend not only on the duration and severity of the condition but also on the age and general condition of the child.

Incidence, prevalence and natural history

It is difficult to describe the precise natural history of the condition because of its fluctuating course and tendency to spontaneous resolution. Such a condition requires assessment of risk factors (Zielhuis *et al.*, 1989). The incidence, i.e. the number of new cases seen per year in 3-year-old children is in the order of 42% but this increases in winter (Fiellau Nikolajsen, 1979). The prevalence or percentage of affected children at any one time is lower and depends on the duration of the condition, which is usually short lived. In 2–7-year-old children it may be in the order of 10–30% (Haggard and Hughes, 1991) but Zielhuis *et al.* (1990b) have shown two points of peak prevalence, initially at about 2 years when approximately 20% of children are affected, and later at 5 years of age. Clearly incidence and prevalence rates depend on the methods used to detect the condition. Most studies now rely on tympanometry and, in some, this is supplemented by otoscopy and audiometry. Rates vary, not only in relation to age but also if particular risk groups are assessed, e.g. in relation to institutional or non-institutional care (Birch and Elbrond, 1986) or whether assessment is made in the winter or summer. Zielhuis, Rach and Van den Broek (1989) using serial tympanometry every 3 months demonstrated a fairly constant improvement rate in effusions of 50% every 3 months with a cumulative rate of 50%. Two-thirds of all cases of effusion, as evidenced by flat tympanograms, had a duration of less than 3 months (Figure 7.1). Previous studies with tympanometry showed incidence rates of 50% in 5–7 year olds in the UK (Brooks, 1976), 30% in Danish 2–4 year olds (Tos and Poulsen, 1979) and 26% in Danish 7 year olds (Lous and Fiellau Nikolajsen, 1981) while Suarez Nieto, Mallaguiza Calvo and Barthe Garcia (1983) confirmed an incidence of 8.7% in 2–10 year olds in Spain. The incidence fitted a logarithmic regression curve with 38.8% in 2 year olds and 1.1% in 11 year olds. Birch and Elbrond (1986) confirmed prevalence peaks at 1 and 5 years of age and they noted a 40% prevalence rate in non-institutionalized children compared with a 70% rate in children cared for in institutions. The prevalence in both groups at 6 years of age was 15%. In the large study in Holland, Rach, Zielhuis and Van den Broek (1986) showed an incidence of 39% in 2 year olds in winter compared with 24% in the summer, and noted that 21% of cases were bilateral. Chalmers *et al.* (1989) confirmed prevalence rates of 10.5% at age 5, 6.5% at 7, 3% at 9 and 2.4% at 11. Zielhuis, Rach and Van den Broek (1989) showed that 23% of 1249 Dutch 2–4-year-old children had persistent type B tympanograms. In Dutch children aged 7½–8 years the prevalence of bilateral otitis media with effusion, as judged by type B tympanograms, was 2.5% while unilateral otitis media with effusion present in 7%. The presence of otitis media with effusion was associated with a mean hearing loss of 20 dB (Schilder, Zielhuis and Van den Broek, 1993).

In Glasgow, studies by Dempster and Mackenzie (1991) of 3–12-year-old children with bilateral disease confirmed that 49% of those with type B tympanograms had a hearing loss of 25 dB or more. It is estimated that 11% of 2–4-year-old children will have a 25 dB hearing loss persisting for 3 or more months (Effective Health Care, 1992).

Our own study of children with persistent bilateral disease, confirmed with otoscopy and tympanometry and observed for 3 months showed that spontaneous resolution without treatment occurred in approximately 20% of cases after 1 year, 30% of cases after 2 years and 60% of cases after 3 years (Maw and Parker, 1988). This is supported by the work of Lieberman and Bartal. (1986) who demonstrated a similar rate of spontaneous resolution in children untreated for 2½ years. These findings reflect the natural tendency for resolution of effusions seen in relation to the time spent on the waiting list (Buckley and Hinton, 1991).

Risk factors

There are racial differences in the incidence of recurrent acute otitis media and otitis media with effusion. Eskimos and American Indians are more frequently affected than American whites. Black children have a lower incidence than white children, and Goycoolea, Goycoolea and Farfan (1988) have shown Easter

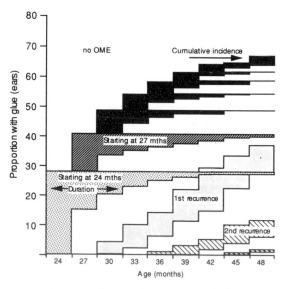

Figure 7.1 Natural history of otitis media with effusion (From Zielhuis, Rach and Van den Broek, 1989)

Islanders of mixed or continental origin have a higher point prevalence of otitis media with effusion than genetically pure native children. Racial variations may be due to anatomical differences in the skull base and eustachian tube or may be genetic.

Certain syndromes and some children with skull base or nasopharyngeal anatomical abnormalities are more likely to have otitis media with effusion, e.g. Down's, Hurler's, Hunter's and fragile X syndromes. Boys are more frequently affected than girls which may be a reflection of anatomical or growth differences or the overall male predominance for childhood infections. Boys have less well pneumatized air cell systems (Tos and Stangerup, 1985) which may be a consequence of tubal dysfunction and more marked middle ear pathology, supporting the environmental rather than the hereditary theory of mastoid pneumatization. Although children with a cleft palate are predisposed to eustachian tube malfunction as a consequence of impaired function of the tensor palati muscle (Stool and Randall, 1967), those with a bifid uvula are not at extra risk of developing otitis media with effusion (Rivron, 1989). Gender, the child's age and seasonal variation are related to the duration of disease and recovery from it (Zeilhuis, Rach and Van den Broek, 1990b). Zeilhuis *et al.* (1989) did not demonstrate a relationship with birthweight nor any effect from passive smoking. Possible relationships have been demonstrated with family size, duration of breast feeding and attendance at public day-care centres (Rassmussen, 1993). However, other studies have suggested that one-third of middle ear effusions may be attributable to passive smoking (Strachan, Jarvis and Feyerabend, 1989) and there appears to be increased admission of children for surgery when parents smoke (Hinton, 1989). Our own work has shown a deleterious effect of smoking on treatment (Maw *et al.*, 1992), whereas others have shown parental smoking to have no effect on the prevalence of otitis media with effusion requiring surgical treatment (Rowe-Jones and Brockbank, 1992; Rassmussen, 1993). These differences may be in part due to the way in which parental smoking is assessed.

The duration of otitis media with effusion following acute otitis media is longer in boys and those with a sibling history of ear infection and in those who are not breast fed (Teele, Klein and Rosner, 1989; Rassmussen, 1993). Mouth breathing posture with a clear nose has been said to account for 20% of the incidence of otitis media with effusion (Van Bon *et al.*, 1989).

The possibility of manipulating risk factors to produce a therapeutic benefit must be considered. However, the relative risk of otitis media with effusion as a consequence of controllable environmental factors is low. Improvements in infant feeding, manipulation of day-care management and advice in respect to parental smoking may have a slight effect on the prevalence of otitis media with effusion.

Aetiology

The main underlying factors for production of otitis media with effusion are a combination of infection and eustachian tube dysfunction. Historically tubal dysfunction has been held as the principal causal factor in the development of otitis media with effusion. However, conclusive scientific evidence to support such dysfunction in relation to otitis media with effusion is lacking. It is possible that the tubal pathology found in otitis media with effusion is a result of rather than a cause of infection in the middle ear. Nevertheless, there is a wide variety of conditions affecting eustachian tube function which may be associated with the development of otitis media with effusion, and these can be considered under three main headings.

> *Eustachian tube dysfunction*
>   Due to palatal abnormalities:
>   cleft palate
>   submucous cleft palate
>   Due to altered mucociliary system:
>   infection
>   allergy
>   immunological factors
>   surfactant deficiency
>   cilial abnormalities
>   hormonal factors
> *Middle ear gas composition*
> *Nasopharyngeal disproportion:*
>   Craniofacial abnormality
>   Adenoids and nasopharynx.

Eustachian tube dysfunction

Palatal problems

It seems likely that during normal childhood development the eustachian tube alters to an adult configuration at about the age of 7 years (Holborow, 1970) and morphological differences in the skull base have been shown to support this (Todd and Martin, 1988) but the tube is not wider in infants and children than in adults (Luntz and Sade, 1988). We have recently demonstrated differences in skull base and nasopharyngeal dimensions in children with otitis media with effusion compared with age and sex matched controls (Maw, Smith and Lance, 1991). The suggestion that tubal dysfunction was a principal cause of the otitis media with effusion was used to account for the universality of the condition in children with cleft palate (Stool and Randall, 1967). Studies of the infective aspects of otitis media with effusion in these cases have not been reported. There is limited evidence of improvement of effusions following palatal repair which attempts to restore the normal mode of function of the tensor palati muscle. Ventilation tube insertion in ears with otitis media with effusion in children with cleft palate is associated with a larger mastoid air cell system than in non-ventilated ears (Robinson *et al.*, 1993). It is unclear whether association of otitis media with effusion with craniofacial abnormalities, syndromic conditions and the racial differences in incidence is due to morphological differences in the nasopharynx, eustachian tube or both (Uhari *et al.*, 1991).

Both functional and mechanical obstruction of the eustachian tube have been said to occur (Bluestone and Beery, 1976). The previously held hydrops ex vacuo theory of the development of effusions suggested that with tubal obstruction a negative pressure developed within the middle ear cleft due to gas absorption. As a consequence it was thought that a sterile transudate formed.

Altered mucociliary system

Infection

The involvement of an inflammatory component originating in the nasopharynx as the cause of the middle ear changes is suggested by demonstration of increased numbers of pathogens in the nasopharynx resembling those found in the middle ear (Hemlin *et al.*, 1991). *Streptococcus pneumoniae, Haemophilus influenzae, Moxarella catarrhalis* and *Streptococcus pyogenes* account for the majority of organisms in both sites. Demonstration of bacterial adherence to nasopharyngeal epithelial cells by pathogenic organisms has been shown by several studies (Stenfors and Raisanen, 1991). Positive bacterial cultures have been demonstrated in up to 50% of middle ear effusions. Bacteria found are similar to those cultured in cases of acute suppurative otitis media (Klein, 1980).

A chronic condition may result from incomplete resolution of acute infection (Mills, Utley and McIntyre, 1984) or treatment of resistant strains of *Haemophilus influenzae* and *Staphylococcus aureus* with pencillin (Mills, Utley and McIntyre, 1985). The surface endotoxin of *Haemophilus influenzae* may be responsible for the induction of otitis media with effusion (De Maria *et al.*, 1984). Whereas endotoxin to *Haemophilus influenzae* was detected in 96% of effusions and bacteria in 38%, relapse of otitis media with effusion occurred in 26% of patients after 1 year and was related to the presence of bacteria in the original effusion and not to the endotoxin (Ovesen, Paaske and Elbrond, 1992).

Stenfors and Raisanen (1992) have shown positive middle ear cultures for *Haemophilus influenzae, Streptococcus pneumoniae* and *Moxarella catarrhalis* in 30% of cases and in 19% there were dormant organisms of *Haemophilus influenzae* and *Streptococcus pneumoniae*. Complement changes and a reduced level of IgG antibodies against *Pneumococcus* have been shown and it is possible that IgE antibodies and immune complexes may be responsible for a secondary

immune response within the middle ear. Furthermore, it has been shown that the act of immunization, by parenteral injection with certain capsular polysaccharides, can prevent the development of otitis media in animal models and in children (Robbins, Schneerson and Szu, 1988). Evidence has accumulated about the importance of prostaglandins, leukotrienes and metabolic arachidonic acid in the production of experimental otitis media with effusion (Jung *et al.*, 1990). Inflammatory cytokines which are host glycoproteins produced by macrophages and other cells mediate the inflammatory reaction and regulate the immune response within the middle ear. While it is likely that nasopharyngeal pathogenic organisms are related to the development of otitis media with effusion, it is possible that the thick mucoid secretions developing within the middle ear may ultimately produce eustachian tube obstruction and could act as a barrier to ascending infection (Stenfors and Raisanen, 1989).

Studies have shown a relationship between viral infection and the incidence of acute otitis media with effusion (Henderson *et al.*, 1982) with a close seasonal relationship between the incidence of the condition and the incidence of respiratory syncytial viral infections.

Allergy

A causative role for IgE-mediated allergic reaction in the development of otitis media with effusion has not been demonstrated, though animal studies have shown that such allergic reactions may intefere with resolution of effusion. Some studies show a high prevalence of allergic conditions in children with otitis media with effusion and improvement in middle ear status following treatment of their allergy (Scadding *et al.*, 1993). Perhaps the increased susceptibility to respiratory infections found in patients with allergy is responsible for the association of otitis media with effusion and atopy.

Immunological factors

The middle ear is an immunologically unique site and in the normal state has few immunocompetent or inflammatory cells, though there are mast cells in the normal tubotympanic mucosa. It is protected from antigenic invasion by the eustachian tube. During episodes of otitis media, immunocompetent cells and inflammatory cells are found in the middle ear mucosa. Alteration of the immune responses within the middle ear system may occur as a result of immediate hypersensitivity, as a cytotoxic response, as a response by the complement system or due to delayed hypersensitivity via a cellular immune mechanism (Lim and De Maria, 1982). Studies have shown that secretory IgA is present in middle ear effusions and that IgA plasma cells are found in the inflamed mucosa of the middle ear cleft, indicating that mucosal immunity operates during infection of the cleft. However, IgG-mediated systemic immunity is the main defence system against bacterial infection of the middle ear.

Otitis media with effusion can be produced by injection with protein antigen into the tympanic cavity of animals systemically immunized with the same antigen, so-called 'immune mediated otitis media'. The immunocomplex is the key factor for the production of effusion (Mogi, 1993). A lower mean IgG2 subclass level has been observed in children with recurrent otitis media compared with otitis free children (Pelton *et al.*, 1988). IgG antibodies and their immune complexes may be the key factor in the generation of the secondary immune-mediated response in the middle ear producing otitis media with effusion (Suzuki *et al.*, 1988). Pathological similarities between rheumatoid arthritis and otitis media with effusion are supported by the finding of rheumatoid factor in 85% of middle ear effusions and in only 8% of serum samples (De Maria *et al.*, 1984). Various forms of reactive arthritis may result from prior localization of bacterial remnants or dormant fastidious bacteria in the affected joint where they act as persisting antigens. Such a phenomenon may also be responsible for otitis media with effusion, in which it is likely that the infectious focus lies close to the middle ear cleft, probably in the nasopharynx (Stenfors and Raisanen, 1992).

Surfactant deficiency

It has been suggested that proteolytic enzyme activity from bacteria causes a deficiency of surfactant in the eustachian tube. Surface active phospholipids which reduce surface tension at the liquid/air interface have been demonstrated in dogs and rabbits by thin layer chromotography (Hills, 1984). However, recent animal and human studies using surfactant for the treatment of otitis media with effusion have produced equivocal results (Kobayashi *et al.*, 1993).

Cilial abnormalities

Otitis media with effusion occurs with the immotile cilia syndrome and particularly with that form of the condition constituting Kartagener's syndrome. Functional reduction in cilial beat frequency occurs with exposure to tobacco smoke and may explain the relationship between passive smoking and otitis media with effusion. However, Wake and Smallman (1992) excluding obvious syndromic cases have shown no difference in cilial beat frequency in otitis media with effusion cases compared with controls. Ears with effusion have been shown to have significantly lower mucociliary clearance than those without (Takeuchi *et al.*, 1990).

Hormonal factors

Hormonal dysfunction with high oestrogen levels and people with hypothyroidism may develop tubal dysfunction sufficient to produce an effusion, although this is very infrequent in children.

There is no increased incidence of otitis media with effusion in patients with mucoviscidosis or fibrocystic disease (Forman-Franco *et al.*, 1979).

Middle ear gas composition

The middle ear cleft may act like a gas pocket (Sade and Luntz, 1990). There are losses and gains from the atmosphere via the eustachian tube and from the circulation by diffusion. Recent mass spectrometry studies in guinea-pigs show middle ear gas partial pressures as follows: P_{N_2} 82.4%, P_{O_2} 7.6%, P_{CO_2} 10%, which is similar to their levels in mixed venous blood and quite dissimilar to atmospheric air.

Middle ear gas deficiency may be secondary, not to eustachian tube input failure, but to excessive loss of middle ear gas by increased diffusion into the blood which is enhanced as a result of the increased vascularization of inflammation. Gas diffusion into the blood may in part explain the negative middle ear pressure developing in chronic inflammatory middle ear disease when there is reduced mastoid pneumatization. The relative contributions of the eustachian tube and diffusion to the steady state gas composition in the middle ear is uncertain (Sade and Luntz, 1993), but these more recent values for middle ear gas composition are similar to those found in previous studies in animals and humans. It has been postulated that there is a chemoreceptor mechanism within the middle ear under neural control, perhaps mediated by stretch receptors in the tympanic membrane (Rockley and Hawkes, 1992). Finally, there has been the suggestion that sniff induced negative pressure changes may lead to the development of negative middle ear pressure and atelectasis (Magnusson, 1989).

Nasopharyngeal disproportion

Craniofacial abnormalities

In Down's syndrome there is an increase in the basal angle of the skull in relation to the cranial cavity. This may be responsible for the resultant nasopharyngeal disproportion and the eustachian tube dysfunction found in the syndrome. It may also explain the relationship in other syndromes with craniofacial abnormalities (Hunter's and Hurler's syndromes). However, the increased susceptibility to infection in these cases may also be a contributory cause of the middle ear change.

Adenoids and the nasopharynx

A survey by Hibbert (1977) showed that 80% of otolaryngologists in the UK advised adenoidectomy as part of the treatment for otitis media with effusion. In 1991 a similar survey showed that 64% advised such treatment (Smith and Maw, 1991). Almost all studies of the nasopharynx and adenoids have been performed with lateral skull radiographs, usually with lateral cephalometry. Physiological variations in the size of the nasopharyngeal airway occur during sleep and during crying, and in relation to position of the mouth and movement of the soft palate during swallowing. Jeans *et al.* (1981) showed that growth of the adenoid outstrips that of the nasopharynx in children aged between 3 and 5 years of age with resultant reduction in the nasopharyngeal airway. Subsequently growth of the nasopharynx increases while the adenoids remain relatively unchanged, and thus the airway increases. Linder-Aronson (1970) confirmed that enlarged adenoids led to mouth breathing and when nasal obstruction was present it was associated with a particular type of facial skeleton. There was agreement between clinical assessment of adenoid size and measurements taken from radiographs. Nasal airflow was lower for larger than smaller adenoids but increased following adenoidectomy. His studies supported the hypothesis that adenoids affect the mode of breathing which then influences the individual's dentition.

There has been correlation of lateral radiographic findings with adenoid size (Hibbert and Whitehouse, 1978) but there are errors due to rotation (Johnson, Murray and Maran, 1983) and due to interobserver variability (Maw, Jeans and Fernando, 1981). The relationship between large adenoids and acute otitis media in young children has been demonstrated (Quarnberg, 1981) and between abnormality of the vomero-ethmoid suture in children with otitis media with effusion (McNicholl, 1983). Relationships between nasopharyngeal dimensions and the presence of otitis media with effusion have been shown (Maw, Smith and Lance, 1991; Uhari *et al.*, 1991).

In children with a repaired cleft palate the improvement in speech following palatal repair was related to adenoid size (Gereau and Shprintzen, 1988).

Clearly morphological differences in the skull base and nasopharynx may be responsible for the underlying changes in the condition of the eustachian tube which are associated with ascending infection from the nasopharynx leading to development of otitis media with effusion.

Clinical presentation

By definition, the quiescent phase of otitis media with effusion has none of the signs and symptoms usually attributed to infection of the middle ear cleft. The most frequent presentation is with covert or overt hearing loss. The hearing fluctuates in severity particularly in relation to seasonal change and the presence or absence of intercurrent infection. When covert in infants and young children it may present with impaired speech and language development (Rapin, 1979). There may be behavioural and scholastic difficulties, but only rarely do younger children themselves complain of hearing difficulty. It is frequently first suspected by parents or detected on routine screening tests, either of hearing by audiometric screening or by assessment of middle ear function with tympanometry. Indirect symptoms also relating to hearing loss, such as insularity, shouting or increasing the volume of the television, are commonly found. Otalgia often occurs, usually as a result of secondary infection of the fluid within the middle ear cleft. Invariably it results from pathogenic bacteria within the nasopharynx which ascend the eustachian tube. It frequently coincides with a minor respiratory tract infection, and sometimes follows sinus infection or an episode of allergic rhinitis. It maybe a sequel to swimming. In some cases the earache is followed by mucoid or mucopurulent otorrhoea.

In some children, hearing impairment may be associated with significant nasal or postnasal obstruction and the latter can be detcted by hyponasality of speech. There may be upper respiratory tract symptoms reflecting non-specific catarrhal conditions, rhinosinusitis, or nasal allergy and, in the latter, there may be lower respiratory tract symptoms, usually reflecting more generalized atopy. Pathological nasal secretions, nasal oedema and minor nasal septal deviations maybe related to negative middle ear pressures and otitis media with effusion (Van Cauwenberge and Kluyskens, 1984). There may be symptoms of obvious palatal abnormality or syndromic conditions with craniofacial abnormality.

Diagnosis

There are five aspects to confirmation of the presence of otitis media with effusion.

The history of hearing loss obtained from parents may not always correctly identify the duration or severity of the condition or they may not be aware of the disability. In a study in a deprived area only 19% of children with bilateral hearing loss comparable to that found in severe glue ear caused parental concern (Watkin, Baldwin and Laoide, 1990).

Otoscopy should be performed with a halogen light source and a pneumatic attachment to the otoscope to give a reasonable degree of specificity but with significantly better sensitivity. Values of 75% and 90% respectively are reported for experienced clincians (Paradise, Smith and Bluestone, 1975; Cantekin, Beery and Bluestone, 1977; Maw, 1979).

Use of an operating microscope with magnification will further improve the diagnostic accuracy. There is considerable variation in the appearance of the tympanic membrane. The colour and loss of translucency range from pale grey or amber to black, or the so-called 'blue drum'. It may be thickened, dull and opalescent or thin and reflective. There may be increased vascularization of radial vessels and an increase in malleolar vasculature. Fluid levels or air bubbles may be visible but the degree of retraction of the pars tensa may be assessed by the extent of splitting and derangement of the light reflex and by the rotation and displacement of the malleus handle, when there is prominence of the lateral process of the malleus.

With progression of the disease there may be indrawing of the pars flaccida to a variable degree and this attic retraction is in some cases associated with erosion of the outer attic wall when the neck of the malleus becomes visible. In part, the degree of retraction of the tympanic membrane reflects the negative middle ear pressure and the reduced mobility of the membrane can easily be assessed with a Seigle's or similar type of pneumatic otoscope. Tuning fork tests may be helpful, particularly in children over 4 years of age. A negative Rinne test is said to predict a hearing loss in excess of 15–20 dB (Yung and Morris, 1981), though our own studies refute this suggestion (Capper, Slack and Maw, 1987). Clinical voice tests failed to detect one-fifth of children with hearing impairment of 20 dB or less (Dempster and Mackenzie, 1992).

Tympanometry was first introduced in Scandinavia, then the UK and later into the USA. It is rapid and reliable, even in infants, and equipment should have a pressure range of − 400 mm to + 200 mm of water in order to distinguish between the established condition and milder forms of the disease. It provides an effective screening test for the detection of negative middle ear pressure but will not always distinguish between a pressure change with or without presence of an effusion. Diagnostic predictability of 84% may be achieved with a simple peak versus no peak pattern of classification. Fiellau Nikolajsen (1983) modified Jerger's (1970) nomenclature, subdividing tympanograms into four types.

Type A – middle ear pressure + 200 to − 99 mm of water
Type C1 – middle ear pressure − 100 to − 199 mm of water
Type C2 – middle ear pressure − 200 to − 400 mm of water
Type B – flat traces without a well-defined compliance maximum.

Dempster and Mackenzie (1991) showed that only 2% of children with a bilateral hearing loss of 25 dB or more did not have flat, type B tympanograms ($P = 0.002$). A type B trace was 93% sensitive in detecting otitis media with effusion which was associated with a 25 dB hearing loss but it was only 76% specific, with a positive predictive value of 49% and negative predictive value of 98%. Development of new microtympanometers and automatic impedance tympanoscopes may aid general practitioners in their ability to diagnose otitis media with effusion. However, they may lack the ability to create a sufficient middle ear pressure (De Melker, 1992) and may lead to over-referral (Maw, 1992). The impedance tympanoscope has been considered unsuited for scientific purposes (Moller and Tos, 1990).

Pure tone audiometry is of only limited diagnostic value for the identification of otitis media with effusion. It does provide some assessment of the severity of the disease and can be used to monitor progress and the effects of treatment. It may be difficult with children under the age of 4 years but they can be tested by the Institute of Hearing Research McCormick automated toy discrimination test and by visual reinforced audiometry (Haggard and Hughes, 1991). Comparisons have been made between pure tone audiometry thresholds and tympanometric findings. Fiellau Nikolajsen (1983) showed dry ears to have a mean hearing threshold of 17 dB, minimal otitis media had 23 dB, moderate otitis media with effusion 29 dB and 'impacted' middle ears 34 dB. Overall, in 79 out of 88 ears tested, the mean hearing threshold averaged 23 dB.

The speech awareness threshold in infants aged between 7 and 24 months with otitis media with effusion was found to be in the order of 25 dB hearing level (Fria, Cantekin and Eichler, 1985). Older chldren from 2 to 12 years of age had mean three frequency pure tone audiometric and speech reception thresholds of 24.5 dB and 22.7 dB respectively.

Comparing the predictive value of pneumatic otoscopy and tympanometry to confirm an immobile tympanic membrane, the presence of a type B tympanometric trace showed values of 88% and 89% respectively, without any improved accuracy when both were used together (Toner and Mains, 1990). However, other recent studies (Finitzo *et al.*, 1992) confirmed tympanometry to have a higher specificity (86%) than otoscopy (58%) compared with sensitivity values of 90% and 93% respectively, reflecting the benefit of tympanometry in the diagnosis of non-effusion states. These differences may reflect clinical experience of the observers.

The 'gold standard' for diagnosis of middle ear effusion is *myringotomy and aspiration of the fluid.* The cause of concern in many studies is the unacceptably high dry tap rate, reaching 34% in some studies (Black *et al.*, 1990). It has been suggested that nitrous oxide anaesthesia displaces middle ear fluid at operation (Gates and Cooper, 1980; Kennedy and Gore, 1982; Marshall and Cable, 1982). A recent study (Rees and Freeland, 1992) showed a 13% dry tap rate with abnormal tympanometry immediately prior to surgery under nitrous oxide anaesthesia. However, it is possible that due to the inability to develop a pressure of in excess of -200 mm of water, there was failure to distinguish between type B and C2 curves.

Management
Medical treatment

All treatment should take into account the known important epidemiological data. There is a high rate of spontaneous resolution of otitis media with effusion. Most episodes are short lived and 50% will resolve within 3 months. Only 5% will have persistent disease for more than a year (Zielhuis, Rach and Van den Broek, 1989).

Longitudinal studies show that there is seasonal variation in the condition. In addition, relapses and remissions may occur several years after onset of the disease and following initial treatment. As with studies of surgical treatment many trials of medical treatment have failed to apply strict and appropriate entry criteria. They have often evaluated outcome measures only in the very short term, frequently on the completion of treatment or usually within a few weeks of completion and seldom longer than 8 months following completion.

A wide variety of medications has been assessed. No improvement was seen following treatment with 0.5% ephedrine hydrochloride nose drops or an antihistimine sympathomimetic amine mixture (Fraser, Mehta and Fraser, 1977). Mucolytics such as bromhexine hydrochloride have not been shown to have a long-term effect (Stewart *et al.*, 1985) and there has been no further report of the effects of gaseous ventilation of the middle ear cleft with sulphur hexafluoride (Andreasson *et al.*, 1983). Though initial studies with autoinflation of the eustachian tube produced equivocal results and more recent attempts with conventional balloons have been ineffective (Brooker and McNeice, 1992), use of more sophisticated autoinflation equipment has been shown to have short-term therapeutic effect (Stangerup, Sederberg-Olsen and Balle, 1992), particularly if there is adequate compliance (Blanshard, Maw and Bawden, 1992, 1993).

The management of associated nasal conditions or nasal allergy may improve eustachian tube malfunction and may alter outcome in some children (Scadding *et al.*, 1993).

More recently, studies have evaluated the effects of antibiotics, either alone or in combination with steroids, anti-inflammatory drugs, decongestants, antihistamines and prostaglandin inhibitors. A recent meta analysis of 10 out of 32 trials carried out between 1980 and 1990, in which there was adequate randomization control and use of either placebo or no drug control, assessed 20 measures of validity. However, the end point was absence of effusion at the first post-treatment assessment. For 1325 children there was a rate of difference of 22.8% (95% CI 10.5–35.1) (Rosenfeld and Post, 1992). The authors concluded that antibiotics have a clinical and statistically significant cure rate but it seems likely that this is only in the short term, bearing in mind the end point analysis. They also noted that children with chronic bilateral otitis media with effusion not related to recent episodes of acute otitis media had lower natural cure rates.

A short-term report of the effectiveness of co-trimoxazole (Marks, Mills and Shaheen, 1981) was not supported by longer-term studies (Marks, Mills and Shaheen, 1983). Of the recent trials of antibiotics alone, Mandel *et al.* (1991) showed a slight benefit at 2 weeks but none at 4 weeks following amoxicillin for 2 weeks, compared with placebo. There was no benefit from erythromycin-sulphisoxazole or cefaclor. The study confirmed previous work demonstrating the short-term benefit from amoxicillin whether alone or in combination with decongestant/antihistamine, though after 2 weeks of antibiotic medication effusions were still present in 69.8% of cases (Mandel *et al.*, 1987). Following treatment for 10 days with amoxicillin and clavulanic acid, compared with amoxicillin alone without placebo, there was a favourable result at 10 days which was not sustained to 4 weeks (Chan *et al.*, 1988).

In another study, amoxicillin and clavulanic acid were prescribed for a month and compared with placebo. Sixty-one per cent of the treated group and 30% of the placebo cases resolved at the end of treatment. The benefit was maintained for 8 months from the end of treatment and there were no differences in tympanograms in either group (Thomsen *et al.*, 1989). The combination of amoxil with prednisolone produced a significant complete or partial recovery from otitis media with effusion in children without oversized adenoids compared with those treated by amoxil alone or placebo (Podoshin *et al.*, 1990). Comparison of trimethoprim with sulphamethoxazole for 4 weeks, prednisolone for 2 weeks and aluminium ibuprofen for 2 weeks with no treatment controls showed better resolution after 2 weeks with the steroid and antibiotic group than controls or those treated with ibuprofen. The difference was smaller at 4 weeks and was not detectable at 12 months (Giebink *et al.*, 1991).

The study of amoxicillin for 2 weeks in combination with a decongestant and antihistamine was said to show twice the resolution in the treatment groups than with placebo to a 4-week end point. The effect was more marked in unilateral cases of a shorter duration and the recurrences after treatment were similar in both groups, though there were more side effects in the treatment group (Mandel *et al.*, 1987). Statistical interpretation of this paper has been the subject of considerable debate (Cantekin, McGuire and Potter, 1990). The combination of antibiotics with naproxen as a prostaglandin inhibitor showed no effect at 30 days on acute otitis media in relation to the occurrence or persistence of subsequent middle ear effusion (Varsano, Valoritz and Grossman, 1989).

None of the studies with oral steroid treatment for otitis media with effusion followed patients for more than a few weeks after discontinuing treatment, but a meta analysis of six trials comparing oral steroids with placebo showed that following 7–14 days of treatment there was a 3.6 times increased likelihood that the ears would be effusion free at the end of therapy. Recent studies with surfactant have shown equivocal results in animal models and in a small number of treated children (Kobayashi *et al.*, 1993).

It seems likely from the results of these studies that a consensus view of the current state of medical treatment for otitis media with effusion is that no medication has been shown to effect a long-term cure. However, with prolonged therapy for several weeks, particularly against beta-lactamase producing organisms using a combination of amoxicillin and clavulanic acid, there is some benefit at the end of treatment which may be sustained in the short term. Furthermore, most of these studies assess tympanometric change rather than hearing gain. Medication is unlikely to correct the hearing disability associated with the condition as rapidly as aspiration of middle ear contents and re-aeration with a ventilation tube.

The development of vaccines against infections of the respiratory tract may hold some hope for improved management in the future. Recent studies with respiratory syncytial virus (RSV) and other viral agents have shown that oral immunization in both human and animal models is highly effective in inducing secretory IgA antibody responses in the upper and lower respiratory tract. Subsequent challenge indicates that enteric immunization with RSV is associated with complete protection against re-infection in the lung though only partial immunity was conferred to the upper airway. Intranasal immunization on the other hand affords complete protection in the upper and lower respiratory tract (Ogra and Nadal, 1993). Similar studies have been carried out in relation to pneumococcal otitis media in animal models (Yoshimura *et al.*, 1993). It may be possible to immunize against *Haemophilus influenzae* B disease and recent studies have shown vaccines to be immunogenic when given to infants at 2, 3 and 4 months. There is thus the potential to treat such infection in the nasopharynx, in the middle ear and in the upper and lower respiratory tracts (Cartwright, 1992).

Hearing aids

No study has yet evaluated the use of a hearing aid as a primary treatment for chronic otitis media with effusion.

Surgical treatment

Introduction

The number of operative procedures on tonsils and adenoids has diminished on a world-wide basis in recent years. Black (1985) showed a reduction of 40% of adenotonsillectomy operations in the UK between 1967 and 1980. In contrast there was a steady increase in the number of myringotomy and ventilation tube insertion procedures during the same period. However, Hospital Inpatient Enquiry data for 1985 show 60 000 such procedures and Hospital Activity data for 1989 shows an almost identical number, so perhaps the rate of myringotomy and ventilation tube operations has reached a plateau. An additional 16% of cases are anticipated to have been carried out in the private sector (Nicholl, Beeby and Williams, 1989). A recent Dutch study showed that at least 18.5% of children aged $7\frac{1}{2}$–8 years had undergone adenoidectomies, 8.7% myringotomies and 11.5% ventilation tubes (Schilder, Zielhuis and Van den Broek, 1993). At ages 3, 5 and 7 years, 1%, 4% and 6% respectively of Swedish children had been treated for otitis media with effusion with tubes (Rassmussen, 1993).

Surgery should only be recommended for persistent disease with significant hearing loss causing symptomatic morbidity. The condition should be observed otoscopically and monitored with tympanometry and hearing tests for at least 3 months prior to listing for operation, and reassessment should be made at a pre-admission clinic to confirm persistence (De Melker, 1992).

Surgical treatment options for otitis media with effusion are either to the ear to drain the fluid and prevent recurrence, or to the nasopharynx in an attempt to induce an effect on eustachian tube function and ascending infection. Myringotomy alone with aspiration of middle ear fluid does not produce long-term benefit. The development of a wide variety of ventilation tubes has followed Armstrong's initial report (1954). Ventilation tubes do not cure the condition but produce temporary improvement in hearing thresholds while they continue to function (Mandel *et al.*, 1992). They may be divided into conventional short-stay tubes, e.g. Shepard or Shah types which remain in place for approximately 12 months, or long-stay tympanostomy tubes which may remain in place for several years. Due to the prolonged course of the disease it is likely that there will be a significant need for re-insertion of short-term tubes before the child eventually outgrows the underlying changes which perpetuate the condition (Curley, 1986). In an effort to alter eustachian tube function and ascending infection, adenoidectomy has been recommended either as a primary or as a secondary treatment procedure. Frequently it is performed in combination with insertion of a ventilation tube. Certain children may require limited surgery to reduce nasal congestion and resolve intrasinus infection. Surveys of management of otitis media with effusion by British consultant otolaryngologists suggest disparity in treatment regimens (Smith and Maw, 1991). Nevertheless, adenoidectomy in combination with myringotomy alone or with ventilation tube insertion was the surgical option recommended by 64% of surgeons.

Myringotomy and short-stay ventilation tube insertion

Myringotomy for aspiration of serous or mucoid effusion can be made in a radial fashion, either in the anteroinferior or anterosuperior quadrants, avoiding excessive damage to the fibrous layer and thus preventing development of a thin triangular scar at the site of incision. Thermal myringotomies offer no significant benefit over the use of a sharp, thin myringotome. In chronic otitis media with effusion the myringotomy incision rapidly heals with re-accumulation of the fluid, and insertion of a ventilation tube or grommet facilitates longer lasting middle ear reventilation. The tube is held with fine forceps by the flange or by the attached wire, but not by the lumen. The edge of the flange is introduced into the incision and the remainder of the tube is pressed into position with a fine needle or with the tip of the myringotome. It is held in place by the tension of the separated fibres of the middle layer. The lumen should be patent after insertion. The procedure should be achieved without any haemorrhage into the middle layer of the tympanic membrane which is known to be associated with the development of tympanosclerosis (Parker, Maw and Powell, 1990). The type of material used and whether or not the tube is in the anterosuperior or inferior quadrants, probably does not affect the time of extrusion. However, tube design, experience of the operator, and whether or not it fits loosely when inserted, do affect extrusion (Mackenzie, 1984; Moore, 1990). Ventilation tubes produce a short-term hearing gain and improvement in speech reception thresholds to 20 dB or less (Gundersen and Tonning, 1976). However, longer-term studies show less satisfactory hearing thresholds (Gundersen, Tonning and Kveberg, 1984). There is no beneficial hearing gain after 12 months (Brown, Richards and Ambegaokar, 1978). Twenty-four months following extrusion of tubes inserted into only one ear in bilateral cases of otitis media with effusion there was no difference in hearing thresholds. Recurrence and persistence of fluid occurred in 30% of treated and non-treated ears (Kilby, Richards and Hart, 1972).

Long-stay ventilation tubes

This variety of tube is designed to remain *in situ* for long periods of time and depends on large intratympanic flanges for sustained retention. They are frequently used in more severely atelectatic tympanic membranes, often following previous treatment with a conventional short-stay tube on one or more occasions. Paparella or Goode type T tubes are most frequently used. They are associated with an increased rate of otorrhoea and with a greater incidence of persistent perforation. The greater complication rate may reflect the use in more severely affected cases. However, even when used for long-term ventilation in barotrauma with healthy tympanic membranes, crusts accumulate around the base of the T tubes giving pressure necrosis and often leading to large and persistent perforations. They do not protect against attic disease (Skinner, Lesser and Richards, 1988).

Adenoidectomy

The rationale for adenoidectomy for treatment of otitis media with effusion was based on the assumption that, in some way, the adenoids affect eustachian tube function. Initially it was thought that a transudate developed within the middle ear cleft by the 'ex vacuo' theory. Such a suggestion is supported by the occurrence of negative middle ear pressure in association with ipsilateral nasal obstruction and by the frequent finding of a unilateral middle ear effusion in association with postnasal space carcinoma involving the eustachian tube cushion. It might be anticipated that adenoidectomy would be more effective in those children presenting with significant symptoms of nasal obstruction, snoring and speech hyponasality. Often these are the cases that are excluded from randomly allocated studies. Recommendation for surgery in children with small, non-obstructive adenoids is based on the premise that they act as a focus of potential ascending eustachian tube infection. There is increasing evidence of a relationship between pathogenic bacteria in the nasopharynx and the subsequent development of otitis media with effusion, possibly involving an immune response. But some studies show no difference in the nasopharyngeal flora in children with otitis media with effusion compared to controls (Maw and Speller, 1985). It is possible that adenoid removal results in an altered nasopharyngeal pressure relationship during swallowing which may affect tubal function.

Tonsillectomy

There would appear to be *no* justification to recommend tonsillectomy for treatment of otitis media with effusion (Maw, 1983; Maw and Herod, 1986).

Randomized controlled trials of surgical treatment

A properly designed, randomized controlled trial is required to show the effectiveness of an intervention. In relation to otitis media with effusion the requirements for such a trial are clearly-defined entry criteria with confirmation of persistent disease on two occasions over a period of not less than 3 months using pneumatic otoscopy and tympanometry. Haggard and Hughes (1991) have extensively reviewed the problems of screening for middle ear disorders with tympanometry. Depending on the criteria used for confirmation of middle ear fluid, referral rates may vary from 9% with the Hertshels criteria, to 32–36% with the ASHA Nashville criteria (Lous, 1987). Investigators using hospital cases for controls should be aware of the high rate of B tympanograms in children in paediatric wards (Wolthers, 1990).

Depending on the age of the child, assessment of hearing thresholds is required by pure tone or free field audiometric testing. Outcome measures should assess change in middle ear status by otoscopy and tympanometry, and should also monitor improvement in hearing thresholds and in those disabilities associated with hearing loss. Studies should take into account the various risk factors and acknowledge the spontaneous remission and relapse rate. Use of matched ears of the same severity of disease should take into account the theoretical possibility that treatment of one ear may affect the condition of the other ear.

The trials reported to date have been the subject of careful appraisal and review (Stephenson and Haggard, 1992). Nineteen randomized controlled trials have reviewed treatment by adenoidectomy, adenotonsillectomy, myringotomy and ventilation tube insertion, either separately or in combination and frequently with one ear used as a control. Almost all of the trials have at least some design problem. These include:

Small numbers (Archard, 1967; Brown, Richards and Ambegaokar, 1978; Rynnel Dagoo; Ahlbom and Schiratzki, 1978; Fiellau Nikolajsen, Falbe-Hansen and Knudstrup, 1980; Bulman, Brook and Berry, 1984; Widemar *et al.*, 1985; Rach *et al.*, 1991)
High dry tap rate (Gates *et al.*, 1987 (32%); Black *et al.*, 1990 (34%))
An unknown dry tap rate (Brown, Richards and Ambegaokar, 1978; Bulman, Brook and Berry, 1984; Bonding and Tos, 1985; Rach *et al.*, 1991)
A short period of follow-up (Richards *et al.*, 1971 (12 months); To, Pahor and Robin, 1984 (12 months); Rach *et al.*, 1991 (6 months); Dempster, Browning and Gatehouse, 1993 (12 months))

Twelve month follow-up studies of ventilation tubes only compared with adenoidectomy plus tube insertion are obviously not long enough to show any extra benefit due to adenoidectomy since most short-stay tubes remain in place for approximately 8–12 months (Gates *et al.*, 1987; Mandel *et al.*, 1989). In some studies there is a high loss to follow up (Black *et al.*, 1990 – 39% loss at 2 years; Paradise *et al.*, 1990 – 47% lost by the third year). Unilateral and bilateral cases may be considered together (Gates *et al.*, 1987). In some studies there is a change in treatment during the study (Mandel *et al.*, 1989) in which tubes eventually replace a myringotomy alone or no treatment. Some studies fail to mention whether observations are made blind (Rynnel Dagoo, Ahlbom and Schiratzki, 1978; Paradise *et al.*, 1990). Exclusion of children with severe nasal obstruction (Rynnel Dagoo, Ahlbom and Schiratzki, 1978) or those with severe hearing loss of over 35 dB (Mandel *et al.*, 1992) result in bias.

In some studies there is no assessment of change in hearing (Roydhouse, 1980) and in other studies some groups have had revision surgery (Lildholt, 1983 – 17% revision tube rate; Maw, 1983; Maw and Herod, 1986 – 26–54% revision rate). In other studies revision surgery has been avoided by use of a hearing aid (Dempster, Browning and Gatehouse, 1993). There is a need for further studies to confirm or refute these uncertainties.

Effects due to adenoidectomy and following ventilation tube insertion

Ventilation tubes have been shown in almost all studies to produce a short-term hearing gain (Maw and Herod, 1986; Black *et al.*, 1990; Dempster, Browning and Gatehouse, 1993). Some studies have shown no difference between the effects of adenoidectomy plus tubes compared to tubes alone at 6 and 12 months (Brown, Richards and Ambegaokar, 1978). Others have shown no difference in hearing thresholds at 2 years between adenoidectomy alone, tubes alone or both in combination (Gates *et al.*, 1987); and some have shown short-term benefit at 3 and 6 months from adenoidectomy and from tubes (Bulman, Brook and Berry, 1984). While tubes are more effective than adenoidectomy alone at 6 months, slightly better hearing thresholds have been reported with both procedures in combination in boys compared with adenoidectomy or tubes alone (Dempster, Browning and Gatehouse, 1993). Though adenoidectomy was not found to produce extra hearing gain over ventilation tubes alone, it produced better normalization of middle ear function (Black *et al.*, 1990). Cases treated with adenoidectomy have been shown to have 40% less time with otitis media compared with controls during the first follow-up year, 37% less time during the second follow-up year, but no differences were found in the third year (Paradise *et al.*, 1990). Greater relapse rates were found in non-adenoidectomy cases which required 9% more tubes (Roydhouse, 1980). There is a clear relationship between effectiveness of adenoidectomy and the age at operation (Maw and Parker, 1993).

The maximum mean improvement in hearing thresholds of the three comparable studies (Maw and Herod, 1986; Black *et al.*, 1990; Dempster, Browning and Gatehouse, 1993) was less than 12 dB at 6 months after surgery. Clearly the clinical significance of this level of improvement requires evaluation in terms of correction of disability. The hearing gain following intervention gradually reduces, partly because of recurrent fluid in the treated group and partly because of spontaneous improvement in the no treatment group. There seems little significant difference between the effects of tube insertion or adenoidectomy. There is, however, significant benefit for the combined procedure in terms of otoscopic clearance, tympanometric change and hearing gain (Maw and Bawden, 1993) (Figure 7.2). A single Shepard tube alone gives a short-lived effect of about 10 months whereas adenoidectomy produces a significantly longer lasting effect for several years (Maw, 1988; Maw and Bawden, 1993). Further studies are required to assess other aspects of disability which result from hearing loss, together with quality of life issues, and the changing need for health care resources following treatment (Facione, 1991). There are obviously important implications in cost–benefit terms for health care purchaser and provider services. Unfortunately meta analysis of 12 randomized controlled trials for surgical treatment for otitis media with effusion has not produced helpful results on which generalized treatment protocols can be recommended (Bodner *et al.*, 1991).

Spontaneous resolution of chronic otitis media with effusion

There are few studies in which severely affected cases which would otherwise have been treated surgically have been followed in the long term and compared with cases submitted to surgical treatment. Thus few comparisons have been made between development of sequelae due to the disease and those which are a consequence of treatment. Our own studies have shown that in cases of persistent otitis media with effusion assessed with otoscopy, tympanometry and audiometry on three occasions during a 3-month period and having a previous history of hearing loss for an average of 18 months, there is a progressive clearance of effusions without any treatment. After 1 year resolution occurs in 20% of such cases, 40% at 2 years, 50% at 3 years, 60% at 4 years, 70% at 5 years, 85% at 7 years and 95% at 10 years (Figure 7.3). There is a commensurate change in tympanometric conversion from flat type B traces to peaked A, C1 or C2 curves. These changes are associated with a progressive hearing improvement of mean six frequency audiometric thresholds from 31.9 dB preoperatively to 28.0 dB in the first year, 23.4 dB in the third year and 18.6 dB

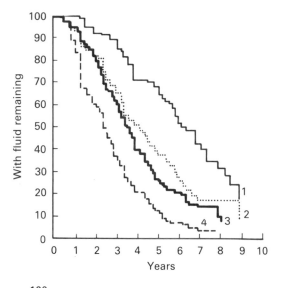

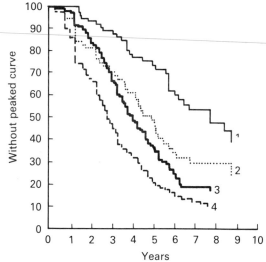

Figure 7.2 Survival analysis data to show otoscopic and tympanometric changes in untreated ears (1) and in ears treated with ventilation tube insertion alone (2) adenoidectomy alone (3) and with both procedures in combination (4) during a 10-year follow up. (From Maw and Bawden, 1993)

in the fifth year with 16.9 dB in the tenth year (Maw and Bawden, 1993). In these cases the median overall duration of the condition without treatment was 6.1 years assessed otoscopically and 7.8 years by tympanometry (Maw and Bawden, 1993) (Figure 7.4).

Prognosis

The outcome of the untreated condition is known to be significantly related to a number of the risk factors

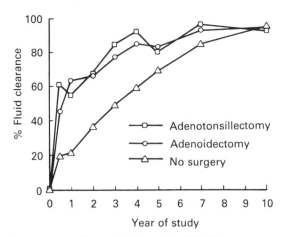

Figure 7.3 Resolution of otitis media with effusion spontaneously in untreated ears (no surgery) and as a result of adenoidectomy and adenotonsillectomy in ears followed for 10 years and assessed otoscopically

for development of the condition. Zielhuis *et al.* (1990) have shown that age, gender and the season are related to duration of the disease and ultimate recovery. There is a relationship between the duration of otitis media with effusion following acute otitis in terms of sibling history of ear infections and those children who have not been breast fed (Teele, Klein and Rosner, 1989).

We have shown that outcome following adenoidectomy is related to some extent in the short term by the degree of postnasal space obstruction, as reflected by the postnasal airway. This is probably related to age and growth (Maw, 1985 a,b). Quarnberg *et al.* (1988) have shown that reduced mastoid pneumatization is a poor prognostic sign for resolution of otitis media with effusion. Changes in middle ear volume demonstrated by impedance measurements following ventilation tube insertion confirm that the smaller the volume the greater the postoperative problems (Suetake *et al.*, 1990). Nakano and Sato (1990) showed similar findings in a comparable study in relation to mastoid pneumatization. These findings may be responsible for the poor prognostic finding in relation to recurrence of effusion in cases with 'glue under pressure' (Salam and Wengraf, 1992). Daly *et al.* (1993) have shown that the otorrhoea following ventilation tube insertion is related to the presence of ear canal and middle ear effusion pathogens. The length of time to tube extrusion is affected by parental smoking and by fever during the first postoperative week. Boys (21%) are more likely than girls (7%) to have repeat tube insertions. Our own work supports the deleterious effect of smoking on outcome following surgery (Maw *et al.*, 1992). Robinson (1988) showed that revision ventilation tube insertion was more likely in those in whom the original operation was performed between July and October and those in which the tube extruded within 6 months, but there was no relationship to gender.

Nevertheless, in unselected cases detected with tympanometric screening the natural history of the untreated condition is usually spontaneous resolution.

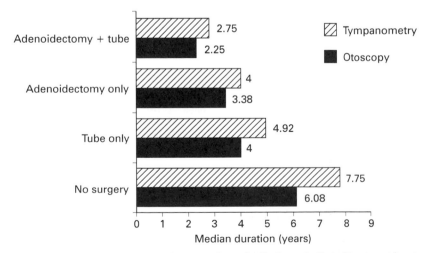

Figure 7.4 Histogram showing duration of untreated otitis media with effusion and effect of treatment by otoscopy and tympanometry. The duration of history of hearing loss from the parents has been added to the 3-month period of preoperative observation and to the duration of observed otitis media with effusion postoperatively. Fluid was said to persist until the ear was reported otoscopically dry or there was persistence of an A, C1 or C2 tympanometric peak on consecutive visits for a period of more than 12 months. The time was taken to be half-way from the interval incorporating the change

The median duration in Dutch children was 3 months or less, the 95th centile was at 12 months. Resolution of otitis media with effusion occurred in about 50% of ears after 3 months, but about half of the ears which recovered had a further episode of otitis media with effusion (Zielhuis, Rach and Van den Broek, 1989) (see Figure 7.1).

Sequelae

Permanent sequelae and disability may occur as a consequence of the disease process or as a result of the effects of treatment. Some are transitory, mild and of little clinical importance but others may be severe, permanent and associated with significant morbidity. Structural and functional changes may develop in the middle ear cleft and in the inner ear. In 964 Dutch 7.5–8-year-old children, 26% had moderate to severe otoscopic abnormalities and 19% had mild abnormalities. Twenty nine per cent had received surgical treatment for various otolaryngological diseases (Schilder, Zielhuis and Van den Broek, 1993). Hearing impairment, even if transitory, may have consequences for speech, language, learning and behaviour.

Middle ear

Scarring, atelectasis and attic retraction

In cases where effusions are left to resolve spontaneously and middle ear reventilation has occurred, there is resolution of the pathological changes in the mucosa of the middle ear cleft. Sequelae are found but only in a small number of cases. There may be tympanic membrane scarring, though tympanosclerosis occurs in less than 5% of untreated, affected ears. Attic retraction and erosion may develop.

In the longer term there may be atrophic changes in the pars tensa or atelectasis which may affect the ossicular chain producing myringoincudostapediopexy. Myringoincudostapediopexy occurs after otitis media with effusion in 0.5% of children aged 5 years, 2.5% aged 7 years and 4.2% aged 16 years. In 40% it is stable, in 36% it fluctuates and in 24% it ultimately resolves (Tos, Stangerup and Larsen, 1992). Apart from tympanosclerosis, these atelectatic tympanic membrane changes and abnormalities in the attic are as common in ears which have not received treatment as in those treated with insertion of ventilation tubes (Larsen, Tos and Stangerup, 1988; Maw, 1989; Tos and Poulsen, 1980; Maw, 1995). It seems that the atelectatic changes in the pars tensa of the tympanic membrane and those seen in the attic relate directly to the severity and duration of the disease and not to treatment. A very slight hearing loss can be demonstrated in association with mild to moderate attic retraction and more marked and permanent hearing loss is associated with atelectasis of the pars tensa. Ventilation tube insertion does not seem to prevent the development of attic retraction. Tube insertion is unlikely to affect the more generalized atelectatic changes and, indeed, if treatment with tubes is repeated it may worsen the situation.

Tympanosclerosis

Almost all studies have shown that approximately 50% of ears treated with ventilation tubes develop some degree of tympanosclerosis (Brown, Richards and Ambegaokar 1978; Tos, Bonding and Poulsen 1983; Maw, 1991). Almost the same degree of sclerotic change can be induced by a single insertion of a tube compared with cases in which tubes are inserted on more than one occasion (Maw, 1991). One tube is able to induce the severest forms of sclerotic change with a horseshoe-shaped plaque almost completely replacing the tympanic membrane. Three and 5 years after tube insertion no hearing impairment can be demonstrated as a consequence of the sclerosis. With longer-term follow up in the most severely affected cases, a loss of 3–4 dB is attributable to the sclerotic change (Maw, 1989). Minor degrees of sclerosis do not seem to be of clinical significance. The tympanosclerosis is clearly due to the insertion of a tube. The incidence and severity of sclerosis decrease if a 'mini' type of tube is inserted, although this is at the expense of earlier extrusion and a greater recurrence of effusion than with conventional tubes (Hampal, Flood and Kumar, 1991). There is increasing evidence that haemorrhage at the time of tube insertion is partly responsible for the sclerotic change (Parker, Maw and Powell, 1990; Dawes *et al.*, 1991). The mass or inertial component of the tube may cause sufficient shear stresses to rupture fibrils within the lamina propria and the sclerosis may be a reparative effect (Lesser, Williams and Skinner, 1988). Other studies have shown that a high partial pressure of oxygen may be toxic to the middle ear mucosa. Felding and Lildholt (1988) have shown that insertion of a ventilation tube increases the intratympanic P_{O_2} by a factor of three. More recently, Hellstrom *et al.* (1993) have shown proliferation of keratinizing squamous epithelium in the development of tympanosclerosis as a consequence of a raised P_{O_2} within the middle ear. Local application of N-acetylcysteine in rabbits with otitis media with effusion reduces the middle ear mucosal inflammation and prevents fibrosis, perhaps by reducing the hyperoxic state within the middle ear (Ovesen, Paaske and Elbrond, 1992).

Otorrhoea

Mucoid or purulent otorrhoea following insertion of a ventilation tube is usually a relatively short-term complication which responds to aural toilet and installation of antibiotic and steroid drops. The use of non-aminoglycoside antibiotic drops will reduce any potential risk to the inner ear through the tube, particularly if a displacement technique is used (Mills, Albizzati and Todd, 1990). Differences in management of this complication by otolaryngologists and general practitioners are recognized in relation to the prescription of oral or topical antibiotics (Robb and Johnston, 1991). Pre-existing bacteria in the effusion in long-standing cases of otitis media with effusion may increase the risk of postoperative infection within the first month following tube insertion (Roos *et al.*, 1990). Removal of the tube in patients with mucopurulent otorrhoea resolved the discharge in 79% of ears within a month (Bingham, Gurr and Owen, 1988).

Perforation

Whereas insertion of short-term Shepard or Shah type tubes are associated with a small risk of permanent perforation (2–3%, Larsen, Tos and Stangerup, 1988; 1.8%, Matt *et al.*, 1991) there is a high rate of perforation following use of long-stay Paparella or Goode type tympanostomy tubes (47.5%, Von Schoenberg, Wengraf and Gleeson, 1989; 21.1%, Prichard *et al.*, 1992; 13.6%, Matt *et al.*, 1991; 6%, Brockbank *et al.*, 1988). Similar rates for Perlee and Paparella type 2 tubes have been reported in a review by Bingham, Gurr and Owen (1988).

Cholesteatoma

Larsen, Tos and Stangerup (1988) recorded development of attic cholesteatoma in 1.7% of ears treated 11–18 years previously with ventilation tube insertion. Implantation cholesteatoma may occur due to insertion of a tube. However, the relationship of cholesteatoma and multiple tube insertions probably reflects the severity of disease in a high risk group rather than the surgery as the cause of epithelial implantation (Herdman and Wright, 1988). This is supported by data from Tayside showing the incidence of cholesteatoma varying between 0.94 and 1.88 (mean 1.32) operations per 10 000 population per year between 1966 and 1986. During the same period there was no change in the incidence of cholesteatoma but a 60-fold increase in the use of ventilation tubes (Padgham, Mills and Christmas, 1989). The rate for cholesteatoma surgery in Liverpool fell between 1960 and 1990, whereas the rate for ventilation tube insertion increased between 1970 and 1990 (Roland *et al.*, 1992).

Inner ear

Both Lim, Kawanchi and De Maria (1990) and Mogi *et al.* (1989) have shown the potential for endotoxins from the middle ear to affect perilymph. Disequilibrium has been demonstrated in 22% of children with otitis media with effusion compared with controls and episodes were related to episodes of otalgia. Resolution occurred in 85% of children after insertion of a ventilation tube (Grace and Pfleiderer, 1990).

Similar improvement in balance on a fixed body sway platform occurred in children with otitis media with effusion after treatment with tubes (Jones *et al.*, 1990). These changes may be self-limiting and without permanent effects on cochlear or vestibular function. We have not shown development of high tone sensorineural hearing loss in our series of children with otitis media with effusion but further studies are required to validate this.

Effects on speech, language, learning and behaviour

There is still only limited evidence of a causal underlying link between otitis media with effusion and clinically significant disablement (Haggard and Hughes, 1991). The developmental effects of otitis media may be due to the associated hearing loss leading directly to poorer language and learning in the early years. However, it may also be that illness other than otitis media is responsible for the developmental effects, or it could be the hearing loss itself leads to degraded input which results in less attention to language (Feagans and Blood, 1993). Studies of the potentially adverse effects of otitis media with effusion on development are complex, time consuming and difficult to control. Chalmers *et al.* (1989), reviewing the Dunedin study with cross-sectional analysis, showed that children with bilateral otitis media with effusion, when compared with tympanometrically normal cases, differed on measures of intelligence at 5 years, verbal comprehension at 3 and 5 years and verbal expression at 3, 5 and 7 years. When a teacher reported behavioural problems, otitis media with effusion was seen to have an effect at 5 years. No significant differences were shown for any of the measures administered at 9 years, or for speech articulation, reading, or parent reported behavioural problems at any age to suggest these abilities may be effected by recurrent bilateral disease before the age of 5 years. Longitudinal analysis showed that while there was a significant difference in intelligence between the groups at 5 years of age, it was not sustained. Disadvantages with respect to language development, speech articulation, reading and teacher reported behavioural problems did persist into mid-childhood years of those children who had bilateral otitis media with effusion at 5. Methodological criticisms of a lack of otological assessment prior to 5 years of age are acknowledged. Other more recent studies have assessed the duration of otitis media with effusion during the first 3 years of life showing reduced scores for cognitive ability, speech and language development, and school performance, in particular with mathematics and reading, at 7 years. Robb, Psak and Pang-Ching (1993) reported reduction in production of consonants in a case of otitis media with effusion followed from 11 to 21 months.

In contrast, the time with otitis media with effusion after the age of 3 years showed no significant effect (Teele *et al.*, 1990). Furthermore, Roberts *et al.* (1991) examined both middle class and low income families and could not detect any difference in language development between $4\frac{1}{2}$ and 6 years of age in children with a history of otitis media with effusion during the first 3 years of life. With a similar group of disadvantaged children there was no relationship between verbal intelligence and academic achievement in the third school year as a consequence of otitis media with effusion in the first 3 years of life. There was a relationship between attentional behaviour in the classroom, orientation and the ability to work alone (Roberts *et al.*, 1989). Feagans and Blood (1993) followed children from 6 months to 3 years of age. Those with more than 20 episodes of otitis per year attending day care were seen to attend less and were more 'off task' during their well sessions than a low otitis group. In an unselected cohort of Danish 7 year olds, Lous (1990) showed an association between a phonological sentence repetitive test and tympanogram type in the better ear. None was found between otological history or pure tone screening. The tympanogram type was found to explain 2–3% of the variation in phonology, compared with the most important background variable which was the mother's social group; itself explaining 4–5% of the variation. Another study showed that at 18 months and 2 years of age both receptive and expressive language were significantly related to average hearing at 6–18 months of age but there was no direct effect of otitis media with effusion on language (Friel-Patti and Finitzo, 1990, 1993). The effects were thought to be indirectly mediated through hearing levels over time. As long as ventilation tubes were in place and patent the hearing was normal and language performance showed no difference when compared with non-otitis media with effusion untreated children. By contrast, children with otitis media with effusion without tubes had statistically poorer language scores if their average hearing levels exceeded 20 dB HL (Friel-Patti and Finitzo, 1993).

To support these studies Rach *et al.* (1991) showed minor non-statistically significant improvements in language scores in relation to verbal expression and comprehension in children following treatment with ventilation tubes compared with untreated controls. Subsequently, Schilder *et al.* (1993) have shown that the association between early otitis media with effusion and changes in language development was no longer present at school age, although some benefit may have resulted from additional speech therapy.

Effects of asymmetrical hearing loss

It is now accepted that children with unilateral hearing loss are significantly disadvantaged (Bess and Tharpe, 1984). Moore, Hutchings and Meyer (1991) have shown an effect of asymmetrical hearing loss leading to long-term or permanent deficits in binaural processing in children and adults. The masking level difference is the psychocoustic measure of sensitivity of the auditory system to subtle intra-aural differences in time and amplitude which relate to the ability of the listener to detect and recognize signals in noisy backgrounds. Small differences in binaural masking level difference in children with otitis media with effusion may lead to difficulties for children in perception of signals in noisy environments. In children with and without a history of otitis media with effusion, Pillsbury, Grose and Hall (1991) showed the masking level differences were abnormally small in the otitis media with effusion group before surgery when hearing loss was present. This sometimes remained small after surgery, when normal hearing had returned. The post-surgery masking level difference was particularly likely to be abnormally reduced in subjects with asymmetrical hearing loss. It is known that sound localization is displaced along a horizontal axis towards the good ear (Morrongiello, 1989).

Summary

Generally speaking the main aim of surgery should be to correct the disability caused by the hearing impairment. This can be achieved by removal of the middle ear effusion. Secondly, surgery may be directed to prevention of recurrence of the effusion in the longer term. Both aims should acknowledge that the condition spontaneously resolves and any complications induced by treatment should not exceed those which develop if the condition is untreated.

In view of the large variation in rates of surgical treatment between districts and regions within the NHS and between different health care services internationally, further studies are required to assess the spontaneous course of the condition in its varying degrees of severity. Studies are also necessary to assess the effects of intervention. Quality of life issues and cost benefit analysis are required in relation both to medical and surgical treatments.

There is a close relationship of the disease to seasonal change and frequently spontaneous resolution occurs in the summer. Consequently, mild forms of the disease, especially in the spring and summer months, require no treatment. There is some evidence that a unilateral effusion may have subtle effects on hearing function, but overall it is probably less detrimental to normal childhood development than if the condition is bilateral. Thus a more conservative treatment regimen may be adopted with unilateral effusions. No satisfactory studies have demonstrated long-term benefit from a wide variety of medical treatments.

Topical and systemic vasoconstrictor medications

and anti-allergy remedies do not effect a long-term cure. Almost all combinations of antibiotics, including those against beta-lactamase producing organisms, have been shown to have a short-lived effect on the condition but do not produce a long-term cure. A transient benefit has been shown with oral steroids. A combination of antibiotics with steroids, anti-inflammatory drugs, decongestants, antihistamines, and prostaglandin inhibitors have all failed to produce a sustained and significant therapeutic effect. There have not been long-term studies to confirm the short-term benefit which has been demonstrated following autoinflation of the eustachian tube. As yet, there has been no benefit from treatment with surfactant nor any significant benefit from antibacterial or antiviral immunization. Evaluation of the use of hearing aids has not been reported. Many of the uncertainties in relation to trials of medical treatment relate to lack of acceptance of either standardized entry criteria or comparable treatment regimens with both short- and long-term outcome measures.

Such limitations also apply to the evaluation of surgical treatment. It is recognized that the best evidence of effectiveness of intervention is a properly designed randomized controlled trial. Of those trials that have been reported in recent years, not all have satisfactory entry criteria or outcome measures and many lack the statistical power to show clinically significant results which are also statistically significant. Surgical treatment options include myringotomy and aspiration alone or in combination with insertion of short- or long-term ventilation tubes. These procedures may be combined with adenoidectomy.

In the past, tonsillectomy was sometimes additionally recommended but has not been shown to be therapeutic (Maw and Herod, 1986). Surgical treatment of other causes of nasal obstruction and removal of nasal and sinus sepsis may also be advised.

There is still a need for further properly controlled studies with sufficient numbers of cases to resolve the many unanswered questions in relation to otitis media with effusion.

References

ARCHARD, J. C. (1967) The place of myringotomy in the management of secretory otitis media in children. *Journal of Laryngology and Otology*, **81**, 309–315

ANDREASSON, L., BYLANDER, A., IVARSSON, A. and TJERNSTROM, O. (1983) Treatment with sulfur hexafluoride in children with serous otitis media. *Archives of Otolaryngology*, **109**, 358–359

ARMSTRONG B. W. (1954) A new treatment for chronic secretory otitis media. *Archives of Otolaryngology*, **59**, 653–654

BESS, F. H., and THARPE, A. M. (1984) Unilateral hearing impairment in children. *Pediatrics*, **74**, 206–216

BINGHAM, B. G. J., GURR, P. A., and OWEN, G. (1988) Tympanic membrane perforation following removal of ventilation tubes in the presence of persistent aural discharge. *Clinical Otolaryngology* **14**, 525–528

BIRCH, L. and ELBROND, O. (1986) Prospective epidemiological study of secretory otitis media in children not attending kindergarten: a prevalence study. *International Journal of Pediatric Otorhinolaryngology*, **11**, 191–197

BLACK, N. (1985) Geographical variations in the use of surgery for glue ear. *Journal of the Royal Society of Medicine* **78**, 641–648

BLACK, N. A., SANDERSON, C. F. B., FREELAND, A. P., and VESSEY, M. P. (1990) A randomized controlled trial of surgery for glue ear. *British Medical Journal*, **300**, 1551–1556

BLANSHARD, J., MAW, A. and BAWDEN, R. (1992) The treatment of otitis media with effusion in children by autoinflation. In: *The New Frontiers of Otorhinolaryngology in Europe*, edited by G. Motter. Bologna: Monduzzi. pp. 31–37

BLANSHARD, J. D., MAW, A. R. and BAWDEN, R. (1993) Conservative treatment of otitis media with effusion by auto-inflation of the middle ear. *Clinical Otolaryngology*, **18**, 188–192.

BLUESTONE, C. D. (1984) Definitions and classifications: state of the art. In: *Recent Advances in Otitis Media with Effusion*, edited by D. J. Lim, C. D. Bluestone, J. O. Klein and J. D. Nelson: Philadelphia: BC Decker Inc, pp. 1–4

BLUESTONE, C. D. and BEERY, Q. C. (1976) Concepts on the pathogenesis of middle ear effusion. *Annals of Otology, Rhinology and Laryngology*, **85**, (Suppl. 25), 182–186

BODNER, E. E., BROWNING, G. G., CHALMERS, F. T. and CHALMERS, T. C. (1991) Can meta-analysis help uncertainty in surgery for otitis media in children. *Journal of Laryngology and Otology*, **105**, 812–819

BONDING, P. and TOS, M. (1985) Grommets versus paracentesis in the management of secretory otitis media: a prospective controlled study. *American Journal of Otolaryngology*, **6**, 455–460

BROCKBANK, M. J., JONATHEN, D. A., GRANT, H. R. and WRIGHT, A. (1988) Goode T-tubes: do the benefits of their use outweigh their complications? *Clinical Otolaryngology*, **13**, 351–356

BROOKER, D. S. and MCNEICE, A. (1992) Auto inflation in the treatment of glue ear in children. *Clinical Otolaryngology*, **17**, 289–290

BROOKS, D. (1976) School screening for middle ear effusion. *Annals of Otology, Rhinology and Laryngology*, **85**, (Suppl. 125), 223–229

BROWN, M. J. K. M., RICHARDS, S. H. and AMBEGAOKAR, A. G. (1978) Grommets and glue ear: a five year follow up of a controlled trial. *Proceedings of the Royal Society of Medicine*, **71**, 353–356

BUCKLEY, G. and HINTON, A. (1991) Otitis media with effusion in children shows a progressive resolution with time. *Clinical Otolaryngology*, **16**, 354–357

BULMAN, C. H., BROOK, S. J. and BERRY, M. G. (1984) A prospective randomized trial of adenoidectomy vs grommet insertion in the treatment of glue ear. *Clinical Otolaryngology*, **9**, 67–75

CANTEKIN, E. I., BEERY, Q. C. and BLUESTONE, C. D. (1977) Tympanometric patterns found in middle ear effusions. *Annals of Otology, Rhinology and Laryngology*, **86**, (Suppl. 41), 16–20

CANTEKIN, E. I. MCGUIRE, T. W. and POTTER, R. L. (1990) Biomedical information, peer review, and conflict of interest as they influence public health. *Journal of the American Medical Association*, **263**, 1427–1430

CAPPER, J. W. R., SLACK, R. W. T. and MAW, A. R. (1987) Tuning fork tests in children (an evaluation of their usefulness). *Journal of Laryngology and Otology*, **101**, 780–783

CARTWRIGHT, K. A. V. (1992) Vaccination against Haemophillus influenzae disease. *British Medical Journal*, **305**, 485–486

CHALMERS, D., STEWART, I., SILVA, P. and MULVENA, A. (1989) Otitis media with effusion in children – the Dunedin Study. *Clinics in Developmental Medicine*, **108**, London: MacKeith Press

CHAN, K. H., MANDEL, E. M., ROCKETTE, H. E., BLUESTONE, C. D., BASS, L. W., BLATTER, M. M., *et al.* (1988) A comparative study of amoxicillin-clavulanate and amoxicillin. Treatment of otitis media with effusion. *Archives of Otolaryngology – Head and Neck Surgery*, **114**, 142–146

CURLEY, J. W. A. (1986) Grommet insertion: Some basic questions answered. *Clinical Otolaryngology*, **11**, 1–4

DALY, K. A., GIEBINK, G. S., MARGOLIS, R. H., LE, C. T., WESTOVER, D. E., JAHN, S. K. *et al.* (1993) Chronic otitis media with effusion (OME) morbidity in a prospective cohort: risk determinants for short term outcomes in children treated with tympanostomy tubes. In: *Recent Advances in Otitis Media*, edited by D. J. Lim. Toronto: Decker Periodicals. pp. 7–11

DAWES, P. J., BINGHAM, B. J., RHYS, R. and GRIFFITHS, M. V. (1991) Aspirating middle ear effusions when inserting ventilation tubes: does it influence postoperative otorrhoea, tube obstruction or the development of tympanosclerosis? *Clinical Otolaryngology*, **16**, 457–461

DE MARIA, T. F., BRIGGS, B. R., LIM, D. J. and OKAZAKI, N. (1984) Experimental otitis media with effusion following inoculation with non-viable H. influenzae. *Annals of Otology, Rhinology and Laryngology*, **93**, 52–56

DE MELKER, R. A. (1992) Treating persistent glue ear in children. *British Medical Journal*, **306**, 5–6

DEMPSTER, J. H. and MACKENZIE, K. (1991) Tympanometry in the detection of hearing impairments associated with otitis media with effusion. *Clinical Otolaryngology*, **16**, 157–159

DEMPSTER, J. H. and MACKENZIE, K. (1992) Clinical role of free-field voice tests in children. *Clinical Otolaryngology*, **17**, 54–56

DEMPSTER, J. H., BROWNING, G. G. and GATEHOUSE, S. G. (1993) A randomised study of the surgical management of children with persistent otitis media with effusion associated with a hearing impairment. *Journal of Laryngology and Otology*, **107**, 284–289

EFFECTIVE HEALTH CARE (1992) The treatment of persistent glue ear in children. Bulletin no 4,. University of Leeds

FACIONE, N. (1991) Quality of life issues in chronic otitis media with effusion: parameters for future study. *International Journal of Pediatric Otorhinolaryngology*, **22**, 167–179

FEAGANS, L. V. and BLOOD, I. M. (1993) The behavioural and language sequelae of otitis media in infants and young children attending day care. In: *Recent Advances in Otitis Media*, edited by D. J. Lim. Toronto: B. C. Decker. pp. 521–523

FELDING, J. H. and LILDHOLT, T. (1988) Direct measurements of middle ear gas composition: clinical implications. In: *Recent Advances in Otitis Media*, edited by D. J. Lim. Toronto: Decker. pp. 86–88

FIELLAU NIKOLAJSEN, M. (1979) Tympanometry in 3 year old children II. Seasonal influence on tympanometric results in selected 3 year old children. *Scandinavian Audiology*, **8**, 181–185

FIELLAU NIKOLAJSEN, M. (1983) Tympanometry and secretory otitis media. *Acta Otolaryngologica*, Suppl. **394**, 1–73

FIELLAU NIKOLAJSEN, M., FALBE-HANSEN, J. and KNUDSTRUP, P. (1980) Adenoidectomy for middle ear disorders: a randomised controlled study. *Clinical Otolaryngology*, **5**, 323–377

FINITZO, T., FRIEL-PATTI, S., CHINN, K. and BROWN, O. (1991) Tympanometry and otoscopy prior to myringotomy: issues in diagnosis of otitis media. *International Journal of Pediatric Otolaryngology*, **24**, 101–110

FORMAN-FRANCO, B., ABRAMSON, A. L., GORVOY, J. D. and STEIN, T. (1979) Cystic fibrosis and hearing loss. *Archives of Otolaryngology*, **105**, 338–342

FRASER, J. G., MEHTA, M. and FRASER, P. M. (1977) The medical treatment of secretory otitis media. Clinical trial of three commonly used regimes. *Journal of Laryngology and Otology*, **91**, 707–765

FRIA, T. J., CANTEKIN, E. I. and EICHLER, A. (1985) Hearing acuity of children with otitis media with effusion. *Archives of Otolaryngology*, **111**, 10–16

FRIEL-PATTI, S. and FINITZO, T. (1990) Language learning in a prospective study of otitis media with effusion in the first two years of life. *Journal of Speech and Hearing Research*, **33**, 18–19

FRIEL-PATTI, S. and FINITZO, T. (1993) Speech-language learning in the first three years in children with tympanostomy tubes for recurrent or persistent otitis media. In: *Recent Advances in Otitis Media*, edited by D. J. Lim. Toronto: B. C. Decker. pp. 523–527

GATES, G. A. and COOPER, J. C. (1980) Effect of anaesthetic gases on middle ear pressure in the presence of effusion. *Annals of Otology, Rhinology and Laryngology*, **89**, (Suppl. 3), part 2, 62–64

GATES, G. A., AVERY, C. A., PRIHODA, T. J. and COOPER, J. C. (1987) Effectiveness of adenoidectomy and tympanostomy tubes in the treatment of chronic otitis media with effusion. *New England Journal Medicine*, **317**, 1444–1451

GEREAU, S. A. and SHPRINTZEN, R. J. (1988) The role of adenoids in the development of normal speech following palate repair. *Laryngoscope*, **98**, 299–303

GIEBINK, G. S., BATALDEN, P. M., LE, C. T., RUSS, J. N., KNOX, J. K., ANDERSON, R. S. *et al.* (1988) Randomised controlled trial comparing trimethoprim sulphamethoxasole, prednisolone, ibuprofen, and no treatment in chronic otitis media with effusion. In: *Recent Advances in Otitis Media*, edited by D. J. Lim. Toronto: Decker. pp. 240–244

GOYCOOLEA, H. G., GOYCOOLEA, M. V. and FARFAN, C. R. (1988) Racial and familial factors in otitis media: a point prevalence study on Easter Island. *Archives of Otolaryngology – Head and Neck Surgery*, **114**, 147–149

GRACE, A. R. and PFLEIDERER, A. G. (1990) Dysequilibrium and otitis media with effusion: what is the association? *Journal of Laryngology and Otology*, **104**, 682–684

GUNDERSEN, T. and TONNING, F. M. (1976) Ventilation tubes in the middle ear; long term observations. *Archives of Otolaryngology*, **102**, 198–199

GUNDERSEN, T., TONNING, F. M., and KVEBERG K. H. (1984) Ventilating tubes in the middle ear. Long term observations. *Archives of Otolaryngology*, **110**, 783–784

HAGGARD, M. and HUGHES, G. (1991) *Screening Children's Hearing. A Review of the Literature and the Implications of Otitis Media*. London: HMSO

HAMPAL, S., FLOOD, L. M. and KUMAR, B. U. (1991) The minigrommet and tympanosclerosis. *Journal of Laryngology and Otology*, **105**, 161–164

HELLSTROM, S., GOLDIE, P., MAGNUSON, K. and FALL, C. (1993) The oxygen level influences the middle ear tissue reaction in ears with perforated tympanic membranes. In: *Recent Advances in Otitis Media*, edited by D. J. Lim. Toronto: B. C. Decker, pp. 334–335

HEMLIN, C., BRAUNDER, A., CARENFELT, C. and WRETLIND, B. (1991) Nasopharyngeal flora in otitis media with effusion. A comparative semiquantitative analysis. *Acta Otolaryngologica*, **111**, 556–561

HENDERSON, F. W., COLLIER, A. M., SANYAL, M. A., WATKINS, J. M., FAIRCLOUGH, D. L., CLYDE, W. A. *et al.* (1982) A longitudinal study of respiratory viruses and bacteria in the aetiology of acute otitis media with effusion. *New England Journal of Medicine*, **306**, 1377–1383

HERDMAN, R. and WRIGHT, J. L. W. (1988) Grommets and cholesteatoma in children. *Journal of Laryngology and Otology*, **102**, 1000–1002

HIBBERT, J. (1977) The current status of adenoidectomy: a survey among otolaryngologists. *Clinical Otolaryngology*, **2**, 239–242

HIBBERT, J. and WHITEHOUSE, G. M. (1978) The assessment of adenoidal size by radiological means. *Clinical Otolaryngology*, **3**, 43–47

HILLS, B. A. (1984) Analysis of eustachian surfactant and its function as a release agent. *Archives of Otolaryngology*, **110**, 3–9

HINTON, A. E. (1989) Surgery for otitis media with effusion in children and its relationship to parental smoking. *Journal of Laryngology and Otology*, **103**, 559–561

HOLBOROW, C. A. (1970) Eustachian tubal function. Changes in anatomy and function with age and the relationship of these changes to aural pathology. *Archives of Otolaryngology*, **92**, 624–626

HOSPITAL ACTIVITY DATA (1989) London: HMSO

HOSPITAL INPATIENT ENQUIRY DATA (1985) London: HMSO

JEANS, W. D., FERNANDO, D. C. J., MAW, A. R. and LEIGHTON, B. C. (1981) A longitudinal study of the growth of the nasopharynx and its contents in normal children. *British Journal of Radiology*, **54**, 117–121

JERGER, J. (1970) Clinical experience with impedance audiometry. *Archives of Otolaryngology*, **92**, 311

JOHNSON, A. P., MURRAY, J. A. M. and MARAN, A. G. D. (1983) Errors in the assessment of nasopharyngeal airway by radiograph. *Journal of Laryngology and Otology*, **97**, 1017–1026

JONES, N. S., RADONMSKI, P., PRICHARD, A. J. N. and SNASHALL, S. E. (1990) Imbalance and chronic secretory otitis media: effect of myringotomy and insertion of ventilation tubes on body sway. *Annals of Otology, Rhinology and Laryngology*, **99**, 477–481

JUNG, T. T., PARK, Y. M., SCHLUND, D., WEEKS, D., MILLER, S., WONG, O. *et al.* (1990) Effect of prostaglandin, leukotriene, and arachidonic acid on experimental otitis media with effusion in chinchillas. *Annals of Otorhinolaryngology*, Suppl. 148, 28–32

KENNEDY, T. L. and GORE, L. B. (1982) Middle ear effusions and the nitrous oxide myth. *Laryngoscope*, **92**, 169–172

KILBY, D., RICHARDS, S. H. and HART, G. (1972) Grommets and glue ear: Two year results. *Journal of Laryngology and Otology*, **86**, 881–888

KLEIN, J. O. (1980) Microbiology of otitis media. *Annals of Otorhinolaryngology*, Suppl. 68, 98

KOBAYASHI, T., YAGINUMA, Y., TOSHIMA, M., SHIGA, N., HOZAWA, K., YOSHIDA, S. *et al.* (1993) Use of surfactant in the treatment of secretory otitis media: a preliminary report.

In: *Recent Advances in Otitis Media*, edited by D. J. Lim. Toronto: Decker. pp. 286–289

LARSEN, P. L., TOS, M. and STANGERUP, S. E. (1988) Progression of drum pathology following secretory otitis media. In: *Recent Advances in Otitis Media*, edited by D. J. Lim. Toronto: Decker. pp. 34–38

LESSER, T. H. J., WILLIAMS, K. R. and SKINNER, D. W. (1988) Tympanosclerosis, grommets and shear stresses. *Clinical Otolaryngology*, **13**, 375–380

LIEBERMAN, A., and BARTAL, N., (1986) Untreated persistent middle ear effusion. *Journal of Laryngology, Otology and Rhinology*, **100**, 875–878

LILDHOLT, T. (1983) Ventilation tubes in secretory otitis media. *Acta Otolaryngologica*, Suppl. 398, 1–70

LIM, D. J. and DE MARIA, T. F. (1982) Pathogenesis of otitis media bacteriology and immunology. *Laryngoscope*, **92**, 278–286

LIM, D. J., KAWAUCHI, H. and DE MARIA, T. F. (1990) Role of middle ear endotoxin in inner ear inflammatory response and hydrops: long term study. *Annals of Otorhinolaryngology*, (Suppl.), **148**, 33–34

LIM, D. J., BLUESTONE, C. D., KLEIN, J. O., NELSON, J. D. and OGRA, P. L. (1993) *Recent Advances in Otitis Media*. Toronto: Decker Periodicals

LINDER-ARONSON, S. (1970) Adenoids. Their effect on mode of breathing and nasal airflow and their relationship to characteristics of the facial skeleton and dentition. *Acta Otolaryngologica*, Suppl. 265, 1–132

LOUS, J. (1987) Screening for secretory otitis media: evaluation of some impedance screening programs for long-lasting secretory otitis media in 7 year old children. *International Journal of Pediatric Otorhinolaryngology*, **13**, 85–97

LOUS, J. (1990) Secretory otitis media and phonology when starting school. *Scandinavian Audiology*, **19**, 215–222

LOUS, J. and FIELLAU NIKOLAJSEN, M. (1981) Epidemiology of middle ear effusion and tubal dysfunction. A one year prospective study comparing monthly tympanometry in 387 non selected seven year old children. *International Journal of Pediatric Otorhinolaryngology* **3**, 303–317

LUNTZ. M. and SADE, J. (1988) Growth of the eustachian tube lumen with age. *American Journal of Otolaryngology*, **9**, 195–198

MACKENZIE, I. J. (1984) Factors affecting the extrusion rates of ventilation tubes. *Journal of the Royal Society Medicine*, **77**, 751–753

MCNICHOLL, W. D. (1983) Otitis media with effusion in children and its association with deformation of the vomero-ethmoid suture. *Journal of Laryngology and Otology*, **97**, 203–212

MAGNUSSON, B. (1989) The sniff theory. *IFOS Conference of Eustachian Tube and Middle Ear Diseasae*, (Abstract) Geneva

MANDEL, E. M., ROCKETTE, H. E., BLUESTONE, C. D., PARADISE, J. L. and NOZZA, R. J. (1987) Efficacy of amoxicillin with and without decongestant-antihistamine for otitis media with effusion in children. *New England Journal of Medicine*, **316**, 432–437

MANDEL, E. M., ROCKETTE, H. E., BLUESTONE, C. D., PARADISE, J. L. and NOZZA, R. J. (1989) Myringotomy with and without tympanostomy tubes for chronic otitis media with effusion. *Archives of Otolaryngology, Head and Neck Surgery*, **115**, 1217–1224

MANDEL, E. M., ROCKETTE, H. E., PARADISE, J. L., BLUESTONE, C. D. and NOZZA, R. J. (1991) Comparative efficacy of erythromycin-sulfisoxazole, cefaclor, amoxicillin or placebo for otitis media with effusion in children. *Pediatric Infectious Disease Journal*, 10, 899–906

MANDEL, E. M., ROCKETTE, H. E., BLUESTONE, C. D., PARADISE, J. L. and NOZZA, R. J. (1992) Efficacy of myringotomy with and without tympanostomy tubes for chronic otitis media with effusion. *Pediatric Infectious Disease Journal*, 11, 270–277

MARKS, N. J., MILLS, R. F. and SHAHEEN, O. H. (1981) A controlled trial of cotrimoxazole therapy in serous otitis media. *Journal of Laryngology and Otology*, 95, 1003–1009

MARKS, N. J., MILLS, R. and SHAHEEN, O. H. (1983) Cotrimoxazole in the treatment of serous otitis media. A follow-up report. *Journal of Laryngology and Otology*, 97, 213–215

MARSHALL, F. P. and CABLE, H. R. (1982) The effect of nitrous oxide on middle ear effusions. *Journal of Laryngology and Otology*, 96, 893–897

MATT, B. H., MILLER, R. P., MEYERS, R. M., CAMPBELL, J. M. and COTTON, R. T. (1991) Incidence of perforation with Goode T tube. *International Journal of Pediatric Otorhinolaryngology*, 21, 1–6

MAW, A. R. (1979) Preliminary findings for inter-observer variability in children with middle ear effusion and adenoids. *Clinical Otolaryngology*, 4, 149

MAW, A. R. (1983) Chronic otitis media with effusion (glue ear) and adenotonsillectomy: prospective randomized controlled study. *British Medical Journal*, 287, 1586–1588

MAW, A. R. (1985a) Age and adenoid size in relation to adenoidectomy in otitis media with effusion. *American Journal of Otolaryngology*, 6, 245–248

MAW, A. R. (1985b) Factors affecting adenoidectomy for otitis media with effusion (glue ear). *Journal of the Royal Society of Medicine*, 78, 1014–1018

MAW, A. R. (1988) Early and late effects of surgery for otitis media with effusion. In: *Recent Advances in Otitis Media*, edited by D. J. Lim. Toronto: Decker. pp.282–286

MAW, A. R. (1989) Tympanic membrane changes following middle ear effusion and after treatment with ventilation tubes. In: *Cholesteatoma and Mastoid Surgery*, edited by M. Tos, J. Thomsen and E. Peitersen. Amsterdam: Kugler and Ghedini. pp.383–386

MAW, A. R., (1991) Development of tympanosclerosis in children with otitis media with effusion and ventilation tubes. *Journal of Laryngology and Otology*, 105, 614–617

MAW, A. R. (1992) Using tympanometry to detect glue ear in general practice. *British Medical Journal*, 304, 67–68

MAW, A. R. (1995) Glue ear in childhood. *Clinics in Developmental Medicine 135*, MacKeith Press, London

MAW, A. R. and BAWDEN, R. (1993) A long term study of spontaneous resolution of severe chronic glue ear in children and the effect of adenoidectomy, tonsillectomy and ventilation tube (grommets). *British Medical Journal*, 306, 756–760

MAW, A. R. and HEROD, F. (1986) Otoscopic impedance and audiometric findings in glue ear treated by adenoidectomy and tonsillectomy. A prospective randomized study. *Lancet*, i, 1399–1402

MAW, A. R. and PARKER, A. (1988) Surgery of the tonsils and adenoids in relation to secretory otitis media in children. *Acta Otolaryngologica*, Suppl. 454, 202–207

MAW, A. R. and PARKER, A. J. (1993) A model to refine the selection of children with otitis media with effusion for adenoidectomy. *Clinical Otolaryngology*, 18, 164–170

MAW, A. R. and SPELLER, D. C. E. (1985) Are the tonsils and adenoids a reservoir for infection in otitis media with effusion (glue ear). *Clinical Otolaryngology*, 10, 265–269

MAW, A. R., SMITH, I. M. and LANCE, G. N. (1991) Lateral cephalometric analysis of children with otitis media with effusion: a comparison with age and sex matched controls. *Journal of Laryngology and Otology*, 105, 71–77

MAW, A. R., JEANS, W. D. and FERNANDO, D. C. J. (1981) Inter-observer variability in the clinical and radiological assessment of adenoid size and the correlation with adenoid volume. *Clinical Otolaryngology*, 6, 317–322

MAW, A. R., PARKER, A. J., LANCE, G. N. and DILKES, M. G. (1992) The effect of parental smoking on outcome after treatment for glue ear in children. *Clinical Otolaryngology*, 17, 411–414

MILLS, R., UTTLEY, A. and MCINTYRE, M. F. (1984) Relationship between acute suppurative otitis media and chronic secretory otitis media: role of antibiotics. *Journal of the Royal Society of Medicine*, 77, 754–757

MILLS, R., UTTLEY, A. and MCINTYRE, M. F. (1985) A bacteriological study of the middle ear and upper respiratory tract in children with chronic secretory otitis media. *Clinical Otolaryngology*, 10, 335–341

MILLS, R. P., ALBIZZATI, C. and TODD, A. S. (1990) Ear drops and grommets. *Clinical Otolaryngology*, 15, 315–319

MOGI, G. (1993) Immunologic and allergic aspects of otitis media. In: *Recent Advances in Otitis Media*, edited by D. J. Lim. Toronto: B. C. Decker. pp. 145–151

MOGI, G., SUZUKI, M., FUJIYOSHI, T., UEYAMA, S. and ICHIMIYA, I. (1989) Influence of middle ear effusion on perilymph. *Acta Otolaryngologica*, Suppl. 457, 116–123

MOLLER, H. and TOS, M. (1990) Point and period prevalence of otitis media with effusion evaluated by daily tympanometry. *Journal of Laryngology and Otology*, 104, 937–941

MOORE, D. R., HUTCHINGS, M. E. and MEYER, S. E. (1991) Binaural masking level differences in children with a history of otitis media. *Audiology*, 30, 91–101

MOORE, P. (1990) Ventilation tube duration versus design. *Annals of Otology, Rhinology and Laryngology*, 99, 722–723

MORRONGIELLO, B. A. (1989) Infants' monaural localization of sounds: effects of unilateral ear infection. *Journal of the Acoustic Society of America*, 86, 597–602

NAKANO, Y. and SATO, Y. (1990) Prognosis of otitis media with effusion in children, and size of the mastoid air cell system. *Acta Otolaryngologica*, Suppl. 471, 56–61

NICHOLL, J. P. BEEBY, N. R. and WILLIAMS, B. T. (1989) Role of the private sector in elective surgery in England and Wales, 1986. *British Medical Journal*, 298, 243–247

OGRA, P. L. and NADAL, D. (1993) Vaccination approaches for infections of the respiratory tract. In: *Recent Advances in Otitis Media*, edited by D. J. Lim. Toronto: B. C. Decker. pp. 222–229

OVESEN, T., PAASKE, P. B. and ELBROND, O. (1992) Local application of N-acetylcysteine in secretory otitis media in rabbits. *Clinical Otolaryngology*, 17, 327–331

PADGHAM, N., MILLS, R. and CHRISTMAS, H. (1989) Has the increasing use of grommets influenced the frequency of surgery for cholesteatoma? *Journal of Laryngology and Otology*, 103, 1034–1035

PARADISE, J. L., SMITH, C. G. and BLUESTONE, C. D. (1975) Tympanometric detection of middle ear effusion in infants and young children. *Paediatrics*, 58, 198–210

PARADISE, J. L., BLUESTONE, C. D., ROGERS, K. D., TAYLOR F. H., COLBORN, D. K., BACHMAN, R. Z. *et al.* (1990). Efficacy of adenoidectomy for recurrent otitis media in children previously treated with tympanostomy tube placement. *Journal of the American Medical Association*, **263**, 2066–2073

PARKER, A. J., MAW, A. R. and POWELL, J. E. (1990) Intratympanic bleeding after grommet insertion and tympanosclerosis. *Clinical Otolaryngology*, **15**, 203–207

PELTON, S. I., TEELE, D. W., REIMER, C. B., DE LANGE, G. G. and SIBER, G. R. (1988) Immunologic characteristics of children with frequent recurrence of otitis media. In: *Recent Advances in Otitis Media*, edited by D. J. Lim. Philadelphia: B. C. Decker Inc. pp. 143–146

PILLSBURY, H. C., GROSE J. H. and HALL, J. W. (1991) Otitis media with effusion in children. Binaural hearing before and after corrective surgery. *Archives of Otolaryngology – Head and Neck Surgery*, **117**, 718–723

PODOSHIN, L., FRADIS, M., BEN-DAVID, Y. and FARAGGI, D. (1990) The efficacy of oral steroids in the treatment of persistent otitis media with effusion. *Archives of Otolaryngology – Head and Neck Surgery*, **116**, 1404–1406

PRICHARD, A. J. N., MARSHALL, J., SKINNER, D. W. and NARULA, A. A. (1992) Long term results of Goode's tympanostomy tubes in children. *International Journal of Pediatric Otorhinolaryngology*, **24**, 227–233

QUARNBERG, Y. (1981) Acute otitis media. A prospective clinical study of myringotomy and antimicrobial treatment. *Acta Otolaryngologica*, Suppl. 375, 1–157

QUARNBERG, Y., MALMBERG, H., RAHNASTO, J. and PALVA, T. (1988) Mastoid pneumatisation and secretory otitis media. In: *Recent Advances in Otitis Media*, edited by D. J. Lim. Philadelphia: B. C. Decker Inc. pp. 127–129

RACH, G. H., ZIELHUIS, G. A. and VAN DEN BROEK, P. (1986) The prevalence of otitis media with effusion in two year old children in the Netherlands. In: *Acute and Secretory Otitis Media*, edited by J. Sade. Amsterdam: Kugler

RACH, G. H., ZIELHUIS, G. A., VAN BAARLE, P. W. and VAN DEN BROEK, P. (1991) The effect of treatment with ventilating tubes on language development in pre-school children with otitis media with effusion. *Clinical Otolaryngology*, **16**, 128–132

RAPIN, J. (1979) Conductive hearing loss effects on children's language development and scholastic skills. *Annals of Otorhinolaryngology*, **88**, (Suppl. 60), 3–12

RASSMUSSEN, F. (1993) Protracted secretory otitis media. The impact of familial factors and day-care center attendance. *International Journal of Pediatric Otorhinolaryngology*, **26**, 29–37

REES, G. L. and FREELAND, A. P. (1992) The effect of anaesthesia on tympanograms of children undergoing grommet insertion. *Clinical Otolaryngology*, **17**, 200–202

RICHARDS, S. H., KILBY, D., SHAW, J. D. and CAMPBELL, H. (1971) Grommets and glue ear: a clinical trial. *Journal of Laryngology and Otology*, **85**, 27–32

RIVRON, R. P. (1989) Bifid uvula: prevalence and association in otitis media with effusion in children admitted for routine otolaryngological operations. *Journal of Laryngology and Otology* **103**, 249–252

ROBB, M. P., PSAK, J. L. and PANG-CHING, G. K. (1993) Chronic otitis media and early speech development: a case study. *International Journal of Pediatric Otorhinolaryngology*, **26**, 117–127

ROBB, P. J. and JOHNSTON, D. (1991) The clinical management of otorrhoea following grommet insertion: a survey of otolaryngologists and general practitioners. *Clinical Otolaryngology*, **16**, 367–370

ROBBINS, J. B., SCHNEERSON, R. and SZU, S. C. (1988) Recent developments of bacterial vaccines related to the preven-

tion of otitis media. In: *Recent Advances in Otitis Media*, edited by D. J. Lim. Philadelphia: B. C. Decker. pp. 210–214

ROBERTS, J. E., BURCHINAL, M. R., COLLIER, A. M., RAMEY, C. T., KOCK, M. A. and HENDERSON, F. W. (1989) Otitis media in early childhood and cognitive, academic and classroom performance of the school-aged child. *Pediatrics*, **83**, 477–485

ROBERTS, J. E., BURCHINAL, M. R., DAVID, B. P., COLLIER A. M. and HENDERSON, F. W. (1991) Otitis media in early childhood and later language. *Journal of Speech and Hearing Research*, **34**, 1158–1168

ROBINSON, P. J., LODGE, S., GOLIGHER, J., BOWLEY, N. and GRANT H. R. (1993) Secretory otitis media and mastoid air cell development. *International Journal of Pediatric Otorhinolaryngology*, **25**, 13–18

ROBINSON, P. M. (1988) Prognostic factors in otitis media with effusion. *Journal of Laryngology and Otology*, **102**, 989–991

ROCKLEY, T. J. and HAWKES, W. M. (1992) The middle ear as a baroreceptor. *Acta Otolaryngologica*, **112**, 816–823

ROLAND, N. J., PHILLIPS, D. E., ROGERS, J. H. and SINGH, S. D. (1992) The use of ventilation tubes and the incidence of cholesteatoma surgery in the paediatric population of Liverpool. *Clinical Otolaryngology*, **17**, 437–439

ROOS, K., GRANSTROM, G., KARLSSON, G., LIND, L., OLLING, S. and REDVALL, U. (1990) Ear discharge after insertion of transmyringeal tubes. *International Journal of Pediatric Otorhinolaryngology*, **20**, 219–223

ROSENFELD, R. M. and POST, J. C. (1992) Meta-analysis of antibiotics for the treatment of otitis media with effusion. *Archives of Otolaryngology – Head and Neck Surgery*, **106**, 378–386

ROWE-JONES, J. M. and BROCKBANK, M. J. (1992) Parental smoking and persistent otitis media with effusion in children. *International Journal of Pediatric Otorhinolaryngology*, **24**, 19–24

ROYDHOUSE, N. (1980) Adenoidectomy for otitis media with mucoid effusion. *Annals of Otorhinolaryngology*, **89** (Suppl. 68), 312–315

RYNNEL DAGOO, B., AHLBOM, A. and SCHIRATZKI, H. (1978) Effects of adenoidectomy: a controlled two year follow up. *Annals of Otorhinolaryngology*, **87**, 272–278

SADE, J. and LUNTZ, M. (1990) Middle ear as a gas pocket. *Annals of Otorhinolaryngology*, **99**, 529–534

SADE, J. and LUNTZ, M. (1993) Dynamic measurement of gas composition in the middle ear: steady state values. *Acta Otolaryngologica*, **113** (Suppl. 3), 353–357

SALAM, M. A. and WENGRAF, C. (1992) Glue under pressure: a bad prognostic sign for recurrence of otitis media with effusion. *Journal of Laryngology and Otology*, **106**, 974–976

SCADDING, G. K., MARTIN, J. A. M., ALLES, R. S., HAWK, L. J. and DARBY, Y. (1993) Letter. *British Medical Journal*, **306**, 455

SCHILDER, A. G. M., ZIELHUIS, G. A. and VAN DEN BROEK P. (1993) The otological profile of a cohort of Dutch 7.5–8 year olds. *Clinical Otolaryngology*, **18**, 48–54

SCHILDER, A. G. M., VAN MAUEN, J. G., ZIELHUIS, G. A., GRIEVINK, E. H., PETERS, S. A. F. and VAN DEN BROEK, P. (1993) Long-term effects of otitis media with effusion on language, reading and spelling. *Clinical Otolaryngology*, **18**, 234–241

SENTURIA, B. H., GESSERT, C. F., CAR, C. D. and BAUMANN, H. S. (1958) Studies concerned with tubotympanitis. *Annals of Otology, Rhinology and Laryngology*, **67**, 440–467

SKINNER, D. W., LESSER, T. H. J. and RICHARDS, S. H. (1988) A

15 year follow up of a controlled trial of the use of grommets in glue ear. *Clinical Otolaryngology*, **13**, 341–346

SMITH, I. M. and MAW, A. R. (1991) Secretory otitis media: a review of management by consultant otolaryngologists. *Clinical Otolaryngology*, **16**, 266–270

STANGERUP, S. E., SEDERBERG-OLSEN, J. and BALLE, V. (1992) Autoinflation as a treatment of secretory otitis media: a randomized controlled study. *Archives of Otolaryngology – Head and Neck Surgery*, **118**, 149–152

STENFORS, L. E. and RAISANEN, S. (1980) Colonization of middle ear pathogens in the nasopharyngeal opening of the eustachian tube during secretory otitis media. *Acta Otolaryngologica*, **107**, 104–110

STENFORS, L. E. and RAISANEN, S. (1991) Is attachment of bacteria to the epithelial cells of the nasopharynx the key to otitis media? *International Journal of Pediatric Otorhinolaryngology*, **22**, 1–8

STENFORS, L. E. and RAISANEN, S. (1992) Occurrence of Streptococcus pneumoniae and Haemophilus influenzae in otitis media with effusion. *Clinical Otolaryngology*, **17**, 195–199

STEPHENSON, H. and HAGGARD, M. (1992) Rationale and design of surgical trials for otitis media with effusion. *Clinical Otolaryngology*, **17**, 67–78

STEWART, I. A., GUY, A. M., ALLISON, R. S. and THOMSON, N. J. (1985) Bromhexine in the treatment of otitis media with effusion. *Clinical Otolaryngology*, **10**, 145–149

STOOL, S. E. and RANDALL, P. (1967) Unexpected ear disease in infants with cleft palate. *Cleft Palate Journal*, **4**, 99–103

STRACHAN, D. P., JARVIS, M. J. and FEYERABEND, C. (1989) Passive smoking, salivary cotinine concentrations and middle ear effusions in seven year old children. *British Medical Journal*, **298**, 1549–1552

SUAREZ NIETO, C., MALLAGUIZA CALVO, R. and BARTHE GARCIA, P. (1983) Aetiological factors in chronic secretory otitis media in relation to age. *Clinical Otolaryngology*, **8**, 171–174

SUETAKE, M., KOBAYSHI, T., TAKASAKA, T. and SHINKAWA, H. (1990) Is change in middle ear air volume following ventilation tube insertion a reliable prognostic indicator? *Acta Otolaryngologica*, Suppl. 471, 73–80

SUZUKI, M., KAWAUCHI, H., UEYAMA, S., FUJIYOSHI, T. and MOGI, G. (1988) Immune mediated otitis media with effusion. In: *Recent Advances in Otitis Media*, edited by D. J. Lim. Philadelphia: B. C. Decker. pp. 191–196

TAKEUCHI, K., MAJIMA, Y., HATTORI, M., HIRATO, K. and SAKAURA, Y. (1990) Quantitation of tubo-tympanic mucociliary clerance in otitis media with effusion. *Annals of Otorhinolaryngology*, **99**, 211–214

TEELE, D., KLEIN, J. and ROSNER, B. (1980) Epidemiology of otitis media in children. *Annals of Otorhinolaryngology*, **89**, Suppl. 68, 5–6

TEELE, D. W., KLEIN, J. O. and ROSNER, B. (1989) Epidemiology of otitis media during the first seven years of life in children in greater Boston: a prospective cohort study. *Journal of Infectious Diseases*, **160**, 83–94

TEELE, D. W., KLEIN, J. O., CHASE, C., MENYUK, P. and ROSNER, B. A. (1990) Otitis media in infancy and intellectual ability, school achievement, speech and language at age 7 years. Greater Boston Otitis Media Study Group. *Journal of Infectious Diseases*, **162**, 685–694

THOMSEN, J., SEDERBERG-OLSEN, J., BALLE, V., VEJLSGAARD, R., STANGERUP, S. E. and BONDESSON, G. (1989) Antibiotic treatment of children with secretory otitis media. A rand-

omized, double-blind, placebo-controlled study. *Archives of Otolaryngology – Head and Neck Surgery*, **115**, 447–451

TO, S., PAHOR, A. L. and ROBIN, P. E. (1984) A prospective trial of unilateral grommets for bilateral secretory otitis media in children. *Clinical Otolaryngology*, **9**, 115–117

TODD, N. W. and MARTIN, W. S. (1988) Relationship of Eustachian tube bony landmarks and temporal bone pneumatization. *Annals of Otorhinolaryngology*, **97**, 277–280

TONER, J. G. and MAINS, B. (1990) Pneumatic otoscopy and tympanometry in the detection of middle ear effusion. *Clinical Otolaryngology*, **15**, 121–123

TOS, M. and POULSEN, G. (1979) Tympanometry in 2 year old children, seasonal influence on secretory otitis media and tubal dysfunction. *Annals of Otology, Rhinology and Laryngology*, **41**, 1–10

TOS, M. and POULSEN, G. (1980) Attic retractions following secretory otitis media. *Acta Otolaryngologica*, **89**, 479–486

TOS, M. and STANGERUP, S. E. (1985) Secretory otitis and pneumatisation of the mastoid process: sexual differences in the size of the mastoid air cell system. *American Journal of Otolaryngology*, **6**, 199–205

TOS, M., BONDING, P. and POULSEN, G. (1983) Tympanosclerosis of the drum in secretory otitis after insertion of grommets. A prospective comparative study. *Journal of Laryngology and Otology*, **97**, 489–496

TOS, M., STANGERUP, S. E. and LARSEN, P. (1992) Incidence and progression of myringoincudoplexy after secretory otitis. *Acta Otolaryngologica*, **112**, 512–517

UHARI, M., NIEMELA, M., HUGGARE, J. and LAUTALA, P. (1991) The associations between nasopharynx dimensions and otitis media in children. In: *Recent Advances in Otitis Media*, 5th International Symposium May, Florida

VAN BON, M. J., ZIELHUIS, G. A., RACH, G. H. and VAN DEN BROEK, P. (1989) Otitis media with effusion and habitual mouth breathing in Dutch preschool children. *International Journal of Pediatric Otorhinolaryngology*, **17**, 119–125

VAN CAUWENBERGE, P. B. and KLUYSKENS, P. M. (1984) Some predisposing factors in otitis media with effusion. In: *Recent Advances in Otitis media with effusion*, edited by D. J. Lim. Philadelphia: B. C. Decker Inc. pp. 28–32

VARSANO, I. B., VOLOVITZ, B. M. and GROSSMAN, J. E. (1989) Effect of naproxen, a prostaglandin inhibitor, on acute otitis media and persistence of middle ear effusion in children. *Annals of Otology, Rhinology and Laryngology*, **98**, 389–392

VON SCHOENBERG, M., WENGRAF, C. L. and GLEESON, M. (1989) Results of middle ear ventilation with Goode's tubes. *Clinical Otolaryngology*, **14**, 503–508

WAKE, M. and SMALLMAN, L. A. (1992) Ciliary beat frequency of nasal and middle ear mucosa in children with otitis media with effusion. *Clinical Otolaryngology*, **17**, 155–157

WATKIN, P. M., BALDWIN, M. and LAOIDE, S. (1990) Parental suspicion and identification of hearing impairment. *Archives of Diseases in Childhood*, **65**, 846–850

WIDEMAR, L., SVENSSON, C., RYNNEL DAGOO, B. and SCHIRATZKI, H. (1985) The effect of adenoidectomy on secretory otitis media. A 2 year controlled prospective study. *Clinical Otolaryngology*, **10**, 345–350

WOLTHERS, O. D. (1990) Tympanometric screening in children on admission to a paediatric ward: a preliminary study. *International Journal of Pediatric Otorhinolaryngology*, **19**, 251–257

YOSHIMURA, H., WATANABE, N., BUNDO, J., SHINODA, M. and MOGI, G. (1993) Oral vaccination for pneumococcal otitis media in animal models. In: *Recent Advances in Otitis*

Media, edited by D. J. Lim. Toronto: B. C. Decker. pp. 161–164

YUNG, M. W. and MORRIS, T. M. O. (1981) Tuning fork tests in diagnosis for serous otitis media. *British Medical Journal,* **283,** 1576

ZIELHUIS, G. A., RACH, G. H. and VAN DEN BROEK, P. (1989) Screening for otitis media with effusion in preschool children. *Lancet,* i, 311–314

ZIELHUIS, G. A., HEUVELMANS-HEINEN, E. W., RACH, G. H. and VAN DEN BROEK, P. (1989) Environmental risk factors for otitis media with effusion in preschool children. *Scandinavian Journal of Primary Health Care,* **7,** 33–38

ZIELHUIS, G. A., RACH, G. H. and VAN DEN BROEK, P. (1990) The natural course of otitis media with effusion in preschool children. *European Archives of Otorhinolaryngology,* **247,** 215–221

ZIELHUIS, G. A., RACH, G. H., BOSCH, A. V. and VAN DEN BROEK, P. (1990) The prevalence of otitis media with effusion: a critical review of the literature. *Clinical Otolaryngology,* **15,** 283–288

8

Acute and chronic suppurative otitis media in children

Roger F. Gray

Suppurative otitis media with its unpleasant symptoms and complications may be a catastrophe for the marvellously structured organ on which much of our appreciation of life and human activity depends. It is the privilege of the otologist to preserve, repair and reconstruct the structure and function of the ear in whatever condition it is found. In children the additional challenge is to prevent acute suppurative otitis media turning into chronic disease.

Acute otitis media

Acute otitis media or acute suppurative otitis media is an episode of inflammation of the middle ear associated with pain, fever, hearing loss and sometimes discharge. Sixty-five to 95% of children will have suffered one or more attacks before the age of 7 years (Claessen *et al.*, 1992).

Aetiology

Spread of infection

Up the eustachian tube

The eustachian tube of young children is relatively incompetent. Most middle ear infections probably occur as a result of ascending infection by this route, usually after an upper respiratory tract infection.

Through a pre-existing perforation of the tympanic membrane

This may be due to a previous infection or trauma. Infection may also enter the middle ear through a ventilation tube.

Blood-borne infection

Middle ear infections may occur during some viral illnesses and predispose to secondary bacterial infection.

Age

There is debate about the peak incidence of acute otitis media with some believing it to be 5–7 years and others who state that it is commonest in pre-school children. The incidence is probably related to the population studied.

Socioeconomic factors

The incidence is said to be highest in low hygiene populations or with overcrowding and malnutrition. Significant associations with acute otitis media were found by Kero and Piekkala (1987) in a regional birth cohort of 5356 infants in Scandinavia. More bouts of acute otitis media were seen in infants with many siblings in crowded day-care facilities where the mother stopped breastfeeding early and where the infant was premature or of low socioeconomic grouping. Fewer bouts of acute otitis media were seen in full-term infants with fewer siblings, longer duration breast-feeding, spacious day-care facilities and high socioeconomic group.

Specific abnormalities associated with acute otitis media

Immunosuppression or immunoparesis, cleft palate and Down's syndrome are all associated with middle ear problems. The principles of treatment are the same as for other children; if medical treatment fails to control the attacks or relieve the hearing loss then surgery (usually ventilation tubes) should be performed. Adenoidectomy must be avoided with open and submucous cleft palates because it may make postnasal escape worse. Otitis media with effusion is almost universal in cleft palate infants and acute otitis media correspondingly frequent. Fifty adolescents who had clefts repaired in infancy were examined and 81% found to have normal hearing and 86% normal middle ear pressures. Half had repeated ventilation tubes and this group had a tendency to tympanosclerotic eardrums (Gordon, Jean-Louis and Morton, 1988). Ovesen and Blegvad-Andersen (1992) found significant pathology in forty-four 11-year-old children with unilateral cleft lip and palate, compared with age matched controls. Hearing impairment was present in 24% compared with 0% in controls and retraction of the pars flaccida in 23% with 6% in controls.

The adenoid pad

A large adenoid pad or a small nasopharynx impede mucociliary flow, and stagnant mucus allows growth of pathogens which would otherwise be washed away. These pathogens lead to ascending infection of the eustachian tube and middle ear. Mucosal oedema prevents drainage. The microbiology of the middle ear flora depends on whether the tympanic membrane is intact. Pus aspirated from the middle ear contains the same organisms as the nasopharynx, with *Streptococcus pneumoniae* predominating in the first year of life and *Haemophilus influenzae* thereafter (Calhoun *et al.*, 1988). When sufficient pressure causes the drum head to give way, discharge takes place and a new route for microorganisms is established through the perforation. *Staphylococcus aureus* and *Pseudomonas aeruginosa*, both commonly found in discharge from perforations and ventilation tubes, are derived from the external skin environment rather than the upper respiratory tract and can be pictured ascending the waterfall like spawning salmon.

Bacteriology of acute otitis media

Karma *et al.* (1987) analysed the fluid from 107 episodes of acute otitis media in 101 infants less than 3 months old. The common pathogens were *Strep. pneumoniae* 19%, *Haemophilus influenzae* 9% and *Branhamella catarrhalis* 7%. A total of one-third of the 107 episodes grew bacteria in culture; half of these organisms were β-lactamase producers. Calhoun *et al.* (1988) looked for bacteria in 908 middle ear effusions in 495 children aged 4 months to 12 years. Twenty per cent of the effusions grew pathogens, over half of which were *Haemophilus influenzae*. The conclusion is that while many attacks may not be bacterial it is impossible to rule out pathogenic bacte-

rial infection when confronted with a child with otalgia.

Nasopharyngeal organisms and acute otitis media

Further evidence of the origin of acute otitis media in children comes from the bacteriology of the nose and the middle ear. Pathogenic bacteria found on nasal swabs in 52 children who subsequently underwent adenoidectomy have been shown by Timon, Cafferkey and Walsh (1991) to correspond closely to organisms found among the lymphoid tissue of the removed adenoid. The pernasal preoperative swabs correctly identified 76% of the pathogens isolated in the adenoid tissue. *Haemophilus influenzae* was the predominant organism in all cultures. Tonsil swabs taken preoperatively had a poor correspondence (38%) with organisms in the depths of removed tonsils.

Middle ear effusions (Karma *et al.*, 1987; Hendrickse *et al.*, 1988; Calhoun *et al.*, 1988) contain *Strep. pneumoniae*, *Haemophilus influenzae* and *Branhamella catarrhalis*. Talaat *et al.* (1989) performed a pre-and postoperative bacteriological study in 50 children with enlarged and infected adenoids and found that the rate of isolation of pathogenic organisms like *Haemophilus influenzae* and *Strep. pneumoniae* decreased markedly after adenoidectomy to fall to the level of pathogens and commensals in 20 healthy controls.

Symptoms and signs

Very young children will not complain of pain but will be cross, irritable and may bang the head on the cot sides. Conversely some children may become very quiet and refuse food, not sleep well or be inconsolable. There may be a history of preceding upper respiratory tract infection or tonsillitis. Pain may be localized to the abdomen. On examination, the young child is febrile, listless and uncooperative with red bulging tympanic membranes. A hearing loss is present though the child is usually too distressed to allow a test of hearing. If the ears discharge it is usually blood-stained initially and this may worry parents. The discharge then becomes mucopurulent.

Investigations

A swab may be taken, though often the result of this does not influence treatment. Mastoid X-rays are only indicated if the acute infection spreads or becomes chronic.

Treatment

Medical treatment

Simple analgesics, such as paracetamol, may be sufficient in mild cases. The role of antibiotics continues to be debated and few rigorous trials have been conducted. In those that have, no definitive conclusions have been reached. Claessen *et al.* (1992) reviewed 50 published studies between 1965 and 1989 and found 13 well constructed trials comparing different antibiotics, though only four used placebo controls. In the USA antibiotics are prescribed in 97.9% of cases and in the Netherlands only in 31% of cases. The ideal antibiotic or even whether to use an antibiotic at all has not been established beyond doubt.

Antibiotic duration and choice

In a double-blind study of 175 patients Hendrickse *et al.* (1988) compared 5-day and 10-day courses of antibiotics for acute otitis media. They found *Strep. pneumoniae* or *Haemophilus influenzae* in 55% of middle ear effusions aspirated before treatment. Cefaclor, 40 mg/kg/day 12 hourly was used. The conclusion of the trial was that in patients with intact tympanic membranes it was not possible to show any advantage by treating for 10 days rather than 5 days. In children with spontaneous purulent discharge a 5-day course did not appear to be sufficient and a 10-day course was more effective. Bluestone (1989) recommended amoxycillin for treatment of acute otitis media and prophylaxis of recurrent attacks. In selected children where amoxycillin seems clinically ineffective and where β-lactamase-producing bacteria are suspected, amoxycillin-clavulanate, cefuroxime and cefixime are advised.

The choice of antibiotic should be guided by the bacteriologist at the local laboratory where swabs are cultured and sensitivities are established as the prevalence of β-lactamase-producing organisms varies from place to place.

Antibiotic prophylaxis in infant acute otitis media

Fauskin (1991) was able to show that while 13 untreated infants had six bouts of acute otitis media over a 4-month period a similar group of 19 infants treated with continuous aminopenicillin or erythromycin had no bouts of acute otitis media. All infants in the trial had suffered their first attack before 3 months of age.

Topical antibiotics

Concern about ototoxicity inhibits general practitioners from prescribing aminoglycoside ear drops. Bickerton, Roberts and Little (1988) questioned 301 general practitioners in Staffordshire. Sixty-six per cent would not give topical treatment when the tympanic membrane was perforated and only 41% would give topical treatment to discharging grommets. The standard teaching of otolaryngologists, that aminoglycoside drops are the most effective treatment for aural discharge and that the risk of ototoxicity is less than the risk of chronic sepsis in causing sensorineural deafness, has not been communicated to general practitioners.

Surgical treatment

Drainage

Occasionally, if the child is very distressed or toxic, a myringotomy incision will allow drainage of pus.

Ventilation tubes

Grommets will usually stop recurrent acute otitis media (Paradise *et al.*, 1990) but sometimes only change its character from episodes of severe fever and pain to episodes of recurrent ear discharge. Discharge may be preferable to pain but does not constitute a complete cure and, in the case of a child with mixed deafness, may make the wearing of hearing aids impossible. Adenoidectomy alone may be preferable for such cases.

Adenoidectomy and acute otitis media

A number of randomized prospective studies have looked at the efficacy of adenoidectomy in relieving otherwise untreated otitis media with effusion (Maw and Herod, 1986; Gates, Muntz and Gaylis, 1992; Maw and Parker, 1993). These studies have demonstrated the effectiveness of the operation over a period of months, but fewer have looked at adenoidectomy and acute otitis media. Paradise *et al.* (1990) took 213 children who had been given ventilation tubes for acute otitis media rather than otitis media with effusion but had relapsed when the tubes came out. Ninety-nine were randomly assigned to adenoidectomy or a control group and 114 assigned according to parental preference. The adenoidectomy group had a more favourable result in the first and second year of follow up with a reduction in the incidence of acute otitis media (28% and 35%) compared with controls.

Tonsillectomy and acute otitis media

No studies specifically address this issue. Maw (1988) found no statistically significant difference in the resolution of otitis media with effusion in response to adenoidectomy alone or adenoidectomy and tonsillectomy combined. His conclusion was that there was no additional benefit from combination of tonsillectomy with adenoidectomy compared with adenoidectomy alone. If these conclusions may be extrapolated to acute otitis media then it is unlikely that tonsillectomy alone will reduce its incidence. One consideration which must not be overlooked however is that bacterial tonsillitis may cause pain to be referred to the ears and mimic acute otitis media even though there are no otoscopic changes or tympanometric abnormalities. Tonsillectomy will then stop the otalgia, and therefore the 'acute otitis media' if it has been misdiagnosed in this way.

The impact of day surgery on acute otitis media

The growth of day surgery facilities in the UK has allowed most children requiring ventilation tubes to go home the same day. This however may discriminate against children requiring adenoidectomy in addition to grommets and who may have to wait longer for more scarce inpatient facilities. Adenoidectomy has been said to be acceptable as a day surgery procedure. Leighton *et al.* (1993b) stated that 78% of 15 minor complications in 62 children occurred within 6 hours of surgery. One major complication (bleeding) occurred within 2 hours of surgery. It is likely that economic pressure will remove more adenoidectomy cases to the day surgery unit in those hospitals that have the facility, and this may increase the proportion of children undergoing adenoidectomy as well as ventilation tubes for acute otitis media.

Complications of acute otitis media

Acute mastoiditis

Classical mastoiditis is described as presenting with pain, fever and swelling behind the ear typically occurring after a middle ear infection. A sagging posterosuperior wall of the deep ear canal (subperiosteal abscess) is seen with the auriscope. Localized tenderness over Macewan's triangle and the sagging wall help to differentiate this dangerous condition from an equally painful but much less dangerous otitis externa. How accurate is this clinical picture today? Nadal *et al.* (1990) reviewed 73 children aged between 4 months and 14 years with acute mastoiditis. The leading four findings in order of frequency were: retroauricular swelling (63 children), tenderness (59 children), erythema (58 children) and protrusion (45 children). Tympanic membrane changes were noted in only 17 (33%) of patients. Thirty-six per cent had subperiosteal abscesses which, when aspirated, cultured organisms in 32 (80%) of samples. Nearly half the children were already taking antibiotics.

Conservative management in less severe cases

Nadal *et al.* (1990) recommended a 48-hour trial of intravenous antibiotics directed against staphylococci and pneumococci if there was not a subperiosteal abscess as those two organisms were the most commonly cultured. Twenty-four patients got better on this management without surgery.

Cortical mastoidectomy

Severe cases with subperiosteal abscess or CNS complications require immediate exploration though delayed exploration is appropriate if conservative treatment fails. Forty-nine out of seventy-three required mastoidectomy in the above series.

Latent or masked mastoiditis

Mastoiditis which has developed despite oral antibiotic therapy has a less dramatic clinical picture and is said to be latent or masked. Garabedian *et al.* (1990) looked at 'protracted otitis' in 118 children and concluded that subacute mastoiditis was a potent factor in failure to improve and should be diagnosed and if necessary operated upon early. Pain, fever and tenderness are less but a fluctuant swelling, indicating a subperiosteal abscess over the mastoid is characteristic. Faye–Lund (1989) described the incidence of mastoiditis in Oslo over a 4-year period and concluded that classical acute mastoiditis was more common than masked disease, the reverse of that expected given that antibiotics are freely available.

Acute mastoiditis and leukaemia

Acute leukaemia may sometimes present with acute mastoiditis or a facial palsy and it is wise to send tissue for histology if exploring an acute mastoiditis. Three leukaemic children undergoing chemotherapy developed 'acute necrotizing otitis media' with severe mastoiditis in a series reported by Arcand, Cerat and Spenard (1989). Immunoglobulin deficiency may lead to the same clinical picture (Castro *et al.*, 1990).

Sigmoid sinus thrombosis and intracranial sepsis

If the outer cortex of the mastoid bone can perforate to allow the formation of a subperiosteal abscess then the inner cortical bone may do the same. Pus lying next to the transverse (lateral) sinus provokes thrombosis, at first sterile and later infected. This condition was formerly deduced from the clinical presentation with irritability and swinging pyrexia occurring as fragments of infected clot detached themselves and entered the circulation. CT scanning will now identify the condition at an earlier stage and is advised in any case of acute mastoiditis with subperiosteal abscess formation. Heitzmann *et al.* (1990) and Oyarzabal, Patel and Tolley (1992) discovered lateral sinus thrombosis in children being scanned for mastoiditis. Fritsch, Miyamoto and Wood (1990) recommended early MRI scanning of cases at risk of sigmoid sinus thrombosis while symptoms are subtle and before they become fulminant.

The management of sigmoid sinus thrombophlebitis involved preventing infected clot spreading in the venous system by ligation of the internal jugular vein in the neck, packing off the vein in the mastoid and evacuation of infected clot from the lumen. The source of infection will have been removed in the course of the mastoidectomy necessary for access to the vein. If an extradural or subdural abscess is present and identified on CT or MRI scan the help of a neurosurgeon will be required (Wackym, Canalis and Feuerman, 1990). Chronic suppurative otitis media is more often the cause of this than acute otitis media (four out of six cases reported by Medwick, Ulhlein and Hallberg, 1949).

Meningitis

Meningitis may occur as a complication of acute otitis media. Gower and McGuirt (1983) reported 85 patients under the age of 20 years with CNS complications of middle ear disease. Sixty-three suffered meningitis after acute otitis media and 13 after chronic suppurative otitis media. The mortality rate was 12%.

Samuel, Fernandez and Steinberg (1986) found 83 cases of meningitis in 335 patients with acute otitis media which had progressed to mastoiditis with a high preponderance of children and young adults and an overall mortality (taken with other intracranial complications) of 14%.

Abnormalities of cochlear morphology, like Mondini's deformity where the middle and apical turns of the cochlea are dilated and fused together, predispose to recurrent meningitis (Herther and Schindler, 1985). Any cause of cerebrospinal otorrhoea may lead to meningitis (Harris, 1978) and the leak must be stopped to remove the risk of further attacks.

Gower and McGuirt (1983) noted that it is the responsibility of the otolaryngologist to keep the paediatricians aware of the ear as a source of infection for the meninges, as otitis media in a child with meningitis is sometimes dismissed as an incidental finding (Rasmussen, Johnsen and Bohr, 1991) rather than recognized as the primary cause.

Sensorineural deafness

Pus within the cochlea results in profound sensorineural deafness. The commonest route is via the cochlear aqueduct from the CSF space around the jugular bulb in cases of bacterial meningitis. This causes soft tissue or new bone to form in the scala tympani, where it is often found during cochlear implant operations. Pus may also enter through the round or oval window when otitis media becomes 'otitis interna' (Brunner, 1949). In either case the sepsis enters the basal or high frequency end of the cochlea and destroys hair cells giving a high frequency hearing loss. Low and mid frequencies often survive unless sepsis spreads to the apex.

Facial palsy

A lower motor neuron facial palsy may be the presenting feature of acute otitis media where immunity is poor (e.g. leukaemia or AIDs) or where the nerve lies outside the bony fallopian tube (dehiscent facial nerve) and the sheath is exposed to pus under pressure. Both these conditions are an indication for urgent surgical drainage, either by a myringotomy or cortical mastoidectomy combined with vigorous antibiotic therapy. Biopsies should be taken if possible, from mastoid mucosa or granulations, carefully avoiding the area of the facial nerve.

Does acute otitis media cause glue ear?

The natural history of acute otitis media is that the drum ruptures and the pus escapes. Giving appropriate antibiotics will destroy the infective organism and may arrest the natural history at the stage of effusion. The child is relieved of pain but may be left with 'glue' ears. Mills (1987) looked at recurrent acute otitis media in general practice diagnosed by tympanometry with pneumatic otoscopy. Forty-one per cent of 58 children had effusions 2 months after their presenting episode and at 3 months this fell to 33%. Significantly more of the children with persistent effusions were in the group which had received cephalexin than in the group with no antibiotics.

Chronic suppurative otitis media

Otitis media with effusion, multiple ventilation tubes, myringostapedopexy, posterior retraction pockets, marginal granulations, accummulation of squamous debris behind any obstruction to the self-cleaning mechanism seem to be stations on a journey which some children make towards serious middle ear disease. Many get off the line without help, but each stage on the list is undesirable and to be avoided if possible. The large numbers that do not progress to cholesteatoma lend credence to the idea that timely intervention by the otologist will arrest the journey in many cases.

Aetiology

Epidemiology

Traditionally the prevalence of chronic suppurative otitis media has been found as a by-product of surveys for hearing loss. The availability of audiologists made this possible in developed countries. The extent of chronic suppurative otitis media in developing countries is only beginning to become known and only a few studies have looked specifically at children.

Chronic suppurative otitis media

Nine of 1485 children (0.6%) were found to have chronic suppurative otitis media after referral to an otologist because of a failed hearing test (Marttila, 1986). Rudin *et al.* (1983) sampled men from the Swedish national census lists and found an incidence of perforations of 1.7% and other major pathological changes in the tympanic membrane (including perforations) of 3.6%. Otorrhoea for more than 1 month was present in 3.2%. The study looked at four age groups to see if disease was less frequent or severe in younger men. The otorrhoea rate for 20 and 30 year olds was 0.8% while for 50 and 60 year olds it was 4.1%. The conclusion was that middle ear disease was not less frequent in the last two decades in Sweden but had become less damaging.

Chronic suppurative otitis media in Israel

Fliss *et al.* (1990) calculated an incidence of 39 per 100 000 in southern Israeli children based on 88 with disease and 76 age matched controls. This is 0.04% and is the lowest figure in the current literature. Significantly increased risk factors were past acute otitis media, parental chronic suppurative otitis media, large families and a high crowding index in large day-care centres.

Chronic suppurative otitis media in Greenland

The incidence reported by Pedersen and Zachau–Christiansen (1988) is about 200 times greater than in Israel. Three-hundred-and-three young people aged between 11 and 20 years had an 8% incidence of chronic suppurative otitis media and 305 aged between 41 and 50 years, an incidence of 2%, although 13% had had active disease in the past.

Chronic suppurative otitis media in South Africa

Halama, Voogt and Musgrove (1986) examined 267 children in a remote South African community and, although 8.2% had otitis media, only one had a perforation with discharge. Scarred tympanic membranes were found in 6.7%.

Chronic suppurative otitis media in the Solomon Islands

Eason *et al.* (1986) found that 3.8% of 3500 children were affected. Of these 65% suffered onset before the age of 18 months and measles, respiratory infections, swimming and malnutrition were identified as the aetiological factors amenable to intervention.

Smoking and chronic suppurative otitis media

There are no published data on the relative incidence of chronic suppurative otitis media in children of smokers, but Maw *et al.* (1992) have shown an increase in the proportion of glue ears in children whose parents smoke. Chemical irritation from passive smoking is associated with mucus hypersecretion and mucosal oedema, both undesirable factors in the eustachian tube and middle ear. Parents of children with chronic suppurative otitis media are asked to stop smoking; there is no deception in saying that treatment will be more likely to be successful.

Systemic conditions associated with chronic suppurative otitis media

Chronic lung disease associated with sepsis such as bronchiectasis or cystic fibrosis predisposes to exacerbations and recurrences of chronic suppurative otitis media particularly if postural drainage techniques put pus in the nasopharynx.

Immunosupression from any cause will impede resolution of active ear sepsis.

The relationship between otitis media with effusion, perforations and cholesteatoma

Eustachian tube obstruction is implicated in the case of otitis media with effusion and in acquired cholesteatoma and it is thus tempting to regard otitis media with effusion as a precursor of cholesteatoma. Is there any evidence? Three-hundred-and-twenty-seven children born in 1975 were followed to age 16, each being examined nine times by Tos, Stangerup and Larsen (1992). The incus protruded through the drum such as to become visible in outline (myringoincudopexy) in 0.5% at 5 years and 4.2% at age 16, after documented episodes of otitis media with effusion. Deguine (1985) reviewed 536 cholesteatomas and found 12 cases where the disease presented in children between the ages of 7 and 12 years who had been treated for otitis media with effusion by repeated ventilation tubes. The age distribution in 1431 cases of cholesteatoma peaked at 20–25 years of age and the first 25 years of life accounted for 31% of cholesteatomas in the series. If a gestation time of 5–10 years is commonplace then many of these must have developed in childhood. Tos (1981) looked at 114 ears in children all of whom had recurrent acute otitis media. One (1%) of these progressed to a dry central perforation and none to cholesteatoma. He also looked at 864 ears in children with secretory otitis media and found three which progressed to dry central perforations and three more to cholesteatoma. In a 10-year ventilation tube study of 65 ears De Saar, Mulder and van den Broek (1992) discovered seven ears (2%) with cholesteatoma which needed surgery. Does the use of ventilation tubes decrease the risk of cholesteatoma? Roland *et al.* (1992) in Liverpool compared the incidence of paediatric cholesteatoma in pre-grommet years 1963–1976 with 1976–1990 (after grommets were introduced). There has been a steady reduction in the cholesteatoma rate but with no lag period which is interesting though the case remains unproved. The conclusion is that otitis media with effusion and chronic tubal dysfunction, both frequent in childhood, cause changes which may predispose in later months or years to cholesteatoma or perforations.

Acute otitis media and chronic suppurative otitis media

While pathogens of the upper respiratory tract exist it will be impossible to prevent children developing attacks of acute otitis media. When the drum head gives way by pressure necrosis and the ear discharges pus it is often a good thing for the patient who is relieved of pain and deafness.

The virtuous circle and the vicious circle

Discharge and healing of the perforation and middle ear is a virtuous circle of events dictated by the classic sequence of acute inflammatory changes. A vicious circle exists when incomplete healing predisposes the ear to further acute episodes and these become so frequent that they merge and appear continuous or chronic. Several things may go amiss in the virtuous circle to create a vicious one. Repeated episodes of acute otitis from infected adenoids in the nasopharynx may overwhelm the drum's capacity to heal. Scar tissue may form in the wrong place, thickening the residual drum head with tympanosclerosis instead of repairing the perforation. Contaminated water may enter the middle ear through the perforation before it has had time to heal. The original organism may be so virulent (streptococcal, scarlet fever), host immunity so low (malnutrition, measles) or both that areas of drum tissue are lost by necrosis and a large hole remains. Sometimes eustachian tube function is so poor that retraction pockets deepen and lose their ability to propel keratin into the self-cleaning system of the ear canal. The accumulation of squamous debris in the depths of a retraction pocket is the beginning of cholesteatoma.

The otologist sees all these things happening and may from time to time be in a position to nudge a patient back into the virtuous circle.

Adenoidectomy for chronic nasopharyngitis, keeping the ear dry while an acute perforation heals, or treating an early infection with ear drops all may be just enough to prevent the development of chronic suppurative otitis media. Ventilation tubes and excision of retraction pockets play a part in arresting the development of cholesteatoma. On a world scale, universal vaccination against measles and the vaccines developed for *Haemophilus influenzae* type B and in due course A, may significantly reduce the incidence of chronic suppurative otitis media and its sequelae.

Bacteriology

Culture from chronic middle ears

A wide range of organisms may be cultured from chronically infected middle ears (Tables 8.1 and 8.2) and each has an intimate relationship with the symptoms and signs, e.g. the odour of *Pseudomonas aeruginosa* (sweaty feet) is quite different from the smell of new baked bread associated with *Monilia*. Similarly the signs of cellulitis and oedema typical of *Streptococcus* contrast strongly with the black deposits of *Aspergillus niger*. The range of organisms suggests that most are opportunistic and a warm dark cul-de-sac like the ear is unlikely to remain uncolonized for long if wetted from outside (washing or swimming) or inside (coryza).

Once established an individual organism or group of organisms tends to flourish for long periods in a chronic ear producing all the symptoms except the conductive deafness due to the perforation or lack of ossicles. Even this may be made worse by oedema, pus and debris. The organisms present in chronic suppurative otitis media aspirate have been counted by Raisanen and Stenfors (1992); 6×10^6 to 6×10^9 are the enormous numbers associated with a symptomatic ear. The organisms present may not be those responsible for the necrosis of the tympanic membrane which occurred months or years before, but each aids the other in perpetuating the symptoms.

Symptoms of chronic ear disease

There may be any combination of discharge, deafness, bleeding, tinnitus, vertigo and pain. Discharge and hearing loss are usually present, and bleeding comes from a polyp or granulation tissue but is rarely as serious as it looks. Tinnitus of a pulsatile type is associated with the blood flow through granulations, but tinnitus of a hissing type implies cochlear damage and may precede vertigo which indicates invasion of the vestibular labyrinth by bacteria or cholesteatoma or both. Deep unremitting pain in the ear is a sinister symptom associated with serious complications. Young children rarely volunteer the symptoms of pain or tinnitus but might admit them if asked; parents are often unaware of anything unusual. Attempts to classify infection by symptoms are useless as the same symptoms (otorrhoea) may indicate a small safe central perforation or dangerously widespread cholesteatoma of the petrous bone.

Table 8.1 Anaerobic bacteria in chronic suppurative otitis media

Palva and Hallstrom (1965)	5% Anaerobic streptococci
Jokipii *et al.* (1977)	33% Anaerobes, 16% *Bacteroides*
Sugita *et al.* (1981)	4% *Peptococcus*, 2% *Bacteroides*
Constable and Butler (1982)	6% *Peptococcus*, 5% *Bacteroides*
Sweeney, Picozzi and Browning	55% *Bacteroides*
Browning *et al.* (1983)	50% Anaerobes
Brook (1985)	81 Anaerobe isolates in 54 children

Table 8.2 Aerobic organisms in chronic suppurative otitis media

Jokipii *et al.* (1977)	*Staphylococcus aureus* 19%	*Escherichia coli* 7%	*Proteus* 5%
Ojala *et al.* (1981)	*Staph. aureus* 22%	*Pseudomonas* 19%	*Proteus* 5%
Constable and Butler (1982)	*Staph. aureus* 29%	*Proteus* 26%	*Pseudomonas* 15%
Sweeney, Picozzi and Browning (1982)	*Proteus* 38%	*Staph. aureus* 16%	*Pseudomonas* 12%
Palva and Hallstrom (1965)	*Pseudomonas* 24%	*Staph. aureus* 13%	*Klebsiella* 9%
Brook (1985)	*Pseudomonas* 29%	*Staph. aureus* 10%	*Klebsiella* 10%

Signs of chronic ear disease

Removal of wax or debris is an essential preliminary, a ring probe, blunt hook or forceps are used to clear a view of the drum head. Examining mother's ears first is a good way of gaining a child's trust. In chronic suppurative otitis media it can then be seen with illumination whether the perforation is in the pars tensa or the pars flaccida. This is how tubotympanic 'safe' disease was distinguished from atticoantral 'unsafe' disease in the early days of otology. The distinction is still valid in situations where specialist equipment is lacking or when introducing a trainee to the concepts of ear disease. Nurse practitioners trained in the use of the head mirror can identify and begin the treatment of a variety of ear disorders in this way.

Using an auriscope, small structures like the lentiform process of the incus touching the drum, the chorda tympani nerve, or if there is a perforation, the ossicular chain and tympanic nerve plexus, can be seen. Wisps of dry cholesteatoma or wet debris may be seen disappearing round corners; the drawback is that it is practially impossible to use a fine sucker or forceps in the ear at the same time. You can look but not touch!

'Siegleization' of the ear still has a place in the consulting room. Alternately compressing and releasing the rubber bulb of the Siegle speculum (or the pneumatic auriscope) will give a good indication of the mobility of the drum head and confirm that perforation has healed. Occasionally a retraction pocket can be temporarily everted. Patients with a labyrinthine fistula will suffer vertigo and nystagmus. The Acoustic Impedence machine elicits much more information about middle ear function and has re-placed the pneumatic auriscope in many clinics; a lightweight hand held version has been usefully combined with an auriscope.

Signs elicited with the microscope

Binocular stereoscopic views of the ear are obtained with axial lighting and a range of magnifications. A power of × 6 is suitable for cleaning the meatus, changing to × 10 for examination of the drum head. The higher powers of × 16 and × 25 are less helpful because the depth of field is too small and one spends more time out of focus than in focus. Suction with an 18 SWG calibre tip allows thorough cleaning of wax or pus and the finer tips, SWG 20 or 22, will pass into the smallest crevices where cholesteatoma might lie concealed. A child can be lifted to the eyepieces and shown a magnified view of a coin to gain his confidence.

Microsuction allows detailed examination of the ear. A crust in the pars flaccida, possibly the subtlest sign in clinical medicine, can be removed to reveal the mouth of an attic cholesteatoma. The whole cholesteatoma may, in favourable circumstances, be sucked out leaving the ear dry for many months. This opens the possibility of conservative management of the disease in children where surgery is refused. Polyps can be gently removed and antiseptic, antibiotic or steroid creams inserted on a gauze wick.

Classification of disease

The purpose of classification is to predict the course of disease and the damage it will do. The otologist needs to know the exact anatomical site of the disease and the pathological process. Suction under the microscope goes further towards this ideal than any other clinical technique. What cannot be known is the posterior limit of the disease, but this may be inferred from the hearing loss, from X-rays, but most of all from what the otologist knows of the natural history of the types of disease listed below.

1 Tubotympanic disease

This is a perforation in the pars tensa with preservation of the fibrous annulus (also known as a central perforation). It is usually associated with bacterial infection of the middle ear mucosa and is thought to be safe.

2 Atticoantral disease

This is a defect in the pars flaccida (Shrapnell's membrane) and is associated with cholesteatoma and therefore unsafe.

3 Marginal perforation or tympanic sinus disease

A posterior defect in the fibrous annulus is also associated with cholesteatoma and is also unsafe.

4 Cholesteatoma in a safe perforation

This is a non-marginal defect in the pars tensa where cholesteatoma can be observed curling under the edge of the perforation and accumulating in the middle ear, and is a contradiction in terms, but is nevertheless unsafe.

Clinical tests of hearing

Whisper tests

The ability of a child to discriminate a whispered voice, conversational voice or shout may be determined from behind. The tragus of the non-test ear is depressed by the surgeon's finger to block the meatus. This limits the distance to the length of an arm but allows each ear to be tested separately. Numbers between 20 and 100 are convenient polysyllables. Browning, Swan and Chew (1989) looked at informal tests of hearing and compared them with pure tone audiometry. They found that 86% of patients with a pure tone loss of clinical significance could be identified by whisper test at 61 cm (2 feet).

Tuning fork tests

The Rinne and Weber tests are still the quickest way of identifying the presence and side of a conductive deafness. A negative Rinne response (hearing better by bone conduction than air conduction) is to be expected in chronic suppurative otitis media unless

the hearing is nearly normal. The false-negative response (beloved by examiners at the Colleges of Surgeons) occurs when the test ear is 'dead' and the patient hears with the opposite ear. The Bárány noise box in the non-test ear removes the false response. It is unwise to operate on an ear for conductive deafness unless the Weber test is referred to that ear and the Rinne test negative. In the same paper as mentioned above Browning, Swan and Chew (1989) found the 256 Hz fork and the loudness comparison method superior to the threshold decay method in identifying conductive deafness in 127 patients who were later proven to have conductive losses on audiometry. A 256 Hz fork identified 48% with a 15 dB loss, 69% with a 20 dB loss and 95% with a 30 dB loss.

Clinical tests of balance

Three clinical tests of balance are useful to judge whether disease, suction or packing has upset the vestibular system. Romberg's test with eyes closed may show that the patient staggers towards the affected ear as the result of a recent paralytic lesion and away from the affected ear with an irritative lesion. Heel/toe walking will be abnormal in a patient who has recently lost labyrinthine function from disease or surgery, or has had it compromised by too tight a pack. Unterberger's stepping test (marching on the spot with eyes closed and arms stretched out in front) demonstrates a tendency to rotate to the side of a weak labyrinth. It is principally a test for long-standing compensated vestibular dysfunction because after an acute loss the patient staggers and cannot complete the test. Complex vestibular function tests are generally unnecessary for the management of chronic suppurative otitis media.

Completing the examination

Examination of the eyes in advanced disease may reveal nystagmus, rectus palsy, or papilloedema. Examination of the neck may show cervical lymphadenopathy, or an abscess in the sheath of sternomastoid (Bezold's abscess). Cranial nerve palsies, particularly the facial nerve, and cerebellar signs must not be missed.

Audiological assessment

In young children behavioural tests will give information about hearing thresholds. In older children a pure tone audiogram with air and bone conduction thresholds is required before a decision can be made about surgery. The surgeon must know which is the better hearing ear, the proportion of the loss that is conductive and the cochlear function that remains in the octaves between 500 Hz and 4000 Hz that are necessary for the discrimination of speech. Two methods of predicting benefit are available: the Glasgow plot (Browning, Gatehouse and Swan, 1991) and the 15/30 dB rule of thumb (Smyth and Patterson, 1985). Both take into account the hearing in the other ear when assessing the potential benefit of middle ear surgery. The pitfall for the surgeon is mistaking a sensorineural loss for a conductive deafness. Even normal bone conduction audiometric thresholds may be a 'shadow curve' derived from the other ear or the audiologist may have mislabelled the left and right ears.

Radiological assessment

Indication for plain films

Plain X-rays of the temporal bone will indicate the position of the tegmen, the sigmoid sinus and the degree of pneumatization. These are all factors which are of interest to the surgeon planning mastoidectomy for cholesteatoma but do not change the management. A less experienced surgeon, however, may wish to refer an anatomically difficult case to someone of more experience once the X-rays have been assessed.

Indications for CT scan of the ear

A CT scan, usually in the axial plane, should be performed if a patient refuses surgery, if there is a threat of complications, or if the patient is referred from another otolaryngologist as a difficult case. Computed tomography gives excellent views of the middle ear in both axial and coronal planes and 1 mm cuts will show cholesteatoma causing bone erosion of the facial nerve canal, the lateral semicircular canal or the cochlea. Leighton *et al.* (1993a) compared CT appearances with operative findings in 20 patients suspected of having cholesteatoma. CT altered the plan of management in 50%.

Magnetic resonance imaging will probably replace CT in due course but at present CT has more to offer except where disease lies at the apex of the petrous bone. MRI shows the relationship to brain more clearly than CT (Phelps and Wright, 1990). Ishii *et al.* (1991) looked at 14 patients suspected of having cholesteatoma on CT and found that cholesteatomas appeared no different to grey matter on T1-weighted spin echo but hyperintense on T2-weighted spin echo. Cholesterol granulomas in two patients appeared hyperintense on both T1 and T2. For the average case, however, CT shows erosion of bone which is the hallmark of cholesteatoma and surgeons navigate by using the bony landmarks which shield the important structures. Both CT and MRI require general anaesthetics in children under 8 years and are not often essential to management.

Differential diagnosis

Langerhans' cell histiocytosis

This is a condition of bone previously called histiocytosis X, Hands–Schüller–Christian disease or Letterer–Siwe disease which occasionally presents with the temporal bone and may erode into the mastoid or ear canal causing an aural polyp. The patient is commonly a child. The diagnosis is made from a biopsy and from the characteristic bony defect seen on an X-ray. Radical mastoidectomy fails to cure or arrest the disease which ebbs and flows and can be partially controlled by systemic steroids. The otologist's role is to help make the diagnosis in combination with a paediatric oncologist and to resist radical surgery (Irving, Broadbent and Jones, 1994). Chemotherapy and radiotherapy have a place in extensive disease. Disease in the ear responds to intralesional steroid injections and mustine ear drops if meatal skin is involved.

Conservative management

Conservative management rests on three foundations: removing debris, identifying and eliminating the associated organism, and ventilating the middle ear if required.

Removing debris

The child lies supine on a couch without a pillow and inclines the head 30° away from the ear under the microscope. The surgeon sits with back straight in a comfortable position on an adjustable stool with wheels. Larger masses of debris can be removed with crocodile microforceps, especially if the mass is dry enough to have an edge which can be grasped. Suction is required to clean the deeper recesses of the canal. Suction is unpleasantly noisy and the child should be warned of this, it should, however, never be painful. An 18 SWG calibre sucker tip greatly reduces the level of noise and is less likely to do damage if it is accidentally applied to a dehiscent facial nerve or a fistula in the membranous labyrinth. There is often difficulty in reaching the back of inaccessible cavities. Two approaches are helpful, first the humble posture of kneeling at the bedside and secondly by viewing the ear from the 'wrong' side of the couch, leaning across the child's chest.

Identifying the organism

Swabs are taken from the depths of the ear canal (special small diameter swabs on a thin wire are available) and carried to the laboratory in a transport medium. It will be necessary to stop the patient taking antibiotics and ear drops for several days if a positive culture is to be obtained. The bacteriologist's recommendation is very helpful in choosing antibiotics or antifungal agents once an organism has been identified. Topical antiseptics are often appropriate and are described in the bacteriology section.

Management of bacterial infection

While elimination of a specific organism from a chronic ear will not be curative, especially in the case of cholesteatoma, it will greatly reduce symptoms and may, in the case of a safe perforation, render the ear quiescent. An uninfected dry ear is a better starting point for tympanoplasty surgery than a smelly wet one. The therapeutic options are reviewed.

Oral antibiotics and aerobic bacteria

Those organisms, such as streptococci, which multiply in tissues, are reached by oral penicillin, which may be dramatically effective in cellulitis of the canal and pinna. *Haemophilus influenzae* multiplies readily in mucosa temporarily devoid of cilia following coryza and responds rapidly to oral amoxycillin or trimethoprim to which the organism is usually sensitive. *Staphyloccocus aureus* causes a secondary otitis externa with oedema round the roots of the hair shafts and may be eliminated by a 2-week course of oral erythromycin or flucloxacillin. Beta-lactamase producing organisms have been identified in 63% of 175 positive cultures from chronic ears (Brook, 1985; Brook and Yocum, 1989), many of which had been previously treated with antibiotics from the penicillin group. Their ability to produce β-lactamase renders them resistant to the semi-synthetic penicillins. *Proteus mirabilis*, *Klebsiella* and *Escherichia coli* are sensitive to oral antibiotics, but frequently fall into this group.

Fourth generation cephalosporins, the fluoroquinolones, particularly ciprofloxacin, have given us oral antipseudomonals for the first time. They are immensely useful with 87% success rates (Van de Heyning, Pattyn and Valcke, 1986; Van de Heyning *et al.*, 1987; Papastavros, Giamarellou and Varlejides, 1989). Malignant otitis externa was cured or controlled by ciprofloxacin 750 mg b.d. in 21 of 23 patients (Sade *et al.*, 1989). Esposito, D'Errico and Montanarro (1990) compared topical with oral treatment of chronic suppurative otitis media, curing more than 85% with ciprofloxacin drops and only 40–60% with oral ciprofloxacin. Resistant strains are however already emerging and at the time of writing it is not licensed for use in children. Some of the quinalone antibiotics (of which ciprofloxacin is one) have significant side effects and temafloxin was withdrawn in 1992 because of haemolytic anaemia, renal failure, and liver damage at the rate of 28 per 100 000 prescriptions. This was far more than for ofloxacin,

norfloxacin, cinoxacin and ciprofloxacin. Organisms which thrive around foreign bodies are largely unaffected by oral antibiotics, hence the failure of medicines to cure discharge from a grommet in children. Topical preparations are needed.

Oral antibiotics and anaerobic bacteria

In the 1980s great interest was expressed in the significance of anaerobic bacteria in chronic suppurative otitis media. The organisms most prevalent in the papers listed in Table 8.1 were *Bacteroides melaninogenicus*, *Bacteroides fragilis* and the microaerophilic *Peptococcus*. The question was, would elimination of anaerobes help to cure chronic suppurative otitis media? Anaerobes were identified as a significant group by Palva and Hallstrom (1965) who isolated *Strep. anaerobicus* in five out of 100 chronic ears. Jokipii *et al.* (1977) recovered anaerobes in 33% of 70 chronic ears. Over half were *Bacteroides* species and present in mixed infections. As many otogenic brain abscesses grow *Bacteroides* it was suggested that chronic ears with anaerobes were more dangerous than those without. Sugita *et al.* (1981) concluded that anaerobes are found where chronic suppurative otitis media due to other causes is well advanced and the middle ear is filled with cholesteatoma or other matter remote from ventilation or a blood supply and are therefore a secondary phenomenon. The anaerobes cultured from chronic ears are all sensitive to metronidazole (Constable and Butler, 1982) but treatment does not cure chronic suppurative otitis media, it merely changes the population of organisms. Browning *et al.* (1983) eliminated anerobes in 15 out of 23 ears, though active discharge continued in each case.

Topical antibiotics

These reach organisms in debris and in mucus more quickly and in greater concentration than oral antibiotics. Gentamicin 0.3% ear drops are the cheapest single preparation and are very effective for a short time against a wide range of organisms, especially *Pseudomonas aeruginosa*. The addition of steroids doubles the cost. A controlled trial (Browning, Gatehouse and Calder, 1988) showed that the addition of a steroid to gentamicin eardrops added nothing to their effectiveness in 80 wet mastoid cavities, where results were no better than in a similar placebo group. Antibiotic resistance to single agents is the argument for mixed antibiotic preparations such as neomycin with polymixin or framycetin, both of the latter showing good employment of antibiotics which are toxic for systemic use. Mixed preparations however are often four times the cost of gentamicin. Compliance is often low as children always need help and the process is labour intensive, especially in a struggling child. Teaching the parent to flush the drops into the deep meatus using the tragus like a piston blends pus and antibiotic which otherwise would lie unmixed. Antibiotic powders applied by the otologist after microsuction are probably better than a single application of drops but are ineffective when puffed into a messy ear at home.

Ototoxicity of eardrops

The balance of opinion amongst bacteriologists and otologists is that a short course of aminoglycoside ear drops in an infected open middle ear carries less risk to hair cell function than the persistent sepsis it will probably cure. Podoshin, Fradis and Ben David (1989) looked at 150 patients with chronic suppurative otitis media over a 10-year period. One-hundred-and-twenty-four patients had been treated with ear drops containing neomycin and 26 with steroid drops. The neomycin group had greater deterioration of hearing over the period of the study than the control group and the patients with longest duration of symptoms had greatest deterioration of hearing in both groups. The possibility of turning a septic ear into a dry one by a short course of aminoglycoside drops and thus doing more good than harm was not considered. This study would suggest that long-term use of aminoglycoside drops in chronic suppurative otitis media is however contraindicated if hearing is still present in the ear in question. Vestibular function is known to be damaged by intratympanic gentamicin and this is used therapeutically in Menière's disease (Lange, 1989), so drops should be used with caution. Ototoxicity from ear drops has yet to be tested in the courts and some pharmaceutical companies write warnings on aminoglycoside-containing ear drops to the effect that they should not be used in the presence of a perforation, passing the responsibility to the physician.

Topical antiseptics

These are used frequently on infected skin elsewhere in the body and are effective. Chlorhexidine cream penetrates 1–2 mm into skin and is particularly potent against staphylococci. It has the drawback of being neurotoxic and must not be deposited on cranial nerves or the meninges. Occasional application to the mould of a hearing aid will prevent otitis externa. Iodine is effective against all organisms and in the form of bismuth iodoform paraffin paste (BIPP) on ribbon gauze is effective in cleaning up infected ears within 10 days. A long inner pack and a short outer pack are recommended. When the otologist is telephoned out of hours to be told that the pack has 'fallen out' he or she may relax if it is the short one! The mixture is hydrophobic and does not absorb body fluids and pus, so that it comes out of an ear smelling medicated even after 3 weeks. Hydrophobic BIPP ribbon gauze packs were compared with Xero-

form hydrophilic dressings in 40 newly fashioned mastoid cavities by Chevretton, McRae and Booth (1991). There were fewer episodes of local and systemic infection and fewer offensive packs in the BIPP group. In the Xeroform group more frequent adverse events required ciprofloxacin and metronidazole to control them. BIPP has remained the favoured packing for mastoidectomy cavities for many decades. About one patient in 100 is allergic to iodine. When the ear swells and weeps copious serum soon after a BIPP pack is put in the diagnosis is obvious and all vestiges of iodine must be removed, the ear smothered with hydrocortisone cream and a strong antihistamine given.

Mercurochrome stains the skin of the meatus and may be applied with a wool dressed probe. It takes several weeks to be absorbed and has the potent antiseptic effect of heavy metals. Mercury poisoning is unlikely from occasional application to the ear, but because of the risk from wide skin application it has been withdrawn from general use and is only available from hospital pharmacies on a named patient basis.

Acetic acid or aluminium acetate drops render the ear too acidic for pseudomonas to survive but make the patient smell of fish and chips! Gentian violet and crystal violet have been found to be carcinogenic and are no longer available. Spirit drops, 70% ethyl alcohol in water, are strongly antiseptic but sting on application. Phenol and clioquinol (Vioform) are used as antiseptic drops or as preservatives in other ear preparations. The antiseptics in glycerol and icthammol (a coal tar fraction) are phenol and cresol. Papastavros, Giamarellou and Varlejides (1989) compared systemic antibiotics to topical treatment with mild antiseptics as preparation for surgery in 119 chronic ears. They reported cure rates of 53% for systemic antibiotics and 40% for topical treatment, and noted that with systemic treatment the emergence of resistant bacterial strains was more frequent and relapses were more common.

Intravenous antibiotics

The most rigorous non-operative treatment that can be offered to the patient with a resistant symptomatic chronic ear is daily suction toilet, dressings and high dose intravenous antibiotics chosen on the advice of a bacteriologist (Kenna *et al.*, 1986; Fliss *et al.*, 1991). Missed doses, so common in home oral therapy, are rare and although this treatment is expensive of hospital time it is very effective. Raas-Rothschild *et al.* (1991) advocated ambulatory intravenous therapy which could mean the use of a syringe pump at home or school. Serum peak and trough levels of antibiotic would need to be measured to avoid ototoxicity if gentamicin is used. Peak levels 1 hour after injection should not exceed 12 μg/ml and trough

levels before the next dose should not exceed 1 µg/ml
(Noone *et al.*, 1974). Intravenous therapy is particularly useful for chronic suppurative otitis media with
threatened complications in immune compromised
patients, such as leukaemics and neutropaenics, or
where otitis media becomes otitis interna with loss of
balance as pus enters the labyrinth.

Antifungal agents

Fungal infection of the middle ear and meatus is
common in chronic suppurative otitis media as
fungi thrive on moist squames and dessicated pus.
Talwar *et al.* (1988) found 49% positive fungal
smears from 286 chronically infected ears. White
felted masses are usually *Monilia* or *Aspergillus flavus*
and black tips to the filaments indicate *Aspergillus
niger*. Itch is the main symptom. Nyastin drops seem
less effective than miconazole creams or packs. Microsuction and an antiseptic are usually as good as an
antifungal agent unless the patient is immune
deficient.

Antituberculous therapy

In countries where tuberculosis is endemic a proportion of chronic ears will contain *Mycobacterium tuberculosis*. Odetoyinbo (1988) reported 23 of 192 (12%)
polyps and biopsies from chronic ears to be positive
for tuberculosis. Ojala *et al.* (1981) found five positive cultures in Finland from 806 chronic ears. It is
also found in the UK (Glover, Tranter and Innes,
1981) and Belgium (De Paep *et al.*, 1989). The
management of the ear is then by antituberculous
therapy, avoiding streptomycin because of its ototoxic properties. Streptomycin is still in regular use
in developing countries because it is one of the cheapest antibiotics. In recent years there has been a
considerable increase in the incidence of tuberculosis
in the USA due to a combination of closure of long-
stay psychiatric institutions and the epidemic of
AIDs.

Prophylactic antibiotics for ear surgery

Carlin, Lesser and John (1987) and John *et al.*
(1988) looked at 71 patients and 130 patients respectively undergoing ear surgery and found no evidence
that systemic prophylactic antibiotics prevented the
development of sepsis in the postoperative period, or
influenced the success rate of myringoplasty
surgery.

Immunosuppression

Children with poor immunity to microorganisms will
require attention to the underlying cause in addition
to local ear treatment. Diabetic otitis, particularly
with *Pseudomonas* needs careful control of blood sugar

as well as strenuous antibiotic therapy. Hypogamma-
globulinaemia may need to be identified and treated
in a child before an ear will dry up. AIDs and drug-
induced immunosuppression in transplant patients
will be less amenable to management but need to be
taken into account when planning the management
of chronic suppurative otitis media.

Management of the hearing loss

Children may present with active chronic suppurative
otitis media who really need improved hearing and
for whom there is no immediate prospect of a surgical
remedy. Sepsis or waiting lists may delay surgery or
the child may be unfit for tympanoplasty. A hearing
aid may make all the difference to the situation but
no audiologist will fit a patient with active chronic
suppurative otitis media unless there is no alternative.
Some children present with two hearing aids and
ears full of pus and debris.

Energetic conservative management with daily
suction and intravenous antibiotics chosen by the
bacteriologist may be needed to control the sepsis
so that the aids may be worn in dry clean ears.
Once active safe chronic suppurative otitis media is
made inactive an occasional smear of antiseptic
cream on the ear moulds helps to keep infection
away. As always with perforations the ears must
be kept dry and 'swimmers' moulds' made by the
audiologist for hair washing and showering often
help.

Bone conduction aids

A bone conductor aid on a spring steel head band
makes an excellent temporary arrangement for a
patient under treatment for otorrhoea who usually
wears an aid. Long-term use is less acceptable as the
device is heavy and uncomfortable. The amplifier
may be a body worn box, but can also be an adapted
postaural aid attached to the other side of the head
band.

Bone anchored hearing aids

If bilateral active chronic suppurative otitis media
cannot be controlled then a bone anchored hearing
aid (BAHA) may be suitable. Attaching an ear level
bone conductor aid to a titanium 4 mm × 4 mm
screw threaded fixture (the Tjellstrom bolt) in the
bone of the skull gives a gain of 15–20 dB over the
conventional bone conductor aid (Tjellstrom, 1990).
In four of the author's patients with bilateral mastoidectomies and chronic resistant discharge under
hearing aids, this system has allowed the ears to
become dry. The skull of a child is thick enough to
carry the titanium fixture from about the age of 4
years.

Clinical presentations and management

Chronic suppurative otitis media with cholesteatoma

The development of cholesteatoma

New evidence for the invagination theory of the development of cholesteatoma and its association with eustachian tube blockage has been found by ear drum photography. Photographs may be used to follow the natural history of an ear disease over a period of time. Christian Deguine's beautiful pictures have in many cases tracked the progress from retraction pocket to infected cholesteatoma and one case is shown in detail with his kind permission (see Plates 6/8/I *a, b*, 6/8/II *a, b*, 6/8/III *a, b*).

Ruedi (1963), an otologist and a pathologist, described in detail the cellular behaviour at the neck of an acquired cholesteatoma sac. The patient was an 11-month-old boy who died from the complications of the ear infection. At the mouth of a large superior marginal perforation there was active proliferation of basal cells in the germinal layer of the epidermis of the adjoining external auditory canal. Cones or finger-like protrusions of proliferating cells were not inhibited by contact with mucous membrane of the middle ear mucosa but were burrowing into the submucosal layer. This layer was inflamed and loose because of either undermining or infection or both.

Posterior retraction pocket accumulating debris

Symptoms

These are usually absent which is why cholesteatoma often develops silently. Retraction is typically seen when examining a child with a history of many grommet insertions or in cases where eustachian tube function is known to be impaired, such as familial airway allergy, cleft palate or Down's syndrome, but often occurs for no obvious reason.

Signs

The pars tensa has an irregularity which can be described as a dent or hollow, if its depths are partially hidden it has become a pocket. The question which must then be asked is, 'is the pocket self-cleaning and passing unwanted surface keratin into the ear canal or is there an accumulation of matter in the pocket'? The area above the lateral process of the malleus or the area near the stapes are the commonest sites, known as attic or posterior marginal pockets respectively. The hearing is normal unless the middle ear is devoid of an air space or the ossicular chain is eroded.

Conservative management

Simple inspection of the area on several occasions may convince the otologist that no accumulation is occurring and that the retraction is unchanged with time. If debris is present and has to be removed by suction or forceps under the microscope then it must be assumed that, left untreated, a cholesteatoma sac will form and deepen into the middle ear cleft. The patient may choose between life-long attendance for microsuction or an operation. The Shah ink spot test can be helpful at this time. Indian ink, on the slimmest of wool tipped probes, is applied to the depths of the retraction. Stained epithelium seen to be migrating down the walls of the ear canal over the following 6 weeks is an indication that the pocket is still self-cleaning. Ink remaining in the retraction over this period suggests that accumulation will take place and that the disease will progress (Shah, 1991).

Surgical management

The retraction pocket is excised and grafted as if it were a perforation using temporalis fascia by the underlay technique. The deep surface of the pocket may need to be gently separated from the ossicles. A ventilation tube should be placed in the unaffected part of the drum if the surgeon considers that the eustachian tube blockage which first caused the retraction is still present. Anything that can be done in the nose or nasopharynx to improve eustachian tube function should be done. Trials of excision and grafting of retraction pockets have not yet reached maturity where they can be compared with auto-inflation or a 'wait and see' policy, but the question must be answered if we are to prevent childhood atelectasis becoming adult cholesteatoma.

Attic retraction pocket accumulating debris

The symptoms and signs are the same as for posterior retractions except for the site of the retraction which is in Shrapnell's membrane. Conservative management is by microsuction if all the debris can be removed without discomfort. Sometimes with the passage of time necrosis of the bone of the outer attic wall (the scutum) occurs and a natural attic cavity forms. When the mouth of this cavity is broad and the bottom shallow the ear may return to a self-cleaning state and the threat of cholesteatoma recedes.

Surgical management

An atticotomy is the smallest surgical procedure that will convert a retraction pocket with a 'bottle neck' into one like the inside of a shallow bowl. The outer attic wall is removed with a drill taking care not to touch the ossicles with the rotating burr head. Careful deliberate cutting of the incudostapedial joint at an early stage is recommended, because if the ossicles are then touched the joint simply separates. It can be reassembled at the end. The operation may be performed by a postaural, endaural or canal approach. The roof of the bony meatus should be made flush with the roof of the attic.

Posterior marginal cholesteatoma

Symptoms

Purulent discharge, which is usually foul smelling, brings the patient to the otologist, often with a preliminary diagnosis of otitis externa. Occasionally dry uninfected disease presents with a hearing loss. In long-standing cases a polyp may be filling the ear canal. Complications, such as vertigo from erosion of the labyrinth or a facial palsy from erosion of the fallopian canal, are more common in countries where a 'running ear' is not thought to require specialist care.

Signs

There is irregularity, collapse or the appearance of a perforation in the posterior half of the pars tensa. Unlike a central safe perforation in the same area, the tympanic annulus is missing and the defect lacks the sharp crescent-like edge that the annulus provides. Debris is seen in the perforation and cannot all be sucked out under the microscope. All this may be hidden behind pus, fleshy granulations or an aural polyp. The use of Siegle's speculum may produce vertigo and nystagmus – a positive fistula test.

Management

Once the diagnosis of cholesteatoma has been made and everything that can be done to improve the ear in an outpatients' visit is complete, plans are made for surgery to eradicate disease. If doubt about the diagnosis exists an examination under anaesthetic is necessary, usually as a day case. Bacteriological, audiological and radiological assessment, if appropriate, are described under separate headings.

Surgical approach

Modified radical mastoidectomy with careful removal of all disease by the use of a drill and microscope under general anaesthesia is the safest and most reliable operation for cholesteatoma, especially if combined with an adequate meatoplasty to make subsequent cleaning of the cavity easy. The trainee otologist should learn this operation early on temporal bones and regard it as the foundation stone of the treatment of cholesteatoma. The place of the more demanding and less reliable canal wall up combined approach tympanoplasty is discussed under a separate heading.

Attic cholesteatoma (see Plate 6/8/IV)

Symptoms

These are the same as for posterior marginal disease.

Signs

The mouth of the cholesteatoma sac is found in the pars flaccida above the short process of the malleus, and also may be obscured by pus, debris or granulations which will need to be removed by suction under microscope before the extent of the disease can be seen.

Management

If cholesteatoma is suspected but not seen in outpatients an examination under anaesthetic as a day case is required. The surgeon may kneel and tilt the microscope head if the attic is difficult to see. When bacteriological, audiological and, if necessary, radiological assessment is complete, an operation to excise the disease is planned. Modified radical mastoidectomy with removal of the posterior bony canal wall is the standard procedure that reaches the disease however extensive and when combined with an effective meatoplasty allows life-long access for outpatient treatment. The place of the more demanding 'inside out' approach and primary obliteration techniques to minimize the size of the cavity are discussed below.

Cholesteatoma arising in a 'safe' perforation (see Plate 6/8/V)

Symptoms

These are indistinguishable from chronic suppurative otitis media without cholesteatoma, hearing loss and discharge.

Signs

The healing edge of a 'safe' pars tensa perforation often presents a feather-like appearance and occasionally exuberant squamous epithelium accumulates on the underside of the margin of the perforation. When any quantity has gathered and cannot escape because it is wedged under the drum remnant a new cholesteatoma exists and will enlarge in the usual way.

Management

If suction clearance does not remove the threat of progressive disease then surgery is indicated. Excision of the drum edges and accumulated disease leaving an open middle ear is the simplest and safest procedure. Restoration of hearing is best left to a second stage when the surgeon can be sure there is no residual or recurrent disease.

Cholesteatoma in a radical cavity

Symptoms

Purulent offensive discharge is the characteristic finding.

Signs

Squamous debris is seen clinging to white cholesteatoma matrix in the depths of a surgical cavity. The ear is resistant to attempts to make it clean and dry by outpatient treatment.

Management

The simplest procedure is a meatoplasty to give better access to the cavity. Revision mastoidectomy with emphasis on lowering the facial ridge, exenterating all mastoid air cells and excising all diseased lining takes more time but may be more successful. Tympanomastoid re-aeration with a long graft reaching from the eustachian tube to the posterior limit of the cavity is another option and obliteration with autologous bone pate or hydroxyl apatite behind a new posterior meatal wall (mastoid reconstruction), is the most demanding of skill and time and still carries risk of recurrence. Any procedure which saves the patient with 'mastoid misery' years of suction toilet for a filthy cavity is a good investment for surgeon and patient. One patient in the author's clinic had 146 separate entries for cavity toilet in the outpatients' records.

Cholesteatoma behind an intact drum

This disease develops silently and, unless found in childhood by an observant doctor or audiologist, may present in middle life with a serious complication. Some 18% of paediatric cholesteatomas in one series of 232 children (Rosenfeld, Moura and Bluestone, 1992) were behind an intact tympanic membrane. The disease is, because of its protected site, uninfected and the tympanic membrane is undamaged except where it is made to bulge by pressure from disease.

The management is surgical excision; the surgeon's difficulty is knowing how far the disease extends. CT readily distinguishes cholesteatoma extending to the petrous apex from a circumscribed deposit in the middle ear. Petrous apex cholesteatoma is the third commonest cause of a mass in the cerebellopontine angle after acoustic neuroma and meningioma. In some cases the disease can be removed through a permeatal tympanotomy; in others a combined approach tympanoplasty is required, and in extensive disease a translabyrinthine approach and the help of a neurosurgeon are needed.

Techniques of cholesteatoma surgery

Anatomical landmarks or path of disease

Macewan (1893) described the surface marking of the mastoid antrum thus allowing generations of surgeons to find the antrum through healthy bone. It was this anatomical approach combined with Neumann's (1930) teaching from Vienna, that there should be systematic evacuation of all mastoid air cells, which led to the large cavity mastoidectomy being the standard treatment for cholesteatoma (Figure 8.1). It is only in recent years that the pendulum has swung the other way and the anatomical approach been exchanged for a 'path of disease' approach in some centres (Figure 8.2). This philosophy means that the postoperative cavity is only as large as the preoperative cholesteatoma. In practical terms this means atticotomy, atticoantrostomy and 'inside-out' small cavity mastoidectomy instead of the troublesome large cavity mastoidectomy or the uncertain safety of the combined approach tympanoplasty. Antibiotics which will kill organisms such as *Pseudomonas* reduce the need to exenterate mastoid air cells with mucosal disease rather than cholesteatoma.

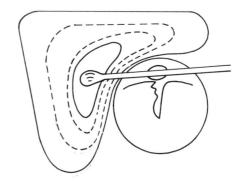

Figure 8.1 Macewan's method of finding the mastoid antrum and then the cholesteatoma

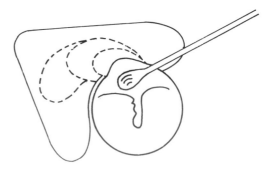

Figure 8.2 Following the path of cholesteatoma with the drill

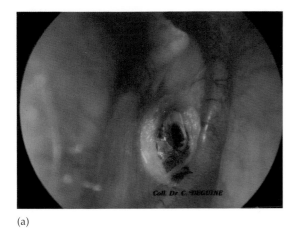

(a)

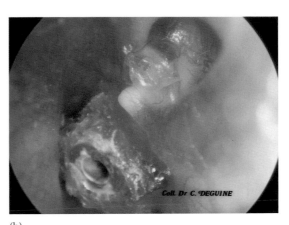

(b)

Plate 6/8/I (*a*) and (*b*) The left and right ears of an 8-year-old child treated by grommet insertion for bilateral 'glue' ear

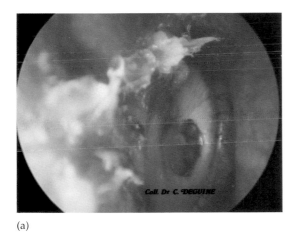

(a)

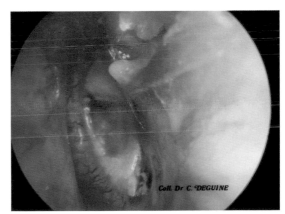

(b)

Plate 6/8/II (*a*) **and** (*b*) The same patient as in Plate 6/8/I at the age of 20 years. There is the appearance of an attic cholesteatoma in the right ear, on the left Shrapnell's membrane appears intact behind a little pale wax

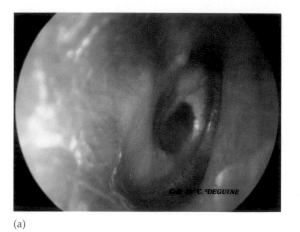

(a)

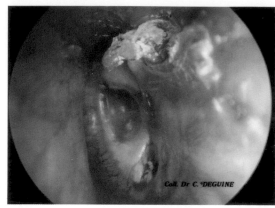

(b)

Plate 6/8/III (*a*) **and** (*b*) The same patient as in Plate 6/8/I at the age of 22 years. The left ear has developed the appearance of an attic cholesteatoma. The right ear has been operated upon by the 'canal wall up' technique of combined approach

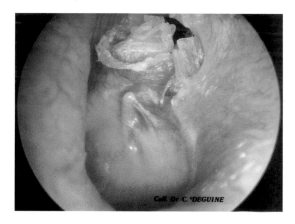

Plate 6/8/IV Attic cholesteatoma

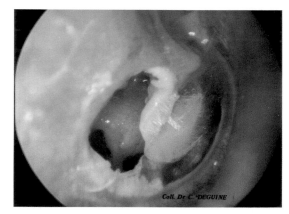

Plate 6/8/V Cholesteatoma arising from the margins of a 'safe perforation' where squamous ingrowth is occurring around the margins of a central perforation

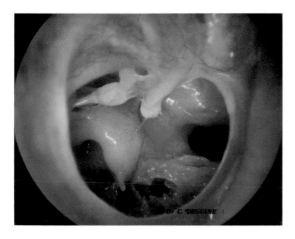

Plate 6/8/VI Subtotal safe perforation showing ossicular chain

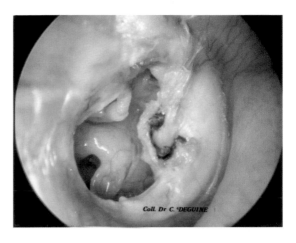

Plate 6/8/VII Extensive tympanosclerosis around a perforation

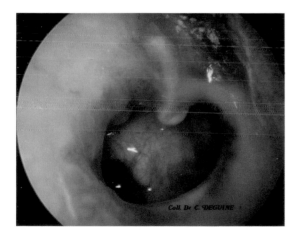

Plate 6/8/VIII Wet perforation, active middle ear infection

The versatile approach

The high quality of training available on temporal bone courses and the unending search for a cure for cholesteatoma has led many surgeons to the point where they offer a range of procedures for this disease. It may be that the answer to the question 'what is the best operation for cholesteatoma?' is whichever is most appropriate to the site and extent of disease (Tos and Lau, 1989b). If the surgeon can offer permeatal tympanotomy, atticotomy, atticoantrostomy, combined approach tympanoplasty and wall down mastoidectomy with meatoplasty, a choice may be made for each situation (Palva, 1993). The difficulty is in knowing beforehand the extent of the disease. Smyth and Brooker (1992) advocated small cavity mastoidectomy, beginning the bone work from inside the bony meatus rather than the outside and stopping the dissection as soon as the posterior limit of the disease is reached. Five-year follow up of 43 patients confirmed their view that this approach produced more stable postoperative ears than the large cavity approach. This technique was described in the 1880s and it has survived as atticotomy or atticoantrostomy over the intervening years but has largely been ignored in the debate about 'wall down' mastoidectomies.

The place of combined approach tympanoplasty in the treatment of paediatric cholesteatoma

This technique of dissecting out cholesteatoma has been described by Gordon Smyth (1962), Claus Jansen (1968) who had been using it for 10 years and then by James Sheehy (Sheehy and Patterson 1967), who described a series followed up for 8 years. An alternative name is the 'wall up' operation to distinguish it from the 'wall down' modified radical mastoidectomy where the posterior bony meatal wall is removed for access to disease. Combined approach tympanoplasty is technically a more demanding procedure than modified radical mastoidectomy and takes more time to learn in the temporal bone laboratory and longer to perform in the operating theatre. The principles of this technique are:

1 Disease is removed from the mastoid and attic and then from the sinus tympani through a slot cut in the posterior canal wall (the facial recess approach), in addition to access down the canal via a Rosen's tympanomeatal flap.
2 The ear drum is returned to its normal position so that cavities in the mastoid and middle ear remain sealed off from the outside and cannot collect wax.
3 The ear canal is left a normal size and shape and its posterior bony wall preserved.

The advantages are that the ear stays dry even with swimming and a hearing aid may be worn without provoking discharge. There is no mastoid cavity to clean in outpatients (a large cavity exists of course but is hidden behind the tympanic membrane and carefully preserved bony canal wall). The disadvantages are that cholesteatoma may persist or recur behind the drum and its associated fascia graft. The combined approach method is suitable for those patients who are settled in the area and have no intention of moving, and furthermore understand the necessity of close follow up.

Contraindications to combined approach tympanoplasty

The combined approach method is contraindicated in patients who have suffered complications of chronic suppurative otitis media, in those who are likely to move out of the area, or fail to comprehend the need for follow up. If the surgeon has a short-term contract or is a locum to a department where combined approach is not usually offered open cavity wall down mastoidectomy is the wisest option. If the disease recurs there may be nothing to see with an auriscope or microscope even though disease has begun to erode the ossicles or labyrinth again. Persistent eustachian tube obstruction often causes the drum head to retract into the attic or sinus tympani and form new corners for debris to accumulate behind. Despite preserving the annulus the hearing is not always better than with modified radical mastoidectomy. Toner and Smyth (1990) reviewed hearing results in 'wall up' and 'wall down' mastoidectomies with obliteration and found the 'wall down' group to have comparable postoperative thresholds.

Adult and paediatric results compared

Recent papers on the relative effectiveness of 'wall up' and 'wall down' mastoidectomies for cholesteatoma now include long-term follow ups of large series allowing some judgements to be made. Austin (1989) compared success rates in 91 'wall down' procedures with 124 'wall up' operations for cholesteatoma. Actuarial tables showing risk of development of residual or recurrent disease were prepared. These showed a 90% success rate for removing cholesteatoma in 'wall down' procedures and 45% success rate for 'wall up' procedures. Tos and Lau (1988) followed up 224 ears which had cholesteatoma surgery for between 3 and 21 years. Ninety-one patients had 'canal wall down' operations and 133 had 'canal wall up' procedures. They found that although cholesteatoma recurrence rate increased with time to 6.3% there was no significant difference between the two surgical methods.

Weiss *et al.* (1992) reported 116 revision operations for recurrent or residual cholesteatoma on average 3.4 years after primary surgery. Sixty-six per cent of the group had undergone 'wall down' surgery and 34% 'wall up' procedures. Palva (1988) revised

43 ears which had had 'wall up' procedures and found 63% had residual or recurrent cholesteatoma. Cholesteatoma clearly may recur after either operation and is visible and relatively safe in the former but invisible and relatively dangerous in the latter.

Charachon, Gratacap and Tixier (1988) described a series of 533 surgical procedures for cholesteatoma, 60% of which were 'wall up' operations. All these were subject to a second operation and 24% of ears had residual or recurrent cholesteatoma.

The modified radical cavity is almost universally wet and smelly in children and they do not readily tolerate suction. Where the surgeon can be sure of long-term follow up the combined approach 'wall up' tympanoplasty seems to be the lesser of two evils. A second look or revision operation at one year is required as the chance of residual or recurrent cholesteatoma is greater than in adults. Rosenfeld, Moura and Bluestone (1992), in 232 children with cholesteatoma treated by either 'wall up' or 'wall down' procedures, found 23% recurrences at first revision operation, rising to 48% at 3 years and 57% at 5 years. Kinney (1988) reported 104 ears with cholesteatoma treated by combined approach tympanoplasty in 1981. After 5 years there was a 7% recurrence rate in adults but a 25% recurrence rate in children. Rigner, Renvall and Tjellstrom (1991) found an incidence of cholesteatoma at 0.4 per 100000 children in Sweden, 19 were operated upon in a 2-year period, 10 by the 'wall up' technique and nine by the 'wall down' procedure. Seven of the 'wall up' group had recurrence and five were then converted to 'wall down' mastoidectomies. If conversion to a modified radical mastoidectomy is to be avoided, a third or even a fourth operation will be required if pearls of cholesteatoma are discovered at revision surgery. Some can undoubtedly be cured of the disease if follow up is stringent, the family compliant and the surgeon diligent.

Otoendoscopy

Hopkins rod rigid endoscopes of less than 3 mm diameter may be passed into the middle ear cleft via the drum or mastoid as a means of discovering whether cholesteatoma has recurred behind the drum head or posterior canal wall. One millimetre flexible endoscopes are available which will pass through the eustachian tube for the same purpose. Dubreuil, Boulud and Dumarest (1991) recommended the mastoid telescope instead of reopening the postaural wound at the second stage of a combined approach tympanoplasty. Filmy adhesions in older children and bony overgrowth in younger ones made for a poor view in the majority of cases and this technique is less practical than it seems.

Problems and solutions with open cavity techniques

Mastoid misery – revision operations and meatoplasty

Years of suppuration despite outpatient visits indicate the desirability of a second operation if the child and parents are willing. Mastoid misery can be quantified in a simple way by a 0 to 3 score for the symptoms of discharge, odour, wax, vertigo and discomfort (Figure 8.3). Zero means never and three means always. A mastoid misery score of 8 or more is most unpleasant and should be addressed by effective revision surgery (Males and Gray, 1991).

Meatoplasty

Meatoplasty may be all that is required and is the least costly procedure in terms of operative time. The ratio of V (the volume of air circulating in the cavity) to S (the surface area of the cavity lining) is thought to be critical to the maintenance of a dry cavity (Portmann and Portmann, 1990). V can be increased by meatoplasty (Osborne, Trerry and Ghandhi, 1985). Revision mastoidectomy with emphasis on lowering the facial ridge, exenterating all mastoid air cells and excising all diseased lining takes more time but may be more successful. Tympanomastoid re-aeration with a long graft reaching from eustachian tube to the posterior limit of the cavity is another option which gives good results in experienced hands but the results of this have not been published. Grafting of the troublesome cavity with autologous epithelium generated by culture of buccal epithelium is advocated by Premachandra et al. (1991).

Obliteration techniques

It is most unwise to use material taken from areas where there is cholesteatoma or tissue that could be contaminated by cholesteatoma.

Cavity obliteration with soft tissue

Mesher (1911) recommended filling the cavity with connective tissue from the back of the auricle and Rambo (1958) advocated a superiorly based flap of temporalis muscle swung into facilitate closure of the canal as a blind pit. Rambo expected the wound to heal by first intention and aimed to eliminate postoperative packs and dressings. The middle ear space however was designed to be mucosal lined and aerated by a functioning eustachian tube. Many who had used Rambo's temporalis muscle flap have adapted his technique to obliterate the cavity while leaving the canal open and packed with a dressing in the usual way.

	Never	Some of the time	Most of the time	Always
	0	1	2	3
Preoperative				
Pain	☐	☐	☐	☐
Wax	☐	☐	☐	☐
Discharge	☐	☐	☐	☐
Smell	☐	☐	☐	☐
Giddiness	☐	☐	☐	☐
Postoperative				
Pain	☐	☐	☐	☐
Wax	☐	☐	☐	☐
Discharge	☐	☐	☐	☐
Smell	☐	☐	☐	☐
Giddiness	☐	☐	☐	☐

A typical questionnaire response total preoperative score = 2 + 1 + 3 + 3 + 1 = 10;

Typical postoperative score = 0 + 1 + 0 + 0 + 1 = 2

Figure 8.3 Males' scale of mastoid misery

Cavity obliteration with hydroxyl apatite

Reconstruction of the posterior canal wall with a preformed hydroxyl apatite prosthesis and hydroxyl apatite granules was advocated by Grote and van Blitterswijk (1986). Hydroxyl apatite is the mineral of natural bone and has no antigenic properties, being invaded over time by osteoblasts and osteoclasts and converted to living bone (Horman and Donath, 1987). It is, however, expensive and the preformed shapes do not always suit the anatomy of the cavity. Its advantage is that a high strong new posterior wall produces a good middle ear space for prosthetic ossicular hearing reconstruction.

Cavity obliteration with autologous bone chips

Fresh bone chips are cut with a burr and recovered from the washings by a filter in the suction tubing. Two teaspoonfuls are sufficient for most cavities and are easily obtained through the usual postaural incision. Care must be taken to collect the bone chips before contaminating the instruments in an infected cavity. Once the cavity is bare and clean it may be filled with a paté made of bone chips (Palva, 1989)

with a little tissue glue behind a fascia graft reinforced with a superiorly based connective tissue flap. The author has used this technique to good effect in 30 cases, achieving better results on the mastoid misery scale than with 30 cavities treated by revision mastoidectomy alone (Irving, Gray and Moffat, 1994). Bone paté obliteration has two advantages over other techniques, the first is that it does not shrink as much as soft tissue and the second is that the materials are to hand and do not have to be purchased from a surgical supplies firm at a cost which may be significant in both developed and developing countries.

Mastoid and middle ear obliteration in a dead ear

Where there is no hearing to preserve and a hearing aid will never be of use the revised cavity may be filled with abdominal fat, the eustachian tube blocked off and the ear canal closed as a blind pit. Violaris and Donovan (1989) described 15 successful cases and Schuknecht and Chandler (1984) 12 with recurrent cholesteatoma, delayed for 9 years in one. The technique is unlikely to be needed in a child but occasionally may prove the answer to a dead wet ear. Long-term follow up will be essential.

Chronic suppurative otitis media without cholesteatoma

The dry central perforation

Symptoms

The complaint is of hearing loss and discharge after swimming or colds. The perforation may be asymptomatic and only found on examination of the ear.

Signs

The appearance with an auriscope is a recognizable perforation with a sharp curved edge most easily seen inferiorly. The structures that can be seen vary with the size, site and angle of the hole; the tip of the long process of the incus and the stapes head are sometime obvious. A source of anxiety for occasional otoscopists is the patch of tympanosclerosis that partially rims the perforation and can be mistaken for cholesteatoma because of its dense white appearance.

Management

The parents make the decision about surgery after hearing what the otologist has to offer. Normal hearing cannot be guaranteed even where the loss is entirely conductive and some improvement may please the otologist, but unless it makes this a useful ear in comparison with the other, the operation confers no social benefit (Browning, Gatehouse and Swan, 1991; Toner, Smyth and Kerr, 1991). A complete closure of the perforation (and therefore an ear safe for swimming) cannot be guaranteed. In a long-term follow up of 605 myringoplasties, Halik and Smyth (1988) indicated 81% closure of perforations. Most patients and surgeons are optimists and myringoplasty surgery remains the commonest middle ear operation. The underlay technique with fresh temporalis fascia gives excellent results in skilled hands. Palva (1987), in 225 ears, had 97% success in closing perforations after one year using temporalis fascia by the underlay technique. Scarifying the undersurface of the anterior and inferior parts of the membrane remnant with a small hook may result in fewer failures than merely excising the rim of the perforation as is usually taught.

The subtotal perforation (see Plate 6/8/VI)

Symptoms

These are hearing loss and discharge after swimming or respiratory infections. Vertigo may occur in cold winds (caloric stimulation).

Signs

Most of the drum head is absent and it is often difficult to see the rim of the perforation in the anterior recess of the ear canal. The ossicular chain should be exposed in this condition but the disease which has led to the necrosis of all three layers of the membrane usually destroys the tenuous parts of the chain as well. The incudostapedial joint is often missing and the malleus handle short and occasionally tethered to the promontory by a fibrous band. The footplate of the stapes always remains but the crura may be absent. The floor of the middle ear is marked by mountainous ridges, spikes and valleys draped in mucosa (a visible part of the pneumatized air cell system) which presents a dramatic and confusing picture to a general practitioner seeing it through a perforation. Some ears with subtotal perforations are characterized by loss of the middle ear structures and some by the presence of masses of tympanosclerosis which feel hard when probed and encase the remnants of the drum and ossicles. It is not known why necrosis dominates in some cases and tympanosclerosis in others.

Management

The parents must decide after understanding what the otologist has to offer. Normal hearing is a rarity after surgery but some improvement can be expected. Closing the perforation is the priority; the ossicular chain may be reconstructed at the first operation or as a second procedure once the graft has been successful (Shelton and Sheehy, 1990). Many techniques are used to recontruct the ossicular chain. A hearing aid (if there is a bilateral loss) is a safe alternative to surgery and may still be required even after two operations if only a moderate hearing result is obtained. This should be discussed with the parents whose expectation may be unduly high.

Burnt out disease with extensive tympanosclerosis
(see Plate 6/8/VII)

Symptoms

Hearing loss and past history of discharge are features.

Signs

Large white rough patches cover what remains of the tympanic membrane; these are rigid or solid when probed.

Management

Medical management is not required if the ear is dry, but the parents may request reconstructive surgery. Surgery is difficult and grafts have no vascular crescent or strips of drum from which to derive a blood supply. Manipulation of a rigid ossicular chain often results in cochlear trauma adding a sensory deafness to the conductive one. A hearing aid is appropriate in most cases.

Active wet perforation, chronic mucosal disease (see Plate 6/8/VIII)

Symptoms

The child complains more of discharge than hearing loss unless the problem is bilateral. Drying the ear up by outpatient treatment is required before a surgical repair. This alone will earn the patient's gratitude as the discharge stains sheets and clothing and is often sufficiently offensive to inhibit social activities, especially swimming. A secondary otitis externa may be painful or itchy.

Signs in the ear

The features of the drum are often obscured by granulations or pus (raspberries and cream) and microsuction or if no microscope, dry mopping with a wool dressed probe is required to see the source of the discharge. Granulations and inflamed mucosa sometimes coalesce into a fleshy mass which occupies the external meatus as an aural polyp. Mucus in the discharge or pulsation of the fluid both indicate a perforation even if one cannot be readily seen, and help to distinguish chronic suppurative otitis media from otitis externa.

Signs in the nose or throat

Perforated ear drums have a natural tendency to dry up. Unremitting discharge in the absence of cholesteatoma suggests something fuelling the flames. Chronic rhinosinusitis, chronically infected adenoids or anatomical abnormalities such as cleft palate may all predispose to chronic otorrhoea.

Management

An outpatient treatment plan of three visits will dry up most ears. On the first visit the nose and sinuses are assessed and bad habits like probing or frequently wetting the ears are corrected. The ear is cleaned by microsuction and a swab sent to discover the infecting organism and its antibiotic sensitivities. The otologist's preferred ear drops are prescribed.

At the second and third visits the ear is cleaned by microsuction again and the antibiotics appropriate to the organism reassessed.

Tympanoplasty in children

Simple techniques

Some simple tympanoplasty techniques can be combined with an examination of the ear under anaesthetic. Needling, or 'bucket handling' the edge of a perforation left after removing a *T* tube will often allow healing by providing a bridge of tissue over the perforation. Adipose plug myringoplasty was advocated by Gross *et al.* (1989).

Results of tympanoplasty surgery in children

Tos and Lau (1989a) described the results of tympanoplasty for non-cholesteatomatous chronic otitis in children aged 2–4 years and in their view there is no age limit below which a perforation should not be closed. Eleven children with cleft palates did well in a series by Vartiainen (1992), who described 68% success in 18 ears of which 11 were non-cholesteatomatous or safe perforations. Hearing results were no different to those obtained in other patients and his conclusion was that cleft palate children should be offered tympanoplasty surgery for the same indications as other children. Hildmann (1989) repaired safe perforations in 185 ears of children up to 14 years with a 9.1% reperforation rate, which is as good a result as expected in adults.

Halik and Smyth (1988), however, found that children less than 10 years of age and with anterior perforations were less likely to have a successful result from surgery. No single factor responsible for the worse results could be identified.

Conclusion

The prevention of pain and deafness and the treatment of chronic ear disease in children is a branch of surgery which has made enormous strides in the last three decades. It is hoped that the brightest and most dextrous of medical graduates will take up this rewarding task.

References

ARCAND, P., CERAT J. and SPENARD, J. R. (1989). Acute otomastoiditis in the leukemic child. *Journal of Otolaryngology*, **18** 380–383

AUSTIN, D. F. (1989) Single stage surgery for cholesteatoma: an actuarial analysis. *American Journal of Otology*, **10**, 419–425

BICKERTON, R. C., ROBERTS, C. and LITTLE, J. T. (1988) Survey of general practitioners' treatment of the discharging ear. *British Medical Journal*, **296**, 1649–1650

BLUESTONE, C. D. (1989) Modern management of otitis media. *Pediatric Clinics of North America*, **36**, 1371–1387

BROOK, I. (1985) Prevalence of β-lactamase-producing bacteria in chronic suppurative otitis media. *American Journal of Diseases in Children*, **139**, 280–283

BROOK, I. and YOCUM, P. (1989) Quantitative bacterial cultures and β-lactamase activity in chronic suppurative otitis media. *Annals of Otology, Rhinology and Laryngology*, **98**, 293–297

BROWNING, G. G., GATEHOUSE, S. and CALDER, I. T. (1988) Medical management of active chronic otitis media: a controlled study. *Journal of Laryngology and Otology*, **102**, 491–495

BROWNING, G. G., GATEHOUSE, S. and SWAN, I. R. (1991) The Glasgow benefit plot: a new method for reporting benefit from middle ear surgery. *Laryngoscope*, **101**, 180–185

BROWNING, G. G., SWAN, I.R. and CHEW, K. K. (1989) Clinical

role of informal tests of hearing. *Journal of Laryngology and Otology*, **103**, 7–11

BROWNING, G. G., PICOZZI, G., SWEENEY, G. and CALDER, I. T. (1983) Role of anaerobes in chronic otitis media. *Clinical Otolaryngology*, **8**, 47–51

BRUNNER, H. (1949) Acute deafness in scarlatina. *Archives of Otolaryngology*, **50**, 589–604

CALHOUN, K. H., NORRIS, W. B., HOKANSON, J. A., STERNBERG, C. M. and QUINN, F. R. (1988) Bacteriology of middle ear effusions. *Southern Medical Journal*, **81**, 332–336

CARLIN, W. V., LESSER, T. H. and JOHN, D. G. (1987) Systemic antibiotic prophylaxis and reconstructive ear surgery. *Clinical Otolaryngology*, **12**, 441–446

CASTRO, R., ROBINSON, N., KLEIN, J. and GEIMEIER, W. (1990) Malignant external otitis and mastoiditis associated with an IgG4 subclass deficiency in a child. *Delaware Medical Journal*, **62**, 1417–1421

CHARACHON, R., GRATACAP, B. and TIXIER, C. (1988) Closed versus obliteration technique in cholesteatoma surgery. *American Journal of Otology*, **9**, 286–292

CHEVRETTON, E. B., MCRAE, R. D. and BOOTH, J. B. (1991) Mastoidectomy packs: Xeroform or BIPP? *Journal of Laryngology and Otology*, **105**, 916–917

CLAESSEN, J. Q. P. J., APPELMAN, C. L. M., TOUW–OTTEN F. W. M. M., de MELKER, R. A. and HORDIJK, G. J. (1992) A review of clinical trials regarding treatment of acute otitis media. *Clinical Otolaryngology*, **17**, 251–257

CONSTABLE, L. and BUTLER, I. (1982) Microbial flora in chronic otitis media. *Journal of Infection*, **5**, 57–60

DEGUINE, C. (1985) Etude multicentrique informatisee comme moyen d'evaluation des resultats de la chirurgie de l'oreille moyenne. *Revue de Laryngologie otologie et Rhinologie (Bordeaux)*, **106**, 355–357

DE PAEP, K., OFFECIERS, F. E., VAN DE HEYNING, P., CLAES, J., and MARQUET, J. (1989) Tuberculosis in the middle ear: 5 case reports. *Acta Oto-Rhino-Laryngologica Belgica* 43, **4**, 321–326

DE SAAR, G. M. A. C., MULDER J. J. S. and VAN DEN BROEK, P. (1992) Sequelae of long-term ventilation tubes. *Clinical Otolaryngology*, **17**, 79–80

DUBREUIL, C., BOULUD, B. and DUMAREST, D. (1991) Value of oto-endoscopy in the follow up treatment of cholesteatoma of the middle ear. *Revue de Laryngologie Otologie et Rhinologie*, **112**, 409–411

EASON, R. J., HARDING, E., NICHOLSON, M. B., NICHOLSON, D., PADA, J. and GATHERCOLE, J. (1986) Chronic suppurative otitis media in the Solomon Islands: a prospective microbiological, audiometric and therapeutic survey. *New Zealand Medical Journal*, **99**, 812–815

ESPOSITO, S., D'ERRICO, G. and MONTANARRO, C. (1990) Topical and oral treatment of chronic suppurative otitis media with Ciprofloxacin. A preliminary study. *Archives of Otolaryngology – Head and Neck Surgery*, **116**, 557–559

FAUSKIN, G. (1991) Acute otitis media in early infancy. Recurrence and prophylaxis. *Acta Paediatrica Scandinavica*, **80**, 418–422

FAYE–LUND, H. (1989) Acute and latent mastoiditis. *Journal of Laryngology and Otology*, **103**, 1158–1160

FLISS, D. M., DAGEN, R., HOURI, Z. and LEIBERMAN, A. (1990) Medical management of chronic suppurative otitis media without cholesteatoma in children. *Journal of Paediatrics*, **116**, 991–996

FLISS, D. M., LEIBERMAN, A., SHOHAM, I. and DAGEN, R. (1991) Chronic suppurative otitis media without cholesteatoma

in children in southern Israel: incidence and risk factors. *Paediatric Infectious Diseases Journal*, **10**, 895–899

FRITSCH, M. H., MIYAMOTO, R. T. and WOOD, T. L. (1990) Sigmoid sinus thrombosis diagnosis by contrasted MRI scanning. *Otolaryngology – Head and Neck Surgery*, **103**, 451–456

GARABEDIAN, E. N., ROELLY, P., LACOMBE, H. and DENOYELLE, F. (1990) Protracted otitis and subacute mastoiditis in children. A prospective study apropos of 118 cases (French: Otites trainantes et mastoidites subaiques de l'enfant. Etude prospective a propos de 188 cas.) *Annales d'Oto-Laryngologie et de Chirurgie Cervico-Faciale*, **107**, 126–131

GATES, G. A., MUNTZ, H. R. and GAYLIS, B. (1992) Adenoidectomy and otitis media (review). *Annals of Otology, Rhinology and Laryngology*, Suppl. 155, 24–32

GLOVER, S. C., TRANTER, R. M. and INNES, J. A. (1981) Tuberculous otitis media – a reminder. *Journal of Laryngology and Otology*, **95**, 1261–1264

GORDON, A. S., JEAN-LOUIS, F. and MORTON, R. P. (1988) Late ear sequelae in cleft palate patients. *International Journal of Pediatric Otorhinolaryngology*, **15**, 149–156

GOWER, D. and MCGUIRT, W. F. (1983) Intracranial complications of acute and chronic infectious ear disease: a problem still with us. *Laryngoscope*, **93**, 1028–1033

GROSS, C. W., BSSILA, M., LAZAR, R. H., LONG, T. E. and STAGNER, S. (1989) Adipose plug myringoplasty: an alternative to formal myringoplasty techniques in children. *Otolaryngology – Head and Neck Surgery*, **101**, 617–620

GROTE, J. J. and VAN BLITTERSWIJK, C. A. (1986) Reconstruction of the posterior canal wall with an hydroxyapatite prosthesis. *Annals of Otology, Rhinology and Laryngology*, Suppl. 123, 6–9

HALAMA, A. R., VOOGT, D. R. and MUSGROVE, G. M. (1986) Prevalence of otitis media in children in a black rural community in Venda (South Africa). *International Journal of Pediatric Otorhinolaryngology*, **11**, 73–77

HALIK, J. J. and SMYTH, G. D. (1988) Long term results of tympanic membrane repair. *Otolaryngology, Head and Neck Surgery*, **98**, 162–169

HARRIS, H. H. (1978) Cerebrospinal otorrhoea and recurring meningitis: report of three cases. *Laryngoscope*, **88**, 1577–1585

HEITZMANN, P., CAPELIER, Y., ROBIER, A., PLOYET, M. J. and BEUTTER, P. (1990) Otogenic thrombosis of the lateral sinus. *Annales d'Otolaryngologie et de Chirurgie Cervico-Faciale*, **107**, 35–41 (English abstract)

HENDRICKSE, W. A., KUSMIESZ, H., SHELTON, S. and NELSON, J. D. (1988) Five vs. ten days of therapy for acute otitis media. *Pediatric Infectious Diseases Journal*, **7**, 14–23

HERTHER, C. and SCHINDLER, R. A. (1985) Mondini's dysplasia with recurrent meningitis. *Laryngoscope*, **95**, 655–658

HILDMANN, H. (1989) Surgery of chronic suppurative otitis media in childhood. *Laryngorhinootologie*, **68**, 193–200

HORMAN, K. and DONATH, K. (1987) Is Hydroxyapatite ceramic an adequate biomaterial in ossicular chain reconstruction? *American Journal of Otology*, **8**, 402–405

IRVING, R. M., GRAY, R. F. and MOFFAT, D. A. (1994) Bone pâté obliteration or revision mastoidectomy a five symptom comparative study. *Clinical Otolaryngology*, **19**, 158–160

IRVING, R. M., BROADBENT, V. and JONES, N. S. (1994) Langerhans cell histiocytosis in childhood, management of head and neck manifestations. *Laryngoscope*, **104**, 64–70

ISHII, K., TAKAHASHI, S., KOBAYASHI, T., MATSUMOTO, K. and ISHIBASHI, T. (1991) MR imaging of middle ear cholesteatomas. *Journal of Computer Assisted Tomography*, **15**, 934–937

JANSEN, C. (1968) The combined approach tympanoplasty (report on 10 years experience). *Journal of Laryngology and Otology*, **82**, 779–793

JOKIPII, A. M., KARMA, P., OJALA, K. and JOKIPII, L. (1977) Anaerobic bacteria in chronic otitis media. *Archives of Otolaryngology*, **103**, 278–280

JOHN, D. G., CARLIN, W. V., LESSER, T. M., CARRICK, D. G. and FIELDER, C. (1988) Tympanoplasty surgery and prophylactic antibiotics: surgical results *Clinical Otolaryngology*, **13**, 205–207

KARMA, P. H., PUKANDER, J. S., SIPILA, M. M., VESIKAN, T. H. and GRONROOS, P. W. (1987) Middle ear fluid bacteriology of acute otitis media in neonates and very young adults. *International Journal of Pediatric Otorhinolaryngology*, **14**, 141–150

KENNA, M. A., BLUESTONE, C. D., REILLY, J. S. and LUSK, R. P. (1986) Medical management of chronic suppurative otitis media without cholesteatoma in children. *Laryngoscope*, **96**, 146–151

KERO, P. and PIEKKALA, P. (1987) Factors affecting the occurrence of acute otitis media during the first year of life. *Acta Paediatrica Scandinavica*, **76**, 618–623

KINNEY, S. E. (1988) Intact canal wall tympanoplasty with mastoidectomy for cholesteatoma: long term follow up. *Laryngoscope*, **98**, 1190–1194

LANGE, G. (1989) Gentamicin and other ototoxic antibiotics for the transtympanic treatment of Meniere's disease. *Archives of Otorhinolaryngology*, **246**, 269–270

LEIGHTON, S. E. J., ROBSON, A. K., ANSLOW, P. and MILFORD, C. A. (1993a) The role of CT imaging in the management of chronic suppurative otitis media. *Clinical Otolaryngology*, **18**, 23–29

LEIGHTON, S. E. J., ROWE-JONES, J. M., KNIGHT, J. R. and MOORE-GILLON, V. L. (1993b) Day case adenoidectomy. *Clinical Otolaryngology*, **18**, 215–219

MACEWAN, W. (1893) *Pyogenic Infective Diseases of the Brain and Spinal Cord*. Glasgow: Maclehare and Sons

MALES, A. G. and GRAY, R. F. (1991) Mastoid misery: quantifying the distress in a radical cavity. *Clinical Otolaryngology*, **16**, 12–14

MARTTILA, T. (1986) Results of audiometric screening in Finnish schoolchildren. *International Journal of Paediatric Otolaryngology*, **11**, 39–46

MAW, A. R. (1988) Tonsils and adenoids, their relation to secretory otitis media. *Advances in Otorhinolaryngology*, **40**, 81–88

MAW, A. R. and HEROD, F. (1986) Otoscopic, impedance and audiometric findings in glue ear treated by adenoidectomy and tonsillectomy: a prospective randomized study. *Lancet*, i, 1399–1402

MAW, A. R. and PARKER, A. J. (1993) A model to refine the selection of children with otitis media with effusion for adenoidectomy. *Clinical Otolaryngology*, **18**, 164–170

MAW, A. R., PARKER, A. J., LANCE, G. N. and DILKES, M. G. (1992) The effect of parental smoking on outcome after treatment for glue ear. *Clinical Otolaryngology*, **17**, 411–414

MEDWICK, J. X., ULHLEIN, A. and HALLBERG, O. E. (1949) Abscess of the cerebellar lobe of otogenic origin: combined otolaryngological and neurosurgical treatment in six cases. *Archives of Otolaryngology*, **50**, 429–439

MESHER, H. P. (1911) A method of filling the excavated

mastoid with a flap from the back of the auricle. *Laryngoscope*, **21**, 1158–1163

MILLS, R. P. (1987) Persistent middle ear effusions in children with recurrent acute otitis media. *Clinical Otolaryngology*, **12**, 97–101

NADAL, D., HERRMANN, P., BAUMANN, A. and FANCONI, A. (1990) Acute mastoiditis: clinical, microbiological and therapeutic aspects. *European Journal of Pediatrics*, **149**, 560–564

NEUMANN, H. (1930) Abscess of the brain. *Proceedings of the Royal Society of Medicine*, **23**, 1045–1049

NOONE, P., PARSONS, T. M. C., PATTINSON, J. R., SLACK, R. C. B., GARFIELD DAVIES, P. and HUGHES, K. (1974) Experience in monitoring gentamicin therapy during treatment of serious gram-negative sepsis. *British Medical Journal*, **1**, 477–481

ODETOYINBO, O. (1988) Early diagnosis of tuberculous otitis media. *Journal of Laryngology and Otology*, **102**, 133–135

OJALA, K., SORRI, M., RIIHIKANGAS, P. and SIPILA, P. (1981) Comparison of pre- and post-operative bacteriology of chronic ears. *Journal of Laryngology and Otology*, **95**, 1023–1029

OSBORNE, J. E., TRERRY, R. M. and GHANDHI, A. G. (1985) Large meatoplasty technique for mastoid cavities. *Clinical Otolaryngology*, **10**, 357–360

OVESEN, T. and BLEGVAD-ANDERSON, O. (1992) Alterations in tympanic membrane appearance and middle ear function in 11 year old children with complete unilateral cleft lip and palate compared with healthy age-matched subjects. *Clinical Otolaryngology*, **17**, 203–207

OYARZABAL, M. F., PATEL, K. S. and TOLLEY, N. S. (1992) Bilateral acute mastoiditis complicated by lateral sinus thrombosis. *Journal of Laryngology and Otology*, **106**, 535–537

PALVA, T. (1987) Surgical treatment of chronic middle ear disease. 1. Myringoplasty and tympanoplasty. *Acta Otolaryngologica*, **104**, 279–284

PALVA, T. (1988) Surgical treatment of chronic middle ear disease. Revisions after tympanomastoid surgery. *Acta Otolaryngologica*, **105**, 82–89

PALVA, T. (1989) Surgical control of the mastoid segment in chronic ear disease *Archives of Otorhinolaryngology*, **246**, 274–276

PALVA, T. (1993) Cholesteatoma surgery today. *Clinical Otolaryngology*, **18**, 245–252

PALVA, T. and HALLSTROM, O. (1965) Bacteriology of chronic otitis media: results of analyses from the ear canal and the operative cavity. *Archives of Otolaryngology*, **82**, 359–364

PAPASTAVROS, T., GIAMARELLOU, H. and VARLEJIDES, S. S. (1989) Preoperative therapeutic considerations in chronic suppurative otitis media. *Laryngoscope*, **99**, 655–659

PARADISE, J. L., BLUESTONE, C. D., ROGERS, K. D., TAYLOR, F. H., COLBORN, D. K., BACHMAN, R. Z. et al. (1990) Efficacy of adenoidectomy for recurrent otitis media in children previously treated with tympanostomy tube placement. Results of parallel randomized and nonrandomized trials. *Journal of the American Medical Association*, **263**, 2066–2073

PEDERSEN, C. B. and ZACHAU-CHRISTIANSEN, B. (1988) Chronic suppurative otitis media and its sequelae in the population of Greenland. *Scandinavian Journal of Social Medicine*, **16**, 15–19

PHELPS, P. D. and WRIGHT, A. (1990) Imaging cholesteatoma. *Clinical Radiology*, **41**, 156–162

PODOSHIN, L., FRADIS, M. and BEN DAVID, J. (1989) Ototoxicity of ear drops in patients suffering from chronic otitis media. *Journal of Laryngology and Otology*, **103**, 46–50

PORTMANN, M. and PORTMANN, D. (1990) Management of open and closed cavities in otology. *Revue de Laryngologie, Otologie, Rhinologie*, **111**, 181–183

PREMACHANDRA, D. J., WOODWARD, B., MILTON, C. M., SERGEANT, R. J. and FABRE, J. W. (1991) Treatment of chronic mastoiditis by grafting of mastoid cavities with autologous epithelial layers generated by in vitro culture of buccal epithelium. *Journal of Laryngology and Otology*, **105**, 413–416

RAAS-ROTHSCHILD, A., LANG, R., SCHABTAI, A., GOSHEN, S. and BERGER, I. (1991) Ambulatory intravenous therapy for chronic suppurative otitis media. *Journal of Pediatrics*, **119**, 160–161

RAISANEN, S. and STENFORS, L. E. (1992) Bacterial quantification – a necessary complement for comprehension of middle ear inflammations. *International Journal of Pediatric Otolaryngology*, **23**, 117–124

RAMBO, J. H. T. (1958) Musculoplasty: a new operation for suppurative middle ear deafness. *Transatlantic American Academy of Ophthalmology and Otolaryngology*, March/April, 166–177

RASMUSSEN, N., JOHNSEN, N. J. and BOHR, V. A. (1991) Otological sequelae after pneumococcal meningitis: a survey of 164 consecutive cases with a follow-up of 94 survivors. *Laryngoscope*, **101**, 876–882

RIGNER, P., RENVALL, U. and TJELLSTROM, A. (1991) Late results after cholesteatoma surgery in early childhood. *International Journal of Pediatric Otolaryngology*, **22**, 213–218

ROLAND, N. J., PHILLIPS, D. E., ROGERS, J. H. and SINGH, S. D. (1992) The use of ventilation tubes and the incidence of cholesteatoma surgery in the paediatric population of Liverpool. *Clinical Otolaryngology*, **17**, 437–439

ROSENFELD, R. M., MOURA, R. L. and BLUESTONE, C. D. (1992) Predictors of residual and recurrent cholesteatoma in children. *Archives of Otolaryngology, Head and Neck Surgery*, **118**, 384–391

RUDIN, R., SVARDSUDD, K., TIBBLIN, G. and HALLEN, O. (1983) Prevalence and incidence of otitis media and its sequelae. The study of men born in 1913–23. *Acta Otolaryngologica*, **96**, 237–246

RUEDI, L. (1963) Acquired cholesteatoma *Archives of Otolaryngology*, **78**, 252–261

SADE, J., WEINBERG, J., BERCO, E., BROWN, M. and HALVEY, A. (1982) The marsupialised (radical) mastoid. *Journal of Laryngology and Otology*, **96**, 869–875

SADE, J., LANG, R., GOSHEN, S. and KITZES-COHEN, R. (1989) Ciprofloxacin treatment of malignant external otitis. *American Journal of Medicine*, **87**, 138s–141s

SAMUEL, J., FERNANDEZ, C. M. and STEINBERG, J. L. (1986) Intracranial otogenic complications – a persisting problem. *Laryngoscope*, **96**, 272–278

SCHUKNECHT, H. F. and CHANDLER, J. R. (1984) Surgical obliteration of the tympanomastoid compartment and external auditory canal. *Annals of Otology, Rhinology and Laryngology*, **93**, 641–645

SHAH, N. (1991) Otitis media and its sequelae. *Journal of the Royal Society of Medicine*, **84**, 581–586

SHEEHY, J. L. and PATTERSON, M. E. (1967) Intact canal wall tympanoplasty with mastoidectomy. A review of eight years experience. *Laryngoscope*, **77**, 1502–1542

SHELTON, C. and SHEEHY, J. L. (1990) Tympanoplasty: review of 400 staged cases. *Laryngoscope*, **100**, 679–681

SMYTH, G. D. L. (1962) A preliminary report on a technique in tympanoplasty designed to eliminate the cavity problem. *Journal of Laryngology and Otology*, **76**, 460–463

SMYTH, G. D. L. and BROOKER, D. S. (1992) Small cavity mastoidectomy. *Clinical Otolaryngology*, **17**, 280–283

SMYTH, G. D. L. and PATTERSON, C. C. (1985) Results of middle ear surgery: do patients and surgeons agree? *American Journal of Otology*, **6**, 276–279

SUGITA, R., SHOZO, K., ICHIKAWA, G., GOTO, S. and FUJIMAKI, Y. (1981) Studies on anaerobic bacteria in chronic otitis media. *Laryngoscope*, **91**, 816–821

SWEENEY, G., PICOZZI, G. L. and BROWNING, G. G. (1982) A quantitative study of aerobic and anaerobic bacteria in chronic suppurative otitis media. *Journal of Infection*, **5**, 47–55

TALAAT, A. M., BAHGAT, Y. S., EL GHAZZAWY, E. and ELWANY, S. (1989) Nasopharyngeal bacterial flora before and after adenoidectomy. *Journal of Laryngology and Otology*, **103**, 372–374

TALWAR, P., CHAKRABARTI, A., KAUR, P., PAHWA, R. K., MITTAL, A. and MEHRA, Y. N. (1988) Fungal infections of ear with special reference to chronic suppurative otitis media. *Mycopathologica*, **104**, 47–50

TIMON, C. I., CAFFERKEY, M. and WALSH, M. (1991) Infection of Waldeyer's rings, the value of pernasal retropharyngeal swabs. *Journal of Otolaryngology*, **20**, 279–822

TJELLSTROM, A. (1990) Osseo-integrated implants for replacement of absent or defective ears. *Clinics in Plastic Surgery*, **17**, 355–366

TONER, J. G. and SMYTH, G. D. (1990) Surgical treatment of cholesteatoma: a comparison of three techniques. *American Journal of Otology*, **11**, 247–249

TONER, J. G., SMYTH G. D. and KERR, A. G. (1991) Realities in ossiculoplasty. *Acta Otorhinolaryngologica Belgica*, **45**, 99–104

TOS, M. (1981) Upon the relationship between secretory otitis in childhood and chronic otitis and its sequelae in adults. *Journal of Laryngology and Otology*, **95**, 1011–1022

TOS, M. and LAU, T. (1988) Attic cholesteatoma. Recurrence rate related to observation time. *American Journal of Otology*, **9**, 456–464

TOS, M. and LAU, T. (1989a) Stability of tympanoplasty in children. *Otolaryngologic Clinics of North America*, **22**, 15–28

TOS, M. and LAU, T. (1989b) Hearing after surgery for cholesteatoma using various techniques. *Auris, Nasus, Larynx*, **16**, 61–73

TOS, M., STANGERUP, S. E. and LARSEN, P. (1992) Incidence and progression of myringo-incudo-pexy after secretory otitis. *Acta Otolaryngologica*, **112**, 512–517

VAN DE HEYNING, P. H., PATTYN, S. R. and VALCKE, H. D. (1986) Ciprofloxacin in oral treatment of ear infections. *Pharmaceutisch Weekblad – Scientific edition*, **8**, 63–66

VAN DE HEYNING, P. H., PATTYN, S. R., VALCKE, H. D. and VAN CAEKENBERGHE, D. L. (1987) The use of Fluoroquinolones in chronic otitis suppurativa. *Pharmaceutisch Weekblad – Scientific edition*, **9** (suppl. S), 87–89

VARTIAINEN, E. (1992) Results of surgery for chronic otitis media in patients with a cleft palate. *Clinical Otolaryngology*, **17**, 284–286

VIOLARIS, N. S. and DONOVAN, R. (1989) Obliteration of the middle ear cleft. *Journal of Laryngology and Otology*, **103**, 43–45

WACKYM, P. A., CANALIS, R. F. and FEUERMAN, T. (1990) Subdural empyema of otorhinological origin. *Journal of Laryngology and Otology*, **104**, 118–122

WEISS, M. H., PARISIER, S. C., HAN, J. C. and EDELSTEIN, D. R. (1992) Surgery for recurrent and residual cholesteatoma. *Laryngoscope*, **102**, 145–151

9

Surgery of congenital abnormalities of the external and middle ears

David W. Proops

A child born with any congenital defect evokes enormous feelings of anxiety and great guilt in the parents. The very obvious congenital abnormality of an ear cannot easily be hidden from the world, especially in the newborn child. The parents of an afflicted individual ask their physician for an explanation and inherent in their questions are further questions about environment and genetics. Was it their fault and what is the chance of a subsequent child being afflicted?

Usually, the medical advisor can offer no explanation to the parents as to why their child is the 1 in 10 000 born with this obvious deformity.

The stage is set for later difficulty, all too often because of parental pressure for treatment, often with unrealistic deadlines and the natural medical desire to act. The first principle must be to manage the parents initially and then manage the child (Proops, 1992).

The developmental anatomy of the external and middle ears

The development of the external, middle and inner ears and temporal bone which houses them involves a complex interaction between the ectoderm, mesoderm and endoderm and the inductive qualities of one on another (Verwoerd, Van Oostrom and Verwoerd-Verhoef, 1982).

The external ear

The auricle

The external ear is divided into the auricle and the external canal. The auricle begins with the appearance of six hillocks around the first pharyngeal groove. Those anterior to the groove are said to be from the first branchial arch and those posteriorly from the second. The lowest hillock anteriorly forms the tragus and the lowest hillock posteriorly forms the antitragus. The intertragal notch is thus the groove between the tragus and the antitragus and is therefore the point of fusion of the anterior and posterior three hillocks (Bowden, 1977). The developing pinna is complete by 20 weeks but moves postcrolaterally by birth and is fully grown at puberty.

The external auditory canal

The external auditory canal is composed of three parts, the tympanic ring, tympanic membrane and the canal itself (Anson, Bast and Richany, 1955). During the second month a solid core of epithelium migrates inwards from the rudimentary pinna towards the first branchial pouch. The tubotympanic recess of the primitive foregut grows outwards to form the middle ear cleft. Where these two meet the trilaminate tympanic membrane forms with its special arrangement and migratory properties. The external auditory canal is bony for its inner two-thirds being composed of the highly developed tympanic ring, the outer one-third is cartilaginous, developed from an inward extension of the pinnal cartilage.

The middle ear and eustachian tube

The middle ear cavity originates from a lateral expansion of the primitive pharynx at the dorsal part of the front three branchial arches. At the same time continuous forward growth of the third branchial arch towards the base of the tongue narrows the proximal part of this lateral expansion of the pharynx to form the pharyngotympanic tube, the precursor of the eustachian tube. As the slit-like cavity of the tubotympanic recess opens up it lies in close proximity to the primitive tympanic membrane.

The ossicular chain originates from the mesenchyme of the front two branchial arches. The most popular explanation is that the first arch contributes to the malleus and incus and the stapes superstructure develops from the second branchial arch. The footplate of the stapes has a double origin, the lateral lamina deriving from the second branchial arch and the inner cartilaginous lamina being derived from the otic capsule. At 16 weeks of embryological development the ossicles are adult in size and shape and each ossifies from a single ossification centre.

As the middle ear cavity expands the ossicles are uncovered and lined with mucosa. The cartilaginous component of the eustachian tube differentiates between the third and fifth month but the osseous part is not formed until the third month after birth (Marquet and Declau, 1988).

Classification of congenital ear abnormalities

Marx (1926) was one of the first to attempt a classification of congenital ear malformations. Since then many authors (Altmann, 1955; Gill, 1969; Marquet, 1971; Nager, 1971; Ombredanne, 1971; Colman, 1974; Pulec and Freedman, 1978) have reviewed and developed their own classifications. These are generally based on a presumed association between the external and middle ear deformities as a basis for decision making about the benefits of surgical intervention.

Marquet's classification (1971) recognized two basic types of atresia. In the first (type I) the atresia is the consequence of abnormal development of the tympanic ring. The facial nerve therefore follows its normal course. The ossicular chain anomalies are minimal and usually the only abnormality is that the lateral two-thirds of the external ear canal may be occluded by fibrous tissue or bone. In other words there has only been a failure of canalization of the external ear canal. This type can be diagnosed radiographically because of the distance between the posterior aspect of the glenoid fossa and the anterior part of the mastoid which is constant and normal.

In the type II atresia, however, the middle ear structures are considerably more affected. There is a loss of space between the posterior part of the glenoid fossa and the anterior part of the mastoid which is therefore situated much closer to the temporoman-

dibular joint than normal. In this situation the facial nerve always follows an abnormal course and in this situation there is almost always an ossicular abnormality of varying severity.

Cremers, Oudenhoven and Marres (1987) refined this classification into three types:

Type I (mild) (Figure 9.1) corresponds to Marquet's type I. The auricle has a normal or nearly normal shape and the external auditory canal is always small and occasionally atretic laterally. The tympanic membrane is smaller than normal with a normal or small tympanic cavity. The middle ear structures may display minor malformations. If there is a fibrous or bony atresia of the external canal then a cholesteatoma may develop.

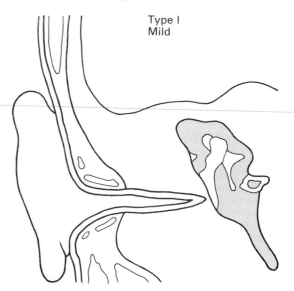

Figure 9.1 Congenital aural atresia type I. Normal external ear, normal middle and inner ear, but narrow or stenotic external canal. This is possibly amenable to conventional surgery

Type II (medium) (Figure 9.2) is the largest group of ear deformities. The auricle is rarely normal and is frequently represented by a rudimentary tag. The canal is either partially or totally aplastic or it may end blindly in a fistulous tract leading to a rudimentary tympanic membrane. An atretic plate forms the lateral wall of the middle ear cavity which is reduced in size. The malleus and incus are deformed and fixed and the facial nerve always takes an abnormal course.

They have also suggested a further subdivision to type IIA and type IIB. In type IIA (Figure 9.2) there is a partial bony stenosis whereas in type IIB (Figure 9.3) there is a total bony stenosis of the full length of the ear canal.

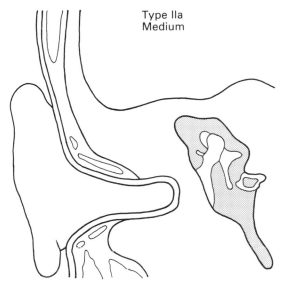

Figure 9.2 Congenital aural atresia type IIA (Cremers). Abnormal external ear and partial stenosis of external ear canal. Normal middle and inner ear

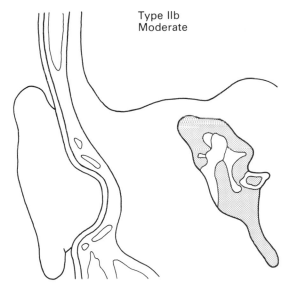

Figure 9.3 Congenital aural atresia type IIB (Cremers). Abnormal external ear, total stenosis of ear canal, probable ossicular abnormalities, normal inner ear

Type III is the most severely affected (Figure 9.4). The auricle is severely malformed or completely absent. The external auditory canal is absent, the tympanic cavity is either very small or missing and the mastoid is not pneumatized. There are often, but not invariably, associated abnormalities of the inner ear and this condition is more commonly encountered as part of a craniofacial syndrome.

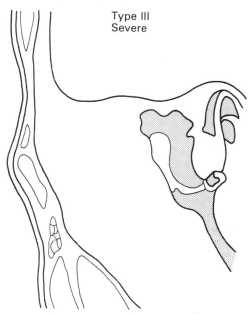

Figure 9.4 Congenital aural atresia type III. Abnormal external ear, abnormal ear canal, abnormally small middle ear space and ossicles, possibly abnormal inner ear

Malformations of the pinna

It is also possible, of course, to devise a classification for the deformities of the various parts of the ear, but it generally serves little purpose except for the pinna, for which a classification may be the basis on which treatment is proposed. Pinna malformations are divided into:

1 Minor malformations (Figure 9.5)
2 Microtia (Figure 9.6)
3 Anotia (Figure 9.7).

Associated anomalies

There are several associated congenital anomalies of the ear.

Position

The set of the ears is easily recognized but less easy to define and may be associated with other syndromes. The degree to which the ear protrudes from the head is variable and an excessive protuberance is called bat or lop ear. This is caused by a disturbance in the curling of the helix between the third and sixth months *in utero*.

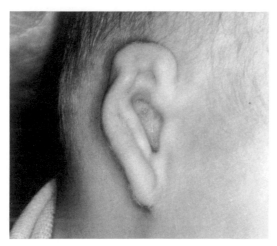

Figure 9.5 Minor ear malformations. Cosmetically acceptable but microtic pinna

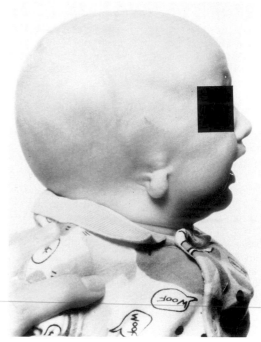

Figure 9.7 Anotia – no obvious external ear or canal – merely a very low set skin tag

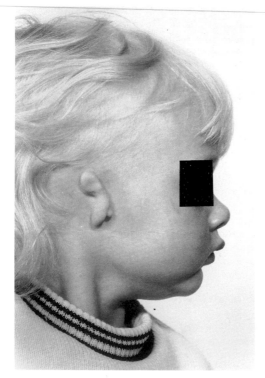

Figure 9.6 Typical microtia, linear folded remnant which is usually too far forward on the face

Form

The darwinian tubercle is present in only a proportion of the population but variations in the form of the lobule, such as adherence, absence and creases, have been associated with sensorineural hearing loss and other somatic disorders.

Auricular appendages

Auricular tags are most frequently located pretragally and they tend to extend along a line from the pinna to the mouth. They may contain elastic cartilage, may go deep and great care should be taken in their excision otherwise the facial nerve may be damaged.

Auricular sinuses and fistulae

These fall into three groups and have different embryological origins (Chami and Apesos, 1989; Prasad, Grundfast and Milmoe, 1990).

1 Fistulae on the anterior margins of the ascending limb of the helix. These are the most common and are the result of incomplete fusion of the first and second branchial arches.
2 Preauricular fistulae between the tragus and the angle of the mouth. These probably represent a failure of fusion of the maxillary and mandibular parts of the first branchial arch.

3 First branchial cleft anomalies which fall into two
groups:

  a Sinuses that run anteriorly under the lobule
  parallel to the ear canal and end blindly
  b Sinuses that arise below the angle of the mandible and run upwards to the cartilage of the
  external ear. There is often a worrying association between type 3b and abnormalities of the
  facial nerve.

The mode of inheritance of ear malformations

Probably the majority of the isolated ear malformations are considered as being sporadic forms of the
first and second arch syndromes. The overall incidence of both the isolated and syndromal types is
between 1 in 5000 to 1 in 10 000 births. There is,
however, a group of syndromes which has congenital
ear anomalies as one of its features. These, of course,
should be familiar to the otolaryngologist (Table
9.1).

Table 9.1 Conditions displaying middle and inner ear
abnormalities

Eponym	Pathological name
Treacher Collins syndrome	Mandibulofacial dysostosis
Apert's syndrome	Acrocephalosyndactyly
Crouzon's syndrome	Craniofacial dysostosis
Cleidocranial dysostosis	
Klippel Feil syndrome	Otocervical syndrome
Goldenhar's syndrome	Oculoauriculovertebral dysplasia
Turner syndrome	Gonadal aplasia
Patau syndrome	Trisomy 13–15 syndrome
Edward's syndrome	Trisomy 18 syndrome
Down's syndrome	Trisomy 21 syndrome
Pierre Robin syndrome	Cleft palate, micrognathia and glossoptosis
Di George syndrome	Third and fourth pharyngeal pouch syndrome

Treacher Collins syndrome (Franceschetti syndrome, mandibulofacial dysostosis)

This is an autosomal dominant syndrome with reduced penetrance. The chief features are hypoplasia
of the facial bones, especially the zygoma and the
mandible. The eyes have an antimongoloid slant
with a coloboma of the lower lid and there may
occasionally be cleft lip and palate. Malformations of
the outer and middle ear are major and a universal

feature but the inner ear is usually spared. The
middle ear cleft is usually dysplastic and the ossicles
absent or dysplastic as a fused mass (Taylor and
Phelps, 1993). A severe conductive hearing loss is
almost universal.

Apert's syndrome (acrocephalosyndactyly)

Major skull deformities are combined with aplasia of
the middle third of the face and syndactyly of the
hands and feet. The ears are low set and dysplastic
with ossicular abnormalities and a high incidence of
perilymph gushers due to a widened cochlear aqueduct (Phelps *et al.*, 1991).

Crouzon's syndrome (craniofacial dysostosis)

This autosomal dominant condition has a very
characteristic facial appearance with marked proptosis due to the shallow orbits. External and middle ear
abnormalities are common.

Cleidocranial dysostosis

A characteristic broad skull with absent clavicles is
associated with stenosis or atresia of ear canal.

Klippel Feil syndrome (otocervical syndrome)

Skeletal anomalies include cervical spina bifida and
scoliosis and the associated conductive hearing loss is
due to ossicular abnormalities.

Goldenhar's syndrome (oculoauriculovertebral dysplasia)

There is unilateral facial abnormality with a small
ramus and body of mandible. There is often a facial
nerve weakness and an associated congenital ear
deformity and conductive hearing loss. The other
findings are dysplasia of the upper vertebral column
and often an epibulbar dermoid at the lateral corneo-
scleral junction.

Further discussion about the mode of inheritance
and the otolaryngological abnormalities in these syndromes is found in Chapters 3 and 4.

Management of congenital ear deformities

The ideal time to start assessing a patient with a congenital ear deformity is within the first few weeks of life. The parents welcome the chance to discuss the problem. It is an ideal opportunity to talk about possible aetiologies, to attempt to allay parental guilt, to discuss the implications of the deformity and to initiate a treatment plan.

The assessment of the child must take account of the other problems if the child has a syndrome. The evaluation of the ear centres on two aspects, cosmesis and the hearing, usually in that order from the parental viewpoint which must be acknowledged and respected.

Investigations

In some centres much reliance is placed upon radiological investigation. Although this will allow classification into one of the three groups suggested by Cremers, this rarely affects management. If the microtia is minor and the ear canal present then radiology will be important to assess suitability for otosurgical approach. If the microtia is marked without the presence of an ear canal, as in Cremers' types II or III, then experience dictates that conventional surgery has a limited role and a more radical approach is indicated (Taylor and Phelps, 1993) (Figure 9.8).

The cosmetic correction of the pinnal deformity is more contentious and is certainly not a matter of urgency. It should not be a high priority until the child becomes aware of it and requests treatment.

The audiological evaluation of the ear can be undertaken early. If the deformity is unilateral the need for this is lessened. The question to be asked is simply, 'is the deafness conductive, sensorineural or mixed?' It is obviously ideal to have symmetrical normal binaural hearing and those so born who lose one ear may have an impairment. However, those born with monaural hearing adapt remarkably well and the benefit to be gained from surgery aimed at giving hearing to an ear that has never experienced normal hearing must be questioned. Smyth (1980) showed that, unless the hearing in the deficient ear can be brought within 15 dB of the good ear, then the patient does not perceive benefit and there is a greater risk of damage to the facial nerve.

For those with bilateral conductive losses the benefits from intervention are overwhelming. After diagnosis the obvious first need of the child is the fitting of a hearing aid. If there is a meatus a conventional behind the ear aid can be tried, but if there is no ear or canal then a conventional bone conducting aid must be used. Young children are remarkably tolerant of a head-band bone conduction aid and nothing is to be gained by delay in fitting. The overriding principle must be to give the child auditory stimulation by whatever means possible. Although there might be parental resistance initially, time spent with the parent and child explaining fully the reasoning is amply repaid by improved compliance later. It also reinforces the professional view that hearing rehabilitation is a greater priority than cosmesis in the young child.

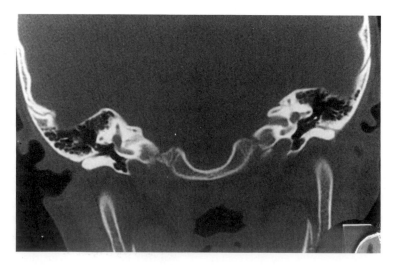

Figure 9.8 Coronal CT scan of patient with bilateral aural atresia. Note the absence of external auditory canals. (By kind permission of Dr Peter Phelps)

Surgical management

This will be discussed in three parts:

1 The classical surgical approaches to the middle ear to produce either a cavity that can be aided or, in more favourable circumstances, will permit near normal hearing by removal of an atretic plate or simple ossiculoplasty
2 The cosmetic reconstruction of the pinna
3 Newer techniques employing implantable devices to facilitate prosthetic rehabilitation or bone conduction hearing aids.

Classical surgical techniques

There are four principal surgical methods for improving the hearing in congenital aural atresia. They are:

1 Fenestration of the lateral canal (Figure 9.9)
2 Type III tympanoplasty (Figure 9.10)
3 Canalplasty (Figure 9.11)
4 Canalplasty with homograft tympanoplasty (Figure 9.12).

Fenestration of the lateral canal (Figure 9.9)

This has the disadvantage that a labyrinthine fistula has to be created and that the mastoid has to be widely exenterated. When there is fixation of the stapes following removal of the incus and the malleus the fenestration can be immediate. Some surgeons prefer a two-stage procedure with a secondary skin graft to reduce the risk of sensorineural deafness.

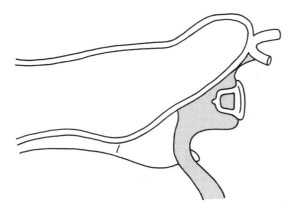

Figure 9.9 Fenestration of the lateral semicircular canal after fashioning of a modified radical mastoidectomy

The type III tympanoplasty (Figure 9.10)

This requires surgical exposure of both the middle ear and the mastoid and its principal disadvantage is an open mastoid cavity with the constant risk of otorrhoea.

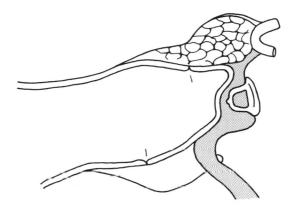

Figure 9.10 Type III tympanoplasty, attempting to obtain direct contact between the stapes and the drum

The canalplasty procedure (Figure 9.11)

This is usually undertaken in the most severe cases and is often combined with the cosmetic surgery for microtia. It is also of course the procedure undertaken in the least severe cases where only a small atretic plate needs removal.

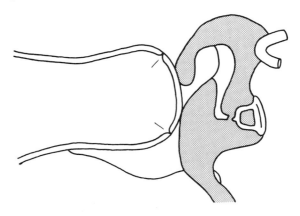

Figure 9.11 Canalplasty suitable only for those with stenotic ear canals but a normal ossicular chain

The canalplasty technique with homograft tympanoplasty (Figure 9.12)

Devised by Marquet (1981, 1988), this theoretically should give the best anatomical and functional result.

Recent worries about the use of homologous material because of the fear of viral transmission may make this obsolete.

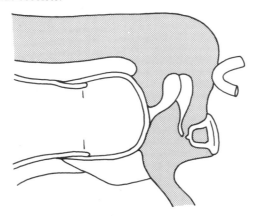

Figure 9.12 Canalplasty with homograph tympanoplasty. This should theoretically fully restore function as long as a mobile stapes is found. However, practical difficulties and anxieties about homograph materials render this a very uncommon procedure

When the only management option was surgical then poor results were seen as an acceptable cost for the relatively few good ones. Cremers, Temissen and Marres (1988) reported that, in their series, 75% of the ears had major anomalies of the ossicular chain. Fixation of the handle of the malleus to an atretic plate occurred in nearly all cases. The average pre-operative threshold for speech frequencies was 43 dB in group IIA and 58 dB in group IIB with complete bony atresia. The postoperative thresholds were 25 dB in group IIA and 38 dB in group IIB, but because of the late complications such as restenosis only 22% of group IIB had a reasonable long-term hearing result.

The purpose of this type of surgery is to create a socially useful level of hearing in the involved ear but in the reported series (which are likely to be the better ones) this is only achieved in 31–71% of patients.

Major complications such as facial nerve damage or sensorineural loss are rarely reported but rates of restenosis and otorrhoea were reported as 33% by Fenner, Wachter and Fisch (1981), 24% stenosis and 18% otorrhoea by Colman (1976) and 10% by Cremers, Temissen and Marres (1988). The level of complexity and complication would make the justification for surgery difficult in a purely unilateral case. This is certainly the view of Bellucci (1981), who stated that surgery should not be attempted if the contralateral ear was normal. In bilateral atresia simpler, safer and more certain forms of modern management would seem best except perhaps for the type I cases. Unilateral atresia is four times more common than bilateral atresia and the type II deformity is by far and away

the most frequent type. The scope then for these more conventional surgical techniques would seem to be very limited indeed. Unfortunately, they continue to be practised.

Surgical reconstruction of the pinna

This is one of the most challenging technical problems in surgery. There are seven suggested criteria that must be met in the reconstruction of an auricle:

1 Correct size
2 Appearance identical to that of the contralateral ear
3 Identical ear-head angles
4 Identical levels of the ears
5 Durability in terms of size and shape
6 Adequate support and soft tissue for moulding
7 Good colour match.

Unfortunately, surgery for malformations of the auricle will affect treatment of the external auditory canal. The decision as to which has precedence differs from patient to patient and may prejudice the hearing result. The main indication for this surgery is the psychological well-being of the patient at the age of 6 years when the ears have almost reached adult size and reconstruction can be started. Walter (1972) and Brent (1980a, b) stressed that surgery should not be carried out earlier because one of the major reconstructive methods includes the autotransplantation of rib cartilage, which may not be large enough to harvest. Brent also believed that a child's major psychological trauma only begins about the seventh year and so recommends 'the summer of the sixth birthday' to be the best starting time. Homologous and alloplastic materials have now largely been abandoned.

In the first step a framework of autologous rib cartilage is placed in a virgin skin pocket. The second step is the transposition of the lobule and the third step is the formation of the tragus from a composite graft from the contralateral auricle. Finally, auricular projection is achieved by placing a skin graft behind the new ear. The increasing refinement of this multistage procedure occasionally gives excellent results. Unfortunately, what appears to the surgeon to be a good cosmetic result rarely seems to please the patient.

Prosthetic management

The use of a prosthesis to replace lost or damaged tissues has a long history from wooden legs to false teeth. The development of modern silicone rubber materials has provided life-like textures and colours, so that the prosthesis can be made indistinguishable from the real ear even to the trained observer. Prosthetic eyes and the nose can be retained by spectacles, but auricular prostheses cannot. Acquired auricular loss is usually traumatic or the result of neoplasia so surgical reconstruction is compromised or not thought worthwhile. The traditional method of retaining these prostheses was by adhesives which were messy and uncertain.

Branemark *et al.* (1977) described the process of osseointegration as the intimate biological connection between living bone and commercially pure titanium. This has now been clinically exploited and developed by Tjellstrom and his team in Gothenburg, Sweden, as a fixture which can carry a prosthesis (Tjellstrom *et al.*, 1985, 1988; Tjellstrom, 1989).

Surgery is performed in two stages. At the first, titanium implants are placed onto the mastoid at predetermined sites. The wound is closed and 3 months allowed to elapse for osseointegration. At a second operation the fixture is exposed and the osseointegration assessed by direct vision. The overlying tissues are greatly reduced and thinned and the vestigial ear removed completely leaving only the periosteum and the skin. An abutment is attached to the fixture which penetrates the skin. When the skin is healed a gold bar superstructure is made to fit the abutment and an auricular prosthesis fashioned by hand to match the other ear in size, colour and position. This is firmly retained on the superstructure by clips and only removed by the patient when going to sleep (Figures 9.13 and 9.14). Each prosthesis will last more than a year, especially if the patient is older and less active. The skin penetrating abutment needs daily cleaning to ensure that the desquamated skin and debris do not accumulate and provoke an inflammatory reaction.

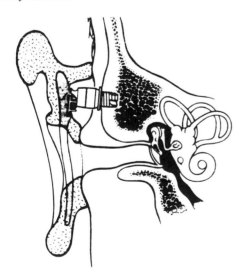

Figure 9.13 Diagram of osseointegrated fixture carrying an auricular prosthesis

This technique is simple, safe and has the highest patient satisfaction. It involves no risk to the hearing or the facial nerve. There are no other scars on the

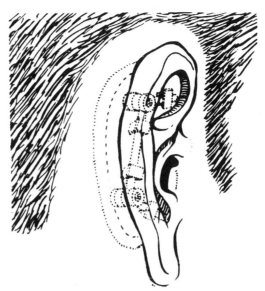

Figure 9.14 Two titanium fixtures implanted within the temporal bone are capped with abutments to which is soldered a gold bar (dotted lines). The auricular prosthesis is located and retained on this gold bar by clips

body and the changes in the skin colour with the seasons can be anticipated by the provision of a winter and summer prosthesis. This technique is especially good for those with bilateral auricular atresia as part of a syndrome as the operation can be performed swiftly under local anaesthesia. This reduces the considerable and recognized anaesthetic risk in these individuals with branchial arch syndromes (Stevenson *et al.*, 1993).

Prosthetic management necessitates a team approach as this work must be planned and coordinated. The Birmingham osseointegrated team is composed of an otolaryngologist, a maxillofacial surgeon, maxillofacial technologists (now known as anaplastologists), audiologists, speech therapist, clinical geneticist and a nurse. There are regular specialized clinics which all members of the team attend. Each clinic is preceded by a planning meeting at which all the team members are encouraged to contribute. Within the clinic a treatment plan is formulated for each patient. This is as follows:

1 Planned assessment by the team
2 The decision
3 Planned surgery
4 Prosthetic rehabilitation
5 Audiological rehabilitation
6 Speech therapy if necessary
7 Follow up including genetic counselling
8 Audit.

The first and major benefit of having set up a special clinic for congenital ear problems is that it allows new patients to meet treated patients. Over the years the team has been impressed by a patient's or parents' excitement at meeting another individual with a similar problem. One of the major difficulties that our patients and their parents suffer is a feeling of isolation. They feel they are the only afflicted individuals in the world. The second advantage of congenital ear deformity clinics is that there are patients at various stages of treatment and this permits both patients and parents to gain a sense of orderliness and planned treatment. This often reduces the patient or parental pressure for immediate action. The most important and overwhelming benefit of such a clinic however is the guiding principal of education, in this context education of the patient by the patient. All patients seen and accepted for our programme do so only after they have met in private another patient with a similar problem, who has completed treatment.

It is an understanding within the programme that when they complete treatment the patient and parents will be asked to discuss their progress and result with the next patient. Doctors, technologists and audiologists can talk endlessly at and with patients, but the level of understanding of what has been said remains woefully low. It is often said that one picture is worth a thousand words. For the patient to see a completed prosthesis with or without a bone anchored hearing aid in position is often the very best form of explanation that any new patient can require. A space is set aside in the clinic for old patients to meet new patients on their own. Privacy is important because there is considerable embarrassment about the congenitally deformed ear. It is vital that neither the surgeon nor any member of the team should be present during this discussion so that there can be no pressure from the enthusiasts. Before a decision to embark on treatment is made a time for reflection is necessary and the patient and the relatives are encouraged to go away and think about what has been seen and heard (Figure 9.15).

The sequence of events can be summarized as follows:

1 Referral to the clinic
2 Attendance at the clinic with the whole team present
3 Surgical, audiological, prosthetic assessment
4 New patient meets old patient in privacy
5 Team discussion – acceptance on the programme
6 Stage one: surgical procedure: placement of fixtures
7 Stage two: 3 months later, skin penetration, placement of abutments, thinning of flap
8 Stage three: one month later, fitting of prosthesis, or bone anchored hearing aid or both
9 Rehabilitation and review
10 Planned replacement programme for both prostheses and bone anchored hearing aid. An assumed life of 2 years for the prosthesis and 3 years for the bone anchored hearing aid.

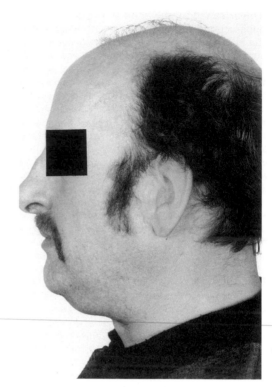

Figure 9.15 The final result, a silastic prosthetic pinna held in place by the titanium fixtures

Bone conduction hearing aids

The principle of bone conduction has been known for many years and indeed bone conduction has been used diagnostically to differentiate between conductive hearing loss and sensorineural hearing loss since the nineteenth century.

Vibratory energy reaching the cochlea causes alternate compression and expansion of the cochlear shell. Compression of the cochlea would not produce inner ear fluid displacement if the cochlear scalae were of equal size and shape. However, the total surface of the contracting walls is lower on the vestibular side than the tympanic side and the oval window is less compliant than the round window, so the cochlear partition is forced downwards.

Bone conduction however cannot be explained by a single phenomenon. Tondorf (1966) identified eight contributing factors.

The development of electrical hearing aids gave rise to the electromagnetic vibrator pressed against the mastoid process held by a steel sprung aid and connected to a body worn processor. The aesthetic appearance was improved with the invention of spectacle aids in which the electrical parts are hidden inside the arms of the spectacles. Unfortunately, this ingenious method rarely pushes the transducer hard enough against the mastoid process. The pressure required to press the transducer to the mastoid to transmit enough energy can cause discomfort and persistent skin irritation.

Dissatisfaction with conventional bone conducting aids led to two significant advances, the American Xomed Audiant bone conductor and the Swedish Nobelpharma bone anchored implant. The Xomed Audiant bone conductor consists of a titanium screw attached to a magnet which is buried subcutaneously. The external part, which can either be at ear level or body worn, contains an electromagnetic induction coil around another magnet which holds it in place over the implanted magnet. Sound is converted to electrical energy which, in the coil, creates a variable electromagnetic field that attracts and repels the implanted magnet, causing the skull and hence the osseous cochlea to vibrate (Gatehouse and Browning, 1990).

Unfortunately, because of the loss of energy through the intervening soft tissue the device has been found to have insufficient power. For the device to be useful the US Food and Drug Administration suggested that the bone conduction average over 0.5 kHz, 1.0 kHz and 2.0 kHz should be no more than 25 dB. The initial hopes for this device (Hough, Himelick and Johnson, 1986) and its refined ear level successor (Hough *et al.*, 1987) have not been borne out in practice. Browning (1990) and Wade, Halik and Chasun (1992) reported the combined British and Canadian experience and found that, although all but one of those surveyed fulfilled the audiological criteria, only half wore the device because of inadequate benefit and to a lesser extent because it was uncomfortable.

The bone anchored hearing aid

The bone anchored hearing aid (BAHA) (Figures 9.16, 9.17, 9.18 and 9.19) is a revolution for those with congenital aural atresia and a severe conductive hearing loss. It is a combination of a Branemark titanium implant and a bone conduction hearing aid. The true bone conducted sound, without the interposition of soft tissues which attenuate and distort a signal, gives excellent quality. The good conductivity of bone and the low attenuation between the ears means that only 2 dB on average are lost between the cochleae, giving the patient binaural, though not stereophonic hearing from one aid.

For children who have bilateral congenital ear deformities attention must be focused early on their hearing loss rather than the cosmetic deformity (Stevenson *et al.*, 1993). Those who do have a meatus and a reasonably shaped ear can be fitted with a conventional aid but for many a bone conducting aid is the only option. This is, of course, uncomfortable

for a child, unsightly for the parents and has its efficiency dependent on the tightness of the band and the thickness of the skin and soft tissues of the mastoid.

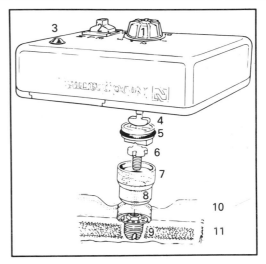

1 Volume control
2 Tone control
3 Microphone
4 Piston
5 Security coupling with O ring
6 Connection screw
7 Titanium coupling
8 Cover screw
9 Titanium fixture
10 Skin
11 Bone tissue

Figure 9.16 Diagram of the bone anchored sound processor

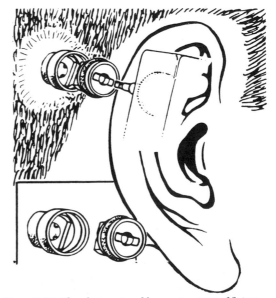

Figure 9.17 The abutment and bayonet system of fixing the bone anchored aid to the special abutment

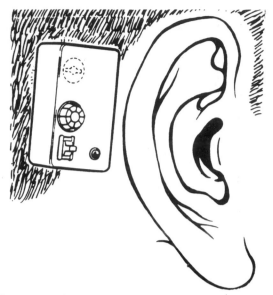

Figure 9.18 The aid *in situ* behind the ear in the hairline

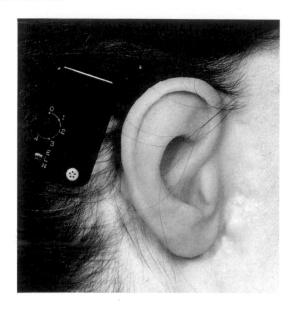

Figure 9.19 A close-up view of the relationship of the auricular prosthesis and bone anchored hearing aid

Because the bone anchored hearing aid is integrally attached to the bone it has no apparent mass to the patient; so having been attached in the morning, the aid is forgotten by the majority of wearers. This means that the wearing time of a bone anchored hearing aid is long with most patients, even children wearing the aid for more than 12 hours per day.

Patient satisfaction is very high because of the quality of the sound, its binaural nature, the comfort and the cosmetic advantage of the aid which can be concealed in the hair. The gain from the aid is such that it acts not only to correct the conductive loss but will also help with a sensorineural loss as well. If the bone conduction level is worse than 45 dB then a body worn bone conduction aid (Superbass) is also available.

Complications are rare. Loss of fixtures occurs in about 10% of patients overall but more especially in children. This can be mitigated against by implanting a spare fixture at primary surgery. The youngest a child can be implanted is between 2 and 3 years of age and the aids themselves of course are subject to the rigours and traumas of childhood.

The results of bone anchored hearing aid fitting can be assessed in terms of surgical success, that is the success rate of long-term integration (Tjellstrom *et al.*, 1983; Cremers, Snik and Beynan, 1992; Mylanus *et al.*, 1994a) and the long-term effects of skin penetration and possible septic complications (Holgers *et al.*, 1988). The results are impressive with 97% of the fixtures being retained and 86% having no significant skin reaction.

The audiological results of the bone anchored hearing aid are superior to the conventional bone conducting hearing aid, especially noticeable in noisy environments. The results compared with air conduction aids are not as good but, nevertheless, patients prefer the bone anchored hearing aid probably because of comfort and binaurality (Hakansson *et al.*, 1990; Cremers, Snik and Beynan, 1992; Mylanus *et al.*, 1994b).

The only problem with this system is its cost but it is universally successful in properly selected patients and of 100 patients with the bone anchored hearing aid in Birmingham all are wearers. This is not true with any other aid.

The future

Individuals will continue to be born with congenital deformity of the ear. Their problems are best evaluated, and their interests best served, by early referral to a multidisciplinary centre where a variety of options can be discussed and full rehabilitative support is available. This should include otolaryngology, maxillofacial or plastic surgery, audiology, maxillofacial prosthetics, speech therapy and genetic counselling.

These patients require time and a life-long commitment which can only be offered by specialized teams offering this service to a large population. These patients and carers deserve the best advice and treatment, sympathy, explanation and help to reduce the inevitable but unnecessary guilt.

References

ALTMANN, F. (1955) Malformation of the auricle and external auditory meatus. *Archives of Otolaryngology*, **54**, 115–139

ANSON, B. J., BAST, T. H. and RICHANY, S. F. (1955) The fetal and early postnatal development of the tympanic ring and related structures in man. *Annals of Ototology, Rhinology and Laryngology*, **64**, 802–833

BELLUCCI, R. J. (1981) Congenital aural malformation diagnosis and treatment. *Otolaryngologic Clinics of North America*, **74**, 119–128

BOWDEN, R. E. M. (1977) Development of the middle and external ear in man. *Proceedings of the Royal Society of Medicine*, **70**, 823–824

BRANEMARK, P. I., HANSSON, B. O., ADELL, R., BREINE, U., LINDSTROM, J., HALLEW, O. *et al.* (1977) Osseointegrated implants in the treatment of the edentulous jaw. *Scandinavian Journal of Plastic Reconstructive Surgery*, **11** (suppl.), 11–16

BRENT, B. (1980a) The correction of microtia with autologous cartilage grafts. I. The classic deformity. *Plastic and Reconstructive Surgery*, **66**, 1–12

BRENT, B. (1980b) The correction of microtia with autologous cartilage graft. II Atypical and complex deformities. *Plastic and Reconstructive Surgery*, **66**, 13–21

BROWNING, G. G. (1990) The British experience of an implantable subcutaneous bone conduction hearing aid (Xomed Audiant). *Journal of Laryngology and Otology*, **104**, 534–538

CHAMI, R. G. and APESOS, J. (1989) Treatment of asymptomatic preauricular sinuses: challenging conventional wisdom. *Annals of Plastic Surgery*, **23**, 406–411

COLMAN, B. H. (1974) Congenital atresia of the ear: the otological problem. Section of Plastic Surgery with section of otology. *Proceedings of the Royal Society of Medicine*, **67**, 1203–1205

COLMAN, B. H. (1976) Congenital deformities of the ear. *The International Otology Workshop*. Chicago

CREMERS, C. W. R. J., OUDENHOVEN, J. M. T. M. and MARRES, E. H. M. (1987) Congenital aural atresia: a subclassification and superficial management. *Clinical Otolaryngology*, **9**, 119–127

CREMERS, C. W. R. J., TEMISSEN, E. and MARRES, E. H. M. A. (1988) Classification of congenital aural atresia and results of reconstructive surgery. *Advances in Otorhinolaryngology*, **40**, 9–14

CREMERS, C. W. R. J., SNIK, A. F. M. and BEYNAN, A. J. (1992) Hearing with bone anchored hearing aids (BAHA HC200) compared to a conventional bone conducting hearing aid. *Clinical Otolaryngology*, **17**, 275–279

FENNER, T., WACHTER, I. and FISCH. U. (1981) Atresia auris congenita, probleme und resultate des opratwen therapie. In: *Aktuelle probleme der otorhinolaryngologie*. Besn: Verlag Hans Hubert

GATEHOUSE, S. and BROWNING, G. G. (1990) The output characteristics of an implanted bone conduction prosthesis. *Clinical Otolaryngology*, **15**, 503–513

GILL, N. W. (1969) Congenital atresia of the ear. *Journal of Laryngology and Otology*, **83**, 1251–1254

HAKANSSON, B., LINDEN, G., TJELLSTROM, A., RINGDALK, A. JACOBSSON, M., CARLSSON, P. *et al.* (1990) Ten years of experience with the Swedish bone anchored hearing aid system. *Annals of Otology, Rhinology and Laryngology*, **99** (Suppl. 151), 1–16

HOLGERS, K. M., TJELLSTROM, A., BJURSTEN, L. M. and ERLANDSON, B. E. (1988) Soft tissue reaction around percutaneous implants. A clinical study of soft tissue conditions around skin penetrating titanium implants for bone anchored hearing aids. *American Journal of Otology*, **9**, 56–59

HOUGH, J., HIMELICK, T. and JOHNSON, B. (1986) Implantable bone conduction device. *Annals of Otology, Rhinology and Laryngology*, **95**, 498–504

HOUGH, J., VERNON, J., MECKEL, M., HIMELICK, T., RICHARD, G. and DORMER, K. (1987) A middle ear implantable device for controlled amplification of sound in the human. A preliminary report. *Laryngoscope*, **97**, 141–151

MARQUET, J. F. (1971) Considerations sur le diagnostic des surdities de transmission par traumatisme de l'oreille. *Acta Otology, Rhinology, Laryngology Belgium*, **25**, 641–644

MARQUET, J. F. (1981) Congenital malformations and middle ear surgery. *Journal of the Royal Society of Medicine*, **74**, 119–128

MARQUET, J. F. (1988) Allografts and congenital aural atresia. *Advances in Otorhinolaryngology*, **40** 15–23

MARQUET, J. F. and DECLAU, F. R (1988). Congenital middle ear malformations. *Acta Otology, Rhinology and Laryngology, Belgium*, **42**, 157–165

MARX, H. (1926) Die Mißbildungen des ohres. In: *Hardback der Hals-Nasen-Ohrenheilkunde*, edited by Denker-Kahler, Vol. VI. Berlin: Springer-Verlag.

MYLANUS, E.A.M., CREMERS, C.W.R.J., SNIK, A.F.M. and VAN DEN BERGE, N.W. (1994a) Clinical results of percutaneous implants in the temporal bone. *Archives of Otolaryngology – Head and Neck Surgery*, **120**, 81–85

MYLANUS, E.A.M., SNIK, A.F.M., JORRITSMA, F.F. and CREMERS, C.R.W.J. (1994b) Audiological results of the bone anchored hearing aid and HC 220. *Ear and Hearing*, **15**, 87–92

NAGER, G. T. (1971) Congenital aural atresia: Anatomy and surgical management. *Birth Defects: Original Article Series*, vol. VII. no. 4

OMBREDANNE, M. (1971) Chirurgie des surdite's congenitales par malformations ossiculaires. *Acta Otology, Rhinology and Laryngology Belgium*, **25**, 37–39

PHELPS, P. D., REARDON, W., PEMBREY, M., BELLMAN, S. and LUXON, L. (1991) X-linked deafness – stapes gushers and a distinctive defect of the inner ear. *Neuroradiology*, **38**, 326–330

PRASAD, S., GRUNDFAST, K. and MILMOE, G. (1990) Management of congenital preauricular pit and sinus tract in children. *Laryngoscope*, **100**, 320–321

PROOPS, D. W. (1992) The child with the congenital ear: manage the parents then manage the child. In: *Congenital Subcanal and Middle Ear Malformation Management*, edited by B. Ars. Basel: Kugler Publications. pp. 27–31

PULEC, J. L. and FREEDMAN, H. M. (1978) Management of congenital ear abnormalities. *Laryngoscope*, **88**, 420–434

SMYTH, G. D. L (1980) Ossiculoplasty in chronic ear disease. *Monographs in Clinical Otolaryngology*. Edinburgh: Churchill Livingstone. pp. 146–174

STEVENSON, D. S., PROOPS, D. W., WAKE, M. J. C., DEADMAN, M. J., WORROLLO, S. J. and HOBSON, J. A. (1993) Osseointegrated implants in the management of childhood ear abnormalities: the initial Birmingham experience. *Journal of Laryngology and Otology*, **107**, 502–509

TAYLOR, D. J. and PHELPS, P. D. (1993) Imaging of ear deformities in Treacher Collins Syndrome. *Clinical Otolaryngology*, **18**, 263–267

TJELLSTROM, A. (1989) Osseointegrated appliances and their

application in the head and neck. *Advances in Oto-rhino-laryngology*, **3**, 39–70

TJELLSTROM, A., ROSENHALL, U., LINDSTROM, J., HALLAM, O. ALBREKTSSON, T. and BRANEMARK, P.I. (1983) Five year experience with skin penetrating bone anchored implants in the temporal bone. *Acta Otolaryngologica*, **95**, 568–575

TJELLSTROM, A., YONTCHEV, E., LINSTROM, J. and BRANEMARK, P.I. (1985) Five years experience with bone anchored auricular prostheses. *Otolaryngology, Head and Neck Surgery*, **93**, 366–372

TJELLSTROM, A., JACOBSSON, M., ALBREKSSON, T. and JANNSON K. (1988) Use of tissue integrated implants in congenital aural malformations. *Advanced Otology, Rhinology and Laryngology*, **40**, 24–32

TONDORF, J. (1966) Bone conduction studies in experimental animals. *Acta Otolarynologica*, Suppl. 213

VERWOERD, C. D. A., VAN OOSTROM, G. and VERWOERD-VERHOEF, H. L. (1982) Otic olacade and cephalic neural crest. *Acta Otolaryngologica*, **91**, 431–435

WADE, P.S., HALIK, J.J. and CHASUN, M. (1992) Bone conduction implants: transcutaneous vs. percutaneous. *Otolaryngology Head and Neck Surgery*, **106**, 68–74

WALTER, C. (1972) Correction of deformities of the auricle. *Archives of Otorhinolaryngology*, **202**, 229–252

10

Management of the hearing impaired child

David A. Adams

There is no doubt that significant hearing loss has important consequences for language acquisition, communication and cognitive, social and emotional development (McClelland *et al.*, 1992). This is particularly true when the onset is in the prelingual period.

Further proof of the difficulties faced by hearing impaired children is the considerable anecdotal evidence that deaf and hard of hearing children fall behind in academic achievement and that they leave school less qualified than their hearing peers, sometimes with no qualifications of any kind. The worrying thing is that there would appear to be no systematically collated government data reporting the achievements of these children at school.

The importance of early detection

Fisch (1983) published a review of the development and maturation of the hearing system in infants and those with a hearing loss. The hearing impaired child may have difficulty with speech perception and have delayed or absent speech and language development. There is no doubt however that many severely hearing impaired children do develop good speech in spite of the restricted function of the auditory channel. It is known that much of the information contained in speech is redundant, since speech contains more information than is needed to understand the message. In a deaf child much of this redundancy is eliminated since it is not heard, though sufficient auditory information may reach the higher centres to allow adequate speech discrimination. Fisch postulated that, for optimum development of speech and language, the auditory pathway must be stimulated from a very early age to allow it and the higher centres to mature properly.

The benefits of early detection and initiation of the

management of deafness have been known for many years (Ewing, 1957). Martin (1982) published a survey of the nine countries which made up the European Economic Community (EEC) at that time. The achievements were far from adequate with 90% of the children not having been diagnosed by their first birthday and as many as 50% not detected until 3 years of age. In most cases there was also a delay in the provision of hearing aids even after the diagnosis had been made, with up to 60% waiting for 12 months or more. This study also demonstrated that more than one half of the children were unable to carry on a meaningful conversation with strangers. Other research further demonstrated the serious developmental consequences of untreated hearing loss in early childhood and also the benefits of early detection and rehabilitation (Markides, 1986; Ramkalawan and Davis, 1992). The effects of middle ear disease such as acute otitis media or otitis media with effusion on language development are less clear. Some authors have suggested that children with these problems have delayed language development (Teele, Klein and Rosner, 1984; Gleason, 1988), although others have suggested caution in attributing language disorders and learning disabilities to middle ear problems (Leviton, 1980; Ventry, 1980). Haggard and Hughes (1991) were of the opinion that inference from indirect evidence together with the best available direct evidence indicated that persistent otitis media with effusion in early childhood does slightly retard the development of language, attention and communication skills.

Present detection policies

Deafness in children is discovered in one of the following ways:

1 The child fails a screening test of hearing
2 The child is known to be 'at risk' of having a hearing loss
3 Parental or professional suspicion
4 A child fails to develop speech and language in the normal way.

Screening tests of hearing

These are discussed in Chapter 6. They are performed in an attempt to identify those children in need of further investigation.

'At risk' children

There are a number of 'at risk' registers giving lists of pathological processes which increase the possibility of the child having a hearing loss. It would appear that one fifth of health districts in the UK already have, or plan to have, some provision for neonatal screening on an 'at risk' basis (Haggard, 1993). This issue is discussed in Chapter 6.

Parental suspicion

It is best to believe parents if they suspect that their child has a hearing problem. They are often wrong but unfortunately occasionally right. Parving (1984) found that, in more than one half of the hearing impaired children in his study group, the parents were the first to suspect a hearing loss. On the other hand, McCormick (1988) and Watkins, Baldwin and Laoide (1990) found that only about one fifth of parents with severely or profoundly deaf children were responsible for initiating the referral. This is discussed further in Chapter 6.

Children who fail to develop speech

Occasionally there are children of 2–3 years of age who present with no speech or very indistinct speech. Some of these children have a hearing loss, though others have specific language disorders, emotional problems or mental retardation. There may be complex combinations of these disorders. There is also no doubt that some of these children have been missed by earlier screening tests.

Future detection policies

At present considerable research is directed towards improving the early detection of deafness. This must use objective electrophysiological methods since reliable behavioural responses are not usually present until 6 months of age. It would appear that the two most promising techniques are those using either evoked response audiometry or evoked otoacoustic emissions. These techniques are discussed further in Chapters 5 and 6.

Management of the child referred for assessment

Children who fail screening tests or are otherwise suspected of having a hearing loss are normally referred to an otolaryngologist or audiological physician for further assessment. Haggard and Pullan (1989) outlined the requirements for a paediatric audiology clinic and suggested that these services, except for screening, should be taken out of the community and based in a hospital. In Belfast, however, community audiology clinics staffed by trained community physicians have successfully provided a service for testing the hearing of children who fail screening tests and for family doctors who would like hearing assessments performed on children. Guidelines have been prepared jointly by these community physicians and local otolaryngologists and describe when it is appropriate to refer a child for further assessment to a hospital clinic.

The aims of the hospital clinic should be as follows:

1 To determine if a hearing loss is present. Many children referred are found to have normal hearing though the number of these has dropped dramatically with the introduction of guidelines for hearing assessment in the community. Reassuringly, there have been no cases of late or missed diagnosis because of the introduction of this second screening tier in the community
2 To decide on the type of hearing loss, whether it is conductive, sensorineural or mixed
3 To determine the severity of the hearing loss
4 To determine, if possible, the age of onset of the hearing loss. Prelingual hearing loss has more serious implications for the child
5 To look for other relevant handicaps.

It is the author's practice to send the parents or care-givers a questionnaire with their initial appointment. This asks the parents to state their main worry about the child and what they think of the child's hearing. There are sections dealing with the pregnancy, postnatal development, ear, nose and throat symptoms and family history. Questionnaires are a notoriously unreliable means of gathering information though they do give parents forewarning of the type of questions they will be asked during the visit to the clinic.

The first part of the assessment must be spent taking a brief, relevant history. The author feels it is better to move quickly to audiological assessment since children become restless and anxious very quickly in unfamiliar surroundings. If necessary a full history, including family history, exposure to pathogens and speech development may be obtained later.

The diagnostic test used depends on the child's chronological and developmental age. The tests are discussed in full in Chapter 5. It is usually possible to establish reliable hearing thresholds at different frequencies. Evoked response audiometry is useful in children under the age of 6 months and those who are handicapped and will not or cannot respond to auditory stimuli in the usual way. It is also good practice to confirm objectively hearing thresholds obtained by free field tests when there is suspicion of sensorineural hearing loss.

All children should have impedence audiometry (tympanometry) performed, especially if free field tests of hearing are used as free field tests might not detect a slight conductive loss. Tympanometry however is not without problems, especially in very young children.

Free field speech discrimination tests are used with children under the age of 4 years. Older children will cooperate for more sophisticated tests of speech discrimination.

The greatest number of children with hearing impairment tested at outpatient clinics will have a conductive hearing loss usually due to otitis media with effusion. The management of these children is discussed in Chapter 7.

It is sometimes necessary to fit children with a conductive loss with hearing aids, particularly if there is a middle or outer ear problem not immediately amenable to surgical or medical treatment (Bergstrom, 1980). This is particularly suitable for children with Down's syndrome where otitis media with effusion is persistent and the ear canals are too small to allow ventilator insertion (Gibbin, 1988).

Children with sensorineural hearing impairments present much greater management problems. Modern techniques including evoked response audiometry, tympanometry and radiology make possible a reliable identification of sites of lesions and hearing thresholds (Parving, 1983, 1985). Accurate identification of hearing thresholds is particularly important when deciding which hearing aids to fit.

The investigation of the cause of deafness, while not having immediate implications with respect to the management of the child's hearing loss, is important. Parents want to know about the risk of subsequent children being born with a hearing loss, and also the risk to future generations. This investigation involves a multidisciplinary approach.

Serological investigations

Deafness due to rubella may be diagnosed from the history and also the presence of specific IgM or IgG antibodies, depending on the child's age. In the neonate rubella-specific IgM is diagnostic. By 6 months of age only 50% of babies have this marker and by 12 months almost all have lost it. It must not be forgotten that rubella antibody is present due to postnatal infection in 5–10% of children under the age of 4 years.

Serological tests for cytomegalovirus, toxoplasmosis and syphilis may be performed. Sutherland (1993) reviewed the usefulness of the TORCH screen (Toxoplasma gondii, rubella, cytomegalovirus, herpes simplex) and concluded that the tests most appropriate for investigation of congenital infection vary depending on the child's age.

Other laboratory tests

The urine of children under the age of 6 months may be examined for cytomegalovirus. Renal disease is sometimes associated with sensorineural deafness. It is therefore useful to screen the urine for blood cells, protein or sugar. Congenital hypothyroidism and Pendred's syndrome are associated with a hearing loss. Fisch (1981) pointed out that effective screening of neonates for congenital hypothyroidism could virtually eliminate this as a cause for deafness. A straightforward means of doing this would be to check the serum thyroxin, although this test is not done routinely in most centres. The simplest approach would be to use the Guthrie test and, if positive, proceed to test the T4 and thyroid stimulating hormone levels.

Radiology

Intracranial calcification is sometimes found in skull X-rays in children with toxoplasmosis. Tomography and CT scanning techniques have limited usefulness in the identification of the aetiology in sensorineural hearing loss but can help localize the lesion and demonstrate structural abnormalities. Lund, Phelps and Beagley (1982) found that a combination of evoked response audiometry and tomography of the ear were useful with reference to surgical reconstruction of the middle ear. With the advent of good CT scanning, tomography is rarely, if ever, indicated. High resolution CT scans are now used routinely to assess children who are being considered for cochlear implantation. It is also useful in children with progressive or fluctuating hearing loss if there is a suspicion of a perilymph fistula.

In some disorders, such as the rare Jervell and Lange-Nielsen syndrome, there are characteristic electrocardiograph findings with prolongation of the Q-T interval and abnormal T waves (Fisch, 1981). Beighton and Sellars (1982) pointed out that this investigation has only a very limited place in the assessment of deaf children.

Assessment by other specialties

Ophthalmological examination is essential in children with a sensorineural hearing loss. The fundal changes in rubella retinopathy are characteristic and can be described as 'pepper and salt' appearance. They may be located in the macular area or at the periphery of the fundus (Wolff, 1973). It is important to remember that the eye lesion may not be detectable by fundoscopy until the child is aged 6 years (Pappas, 1985) though it is possible to detect the lesions earlier by using electroretinography (Chan, 1994). Parving (1985) stated that combined serological and ophthalmological examination is necessary for the assessment of rubella deafness. Fisch (1981) summarized the ocular findings in Usher's, Cockayne's, Lawrence-Moon-Biedl and Refsum's syndromes.

An assessment of visual acuity may also be important when considering the educational management of the hearing impaired child.

The hearing impaired child may be referred for further assessment either to a paediatrician or a paediatric neurologist, especially if there is evidence of head and neck abnormalities or delayed growth and development in any sphere.

If the hearing loss is not obviously due to an environmental factor it should be assumed until proven otherwise that it has a genetic basis. These children and their parents should be referred to a medical geneticist, though all doctors dealing with these children should have a working knowledge of genetically transmitted deafness. This is further discussed in Chapter 3.

Chan (1994) summarized the essential investigations of a deaf child. These included thyroid function tests, fluorescent treponemal antibody (FTA) absorption test (for syphilis), urinalysis and tests for rubella and cytomegalovirus (either by obtaining a positive viral culture during the first week of life or by using serial IgG measurements). He suggested that a metabolic work up was not useful because the underlying disorders usually manifest clinically at an early stage. A CT scan is useful if the hearing loss is progressive, fluctuating or asymmetrical. Autoimmune screening is only useful if there is rapidly progressive hearing loss.

Parents' reaction to the diagnosis

Much has been written about the parents' response to the diagnosis (Boothroyd, 1982; Tucker and Nolan, 1984). The impact is usually devastating and the sequence of reactions is very like that found in mourning.

Shock

This is a natural defence mechanism which protects the individual from information which he does not want to hear. There is a profound sense of loss, in that the child is handicapped and therefore abnormal. There is very little point in giving detailed information to parents in this state. They cannot take any of it in. It is important that the parents are shown that there is a team of professional people available immediately

to help. In Belfast this is achieved by having a peripatetic teacher and a social worker for the deaf at the diagnostic clinic. Written information is also given to the parents to take home and read.

Denial

The protective effects of shock wear off. The parents question the diagnosis and produce 'evidence' that the child can hear. Some parents seek second, third or even fourth opinions, often taking the child to many different clinics in the hope that someone will say that the child's hearing is normal.

Anger

Parents sometimes ask why this disaster should have happened to them. Tucker and Nolan (1984) cited an example in which the mother blamed her husband for the child's hearing impairment. Some parents become hostile and bitter and their anger may be directed at the clinician. Patient support and willingness to listen often helps parents through this stage.

Acceptance and constructive action

Eventually the parents acknowlege the child's hearing loss and accept that the child, though handicapped, can and must be helped. This involves the parents learning about deafness and how it affects the child's development and education.

The author would agree with Tucker and Nolan's observation that parent adaptation does not always follow the predictable sequence of events as outlined above. Most parents do eventually adapt to the child's deafness. Some continue to deny the existence of the handicap and others remain angry and bitter.

Other parental responses are observed. Parents may have suspected for some time that the child is deaf and with the diagnosis comes a sense of relief that at last their suspicions are believed and action will be taken to help their child. There is also relief that the child is not brain damaged.

Parents of deaf children often feel isolated and inadequate. This can be lessened by immediate contact with counselling and supporting services who should provide ready access for help and information as required. Local parent support groups allow the parents of newly diagnosed children to discuss their problem with others who have been through the initial traumas. Branches of various organizations such as the Royal National Institute for Deaf People (RNID) and the National Deaf Children's Society have regular educational meetings for parents, and act as a forum for the exchange of information and ideas. The Belfast branches of the National Deaf Children's Society and the Royal National Institute for Deaf People have information racks in the waiting area of outpatient clinics and parents are encouraged to take leaflets from these.

Tucker and Nolan (1984) discussed the theory and practice of counselling and pointed out that the counsellor's professional background is unimportant. The essential in any person undertaking this task is that they be knowledgeable in all aspects pertaining to the child's management. Parents come into contact with many different professionals – otologists, audiological physicians, peripatetic teachers, audiological scientists, medical technical officers, social workers for the deaf, hearing therapists, speech therapists and educational psychologists. Each has expertise in some aspect of management of the hearing impaired child and often this expertise overlaps. It is important that each understands their role and also the role of the others. Snashall (1990) emphasized the need for a multidisciplinary team approach but regretted the presence of interprofessional jealousies and felt that these had detracted from the development of paediatric audiology services.

Parents must be given sufficient information which is intelligible and relevant. Enright and O'Connor (1982) emphasized the importance of peripatetic teacher counselling to families of preschool children. Good relationships between teachers and parents may contribute significantly towards making more effective the educational guidance provided and this relationship allows parents to exercise a central role in their child's progress. Parents, unfortunately, are often given conflicting advice, especially about forms of education whether oral or total communication. Some professionals have fixed ideas about which type of hearing aid is best and refuse to have anything to do with the others. More recently, there has been controversy about who should have cochlear implants and the best age for performing the procedure. Such conflicts should be avoided since they merely add to the parents' insecurity and may cause a lack of confidence in the professionals involved. The medical profession have, in general, a reputation for being abrupt and having little time to spare to discuss problems with parents. Tucker and Nolan pointed out that medical people are usually trained to an action-orientated approach and sometimes lack the skills in other essential areas such as information-giving and support.

There is a need for a clear team approach and there must be a flexible interchange of ideas and information. It is essential that the parents are seen as part of the team and management decisions are not made without consultation and explanation. Once the parents' confidence is lost it is difficult to regain. Having a deaf child causes enormous stress within the family and other children may feel that they are not getting as much attention. Sometimes one parent may feel neglected. Worries about the child's education are very real since there may not be a suitable local school. There is no doubt that having a deaf child throws a considerable financial burden on the family. These parents need good counselling and support throughout the child's development.

Concern has been expressed about interference with parent–child bonding, especially in neonates and young babies. Taylor (1985) emphasized the fine balance between the need for parental awareness when hearing loss is suspected and the fear of interference with bonding. He reported the results of a questionnaire sent out to families of hearing impaired children. About 20% of parents who replied would rather not have known about the child's hearing loss within the first week of life, the most common reason given was that parents would have preferred to establish a bond with their child before undertaking the task of managing a deaf child. Some parents felt that they would rather not know because they felt there was nothing could be done with the child at such an early age. There is clearly a need for improved awareness and better education of both parents and professionals if deafness is to be detected and managed early.

Subsequent management of the hearing impaired child

The mainstays of management of a child with sensorineural hearing loss are:

1 Appropriate hearing aid selection
2 Promotion of the development of language and communication skills and, if possible, speech development.

It is rare for a child to be born totally deaf and every attempt should be made to reach the residual hearing by the use of the high-powered hearing aids which are currently available. Commonly the only residual hearing is for low frequency sounds and hearing aids which extend the low frequency responses can be used. It is the hope of most professionals and parents that the child will develop intelligible speech, although there are those who feel that is is more important that the child should develop a language system and if this is by manual means then so much the better.

The establishment of the technique of cochlear implantation has revolutionized the management of the severely or profoundly hearing impaired child. This is discussed further in Chapter 11.

Hearing aids

Sensorineural hearing loss in children cannot be corrected to normal by any form of medical or surgical treatment. The role of the cochlear implant has been mentioned. Similarly some conductive losses due to congenital abnormalities of the external or middle ear are not suitable for surgical treatment. These children should also be considered for the fitting of hearing aids. A full discussion of hearing aids is to be found in Volume 2. The following is limited to the particular problems found with children.

Types of hearing aids

Hearing aids currently available are of two types, personal aids and aids not entirely worn on the listener (Tucker and Nolan, 1984).

Personal hearing aids

A variety of different personal hearing aids can be bought from several commercial firms. In the UK the National Health Service (NHS) supplies a wide range of such aids free of charge. It is, however, possible for an NHS consultant to prescribe certain aids outside this range if it is considered that there is no NHS aid sufficient to meet the child's needs. There are two groups of NHS aids, the body worn (BW) aids and the behind-the-ear (BE) aids (Figure 10.1).

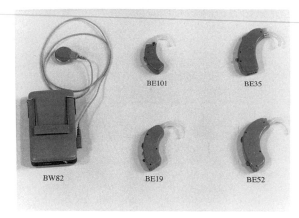

Figure 10.1 The range of NHS hearing aids

Body worn aids (BW)
  BW 61 (low/medium power)
  S 1594 (which replaced BW 81, high power)
Behind-the-ear aids (BE)
  BE 10 series (low power)
  BE 30 series (medium power)
  BE 50 series (high power)

The range of aids is such that a suitable aid can be found to fit most children's requirements. However, it must not be forgotten that the NHS range has been designed chiefly for adults, the powerful behind-the-ear aids are too big for most small children's ears. In-the-ear or conchal hearing aids are not currently available routinely through the NHS, but can be prescribed if appropriate. It is the author's feeling that, because of budgetary constraints, they should be reserved at present for children who cannot wear either body worn or postaural hearing aids, in other

words children with deformities of the pinna. It is hoped that they will become more widely available through the health service within the next few years. It must be remembered that they are not suitable for children with severe to profound losses.

Bone conduction hearing aids are available for children with deformed external ears or severe, recurrent ear infections which prohibit the insertion of ear moulds. The bone conductor can be used in conjunction with the conventional body worn aid, though a better cosmetic result is achieved by using a postaural hearing aid on a head band with an output receiver wired to the bone conductor (Figure 10.2).

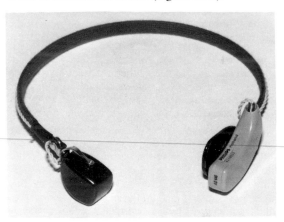

Figure 10.2 A bone conductor aid

The introduction of bone anchored hearing aids (Chapter 9) has revolutionized the management of these children. These hearing aids, however, are not suitable for children who are very young and whose skull bones are not sufficiently thick to accept the osseointegrated screw.

Aids not entirely worn by the listener

The greatest disadvantage of conventional hearing aids is their inability to distinguish between speech sounds and the unwanted background noise which tends to mask speech. This is referred to as the signal-to-noise ratio of the system. The problem is made worse by reverberation due to sound reflections off walls, ceilings, floor and furnishings and will cause the relatively strong vowel sounds to persist and mask the weaker consonants, which contain most of the information in speech (John, 1957).

With most hearing aids the signal-to-noise ratio is a function of the distance between the sound source and the listener. Classrooms tend to be very noisy so that children seated away from the teacher will be at a disadvantage in that the background noise will mask the teacher's voice. This problem can be overcome by either improving the environmental conditions or by using aids primarily supplied by Education Authorities.

Speech trainer

The child wears headphones connected to an amplifier. Controls on the amplifier allow adjustment of gain and frequency response. The teacher or parent uses a microphone connected directly to the amplifier. This useful device has a low signal-to-noise ratio since the microphone is close to the speaker's mouth. In addition, since feedback is reduced because of the distance between microphone and headphones, it is possible to achieve high levels of amplification with profoundly deaf children. It is most useful for short periods of intensive speech and language teaching.

Group hearing aid

The principle is very similar to that of the speech trainer except that several children are connected to one teacher and to each other. Each child's 'station' has an amplifier which allows individual adjustment of output and frequency response. Tucker and Nolan (1984) described this system's benefits and drawbacks, the chief of which is lack of mobility for both children and teacher.

Radio hearing aids

Frequency modulated (FM) radio systems allow the child to be fully mobile within a fairly large area while retaining the good signal-to-noise ratio of group aids. The teacher or parent wears a microphone transmitter and the child a receiver so that no matter where the child is in a room the person using the microphone will seem to be speaking almost directly into the child's ears.

There are two types of radio aid (Nolan, 1983a):

1 The body worn receiver/hearing aid. This can be used either as an ordinary body worn aid or as an FM system.
2 The audio-input system, used in conjunction with the child's personal hearing aids. This type of FM system can be plugged into the child's personal body worn or behind-the-ear aids as required. The advantage of this system is that the child need only wear one set of aids and does not have to change between the body worn receiver/aid and personal aids.

The chief drawback of both types of FM system is that only the teacher has a radio transmitter and therefore interaction between pupils is limited. In the UK one third of these radio aids are supplied by charitable sources or paid for by parents (McCormick, Bamford and Martin, 1986). The NHS has no policy of central provision for radio aids though a departmental circular (C331) does allow an otologist or audiological physician to supply these aids if money is available locally within the health system.

Infrared hearing aid systems

The FM radio signals from the teacher's transmitter pass easily through walls and doors into adjacent areas. This gives rise to problems if children in a nearby classroom are using a system on the same frequency. The infrared system overcomes this difficulty since the infrared waves are contained by the boundaries of any room in which the system is used. Problems do occur in bright sunlight which can produce noise in the system.

Loop system

Input from the teacher's microphone is amplified and transmitted either directly around an electromagnetic loop installed on the classroom walls, or by means of an FM system to a loop worn around the child's neck. Tucker and Nolan (1984) listed the drawbacks of the loop system, including spill-over into adjacent classrooms, unpredictable frequency response and weak or dead spots with the classroom loop. These authors pointed out that most of the drawbacks are eliminated by using the personal neck loop with an FM receiver.

Problems with hearing aid selection in children

There are two main areas of difficulty with hearing aid fitting because:

1 There is often limited information about the extent of the child's hearing loss
2 Young children cannot say which aid, or settings on the aid, they prefer.

Young children present particular problems in respect of information about the hearing loss. Standard free field distraction test stimuli give a reasonable estimate of thresholds at different frequencies. These stimuli can be supplemented by using warble tones or narrow band noise. Information about children too young for distraction testing can be obtained by evoked response audiometry, though it is usually difficult to get measurements of low frequency thresholds by this technique.

It is important to estimate the dynamic range of residual hearing. This is the difference between threshold and loudness discomfort level. If the child receives frequency aided stimulation greater than the loudness discomfort level, there is a risk that the aids might be rejected. One means of estimating loudness discomfort level is to examine the stapedial reflex, though in many cases this is not present because of the severity of the deafness. Tucker and Nolan (1984) described an electroacoustical method of estimating loudness discomfort using an earmould receiver and watching the child's responses to increasing stimulation at different frequencies.

Most profoundly deaf children do have some residual hearing, usually for the low frequencies. In the newly diagnosed child there is no way of predicting how useful this will be, if at all, in helping speech discrimination. Every effort, however, must be made to use this residual hearing in an attempt to obtain communication. Rees and Velmans (1993) described how frequency transposition hearing aids greatly enhanced the auditory discrimination of consonants in a group of deaf children they studied. Frequency transposition takes the information from the consonant end of the speech spectrum and transposes it to the low frequency vowel end. These hearing aids, however, tend to be very expensive and their value has not yet been conclusively demonstrated.

Having obtained as much information as possible about the child's hearing it is then essential to select appropriate aids and to adjust their output and frequency responses as necessary to suit the child's needs. As with adults there are two main ways of choosing an aid.

The empirical (selective) method

The child is given several different aids in turn for trial. The problem with this method is that young children cannot say which aid is best. It is possible, by carrying out free field tests, including speech if the child is old enough, to gain a partly subjective impression of the relative merits of each aid.

The theoretical (prescriptive) method

Information about various parameters such as the child's thresholds at each frequency, most comfortable listening level and speech discrimination scores allows a prediction of best amplification characteristics for that child. This permits a suitable hearing aid to be chosen. Many different formulae are available which calculate theoretical settings for the frequency response and gain of the aids. It must not be forgotten that the hearing aid performance in a test box with a 2 cc coupler is not an accurate reflection of the aid's performance in the human ear. Modifications to the frequency response occur due to variations in earmould parameters and the resonance effect of the ear canal.

Considerable interest has been focused on the use of insertion gain measurements in young children as a means of predicting the help from hearing aid fitting. Concern was expressed about the reliability of such methods in children but Westwood and Bamford (1992) published work that suggested that probe tube microphone measurements were feasible, repeatable and reliable in infants. Snik and Hymbergen (1993) used insertion gain technology to evaluate prescriptive rules for fitting hearing aids to children and decided that the prescriptive rule they studied

(the half gain rule) was suitable. They emphasized, however, that such rules must be used together with structured audiolgical evaluations by experienced staff.

As the child becomes older the hearing aids, or the settings of the controls, may need to be changed as more information about the child's hearing becomes available. There are also children, particularly those with hereditary deafness, in whom the hearing may deteriorate.

Hearing aids are usually fitted to each ear, except when low and middle frequency hearing are normal or only slightly impaired when a unilateral aid, perhaps with vented mould is suitable. Amplification of these frequencies may introduce distortion of the perceived speech signal.

There are many advantages to binaural fitting:

1 Improved localization of the sound source
2 Improved hearing in background noise
3 A binaural summation effect giving better amplification.

Green (1988) provided a useful summary of the process of hearing aid selection and evaluation for preschool children:

- The hearing impairment disability should be measured
- Specification of the aerodynamic and electroacoustic characteristics required to provide optimum benefit to the particular child need to be assessed
- A hearing aid is selected with the required characteristics
- The performance of the hearing aid when worn by the child is evaluated
- There must be modifications of the selected hearing aid, if necessary, to bring the achieved performance in line with the required performance.

There has been some controversy over the relative merits of behind-the-ear or body worn aids. The power outputs of both are equivalent. It is generally agreed that behind-the-ear aids give a more natural sound environment because sound reception is at ear level, in addition, they are free of clothes rub, give improved localization over the body worn aids and are cosmetically more acceptable. It has been argued that they are more easily removed and thrown away by young children. This can be avoided by taping the aid to the back of the ear, by using double-sided sticky tape or by using a commercially available rubber ring which fits around the ear. Children with a body worn aid can pull the cord and displace the receiver from the ear, though this can be minimized by feeding the cord around the child's back and through a harness up to the ear. The body baffle effect with body worn aids improves the frequency response below 600 Hz by 5 dB (Wald, 1976). This may be useful in children with low frequency hearing only, but can be a disadvantage in a child with a flat loss. In these children, the masking effects of the powerful low frequency vowel sounds on the weaker consonants would be enhanced by the body baffle effect.

The most significant limitation of all types of powerful hearing aids is acoustic feedback (Nolan, 1983b). This is most likely to occur when the microphone of the hearing aid is close to the receiver or ear mould. Body worn aids are therefore less susceptible to this problem since they are worn on the chest. Good fitting ear moulds are essential if powerful behind-the-ear aids are to be used (Nolan, 1988). The impression should be obtained by the syringe technique after putting a small sponge tamp into the child's external ear. Children need to have ear moulds made at regular intervals as the external auditory canal grows.

It is important that the parents check the child's hearing aid daily and this is most easily carried out using a Stetaclip (Figure 10.3). The hearing aid is attached by hollow plastic tubing (behind-the-ear aid) or by plugging the receiver into the Stetaclip (body worn aid). This allows detection of a failed battery and other faults in the hearing aid, though it is admittedly a fairly crude check. Many schools and peripatetic teachers of the deaf have access to a hearing aid test box which will allow accurate assessment of the hearing aid function.

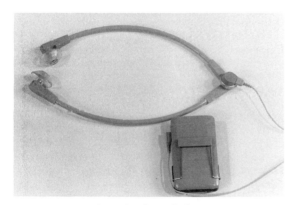

Figure 10.3 Stetaclip with aid attached

Cochlear implants

Cochlear implantation in children is now an established technique in the UK, although there has been some concern expressed by organizations involved with deaf children and adults. The subject is discussed in Chapter 11.

The education of hearing impaired children

The ideal outcome is a child with good speech who can progress normally through the education system and integrate fully into a society which communicates mainly by the oral–aural channel. In the author's experience this is possible even with profoundly deaf children, though with this group it is the exception rather than the rule. The advent of cochlear implants for deaf children may well change this. It is important also to be aware of the sensitivities of the 'deaf community' who do not see oral speech as an essential to be aimed at. Conrad (1980) investigated the reading, lipreading, speech intelligibility and 'inner speech' in a large group of 15–16 year olds with either partial or severe hearing loss. He found that between 50% of children with a severe hearing loss and 25% of the partially hearing had no reading comprehension at all. In addition, the severely deaf had poor lipreading ability, poor speech and poor 'inner speech'.

A survey of children in the European community with an average loss of greater than 50 dB showed that more than half of children were unable to carry on a meaningful conversation with a stranger (Martin, 1982).

A child's ability to acquire normal, or intelligible speech depends on several factors:

1 The extent of the hearing loss. This must take into account the pattern of the hearing loss, whether it is flat or ski-slope shaped
2 The child's ability to use the residual hearing. In some cases the residual hearing, even with amplification, is insufficient for speech discrimination
3 The time of onset of the hearing loss, whether present at birth or developing later in childhood
4 The child's personality and motivation
5 The child's intelligence
6 Sufficient exposure to communication systems, especially speech. This requires considerable motivation on the part of the parents. It also includes the early fitting of hearing aids and perhaps cochlear implantation.

Galloway *et al.* (1990) looked at some of the linguistic characteristics of a population of hearing impaired children in Manchester. They found that, although the degree of heterogeneity in hearing impaired children made the study difficult to perform, there were nonetheless important influencing factors which determined how good the child's speech might be; the most important being the degree of hearing loss, age, intelligence and sex. Females on average were better than males.

Preschool children

Enright and O'Connor (1982) examined the role of the peripatetic teachers of the deaf in preschool education of hearing impaired children. A major part of the task involves giving information, support and encouragement to parents, in addition to teaching language skills to the child. Parents are shown how to develop these skills and how best to use the child's residual hearing.

Kernohan, Lucas and Muter (1981) listed the information which should be given to parents:

1 An explanation of the child's hearing loss with special reference to the frequencies involved
2 The differences between vowels and consonants and the importance of each to speech
3 The effects of amplification on speech and which parts of speech the child is likely to receive
4 The effects of background noise
5 How to look after the hearing aids
6 The importance of talking normally to the child.

Most of the information in speech is contained in transitions between phonemes, speech rhythm and with intonation patterns. In the hearing impaired child this information is vital and is lost if the child is spoken to in an artificial or exaggerated manner.

School age children

At present hearing impaired children may be placed in one of several types of school situation:

1 Ordinary classrooms, using hearing aids
2 Ordinary classrooms, with hearing aids and regular help from peripatetic teachers of the deaf
3 Ordinary classrooms for part of the day, the remainder of the time being spent in an attached partial hearing unit
4 A partial hearing unit only, staffed by specialist teachers of the deaf
5 A school for the profoundly deaf
6 Other schools, such as speech and language units and schools for children with additional handicaps.

There is a move towards integration of children with hearing loss into ordinary schools and although this may have many admirable features, the author is worried that some children with hearing impairments struggle to keep up. Markides (1989) investigated the use of individual hearing aids by hearing impaired children in a number of settings and found that hearing impaired children in ordinary schools used hearing aids poorly in comparison with children in schools for the hearing impaired or deaf. He felt there were two reasons for this. First, ordinary classrooms are much noisier than the classrooms found in schools for hearing impaired children and second, the resident teacher of the deaf had insufficient time to monitor hearing aid usage in children in ordinary schools.

Legislation

The Education Act 1976 amended the 1944 Act and required Local Education Authorities to make provision for the education of handicapped pupils in ordinary county and voluntary schools as well as in special schools. The trend towards integration was further encouraged by a report (Warnock Report) from the Department of Education and Science (1978). This provided an overview of the then existing provisions and made proposals for future policy. It highlighted the importance of parental involvement in the general management of the hearing impaired child, especially in the preschool years.

The Education Act (1981) is largely based on the proposals of the Warnock Report. The Act abolished the use of existing categories of handicap (educationally subnormal, maladjusted, partially hearing and deaf) and replaced them with a 'statement'. A statement is produced for each affected child and details the child's needs. It also lists the facilities and resources, including the school placement, necessary to meet these needs. The statement is prepared from evidence submitted by the various people in contact with the child, including the parents, teachers of the deaf, educational psychologists, clinical medical officers, otologists and audiological physicians.

The Act encouraged the trend towards integration of the handicapped into ordinary schools.

The 1981 Act has been criticized by many. It introduces complex referral, assessment and appeal procedures which increase administrative time and costs. With resources already stretched, this reduces the amount of time spent on educating these children (Reeves, 1983). There is also no doubt in the author's mind that statements produced sometimes reflect what is available rather than attempting to meet the child's needs.

The Education Act (1993) and the accompanying Code of Practice set out the responsibilities of schools, local education authorities (LEAs), NHS and Social Services in relation to children with special educational needs. Children about to leave school should have a transition plan using information from relevant professionals, including the careers service.

Communication methods in the education of deaf children

Arguments about which method of education is best for hearing impaired children have been going on for years. Llewellyn-Jones (1986) gave a brief account of the history. In the early 1800s the predominant method of communication was a combined system using speech, finger spelling and signing simultaneously. By the 1870s oralism was being increasingly used in Europe and at the International Congress in the Education of the Deaf in Milan in 1880 oralism was endorsed as a method of choice. In Britain in 1889 a Royal Commission recommended that a child should have the full opportunity of being educated in the oral system. The move towards oralism in schools was resisted by the British Deaf and Dumb Association (now the British Deaf Association) who fought to retain the combined systems.

The Lewis Report in 1968 found that, although British schools claimed to prefer oralism, over three-quarters of them used some form of signs or manual communication. As a result of this report some schools in the late 1960s and early 1970s began to use a variety of sign systems as educational aids. This move towards combined systems continued.

Figures published by the National Deaf Children's Society show that in the UK 47% of special schools and 13% of partial hearing units now nominally use combined speech and signing systems.

Auralism

Children educated in this system use only speech and lipreading as a means of communication. Signing of any sort is strongly discouraged or even prevented. Listening and speaking require considerable effort and concentration by the severely hearing impaired child, signing is much easier. Oralists argue that the ability of the child to develop speech is inhibited if the child is allowed to communicate by signing. The normal hearing child is thought to understand a significant amount of language by about the age of 12 months and 80% of this language development is acquired by 3 years. Oralism assumes that the brain of the hearing impaired child remains capable of learning speech and language to at least puberty, and perhaps beyond (Lenneberg, 1967).

Many others subscribe to the view that there is a 'critical period' for most children during the first few years of life during this language development. If these children are not taught communication skills within this period they may never acquire it. The National Aural Group (NAG) was set up in 1980 to promote natural oralism/auralism.

Finger spelling

This, on its own is a slow means of communication.

Cued speech

Some speech sounds M, P, B or K, D, L, cannot be distinguished by lipreading alone. Cued speech uses eight different hand shapes in four different positions close to the speaker's mouth to enable the child to discriminate the lip movement. It was developed as an aid to teaching English to deaf children, and not as an exclusive signing system.

Signing systems (manualism)

British sign language

This is the communication system favoured by most profoundly deaf adults. It is a completely separate language with its own vocabulary, syntax and grammar. It has no written form. Most signs do not come from English words nor can they be readily translated in a one-to-one fashion.

Signed English

True (exact) signed English uses signs taken from British sign language and is the representation, with sign, of every facet of spoken English. All the vocabulary, gender, plurals, tenses etc. are present.

Another more popular version, sign supported English, uses signing in English word order, but with fewer signs, together with speech.

Paget-Gorman sign system

This was developed as a means of accurately reflecting spoken and written English. It has a large vocabulary of invented signs with provision for indicating grammatical structures such as word endings and tenses. It is rarely used in schools for the deaf.

Maketon

This signing system, based largely on gestures and simple signs, is used with some children with learning difficulty.

Total communication

Total communication is the use of any and all modes of communication and involves using a combination of speech, gestures, formal signing, finger spelling, speech reading (lipreading), reading and writing. Conrad (1980) postulated that, in very deaf children, exclusive use of spoken language fails to provide sufficient linguistic stimulation to the child's brain, parts of which may then undergo functional and perhaps even physical atrophy.

Supporters of total communication argue that providing sensory input through different channels, auditory and visual, enhances the possibility of language development. This must be understood as being language in its widest sense, since language may be thought of as a system of symbols and rules for communication.

Speech is one mode of language. It has been argued that total communication impairs speech development. Taylor (1985), in a survey of different schools, produced evidence that oral-only schools are more likely to succeed in developing the most normal speech aspects of language. Nix (1983) reviewed various studies of communication systems and suggested that simultaneous oral/manual communication is beneficial, but that stimulation of the two channels together did not produce such good results as oralism alone. On the other hand, Dee, Rapin and Ruben (1982) demonstrated that total communication facilitated speech development and did not inhibit it.

There are problems comparing results claimed for oralism and total communication. It is often difficult to know which parameters are being assessed, since intelligible speech is not always a measure of language development. There is no standardization of teaching practice. In many schools total communication is not total, but sacrifices speech in the interests of signing. One of the difficulties encountered with total communication is that total synchrony of speech and signing is impossible. It is difficult to sign quickly enough so as not to interrupt normal speech flow. Normal speech patterns contain information which is highly redundant to the normal hearing person, but essential to those with a hearing loss.

Total communication aims not only to stimulate language development, but also to provide a reliable system by which the child can communicate with teachers, parents, classmates and an increasing number of the population who are learning to sign. The child is hopefully 'bilingual' and has a flexible means of communication for use in different situations.

Arnold (1982), in a reply to Conrad's paper, pointed out that there was no evidence that any approach yet devised has successfully been used to educate the majority of severely deaf children.

Recent legislation gives parents a central role in the education of their hearing impaired child. Parents must therefore be given a balanced and informed view of the different communication methods available. Professionals must not force their opinions on parents.

There are many problems in the management of the deaf child. There is a need for more information about the extent of the child's hearing loss and the implications of this for the selection of suitable amplification. It is obvious that no single type of education system meets the needs of all deaf children, but the decision about which type is best for a particular child remains a problem. It is clear, however, that the early identification and an enthusiastic approach to management will considerably improve the child's future.

References

ARNOLD, P. (1982) Oralism and the deaf child's brain: a reply to Dr Conrad. *International Journal of Pediatric Otorhinolaryngology*, **4**, 275–286

BEIGHTON, P. and SELLARS, S. (1982) Inherited deafness – diagnostic evaluation, screening and genetic management. In: *Genetics and Otology*. Edinburgh: Churchill Livingstone. pp. 98–104

BERGSTROM, L. (1980) Continuing management of conductive hearing loss during language development. *International Journal of Pediatric Otorhinolaryngology*, **2**, 3–9

BOOTHROYD, A. (1982) *Hearing Impairments in Young Children*. Englewood Cliffs: Prentice Hall

CHAN, K. H. (1994) Sensorineural hearing loss in children classification and evaluation. *Otolaryngological Clinics of North America*, **27**, 473–486

CONRAD, R. (1980) Let the children choose. *International Journal of Pediatric Otorhinolaryngology*, **1**, 317–329

DEE, A., RAPIN, I. and RUBEN, R. J. (1982) Speech and language development in a parent-infant total communication programme. *Annals of Ctology, Rhinology and Laryngology*, **91**, (suppl. 97), 62–72

DEPARTMENT OF EDUCATION AND SCIENCE (1978) *Special Educational Needs. Report of the Committee of Enquiry into the Education of Handicapped Children and Young People (Warnock Report)*. London: HMSO

ENRIGHT, F. P. and O'CONNOR, D. J. (1982) A profile of counselling skills applied in the pre-school setting by peripatetic teachers of the deaf. *Journal of the British Association of Teachers of the Deaf*, **6**, 94–100

EWING, I. R. (1957) Screening tests and guidance clinics for babies and young children. In: *Educational Guidance and the Deaf Child*, edited by A. W. G. Ewing. Manchester: Manchester University Press. pp. 21–43

FISCH, L. (1981) Syndromes associated with hearing loss. In: *Audiology and Audiological Medicine*, vol. II, edited by H. Beagley. Oxford: Oxford University Press. pp. 595–639

FISCH, L. (1983) Integrated development and maturation of the hearing system. A critical review article. *British Journal of Audiology*, **17**, 137–154

GALLOWAY, C., APLIN, D. Y., NEWTON, V. E. and HOSTLER, M. E. (1990) The GMC project: some linguistic and cognitive characteristics of a population of hearing impaired children. *British Journal of Audiology*, **24**, 17–27

GIBBIN, K. P. (1988) Otological considerations in the first five years of life. In: *Paediatric Audiology 0–5 years*, edited by B. McCormick. London: Whurr. pp. 37–68

GLEASON, J. B. (1988) Otitis media with effusion and the development of language. In: *Proceedings of the Third International Symposium: Recent Advances in Otitis Media*, edited by D. J. Lim, C. D. Bluestone, J. O. Klein and J. D. Nelson. Philadelphia: Decker. pp. 373–376

GREEN, R. (1988) Hearing aid selection and evaluation for pre-school children. In: *Paediatric Audiology 0–5 years*, edited by B. McCormick. London: Whurr. pp. 303–325

HAGGARD, M. P. (1993) *Research in the Development of Effective Services for Hearing Impaired People*. London: Nuffield Provincial Hospital's Trust

HAGGARD, M. P. and HUGHES, E. A. (1991) *Screening Children's Hearing*. London: HMSO

HAGGARD, M. P. and PULLAN, C. R. (1989) Staffing and structure for paediatric audiology services in hospital and community units. *British Journal of Audiology*, **23**, 99–116

HAMILTON, P. (1972) Language and reading skills in children with impaired hearing in ordinary schools. *MSc Thesis*. Manchester: University of Manchester

JOHN, J. E. J. (1957) Acoustics in the use of hearing aids. In: *Educational Guidance and the Deaf Child*, edited by A. W. G. Ewing. Manchester: Manchester University Press. pp. 160–175

KERNOHAN, G., LUCAS, G. and MUTER, V. (1981) Education of the hearing-handicapped child. In: *Audiology and Audiologi-*

cal Medicine, vol. II, edited by H. Beagley. Oxford: Oxford University Press. pp. 663–684

LENNEBERG, E. H. (1967) *Biological Foundations of Language*. New York: Wiley

LEVITON, A. (1980) Otitis media and learning disorders. *Journal of Developmental and Behavioural Paediatrics*, **1**, 58–63

LLEWELLYN-JONES, P. (1986) *A Language for Ben. Early Communication – a Parent's Choice*. London: Tyne Tees Television

LUND, V. J., PHELPS, P. D. and BEAGLEY, H. A. (1982) Evoked response audiometry and tomography – complementary procedures for the assessment of the deaf infant. *International Journal of Pediatric Otorhinolaryngology*, **4**, 95–106

MCCLELLAND, R. J., WATSON, D. R., LAWLESS, V., HOUSTON, H. G. and ADAMS, D. A. (1992) Reliability and effectiveness of screening for hearing loss in high risk neonates. *British Medical Journal*, **304**, 806–809

MCCORMICK, B. (1988) *Screening for Hearing Impairment in Young Children*. London: Chapman and Hall

MCCORMICK, B., BAMFORD, J. and MARTIN, M. (1986) *The Provision of Radio Hearing Aids for Children*. London: RNID

MARKIDES, A. (1986) Age at fitting hearing aids and speech intelligibility. *British Journal of Audiology*, **20**, 165–168

MARKIDES, A. (1989) The use of individual hearing aids by hearing impaired children: a long-term survey 1977–1981. *British Journal of Audiology*, **23**, 123–132

MARTIN, J. A. M. (1982) Diagnosis and communicative ability in deaf children in the European community. *Audiology*, **21**, 185–196

NIX, G. W. (1983) How total is total communication? *Journal of the British Association of Teachers of the Deaf*, **7**, 177–181

NOLAN, M. (1983a) Radio hearing aid systems. *Journal of the British Association of Teachers of the Deaf*, **7**, 105–121

NOLAN, M. (1983b) Acoustic feedback – causes and cures. *Journal of the British Association of Teachers of the Deaf*, **7**, 13–17

NOLAN, M. (1988) Earmoulds. In: *Paediatric Audiology 0–5 years*, edited by B. McCormick. London: Whurr. pp. 325–347

PAPPAS, D. G. (1985) *Diagnosis and Treatment of Hearing Impairment in Children. A Clinical Manual*. London: Taylor and Francis

PARVING, A. (1983) Aetiological diagnosis in the hearing impaired child – clinical value and application of a modern examination programme. *International Journal of Pediatric Otorhinolaryngology*, **5**, 159–165

PARVING, A. (1984) Early detection and identification of congenital/early acquired hearing disability. Who takes the initiative? *International Journal of Pediatric Otorhinolaryngology*, **7**, 107–117

PARVING, A. (1985) Hearing disorders in childhood, some procedures for detection, identification and diagnosis evaulation. *International Journal of Pediatric Otorhinolaryngology*, **9**, 31–57

RAMKALAWAN, T. W. and DAVIS, A. C. (1992) The effects of hearing loss and age of intervention on some language metrics in young hearing impaired children. *British Journal of Audiology*, **26**, 97–108

REES, R. and VELMANS, M. (1993) The effects of frequency transposition on the untrained auditory discrimination of congenitally deaf children. *British Journal of Audiology*, **27**, 53–60

REEVES, K. (1983) The Education Act, 1981. The influence of government and legislation on the education of the hearing impaired. *Journal of the British Association of Teachers of the Deaf*, **7**, 170–197

SNASHALL, S. (1990) Paediatric audiological medicine: policy and perspectives. *British Journal of Audiology*, **24**, 289–291

SNIK, A. F. M. and HAMBERGEN, G. C. H. J. (1993) Hearing aid fitting of pre-school and primary school children: an evaluation using the insertion gain. *Scandinavian Audiology*, **22**, 245–250

SUTHERLAND, S. (1993) A reassessment of TORCH screening. *Journal of Audiological Medicine*, **2**, 64–74

TAYLOR, I. G. (1985) Hearing impaired babies and methods of communication. *Ear and Hearing*, **6**, 25–28

TEELE, D. W., KLEIN, J. O. and ROSNER, B. A. (1984) Otitis media with effusion during the first years of life and development of speech and language. *Paediatrics*, **74**, 282–287

TUCKER, I. and NOLAN, N. (1984) *Educational Audiology*. Beckenham: Croom Helm

VENTRY, I. M. (1980) Effects of conductive hearing loss: fact or fiction. *Journal of Speech and Hearing Disorders*, **45**, 143–156

WALD, Z. J. (1976) The coupler measurement of hearing aid gain – some reservations: *MSc Thesis*. Manchester: University of Manchester

WATKINS, P. M., BALDWIN, M. and LAOIDE, S. (1990) Parental suspicion and identification of hearing impairment. *Archives of Disease in Childhood*, **65**, 846–850

WESTWOOD, G. F. S. and BAMFORD, J. S. (1992) Probe tube measurements with very young infants. *British Journal of Audiology*, **26**, 143–151

WOLFF, S. M. (1973) The ocular manifestations of congenital rubella. *Journal of Pediatric Ophthalmology*, **10**, 101–141

11

Cochlear implantation in children

Kevin P. Gibbin

> When I was an ordinary boy I changed my hearing because at first I could hear but now my hearing has stopped working so I changed from an ordinary boy into a deaf boy. But now my hearing has started to work because I have got my implant so I can hear lots of things but I have still changed because my hearing aid still doesn't make me into an ordinary boy because I am still deaf and I can't hear without my implant. DB

Cochlear implantation has now become established as a means of treating profound deafness both in adults and in children. While there are many similarities between the needs of children and adults there are many differences in the requirements for treating children, relating particularly to their habilitation and rehabilitation needs.

Profound deafness in an adult can have disastrous consequences; in children it can be catastrophic whether congenital in origin or acquired, the latter most commonly due to meningitis. In acquired deafness speech and language development may be arrested, reversed or even lost; in cases of congenital profound sensorineural hearing loss a child may fail to develop any spoken language and will be denied access to the world of the hearing even with the most powerful conventional hearing aids. It is in these cases, both congenital and acquired, that cochlear implantation may be considered.

Types of cochlear implant

Broadly speaking there are two main types of cochlear implant: *intracochlear* ones in which the stimulating electrodes are implanted within the lumen of the cochlea in the scala tympani and which are typically multichannel; and the *extracochlear* device, typically single channel, in which the active electrode is implanted in the region of the round window. In addi-

tion to the stimulating electrode(s), there are several other components to an implant system including the receiving microphone, the signal processor and a means of transmitting the signal from the processor to the implanted receiver/electrode package.

In adults and in children most experience has been gained using the multichannel intracochlear device produced by the Nucleus Corporation of Australia, commonly known as the Nucleus device. Much of this chapter will reflect the use of this particular implant system which has been fitted to over 500 children in Europe alone. The Nucleus device was approved for use in children by the United States Food and Drug Administration in June 1990 (Staller, 1991).

In brief the Nucleus cochlear implant comprises a receiver/electrode package which is implanted in the postaural region, the electrode array being led through a posterior tympanotomy for implantation into the cochlea. One of two routes into the cochlea may be used, either through the round window membrane or via a separate cochleostomy on the promontory.

The external components of the implant comprise the receiving microphone worn over the ear which is in turn connected to the speech processor, a body-worn device rather like a body-worn hearing aid. From the speech processor a connecting lead passes to a small transmitter coil held magnetically over the implant package and which transmits an electromagnetic signal to the implanted receiver. The Nucleus device is fully described by Patrick and Clark (1991).

In addition to the Nucleus device many other systems are available, both multichannel and single channel; the former include the Ineraid system, the LAURA system from Belgium, the French MXM Digisonic system and the Clarion device from the American company Mini Med Technologies (Schindler and Kessler, 1992). Single channel devices include the UCH/RNID device developed at University College Hospital, London, the MXM Monosonic and the MED-EL system from Austria.

Background to cochlear implantation in children

Cochlear implantation is a relatively new method of treatment following seminal work by House (1976), Simmons (1966), Michelson (1971) and others. In the 1970s cochlear implantation achieved prominence in the media in various countries, but it was not until the 1980s that implants were used in children. The House Ear Institute started its children's programme in the summer of 1980 and by 1983 had carried out 63 operations. At the same stage in France 15 teenagers and five children under the age of 12 years had received implants, while in Australia Dr Richard Dowell had stated that children were not being implanted. During a panel discussion at the same conference, the 10th Anniversary Conference on Cochlear Implants: An International Symposium (Schindler, 1984), doubts were raised about the use of cochlear implants in deaf children.

By 1985 cochlear implantation had come to be recognized as a method of treating profound deafness in children (Berliner, Eisenberg and House, 1985; Simmons, 1985), although the dilemmas were being recognized.

The first child to undergo cochlear implantation in the UK received his implant in 1987 (Booth *et al.*, 1989); the child, a patient of the author, sustained a minor head injury with a brief period of loss of consciousness in 1986. It was only after considerable debate that he received a single channel UCH/RNID implant (McCormick, 1991). The second child in the UK to undergo this treatment was also a Nottingham child who had meningitis at the age of 2 years and 8 months; he subsequently received a Nucleus multichannel device in 1989.

During this period in the UK there was much debate about the propriety of carrying out paediatric cochlear implantation, with great caution being urged by the National Deaf Children's Society. At a conference in 1989 many of these issues were discussed by Graham (1990) who concluded, first that children under the age of 2 years should not be implanted and that there should be an upper age limit, say 6 or 7, for implanting prelingually deaf children. Secondly, there should be an adequate period of conventional acoustic amplification and thirdly, that an extracochlear device should be used in order to avoid possible damage to the cochlea.

The psychosocial implications of cochlear implants in children have been discussed by Evans (1989) and by Kessler and Owens (1989). Evans raised the question of informed consent for paediatric procedures

and noted that in the USA the age of consent for surgical treatment varies from state to state. In the UK the age of consent for surgery is 16 years. However, the majority of children likely to benefit from cochlear implantation will be found in the first 5 years of life and therefore the onus rests on the parents to give consent – *informed* consent. Evans recognized the need for a strong family support system, echoing the thoughts of many others (Tiber, 1985; Downs *et al.*, 1986; Boothroyd, 1987; Nienhuys *et al.*, 1987).

Another concern raised by Evans was the conspicuousness of the external components of the system which might result in feelings of difference and isolation, especially in adolescents.

Kessler and Owens (1989) raised other issues including emotional and psychological considerations and the need for proper counselling. Much of their advice remains true today. Other factors they discussed included the age of onset of the deafness and parental hearing, stressing that different considerations apply in the case of children of deaf parents compared with those of hearing ones. Much of the emotion aroused in considering cochlear implantation in children has centred on the wishes of deaf parents who wish their child to be part of the deaf community. They also considered that the outlook for congenitally deaf children appeared to be rather discouraging in the light of work by Ruben (1986), who felt that the critical period for speech perception ranges from birth to the twelfth through the eighteenth month postnatally. Modern experience has now shown that this is not the case. This will be discussed later, although it appears that congenitally deafened teenagers do less well, with a low patient satisfaction rate and a high non-user rate (O'Donoghue, 1992).

It is now clear that cochlear implantation can be of benefit to congenitally deaf children as well as those with acquired hearing loss but that special considerations apply in all children (Gibbin, 1992). This raises the issue of the need for a special paediatric implant programme with a team of professionals familiar with all aspects of paediatric otology and audiology and including teachers of the deaf, medical physicists and paediatric speech and language therapists.

The paediatric cochlear implant team

It is evident that the paediatric cochlear implant team requires one or more surgeons skilled in paediatric otology, but it is also clear to those working in this field that it is necessary to integrate the skills of many other health care professionals, both in the implant centre and in the child's home area. Because of the need to bring together these various professionals and because there is the need for such a team to develop its skills, it is appropriate that cochlear implantation in children should only be carried out in a limited number of centres. Kileny, Kemink and Zimmerman-Phillips (1991) have discussed the resource implications of paediatric cochlear implantation, noting that it is a complex area. They observed that most of the surgical experts in this area are individuals who have subspecialized in otology or otoneurosurgery. They also observed that the audiologists need to have training and expertise in a difficult combination of areas: diagnostic audiology, paediatric audiology, electrophysiology, rehabilitational audiology and educational audiology. Kveton and Balkany (1991) on behalf of the American Academy of Otolaryngology – Head and Neck Surgery Subcommittee on Cochlear Implants observed that 'the complex assessment, rehabilitation and counselling should be performed by centers with the multidisciplinary staffs necessary'. Cochlear implantation in children is likely to be located in a limited number of centres and therefore many children will have to travel to their nearest centre which may be many miles from their homes.

The team may be considered in two broad groups, those members at the implant centre and those in the child's home town, including local health and educational professionals as well as parents, immediate family and friends and others who have day-to-day involvement with the child. There are obvious logistic difficulties but these are surmountable. The main point to stress in this respect is that there should be direct contact between the professionals at the implant centre and those in the child's home area. While much of this can be achieved by written and telephone communication it is of immeasurable benefit for those workers from the implant centre to visit the child and his carers in the home surroundings. The outreach element of the paediatric cochlear implantation team can be seen as an essential component of the whole, even though it is potentially very time consuming.

The key members of the implant centre team may be listed as follows:

- Surgeon(s)
- Audiological scientist(s)
- Teacher(s) of the deaf
- Medical physicist(s)
- Speech and language therapist(s)
- Administrator.

In addition the surgeons will work closely with their radiological colleagues and paediatric nursing staff both in the clinic, ward and operating theatre areas. Finally, it is of great benefit to have direct access to psychological advice and support from social workers for the deaf.

The team in the child's home area will consist of most of the above with the addition of the mainstream teachers and others who come into daily contact with the child. It is particularly important

that the child has contact with a local otologist who is familiar with the child's medical history and who has an awareness of the implications of cochlear implantation. This will ensure that any day-to-day medical problems may be dealt with locally without the need for the child and parents to travel to the implant centre.

One of the other benefits of having contact with the child's local professionals is that it provides an opportunity for the implant centre team to gain more insight into the local circumstances and the child's everyday life and educational requirements. It helps ensure that the (re)habilitation programme can be geared to the child's needs and established communication skills.

With such a diverse spread of skills it is of paramount importance that the various activities are coordinated both from the child's viewpoint but also because of the need to utilize those skills to their optimum. Coordination and administration of the implant programme is therefore an extremely important function.

Indications for cochlear implantation in children – candidacy issues

The question as to which child should receive a cochlear implant involves consideration of a variety of factors, audiological, medical (including radiological) and the child's ability to develop his or her communication skills. The child should have no other significant learning difficulties and should be considered psychologically stable. Parental expectation should be realistic and there should be strong support at home and locally. There should be the commitment of the local services to work with the implant team.

It is now apparent that many, if not most, young children with profound sensorineural hearing loss may be considered as candidates for cochlear implantation, whether their hearing loss be congenital or acquired. Information is now accumulating that both groups of children are likely to benefit from this procedure. The Children's Hearing Institute in New York has introduced the ChIP – Children's implant profile–as a means of determining which children may expect to receive benefit from a cochlear implant (Hellman *et al.*, 1991). Eleven factors are assessed: chronological age, duration of deafness, medical/ radiological findings, multiple handicapping conditions, functional hearing level, speech–language abilities, family structure and support, parent–child expectations, education environment, availability of support services, and cognitive learning style. A descriptive account of the various factors is given allowing appropriate scoring. The factors are graded along a continuum varying from 'no concern' to 'great concern'. All are taken into account when deciding an individual child's suitability for implantation and likelihood of obtaining benefit. Assessment of these factors also helps in planning postoperative rehabilitation.

Perhaps one of the most important considerations is to avoid implanting an ear which has sufficient residual hearing to gain benefit from conventional acoustic amplification. It is essential that any child considered for possible cochlear implantation should have had an adequate trial of *appropriate* conventional amplification for a sufficiently long period. The National Institutes of Health in the USA recommended in 1988 'A minimum of a six month trial with appropriate amplification and rehabilitation'. The other prerequisite is that training should be provided (Boothroyd, 1989). This issue is explored by Brookhouser, Worthington and Kelly (1990) who noted that it is inappropriate to categorize severely hearing-impaired children with those having profound losses.

Rickards *et al.* (1990) noted that the audiological assessment aims first to establish an accurate assessment of hearing threshold levels, second to evaluate the hearing aid system and third to determine how effectively the residual hearing is being used. Both unaided and aided auditory thresholds should be measured.

The Nottingham Paediatric Cochlear Implant Team's audiological guidelines state that the hearing loss should be profound or total and there must be clear lack of hearing aid benefit over a period of months. Measures should include sound-field warble-tone threshold determination obtained in the absence of any conductive overlay with the most powerful hearing aids and well fitting moulds. These aided responses should be greater than 60 dB(A) across the frequency range from 500 Hz to 4 kHz. Figure 11.1

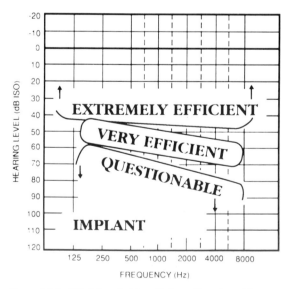

Figure 11.1 Aided threshold prediction of hearing aid benefit in children and the place of cochlear implants

illustrates results from the Nottingham Children's Hearing Assessment Centre showing benefit of hearing aid use and indicating the possible role of cochlear implants.

This compares with the criteria used in Melbourne (Rickards *et al.,* 1990). The child should have a profound to total bilateral sensorineural hearing loss showing no significant usable hearing. This would normally mean hearing levels of 95 dB HL or greater, although slightly better hearing may be present at 250 Hz and lower. The child should demonstrate at the end of the preoperative training period an inability to acquire speech and language through audition with the hearing aid or tactile aid.

Staller, Beiter and Brimacombe (1991) noted that it can be difficult to define precisely what is meant by lack of benefit from acoustic amplification because benefit must be considered in the light of each child's particular circumstances and environment as well as the level of performance that might reasonably be expected from the implant. They recommended the administration of a variety of open- and closed-set speech materials. If a child demonstrates significant open-set word recognition or significant above-chance performance on closed-set word identification tests then he or she is not considered to be an implant candidate.

In assessing any child for possible implantation the question of a conductive component to the hearing loss arises. Both audiologist and otologist need to be alert to this possibility as even a relatively minor additional loss due to a middle ear effusion may be sufficient to convert a sensorineural hearing loss that would be potentially aidable to one that is too great to benefit from even the most powerful of hearing aids. The conductive loss should be eliminated and further assessment should then be carried out.

From the Nottingham experience children are more likely to be found unsuitable on audiological grounds with inadequate trial of suitable amplification or hearing better than the recommended thresholds. Therefore this assessment is the first to be carried out (Figure 11.2), although this is not the case with all programmes; some programmes undertake the medical evaluation first (Staller, Beiter and Brimacombe, 1991).

The next issue is therefore one of medical suitability. This may be considered on the basis of otological, radiological and general medical suitability.

A general medical and otological history is needed with particular reference to frequency and degree of upper respiratory infection, ear infections, middle ear effusions and their treatment. The most common complicating factor in childhood sensorineural deafness is the presence of otitis media with effusion. This may add an additional 30 dB hearing loss to any preexisting loss and confound the audiological assessment. If found it should be treated by carrying out myringotomy and inserting a ventilating tube in

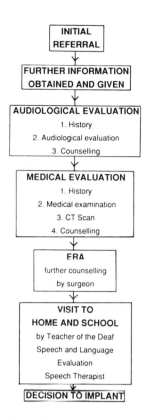

INITIAL
REFERRAL

FURTHER INFORMATION
OBTAINED AND GIVEN

AUDIOLOGICAL EVALUATION
1. History
2. Audiological evaluation
3. Counselling

MEDICAL EVALUATION
1. History
2. Medical examination
3. CT Scan
4. Counselling

ERA
further counselling
by surgeon

VISIT TO
HOME AND SCHOOL
by Teacher of the Deaf
Speech and Language
Evaluation
Speech Therapist

DECISION TO IMPLANT

Figure 11.2 The Nottingham schema for the preoperative evaluation and selection of children for cochlear implantation

order to obtain a true picture of the child's cochlear function. The ventilator will need to be removed before cochlear implantation. An effusion may also predispose a child to recurrent acute otitis media. Any child with such a history will need careful evaluation including assessment of the upper respiratory tract. Adenoidectomy may be required if it is felt that adenoidal hypertrophy or adenoiditis are aetiological factors. Other upper respiratory tract infections will need appropriate treatment.

Other otological conditions detected will of course need attention. A perforated tympanic membrane is a contraindication to implantation in that ear as is the presence of attico-antral disease including cholesteatoma. A perforation may require repair by tympanoplasty before the final decision to implant can be taken.

The medical history may help to reveal the cause of the deafness, whether it is congenital or acquired and whether there may be any cochlear abnormalities. In cases of congenital deafness the possibility of cochlear malformations may arise, the commonest of these being the Mondini deformity. Marked narrow-

ing of the internal meatus may result in lack of auditory response to electrical stimulation in children with cochlear implants as discussed by Shelton *et al.* (1989).

The commonest single cause of acquired profound hearing loss in childhood is meningitis with a prevalence of somewhere in the region of 1 in 12 000 to 1 in 15 000 of the population, though the figure could be larger than this (Davis and Wood, 1992).

Discussion of profound deafness due to meningitis raises several issues, perhaps the most important of which is that of *labyrinthitis ossificans*, new bone growth within the lumen of the cochlea. In cochlear implant procedures new bone growth has been found in the scala tympani in up to 35% of children (Luxford and House, 1987). It is suggested that cochlear sepsis is responsible for the hearing loss (Kay, 1991) and it is probable that this stimulates the new bone formation. The route of spread of the infection has been described by Perlman and Lindsay (1939) and in a study of 24 temporal bones with labyrinthitis ossificans Green, Marion and Hinojosa (1991) showed that the most frequent location for this is the scala tympani of the basal turn of the cochlea. They also demonstrated reduced spiral ganglion cell counts. Radiographic evidence of ossification can be found as early as 2 months after meningitis (Novak *et al.*, 1990) indicating that the intracochlear process probably begins much earlier.

Paparella and Sugiura (1967) have shown a variable degree of fibrosis within the perilymph which may then proceed to ossification. The process usually extends from base to apex but may involve any part of the labyrinthine apparatus (Hoffman, Brookler and Bergeron, 1979; Swartz *et al.*, 1985).

In children with profound deafness due to meningitis it is important to identify impending ossification at as early a stage as possible with CT scanning being carried out at 1–2 months after onset. If ossification is identified at this stage early implantation may be advised in order to improve the chances of satisfactory implantation of a multichannel electrode array (Novak *et al.*, 1990). House (Miyamoto *et al.*, 1991) proposed to carry out the surgery sooner than 4 months after the meningitis.

While early implantation in these children may be desirable, a related issue that must be addressed is the possibility of recovery of hearing after meningitis. Balkany (Miyamoto *et al.*, 1991) reported one child whose hearing had recovered 6 months after the meningitis and Brookhouser and Auslander (1989) reported three children with deafness due to meningitis who recovered some hearing up to 25 months after contracting meningitis. McCormick *et al.* (1993) reported partial recovery of hearing 14 months after onset of meningitis in a patient who had a cochlear implant. However, they recommended a period of 6 months after meningitis should be enough to detect most cases of spontaneous recovery. This period would also allow for a period of adjustment by the parents before an informed decision could be made.

Radiological assessment

Imaging of the temporal bone and neural pathways is an essential component of the preoperative evaluation. Balkany, Dreisbach and Seibert (1986) described the use of thin-section high resolution CT to evaluate the temporal bone. The evaluation included:

1 The thickness of the parietal bone
2 The degree of pneumatization of the mastoid
3 Measurement of the size of the facial recess
4 Description of the size and orientation of the round window niche
5 The patency of the basal turn of the cochlea.

Phelps, Annis and Robinson (1990) reviewed their experience with 165 patients using high resolution CT with thin (1 mm) cuts in axial and coronal planes and discussed the possible use of magnetic resonance imaging (MRI) to show that the inner ear is fluid filled. They suggested that the more severe type of dysplasias with an amorphous cochlear sac and risk of cerebrospinal fistula are not suitable as it is doubtful if there is a cochlear nerve in these cases. Harnsberger *et al.* (1987) used the information from CT to:

1 Exclude patients in whom multichannel implantation would be most likely to be unsuccessful
2 Help select the better ear for implantation
3 Provide a preoperative picture of normal variants and avoidable surgical pitfalls.

Their experience of MRI suggested that it could not routinely demonstrate cochlear nerve size but that it can address the issue of cochlear patency.

Using thin section tomography, high resolution CT and MRI, Yune, Miyamoto and Yune (1991) demonstrated signs of sclerosing labyrinthitic or labyrinthitis ossificans in 33 of 45 postmeningitic patients (73%). They also demonstrated three other inner ear deformities sufficient to explain congenital deafness.

Using CT, Shelton *et al.* (1989) suggested a new explanation for lack of auditory response to electrical stimulation in children with cochlear implants – a very narrow internal auditory canal, 1–2 mm in diameter and the probable absence of the auditory nerve. After analysing results in eight children with this anomaly they believed that a very narrow internal auditory canal on high resolution CT in patients with congenital profound sensorineural hearing loss is a contraindication to implantation.

Seicshnaydre, Johnson and Hasenstab (1992) compared preoperative CT interpretations with the surgical findings in 34 children undergoing implant surgery. They found abnormal CT scans in 22 of 31 patients (71%); 92% of patients with deafness following meningitis demonstrated abnormality, compared with 59% of patients with congenital loss. The abnormalities included narrowing of the basal turn of the cochlea, bony lip at the round window, a widened cochlear aqueduct and cochlear ossification. In the latter case, of five scans read as showing ossification four were confirmed at surgery. Of 26 scans negative for ossification one ossified cochlea was found at surgery, a 4% false negative rate. Bath *et al.* (1993) showed a high degree of accuracy in predicting cochlear patency (87%) in patients with a normal inner ear on CT. However, in 15% of cases, the degree of ossification was significantly underestimated causing difficulties at the time of surgery. Figure 11.3 shows a high resolution CT of a patent cochlear duct; it also shows fluid in the middle ear. Figure 11.4 shows ossification of the cochlea.

Takahashi, Sando and Takagi (1990) have advocated the use of three-dimensional reconstruction of the temporal bone to aid multiple channel implant surgery. Laszig *et al.* (1988) recommended using high resolution (HR) CT in conjunction with MRI. Where they had used both methods they did not experience any surprises as to the real status of the cochlea at surgery. They advocated an extracochlear back-up device if these methods of choice are not available.

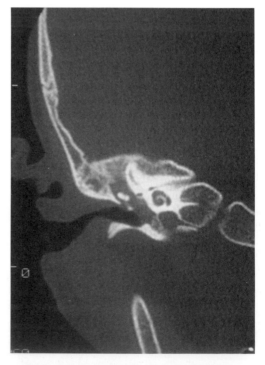

Figure 11.3 High resolution CT scan to show patent cochlear duct. Note the fluid within the middle ear. (Courtesy Drs I. Holland and T. Jaspan)

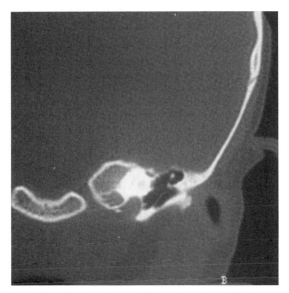

Figure 11.4 High resolution CT scan showing ossification of the cochlea. (Courtesy Drs I. Holland and T. Jaspan)

Medical assessment

The general medical assessment is an equally important element of the examination of a child for cochlear implantation. Children undergoing cochlear implantation require typically two general anaesthetics and should therefore be fit enough for this, bearing in mind that the actual implant surgery takes between 3 and 4 hours, allowing for time for the electrophysiological and other recordings to be carried out. Children with other major system problems such as cardiovascular disease need not be excluded from consideration for implantation; however, if such disease is present it will need careful evaluation in conjunction with both a paediatric physician and also the anaesthetist with whom the surgeon will be operating. Such close liaison is inherent in all paediatric surgical practice.

A much more difficult problem is that of the child with developmental delay. It is essential to recognize that children for implantation need to be able to cooperate with the tuning and rehabilitation process. The advice and opinion of a developmental paediatrician or paediatric neurologist may be necessary.

Formal psychological assessment may be necessary in only a limited number of children for implantation. The otologist(s) in the implant team will have a wide experience of paediatric medical practice and if there is doubt about a child's psychological suitability for surgery will liaise with other members of the team who will also have great experience of the problems encountered by deaf children. If doubts remain then referral to a child psychologist may be required.

Electrophysiological and other assessment

Once the child has been assessed audiometrically and medically and no contraindication has been detected, it is usually possible to assume that an offer to implant the child will be made in due course. However, it is important to ratify the subjective audiological assessment with objective tests. As a routine each child undergoes brain stem evoked response audiometry which is usually performed with sedation. It is expected that this will show no evidence of residual hearing and will confirm the subjective tests. Behavioural promontory stimulation is not usually carried out in young children (Shallop, 1993). The major disadvantage of such testing, including electrically evoked brain stem and stapedius responses in children, is that a general anaesthetic is required. In the author's department a research project uses such tests immediately pre-implantation in order to try to determine which ear is to be implanted where no guidance can be obtained from other preoperative assessment.

The final phase of the preoperative assessment is for the rehabilitation staff and the speech and language therapist to visit the home and, where relevant, the child's school. This is an important element of the assessment as it allows personal contact with those who are going to be dealing with the child in his own area as well as permitting an evaluation of the nature and degree of support likely to be provided postoperatively and whether the child has been brought up in an oral aural setting or one in which signing has been extensively used in a total communication environment.

Counselling

One of the most important elements in any paediatric cochlear implant programme is that of counselling parents and others responsible for a child being considered for an implant. This cannot be stressed too highly. It is the responsibility of all members of the implant team to ensure that parents (or guardians) in particular understand the implantation process and that their expectations are realistic and well founded. It is paramount that they should realize that a cochlear implant does not produce a normally hearing child but rather that an implant is a very sophisticated hearing aid, without which the child remains deaf. They should be aware at all stages right up to surgery that implantation may not prove possible, although with increasing experience in individual teams the likelihood of this occurring will diminish. The parents need to be aware that implantation requires a major commitment from themselves and that it is a long-term process with improvements in the child's communication skills developing over years.

A full and honest account of the team's results to date is an essential element in the counselling process, as well as a sensible account of the risks of the surgery itself. The cochlear implant surgeon will be guided by all his team colleagues in the decison to implant and will expect their support in counselling parents before the operation; indeed the final decision to implant will be a team one, but it is the surgeon who carries ultimate clinical responsibility for the care of the child. He must therefore be intimately involved in the whole decision-making process.

In addition to providing verbal support and counselling to parents it is helpful to be able to provide written information and many centres make available such literature. This allows the parents the opportunity to reflect fully on what has been said to them.

Particular sensitivity is required in dealing with the parents of children whose deafness has been as a result of meningitis. Much, if not all, of their previous dealings with hospitals will have occurred during the course of a potentially life-threatening illness. The parents need to be firmly reassured about the possible risks of the implant predisposing their child to further bouts of such infection.

Special aspects of implantation in children

Four particular aspects need to be addressed and may well result in questions from parents and others. The first involves the question of skull growth and the implanted device. Eby and Nadol (1986) have shown, using plain skull radiographs, that maximum postnatal skull growth occurs in the first 2 years. This agreed with the findings of O'Donoghue *et al.* (1986) who used measurements on CT scans and showed that 50% of skull growth occurred in the first 2 years. In another study, using direct measurements on the surface of temporal bones, Simms and Neely (1989) showed that the average growth per year, recorded in percent of the maximum growth per year, was 6.5% per year for ages 4 years or younger and 1.4% per year for those over 4. The greatest change (9.5% per year) occurred from birth to 2.5 years of age.

A second issue especially relevant to children is that of acute otitis media subsequent to implantation. While animal studies have shown that the implant could act as a conduit for the spread of infection from the middle ear to the labyrinth (Jackler, O'Donoghue and Schindler, 1986) there have been no reports to date of labyrinthitis or meningitis following implantation in children. Shepherd, Franz and Clark (1990) have investigated this and concluded that the implanted cochlea is able to resist the spread of infection nearly as effectively as a non-implanted one. There

is, however, a vulnerable period during the healing process after implantation and they recommend antibiotic prophylaxis during this period. In a survey of 26 cochlear implant patients carried out by House, Luxford and Courtney (1985) no change was seen in the pattern of incidence or severity of otitis media after implantation and none of the children developed meningitis or other evidence of inner ear infection. This has also been the experience in Nottingham in over 40 implanted children.

The possible long-term effects of electrical stimulation of the cochlea present a third consideration when implanting children. This matter has been reviewed by Shepherd, Franz and Clark (1990) who have carried out both electrophysiological testing and histological examination of cats subjected to chronic electrical cochlear stimulation. They concluded that chronic electrical stimulation does not adversely affect residual auditory nerve fibres nor the cochlea in general.

The fourth issue is of the longevity of the implanted device and the results of reimplantation should there be failure of the implanted package. Patrick *et al.* (1990) reported only one hermetic device failure in 2000 implants using the Nucleus device. To date there have been six device failures in children implanted with the Nucleus device in Europe. Parisier *et al.* (1991) reported the results of 15 reinsertions, eight in which a 3M/House device was replaced with a further 3M/House implant, five in which a 3M/House device was replaced with a Nucleus implant and two in whom a Nucleus device failed and was replaced with a similar device. They found that reinsertion has not proved to be technically problematic. Gantz, Lowder and McCabe (1989) noted that replacement of intracochlear electrodes did not result in clinically apparent degeneration of auditory performance and in a single case study, Chute *et al.* (1992) showed that explantation/reimplantation was technically feasible with no adverse effects on the patient's ability to utilize a more sophisticated device.

A more difficult problem related to device failure in children is the ability to recognize it. This is an area where the skill and experience of the rehabilitation and scientific staff, coupled with alertness by the parents and others, is of paramount importance as otherwise such an event may not be detected for a considerable period of time. The use of electric brain stem response audiometry (EBRA) may prove invaluable and, in the case of the Nucleus device, an integrity test may be carried out, looking for the signal artefact in response to electrical stimulation.

The surgery and postoperative period: surgical and safety considerations

The surgery of cochlear implantation in children differs from that in adults in a number of ways.

First it is essential to recognize the role of the parents in giving consent for the operation. This has been discussed in the section on counselling. In the immediate preoperative period the parents should be given further opportunity to have any remaining questions answered. As with all paediatric surgery it is necessary to prepare the child properly and, where appropriate, to involve the child in what is about to happen subject, of course, to parental wishes. The child can be given specially prepared booklets with simple text and diagrams describing the time in hospital. Typically cochlear implantation involves a 3–4 day stay in hospital and it is helpful if suitable facilities can be provided for the parents to stay within the hospital during this time.

A number of surgical incisions has been used for cochlear implantation including an inverted U in the postauricular region, a C-shaped incision, an inverted L or hockey stick, or an extended endaural incision. It is the Nottingham practice to use the extended endaural approach (Figure 11.5). To date no flap complications have been encountered with this incision in over 50 cases. Meticulous haemostasis is essential and it is our practice not to raise a separate

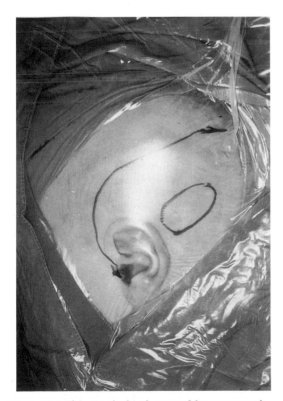

Figure 11.5 Showing the head prepared for surgery with the incision and site of the implant marked

periosteal flap. In children thinning of the flap is not required.

Once the flap has been raised a cortical mastoidotomy is carried out and the bed for the implant then prepared, anchorage points for the implant package also being prepared. Caution must be exercised as the squamous temporal bone in children can be very thin, sometimes less than 2 mm in places. The bone is typically softer in children than in adults. A posterior tympanotomy is then carried out giving access to the round window area and the promontory. Two possible routes are available for inserting the intracochlear electrode array – either via the round window membrane or via a separate cochleostomy on the promontory. In Nottingham the latter route is used. Once inserted the electrode array is secured using dental cement and Dacron ties, the receiver package being anchored with nylon ties through the squamous temporal bone. The cochleostomy is sealed with a small piece of muscle taken at the start of the operation.

At this stage during the operation it is invaluable to carry out recording of the electrically induced stapedius reflex, which is assessed by visual observation, and electrically induced brain stem evoked response audiometry. While relatively time consuming during the operation these two measures can be used at the time of the initial switch-on and tuning to give an indication of likely levels required for the C (comfort) levels and T (threshold) levels respectively. This can save a considerable period of time at the switch-on and help avoid giving the child too great a stimulus. An additional benefit of these recordings is to be able to reassure the parents that not only has the implant been successfully inserted but also that it is working.

The whole operative period is covered with a broad-spectrum antibiotic, initially by injection and then by mouth. In addition the wound is irrigated with a tetracycline solution. Suture removal in children can be distressing and therefore it is better to use subcuticular sutures in order to avoid this. After the operation a firm head dressing is applied and left on for 48 hours in order to help reduce the risk of haematoma formation; drains are not used. Most children require only mild analgesia and dizziness has not proved to be a problem.

Once the dressing has been removed postoperative radiographs may be taken using a reversed Stenver's view to demonstrate the position of the electrodes (Figure 11.6). This X-ray may be invaluable at later stages if, for example, the child suffers a head injury or there is change in the performance of the device. In addition, it has been suggested that insertion depth as determined by X-ray studies has a strong correlation with open-set speech discrimination (Marsh *et al.*, 1993).

At this stage the child is allowed home, parents being reminded about the possible medical hazards

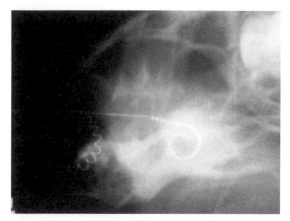

Figure 11.6 Postoperative X-ray showing full insertion of the electrode array. (Courtesy of Drs I. Holland and T. Jaspan)

associated with implantation, including the need to avoid the use of monopolar diathermy and magnetic resonance imaging. It is the Nottingham practice to provide a MedicAlert bracelet or necklace. Close liaison is established with the local otolaryngologist and arrangements made for the child to return to the implant centre for initial switch-on and tuning approximately one month after surgery.

In experienced hands surgical complications should be few. Clark, Cohen and Shepherd (1991) reported an overall incidence of complications of 6.8%. They had a total of five facial palsies out of 548 children. The most common complications were related to the flap and to electrode placement. The complication rate in children compares favourably with that in adults, Cohen, Hoffman and Stroschein (1988) reporting a 12% complication rate in 459 adults. Of 46 children operated on to date in the Nottingham programme three major complications have occurred: one child developed pain on stimulation coupled with failure of response. This child had had the electrode array implanted in a gutter drilled onto the promontory as the cochlea was completely obliterated. A second child developed a deep retraction pocket with cholesteatoma, a complication also reported by Webb *et al.* (1991). A third child has recently experienced total device failure and been successfully reimplanted with another Nucleus device without undue difficulty. In the Nottingham series one operation was abandoned due to total ossification and it is now our practice to have a single channel extracochlear device available to deal with this contingency.

Surgery and ossification

If there is limited basilar obliteration due to new bone growth then it may be possible to continue drilling until a lumen is visualized and then insert the electrode array. Balkany, Gantz and Nadol (1988) have shown a 93% success rate for insertion greater than 20 mm in ears with obliteration of the basal turn. Lehnhardt (1992) drilled anteroinferiorly to the round window niche, if the ossification is severe, drilling may be continued forwards to a depth of no more than 8–10 mm or until the carotid artery is visible. In cases of total obliteration Gantz, McCabe and Tyler (1988) have advocated a radical mastoidectomy with a drill-out well beyond the basal turn of the cochlea. They attempt to create a channel for the electrode lead so that it can wrap around the modiolus.

Switch-on

Before the external components of the implant are fitted and switched on the child is checked medically to ensure that the wound has healed fully and that the middle ear is healthy. The switch-on can be an emotional and relatively traumatic time for the parents. Many children exhibit signs of distress at this point and parents need to be forewarned that this may happen. It is usually short-lived. The actual stimulus levels to be used initially are based on the intraoperative recordings with correction factors being applied as described by Mason *et al.* (Nottingham unpublished data). Shallop *et al.* (1991) have shown that electric brain stem response audiometry threshold current level is consistently near the behavioural comfort level rather than the patient's behavioural threshold level.

The objective of device programming is to obtain behavioural measures of threshold and comfortable loudness for each electrode pair. These stimulation levels are stored in the random access memory within the speech processor and are referred to as the *MAP*. The first session may only achieve switch-on of a limited number of channels. Comfortable loudness levels should be set conservatively so that unpleasant experiences are avoided for the child. The initial switch-on and tuning with a limited amount of rehabilitation is spread over a 2-day period. Programming is time consuming; the mean time spent on this activity in Nottingham is 27 hours in the first year and 10 hours in the second, with younger children requiring a longer time. With children a simple test of speech can be used to assess how appropriate the MAP settings are and liaison with rehabilitation staff can provide further guidance. Reprogramming may be necessary as the MAP changes with time after implantation.

Rehabilitation and subsequent assessments

Once a MAP has been produced the rehabilitation process starts and the child's functional level will determine subsequent management. Three categories may be recognized:

- Preverbal – children with effectively none of the normal early communication skills
- Transitional – children who have started to use sound meaningfully for communication
- Functional language – children using spoken language for communication.

Tait (1987) has identified five stages through which children pass in making the transition from preverbal communication to the beginnings of conversational competence using a technique of video analysis. The various stages are as follows:

1 Disengaged: the child's visual attention is not on the speaker but on other activities
2 Engaged: the child starts to look at the speaker or at the object of the discourse
3 Structured looking: the child now starts to look at the speaker and takes his 'turn' in conversation
4 Structured vocalization: vocalizations become more word-like and are more likely to take place in turns
5 Equal conversational partnership: the child now demonstrates initiative and autonomy in the conversation.

Using these techniques it is possible to monitor the progress and development of both preverbal children and those in the transitional stage of language development.

In children with some functional language assessment is probably easier and more straightforward using a variety of established techniques in testing prosodic and closed-set speech and open-set word recognition. Staller, Beiter and Brimacombe (1991) have reviewed the various speech and language assessments to be used, commenting that standardized instruments should be used.

Results

The results of cochlear implantation may be presented in a variety of ways. One method is to use the implant-aided response levels of children to pure tone or warble tones. Figure 11.7 shows warble tone reponses with the implant of the first 23 children in the Nottingham series. This may be compared with the criteria for implantation as shown in Figure 11.1. An alternative method of assessing benefit is to use measures of hearing performance. Figure 11.8 demonstrates the performance of the children in the Nottingham Programme to date. It can be seen that there is progressive improvement of performance with time, but even at initial tuning there is an immediate demonstration of benefit. Figure 11.9 indicates that prelingually deaf children develop listening skills more slowly than those who have functional language but that with time the two groups attain similar benefits from implantation.

These results compare favourably with more detailed studies of various aspects of speech perception and production. For example Staller (1990) showed that after 12 months' experience with the Nucleus Multichannel device significant improvements in auditory alone speech perception were seen in 66% of subjects tested on prosodic and closed-set measures and by 46% on open-set word recognition. In a group of 51 children implanted with the 3M/House single channel device at a mean age of 6.2 years and with a mean age of 9.2 years at testing, Berliner *et al.* (1989) showed that 52% had some open-set performance on word identification and 41.5% did so on sentence comprehension.

Waltzmann, Cohen and Shapiro (1992) have shown that congenitally and prelinguistically deaf children obtain significant benefit from cochlear implantation and that the improvement does not appear to plateau within a 2 year period. Their data support the view that early implantation of prelingually and congenitally deaf children is advisable and desirable in order to foster linguistic development. This work is supported by Osberger, Maso and Sam (1993) who have shown that subjects with early onset of deafness, who received their implant before the age of 10 years, demonstrated the highest speech intelligibility whereas those who received their implant after 10 years of age had the poorest speech intelligibility. Osberger and her colleagues also compared the results of implant users with children using hearing aids, the latter being grouped into three categories:

- Gold hearing aid users – children with unaided auditory thresholds of 90–100 dB HL between

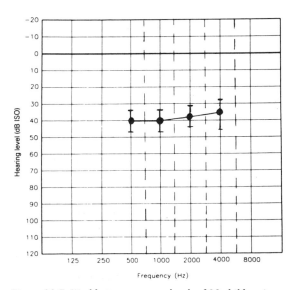

Figure 11.7 Warble-tone response levels of 23 children in the Nottingham Programme using the Nucleus device

Before implant (N = 40)	Category of performance	0 months (N = 40) (at initial tuning)	6 months (N = 32)	12 months (N = 25)	24 months (N = 15)	36 months (N = 6)
	Use of telephone with known speaker		1		1	2
	Understanding of conversation without lipreading		1	1	6	3
	Understanding of common phrases without lipreading				5	
	Discrimination of some speech sounds without lipreading	6	18	23	3	1
	Identification of environmental sounds		7	1		
	Response to speech sounds (e.g. 'go')	17	5			
2	Awareness of environmental sounds	17				
38	No awareness of environmental sounds					

Nottingham Paediatric Cochlear Implant Programme (August 1993): number of children achieving each category

Figure 11.8 Performance in young children before and after cochlear implantation showing the progressive improvement with time

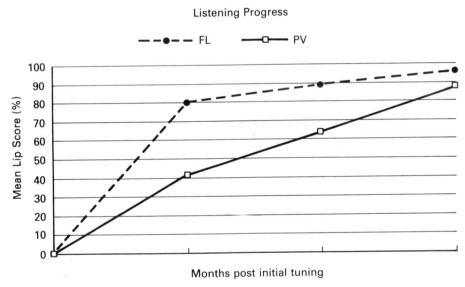

Listening Progress

Figure 11.9 Listening progress in young children after cochlear implantation. FL = Functional language; PV = preverbal

500 and 2000 Hz and aided thresholds of 30–55 dB HL
- Silver hearing aid users – unaided thresholds of 100–110 dB HL between 500 and 2000 Hz and aided thresholds greater than 55 dB HL above 1000 Hz
- Bronze hearing aid users – unaided thresholds greater than 110 dB HL, probably receiving only vibrotactile information, and with negligible hearing aid benefit.

Osberger, Maso and Sam (1993) noted that the scores of the highest performing children with the Nucleus implant are now approaching those of the gold hearing aid users with average speech intelligibility scores similar to the silver hearing aid users.

It is becoming apparent that postlingually deafened children gain benefit from an implant at an earlier stage after implantation than prelingually deaf children. Fryauf-Bertschy *et al.* (1992) showed that postlingually deafened children exhibited significantly improved performance on open- and closed-set tests of word recognition after 6 months compared with congenitally deaf children who did not exhibit measurable improvement on speech perception tests until after 12 months or more of implant use. After 12–24 months of use some congenitally deaf children demonstrated limited open-set word recognition. This work supports that of Osberger *et al.* (1991) who showed that children who went deaf after the age of 5 years demonstrated significantly better speech perception abilities than those who were either congenitally deaf or who became deaf during the first 3 years of life. Indeed, within the latter group, there were no differences in speech perception between those congenitally deaf and those with an acquired deafness. Similar results have been reported by Staller *et al.* (1991) who also noted that the mode of communication used did not appear to have a significant effect on the performance tests used in their investigation.

Geers and Moog (1991) and Moog and Geers (1991) concluded that training in auditory skills is required to improve speech and language skills and that the auditory advantage conferred by an implant should become apparent in more dramatic differences in spoken language development when 2 and 3 year post-implant results are examined. They felt that it is too early to expect significant differences in spoken language after less than 1 year of implant use. They also stressed that parents and teachers need to learn techniques for monitoring the devices and for capitalizing on their features for maximum benefit for the child. However, Miyamoto *et al.* (1993) have produced data which show that communication mode does not appear to account for large differences in speech perception performance among prelingually deafened children receiving a multichannel cochlear implant. Of a group of 19 prelingually deaf children, those in an oral communication setting obtained significantly higher scores on only two out of 13 speech perception measures compared with those who used total communication. They showed also that performance with a multichannel implant is not strongly influenced by age of onset of deafness when deafness occurs before the age of 3 years, children with congenital deafness having the potential to obtain the same benefit as those with an acquired loss.

Another factor to be considered in assessing the results of cochlear implantation is whether the implant is single or multichannel. This issue has been addressed by Miyamoto *et al.* (1992). In speech perception and production tests, children with a multichannel implant continued to show improvement after 2 or more years whereas those with a single channel device (3M/ House) reached a plateau by 1.5 years post-implant. Changes in language were limited over time with no obvious difference in performance as a function of type of implant.

There remains the possibility in cases of acquired deafness due to meningitis that other factors may be present causing cognitive deficits that might prevent the perception and production of spoken language. The Nottingham Paediatric Cochlear Implant Group has experience of one such case in which a child deaf after meningitis developed good awareness of environmental sounds but failed to develop any spoken language even 3 years after implantatation. Such a deficit would probably have remained unrecognized if he had not received an implant.

Conclusions

Cochlear implantation is now established as a means of managing profound deafness in children. There are still many issues to be resolved but William House (1991) summed up the status of cochlear implantation in children: 'The future is not in the adult programme, but in the continued expansion of the children's programme'.

References

BALKANY, T. J., DREISBACH, J. N. and SEIBERT, C. E. (1986) Radiographic imaging of the cochlear implant candidate. *Otolaryngology – Head and Neck Surgery*, **95**, 592–597

BALKANY, T. J., GANTZ, B. J. and NADOL, J. B. J. (1988) Multichannel cochlear implants in partially ossified cochleas. *Annals of Otology, Rhinology and Laryngology*, **97**, 3–7

BATH, A. P., O'DONOGHUE, G. M., HOLLAND, I. M. and GIBBIN, K. P. (1993) Paediatric cochlear implantation: how reliable is computed tomography in assessing cochlear patency? *Clinical Otolaryngology*, **18**, 475–479

BERLINER, K., EISENBERG, L. S. and HOUSE, W. F. (1985) The cochlear implant: an auditory prosthesis for the profoundly deaf child. *Ear and Hearing*, **6**, 1s–69s

BERLINER, K. I., TONOKAWA, L. L., DYE, L. M. and HOUSE, W. F. (1989) Open-set speech recognition in children with a single channel cochlear implant. *Ear and Hearing*, **10**, 237–242

BOOTH, C. L., READ, T. E., ARCHBOLD, S. DYAR, D., MORGAN, C. and GRAY, R. F. (1989) Case study of a post-lingually deafened child with a UCH/RNID single channel cochlear implant. *Journal of Laryngology and Otology*, Suppl. 18, 50–54

BOOTHROYD, A. (1987) Management of profound sensorineural hearing loss in children: possibilities and pitfalls of cochlear implants. *Annals of Otology, Rhinology and Laryngology*, **96** (Suppl. 128), 84

BOOTHROYD, A. (1989) Hearing aids, cochlear implants and profoundly deaf children. In: *Cochlear Implants in Young Deaf Children*, edited by E. Owens and D. K. Kessler. Boston: College Hill Press. pp. 81–99

BROOKHOUSER, P. E. and AUSLANDER M. C. (1989) Aided auditory thresholds in children with post-meningitic deafness. *Laryngoscope*, **99**, 800–808

BROOKHOUSER, P. E., WORTHINGTON, D. W. and KELLY, W. J. (1990) Severe versus profound sensorineural hearing loss in children: implications for cochlear implantation. *Laryngoscope*, **100**, 349–356

CHUTE, P. M., HELLMAN, S. A., PARISIER, S. C., TARTTER, V. C. and ECONOMOU, A. (1992) Auditory perception changes after reimplantation in a child implant user. *Ear and Hearing*, **13**, 195–199

CLARK, G. M., COHEN, N. L. and SHEPHERD, R. K. (1991) Surgical and safety considerations of multichannel cochlear implants in children. *Ear and Hearing*, **12**, (Suppl), 15s–24s.

COHEN, N. L., HOFFMAN, R. A. and STROSCHEIN, M. (1988) Medical or surgical complications related to the Nucleus multichannel cochlear implant. *Annals of Otology, Rhinology and Laryngology*, **97**, (Suppl. 135), 8–13

DAVIS, A. and WOOD, S. (1992) The epidemiology of childhood hearing impairment: factors relevant to planning of services. *British Journal of Audiology*, **26**, 77–90

DOWNS, M. P., CAMPOS, C. T., FIREMARK R., MARTIN, E. and MYRES, W. (1986) Psychosocial issues surrounding children receiving cochlear implants. *Seminars in Hearing*, **7**, 383–405

EBY, T. L. and NADOL, J. B. (1986) Postnatal growth of the human temporal bone. Implications for cochlear implants in children. *Annals of Otology, Rhinology and Laryngology*, **95**, 356–364

EVANS, J. W. (1989) Thoughts on the psychosocial implications of cochlear implantation in children. In: *Cochlear Implants in Young Deaf Children*, edited by E. Owens and D. K. Kessler. Boston: College Hill. pp. 307–314

FRYAUF-BERTSCHY, H., TYLER, R. S., KELSAY, D. M. and GANTZ, B. J. (1992) Performance over time of congenitally deaf and postlingually deafened children using a multichannel cochlear implant. *Journal of Speech and Hearing Research*, **35**, 913–920

GANTZ, B. J., MCCABE, B. F. and TYLER, R. S. (1988) Use of multichannel cochlear implants in obstructed and obliterated cochleas. *Otolaryngology – Head and Neck Surgery*, **98**, 72–81

GANTZ, B. J., LOWDER, M. W. and MCCABE, B. F. (1989) Audiologic results following reimplantation of cochlear implants. *Annals of Otology, Rhinology and Laryngology*, **98**, 12–16

GEERS, A. E. and MOOG, J. S. (1991) Evaluating the benefits of cochlear implants in an education setting. *American Journal of Otology*, **12**, (Suppl.) 116–125

GIBBIN, K. P. (1992) Paediatric cochlear implantation. *Archives of Disease in Childhood*, **67**, 669–671

GRAHAM, J. (1990) Cochlear implants for children? Conclusions. In: *Current Approaches. Clinical Developments in Cochlear Implants*, edited by M. P. Haggard. London: Duphar Laboratories Ltd. pp. 82–85

GREEN, J. D., MARION, M. S. and HINOJOSA, R. (1991) Labyrinthitis ossificans: histopathologic consideration for cochlear implantation. *Otolaryngology – Head and Neck Surgery*, **104**, 320–326

HARNSBERGER, H. R., DART, D. J., PARKIN, J. L., SMOKER, W. R. K. and OSBORN, A. G. (1987) Cochlear implant candidates: assessment with CT and MR Imaging. *Radiology*, **164**, 53–57

HELLMAN, S. A., CHUTE, P. M., KRETSCHMER, R. E., NEVINS, M. E., PARISIER, S. C. and THURSTON, L. C. (1991) The development of a children's implant profile. *American Annals of the Deaf*, 77–81

HOFFMAN, R., BROOKLER, K. and BERGERON, R. (1979) Radiologic diagnosis of labyrinthitis ossificans. *Annals of Otology, Rhinology and Laryngology*, **88**, 253–257

HOUSE, W. F. (1976) Cochlear implants. *Annals of Otology, Rhinology and Laryngology*, **85**, (Suppl. 27), 3–6

HOUSE, W. F. (1991) Cochlear implants in children: past and present perspectives. *American Journal of Otology*, **12**, (Suppl.), 1–2

HOUSE, W. F., LUXFORD, W. M. and COURTNEY, B. (1985) Otitis media in children following the cochlear implant. *Ear and Hearing*, Suppl. 1, 24–26

JACKLER, R. K., O'DONOGHUE, G. M. and SCHINDLER, R. A. (1986) Cochlear implantation. Strategies to protect the implanted cochlea from middle ear infection. *Annals of Otology, Rhinology and Laryngology*, **95**, 66–70

KAY, R. (1991) The site of the lesion causing hearing loss in bacterial meningitis: a study of experimental streptococcal meningitis in guinea-pigs. *Neuropathology and Applied Neurobiology*, **17**, 485–493

KESSLER, D. K. and OWENS, E. (1989) Conclusions: Current considerations and future directions. In: *Cochlear Implants in Young Deaf Children*, edited by E. Owens and D. K. Kessler. Boston: College Hill. pp. 315–330

KILENY, P. R., KEMINK, J. L. and ZIMMERMAN-PHILLIPS S. (1991) Cochlear implants in children. *American Journal of Otology*, **12**, 144–146

KVETON, J. and BALKANY, T. J. (1991) Status of cochlear implantation in children. *Journal of Pediatrics*, **118**, 1–7

LASZIG, R., TERWEY, B., BATTMER, R. D. and HESSE, G. (1988) Magnetic resonance imaging (MRI) and high resolution computertomography (HRCT) in cochlear implant candidates. *Scandinavian Audiology*, Suppl. 30, 197–200

LEHNHARDT, E. (1992) Surgical procedure for cochlear implants. In: *Debrett's Book of Surgery*, edited by L. Paine. London: Sterling Publications Ltd. pp. 101–106

LUXFORD, W. M. and HOUSE, W. F. (1987) House 3M cochlear implant: surgical considerations. International Cochlear Implant Symposium and Workshop, Melbourne, 1985, edited by G. M. Clark, and P. A. Busby. *Annals of Otology, Rhinology and Laryngology*, **96**, (Suppl. 128), 12–14

MCCORMICK, B. (1991) Paediatric cochlear implantation in the United Kingdom – a delayed journey on a well marked route. *British Journal of Audiology*, **25**, 145–149

MCCORMICK, B., GIBBIN, K. P., LUTMAN, M. E. and O'DONOGHUE, G. M. (1993) Late partial recovery from meningitic deafness after cochlear implantation: a case study. *American Journal of Otology*, **14**, 610–612

MARSH, M. A., XU, J., BLAMEY, P. J., WHITFORD, L. A., XU, S. A., SILVERMAN, J. M. et al. (1993) Radiologic evaluation of multichannel intracochlear implant insertion depth. *American Journal of Otology*, **14**, 386–391

MICHELSON, R. P. (1971) Electrical stimulation of the human cochlea. *Archives of Otolaryngology*, **93**, 317–323

MIYAMOTO, R. T., MADDOX, H. E., BALKANY, T. J., HOUSE, W. F., LUETJE, C. M., LUXFORD, W. M. et al. (1991) Medical and surgical issues. *American Journal of Otology*, **12**, (Suppl.), 18–21

MIYAMOTO, R. J., OSBERGER, M. J., ROBBINS, A. M., MYRES, W. A., KESSLER, K. and POPE, M. L. (1992) Longitudinal evaluation of communication skills of children with single-or multichannel cochlear implants. *American Journal of Otology*, **13**, 215–222

MIYAMOTO, R. T., OSBERGER, M. J., ROBBINS, A. M., MYRES, W. A. and KESSLER, K. (1993) Prelingually deafened children's performance with the Nucleus multichannel cochlear implant. *American Journal of Otology*, **14**, 437–445

MOOG, J. S. and GEERS A. E. (1991) Educational management of children with cochlear implants. *American Annals of the Deaf*, **136**, 69–76

NATIONAL INSTITUTES OF HEALTH (1988) *Consensus Development Conference Statement*. Vol 7, no. 2, May 4, 1988

NIENHUYS, T. G., MUSGRAVE, G. N., BUSBY, P. A., BLAMEY, P. J., NOTT, P., TONG, Y. C. *et al.* (1987). Educational assessment and management of children with multichannel cochlear implants. *Annals of Otology, Rhinology and Laryngology*, **96**, (Suppl. 128), 80–82

NOVAK, M. A., FIFER, R. C., BARKMEIER, J. C. and FIRSZT, J. B. (1990) Labyrinthine ossification after meningitis: its implications for cochlear implantation. *Otolaryngology – Head and Neck Surgery*, **103**, 351–356

O'DONOGHUE, G. M. (1992) Cochlear implants in children. *Journal of the Royal Society of Medicine*, **85**, 655–658

O'DONOGHUE, G. M., JACKLER, R. K., JENKINS, W. M. and SCHINDLER, R. A. (1986) Cochlear implantation in children: the problem of head growth. *Otolaryngology – Head and Neck Surgery*, **94**, 78–81

OSBERGER, M. J., TODD, S. L., BERRY, S. W., ROBBINS, A. M. and MIYAMOTO, R. T. (1991) Effect of age at onset of deafness on children's speech perception abilities with a cochlear implant. *Annals of Otology, Rhinology and Laryngology*, **100**, 883–888

OSBERGER, M. J., MASO, M. and SAM, L. K. (1993) Speech intelligibility of children with cochlear implants, tactile aids or hearing aids. *Journal of Speech and Hearing Research*, **36**, 186–203

PAPARELLA, M. and SUGIURA, S. (1967) The pathology of suppurative labyrinthitis. *Annals of Otology, Rhinology and Laryngology*, **76**, 554–586

PARISIER, S. C., CHUTE, P. M., WEISS, M. H., HELLMAN, S. A. and WANG, R. C. (1991) Results of cochlear implant reinsertion. *Laryngoscope*, **101**, 1013–1015

PATRICK, J. F. and CLARK G. M. (1991) The Nucleus 22-channel cochlear implant system. *Ear and Hearing*, **12**, (Suppl.), 3s–9s

PATRICK, J. F., SELIGMAN, P. M., MONEY, D. K. and KUZMA, J.A. (1990) Engineering. In: *Cochlear Prostheses*, edited by G. M. Clark, Y. C. Tong and J. F. Patrick. London: Churchill Livingstone. pp. 99–124

PERLMAN, H. B. and LINDSAY, J. R. (1939) Relation of the internal ear spaces to the meninges. *Archives of Otolaryngology*, **29**, 12–23

PHELPS, P. D., ANNIS, J. R. and ROBINSON, P. J. (1990) Imaging for cochlear implants. *British Journal of Radiology*, **63**, 512–516

RICKARDS, F. W., DETTMAN, S. J., BUSBY, P. A., WEBB, R. L., DOWELL, R. C., DENNEHY, S. E. *et al.* (1990) Preoperative evaluation and selection of children and teenagers. In: *Cochlear Prostheses*, edited by G. M. Clark, Y. C. Tong and J. F. Patrick. London: Churchill Livingstone. pp. 135–152

RUBEN, R. J. (1986). Unsolved issues around critical periods with emphasis on clinical application. *Acta Otolaryngologica*, Suppl. 429, 61–64

SCHINDLER, R. A. (1984) *Tenth Anniversary Conference on Cochlear Implants – An International Symposium*. New York: Raven Press

SCHINDLER, R. A. and KESSLER, D. K. (1992) Preliminary results with the clarion cochlear implant. *Laryngoscope*, **102**, 1006–1013

SEICSHNAYDRE, M.A., JOHNSON, M. H. and HASENSTAB, M. S. (1992) Cochlear implants in children: reliability of computed tomography. *Otolaryngology – Head and Neck Surgery*, **107**, 410–417

SHALLOP, J. K. (1993) Objective electrophysiologic measures from cochlear implant patients. *Ear and Hearing*, **14**, 58–63

SHALLOP, J. K., VAN DYKE, L., GOIN, D. W. and MISCHKE, R. E. (1991) Prediction of behavioral threshold and comfort values for Nucleus 22-channel implant patients from electrical auditory brain stem response test results. *Annals of Otology, Rhinology and Laryngology*, **100**, 896–898

SHELTON, C., LUXFORD, W. M., TONOKAWA, L. L., LO, W. W. M. and HOUSE, W. M. (1989) The narrow internal auditory canal in children: a contra-indication to cochlear implants. *Otolaryngology, Head and Neck Surgery*, **100**, 227–231

SHEPHERD, R. K., FRANZ, B. K. -H. G. and CLARK, G. M. (1990) The biocompatibility and safety of cochlear prostheses. In: *Cochlear Prostheses*, edited by G. M. Clark, Y. C. Tong and J. F. Patrick. London: Churchill Livingstone. pp. 69–98

SIMMONS, F. B. (1966) Electrical stimulation of the auditory nerve in man. *Archives of Otolaryngology*, **84**, 2–54

SIMMONS, F. B. (1985) Cochlear implants in young children: some dilemmas. *Ear and Hearing*, **6**, 61s–62s

SIMMS, D. L. and NEELY, J. G. (1989) Growth of the lateral surface of the temporal bone in children. *Laryngoscope*, **99**, 795–799

STALLER, S. J. (1990) Perceptual and production abilities in profoundly deaf children with multichannel cochlear implants. *Journal of the American Academy of Audiology*, **1**, 1–3

STALLER, S. J. (1991) Foreward. *Ear and Hearing*, **12**, (Suppl.), 1s

STALLER, S. J., BEITER, A. L. and BRIMACOMBE J. A. (1991) Children and multichannel cochlear implants. In: *Cochlear Implants; a Practical Guide*, edited by H. Cooper. London Whurr Publishers Ltd. pp. 283–321

STALLER, S. J., BEITER, A. L., BRIMACOMBE, J. A., MECKLENBURG, D. J. and ARNDT, P. (1991) Pediatric performance with the Nucleus 22-channel cochlear implant system. *American Journal of Otology*, **12**, (Suppl.), 126–136

SWARTZ, J. D., MANDELL, D. M., FAERBER, E. N., POPKY, G. L., ARDITO, J. M., STEINBERG, S. B. *et al.* (1985) Labyrinthine ossification etiologies and CT findings. *Radiology*, **157**, 395–398

TAIT, M. (1987) Making and monitoring progress in the pre-school years. *Journal of the British Association of Teachers of the Deaf*, **5**, 143–153

TAKAHASHI, H., SANDO, I. and TAKAGI, A. (1990) Computer aided three-dimensional reconstruction and measurement for multiple-electrode cochlear implant. *Laryngoscope*, **100**, 1319–1322

TIBER, N. (1985) A psychological evaluation of cochlear implants in children. *Ear and Hearing*, **6** (Suppl.), 48s–51s

WALTZMANN, S. B., COHEN, N. L. and SHAPIRO, W. H. (1992) Use of a multichannel cochlear implant in the congenitally and prelingually deaf population. *Laryngoscope*, **102**, 395–399

WEBB, R. L., LEHNHARDT, E., CLARK, G. M., LASZIG, R., PYMAN, B. C. and FRANZ, B. K. -H. G. (1991) Surgical complications with the cochlear multiple-channel intracochlear implant: experience at Hannover and Melbourne. *Annals of Otology, Rhinology and Laryngology*, **100**, 131–136

YUNE, H. Y., MIYAMOTO, R. T. and YUNE, M. E. (1991) Medical imaging in cochlear implant candidates. *American Journal of Otology*, **12**, (Suppl.), 11–17

12

Vestibular disorders

Alexander W. Blayney

The vestibular apparatus begins its formation on days 30–31 of intrauterine life and on day 49 its morphogenesis is complete, although the semicircular canals continue their dimensional development (Pignataro *et al.*, 1979). Between the 12th and 24th week of gestation, the connections of the labyrinth to the oculomotor nuclei in the brain stem develop and brain stem oculomotor reflexes are initiated. The vestibular nerve is the earliest cranial nerve to achieve full myelination, by the age of 16 weeks (Eviatar and Eviatar, 1988). The vestibular system becomes active by the eighth or ninth month of gestation, being responsible in part for the startle responses during fetal life (Holt, 1975). It is, therefore, the first sensory system to develop, ahead of the visual, auditory and proprioceptive systems to which it is inextricably linked. At birth the change from an intrauterine fluid milieu to a gravity-dependent environment necessitates a series of developmental steps to achieve an upright position and posture. Development thus occurs in a cephalocaudal direction so that the infant first acquires the ability to support and control the head; then as the spinal musculature develops the baby learns to sit, then begins to use the limbs, the arms first and then the legs, learning to crawl and creep and finally to walk (Sidebotham, 1988). This period of development is accompanied by marked vestibular activity, adaptation and maturation aided by both proprioceptive and visual stimuli in the acquistion of balance, control and movement.

Basic neuroanatomy

The labyrinth consists of three semicircular canals, the utricle and the saccule. The peripheral vestibular nerve endings are located on the hair cells of the maculae of the utricle and saccule and in the cristae of the ampullae of the semicircular canals (Gatz, 1974).

Rotational head movement or angular acceleration is thought to be primarily sensed by the semicircular canals, while linear acceleration and gravitational motion are detected by the otolithic organs, namely the maculae of the utricle and saccule, of which the utricle plays the greater part (Dohlman, 1981; Glasscock, Cueva and Thedinger, 1990).

Information regarding both movement and position of the head in space is relayed via the vestibular nerves to the vestibular nuclei in the brain stem. From here connections are made to the other relevant systems concerned with equilibrium, movement and spatial orientation:

1 A few fibres pass directly from the nuclei to the cerebellum ending in the cortex of the flocculonodular lobe.
2 The fastigio bulbar tract arises from the cerebellum, its fibres terminating in the vestibular nuclei and on the hair cells of the labyrinth. An additional efferent component arises in the lateral vestibular nucleus and ends on the vestibular hair cells, thus exerting a modulating influence on the receptors of the membranous labyrinth.
3 From the vestibular nuclei labyrinthine impulses are transmitted to the motor neurons in the anterior horns of the spinal cord through the vestibulospinal tract, reinforcing local myotactic reflexes in the extensor muscles of the trunk and extremities producing support for the body in the maintenance of upright posture.
4 Fibres from the vestibular nuclei ascend via the medial longitudinal fasciculus and constitute the vestibulomesencephalic tract, which is distributed to the cranial nerves supplying the ocular muscles (Eviatar and Eviatar, 1978).

5 Central connections are to the reticular formation and basal ganglia while the vestibular system is represented cortically at the level of the posterior superior gyrus of the temporal lobe. From here it is suggested that inhibitory and facilitatory reflexes are transmitted to the lower vestibular centres (Cantor, 1971).

Thus labyrinthine, visual and somatosensory inputs converge within the 'central vestibular system' in order to subserve dynamic spatial orientation and to control eye movements, posture and locomotion. This integration of both vestibular and motor responses is believed to occur at the level of the red nucleus (Brandt, Dieterich and Büchele, 1986).

Development and maturation of vestibular function

At birth the labyrinth is morphologically complete but functionally immature (Pignataro *et al.*, 1979). The responses of children to vestibular stimulation are not only different from those of adults but even differ within the childhood age span with the most marked maturational changes taking place in pre-school children (Ornitz *et al.*, 1979). The development of vestibular-based function can be divided into two main categories:

1 General motor development as it pertains to posture
2 Specific development of stable vision in the presence of head movement.

While motor milestones and developmental reflexes are more the terrain of the developmental paediatrician, an understanding of such processes is essential for the otolaryngologist with an interest in paediatric disorders. A basic account of the postural reactions and vestibulocular physiology is given as a background, against which the clinical disorders will be considered later.

Posture

When the newborn baby is held ventrally suspended with a hand under the abdomen, the head will drop down. By 6 weeks the baby can hold it in the plane of the body and by 12 weeks above that plane for prolonged periods.

When the baby is pulled to a sitting position the initial lack of head control is obvious as the head lags behind and then flops forward, but by 16 weeks head control is such that the baby can look around while sitting. By 36 weeks the infant can sit unsupported for several minutes. The baby now attempts to crawl and at 1 year crawls on hands and knees, shuffles on the buttocks and pulls himself to standing holding onto furniture.

At 15 months most babies can walk alone with uneven steps, feet apart, arms slightly flexed and held above head or shoulder level for balance (Sheridan, 1975; Illingworth, 1983; Sidebotham, 1988).

As many of the earliest activities of infants are concerned with overcoming the influences of gravity, a sequence of neurological chain reactions develops, such that an initial movement makes it easier for certain other movements to follow. In addition to the kinaesthetic stimuli, visual, auditory and sensori-motor links develop to provide information which reveals the results of previous movements and enables the brain to assimilate and modify future locomotion (Holt, 1975).

The reader is referred to the above authors for a complete account of this dynamic sequential change in posture and movement. A selected number of responses will be described to demonstrate the maturational changes that occur in infancy and early childhood.

Postural reactions

In the small infant up to the age of 4 months the principal reactions are primarily tonic neck responses. The Moro reflex is the best known of these and is performed by supporting the baby along the examiner's hand and forearm with the head slightly ventro-flexed. The head is permitted to drop backwards through about 30° in relation to the trunk. Sudden bilateral extension of the upper limbs is followed by flexion. A similar response may be obtained by jarring the cot suddenly. A variation of this test, suggested by Eviatar and Eviatar (1978), prevents head movement thus eliminating proprioceptive input from the neck muscles. The infant is held horizontally on the examiner's forearms and motion is induced by the examiner dropping from the standing position to the crouching position by bending the knees. The appropriate response for the baby is slight dorsiflexion of the head and abduction and extension of the arms with fanning of the hands (Figure 12.1).

The *doll's eye response* is usually demonstrable in full-term babies during the first 2 weeks of life, persisting longer in the premature infant (Eviatar and Eviatar, 1974). With the baby held at arm's length facing towards the examiner, rotation of the baby around the examiner's axis produces deviation of the eyes and head opposite to the direction of rotation. This eye deviation represents vestibular activity, but lacks the fast component of nystagmus generated by the saccadic system which is still immature at birth. As the child matures nystagmus occurs, with the quick component in the direction of the rotation (Figure 12.2).

Between 4 and 6 months the primitive tonic neck reflexes are gradually replaced by the righting responses, depending on the maturity of the individual. For example, from 4 months the infant will tilt the

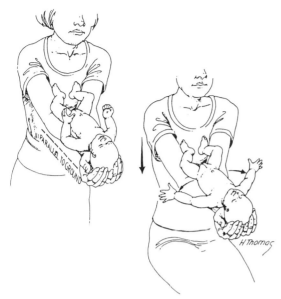

Figure 12.1 Moro reflex variation. (Reproduced from Electronystagmography and vestibular testing in children, in: *Otologic Medicine and Surgery* edited by P. W. Alberti and R. J. Ruben, New York: Churchill Livingstone, 1988 by kind permission of the authors, editors and publishers)

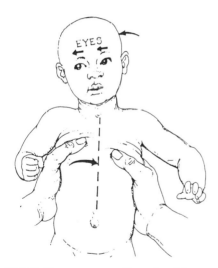

Figure 12.2 Doll's eye response. (Reproduced from Electronystagmography and vestibular testing in children, in: *Otologic Medicine and Surgery* edited by P. W. Alberti and R. J. Ruben, New York: Churchill Livingstone, 1988 by kind permission of the authors, editors and publishers)

head to maintain it vertical if the trunk is tilted through 30° (oblique suspension). At 5 months this manoeuvre is accompanied by the lower limbs moving away from the side to which the infant has been tilted (Snashall, 1987; MacKeith and Robson,

1970). These responses are variously described as head righting, propping, hopping and buttress reactions (Figure 12.3) and are elicited by rapidly changing the centre of gravity of the infant, thus initiating a vestibular response which induces head righting, whereby the mouth and eyes become horizontal to the ground (Eviatar and Eviatar, 1978).

These reflexes result from the integration of visual, proprioceptive and vestibular stimuli at the level of the red nucleus. Ideally they are best assessed with the infant or child blindfolded so as to reduce visual input, or optical righting reflexes.

While these responses may form the basis of future postural control, e.g. the 'propping reaction' in the maintenance of equilibrium in sitting and the 'hopping reaction' aiding in the acquistion of walking balance (Eviatar and Eviatar, 1978), there is also a basic protective reaction which may be demonstrable at this age and which may persist throughout life. This is termed the 'parachute reaction' and is felt to represent visual-vestibular interaction (Wenzel, 1978). In the downward parachute, the baby is held in vertical suspension and moved suddenly downwards. Up to 5 months of age this elicits the Moro response, but above this age the lower limbs extend and abduct. Finally, such responses must be interpreted in the light of the child's development as a whole, as the parameters of development, motor, vision and fine movements, hearing and speech, social behaviour and spontaneous play, may not concurrently proceed at equal rates (Sheridan, 1975). With age the child will be better able to cooperate with the clinical tasks and electrophysiological investigations which will be described later in the chapter.

Stability of vision

Vestibular and optic reflexes permit us to keep the eyes fixed on stationary objects while the head and body are in motion. Movement of the head to the right, for example, causes a relative flow of endolymph in the horizontal semicircular canals directed to the left, due to fluid inertia, which makes it lag behind the movement of the head (Eviatar and Eviatar, 1978). Vestibular impulses, sent to the abducens and oculomotor nuclei, induce a slow movement of the eyes to the left in order to counteract head movement and maintain the original field of vision. As the eyes reach maximal deviation, they quickly jerk back to the mid position. A rapid sequence of such movements consisting of both slow movements and quick jerks is termed nystagmus and represents the objective visual evidence of vestibular-optic activity, from which we indirectly glean information about the physiology and pathology of these pathways. The direction of nystagmus is designated in accordance with the direction of the fast component.

There are thus two systems involved in the generation of these movements:

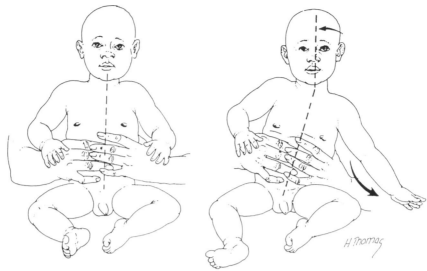

Figure 12.3 Buttress reaction. (Reproduced from Electronystagmography and vestibular testing in children, in: *Otologic Medicine and Surgery* edited by P. W. Alberti and R. J. Ruben, New York: Churchill Livingstone, 1988 by kind permission of the authors, editors and publishers)

1 The *smooth pursuit system*, or visual tracking, which can be seen during the slow phase of nystagmus when a person tries to follow a slow-moving target (30°/s)
2 The *saccadic system* which generates all fast eye movements, including the fast component of nystagmus and microsaccades involved in fixation. The saccadic system is used when the target movement becomes too fast to track by the slow pursuit system. It has a short latency period (200 ms) and can initiate very rapid eye movements.

A third system, termed *vergence*, functions to turn the eyes towards or away from each other in order to follow an object as it moves closer or further away (Gay *et al.*, 1974; Gilligan *et al.*, 1981).

Vestibular responses to an equivalent stimulus, be it rotational or caloric, are markedly different between adults and children in whom the vestibular system is still maturing functionally (Jongkees and Gasthuis, 1973). Electronystagmography (ENG) is routinely used in combination with perrotatory and caloric tests to demonstrate more accurately, assess and quantify the nystagmic response to these tests. Thus the vestibulo-ocular activity emanating from the two labyrinths may be compared and the different responses from birth to adulthood obtained.

Developmental responses to rotational and caloric stimulation

In neonates rotation is most conveniently achieved by holding the infant at arm's length in vertical suspension, while the examiner rotates about her own axis, with the infant on the circumference looking inwards. The eyes will open and deviate in the direction opposite to that of the rotation (Snashall, 1987). For the first few weeks of life there will be deviation alone, followed at 4–6 weeks by the superimposition of visible nystagmus (Groen, 1965).

Various methods have been used to induce nystagmus in neonates, infants and small children. These have included electrically rotating tables (Pendleton and Paine, 1961), torsion swing and calorics (Eviatar and Eviatar, 1979; Eviatar *et al.*, 1979), an electromechanically controlled rotating chair (Goebel and Aust, 1978; Aust and Goebel, 1979) and impulsive acceleration (Tibbling, 1969).

Given the different methodologies employed, a pattern of development becomes apparent. Vestibular function is present at birth, increases in strength to 6–9 months of age and exhibits its greatest degree of responsiveness from 6–12 months. Thereafter a relatively rapid decline in activity occurs to 30 months of age followed by a more gradual decrease in reactivity levels until adult values are reached by 10–14 years (Ornitz, 1983). Of interest is the fact that premature or small for gestational age babies, whose nystagmic responses initially lag behind the norm, show a similar response rate by 6 months (Eviatar, Eviatar and Naray, 1974).

Development of vestibular function therefore is accompanied by high levels of vestibular stimulation (Henriksson, 1955) and peripheral activity (Weeks, 1979) coupled with the gradual imposition of central inhibition (Groen, 1963), cerebellar control (Hood, 1980) and central vestibular adaptation (Ornitz *et al.*, 1979).

Thus heightened vestibular reactivity in the infant and toddler may be related to the development of postural control during a period of rapid acquistion of new motor skills. Further research is required to elucidate the visual–vestibular interactions that accompany these vestibular developments (Ornitz *et al.*, 1974; Wenzel, 1978; Kenyon, 1991).

Clinical disorders

Young children are unable to provide the clinician with an accurate history of the vertigo or dysequilibrium. In many instances reliance must be placed upon an observant parent for a description of the specific attack or recurrent events.

Most otolaryngologists do not have a detailed knowledge of developmental paediatrics. As many of the conditions producing dysequilibrium in childhood are not specifically otological in their aetiology, it is recommended that the approach to the vertiginous child should be multidisciplinary, involving close co-operation between otologist, paediatrician, paediatric neurologist and ophthalmologist. Such an approach should permit more accurate diagnosis and in terms of outcome allow one to:

1 Recognize and if necessary treat those conditions which can be identified with a reasonable degree of certainty
2 Exclude serious underlying conditions
3 Follow up the child until diagnosed or the symptom has settled
4 Reassure the parents and child (Blayney and Colman, 1983).

History taking

The importance of the history cannot be overemphasized, as physical examination frequently reveals no abnormality in these children. Attacks of vertigo may start before the age of 2 years, with the child suddenly crying out and dropping to the floor, crawling, or clinging to the parent's leg for support until the acute episode has waned. This may occur quite quickly with rapid resumption of play or alternatively ataxia may be observed. Pallor, sweating or vomiting may accompany the more severe attack. Vertigo should be suspected if the child lies face down wedged against the side of the cot with the eyes closed, not wanting to be moved (Farmer, 1964).

An accurate history may be forthcoming such as, 'the skies are falling, the world is going around', (Snashall, 1987) or 'the walls are falling in' (Blayney and Colman, 1983). Headache may be present if the attack is accompanied by screaming.

As in the adult a full description of the attack should be eludicated including age and speed of onset, frequency, periodicity, duration, speed and manner of recovery, associated loss of consciousness, amnesia, lassitude, postictal sleep or drowsiness, wetting, precipitating or aggravating factors and sequelae.

Specific areas to be explored

Ear disease

Are the attacks of vertigo associated with otological symptoms such as hearing loss or tinnitus? Has there been a recent episode of acute suppurative otitis media or an exacerbation of serous otitis/ glue ear? Is there a recent history of offensive otorrhoea, exertion, barotrauma, or head injury involving the ear or resulting in clear or bloody discharge from the ear? Has the child had recent measles or mumps with otological involvement, or has the child been inoculated against these diseases?

Eye symptoms

Is there a history of photophobia, ocular palsy, nystagmus or visual aura?

CNS symptoms

Are the attacks associated with motor or speech problems, bizarre movements, hemiparesis or paraesthesiae? Has the child's development been normal or were the milestones delayed? Are school performance and learning ability within the normal range? Is the child spatially disorientated in the dark, afraid of swings or roundabouts, or does motion sickness pose a problem? Has there been a recent head injury or does the child get intermittent torticollis?

Infection

Has the child had meningitis, or has there been a reluctance to mobilize following the acute phase of a viral illness suggestive of labyrinthine involvement. Labyrinthitis usually occurs in relation to the acute phase of a viral illness as opposed to cerebral ataxia which presents 7–10 days after the event.

Past history

Does the child suffer from any renal or endocrine disease, any physical deformity, serious medical disorder, or psychological disturbance which might have a bearing on his condition? Is the child taking phenytoin for epilepsy control, amitriptyline for enuresis or piperazine for threadworm infestation? Has the child been exposed to the potentially ototoxic effects of aminoglycosides as a consequence of maternal treatment for severe infection during pregnancy, or for personal treatment of perinatal sepsis?

Family history

Is there a family history of migraine, epilepsy, deafness, endocrine or renal disease? Infections which cross the placental barrier, such as syphilis must be considered, as more than one sibling may be affected.

Finally, an attempt is made to define whether the dysequilibrium is due to a primary vestibular defect as opposed to ataxia due to CNS disease (Beddoe, 1977). It is important to distinguish delay and arrest in motor and postural function from deterioration, as the latter is more likely to denote posterior fossa disease (Curless, 1980).

Physical examination

This should include otolaryngological, neurological and developmental examination:

1 Complete otolaryngological examination
2 Neurological examination: including hand–eye coordination, cranial nerves, tendon reflexes, tone, developmental abnormalities, congenital defects and syndromes, abnormal movements
3 Vision and eye movements: visual acuity, ophthalmoscopy, heterochromia, nystagmus, cover test for latent strabismus, pursuit, convergence
4 Postural control: righting reflexes, positional nystagmus, heel-toe walking, Romberg's test, hopping, kicking a ball, gait, stance
5 General examination: congenital defects, pigmentation, musculoskeletal defects, heart sounds.

Investigations

These should be selected in a logical manner, the clinician's own judgement determining which child requires full vestibular assessment and radiological investigation to make or exclude a certain diagnosis.

Auditory tests

Pure-tone audiometry should be performed in all children capable of providing reliable responses, supported by speech discrimination and tympanometry.

Electrophysiological tests

An EEG should be done in all children presenting with persistent or progressive dysequilibrium. Likewise evoked response audiometry may readily be included in the scheme of investigation.

Blood tests

Serology

Screening for congenital syphilis is mandatory in all children with progressive cochlear or vestibular dysfunction in the first or second decade. Viral screening is useful if congenital deafness is present. Full blood count and ESR is routine. An autoimmune profile is indicated if fluctuating hearing loss is present.

Blood chemistry

Sugar, creatinine, calcium phosphate, electrolytes, T3 and T4 are advocated.

Radiological

Skull, sinuses and mastoid X-rays as indicated, but in reality most children presenting with a vestibular disorder will now undergo a CT scan or MRI in order to rule out any potential intracranial pathology or aid in its localization and assessement. Inner ear abnormalities associated with vestibular dysfunction may be revealed.

Urinalysis

Estimation of urinary protein, sugar and red blood cells is carried out.

Vestibular tests

Snashall (1993) emphasized that there is still a need for the classical tests of vestibular function. Most of the lesions causing vertigo are in the inner ear and are therefore not demonstrable by imaging techniques or evoked response testing.

With the increasing awareness of the vertigo syndromes in childhood, there is a need for a better understanding of vestibular function and objective measurement of it. Thus electronystagmography (ENG) has been applied to the different tests of vestibular function in childhood in order to try to establish objective reproducible results for the various tests at different ages. As the methodology of testing varies significantly between laboratories, the parameters of testing need to be taken into account when comparing results. Each laboratory needs to establish its own baseline values for the different tests involved.

ENG permits evaluation of vestibular function without the influence of visual and proprioceptive input. As a result of stimulation, changes in the magnetic field generated by eye movements are picked up by two electrodes placed bitemporally. Amplification of this potential is used to produce displacement on a pen recording strip, which in turn acts as a permanent record of the eye movements that have taken place. Mathematical calculations of the nystagmus frequency, amplitude and velocity can subsequently be performed.

Factors affecting vestibular testing in infants and children

1 Eye closure inhibits nystagmus (Tjernstrom, 1973). This is considered to result from vertical eyeball deviation (Bell's phenomenon). Optimum results for vestibular induced nystagmus are obtained with eyes open in the dark.
2 Mental tasking, e.g. mental arithmetic, has a releasing effect on horizontal nystagmus.
3 Maintenance of attention during test procedure. It is difficult to maintain the child in a constant state of alertness. The child may fall asleep, as often happens during torsion swing stimulation (Pignatoro *et al.*, 1979). Testing infants midway between meals and appeasing them with a drink may help, as does the recitation of nursery rhymes by the technician in order to maintain alertness (Eviatar and Eviatar, 1979). Ornitz *et al.* (1979) suggested the use of an infrared TV system and EEG monitoring in absolute darkness to aid the acquistion of an optimum trace.
4 Anatomical: narrow external canals may lead to inequalities in caloric irrigation and thus variable results. Maintenance of the child's head in the correct position throughout the course of a caloric or rotational test may likewise prove difficult.
5 Neurological immaturity of eye movement control:
  a Defective stability of gaze produces excessive miniature random eye movements of the drift variety which are particularly evident with the eyes closed and to a lesser extent open in the dark (Carpenter, 1977). This may make interpretation of ENG traces in children difficult (Snashall, 1983).
  b Saccadic movements are present at birth but not accurate until later, infants frequently requiring more than one saccade to reach their target and they may overshoot (Bower, Broughton and Moore, 1971).
  c Smooth pursuit is possible only at low velocities, reflecting foveal immaturity (Kremenitzer *et al.*, 1979). At greater velocities, catching-up saccades are required (Herman, Maulucci and Stuyck, 1982).
  d Infant optokinetic nystagmus differs strikingly from that of adults in that tonic ocular deviation is in the direction of field movement rather than away from it, i.e. in the direction of the slow phase as opposed to the fast one, as in adults (Kremenitzer *et al.*, 1979).
  e Visual stimulation alone causes a sensation that is perceptually identical to that produced by rotation. Vision therefore not only provides an image of the surrounding environment but also aids exteroceptive self-orientation. Peripheral retinal vision is believed to subserve this spatial orientation activity and is independent of the direction of eye movement (Brandt, Dichgans and Koenig 1973; Brandt, Wist and Dichgans, 1975). This complex visual–vestibular interaction in the acquistion of motor skills increases with maturity.
  f Inexperience with test procedures and difficulty in cooperation.

The methodology must therefore be adapted to take into consideration the effect of inattention and immaturity on performance and the resultant ENG trace obtained. As with adults, a quantitative measurement of the vestibular response to stimulation requires recording conditions that are properly controlled for the state of arousal, the effects of visual input and eye closure, proper head position, contamination by artefact due to muscle tension, head movement and adventitious eye movements (Ornitz, 1983).

In attempting to define the presence or absence of normal vestibular function in an infant or child, a selection of different procedures may be used depending upon the patient's age and potential for cooperation. The result obtained therefore reflects the summation of the responses demonstrated by the different test methods. The proposed methods of testing described below represent the broad approach of a number of investigators in this field.

Calibration, gaze and ocular dysmetria

According to Cyr (1980), calibration of the recording unit, as well as gaze testing, can be accomplished with the use of a standard light bar in 3–4 year olds, while painted lamp shades with cartoon characters and an option for motion or light have proved effective in children down to the age of 6 months. The child's eyes will follow the light back and forth giving a calibration trace. Gaze testing can be performed to the right and left by stabilizing the head and alternating the activity of the light sources. In the infant, eye tracking can be accomplished by what Cyr (1980) describes as the modified 'doll's head' manoeuvre. The infant lies in the parent's arms, in a rocking chair, gazing at a lighted toy dangling above him. This permits evaluation of centre gaze and demonstrates pathological nystagmus if present. By gently rocking the chair, the head 'rotates' around the eyes creating a sinusoidal trace on ENG. While basic in its concept, this method may yield information regarding disconjugate eye movements, ocular muscle pathology or visual pursuit pathology above 5–6 months of age.

Positional testing

Positional testing can be performed in infants and children as in adults. The method of testing will obviously take into account the patient's age, an infant being tested on a table or held in the parent's arms, while an older child may cooperate independently. Testing is performed, if possible, in the prone, supine and lateral positions and in the infant with the head supported looking straight ahead and turned to the left and right. While Eviatar and Eviatar (1988) propose that such testing be performed with the patient blindfolded, this may prove unacceptable to the young patient and an alternative method would be to test the infant in the dark (in order to abolish visual suppression), monitoring the degree of alertness using an infrared viewer (Snashall, 1987).

Optokinetic tracking (OKN)

Optokinetic tracking can be measured in very young children with a drum that fits over the child's head and fills a good portion of the child's visual field (Cyr, 1980).

A hand-held drum may just test the visual pursuit system and as this is not myelinated until the fourth or fifth month of life it is not surprising that an OKN test with a hand-held drum yields poor results below this age and frequently even with older children (Snashall, 1987).

Projected cartoon characters or a filmstrip moving from right to left and vice versa at speeds ranging from 4°/s to 30°/s may be more applicable to 3–4 year olds, while older children may respond to the presentation of vertical or horizontal lines in sequence, as would an adult (Eviatar and Eviatar, 1988).

Abnormalities may be related to ocular problems, visual field defects due to damage to optic tracts or radiations, and frontal or cerebellar lesions. It is worth remembering that the pathways subserving optokinetic nystagmus are different from those for vestibular nystagmus.

Perrotational tests

Rotation responses, either to sinusoidal harmonic rotation or to ramp acceleration and deceleration are feasible in children (Snashall, 1987). Once perrotatory nystagmus is elicited, its quality remains unchanged regardless of age and level of central nervous system maturation. This 'all or none' phenomenon represents the vestibular response to threshold physiological bilateral labyrinthine stimulation (Eviatar and Eviatar, 1979).

Both Cyr (1980) and Eviatar and Eviatar (1978) suggest that perrotatory nystagmus is best produced by the use of a torsion swing which provides alternating angular acceleration of 180° to the right and left at a rate of 10 revolutions/60 s. Several commercial systems are now available. Testing is performed with the child sitting upright in the chair or on a parent's lap, the head flexed 30° forwards to align the horizontal semicircular canals parallel with the ground. By rotating the chair alternatively to the left and right

through a 180° arc, a cupular deviation in an ampullopetal and ampullofugal direction occurs producing nystagmus in opposite directions with each half cycle of rotation.

A right-beating nystagmus burst is recorded when the chair swings to the right and a left-beating nystagmus when the chair swings to the left. The number of beats that occur in each direction are calculated for a given period of time. According to Eviatar and Eviatar (1979), the most reliable variables for the method used appear to be the speed of the slow component and the number of beats per 10 s. The total duration of nystagmus is a valid measure of intensity of response but is subject to much greater variability.

In a normal response an approximately equal number of nystagmic beats should occur in both directions. If the number of beats in one direction exceeds that in the other direction by 25%, this is considered to represent a directional preponderance in favour of the greater side. In the very young infant, a nystagmic response may be replaced by a sinusoidal curve denoting the conjugate eye movement in the direction opposite the direction of rotation (doll's eye movement). Nystagmic beats may become superimposed upon this trace until a standard alternating nystagmic pattern is attained.

A directional preponderance is seen in the presence of a central lesion or labyrinthine imbalance. Cyr (1980) makes the point, however, that if a child has a unilateral direction-fixed nystagmus, perrotatory testing will have the effect of producing a summation of the spontaneous nystagmus and the ipsilateral rotation-induced nystagmus in one direction, while apparently negating the spontaneous nystagmus when rotation is induced in the other direction to it. This could falsely lead one to conclude that a unilateral lesion is present.

Torsion swing testing is not an unpleasant experience for children, it may even be enjoyable. Three hundred and sixty degrees rotation on the Bárány chair may, on the contrary, be a sickening affair. In certain instances, however, of inner ear anomaly associated with a lack of lateral semicircular canals, a lack of perrotatory nystagmus on Bárány rotation testing may indicate a more marked developmental delay than in those cases where nystagmus is elicited by both damped rotation and Bárány testing (Tsuzuku and Kaga, 1991).

Huygen *et al.* (1993) described a study of the vestibulo-ocular reflex in pupils at a school for hearing-impaired children. They used a velocity step (VS) test rather than the older Bárány technique.

Caloric tests

The ice-cold caloric test is a crude non-physiological method of driving the labyrinth in a way totally different from everyday normal physiological function. It is probably unpleasant for the infant and therefore should be reserved for cases where serious doubt exists regarding vestibular function, such as abnormal responses to torsion swing, ototoxic drug exposure, delayed head and postural control and congenital deafness. With age there tends to be a higher frequency of nystagmus, a higher amplitude of beats and a higher speed of the slow component in response to both the ice-cold caloric test and perrotatory stimulation, reaching a plateau at about 18–24 months (Eviatar and Eviatar, 1979). Snashall (1987) recommends that a DC machine should be utilized for recording ENG responses to both caloric and perrotatory tests as this tends to diminish the likelihood of adventitious eye movements which may occur with an AC machine.

Eviatar and Eviatar (1988) propose that this test should be performed with the infant blindfolded in the supine position, using irrigation with ice-cold water lasting 10 s (spout temperature 5°C). The nystagmus towards the opposite ear is present in the vast majority of full-term infants, but in only 20% of premature and small for gestational date (SGA) babies within the first 3 months. As soon as a response is obtained, the baby is turned prone, thus reversing the nystagmus and confirming the presence of an active labyrinth.

A unilaterally depressed response suggests an ipsilateral hypoactive labyrinth. Bilateral suppression may indicate sleep or drowsiness or may accompany ototoxic drug exposure. Middle ear infection may produce an 'exaggerated' response.

In very premature infants the ice-cold caloric test produces lateral deviation of the ipsilateral eye towards the stimulated ear. Medial deviation of the contralateral eye, however, may not occur, thus demonstrating disconjugate movement suggestive of an internuclear ophthalmoplegia. This is considered to be secondary to immaturity of the medial longitudinal fasciculus (Donat, Donat and Lay, 1980).

By 36 months of age most children will accept a bithermal caloric test. As with other vestibular tests acceptance of the test is helped by the display of a photograph of a child wearing electrodes (Snashall, 1987).

The Jongkees formula (Jongkees and Philipszoon, 1964; Jongkees and Gasthuis, 1973) may be used to determine labyrinthine or directional preponderance (RW = right ear warm water, RC = right ear cold water, LW = left ear warm water, LC = left ear cold water).

Labyrinthine preponderance:

$$\frac{(RW + RC) - (LW + LC)}{(RW + RC) + (LW + LC)} \times 100 > 14\%$$

Directional preponderance:

$$\frac{(RW + LC) - (LW + RC)}{(RW + LC) + (LW + RC)} \times 100 > 18\%$$

The presence of directional preponderance in children is strongly suggestive of central vestibular pathology. Labyrinthine preponderance correlates with the presence of peripheral organ disease or an VIIIth nerve lesion. Labyrinthine preponderance is considered synonymous with a hypoactive labyrinth. The combination of both directional and labyrinthine preponderance in a young patient is suggestive of a central lesion, though a peripheral one cannot be ruled out (Eviatar and Wassertheil, 1971).

Another variation of the caloric test uses a closed loop system attached to an ear probe with an inflatable silicone balloon on the end. Water can thus circulate within the balloon at different temperatures and at a fixed flow rate. Because it is a closed system, simultaneous binaural bithermal irrigation and testing may be performed (Brookler, 1976). As both labyrinths are stimulated simultaneously this rules out interaural variability in testing. Stimulation of one labyrinth negates stimulation of the other and therefore little vertigo is experienced. This test shows that the labyrinthine activity is equal, but one side needs to be independently tested to ensure that the system is active and not, for example, bilaterally hypoactive (Cyr, 1980).

Other tests

Three other tests are worth mentioning in this category and while not widely used in paediatric practice can readily be performed in the older and more cooperative child.

Vestibulospinal stability test

This investigation basically consists of the Romberg test performed on a platform with computer-controlled assessment of centre of mass determinations (Black *et al.*, 1977). It may be employed objectively and quantitatively to study spatially disorientated subjects. A minimum patient time is required (2 minutes), the procedure is non-invasive and can be done as soon as the child is capable of cooperating (and standing still).

Dynamic posturography

The maintenance of balance depends upon input from the three sensory modalities: visual, vestibular and somatosensory. Vestibular input is referenced to gravity, while both somatosensory and visual input are influenced by earth-based support surface and visual surrounds. Dynamic posturography uses a movable platform designed to isolate the relative contributions of visual, somatosensory and vestibular feedback in the maintenance of balance, thus highlighting where the defect lies (Mirka and Black, 1990).

The pressure receptors of the feet and the proprioceptive system are of major importance in compensating for the vestibular defect in children with congenital or early acquired bilateral vestibular loss (Enbom, Magnusson and Pyykkö, 1991).

Harmonic acceleration

This consists of a computer-controlled chair system which produces sinusoidal harmonic acceleration (0.01–0.16 Hz). It may be more accurate and less aversive than ENG/rotation/calorics and is also applicable to the study of the vestibulo-ocular reflex arc. While providing reliable information regarding vestibular function, like simultaneous binaural bithermal irrigation it does not localize peripheral abnormalities in terms of an 'involved ear', but rather tests the system as a whole (Staller, Goin and Hildebrandt, 1986).

Causes of vertigo in childhood

The conditions causing vertigo in childhood may be classically described as being either peripheral or central in origin (Table 12.1). In the vestibular system a lesion is conventionally described as peripheral when the site of the lesion is either at the level of the end organ or the first vestibular neuron. A central disorder indicates a lesion above the first vestibular neuron.

Table 12.1 Causes of vertigo in childhood

Peripheral causes	Central causes
Congenital vestibular defects	Congenital skull anomalies
Wax	Migraine-related disorders:
Otitis media with effusion (glue ear)	paroxysmal torticollis of infancy (PTI)
Infection:	benign paroxysmal vertigo
suppurative otitis media	of childhood (BPVC)
cholesteatoma	basilar artery migraine
labyrinthitis	Infection
Trauma	Trauma
Benign paroxysmal positional vertigo (BPPV)	Neoplasia
	Demyelination
Perilymph fistula	Seizure disorders (epilepsy)
Ototoxic drugs and irradiation	Hereditary cerebellar ataxias
Vestibular neuronitis	Hereditary disease of the
Menière's disease	peripheral and cranial nerves

Other causes
Metabolic: hyperlipidosis, hypothyroidism, anaemia, diabetes mellitus
Psychosomatic: hyperventilation
Vestibular disorders associated with abnormal development, behaviour and learning ability
Motion sickness

While the division into peripheral and central causes is convenient, certain conditions may present in either terrain, e.g. infection may spread from the periphery (middle ear) to produce a peripheral labyrinthitis or from a central focus (meningitis) via the cochlear aqueduct again producing a peripheral labyrinthitis. Trauma to the head and ear again may produce both peripheral and central manifestations.

Table 12.2 describes the causes of vertigo in a series of 27 children, with an age range of 18 months – 15 years, who presented to an ENT clinic over an 18 month period (Blayney and Colman, 1984). Snashall (1986) reported a series in which the distribution of diagnoses were very similar.

Table 12.2 Causes of vertigo in 27 children aged 18 months–15 years

Diagnosis	No. cases
Serous otitis/glue ear	5
Benign paroxysmal vertigo	5
Post-traumatic vertigo	1
Labyrinthine fistula	1
Labyrinthitis	3
Migraine	2
Epilepsy	1
Tumour	1
Undiagnosed	8
Total	27

Peripheral causes

Congenital vestibular defect

A congenital vestibular defect frequently accompanies sensorineural hearing loss in childhood. It is often overlooked in the assessment of the child, as the more definitively measurable deafness takes precedence. While vestibular hypofunction may contribute to the handicap of Down's syndrome (Zarnoch, 1980), vestibular dysfunction may only be suspected if frank vertigo or dysequilibrium results in investigation which reveals an anatomical abnormality of the vestibular system on CT scanning (Brama, 1985). Gradual loss of vestibular activity in a child may be asymptomatic even when monitored over a period of time. Disorientation in the dark may prove the only disability (Longridge, 1989). Children with bilateral congenital or early acquired vestibular loss compensate for this loss more by somatosensory input than by visual input as occurs in adults (Magnusson, Enbom and Pyykkö, 1991).

It has been suggested that children with congenital sensorineural deafness should have vestibular investigations. Sandberg and Terkildsen (1965) showed fair correlation between the degree of hearing loss and the vestibular response. The vestibular function was normal in 80% of patients with a hearing level better than 90 dB and in only 20% when the loss was greater than 98 dB. Brookhouser, Cyr and Beauchaine (1982) suggested that mental alerting was necessary with this group to prevent central suppression and that by using the Jendrassik manoeuvre with the tandem Romberg, a high degree of correlation was demonstrated with those children who had vestibular hypoactivity on ENG. The identification of a vestibular defect allowed for counselling with regard to sport and recreational activities. Unfortunately, there is a lack of significant correlation between auditory brain stem responses and vestibular tests during the first year of life, i.e. at a time when such information would be useful (Brookhouser *et al.*, 1991)

Delay in motor development suggests a variety of disabilities such as cerebral palsy, mental retardation and minimal brain dysfunction. Failure correctly to identify a peripheral vestibular lesion may lead to increased anxiety in the parents, or even a misdiagnosis of neurological impairment (Kaga *et al.*, 1981). In order to avoid this error in the case of hearing impaired children who have 'floppy' heads, or who are late walkers, Rapin (1974) emphasized that all deaf children should routinely undergo vestibular testing. It must be remembered that children with spastic cerebral palsy may yield no response to damped-rotation testing, but that vestibular responses appear at a later stage and increase as the children develop (Takiguchi *et al.*, 1991).

Vestibular dysfunction forms part of the picture of a number of rare conditions encountered in childhood including: Waardenburg's syndrome (Schweitzer and Clack, 1984), Hurler's syndrome (Friedmann *et al.*, 1985) and Usher's syndrome, (Kumar, Fishman and Torok, 1984; Karjalainen *et al.*, 1985; Möller *et al.*, 1989). In Waardenburg's syndrome 30% of patients have congenital vestibular failure, in Hurler's syndrome the lesion affects the vestibulocochlear nerve, while in Usher's syndrome congenital severe hearing loss, absent vestibular responses and the early onset of retinitis pigmentosa distinguish type I from type II, in which the vestibular responses are normal.

Wax

Impacted wax may cause dysequilibrium. The exact cause is unknown, but an articulate child may well remark on the cessation of the symptom following removal of an impacted bolus.

Otitis media with effusion

The occurrence of vertigo or dysequilibrium in childhood, related to eustachian tube dysfunction or middle ear effusion, is infrequently alluded to during the standard paediatric otolaryngological history-taking process (Clinical Otolaryngology, 1978; Blayney and

Colman, 1983). According to Snashall (1987) 50% of children with serous otitis media may have some balance disorder.

The degree of dysequilibrium experienced by the child varies and may not parallel the clinical findings, often being absent even in the most intractable case of otitis media with effusion.

Episodes may take the form of 'falling all over the place', 'walking clumsily' or 'walking into things'. The child may trip easily, or even fall when walking on a flat surface. Less frequently the symptom may amount to true rotational vertigo.

The dizziness accompanying glue ear settles following myringotomy and grommet insertion (Golz *et al*, 1991). Indeed the presence of dizziness may be an added indication for grommet insertion in cases of otitis media with effusion. If the dysequilibrium does not settle following grommet insertion then another aetiology should be suspected.

The precise mechanism of this symptom remains uncertain and the middle ear abnormality may vary from mild eustachian tube dysfunction to dense glue ear with superadded infection. In the former the unsteadiness may be due to transient negative middle ear pressure changes, associated with displacement of the round window membrane, leading to secondary movement of perilymph. In the latter it may be due to a serous labyrinthitis secondary to the episodic superadded infection of a middle ear effusion (Blayney and Colman, 1983).

Infection

Suppurative otitis media, cholesteatoma and labyrinthitis

The occurrence of acute suppurative labyrinthitis secondary to acute suppurative otitis media or bony invasion of the labyrinth by cholesteatoma producing fistula formation is well recognized. Pain may be present.

Bacterial infection is transmitted to the labyrinth via the middle ear or alternatively from meningeal infection via the cochlear aqueduct. Any child with a persistently discharging ear or attic disease in association with vertigo should have a fistula test performed. Early exploration must be considered if there is not a rapid response to antibiotic treatment.

Meningitis caused by *Streptococcus pneumoniae* or pneumococcal meningitis is associated with purulent otitis media in 20–30% of cases, with deafness occurring in 30% of the survivors (Nadol, 1978; Bohr, Hansen and Jessen, 1983; Dodge, Davis and Feigin, 1984). Rasmussen, Johnsen and Bohr (1991) suggest that preadmission treatment with antibiotics in cases of suspected 'otogenic meningitis', appeared to protect from acousticovestibular damage and did not hamper the diagnosis by lumbar puncture. As deafness due to meningitis is accompanied by loss of vestibular function in 66% of cases (Arnvig, 1955) early treatment of suspected bacterial meningitis may result in less auditory and vestibular damage.

Infection with congenital syphilis presents with deafness, tinnitus and vertigo in a pattern not dissimilar to hydrops (Wilson and Zoller, 1981). Viral labyrinthitis is the most common labyrinthine infection. Two general patterns of viral infection occur:

1 An endolymphatic labyrinthitis secondary to viraemia via the stria vascularis in rubella, mumps, rubeola and cytomegalovirus (CMV)
2 A perilymphatic infection secondary to meningeal, perineural or endoneural spread is seen in varicella-zoster (Strauss and Davis, 1973).

The part played by the viruses mumps, measles and varicella is well recognized in the genesis of sudden deafness in both adults and children (Rowson, Hinchcliffe and Gamble, 1976; Tieri *et al.*, 1984). In children the diagnosis may be missed at the time of the original infectious disease, as the child may be too young to describe the hearing loss and the lack of mobility may be ascribed to the illness itself rather than to vertigo as such. The vertigo may subside in a few days without recognition of labyrinthine involvement. Subsequent caloric weakness may be demonstrated even in the absence of vertigo (Hydén, Odkvist and Kylén, 1979). Involvement of both cochlear and vestibular structures is seen in the early stages of viral labyrinthitis histopathologically, with saccule degeneration and sloughing of the otolithic membrane specifically noted in the vestibular labyrinth (Karmody, 1983).

With the introduction of vaccination programmes against measles, mumps and rubella, cytomegalovirus may become the most significant cause of congenital and/or viral induced deafness in the future. Consideration should be given to routine vestibular testing in those children suspected of having sustained a significant hearing loss as a result of viral infection. In children who are deaf as a result of rubella infection the caloric test may be normal, though rotational tests may show impairment (Huygen *et al.*, 1993).

Trauma

Peripheral hearing loss and vertigo can follow head trauma either with or without a fracture of the temporal bone. Fractures of the temporal bone have been divided into transverse and longitudinal types (Vartiainen, Karjalainen and Karja, 1985). A longitudinal fracture usually bypasses the inner ear, but crosses the middle ear causing a conductive hearing loss as a result of haemotympanum or rupture of the tympanic membrane and/or injury to the ossicular chain. Ossicular damage usually involves dislocation of the incus or fracture of the stapedial crura (Hough, 1969; Podoshin and Fradis, 1975). A transverse fracture may, on the other hand, involve the inner ear producing a significant sensorineural deafness which manifests shortly after the accident.

Vartiainen, Karjalainen and Karja (1985) reported a series of 199 children who had sustained head injuries. Ten children had a haemotympanum with a conductive hearing loss of which nine spontaneously recovered over a 6-month period. Seven per cent had a persistent sensorineural deafness probably attributable to inner ear haemorrhage, caused by intracranial pressure waves spreading through the open cochlear aqueduct into the inner ear.

While persistent vertigo of central origin is uncommon following head injury in children, two peripheral causes must be considered if vertigo continues in a child following such an event. The possibility of a perilymph fistula (particularly if associated with a hearing loss) may warrant an exploratory tympanotomy. If the vertigo is definitely positional in nature benign paroxysmal positional vertigo may be the underlying aetiology (see below).

Benign paroxysmal positional vertigo

Benign paroxysmal positional vertigo is a purely peripheral labyrinthine phenomenon as opposed to benign paroxysmal vertigo which is considered to represent a central lesion.

In a series of 240 cases with benign paroxysmal positional vertigo, 17% were attributed to head trauma and 15% to neurolabyrinthitis (Baloh, Honubria and Jacobson, 1987). As both these events may affect children as well as adults, it is not surprising that in a series of 115 patients with benign paroxysmal positional vertigo 9% were in the age group 11–12 years (Eadie, 1967).

Benign paroxysmal positional vertigo is characterized by a burst of nystagmus (and associated vertigo) elicited by rapidly altering the position of the head from the upright position to a head-hanging position with the affected ear undermost (i.e. directed towards the floor). After an initial brief lag phase, a rotatory nystagmus starts with the fast component directed towards the floor. This abates after 30–40 seconds and on repetition is noted to fatigue. Accompanying nausea or vertigo may result in cessation of the manoeuvre.

Most commonly seen after head trauma in children this condition settles in time, the child's ability to adapt and compensate being more rapid than the adult.

As the condition is thought to result from cupulolithiasis (Schuknecht and Ruby, 1973), the surgical treatment of posterior ampullary nerve section (Gacek, 1978) may be considered in adults but is rarely indicated in children. Physiotherapy entailing the manoeuvre of Semont may be useful in refractory cases of childhood benign paroxysmal positional vertigo (Hausler and Pampurik, 1989), but should be performed with caution.

Perilymph fistula

A perilymph fistula is an abnormal communication between the fluids surrounding the membranous labyrinth and the middle ear space. A fistula can occur either in the semicircular canals, the vestibule, or the cochlea. Because of the potential hazards of meningitis, permanent hearing loss and occasionally incapacitating vestibular symptoms, early recognition and prompt repair of the perilymph leak is mandatory (Althaus, 1981).

Although audiometric, vestibular and radiographic studies can be helpful, there is no way of proving the presence or absence of a fistula without directly viewing the middle ear. Therefore a high index of suspicion, a carefully taken history and an understanding of both the pathophysiology and possible anatomical anomalies associated with the presence of a fistula in a child are essential.

Any child presenting with a history of recurrent meningitis and/or labyrinthitis, sudden, fluctuating or progressive sensorineural deafness and/or symptoms of dysequilibrium, potentially has a perilymph fistula and should be investigated accordingly (Grundfast and Bluestone, 1978; Supance and Bluestone, 1983).

Certain features in the history are worth elucidating, namely: a history of head injury (with or without skull fracture), penetrating ear injury, slapping injury, barotrauma (including a history of exertion, straining, laughing, sneezing, jumping, blowing a wind instrument, Valsalva manoeuvre or air flight prior to the event), or a history of a sudden 'pop' in the ear.

Nenzeilus (1951) gave an account of a 15 month-old-child with an aplastic ear and otitic meningitis who was shown to have a fistula ending on the promontory. The main interest in this subject, however has been driven by the events surrounding stapes surgery, its complications and the occurrence of the so-called 'stapes gusher'.

Althaus (1981) presented a number of logical physiological and anatomical concepts in an attempt to understand better the genesis of such fistulae. It would appear that the cochlear aqueduct is the principal source of pressure transfer from the cranial cavity to the perilymphatic space and may be important in the genesis of round window membrane rupture in humans (Harker, Norante and Ryu, 1974). Kobrak (1934) demonstrated that both positive and negative changes in intracranial pressures caused a change in perilymph pressure. The cochlear aqueduct originates internally in an orifice on the medial wall of the scala tympani near the origin of the latter and terminates on the undersurface of the petrous portion of the temporal bone in the superior border of the jugular fossa, between the jugular bulb and the inferior surface of the internal auditory canal.

The cochlear aqueduct is open in the fetus and young child and is filled with a meshwork of arachnoidal connective tissue in the adult. A temporal bone study indicates that this aqueduct is open in 75% of individuals under the age of 21 years but only in 32% of the elderly (Wtodyka, 1978). Other potential routes by which the CSF could enter either the perilymph or vestibule respectively are via the vestibular aqueduct or the internal auditory canal (Rockett, 1969).

Specific abnormalities have been reported in relation to the development of fistulae in children including:

1 An abnormal stapes with a straight anterior crus joining the central portion of the footplate rather than the anterior edge with a fistula visible anteriorly (Grundfast and Bluestone, 1978)
2 An abnormal stapes with the posterior crus joining the footplate centrally and a fistula situated in the posterior half of the footplate, the anterior crus being normal (Pashley, 1982)
3 A fistula situated centrally between the two crura.

Where the round window is concerned, Pashley (1982) reported the finding of a malformation of the round window niche such that the round window appeared to be funnel-shaped, approximately three times normal size and extended deeply into the temporal bone. While linear tears and severe disruption of the round window membrane have been reported, marginal defects are usually the rule (Goodhill, 1976). Fistulae have also been reported in children in the region of the geniculate ganglion (Harrington and Birck, 1967) and Hyrtl's fissure (Gacek and Leipzig, 1979), the bony cleft just below the round window niche which extends under the cochlea towards the cranial fossa.

Thus certain physiological and anatomical factors can render a child more susceptible to develop a fistula. Radiologically, the finding of a shortened cochlear coil, a dilated semicircular canal system and a widened inner ear vestibule renders a patient prone to fistula development (Parisier and Birkin, 1976). Pullen (1972) detected a common anatomical variation in the cases of round window membrane rupture, namely an abnormal angulation of the round window such that it was visible and angled less than one would expect. Other authors including Clark, De Santo and Facer (1978) and Illum (1972) have described temporal bone anomalies and otic capsule CSF or perilymph fistulae in children with Klippel-Feil syndrome, Pendred's syndrome, craniosynostosis and Mondini dysplasia. It would appear that certain anatomical and physiological variations render certain individuals susceptible to the effects of implosive (alteration in tubotympanic pressure) or explosive (alteration in CSF pressure) barotrauma which places them at risk of fistula formation.

Clinically, the definitive diagnosis of perilymph fistulae can be made only by tympanotomy. Various investigative tests have been tried in an attempt to identify more accurately such fistulae:

1 The Tullio phenomenon was considered to be positive if the patient experienced vertigo or loss of balance after presentation of a 95 dB tone (at 500 Hz) for a duration of not longer than 3 seconds. In a series of 54 patients, in whom free-flowing fistulae were found at surgery, 12% demonstrated the Tullio phenomenon (Fox, Balkany and Arenberg, 1988).
2 Postural audiometry was reported to be positive in 11 patients out of 14 who underwent exploratory tympanotomy (Flood *et al.*, 1985). In the test a minimum hearing gain of 10 dB in at least two frequencies on pure tone audiometry is considered positive after the patient has lain horizontally with the affected ear uppermost for 30 minutes. This works on the basis that an air column that has been locked in the labyrinth is released thus reversing the conductive loss encountered in such cases particularly in relation to post-stapedectomy fistulae (Goodhill, 1967).
3 A positive fistula test was found strongly to indicate a perilymph fistula but was more often negative than positive in ears with fistulae demonstrated by surgery (Vartiainen *et al.*, 1991).
4 Magnetic resonance imaging is not of proven value in the diagnosis of perilymphatic fistulae in humans (Morris, Kil and Carvlin, 1993).
5 Gibson (1992) described the use of electrocochleography (E/COCHG). When the electrocochleographic changes were clear cut the diagnosis of fistula was very accurate. The investigation was less useful when the changes were equivocal.
6 Fibreoptic and rigid endoscopes may be used to visualize the middle ear. Poe, Rebeiz and Pankratov (1992) failed to demonstrate fistulae in 20 patients suspected of having the problem.
7 Most now agree that the combination of ENG and impedence audiometry (tympanometry) is the most efficacious method of demonstrating fistulae. Having achieved a seal in the test ear, the pressure is increased to 200 mm, held at this level for approximately 15 seconds, and then rapidly reduced to − 400 mm. ENG recording is made throughout the procedure which is repeated three times with visual inspection for rotary nystagmus. ENG recording of nystagmus is established so long as the pressure is maintained on the test ear and the results can be repeated on retest (Daspit, Churchill and Linthicum, 1980).
8 While most fistula tests are based upon the vestibulo-ocular reflex, a new fistula test has been developed based upon the vestibulospinal responses. Systematic removal of both visual (by blind-folding) and support-surface orientation references (by placing on a moving posture platform) are performed, thus leaving the subject solely with

vestibular control of postural reflexes. Patients with perilymphatic fistulae demonstrate an increased (sometimes phase-locked) postural sway in response to sinusoidal changes in external canal pressures (Black *et al.*, 1987).

While definitive information can be gleaned from the different investigations described above, the compliance of each child will be variable and certain tests, such as the latter, may prove impossible. Thus surgical exploration of the child's ear is useful for both diagnosis and treatment.

A meticulous and patient approach to surgery is required (Althaus, 1981) with inspection of the oval window region at high magnification, with the patient in the head-down Trendelenburg position. It may be necessary to drill off some of the bony overhang of the round window niche to expose the annular ligament of the round window membrane. Pledgets of Gelfoam are used to dry up completely the suspicious areas before inspecting for the fistula. The laser and autologous fibrin glue may be used to seal the area of the suspected fistula more accurately (Black *et al.*, 1991).

Useful review articles describing the aetiology, diagnosis and management of perilymph fistulae are provided by Calhoun and Strunk (1992); Davis (1992); Kohut (1992) and Weider (1992).

Finally it is worth noting that even after successful identification and sealing of such a fistula the hearing result may not be substantially altered by the procedure.

Ototoxic drugs and irradiation

The part played by the use these agents in both hearing and vestibular disorders in childhood remains to be elucidated.

Animal experimentation demonstrates the effect of the various agents on the developing vestibular system. The earlier the developing labyrinth is exposed to irradiation, the more severe will be the malformation of the crista ampullaris. The most vulnerable time for exposure to irradiation is on the twelfth and thirteenth gestational days. Less severe malformations occur following exposure on the sixteenth gestational day (Hultcrantz and Anniko, 1984). Several species undergo age-dependent changes in susceptibility to noise-induced and drug-induced hearing loss, which may be extrapolated to include the vestibular system (Prieve and Yanz, 1984).

Kanamycin is known primarily to affect hearing. Gentamicin, amikacin and tobramycin are mainly vestibulotoxic. Aminoglycosides and especially gentamicin and kanamycin are widely used in newborns for neonatal sepsis. While it would appear that the cochlear and vestibular nerves may be affected at different rates in relation to dosage, duration of treatment, renal function and the patient's age, the evidence in clinical terms is still contradictory (Eviatar and Eviatar, 1981).

A prospective controlled evaluation of auditory function in neonates given netilmicin or amikacin revealed no significant difference in the incidence of hearing impairment when compared with age- and sex-matched controls. There was a high incidence of transient auditory abnormalities in this intensive care population (Finitzo-Hieber, McCracken and Brown, 1985). While Elfving, Pettay and Raivo (1973) demonstrated the occurrence of damage to the hearing and/or vestibular function in six out of 28 children who underwent a follow-up study of their cochlear, vestibular and renal function following gentamicin therapy in the newborn period, it was felt that ototoxicity could be incriminated in only two of the six cases, other obvious factors accounting for the dysfunction in the remaining cases. In a study of 347 children of whom 234 had received either gentamicin or kanamycin no significant abnormalities were found on audiometric, vestibular or psychometric evaluation in a controlled 4-year follow-up (Finitzo-Hieber *et al.*, 1979).

On the other hand, Camarada *et al.* (1981) performed a retrospective study of 52 patients treated during childhood with potentially ototoxic drugs. Impairment of vestibular function without remarkable hearing loss was demonstrated in four subjects who had been treated with streptomycin during childhood. While most subjects showed a dysfunction of equilibrium, 19 showed a considerable deambulation delay. Kastanioudakis *et al.* (1993) described hearing loss and vestibular dysfunction in a group of children treated with streptomycin, though the severity and clinical manifestations of the vestibular dysfunction are not detailed. Eviatar and Eviatar (1982) demonstrated that there may be a delay in development of head control and vestibular responses in infants treated with aminoglycosides resulting in retarded motor development and postural difficulties. Forty-three infants were treated with aminoglycosides for suspected neonatal sepsis, 17 had been treated with gentamicin alone or in combination with amikacin or tobramycin and 26 had been treated with kanamycin alone. Positional nystagmus was found in six patients in the kanamycin group and 10 of the gentamicin group.

The first diagnostic sign of static encephalopathy is often delayed head control and is most strikingly correlated with atonic diplegia or the dysequilibrium syndrome of cerebral palsy. When delayed milestones appear to be the major problem, vestibular studies may uncover dysfunction to explain the delay and avoid the erroneous and devastating diagnosis of brain damage. The availability of a prospective longitudinal study which provides data on maturation of the vestibular responses in infants of different gestational ages and birthweights should permit the correlation of quality of responses in the various gestational groups with different stages of head and postural control.

Thiringer *et al.* (1984) identified the risk factors for the development of sensorineural deafness in preschool children. These factors may well be applied to the vestibular system also:

1 Hereditary tendency to deafness
2 Rubella / virus infection in pregnancy
3 Malformations of the ear, face, syndrome-like appearance, chromosome defects and alcohol fetopathia
4 Asphyxia requiring more than 10 minutes resuscitation and / or intensive care therapy
5 Low birthweight
6 Neonatal sepsis / meningitis.

As more potentially ototoxic drugs are used in the treatment of neonatal sepsis, it may well be that a combination of such drugs or prolonged usage (25–45 days) may pose a significant risk of vestibular damage as well as cochlear loss. Children in this broad risk category will require long-term follow up from a vestibular point of view as well as the obvious necessity for hearing assessment.

Vestibular neuronitis

First described by Dix and Hallpike in 1952, this condition is thought to be due to a lesion sited in the vestibular pathways at some point central to the labyrinth (Harrison, 1962b).

Typically, vestibular neuronitis consists of a major attack of vertigo accompanied by vomiting and autonomic disturbance. Caloric tests reveal unilateral or bilateral canal paresis, while cochlear function is normal. There is frequently a history of a prodromal febrile illness. Approximately 50% of those affected have one attack only. The other 50% may have subsequent attacks but these usually decrease in both frequency and severity over a 6–12 month period. With a resolution of the condition the caloric responses return to normal.

While Harrison (1962b) has reported on the possible association between epidemic labyrinthitis, 'epidemic vertigo' and vestibular neuronitis, Shirabe (1988) has proposed that vestibular neuronitis may represent a form of polyneuritis.

Vestibular neuronitis appears to be a disease of young adults, though children are also known to be affected (Eviatar and Eviatar, 1977; Snashall, 1987; Shirabe, 1988). In Shirabe's series of 177 children with vertigo, six had vestibular neuronitis, all were boys and showed neuro-otological findings that suggested not only unilateral dysfunction, but also bilateral disorders or partial lesions of the central vestibular system. As with patients described by Gates (1980) they recovered quickly with a return to normality within 2–4 weeks.

The proceedings of the 1991 international symposium on vestibular neuronitis detail many different aspects of this subject (Sekitani and Harada, 1993).

Menière's disease

Menière's disease is traditionally a disease of adults, 75% of those suffering from the affliction being between 30 and 60 years of age (Harrison and Naftalin, 1968). Over the years, however, various authors have reported the occurrence of Menière's disease in children and adolescents (Crowe, 1938; Simonton, 1940; Ombredanne and Aubry, 1941; Parving, 1976; Meyerhoff, Paparella and Shea, 1978; Sadé and Yaniv, 1984; Filipo and Barbara, 1985). It is suggested that between 3% and 7% of those suffering with the disease are children or adolescents (Meyerhoff, Paparella and Shea, 1978; Filipo and Barbara, 1985).

Menière's disease is a clinical entity consisting of recurrent attacks of vertigo, frequently truly rotational in nature, accompanied by nausea and vomiting, progressive sensorineural and fluctuating hearing loss of a cochlear type, and tinnitus. Prior to an attack there may be a feeling of pressure in the involved ear. Nystagmus may be seen if the patient is examined in the throes of an attack or for a certain period afterwards, depending on the severity of the attack.

While the precise pathogenesis remains speculative (Sadé, 1981) it is considered, in its pure form, to be associated with endolymphatic hydrops and a low frequency hearing loss.

If one is to be accurate in making a diagnosis of true Menière's disease in a child, it is imperative that a precise definition of the disease be adhered to. The custom of using Menière's syndrome, or pseudo-menière's, to describe a patient with symptoms suggestive of Menière's disease, is inaccurate and may include a variety of conditions superficially similar, but with a wide spectrum of possible underlying aetiologies. In support of this argument is the fact that a number of children labelled as having Menière's disease in previous reports had antecedent histories suggestive of mumps, meningitis or viral labyrinthitis. In these children the diagnosis of a vestibulopathy of unknown aetiology might have been more accurate.

Meyerhoff, Paparella and Shea (1978) advocated a complete and thorough work-up in such children before labelling them as cases of Menière's disease. The test battery will include a complete audiovestibular and otoneurological screening including a glycerol test if the child will tolerate it, coupled with investigation aimed at identifying any abnormality of adrenal, thyroid or pituitary function, metabolic abnormality such as diabetes mellitus, autoimmunity, allergy, trauma, syphilis, perilymph fistula and congenital abnormalities of the skull base and temporal bone. In relation to the latter, there has been recent interest in the vestibular aqueduct and its association with endolymphatic hydrops and vertigo. Rizvi and Smith (1981) reported that there is a statistically significant reduction in the mean lengths and lateral diameters of the vestibular aqueducts of ears showing endolymphatic hydrops.

At the other end of the scale, Valvassori and Clemis (1978) reported the occurrence of a large vestibular aqueduct in 1.5% of temporal bones in patients undergoing tomographic investigation because of hearing loss and vertigo. Hill, Freint and Maffe (1984) described a 16 year old with enlargement of his vestibular aqueduct associated with vertigo and hearing loss whose vestibular symptoms responded to a no-added salt diet.

Infants who are seen by a paediatrician when they present with a vomiting crisis, can hardly complain of vertigo, thus nystagmus can frequently be missed (Sadé and Yaniv, 1984). Parents and paediatricians will naturally tend to associate vomiting with a gastrointestinal or metabolic disorder rather than an inner ear problem (Filipo and Barbara, 1985).

A high index of suspicion in those dealing with children and adolescents, together with a complete series of investigations will serve to identify more accurately those few cases of Menière's disease that present amid a myriad of other general and labyrinthine pathology. Filipo and Barbara (1985) have found the glycerol test useful in both diagnosis and the identification of those who will respond to diuretic treatment.

Suggested treatments include low-salt diet, diuretics, labyrinthine sedatives, vasodilators, anticholingergics and antihistamines. Finally, failure to respond to medical therapy in children with significant interference with everyday activities may be an indication for operative intervention such as mastoidectomy and endolymphatic sac drainage (Meyerhoff, Paparella and Shea, 1978).

Central causes

Congenital skull anomalies

Vertigo may result from pressure on, and stretching of, the cerebellum, brain stem and lower cranial nerves by structural abnormalities of the upper cervical vertebrae and foramen magum. Upward displacement of the floor of the posterior fossa and narrowing of the foramen magnum occurs in the familial disorder, platybasia. Neurological symptoms including progressive spasticity, incoordination, nystagmus and weakness of the lower cranial nerves appear in the second or third decade. Platybasia may be associated with other central nervous system abnormalities such as the Chiari malformations.

The Chiari malformations

The Chiari malformations are characterized by cerebellar elongation and protrusion through the foramen magnum into the spinal cord. In type 1 malformation the cerebellar herniation exists alone or with malformations of the base of the skull such as platysbasia, basilar impression, or Klippel-Feil syndrome. Often asymptomatic in childhood it may become clinically apparent in adolescence with hydrocephalus, signs of cervical cord compression, suboccipital headache, vertigo, laryngeal paralysis and progressive cerebellar signs. Downbeating vertical nystagmus may occur. Other central vestibular signs found on electronystagmographic recording such as saccadic smooth pursuit, optokinetic disruption, ocular dysmetria and failure of fixation suppression are present, but are not diagnostic of Chiari malformation (Chait and Barber, 1979; Snashall, 1987).

Type 2 Chiari malformation is the most common form of this condition, comprising type 1 malformation together with non-communicating hydrocephalus and lumbosacral spina bifida.

Type 3 may have features of types 1 and 2 with occipital cranial bifidum or cervical spinal bifida.

Types 2 and 3 present early in childhood with widespread neurological abnormalities, whereas type 1 may present with vertigo or ataxia in adolescence, or simply a failure to learn to cycle or partake in sport that demands balance and coordination. Diagnosis is by CT scanning or MRI of the skull base (Snashall, 1987).

Klippel-Feil syndrome, characterized by fusion and reduction in number of the the cervical vertebrae causes variable neurological symptoms and may be associated with congenital deafness and other malformations.

Migraine-related disorders

Headache is a common symptom in children, occurring in up to 21.4% of 11 year olds (Del Bene, 1982). Migraine is less common but is believed to occur in 3.6% of children. Although one equates migraine in adulthood with headache alone (common migraine) or with headache and neurological symptoms (classical migraine), in childhood the manifestations are much more varied and the headache does not necessarily play as prominent a part (Watson and Steele, 1974).

It is accepted that classical migraine is a vascular disorder associated with vasospasm of vessels supplying the central nervous system and is responsible for the neurological symptoms, followed by vasodilatation of extracranial vessels responsible for the headache. The cause of the disruption to the autoregulation of the cerebral blood flow, which is normally quite constant, is unknown. There is some evidence that there is abnormal production of vasoactive substances causing reduced regional circulation with a sterile inflammatory response and in some cases oedema (Parker, 1989).

The realization that migraine can be associated with, or form the underlying pathophysiology of a number of paediatric conditions has become more readily recognized. Analysis of data from observations of migrainous children shows certain clinical symptoms such as motion sickness, cyclic vomiting, recurrent abdominal pain, limb or growing pains, dizziness, sleeping troubles and hyperactivity, which may accompany or frequently precede the development of the classical migraine headache (Del Bene, 1982). These may be termed migraine 'risk' factors, precursors, equivalents or variants (Parker, 1989). Paroxysmal torticollis of infancy, benign paroxysmal vertigo and basilar artery migraine merit description.

Paroxysmal torticollis of infancy

Paroxysmal torticollis of infancy is a relatively uncommon condition that was first described by Snyder (1969). The onset of the illness is in early infancy in the majority of cases and consists of episodes during which the head is tilted to one side and often slightly rotated to the opposite side. This torticollis is frequently present on wakening. The attacks last from minutes to days and may be associated with nausea, pallor, vomiting and agitation. These symptoms then abate followed by a resolution of the torticollis until the next attack occurs. The main clinical features of the condition are listed below (Sanner and Bergström, 1979):

- Paroxysmal occurrence of head-tilting and retraction
- Curvature of the trunk
- Extension pattern of one leg
- Usually more abnormal posture in supine and upright positions
- Sometimes distress and abnormal rolling of the eyes at onset of attacks
- Regular periodicity of attacks for a long time
- Duration of attacks: hours to days
- Onset: within the first year or two of life
- Recovery from 1 to 5 years of age
- Female preponderance

The aetiology is unknown but the site of the dysfunction is considered to be the brain stem or cerebellum, the paroxysmal nature being explained by vascular or metabolic disturbances (Sanner and Bergström, 1979).

While Snyder (1969) reported that the vestibular tests were abnormal in the vast majority of cases, later reports (Sanner and Bergstrom, 1979; Parker, 1989) suggested that it is not easy to evaluate properly nystagmus in children without ENG and analysis of such vestibular testing in recent literature would indicate that caloric tests were normal in paroxysmal torticollis of infancy in 62% of those tested (Parker, 1989).

Some older children, with speech, described vertigo and demonstrated ataxia during attacks when able to walk. This suggests the progression of the condition to that of benign paroxysmal vertigo of childhood. The actual clinical presentation probably just manifests the developmental stage or maturation of the nervous system (Dunn and Snyder, 1976).

Benign paroxysmal vertigo of childhood

Benign paroxysmal vertigo of childhood is a relatively rare condition probably underestimated in its frequency due to the difficulty of both evaluating and classifying dizziness in children. First described by Basser (1964), benign paroxysmal vertigo of childhood is characterized by sudden brief attacks of dizziness occurring when standing or lying, is unrelated to position and is possibly associated with pallor, nausea and even vomiting. During an attack the child may clutch at the parent or remain absolutely still until the episode has waned. There is then resumption of play or activity as if nothing had happened. The condition is usually seen in the first 4 years of life but can occur up to the age of 10. The attacks are said to occur in 4–6-week cycles but this can be variable. The final outcome as its name suggests, is benign, usually settling within a few months or a few years. In a series of 17 such cases reported by Koenigsberger *et al.* (1970) it was noted that all children were bright and frequently very articulate and importantly none appeared sleepy or lethargic after an attack. There was no clouding of consciousness during or after the episode and no evident postictal depression or amnesia (Chutorian, 1972).

Investigations in these children are invariably normal in terms of neuro-otological tests, audiology, electroencephalography, haematology and serology.

Caloric testing

Basser, in his original report (1964), stated that the one outstanding abnormal finding in these children was disordered vestibular function in the form of moderate, severe, or complete canal paresis, which was either unilateral or bilateral. Koenigsberger *et al.* (1970), in establishing a range of normal values for the duration of nystagmus in young children, found that the results for children with benign paroxysmal vertigo of childhood differed from the norm by more than two standard deviations and uniformly reflected canal paresis. Others reported similar abnormal calorics in children with the condition (Chutorian, 1972; Watson and Steele, 1974; Dunn and Snyder, 1976; Koehler, 1980). These findings therefore suggested a peripheral aetiology for benign paroxysmal vertigo in childhood.

More recent reports, however, demonstrate an ever increasing number of normal caloric tests in these children (Eeg-Olofsson *et al.*, 1982; Mira *et al.*, 1984; Lanzi *et al.*, 1986; Finkelhor and Harker, 1987; Parker, 1989). The variable caloric responses obtained by different authors indicate the difficulty in obtaining standardized results from children whose vestibular systems are developing and also represents the wide variability in the methodology of testing such children (Eeg-Olofsson *et al.*, 1982; Blayney and Colman, 1984).

Just as the progression from paroxysmal torticollis of infancy to benign paroxysmal vertigo in childhood has been reported by Dunn and Snyder (1976) the association between benign paroxysmal vertigo in childhood and migraine has been highlighted by others. Lanzi *et al.* (1986) reported that headache provocation tests were positive in 10 out of 15 children suffering from benign paroxysmal vertigo in childhood, while Koehler (1980) reported a series of eight children with benign paroxysmal vertigo in childhood, all of whom had a positive family history of migraine. Watson and Steele (1974) reviewed 286 children with migraine syndrome and found that 66 of these children were unsteady before or during an attack. Of these 43 had classical migraine headache accompanying the vertigo, while 23 were considered to suffer from a migraine equivalent, i.e. vertigo without the headache.

As with any syndrome that relies entirely on clinical observation for diagnosis, there may be more than one cause. Dunn and Snyder (1976) suggested that a food allergy should be considered in all cases. Many, however, consider a migrainous pathophysiology as the most likely cause, with a vascular disturbance of the posterior circulation and ischaemia of the labyrinth and vestibular nuclei (Fenichel, 1967; Eeg-Olofsson *et al.*, 1982; Curatolo and Sciaretta, 1987; Finkelhor and Harker, 1987).

Basilar artery migraine

Basilar artery migraine was defined by Bickerstaff (1961). The syndrome frequently affects adolescent females and occurs against a positive family background. The onset of each attack is sudden and the episode usually includes visual manifestations, vertigo, gait ataxia, dysarthria and tinnitus in varying combinations. Headache, which may be occipital, often follows the disappearance of the other symptoms and many patients have more typical vascular headaches between the episodes. In Golden and French's (1975) series of eight children with basilar artery migraine six were under 4 years of age, the youngest being only 7 months.

Diagnosis of the migraine syndrome in children is difficult as one is relying on the patient's limited ability to provide a lucid history about the extent and variation of the symptoms present. Thus objective manifestations or equivalents such as head-banging, cyclical vomiting or recurrent abdominal pain may provide the necessary clue to a migrainous pathophysiology.

In the infant an attack may start with progressive lethargy, anorexia and photophobia. This is followed by a period of disturbed sleep during which the infant chooses to 'stabilize' himself wedged motionless against the side of the cot. Picking up the child may induce vomiting. The presence of headache may be deduced from the fact that the child clutches its head or pulls its hair in desperation. Other symptoms such as ataxia, slurring of speech, diplopia, bilateral limb weakness, bilateral paraesthesiae and/or visual field defects, are just as likely to be present in the infant or child, as in the adult but may be more difficult to elicit, depending on the child's communicative ability.

Eviatar (1981) noted that vestibular testing revealed abnormalities on bithermal calorics in 16 out of 20 children with basilar artery migraine. Of these seven had labyrinthine preponderance, four had directional preponderance and five had combined labyrinthine and directional preponderance. Four children had normal calorics.

While directional preponderance is found in patients with temporal lobe tumours or vertiginous epilepsy, in basilar artery migraine it is suggested that ischaemia in the territory of the posterior temporal branches of the posterior cerebral arteries may be responsible. Labyrinthine preponderance on the other hand generally indicates peripheral dysfunction of the labyrinth and it is difficult to relate this finding to a condition which, by its nature, is centrally situated. Harker and Rassekh (1987) reported normal calorics in five cases of basilar artery migraine in this age group. It may well be that the caloric results correlate with the severity of the clinical presentation.

Auditory function has been found to be normal in most cases tested (Eviatar, 1981; Harker and Rassekh, 1987).

As the degree of spasm and the patterns of vascular involvement are probably very variable, so the precise presentation and symptomatic involvement vary accordingly. Thus, locating the source of the vertigo is speculative though one could surmise that if associated with fluctuating hearing, involvement of the internal auditory artery would seem likely. While the presence of visual symptoms would point towards the posterior cerebral artery as the cause of the vertigo, the absence of both visual and auditory symptoms would tend to indict the brain stem region (Parker, 1989).

Infection

The association between meningitis and labyrinthitis, as a result of the spread of infection from the meninges via the cochlear aqueduct to the labyrinth, has already been alluded to earlier in this chapter. Ascending infection through the internal acoustic meatus (Eavey *et al.*, 1985) or in the blood to the acousticovestibular organs are alternative modes of spread.

Ataxia may be a presenting feature of meningitis in infants, even prior to diagnosis, or may develop during the course of such an illness, in particular if the causative organism is *Haemophilus influenzae* (Schwartz, 1972). Of 94 patients who were followed up after pneumococcal meningitis, 23 were found to have otological sequelae: 17 had hearing losses, seven had tinnitus and nine had vertigo (Rasmussen, Johnsen and Bohr, 1991). Symptomatic dizziness can persist in the absence of deafness and be associated with central manifestations. Eviatar and Eviatar (1977) identified post-meningitis dizziness in three of a series of 50 children presenting with vertigo.

While viral infections are usually associated with a 'peripheral' labyrinthitis, Mangabeira-Albernaz and Malavasi Gananca (1988) reported a series of patients who presented with intense vertigo and signs of central vestibular involvement following a viral infection. Symptomatically improving over a 3–4 month period, their central signs persisted for 6–12 months. The condition responded to corticosteroids, but was exacerbated by vestibular depressor drugs. Brain stem encephalitis gives rise to either vertigo or ataxia. The symptom is persistent and is accompanied by fever and neurological signs such as supranuclear or internuclear ophthalmoplegia, vertical nystagmus and directional preponderance of induced nystagmus (Ellison and Hanson, 1977; Curless, 1980; Fried, 1980).

Cerebellar encephalitis may present with a similar picture and is distinguished from acute cerebellar ataxia by the identification of a causative organism (Menkes, 1985). Acute cerebellar ataxia is more common in the first 3 years of life and follows 7–21 days after a non-specific infectious illness. There is a sudden truncal ataxia with other neurological symptoms and signs. In the very young child it may be difficult to distinguish from acute labyrinthitis. Symptoms may persist for months and although it is a self-limiting condition, there are sometimes permanent sequelae.

Trauma

Dizziness and vertigo of central origin are relatively rare sequelae in the postconcussion syndrome in children. Because of the differences between children's and adult's tissues, e.g. bone flexibility, the severity and after-effects of children's head injuries probably differ from those in adults (Vartiainen, Karjalainen and Karja, 1985).

Freytag (1963) examined autopsy samples from 1213 people with head injuries and found that while the basal ganglia, midbrain and pons were frequently damaged in adults, surprisingly there were often no signs of injury to the midbrain in young children, except in connection with a major increase in intracranial pressure.

Plasticity of the vestibular system and a ready ability to compensate, may thus account for the low incidences of persistent dysequilibrium in children following closed head injury considering the frequency of this event in children. Vertigo developing days or weeks after a closed head injury is suggestive of a contracoup injury to the temporal lobe vestibular cortex as it strikes the sphenoid ridge (Busis, 1983).

Neoplasia

Lesions of the VIIIth cranial nerve give rise to progressive deafness, tinnitus and imbalance. In childhood and adolescence, however these symptoms are more likely to be due to progressive, genetic, infective, or hydropic disorders of the labyrinth (Snashall, 1987).

Benign cerebellopontine angle tumours do occasionally occur in children. Each case of asymmetrical progressive sensorineural deafness or imbalance should therefore be investigated in a child, as it would be in an adult.

More ominous in presentation, however, is the child with progressive, persistent vertigo or observable ataxia. There may be no history of a preceding pyrexial illness or of associated otological symptoms. The progressive nature of the condition, however, points towards a posterior fossa neoplasm and MRI is strongly indicated.

The presence of other neurological symptoms and signs, particularly disorders of eye movement control are suggestive of a central rather than a peripheral aetiology (Curless, 1980; Hood, 1980).

Demyelination

Multiple sclerosis is an unusual diagnosis in children. The incidence of the condition, however, is probably similar to that in adults (Molteni, 1977; Menkes, 1985). As the diagnosis usually depends upon a long period of observation, the condition is more likely to occur after, rather than before puberty. With the application of objective vestibular testing, increased and earlier diagnosis may be possible in the future.

Seizure disorders

Seizures may give rise to vertigo in three ways. The most common method is when the vertigo forms part of the aura of a grand mal fit and is easy to distinguish from other causes (de Jesus, 1980). The other two specific varieties are vestibulogenic (Behrman and Wyke, 1958) and vertiginous (Alpers, 1960) of which the latter is the more frequent.

Vestibulogenic epilepsy, a form of reflex epilepsy, is a rarity (Chutorian, 1972). It is said to be precipitated by stimulation of the labyrinth, producing activation of hyperexcitable neurons both in the brain stem and reticular system resulting in a convulsion (Beddoe, 1977). This type of attack can be seen during caloric stimulation, at which time an abnormal EEG may be obtained. At other times the EEG is normal.

Vertiginous epilepsy, or temporal lobe epilepsy with a vertiginous component is more commonly seen (Chutorian, 1972). Dizziness may be the sole feature of the aura of motor cortical epilepsy or that affecting the basal ganglion or red nucleus area. It may precede the occurrence of frank seizures by a few years. The clinical features of vertiginous epilepsy are: episodic vertigo possibly accompanied by headache, nausea and vomiting, which may progress to loss of consciousness with or without a seizure. Postictal unsteadiness does not occur (Harrison, 1962a).

The diagnosis is not difficult if vertigo followed by a fully fledged fit is associated with an abnormal EEG. More difficult to recognize is the condition in which the seizure itself is accompanied by a brief loss of consciousness or amnesia for the event. In this case an interictal EEG may reveal an abnormality and point towards the diagnosis. Eviatar and Eviatar (1977) reported that, of 42 cases of central vertigo in childhood, 25 were caused by vertiginous epilepsy. In those with mainly focal abnormalities on EEG testing, the results of ENG calorics were abnormal, while in those with diffuse EEG changes, normal vestibular responses were found. Vertiginous seizures should be distinguished from minor motor seizures in which balance may be lost as a result of muscle contraction and from myoclonic-astatic epilepsy of early childhood (Bower, 1981).

The incidence of vertiginous epilepsy in childhood is much higher in some series (Eviatar and Eviatar, 1977) than others (Blayney and Colman 1984; Snashall, 1986). This largely reflects the referral pattern in a specific region and the recognized expertise of the specialist clinics. Snashall (1987) cautioned against the assumption that vertigo with an abnormal EEG automatically represents vertiginous epilepsy.

Finally, children occasionally present with headache or abdominal pain. Headache may, in certain instances, be the sole presentation of a seizure disorder (Swaiman and, Frank, 1978). Recurrent abdominal pain, though more commonly representing part of the 'periodic syndrome' or 'cyclical vomiting' a migraine equivalent, may be deemed an epileptic variant on follow up (Papatheophilou, Jeavons and Disney, 1972).

Hereditary cerebellar ataxias

Heredodegenerative diseases that involve the cerebellum and begin in childhood are uncommon (Snashall, 1987). They present with slowly progressive ataxia as do posterior fossa tumours and the latter must be excluded by an MRI scan before the diagnosis can be made.

The most frequent cerebellar degenerations are ataxia telangiectasia, Friedreich's ataxia with congenital deafness and Refsum's disease, which presents with cerebellar ataxia, deafness, retinitis pigmentosa and polyneuritis. Inherited as an autosomal recessive condition, Refsum's disease causes progressive difficulty in walking, as a result of night blindness, cerebellar ataxia and vestibular dysfunction. The onset is usually between 4 and 7 years of age. It is due to an underlying disorder of lipid metabolism, is detected by the presence of lipiduria and raised phytanic acid. It responds to a phytol-free diet as this lowers the serum phytanic acid level (Menkes, 1985).

Acute intermittent familial cerebellar ataxia is a self-limiting disease inherited as a dominant trait with variable penetrance. The disorder gives rise to acute episodes of ataxia beginning in the first 2 years of life and usually ceasing around the age of 15 years. The clinical picture in the juvenile form consists of sudden onset of gait and truncal ataxia, usually with upper limb ataxia, intention tremor and dysarthria or aphonia. Occasionally there is headache, vomiting, nystagmus or seizures. In childhood the attacks last about 4 weeks and leave no residual neurological symptoms or signs. With maturity, the attacks decrease in both severity and duration, the patient being symptom-free between attacks. There have been no underlying biochemical abnormalities detected in the condition, which is considered to be triggered by such factors as viral infections, ascariasis and psychological trauma (Hill and Sherman, 1968).

Hereditary disease of the peripheral and cranial nerves

The most common heredodegenerative condition is Charcot-Marie-Tooth disease. Peroneal muscular atrophy is the usual presentation of this disease (Menkes, 1985), but congenital sensorineural deafness is present in a proportion of cases (Cornell, Sellars and Beighton, 1984). As the deafness is retrocochlear it is likely to be accompanied by vestibular weakness.

Neurofibromatosis affects both peripheral and cranial nerves. The optic nerve is the commonest and earliest site of involvement, bilateral acoustic neuromas are less common. The presence of seizures in early childhood associated with café-au-lait spots, with or without subcutaneous neurofibromas, raises the possibility of intracranial tumours (Menkes, 1985).

Congenital nystagmus is a recessive trait in which there is fine and rapid nystagmus, usually pendular and generally asymptomatic.

A familial disorder has been described by White (1969), which consists of recurrent attacks of nystagmus, vertigo and ataxia, with an onset in early childhood and a good prognosis in relation to abatement of symptoms. Unlike congenital nystagmus it appears to be due to a single autosomal dominant trait.

Other causes

Metabolic causes of vertigo

The occurrence of vertigo in a variety of metabolic disorders in childhood such as diabetes, hyperinsulinism, adrenal insufficiency and hyperthyroidism has been recognized by paediatricians for many years (Eviatar and Eviatar, 1980). Anaemia may also produce a non-specific form of dysequilibrium, more frequently referred to by the patient as giddiness or light-headedness, as opposed to true vertigo.

Hyperlipidosis and in particular hyperlipoproteinaemia type II may develop in infancy and can be associated with inner ear disease (Pillsbury, 1981).

Occlusive disease of the vertebro-basilar arterial system in childhood can produce vertigo but other CNS signs such as dysarthria, hemiparesis and ocular palsies are also present (Ouvrier and Hopkins, 1970).

Hypothyroidism and congenital deafness (Pendred's syndrome) may present with episodic vertigo, tinnitus, sensorineural hearing loss and vomiting, suggestive of Menière's disease (Das, 1987).

Psychosomatic dizziness and hyperventilation

These disturbances may present as vestibular disorders and must be distinguished from organic disease. In the school-age child, problems of anxiety, social adaptation and academic pressure may manifest themselves in many ways, and sometimes as dizziness. In preschool children, psychosomatic disorders are uncommon, the older the child at the onset of symptoms the more likely it is to be psychogenic (Beddoe, 1977).

Two groups are most at risk: those under excessive social pressure to achieve, and adolescent females (Fried, 1980).

The symptom of dizziness rarely occurs as an isolated entity in children with psychosomatic illness, but frequently accompanies hyperventilation, nausea, headache, palpitations, faintness and visual disturbance. The patient may also complain of paraesthesiae and circumoral tingling. Diagnosis is facilitated by precisely reproducing the symptoms with hyperventilation but none of the other manoeuvres in the dizziness simulation battery (Pincus, 1978).

It is important to distinguish this group from those who may hyperventilate but have underlying psychiatric disorders as well. In these patients the dizziness may be equated with 'loss of energy', 'mental fuzziness' or 'difficulty thinking' (Drachman and Hart, 1972).

Vestibular disorders associated with abnormal development, behaviour and learning ability

Vestibular dysfunction has been reported to occur in a number of conditions, even though overt vestibular symptoms and signs are not present. Delayed vestibular responsiveness and motor development in Down's syndrome and cerebral palsy in infants (Kravitz and

Boehm, 1971), abnormal nystagmus in girls with idiopathic scoliosis (Asaka, 1979), abnormal postrotatory nystagmus in children with minor neurological impairments (Steinberg and Rendle-Short, 1977) and vestibular hypofunction in children with learning disability (de Quiros, 1976) represent a selection of such disabilities in which vestibular dysfunction has been implicated.

While vestibular deficits seemingly occur in children with autism (Colbert, Koegler and Markham, 1959), schizophrenia (Silver and Gabriel, 1964) and Down's syndrome, it may well be that in autism the deficient nystagmus response can be attributed to a disorder of visual–vestibular interaction (Tjernstrom, 1973). In schizophrenia the defect may lie in the vestibulospinal mechanism and in Down's syndrome global motor delay may be the responsible factor (Ornitz, 1983). In the normal infant vestibular self-stimulation in the form of swaying, body-rocking and head-banging begin in the first year of life. While such behaviour also occurs in autistic and retarded children, body rocking, in particular, by providing vestibular sensations through self-stimulation may be associated with early motor development (Sallustro and Atwell, 1978; Clark, Kreutzberg and Chee, 1977). In view of the fact that children with learning disability also demonstrated inadequate vestibular function (Ayres, 1978), it was proposed that vestibular stimulation, as measured by postrotatory nystagmus, might be used to activate dormant pathways. These could then be used by other sensory integrative processes (Ottenbacher, 1982). Learning disability is multifactorial, however, and the neuropathological findings are frequently more widespread than the vestibular system and its connections (Fuller, Guthrie and Alvord, 1983). Disorders of eye movement control and vestibular sensitivity do occur in children with developmental, learning and behavioural problems but, in any study of such children, comparison with age-matched controls and careful control of the variables such as lighting and mental alerting are advisable (Ornitz, 1983; Snashall, 1983).

Motion sickness

Motion sickness, a form of physiological vertigo, usually implies a mismatch between inputs from the sensory systems subserving static and dynamic spatial orientation as well as posture, visual, vestibular and somatosensory stimuli (Brandt and Daroff, 1980).

Motion sickness is thought to occur when the brain receives conflicting information about body motion from visual and vestibular receptors and proprioceptors. The intensity of the vertigo experienced is a function of the magnitude of the mismatch (Ruckenstein and Harrison, 1991).

Sharma (1980) found that 16.6% of male and 29.2% of female children were affected. Children are most susceptible to motion sickness from 2 years to 12 years of age with a subsequent gradual decrease in symptoms (Lentz and Collins, 1977). Motion sickness has been reported during childhood in up to 60% of migraine sufferers (Pearce, 1971). Kuritzky, Ziegler and Hassanien (1981) reported that, while motion sickness was significantly more frequent in classical migraine patients, there was no significant increase in the incidence of childhood motion sickness in any of the migraine groups when compared with controls.

While the sensory conflict theory helps to explain the genesis of motion sickness, it does not explain the differences in individual susceptibility to the condition, or map out the central neural structures involved (Ruckenstein and Harrison, 1991). Groen (1963) makes a case for the development of a central inhibitory mechanism, whose efficacy and maturation vary from individual to individual.

Infants under the age of 2 years rarely suffer from motion sickness, either because they travel supine or because their visual input is limited (Money, 1970). Girls may be more prone to motion sickness because their degree of vestibular stimulation or adaptation may be less than that experienced by boys of the same age (Deich and Hodges, 1973).

As one progresses from childhood to adolescence, field dependency (relying on visual clues for orientation in space) and motion sickness decrease in incidence and field independence (relying on internal clues) comes to the fore (Deich and Hodges, 1973).

Differential diagnosis

Paroxysmal disorders

In children, as in adults, the diagnosis of apparent vertigo has two aspects: the differential diagnosis, or the separation of vertigo from conditions which may resemble it, and the diagnosis of the cause of the vertigo (Collins, 1983).

While Britton and Block (1988) suggest that the evaluation of 'the dizzy paediatric patient' is the responsibility of the otolaryngologist, there are certain paroxysmal disorders more frequently encountered by the paediatrician or paediatric neurologist which may require their expertise for diagnosis.

'Subtle seizures' and various forms of syncope may necessitate joint consultation to define more accurately the diagnosis. As epilepsy may account for a significant proportion of cases of dysequilibrium in childhood (Eviatar and Eviatar, 1977), the main differential diagnosis lies between a seizure disorder, syncope and an 'otological' condition (Aust, 1991). Thus EEG evaluation is frequently necessary, unless the diagnosis is obvious.

Certain paroxysmal disorders should be differentiated from peripheral and central disorders of vestibular function.

Breath-holding spells and seizures have a peak incidence between 2 and 3 years of age. Sudden fear, frustration or trauma may precipitate the attack, which lasts for 2–20 seconds, is initiated by a Valsalva manoeuvre and consists of crying, exhalation, cyanosis and limpness. The child regains consciousness, is transiently confused and then recovers (Hutchison, 1972).

In a second, less common form of breath holding, an unexpected painful stimulus precipitates sudden limpness, pallor, loss of consciousness and apnoea. The child may quickly regain consciousness or progress to opisthotonus and seizures. Diagnosis is by the ocular compression test which induces cardiac asystole for more then 2 seconds in 35% of cases. There is a positive family history in 30% and the EEG between attacks is normal (Snashall, 1987).

Recurrent syncope is seen in infants and adolescents. Usually it is a reaction to emotional stress, mild hypoglycaemia and environmental factors, but the possibility of cardiac syncope should be considered. This is particularly the case with children with congenital deafness, who may be expected to have episodic vertigo. The surdo-cardiac syndrome is familial and produces congenital deafness, a prolonged Q-T interval, fainting and sudden death. The attacks begin in infancy.

Infantile spasms occurring in mentally handicapped infants are associated with an abnormal EEG which is diagnostic. Myoclonic-astatic epilepsy of early childhood is similar to infantile spasms but occurs in children over the age of 2 years. In such a 'drop-attack' the child is suddenly flung forwards or backwards as if pushed violently (the myoclonic attack) or suddenly collapses due to loss of muscle tone (the astatic attack). Consciousness may be lost momentarily (Bower, 1981; Hutchison, 1972).

Night terrors may be confused with positional vertigo or basilar artery migraine occurring at night. Night terrors occur in the first 3 hours of deep, non-REM sleep. The child suddenly sits bolt upright, screaming with terror, and remains unaware of the surroundings for 10–20 minutes before dropping back into quiet sleep (Snashall, 1987).

Management of vertigo

As childhood vertigo is self-limiting in many instances, treatment may only be necessary in a specific number of circumstances.

Medical

Motion sickness

Motion sickness in the child results from a mismatch of inputs from the sensory systems subserving static and dynamic spatial orientation and posture (Brandt and Daroff, 1980). Positioning of the child in the vehicle with a clear view of the surroundings may help to avoid this mismatch between visual and vestibular information. Vestibular sedatives such as dimenhydrinate and transdermal hyoscine may be effective.

Benign paroxysmal vertigo

Benign paroxysmal vertigo usually requires little more than reassurance, but in persistent cases dimenhydrinate may be helpful.

Migraine

Exclusion of known precipitants such as chocolate, cheese, oranges, tomato derivatives and 'E factor'-containing foodstuffs may alleviate the symptoms. Failing these, dietary steps, antihistamines and beta blockers have been advocated (Britton and Block, 1988).

Seizure disorders

Seizure disorders, if accompanied by vertigo may need adjustment of the antiepileptic regimen to achieve control of the vertigo.

Menière's disease

Rare in childhood, it would appear that this condition is more difficult to treat in children than in adults as there is poor compliance with routine medication (Snashall, 1987). Low-salt diet, diuretics and betahistine may be used in conjunction with antihistamines. While many children will not require regular treatment, the occasional one will need to be considered for surgical intervention.

Surgical

Surgical treatment is indicated in those children whose vertigo is caused by:

1 Persistent glue ear in whom a grommet may correct the fluctuations in middle ear pressure
2 A labyrinthine fistula with a fluctuating or deteriorating sensorineural reserve, when an exploratory tympanotomy is indicated
3 Post-traumatic labyrinthine dysfunction with a non-hearing ear and recurrent troublesome vertigo, in which a three-canal labyrinthectomy may lead to a resolution of the vertigo
4 Operable cerebellopontine angle/brain stem or posterior fossa tumours or lesions
5 Exploratory mastoid and/or middle ear surgery in a child with a suspected lateral semicircular fistula secondary to cholesteatoma, or in whom recurrent meningitis or the combination of labyrinthitis and meningitis suggests the possibility of an abnormal

communication between the middle ear/mastoid
and the meninges or labyrinth/inner ear and internal auditory canal
6 Endolymphatic sac surgery may rarely be considered in the child with intractable vertigo due to
Menière's disease.

Psychological support

Frequently overlooked, this aspect of management is
important particularly in relation to reassurance of
both parents and patient. A positive approach should
be adopted as in many instances the symptom will
decrease both in severity and frequency with the
passage of time. Adolescent females most often need
firm reassurance in order to resume normal mobility
(Snashall, 1987).

References

ALPERS, B. J. (1960) Vertiginous epilepsy. *Laryngoscope*, **70**,
631–637
ALTHAUS, S. R. (1981) Perilymph fistulas. *Laryngoscope*, **91**,
538–562
ARNVIG, J. (1955) Vestibular function in deafness and severe
hardness of hearing. *Acta Oto-Laryngologica*, **4**, 283–288
ASAKA, Y. (1979) Idiopathic scoliosis and equilibrium disturbance. *Nippon Seikeigekagakkai Zasshi*, **53**, 963–977
AUST, G. (1991) Gleichgewichtsstörungen und ihre Diagnos-
tik Kindersalter. *Laryngology, Rhinology, Otology (Stuttgart)*, **70**, 533–537
AUST, G. and GOEBEL, P. (1979) Vestibulookuläre Gleichge-
wichtsreaktionen beim Säugling und Kleinkind. *Laryngol-
ogy, Rhinology, Otology (Stuttgart)*, **58**, 516–521
AYRES, A. J. (1978) Learning disabilities and the vestibular
system. *Journal of Learning Disabilities*, **11**, 18–29
BALOH, R. H., HONUBRIA, V. and JACOBSON, K. (1987) Benign
positional vertigo. *Neurology*, **37**, 371–378
BASSER, L. S. (1964) Benign paroxysmal vertigo of childhood.
Brain. **87**, 141–152
BEDDOE, G. M. (1977) Vertigo in childhood. Symposium of
pediatric otorhinolaryngology. *Otolaryngologic Clinics of
North America*, **10**, 139–144
BEHRMAN, S. and WYKE, B. D. (1958) Vestibulogenic seizures.
Brain, **81**, 529–541
BICKERSTAFF, E. R. (1961) Basilar artery migraine. *Lancet*, i,
15–17
BLACK, F. O., O'LEARY, D. P., WALL, C. and FURMAN, J. (1977)
The vestibulo-spinal stability test: normal limits. *Transac-
tions of American Academy of Ophthalmology and Otolaryngol-
ogy*, **84**, 549–560
BLACK, F. O., LILLY, D. J., NASHNER, L. M., PETERKA, R. J. and
PESZNECKER, S. C. (1987) Quantitative diagnostic test for
perilymph fistulas. *Otolaryngology-Head and Neck Surgery*,
96, 125–134
BLACK, F. O., PESZNECKER, S., NORTON, T., FOWLER, L., LILLY, D.,
SHUPERT, C. *et al.* (1991) Surgical management of peri-
lymph fistulas, a new technique. *Archives of Otolaryngology, Head and Neck Surgery*, **117**, 641–648
BLAYNEY, A. W. and COLMAN, B. H. (1983) The dizzy child.
Proceedings of the Irish Otorhinolaryngological Society, –

24th Annual Meeting, 1983, edited by J. Byrne. Published
1984, pp. 55–61
BLAYNEY, A. W. and COLMAN, B. H. (1984) Dizziness in
childhood. *Clinical Otolaryngology*, **9**, 77–85
BOHR, V., HANSEN, B. and JESSEN, O. (1983) 875 cases of
bacterial meningitis Part 1. clinical data, prognosis and
the role of specialised hospital departments. *Journal of
Infection*, **7**, 21–30
BOWER, T. G., BROUGHTON, T. and MOORE, M. K. (1971) Development of the object concept as manifested in changes in
the tracking behaviour of infants between 7 and 20
weeks of age. *Journal of Experimental Child Psychology*, **11**,
182–193
BOWER, B. (1981) Fits and other frightening or funny turns
in young children, *Practitioner*, **225**, 297–304
BRAMA, I. (1985) Congenital neural hearing loss due to
inner ear malformation. *Journal of Laryngology and Otology*, **99**, 293–295
BRANDT, T. and DAROFF, R. B. (1980) The multisensory physiological and pathological vertigo syndromes. *Annals of
Neurology*, **7**, 195–203
BRANDT, T., DICHGANS, J. and KOENIG, E. (1973) Differential
effects of central versus peripheral vision on egocentric
and exocentric motion perception. *Experimental Brain Research*, **16**, 476–491
BRANDT, T., WIST, E. R. and DICHGANS, J. (1975) Foreground
and background in dynamic spatial orientation. *Perception
and Psychophysics*, **17**, 497–503
BRANDT, T., DIETERICH, M and BUCHELE, W. (1986) Postural
abnormalities in central vestibular brain stem lesions.
Disorders of Postures and Gait, edited by W. Bles and T.
Brandt. Amsterdam: Elsevier; pp. 141–156
BRITTON, B. H. and BLOCK, L. D. (1988) Vertigo in the paediat-
ric and adolescent age group. *Laryngoscope*, **98**, 139–146
BROOKHOUSER, P. E., CYR, D. G. and BEAUCHAINE, K. A. (1982)
Vestibular findings in the deaf and hard of hearing.
Otolaryngology – Head and Neck Surgery, **90**, 773–777
BROOKHAUSER, P. E., CYR, D. G., PETERS, J. E. and SCHULTE, L. E.
(1991) Correlates of vestibular evaluation results during
the first year of life. *Laryngoscope*, **101**, 687–694
BROOKLER, K. (1976) The simultaneous binaural bithermal:
a caloric test utilising electronystagmography. *Laryngo-
scope*, **96**, 1241–1250
BUSIS, S. N. (1983) Vertigo. In: *Pediatric Otolaryngology*, edited
by C. D. Bluestone and S. E. Stool. Philadehia: W. B.
Saunders, pp. 261–270
CALHOUN, K. H. and STRUNK, C. L. (1992) Perilumph fistula.
Archives of Otolaryngology, Head and Neck Surgery, **118**,
693–694
CAMARADA, V., MORENO, A. M., BOSCHI, V., DI CARLO, A.,
SPAZIANI, G. and SAPONARA, M. (1981) Vestibular ototoxi-
city in children: a retrospective study of 52 cases.
International Journal of Pediatric Otorhinolaryngology, **3**,
195–198
CANTOR, F. K. (1971) Vestibular-temporal lobe connections
demonstrated by induced seizures. *Neurology, Minneapolis*,
21, 507
CARPENTER, R. H. S. (1977) *Movement of the Eyes*. London:
Pion Ltd. p. 96
CHAIT, G. C. and BARBER, H. O. (1979) Arnold-Chiari malformation – some neurological features. *Journal of Laryngology and Otology*, **8**, 65–79
CHUTORIAN, A. (1972) Benign paroxysmal vertigo of childhood. *Developmental Medicine and Child Neurology*, **14**,
513–515
CLARK, D. L., KREUTZBERG, J. R. and CHEE, F. K. W. (1977)

Vestibular stimulation influence on motor development in infants. *Science*, **196**, 1228–1229

CLARK, J. L., DE SANTO, L. W. and FACER, F. W. (1978) Congenital deafness and spontaneous CSF otorrhoea. *Archives of Otolaryngology*, **104**, 163–166

CLINICAL OTOLARYNGOLOGY (1978) Vertigo and glue ear in children. 3, 198–200

COLBERT, E. G., KOEGLER, R. R. and MARKHAM, C. H. (1959) Vestibular dysfunction in childhood schizophrenia. *Archives of General Psychiatry*, **1**, 600–617

COLLINS, K. J. (1983) Vertigo and dizziness in childhood: clinical aspects of diagnosis. *Journal of the Otolaryngological Society of Australia*, **5**, 209–211

CORNELL, J., SELLARS, S. and BEIGHTON, P. (1984) Autosomal recessive inheritance of Charcot-Marie-Tooth disease associated with sensorineural deafness. *Clinical Genetics*, **25**, 163–165

CROWE, S. J. (1938) Menière's disease: study based on examinations made before and after divisions of vestibular nerve. *Medicine*, **17**, 1

CURATOLO, P. and SCIARETTA, A. (1987) Benign paroxysmal vertigo and migraine. *Developmental Medicine and Child Neurology*, **29**, 405–406

CURLESS, R. G. (1980) Acute vestibular dysfunction in childhood, central versus peripheral. *Child's Brain*, **6**, 39–44

CYR, D. G. (1980) Vestibular testing in children. *Annals of Otology, Rhinology and Laryngology*, **74** (suppl.), 63–69

DAS, V. K. (1987) Pendred's syndrome with episodic vertigo, tinnitus and vomiting and normal bithermal caloric responses. *Journal of Laryngology and Otology*, **101**, 721–722

DASPIT, C. P., CHURCHILL, D. and LINTHICUM, F. H. (1980) Diagnosis of perilymph fistula using ENG and impedence. *Laryngoscope*, **90**, 217–223

DAVIS, R. E. (1992) Diagnosis and management of perilymph fistula: the University of North Carolina approach. *American Journal of Otology*, **13**, 85–89

DEICH, R. F. and HODGES, P. M. (1973) Motion sickness, field dependence and levels of development. *Perceptual and Motor Skills*, **36**, 1115–1120

DE JESUS, C. P. V. (1980) Neurologic aspects of vertigo. *Ear, Nose and Throat Journal*, **59**, 366–376

DEL BENE, E. (1982) Multiple aspects of headache risk in childhood. *Advances in Neurology*, **33**, 187–193

DE QUIROS, J. B. (1976) Diagnosis of vestibular disorders in the learning disabled. *Journal of Learning Disabilities*, **9**, 39–45

DIX, M. R. and HALLPIKE, C. S. (1952) The pathology, symptomatology and diagnosis of certain common disorders of the vestibular system. *Proceedings of the Royal Society of Medicine*, **45**, 341–354

DODGE, P. R., DAVIS, H. and FEIGIN, R. D. (1984) Prospective evaluation of hearing impairment as a sequela of acute bacterial meningitis. *New England Journal of Medicine*, **311**, 869–874

DOHLMAN, G. F. (1981) Critical review of the concept of cupular function. *Acta Oto-Laryngologica*, Suppl. 376, 1–3

DONAT, J. F. G., DONAT, J. R. and LAY, K. S. (1980) Changing response to caloric stimulation with gestational age in infants. *Neurology*, **30**, 776–778

DRACHMAN, D. A. and HART, C. W. (1972) An approach to the dizzy patient. *Neurology*, **22**, 323–334

DUNN, D. W. and SNYDER, C. H. (1976) Benign paroxysmal vertigo of childhood. *American Journal of Diseases of Children*, **130**, 1099–1100

EADIE, M. J. (1967) Paroxysmal positional giddiness. *Medical Journal of Australia*, **1**, 1169–1173

EAVEY, R. D., GAO, Y. Z., SCHUKNECHT, H. F. and GONZALEZ-PINEDA, M. (1985) Otologic features of bacterial meningitis of childhood. *Journal of Pediatrics*, **106**, 402–409

EEG-OLOFSSON, O., ODKVIST, L., LINDSKOG, V. and ANDERSON, B. (1982) Benign paroxysmal vertigo in childhood. *Acta Oto-Laryngologica*, **93**, 282–289

ELFVING, J., PETTAY, O. and RAIVIO, M. (1973) A follow-up study on the cochlear, vestibular and renal function in children treated with gentamicin in the newborn period. *Chemotherapy*, **18**, 141–153

ELLISON, P. H. and HANSON, P. A. (1977) Herpes simplex: a possible cause of brainstem encephalitis. *Pediatrics*, **59**, 240–243

ENBOM, H., MAGNUSSON, M. and PYYKKO, I. (1991) Postural compensation in children with congenital or early acquired vestibular loss. *Annals of Otology, Rhinology and Laryngology*, **100**, 472–477

EVIATAR, L. (1981) Vestibular testing in basilar artery migraine. *Annals of Neurology*, **9**, 126–130

EVIATAR, L. and EVIATAR, A. (1977) Vertigo in children: differential diagnosis and treatment. *Pediatrics*, **59**, 833–838

EVIATAR, L. and EVIATAR, A. (1978) Neurovestibular examination of infants and children. *Advances in Oto-Rhino-Laryngology*, **23**, 169–191

EVIATAR, L. and EVIATAR, A. (1979) The normal nystagmic response of infants to, caloric and perrotatory stimulation. *Laryngoscope*, **89**, 1036–1045

EVIATAR, L. and EVIATAR, A. (1980) Vertigo in children and adolescents; a diagnostic approach. In: *Pediatric Otorhinolaryngology*, edited by B. Jazbi. New York: Appleton-Century-Crofts, Prentice-Hall Inc. pp. 29–39

EVIATAR, L. and EVIATAR, A. (1981) Aminoglycoside ototoxicity in the neonatal period: possible aetiological factor in delayed postural control. *Otolaryngology–Head and Neck Surgery*, **89**, 818–821

EVIATAR, L. and EVIATAR, A. (1982) Development of head control and vestibular responses in infants treated with aminoglycosides. *Developmental Medicine and Child Neurology*, **24**, 372–379

EVIATAR, L. and EVIATAR, A. (1988) Electronystagmography and vestibular testing in children. In: *Otologic Medicine and Surgery*, Vol. 1 edited by P. W. Alberti and R. J. Ruben. New York: Churchill Livingstone. pp. 507–521

EVIATAR, A. and WASSERTHEIL, S. (1971) The clinical significance of directional preponderance concluded by electronystagmography. *Journal of Laryngology and Otology*, **85**, 335

EVIATAR, L., EVIATAR, A. and NARAY, I. (1974) Maturation of neurovestibular responses in infants. *Developmental Medicine and Child Neurology*, **16**, 435–446

EVIATAR, L., MIRANDA, S., EVIATAR, A., FREEMAN, K. and BORKOWSKI, M. (1979) Development of nystagmus in response to vestibular stimulation in infants. *Annals of Neurology*, **5**, 508–514

FARMER, T. W. (1964) *Pediatric Neurology*. New York: Harper and Row Inc.

FENICHEL, G. M. (1967) Migraine as a cause of benign paroxysmal vertigo of childhood. *Journal of Pediatrics*, **71**, 114–115

FILIPO, R. and BARBARA, M. (1985) Juvenile Menière's disease. *Journal of Laryngology and Otology*, **90**, 817–821

FINITZO-HEIBER, T., MCCRACKEN, G. H. and BROWN, K. C. (1985)

Prospective controlled evaluation of auditory function in neonates given netilmicin or amikacin. *Journal of Pediatrics*, **106**, 129–136

FINITZO-HEIBER, T., MCCRACKEN, G. H., ROESER, R. J., ALLEN, D. A., CHRANE, D. F. and MORROW, T. (1979) Ototoxicity in neonates treated with gentamicin and kanamycin: results of a four-year controlled follow-up study. *Pediatrics*, **63**, 443–450

FINKELHOR, B. K. and HARKER, L. A. (1987) Benign paroxysmal vertigo of childhood. *Laryngoscope*, **97**, 1161–1163

FLOOD, L. M., FRASER, G., HAZELL, J. W. P. and ROTHERA, M. P. (1985) Perilymph fistula. Four year experience with a new audiometric test. *Journal of Laryngology and Otology*, **99**, 671–676

FOX, E. J., BALKANY, T. J. and ARENBERG, K. (1988). The Tullio phenomenon and perilymph fistula. *Otolaryngology–Head and Neck Surgery*, **98**, 88–89

FREYTAG, E. (1963) Autopsy findings in head injuries from blunt forces. *Archives of Pathology*, **75**, 402–413

FRIED, M. P., (1980) The evaluation of dizziness in children. *Laryngoscope*, **90**, 1548–1560

FRIEDMANN, I., SPELLACY, E., CROW, J. and WATTS, R. W. E. (1985) Histopathological studies of the temporal bones in Hurler's disease (mucopolysaccharidosis (MPS) IH). *Journal of Laryngology and Otology*, **99**, 29–41

FULLER, P. W., GUTHRIE, R. D. and ALVORD, E. C. (1983) A proposed neuropathological basis for learning disabilities in children born prematurely. *Developmental Medicine and Child Neurology*, **25**, 214–231

GACEK, R. (1978) Further observations on posterior ampullary nerve transection for positional vertigo. *Annals of Otology, Rhinology and Laryngology*, **87**, 300–305

GACEK, R. and LEIPZIG, B. (1979) Congenital cerebrospinal otorrhoea. *Annals of Otology, Rhinology and Laryngology*, **88**, 358–365

GATES, G. A. (1980) Vertigo in children. *Ear, Nose and Throat Journal*, **59**, 358–365

GATZ, A. J. (1974) *Manter's Essentials of Clinical Neuroanatomy and Neurophysiology*. Philadelphia: Davis

GAY, A. J., NEWMAN, N. M., KELTER, J. L. and STROUD, M. H. (1974) *Eye Movement Disorders*. St Louis: C. V. Mosby Co.

GIBSON, W. P. (1992) Electrocochleography in the diagnosis of perilymph fistula: intraoperative observations and assessment of a new diagnostic office procedure. *American Journal of Otology*, **13**, 146–151

GILLIGAN, M. B., MAYBERRY, W., STEWART, L., KENYON, P. and GAEBLER, C. (1981) Measurement of ocular pursuits in normal children. *American Journal of Occupational Therapy*, **35**, 249–255

GLASSCOCK, M. E. III, CUEVA, R. A. and THEDINGER, B. A. (1990) *Handbook of Vertigo*. New York: Raven Press

GOEBEL, P. and AUST, G. (1978) Ein Vergleich der Entwicklung der Nystagmusfrequenz nach vestibulärer Stimulation mit der motorischen Entwicklung in der ersten Lebensjahren. *Archives of Oto-Rhino-Laryngology*, **220**, 265–276

GOLDEN, G. S. and FRENCH, J. H. (1975) Basilar artery migraine in young children. *Pediatrics*, **56**, 722–726

GOLZ, A., WESTERMAN, S. T., GILBERT, L. M., JOACHIMS, H. Z. and NETZER, A. (1991) Effect of middle ear effusion on the vestibular labyrinth. *Journal of Laryngology and Otology*, **105**, 987–989

GOODHILL, V. (1967) The conductive loss phenomenon in post-stapedectomy perilymphatic fistulae. *Laryngoscope*, **77**, 1179–1190

GOODHILL, V. (1976) Labyrinthine membrane ruptures in sudden sensorineural hearing loss. *Proceedings of the Royal Society of Medicine*, **69**, 565–572

GORMAN, J. J., COGAN, D. C. and GELLIS, S. S. (1957) An apparatus for grading the visual acuity of infants on the basis of optokinetic nystagmus. *Pediatrics*, **19**, 1088–1092

GROEN, J. J. (1963) Postnatal changes in vestibular reactions. *Acta Oto-Laryngologica*, **56**, 390–397

GROEN J. J. (1965) Central regulation of the vestibular system. *Acta Oto-Laryngologica*, **59**, 211–218

GRUNDFAST, K. M. and BLUESTONE, C. D. (1978) Sudden or fluctuating hearing loss and vertigo in children due to perilymph fistula. *Annals of Otology, Rhinology and Laryngology*, **87**, 761–770

HARKER, L. A. and RASSEKH, C. H. (1987) Episodic vertigo in basilar artery migraine. *Otolaryngology–Head and Neck Surgery*, **96**, 239–250

HARKER, L. A., NORANTE, J. D. and RYU, J. H. (1974) Experimental rupture of the round window membrane. *Transactions of the American Academy of Ophthalmology and Otolaryngology*, **78**, 448–452

HARRINGTON, J. W. and BIRCK, H. G. (1967) Recurrent meningitis due to congenital petrous fistula. *Archives of Otolaryngology*, **85**, 572–575

HARRISON, M. S. (1962a) Vertigo in childhood. *Journal of Laryngology and Otology*, **76**, 601–616

HARRISON, M. S. (1962b) 'Epidemic vertigo' – vestibular neuronitis, a clinical study. *Brain*, **85**, 613–619

HARRISON, M. S. and NAFTALIN, L. (1968) *Menière's Disease*. Springfield Illinois: Charles C. Thomas

HÄUSLER, R. and PAMPURIK, J. (1989) Die chirurgische und die physiotherapeutische Behandlung des benignen paroxysmalen Lagerungsschwindels. *Laryngology, Rhinology, Otology (Stuttgart)*, **68**, 342–346

HENRIKSSON, N. G. (1955) The correlation between the speed of the eye in the slow phase of nystagmus and vestibular stimulus. *Acta Oto-Laryngologica*, **45**, 2

HERMAN, R., MAULUCCI, R. and STUYCK, J. (1982) Development and plasticity of visual and vestibular generated movements. *Experimental Brain Research*, **47**, 69–78

HILL, J. H., FREINT, A. J. and MAFFE, M. F. (1984) Enlargement of the vestibular aqueduct. *American Journal of Otolaryngology*, **5**, 411–414

HILL, W. and SHERMAN, H. (1968) Acute intermittent familial cerebellar ataxia. *Archives of Neurology*, **18**, 350–357

HOLT, K. S. (1975) Movement and child development. How and why children move. *Clinics in Developmental Medicine*, 55, Philadelphia: Lippincott

HOOD, J. D. (1980) Unsteadiness of cerebellar origin: investigation into its cause. *Journal of Laryngology and Otology*, **94**, 865–876

HOUGH, J. V. D. (1969) Restoration of hearing loss after head trauma. *Annals of Otology*, **78**, 210–226

HULTCRANTZ, M. and ANNIKO, M. (1984) Malformation of the vestibular organs following low dose gamma irradiation during embryonic development. *Acta Oto-Laryngologica*, **97**, 7–17

HUTCHISON, J. H. (1972) *Practical Paediatric Problems*, 3rd ed. London: Lloyd-Luke Ltd. pp. 493–498

HUYGEN, P. L. M., VAN RIJN, P. M., CREMERS, C. W. R. J. and THEUNISSEN E. J. J. M., (1993) The vestibulo-ocular reflex in pupils at a Dutch school for the hearing impaired; findings relating to acquired causes. *International Journal of Pediatric Otorhinolaryngology*, **25**, 39–47

HYDÉN, D., ODKVIST, L. and KYLÉN P. (1979) Vestibular symptoms in mumps deafness. *Acta Oto-Laryngologica*, Suppl. 360, 182–183

ILLINGWORTH, R. S. (1983) *The Normal Child*, 8th edn. Edinburgh: Churchill Livingstone

ILLUM, P. (1972) The Mondini type of cochlear malformation. *Archives of Otolaryngology*, **95**, 305–311

JONGKEES, L. B. W. and GASTHUIS, W. (1973) La fonction de l'organe vestibulaire du nouveau-né et de l'enfant. *Journal Français d'Oto-Rhino-Laryngologie*, **22**, 97–101

JONGKEES, L. B. W. and PHILIPSZOON, A. J. (1964) Electronystagmography, *Acta Oto-Laryngologica*, Suppl. 189, 7–11

KAGA, K., SUZUKI, J-I., MARSH, R. R. and TANAKA, Y. (1981) Influence of labyrinthine hypoactivity on gross motor development of infants. *Annals of the New York Academy of Science*, **374**, 412–420

KARJALAINEN, S., TERASVIRTA, M., KARJA, J. and KAARAINEN, H. (1985) Usher's syndrome type III: ENG findings in four affected and six unaffected siblings. *Journal of Laryngology and Otology*, **99**, 43–48

KARMODY, C. S. (1983) Viral labyrinthitis: early pathology in the human. *Laryngoscope*, **93**, 1527–1533

KASTANIOUDAKIS, J., SKEVAS, A., ASSIMAKOPOULOS, D. and ANASTASOPOULOS, D. (1993) Hearing loss and vestibular dysfunction of the childhood from the use of streptomycin in Albania. *International Journal of Pediatric Otorhinolaryngology*, **26**, 109–115

KENYON, G. S. (1991) Vestibular evolution. In: *Current Approaches to Vertigo*, Dorchester: Henry Ling Ltd. pp. 26–37

KOBRAK, H. (1934) Untersuchungen uber den Zusammenhang Zwischen Hirndruck und Labyrinthdruck. Beitr. Prakt. Theoret. Hals-Nasen-Ohrenheilk, **31**, 212 219

KOEHLER, B. (1980) Benign paroxysmal vertigo of childhood. *European Journal of Pediatrics*, **134**, 149–151

KOENIGSBERGER, M. R., CHUTORIAN, A. M., GOLD, A. P. and SCHVEY, M. S. (1970) Benign paroxysmal vertigo of childhood. *Neurology*, **20**, 1108–1113

KOHUT, R. I. (1992) Perilymph fistulas. Clinical criteria. *Archives of Otolaryngology, Head and Neck Surgery*, **118**, 687–692

KRAVITZ, H. and BOEHM, J. J. (1971) Rhythmic habit patterns in infancy: their sequence, age of onset and frequency. *Child Development*, **42**, 399–413

KREMENITZER, J. P., VAUGHAN, H. G., KURTZBERG, D. and DOWLING, K. (1979) Smooth pursuit eye movements in the newborn infant. *Child Development*, **50**, 442–448

KUMAR, A., FISHMAN, G. and TOROK, N. (1984) Vestibular and auditory function in Usher's syndrome. *Annals of Otology, Rhinology and Laryngology*, **93**, 600–608

KURITZKY, A., ZIEGLER, D. K. and HASSANIEN, R. (1981) Vertigo, motion sickness and migraine, *Headache*, **21**, 227–231

LANZI, G., BALOTTIN, U., FAZZI, E., MIRA, E. and PIACENTINO, G. (1986) Benign paroxysmal vertigo in childhood: a longitudinal study. *Headache*, **26**, 494–497

LENTZ, J. M. and COLLINS, W. E. (1977) Motion sickness and susceptibility and related behavioural characteristics in men and women. *Aviation Space and Environmental Medicine*, **48**, 316–322

LONGRIDGE, N. S. (1989) Progressive vestibular failure in childhood. *Acta Oto-Laryngologica*, Suppl. 468, 373–377

MACKEITH, R. C. and ROBSON, P. (1970) Postural reactions in the first year of life. *Update*, **2**, 1275–1282

MAGNUSSON, M., ENBOM, H. and PYYKKÖ, I. (1991) Postural compensation of congenital or early acquired vestibular

loss in hearing disabled children. *Acta Oto-Laryngologica*, Suppl. 481, 433–435

MANGABEIRA-ALBERNAZ, P. L. and MALAVASI GANANÇA, M. (1988) Sudden vertigo of central origin. *Acta Oto-Laryngologica*, **105**, 564–569

MENKES, J. H. (1985) *Textbook of Child Neurology*. Philadelphia: Lea and Febiger

MEYERHOFF, W. L., PAPARELLA, M. M. and SHEA, D. (1978) Ménière's disease in children. *Laryngoscope*, **88**, 1504–1511

MIRA, E., PIACENTINO, G., LANZI, G., BALOTTIN, U. and FAZZI, E. (1984) Benign paroxysmal vertigo in childhood: a migraine equivalent. *ORL: Journal of Otorhinolaryngology and its Related Specialties*, **46**, 97–104

MIRKA, A. and BLACK, F. O. (1990) Clinical application of dynamic posturography for evaluating sensory integration and vestibular dysfunction. *Neurologic Clinics*, **8**, 351–359

MÖLLER, C. G., KIMBERLING, W. J., DAVENPORT, S. L. H., PRILUCK, I., WHITE, V., BISCONE-HALTERMAN, K. et al. (1989) Usher's syndrome: an otoneurologic study. *Laryngoscope*, **99**, 73–79

MOLTENI, R. A. (1977) Vertigo as a presenting feature of multiple sclerosis in childhood. *American Journal of Diseases in Children*, **131**, 553–554

MONEY, K. E. (1970) Motion sickness. *Physiological Reviews*, **50**, 1–39

MORRIS, M. S., KIL, J. and CARVLIN, M. J. (1993) Magnetic resonance imaging of perilymphatic fistula. *Laryngoscope* **103**, 729–733

NADOL, J. B. (1978) Hearing loss as a sequela of meningitis. *Laryngoscope*, **88**, 739–755

NENZEILUS, C. (1951) On spontaneous cerebrospinal otorrhoea due to congenital malformations. *Acta Oto-Laryngologica*, **39**, 341–328

OMBREDANNE, M. and AUBRY, M. (1941) Syndrome de Ménière chez un enfant de 13 ans. Section intracranienne de nerf auditif. Guerison depuis 3 ans. *Bulletin de la Société de Pediatrie de Paris*, **38**, 193

ORNITZ, E. M. (1983) Normal and pathological maturation of vestibular function in the human child. In: *Development of Auditory and Vestibular Systems*, edited by R. Romand. New York: Academic Press Inc. pp. 479–536

ORNITZ, E. M., BROWN, M. B., MASON, A. and PUTNAM, N. H. (1974) The effect of visual input on post-rotatory nystagmus in normal children. *Acta Oto-Laryngologica*, **77**, 418–425

ORNITZ, E. M., ATWELL, C. W., WALTER, D. O., HARTMANN, E. E. and KAPLAN, A. R. (1979) The maturation of vestibular nystagmus in infancy and childhood. *Acta Oto-Laryngologica*, **88**, 244–256

OTTENBACHER, K. (1982) Patterns of postrotatory nystagmus in three learning disabled children. *American Journal of Occupational Therapy*, **36**, 657–663

OUVRIER, R. and HOPKINS, I. (1970) Occlusive disease of the vertebrobasilar arterial system in childhood. *Developmental Medicine and Child Neurology*, **12**, 186–192

PAPATHEOPHILOU, R., JEAVONS, P. M. and DISNEY, M. E. (1972) Recurrent abdominal pain: a clinical and electronystagmographic study. *Developmental Medicine and Child Neurology*, **14**, 31–44

PARISIER, S. C. and BIRKIN, E. A. (1976) Recurrent meningitis secondary to idiopathic oval window CSF leak. *Laryngoscope*, **86**, 1503–1515

PARKER, W. (1989) Migraine and the vestibular system in

childhood and adolescence. *American Journal of Otology*, 10, 364–371

PARVING, A. (1976) Menière's disease in childhood. *Journal of Laryngology and Otology*, 90, 817–821

PASHLEY, N. R. T. (1982) Simultaneous round and oval window fistulae in a child. *Annals of Otology, Rhinology and Laryngology*, 91, 332–335

PEARCE, J. (1971) *General Review of Some Aetiological Factors in Migraine*. New York: Springer Verlag. pp. 1–7

PENDLETON, M. E. and PAINE, R. S. (1961) Vestibular nystagmus in newborn infants. *Neurology*, 11, 450–458

PIGNATARO, O., ROSSI, L., GAINI, R., OLDINI, C., SAMBATARO, G. and NINO, L. (1979) The evolution of the vestibular apparatus according to the age of the infant. *International Journal of Pediatric Otolaryngology*, 1, 165–170

PILLSBURY, H. C. (1981) Metabolic causes of hearing loss and vertigo. *Otolargyngologic Clinics of North America*, 14, 347–354

PINCUS, J. H. (1978) Hyperventilation syndrome. *British Journal of Hospital Medicine*, 19, 312–313

PODOSHIN, L. and FRADIS, M. (1975) Hearing loss after head injury. *Archives of Otolaryngology*, 101, 15–18

POE, D. S. REBEIZ, E. E. and PANKRATOV, M. M. (1992) Evaluation of perilympathic fistulas by middle ear endoscopy. *American Journal of Otology*, 13, 529–533

PRIEVE, B. A. and YANZ, J. L. (1984) Age-dependent changes in susceptibility to ototoxic hearing loss. *Acta Oto-Laryngologica*, 98, 428–438

PULLEN, F. N. (1972) Round window membrane rupture: a cause of sudden deafness. *Transactions of the American Academy of Ophthalmology and Otolaryngology*, 76, 1444–1450

RAPIN, I. (1974) Hypoactive labyrinth and motor development. *Clinical Pediatrics*, 13, 922–937

RASMUSSEN, N., JOHNSEN, N. J. and BOHR, V. A., (1991) Otologic sequelae after pneumococcal meningitis: a survey of 164 consecutive cases with a follow-up of 94 survivors. *Laryngoscope*, 101, 876–882

RIZVI, S. S. and SMITH, L. E. (1981) Idiopathic endolymphatic hydrops and the vestibular aqueduct. *Annals of Otology, Rhinology and Laryngology*, 90, 77–79

ROCKETT, F. X. (1969) Pantopaque visualisation of a congenital dural defect of the internal auditory meatus. *Acta Radiologica* (special issue), 9, 83–90

ROWSON, K., HINCHCLIFFE, R. and GAMBLE, D. R. (1976) The role of viruses in acute auditory failure. *British Journal of Audiology*, 10, 107–109

RUCKENSTEIN, M. J. and HARRISON, R. V. (1991) Motion sickness. Helping patients tolerate the ups and downs. *Postgraduate Medicine*, 89, 139–144

SADÉ, J. (1981) Menière's disease. *Journal of Laryngology and Otology*, 45, 261

SADÉ, J. and YANIV, S. (1984) Menière's disease in infants. *Acta Oto-Laryngologica*, 97, 33–37

SALLUSTRO, F. and ATWELL, C. W. (1978) Baby rocking, head banging and head rolling in normal children. *Journal of Pediatrics*, 93, 704–708

SANDBERG, L. E. and TERKILDSEN, K. (1965) Caloric tests in deaf children. *Archives of Otolaryngology*, 81, 350–355

SANNER, G. and BERGSTRÖM, B. (1979) Benign paroxysmal torticollis in infancy. *Acta Pediatrica Scandinavica*, 68, 219–223

SCHUKNECHT, H. and RUBY, R. (1973) Cupulolithiasis. *Advances in Otorhinolaryngology*, 20, 434–443

SCHWARTZ, J. F. (1972) Ataxia in bacterial meningitis. *Neurology*, 22, 1071–1074

SCHWEITZER, V. G. and CLACK, T. D., (1984) Waardenberg's syndrome: a case report with CT scanning and cochleovestibular evaluation. *International Journal of Pediatric Otorhinolaryngology*, 7, 311–322

SEKITANI, T. and HARADA, Y. (eds). (1993) Vestibular neuronitis. Proceedings of an international symposium on vestibular ganglia and vestibular neuronitis. Yamaguchi, Japan 14–16 September 1991. *Acta Otolaryngologica*, Suppl. 503, 1–208

SHARMA, K. (1980) Susceptibility to motion sickness. *Acta Geneticae Medicae et Gemellologiae (Roma)*, 29, 157–162

SHERIDAN, M. D. (1975) *Children's Developmental Progress*, 3rd edn. Windsor, NFER Publishing Company. pp. 12–13

SHIRABE, S. (1988) Vestibular neuronitis in childhood. *Acta Oto-Laryngologica*, Suppl. 458, 120–122

SIDEBOTHAM, P. (1988) Balance through the ages of man. *Journal of Laryngology and Otology*, 102, 203–208

SILVER, A. A. and GABRIEL, H. P. (1964) The association of schizophrenia in childhood with primitive postural control and decreased muscle tone. *Developmental Medicine and Child Neurology*, 6, 495–497

SIMONTON, K. M. (1940) Menière's symptom complex: a review of the literature. *Annals of Otology, Rhinology and Laryngology*, 49, 80

SNASHALL, S. E. (1983) Vestibular function tests in children. *Journal of the Royal Society of Medicine*, 76, 555–559

SNASHALL, S. E. (1986) Vertigo in children. In: *Current Approaches to Vertigo*. Eastbourne: Duphar Laboratories Ltd. published by Transmedica Europe Ltd. pp. 37–41

SNASHALL, S. E. (1987) Vestibular disorders. In: *Scott-Brown's Otolaryngology*, 5th ed., vol. 6, *Paediatric Otolaryngology*, edited by J. N. G. Evans, pp. 194–217. London: Butterworths

SNASHALL, S. (1993) Vestibular testing: the current position (Editorial). *Journal of Laryngology and Otology*, 107, 481–482

SNYDER, C. H. (1969) Paroxysmal torticollis in infancy. *American Journal of Diseases in Children*, 117, 458–460

STALLER, S. J., GOIN, D. W. and HILDEBRANDT, M. (1986) Pediatric vestibular evaluation with harmonic acceleration. *Otolaryngology – Head and Neck Surgery*, 95, 471–476

STEINBERG, M. and RENDLE-SHORT, J. (1977) Vestibular dysfunction in young children with minor neurological impairment. *Developmental Medicine and Child Neurology*, 19, 639–651

STRAUSS, M. and DAVIS, G. L. (1973) Viral disease of the labyrinth. A review of the literature and discussion of the role of cytomegalovirus in congenital deafness. *Annals of Otology, Rhinology and Laryngology*, 82, 577–583

SUPANCE, J. S. and BLUESTONE, C. D. (1983) Perilymph fistulas in infants and children. *Otolaryngology – Head and Neck Surgery*, 91, 663–671

SWAIMAN, K. F. and FRANK, Y. (1978) Seizure headaches in children. *Developmental Medicine and Child Neurology*, 20, 580–585

TAKIGUCHI, T., HONDA, M., KAGA, K., OGAWA, T. and GOTO, S. (1991) Results of damped-rotation tests in brain damaged infants and children. *Acta Oto-Laryngologica*, Suppl. 481, 536–542

TIBBLING, L. (1969) The rotatory nystagmus response in children. *Acta Oto-Laryngologica*, 68, 459–467

TIERI, L., MASI, R., MARSELLA, P. and PINELLI, V. (1984) Sudden deafness in children. *International Journal of Pediatric Otorhinolaryngology*, 7, 257–264

THIRINGER, K., KANKUNEN, A., LIDÉN, G. and NIKLASSON, A. (1984) Perinatal risk factors in the aetiology of hearing loss in preschool children. *Developmental Medicine and Child Neurology*, **26**, 799–807

TJERNSTROM, O. (1973) Nystagmus inhibition as an effect of eye closure. *Acta Oto-Laryngologica*, **75**, 408–418

TSUZUKU, T. and KAGA, K. (1991) The relation between motor function development and vestibular function tests in four children with inner ear anomaly. *Acta Oto-Laryngologica*, Suppl. 481, 443–446

VALVASSORI, G. E. and CLEMIS, J. D. (1978). The large vestibular aqueduct syndrome. *Laryngoscope*, **88**, 723–728

VARTIAINEN, E., KARJALAINEN, S. and KARJA, J. (1985) Auditory disorders following head injury in children. *Acta Oto-Laryngologica*, **99**, 529–536

VARTIAINEN, E., NUUTINEN, J., KARJALAINEN, S. and NYKÄNEN (1991) Perilymph fistula – a diagnostic dilemma. *Journal of Laryngology and Otology*, **105**, 270–273

WATSON, P. and STEELE, J. C. (1974) Paroxysmal dysequilib-rium in the migraine syndrome of childhood. *Archives of Otolaryngology*, **99**, 177–179

WEEKS, Z. R. (1979) Effects of the vestibular system on human development Part 1. Overview and effects of stimulation. *American Journal of Occupational Therapy*, **33**, 376–381

WEIDER, D. J. (1992) Treatment and management of perilymphatic fistula. *American Journal of Otology*, **13**, 158–166

WENZEL, D. (1978) The development of the parachute reaction: a visuo-vestibular response. *Neuropediatrie (Stuttgart)*, **9**, 351–359

WHITE, J. C. (1969) Familial periodic nystagmus, vertigo and ataxia. *Archives of Neurology*, **20**, 276–280

WILSON, W. R. and ZOLLER, M. (1981) Syphilitic otitis. *Annals of Otology, Rhinology and Laryngology*, **90**, 21–25

WTODYKA, J. (1978) Studies on cochlear aqueduct patency. *Annals of Otology, Rhinology and Laryngology*, **87**, 22–28

ZARNOCH, J. M. (1980) Vestibular characteristics of the Down's population. *Seminars in Speech, Language and Hearing*, **1**, 87–97

13

Speech and language

Sylvia Thompson

The term 'communication' is a rather broad, yet useful one, to cover the vast area of human skills connected with sending and receiving of messages between individuals or groups of individuals which forms the heart of human interaction.

As, in this situation, this writer communicates by writing, and you receive the message by reading, a very complex set of skills is in play; yet these skills are taken so much for granted that it is only when they break down, in the case of adults, or fail or are slow to develop, in the case of children, that the full extent of the complexity of communication is realized, and the potentially devastating effects such disorders can have on the normal development of a child is understood.

What follows then, is a journey through the various stages of development, highlighting the potential areas for problems or breakdown, so that the practitioner will have some useful 'rules of thumb' to use in work with children. Thus, knowing when to get alarmed, when to reassure, when to seek further specialist help or when and how to do some, or all of these things, on the occasion of the child meeting you with such problems will be another positive step in the therapeutic process.

Terminology

The explanation of a few terms will be useful and, as in other areas, there are trends in the use of terms, so some old and new terms are given.

Communication: concerned with ways in which the individual intentionally influences the behaviour of others (Kiernan and Reid, 1987).

Language: a way in which the individual internalizes and codifies aspects of experience.

1 Comprehension/reception/receptive language: the understanding of spoken, written, signed, or symbolic aspects of language.
2 Production/expression/expressive function: the spoken word, sign, symbol or written word.
3 Semantics: the aspect of language that governs the meaning of words and word combinations.

Voice: its characteristics are quality, pitch, loudness, resonance; all of which vary according to the age, size, sex, etc. of the speaker.

Fluency: includes aspects of rate, rhythm, and conversely in their absence, non-fluent patterns such as stammering and cluttering.

Sound production

1 Articulation: primarily the movement of the tongue, lips, and palate, all of which need to co-articulate at the correct speed and precision, to produce intelligible speech.
2 Phonology: rules governing the production of sounds, over which the child gradually gains control; this means learning to put endings on words, to produce consonant strings, for example 'str' in 'string'.

The development of speech

At birth, given good lungs and gross movements of lips and tongue, the new baby can communicate very effectively (and loudly too!). However, much of this communication is unintentional, and it is only due to the consistent response of carers to this early sound, or rather noise making, that the cries indicating 'hunger', 'pain', etc. begin to differentiate. The norm is that at 1–2 months there is a special cry for hunger. A question to ask is: Does the child cry in a different way when he is wet or hungry etc.? What about his sucking, eating or drinking skills, are any problems apparent?

Warning signs

- A quiet baby or a baby with no differentiated cries.
- A lack of response to sounds, especially the human voice.
- Problems noted with the lips, or the tongue during feeding, i.e. swallowing, use of teat, bottle etc.
- Problems in the baby's interaction with carers, i.e. unusual eye contact, lack of response to touch etc.

Between the stage of frequent crying (about 1 month), and the child using some plural forms correctly in speech (about 36 months), the child has made huge gains in the development of *productive* language skills. Similarly, the child who gives a startle response to loud sudden noises (about 1 month), and the child who demonstrates an understanding of prepositions (e.g. on, under, front, behind), has made a journey in the development of *receptive* language skills, but breakdown or delay may occur at any point along the way.

Language has traditionally been subdivided into the 'productive' and 'receptive' aspects. Though a somewhat artificial division, it is nonetheless useful in terms of examination or study, provided the interrelationship or interconnection is realized. The following assumes the productive–receptive format.

Some stepping stones in the development of receptive language skills

The baby or child:

- Responds to sound: stops activity
- Is quieted by a familiar voice
- Responds to voice by smiling
- Watches the lips and mouth of a speaker
- Raises arms in response to outstretched arms
- Looks around in search of a speaker
- Responds to an angry voice by crying and a pleasant voice by smiling
- Recognizes and responds to own name
- Stops or withdraws in response to a 'No' 50% of the time
- Listens to own vocalization
- Stops activity when name is called
- Has some comprehension of symbolic gestures and intonation patterns, e.g. 'no-no', 'hot', own name
- Will look at pictures for one minute, if they are named
- Differentiates between family and strangers
- Responds rhythmically to music

- Appears to understand simple questions, e.g. 'Where's the ball?'
- Likes rhymes and simple songs
- Understands object names and actions within routines only (8–12 months)
- Understands some people's names (12–18 months)
- Understands some common objects within a visual field (18 months)
- Recognizes two familiar objects from a group of four familiar objects (19–24 months)
- Can follow a few simple commands, e.g. 'Give me the block'
- May understand a simple question that is answered by 'yes' or 'no', e.g. 'Want milk?'

With age, the baby shows a growing comprehension of 'wh . . .' questions, e.g. 'what?' ($2 - 2\frac{1}{2}$ years), 'whose?' 'why', 'how many?', 'how often?', 'when?' ($5\frac{1}{2}$ years), and such concepts as 'in'; 'on'; 'under'; 'in front of', 'behind', 'through', 'middle', etc.

The language environment, and the effects of the home, parents, siblings, TV, books, school, teachers, friends and 'the street', will have a very big influence on the development of language production and comprehension in the growing child.

Breakdown

Breakdown may occur at any point along the way.
Some potential problems include:

1 Hearing status, varying from a fluctuating conductive loss, to a severe to profound degree of sensorineural hearing loss.
2 Significant attention problems.
3 Difficulties related to understanding of connected speech (i.e. sentences, or the syntax, grammar, etc.)

Questions should be asked about:

1 The history of ear and hearing problems.
2 The type of language input, e.g. bilingual, monolingual.
3 The ability to listen (to sit still for any length of time) to a story.

Some stepping stones in the development of productive language skills

The baby's vocal behaviour:

- Basic biological noises (Crystal, 1986)
- Crying, vowels and -ng with some pitch changes
- Sounds that are produced with reflex activities
- A special cry for hunger
- Cooing, gurgling and squeals
- Predominating sounds:

a *Nasal sounds*: tension in the facial and oral area results in a tense palate nasalization effect
b *Vowels*: open tract with minimal tongue movement
c *Velars*/k, g/: lying back relaxed after feeding with tongue lolling back in mouth, the back of the tongue moves towards the palate

- The infant responds to the adult 'vocal contagion' (2–4 months), i.e. the infant may increase vocalizing if speech or sounds are being made around her
- Babbling: single syllable /p, b or m/ plus a vowel; double syllable

The baby or child:

- Responds with a vocalization when called by name
- Can play speech-gesture games like 'pat-a-cake', 'peek-a-boo'
- Uses facial and arm gestures to accompany vocalization
- Tries out different pitches
- Copies melody pattern of familiar phrases, e.g. greetings
- Uses jargon
- Waves bye-bye, shakes head to some questions
- Tries to name a familiar object on seeing it again
- Sometimes uses 'uh oh'
- 'Talks' to self in a mirror
- Vocalizes in varied jargon patterns while playing alone
- Initiates speech-gesture games like 'peek-a-boo'
- Uses some true words in jargon utterances
- Uses single true words along with gestures for wants and needs
- Begins repeating words heard in conversation (8–12 months)
- May use as first words: dada, mama, down, box, bye-bye, more, no, stop, there, away, all gone, turn, baby (indicating possession).

These first words are actually word approximations. The first word may be 'Mama' due to parent's response, appearing as early as 8–9 months, or up to 12–15 months. Boys are reputed to be later than girls, but mothers appear to talk less to boys. The first 50 words usually emerge before the child puts two words together. Mother/father–child routines are important here, e.g. games like 'pat-a-cake', 'peek-a-boo' etc.

Phonological processes

These allow the child to produce her first words:
a The child omits the ends of words.
b Repeats the syllable (i.e. phonetic reduplication– 'wa-wa' for 'water')
c Reduces clusters, e.g. 'spoon' becomes 'boon'
   The above processes gradually drop out and speech becomes more intelligible by 2–3 years of age.

Development continues as follows:
The child:

- Uses successive single words with phrases in between.
- Imitates environmental sounds during play, e.g. motors, animals.
- May pull a person to show some object, person or situation.
- Uses two words together, e.g. agent-action (nearer to 2 years of age).
- Uses 'in' 'on' '-ing' verb ending, and maybe some plurals.
- Uses three word phrases and uses irregular past tense, possessive.
- Uses four word phrases (3–4 years) and uses 'the', 'a'

The mean length of utterance is related to age at this stage. The child gradually acquires the regular past tense, use of the auxiliary verb system and use of complex sentences, e.g. 'Can I do it when we get home?', 'I guess she's sick'. Studies show how parents modify their speech patterns to their young children learning language. Immaturity of the sound system gradually reduces. An average 4 year old has a complete sound system and syntax repertoire and is using complete and complex sentences to comment on topics such as family, pets, school, etc.

Problems

Problems which may present are:

1 Physical problems associated with the oral musculature, as in cerebral palsy, cleft palate and various syndromes.
2 Hearing difficulties varying from a fluctuating conductive loss to a severe to profound degree of sensorineural loss.
3 Lack of appropriate stimulation input and reinforcement.
4 Significant cognitive limitations.
5 Severe attention difficulties.
6 Social or interactive difficulties.

Questions should be asked about:

1 The development of feeding and drinking skills (including swallowing).
2 The child's response to speech games.
3 The child's interest in communication.

Voice problems in childhood

Children, like adults, can present with a wide range of voice problems. However, with an understandable emphasis on intelligibility of speech and normal language, parents, teachers, and the various professionals coming into contact with the child may not be concerned or aware of the existence of a voice problem, and thus may not realize that intervention is possible or necessary.

Some essential and basic points on the characteristics of a normal voice and a problem voice will therefore give a useful basis so that voice problems can be identified, evaluated and diagnosed, and appropriate treatment instituted.

Characteristics of a normal voice (Wilson, 1979)

1 Pleasing voice quality.
2 Proper balance of oral and nasal resonance.
3 Appropriate loudness.
4 A model frequency level, suitable for age, size and loudness.
5 Appropriate voice inflections, involving pitch and reinforcement.

The rate of speaking should be such that it does not interfere with these five essential characteristics.

Characteristics of a problem voice (Wilson, 1979)

1 Disturbed voice quality, caused by laryngeal dysfunction and characterized by hoarseness, harshness or breathiness.
2 Hypernasality and hyponasality, caused by improper balance of oral and nasal resonance.
3 A voice too soft to be heard easily, or so loud it is unpleasant.
4 A modal frequency level too high, or too low for age, size and sex.
5 Inappropriate inflections of pitch and loudness.

If the rate of speaking is too fast, or too slow, it may interfere with adequate voice production.

Classifications of voice problems

Voice quality problems

Disturbance may occur in the laryngeal tone, usually associated with sound generated at the level of the vocal cords. This can result in harshness, breathiness, hoarseness or exclusive or excessive use of vocal fry. This latter is a vocal quality of unsustained phonation due to the restricted amplitude of vocal fold oscillation. It is often heard as a change in phonation towards the end of phrases or sentences.

Resonance problems

These include hypernasality and hyponasality.

Loudness problems

The voice can be too loud or too quiet.

Pitch problems

These include a modal frequency level that is too high, or too low; a narrow pitch range; or too many pitch breaks and a pitch too high, too low in specific situations.

The causes of voice problems (Table 13.1)

The causes of voice problems fall into four general categories:

1 Organic
2 Organic changes due to vocal abuse and vocal misuse
3 Functional
4 Factors contributing to the voice problem.

The child presenting with a voice problem is best served by a multidisciplinary team, such as typically exists for cleft palate, and paediatric audiology. As well as the expected members of such a team, an otolaryngologist, a speech-language therapist and audiologist, input may be necessary from the fields of paediatrics, neurology, psychiatry, psychology, social work, education, dentistry, allergy, radiology and plastic surgery.

All the problems identified thus far should be managed within the skill mix of such a team and are best managed in a specialist clinic, or a setting where such team members work in close liaison with one another. In this way, diagnosis and treatment of voice problems in children can proceed in an efficient and effective manner.

The goals of the speech-language therapist working in the area of childhood voice problems are:

1 To prevent problems developing.
2 To act as a member of a team contributing towards appraisal and diagnosis.
3 To offer a voice therapy programme to modify or eliminate the voice problems.

Many voice disorders in adults began in childhood, so early intervention is always recommended.

Problems in sound production

The child whose speech and language skills are developing normally usually has speech which is intelligible, even to strangers, by 3 years of age. In contrast, it is often just at this age that the prob-

Table 13.1 Causes of voice problems

Cause	Level	Vocal quality	Physical aspect
Organic	Larynx	May be harsh, breathy, hoarse, or at an inappropriate pitch	Structural anomalies e.g. laryngeal webs, cord pathology, absence of a structure (e.g. epiglottis) Vocal cord paralysis Laryngeal growths: papilloma, cyst, laryngocoele Laryngeal trauma
	Velopharynx and oral area	Hypernasal	Velopharyngeal insufficiency e.g. cleft palate, short hard and/or soft palate, abnormally capacious pharynx, velar paralysis, submucous cleft palate, adenoidectomy
	Nose	Hyponasal	Obstruction in nasal or nasopharyngeal passages due to: deviated septum, bilateral turbinate hypertrophy, nasal polyps, enlarged adenoid tissue, allergic or inflammatory swelling of mucosa, traumatic injuries On a functional basis: poor motor coordination, congenital dyspraxia, faulty habits of verbal behaviour
	Hearing mechanism		Abnormal pitch (e.g. too high), inappropriate loudness, hyper/hyponasality, defective laryngeal tone: breathiness, harshness; hard glottal attack, monotony in rhythm, rate and pitch, hollow or non-resonant quality

Cause	Types of abuse	Organic changes
Organic changes due to vocal abuse	Shouting, screaming, cheering Strained vocalizations Excessive talking Explosive vocalizations and abrupt glottal attack Throat clearing and coughing	Vocal nodules Nodules Polyps Dysphonia plicae ventricularis
Organic changes due to vocal misuse	Abuse of pitch and loudness, e.g. talking in noise	Hyperkeratosis Non-specific laryngitis

Cause	Vocal quality	Due to
Functional	May be hoarse, harsh, breathy hypernasal too loud or too quiet aphonic	Disturbed mutation Psychological factors Imitation Faulty learning

Cause	Vocal quality	Physical conditions

Contributing causes	Hoarse, husky, high-pitched, voice-breaks	Glandular conditions
		Allergies
		Upper respiratory conditions
		  chronic pharyngitis
		  sinusitis
		  deviated nasal septum
		Premenstrual and menstrual problems

lems of 'unclear' speech or poor pronunciation are noted, perhaps at nursery school, by the child-minder, by the health visitor (nurse), the family doctor, or sometimes by the parents themselves, with a resulting referral to the local speech and language therapist.

Categories of problems

The disorders or problems of sound production can be described or divided into two categories. A problem at the *phonetic level* which involves an inability, or difficulty in the production of speech, usually as a result of some organic deficiency in the speech mechanism; or a problem at the *phonological level* which involves an abnormal, inadequate, or disorganized system of sound patterns, evidenced by deviations in the spoken medium of language. However, it must be noted that problems at both levels may also coexist in a child with for example a cleft palate or a hearing impairment.

More importantly, problems in sound production may simply form one part of an overall disordered system rather than existing in isolation, occurring alongside other difficulties in expressive language skills and/or language comprehension skills.

Causes

Phonetic level

Normal production of speech requires accurate and rapid movements of the lips, tongue, and soft palate. Therefore difficulty in such movement, and/or control of these movements may result in a speech problem. The causes are numerous and include conditions such as cleft lip and/or palate, cerebral palsy, unusual or abnormal structures involved, as in particular syndromes (e.g. Down's syndrome; Pierre-Robin syndrome), or traumatic injury.

In cerebral palsy there is a clearly observable neuromuscular impairment, though the degree of severity will vary, leading to *dysarthria*, a problem of accuracy, mobility, control, timing and coordination of the movements of the speech musculature.

Phonological level

The cause of the problem at this level is somewhat more elusive, but it has been described as a 'neurolinguistic dysfunction at the phonological level of cortical representation and organisation of the language system' (Grunwell, 1982).

Management

The role of the speech and language therapist in this area has long been recognized and acknowledged. Early intervention is always recommended as progress can vary from very rapid to lengthy and continuing, with some children requiring special educational provision within a special unit catering for specific language disorders. Any suggestion of a 'wait and see' approach by professionals other than the speech and language therapist is strongly discouraged.

As an integral part of the diagnostic process, hearing testing will be crucial, not only to eliminate the presence, though unlikely, of a sensorineural loss, but more likely, the possible presence of a conductive loss, persistent or fluctuating.

Feeding skills

In the event that babies or young children with a neurological involvement may present at an otolaryngological clinic, it may be helpful to be aware of the general concerns that often surround the issue of feeding.

Such children may have some, or all of the following limiting movements: an inefficient sucking pattern, jaw thrust, tonic bite reflex, jaw clenching, exaggerated tongue protrusion or retraction, low tone in the lips, lip retraction, or lip pursing (Evans-Morris and Dunn Klein, 1987).

It is clear that the normal development of oral speech and language skills will be greatly hindered in such children and that specific feeding strategies will be required to limit the potentially devastating effects on normal movements of the speech articulators.

The feeding process is a complicated one, involving the mouth, jaw, teeth, neck, shoulders, trunk, sitting skills, the digestive system, the environment, communication, and a relationship to the feeder. Therefore, it is evident that a team approach to management is crucial, involving the child, parents, feeding therapist, speech and language therapist, physiotherapist, occupational therapist, doctor, nutritionist, dietician, teacher, and dentist.

Developmental dyspraxia of speech

In the case of a young child (not more than 2 years old) without single words, or with words which are grossly unintelligible, it may very well be important to consider the possibility of a motor problem in the oral area. The child may lack the motor control and organization necessary to produce speech sounds. A review of the child's history may indicate difficulties in the area of feeding, e.g. in the move to solid foods, drooling and choking may also be reported. Even if the problem is mild in nature or degree, it may be an early warning of something that will later present significant difficulties for planning the motor movements for oral speech. Such a problem at the central planning stage may be diagnosed as a developmental dyspraxia of speech.

Problems of fluency

'Nonfluency is best characterised as a developmental disorder where multiple etiological factors are likely to play a role in determining onset' (Rustin, 1987).

The view that stuttering is caused by a multiplicity of factors is hard to dispute given our present knowledge. These factors may be language based, environmentally induced, or inherited. It is the interaction of these factors with the child and the family that will largely determine how communication develops. It is thought that the ways in which the family and significant others construe stuttering are influential in its development or failure to develop (Hayhow and Levy, 1985).

Stuttering relates to a complex interaction between the child's environment and the skills and abilities the child brings to that environment (Conture and Caruso, 1987).

In light of the above, it can be seen that a 'hands off' approach is not a good policy when dealing with fluency problems in young children, as this is really a valuable opportunity to practise prevention through early intervention. Early referral to a speech and language therapist is much more advisable, as it is the role of the therapist to differentiate between normal non-fluency and the dysfluency associated with the young stutterer.

Normal non-fluency is observed in children between 2 and 6 years of age, when a child may repeat sounds, syllables or whole words when speaking. The amount of repetition will vary from child to child, and from one situation to another. It may last from several weeks to several months; it may disappear altogether for a time, and then reappear later. Eventually, it will disappear completely.

In contrast, dysfluency characteristic of the young stutterer is marked by 'The occurrence of audible prolongations and double unit repetitions together with the overall frequency of repetitions and prolongations' (Rustin, 1987).

Therefore, during the first visit to a speech and language therapist, it is not unusual for both a parental interview and a child assessment to take place. During the assessment with the child the therapist may introduce several fluency techniques to try to determine whether this is a case of normal non-fluency or otherwise. Ultimately the therapist wants a profile of the cognitive, linguistic, social and emotional components of the child's stuttering, in order to plan appropriate intervention. With a very young child, such intervention will normally be with the parents themselves, and only later will it involve any direct work with the child.

Those families where the fluency is determined to be within normal limits, and where there are no other complicating or predisposing factors, may be advised to attend for counselling sessions, to inform them about the nature and development of normal speech and to monitor periodically the development of the child's speech (Rustin, 1991).

Problems in the use of language or pragmatics

Pragmatics is the study of language in its context of use: 'The roots of communication lie in the first relationships we make; in the first smile, even the first reflex grasp of the newborn baby's finger … with clear evidence of turntaking and synchronisation in communication even in the first few weeks between adults and babies' (Mittler, 1988).

This develops from birth to 4 years and beyond, and in the area of response to communication (Dewart and Summers, 1988): from the infant smiling in recognition of the familiar words in an action game, e.g. 'round and round the garden', to the young child of 4 years or older, who is beginning to understand riddles. Other areas of such development are *communicative intention* and *interaction* and *conversation*.

This area of communication skills is clearly seen at its most disordered in children on the autistic continuum. Such children may have normal or near normal articulation and phonological skills, and also some language skills (e.g. phrases and sentences), but may have no affective use of these skills.

It is a crucial area of assessment for a speech and language therapist facing a child with a language problem. Such an assessment gives an overall picture of the child as a communicator, and not just in the clinic or assessment centre. This dynamic process of exploration naturally involves parents and other carers, who are invited to share the knowledge they have about communicating with the child.

Problems related to cleft lip and palate
The size of the problem

In the UK there are around 15 000 children each year who require help because of communication difficulties related to cleft palate (Enderby and Philipp, 1986).

There is a continuum of degree of severity of cleft ranging from mild to severe. In the mildest forms there may be a submucous cleft of the soft palate or slight notching of the vermilion border of the upper lip. In the severest form there may be complete bilateral clefts of the lip and alveolus.

The likelihood of long-term communication difficulties is most likely, though not inevitable, in those children at the severe end of the continuum. Stengelhofen (1989) listed the other factors which will affect the development of adequate and acceptable communication:

- The timing and outcome of surgery
- The presence or absence of other handicapping conditions
- The child's intellectual potential
- The child's ability to adapt to adverse factors
- The family support available.

The management team

It is now standard practice for a child with a cleft palate to be managed by a team. The typical members of such a team are a plastic surgeon, an orthodontist, a paediatrician, an otolaryngologist, a speech-language therapist, an audiologist, the parents, and nursing staff. The involvement of some team members may continue well into the child's teenage years. These children with long-standing problems, leading to deficits in their communication skills, make up about 40% of the original population.

Related velopharyngeal problems

Other problems which may impact on velopharyngeal function are:

Velopharyngeal competence or incompetence following adenoidectomy. This highlights the need for a team evaluation prior to such surgery, especially in the older child.

Congenital palatopharyngeal incompetence due to either palatopharyngeal disproportion, or congenital suprabulbar paresis.

Problems associated with hearing impairment

Communication difficulties in the child with a hearing impairment may exist, depending on the type and extent of hearing loss, the age detected, and the presence or otherwise of associated problems.

Speech problems

If the child with the hearing impairment has an intact speech-sound production mechanism, then that child is capable of producing the whole range of sound types within the total human speech repertoire, but may be unable to develop or maintain a normal and intelligible pattern of speech because the hearing impairment prevents the monitoring of speech production via the auditory feedback loop (Grunwell, 1982). The problem may exist at both phonetic and phonological levels.

Voice problems (see also under Voice section)

The child may present with vocal problems of excessive or inadequate loudness, abnormal pitch, e.g. a monotonous pitch, rate and rhythm, resonance and laryngeal tone. This again will vary according to the type and degree of loss.

Language problems

A child with a hearing impairment may be expected to show signs of language delay. However this will be very closely related to the degree and type of deafness, and the age at which this was detected. For example, a child with profound sensorineural loss, born to deaf parents, may be a very fluent communicator in sign language, but may exhibit severe oral language delay, whereas a child with a fluctuating conductive loss may show significant deficits in the development of speech and language skills (Bamford and Saunders, 1991).

It is clear that normal hearing, including normal function of the middle ear, is an integral part of a normally developing set of oral communication skills, and that any degree of impairment needs to be monitored very carefully, with intervention at the earliest opportunity to prevent or limit delay or disorder.

References

BAMFORD, J. and SAUNDERS, E. (1991) Hearing impairment. Auditory perception and language disability. In: *Studies in Disorders of Communication*, 2nd edn. London: Whurr Publishers

CONTURE, E. G. and CARUSO, A. J. (1987) Assessment and diagnosis of childhood dysfluency. In: *Progress in the Treatment of Fluency Disorders*, edited by L. Rustin, H. Purser and D. Rowley. London: Taylor and Francis. pp. 84–104

CRYSTAL, D. (1986) *Listen to Your Child. A Parent's Guide to Children's Language*. Harmondsworth: Penguin

DEWART, H. and SUMMERS, S. (1988) *The Pragmatics Profile of Early Communication Skills*. Windsor: NFER-Nelson

ENDERBY, P. and PHILIPP, R. (1986) Speech and language handicap: towards knowing the size of the problem. *British Journal of Disorders of Communication*, **21**, 151–165

EVANS-MORRIS, S. and DUNN KLEIN, M. D. (1987) *Pre-feeding Skills. A Comprehensive Resource for Feeding Development*. Tucson, Arizona: Therapy Skill Builders

GRUNWELL, P. (1982) *Clinical Phonology*. London: Croom Helm

HAYHOW, R. and LEVY, C. (1985) *Working with Stuttering*. Windsor: Winslow Press

KIERNAN, C. and REID, B. (1987) *Pre-verbal Communication Schedule* (manual). Windsor: NFER-Nelson

MITTLER, P. (1988) Foreword. In: *Communication before Speech*, edited by J. Coupe and J. Goldbart. London: Croom Helm

RUSTIN, L. (1987) The treatment of childhood dysfluency through active parental involvement. In: *Progress in the Treatment of Fluency Disorders*, edited by L. Rustin, H. Purser and D. Rowley. London: Taylor and Francis. pp. 166–180

RUSTIN, L. (1991) *Parents, Families and the Stuttering Child*. Kibworth: Far Communications

STENGELHOFEN, J. (ed.) (1989) The nature and cause of communication problems in cleft palate. In: *Cleft Palate. The Nature and Remediation of Communication Problems*. London: Churchill Livingstone. pp. 1–30

WILSON, D. K. (1979) *Voice Problems in Children*, 2nd edn. London: Williams and Wilkins

14

Foreign bodies in the ear or nose

A. P. Walby

Foreign bodies in the ears or nose of children have usually been placed there deliberately, and deserve mention both because they may be difficult to diagnose, and also to remove.

Foreign bodies in the ear

Aetiology

Foreign bodies enter the ear most commonly through the external auditory meatus, although penetrating injuries may also be responsible possibly with more serious immediate medical consequences. Surgery may be responsible for the presence of foreign material. Inexpert use of spring-loaded ear-piercing instruments for insertion of earrings may lead to an earring backing becoming embedded in the ear lobe or helix (Muntz, Pa-C and Asher, 1990).

Young children more commonly insert objects in their ears than babies or older children, and they may also insert them into the ears of their sibs. Insertion has a greater incidence in mentally retarded children and they will commonly repeat the episode.

Site of the foreign body

Inserted foreign bodies are usually found in the external auditory meatus. There is a slight constriction at the junction of the cartilaginous and bony canals and most foreign bodies will lodge just lateral to this. They may however be impacted at the constriction, or lie beyond it. It is more common for the object to lie in the external auditory canal than to pass through the tympanic membrane into the middle ear, but passage through the tympanic membrane to lie in the middle ear may occur. Even more serious penetrating injury is caused by those foreign bodies which lodge in the inner ear after passage through the external ear canal and the middle ear.

Inserted foreign bodies are more likely to be placed in the right ear by right-handed people and vice-versa.

Types of foreign body

The term foreign body relates to material which should not be there, and excludes naturally occurring substances such as cerumen or an accumulation of desquamated epithelium. Foreign bodies may be inanimate or animate.

Inanimate

Everyday materials such as beads and stones are common objects inserted into children's ears, and paper and other vegetable matter are often found by children however carefully parents try to prevent the availability of materials.

Middle ear ventilating tubes after extrusion from the tympanic membrane may come to lodge across the canal and cause symptoms. Surgically implanted middle ear prostheses may extrude into the external auditory canal. Silicone material used for taking an impression of the ear canal for a hearing aid can remain in the ear canal or occasionally rupture the tympanic membrane and remain in the middle ear (Schimanski, 1992). Button batteries inserted into the ear canal cause problems and will be discussed later.

Animate

Insects may enter the external auditory canal.

Pathology

A foreign body in the external auditory meatus for a short time will probably not cause any tissue reaction, especially if the squamous epithelium is undamaged. If the entry goes unnoticed, prolonged presence may cause obstruction of cerumen clearance and the hygroscopic property of vegetable matter may allow the foreign body to swell and enable a bacterial otitis externa to develop. Inflammation and oedema of the skin of the external auditory canal, with discharge and swelling in the canal laterally, may obscure the foreign body.

Alkaline button batteries may mimic a malignant otitis externa by causing extensive liquefactive necrosis of surrounding tissue by leaking an alkaline electrolyte solution. Skin, bone, and tympanic membrane necrosis with facial nerve paralysis have been reported (McRae, Premachandra and Gatland, 1989).

A foreign body penetrating the tympanic membane may cause a ragged perforation which will probably heal spontaneously in about 6 weeks, although the larger the perforation the less likely it is to heal. A foreign body reaching the tympanic membrane even without perforation raises the possibility of trauma being transmitted to the cochlea by ossicular disturbance. The ossicles may be subluxed, dislocated, or fractured with ensuing conductive deafness and, if the stapes is displaced, trauma to the cochlea is likely with the hydraulic effect leading to sensorineural deafness particularly in the high frequencies. Loss of perilymph will probably lead to a severe sensorineural deafness and acute vertigo, with the likely development of a bacterial labyrinthitis.

Symptoms and signs

The child may present with pain or bleeding from the ear possibly with deafness or vertigo if the foreign body insertion or an attempt at removal is traumatic. If insertion is unnoticed there may be no symptoms. Late presentation may be associated with the pain and discharge of an otitis externa and often a conductive deafness. The foreign body will cause a conductive deafness only if it completely occludes the external ear canal.

On examination the foreign body will usually be visible in the external auditory canal, and its proximity to the tympanic membrane should be assessed. It may be obscured by wax or discharge or oedema of the canal. Examination on a couch using the operating microscope is usually required for adequate assessment. If the object lies anteriorly in the tympanic sulcus it may not be visible because of the curve of the ear canal. Water may be instilled into the ear

canal and the water level adjusted to use the surface as a concave lens thus making the tympanic sulcus visible (Peltola and Saarento, 1992). This would only be possible in older children.

A penetrating foreign body protruding from the meatus should not be removed initially if there is evidence of inner ear damage. Radiological assessment of the depth of penetration will assist in management.

Diagnosis

The diagnosis of a foreign body in the ear is usually straightforward. The child may attend with the complaint or the parent is aware that a foreign body has been inserted. As the foreign body is usually visible, it is only when it is obscured by a consequent otitis externa that the differential diagnosis from an unrelated otitis externa needs to be made.

Management

Many objects may be flushed out of the ear canal by syringing with water at body temperature, but this may not be tolerated by a child. There is a risk that a hygroscopic foreign body may swell on syringing and become impacted. The child may not sit or lie still to allow proper examination or removal of the object, and there is the danger that inadequate restraint of the child will allow her to move her head while an instrument is in the ear with consequent injury. If an initial attempt to remove a foreign body is unsuccessful because of a frightened moving child, or if pain is induced, the patient should have the removal performed under general anaesthetic. The procedure need not be done as an emergency, except in the case where the object is protruding and further damage could be caused by touching it, but the patient treated on the next available operating list. Button batteries should be removed urgently because of the risk of tissue necrosis.

In children aged 4 years or older it is usually possible to gain the confidence of the child and either remove the object with a hook or forceps while the child is sitting in the chair. The child may not even notice the object being removed. The surgeon's hand using the instrument must rest on the child's head so that if pain is induced even momentarily any head movement will safely carry the instrument as well, and avoid trauma to the ear canal skin or tympanic membrane (Figure 14.1). With the child's head on a couch and the use of the operating microscope, movement carries the risk of trauma to the ear because the movement may be towards the instrument. The instrument cannot move because of the microscope and this may allow the child to impale the instrument

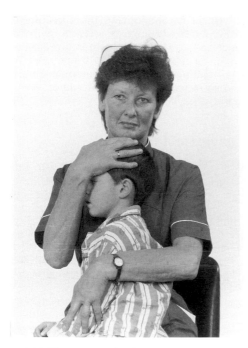

Figure 14.1 The position of a child for removal of a foreign body from the ear

in the ear, so the child must be asked to lie still. This may be difficult for a child in the foreign surroundings of a darkened room with a microscope looming overhead and instrumentation of the ear, but it is frequently successful if the confidence of the child is gained first. Vegetable matter can break up on removal and may be better managed with suction aspiration. The child needs to be warned of the noise of the suction in the ear. Demonstrating the effect of suction on the skin of the child's hand often puts her at ease.

A spherical object such as a bead may lodge in the hourglass-shaped ear canal, and in this case it is impossible to insert a probe beyond the object. Suction may permit removal of the bead. It may also be possible to use a super-glue (cyanoacrylate) to stick a probe to the bead and so pull it out (Pride and Schwab, 1989), but these objects often require removal under general anaesthetic, especially if the object has been pushed beyond the narrowest midportion of the canal.

Foreign bodies which have induced a tissue reaction with swelling of the ear canal often require removal under anaesthetic, with subsequent treatment of the otitis externa by topical antibiotic drops. Middle ear infection following perforation of the tympanic membrane will need systemic antibiotic treatment or antibiotic eardrops if the cochlea has not been breached.

Foreign bodies in the nose
Aetiology

Foreign bodies may enter the nose by several different means:

1 The anterior naris
2 The posterior naris, during vomiting, coughing, regurgitation, or in patients with palatal incompetence – when the foreign body will consist of stomach, oesophageal or mouth contents, and occasionally a roundworm (ascaris)
3 Penetrating wounds and nasal surgery
4 A palatal perforation, as in cleft palate, or following a gumma of the hard palate or surgery of the palate for malignant disease
5 Sequestration of bone *in situ* after trauma (which may be operative), or syphilis
6 Calcification *in situ* of inspissated mucopus or around foreign material can lead to the formation of a rhinolith.

Incidence

The foreign body may be any small object encountered by the child, and it will usually be introduced through the anterior naris. Children with cleft palate will have food from the mouth entering the nose, and occasionally other foreign material which the child is exploring with the mouth.

Children may also be the victims of penetrating injuries caused by bullets, shrapnel or propelled debris which lodge in the nose.

Operations on the nose may leave behind swabs, particles of tissue, or instruments.

Children of low socioeconomic groups living in tropical climates may be the victims of myiasis which is a disease due to flies or their larvae, particularly if they already suffer from debilitating disease.

Older children with foreign bodies in the nose are usually mentally disturbed.

Site of the foreign body

The foreign body may lie in any part of the nasal fossa, but those which are seen by an otolaryngologist are usually beyond the constriction at the nasal vestibule.

Types of foreign body

Foreign bodies in the nose may be inanimate (vegetable, mineral, sequestra, rhinoliths, or arising from surgery), or occasionally animate.

Inanimate

Vegetable foreign bodies are commonly peas, beans, dried pulses, nuts, paper, cotton wool, and pieces of pencil. Mineral matter may be parts from metal and plastic toys, washers, nuts, nails, screws, buttons, sponge, studs, plasticine, pebbles, beads, etc. Button batteries may be placed in the nose. After surgery pieces of polyps, bone, cartilage, swabs, instruments, or packs may be left behind. Sequestra occur in syphilis or neoplasm, or after trauma. An aberrant tooth may occasionally come to lie in the floor of the nose. Rhinoliths may be formed by concretions of varying materials.

Animate

Screw worms and their larvae, maggots and black carpet beetles may all infest the nose (myiasis) in tropical climates, and occasionally a roundworm may be coughed or regurgitated through the posterior naris.

Pathology

Some foreign bodies are inert and may remain in the nose for years without mucosal changes. Many however lead to inflammation and infection of the mucous membrane which, in turn, leads to foetid mucopurulent discharge and epistaxis. These symptoms are normally unilateral, except with animate infestations. Ultimately granulation tissue is formed, and there may be ulceration of the mucosa, and occasionally necrosis of bone or cartilage. Button batteries may result in destruction of the nasal septum (Fosarelli *et al.*, 1988).

These changes impact the foreign body, which may not be visible on either anterior or posterior rhinoscopy because of surrounding oedema, granulations and discharge. This is particularly so with vegetable foreign bodies which not only absorb water from the tissues and swell, but also evoke a very brisk inflammatory reaction. Occasionally the inflammatory reaction is sufficient to produce toxaemia.

Sharp foreign bodies may occasionally penetrate the sinuses and cause sinusitis.

If a foreign body is buried in granulations or firmly impacted, it may act as a nucleus for concretion, i.e. it receives a coating of calcium, magnesium phosphate and carbonate and becomes a *rhinolith*. Occasionally this process may occur round an area of inspissated mucopus, or even a blood clot. Rhinoliths usually form near the floor of the nose and are radiopaque.

Maggots and screw worms attack both nasal cavities and may give rise to a severe inflammatory reaction. During maturation larvae burrow into the tissues. The mature larva of the screw worm has rings around its body giving the appearance of a screw. If untreated they may attack nasal bone and cartilage and also involve the sinuses, orbits, adjoining skin, meninges, and brain (Gupta and Nema, 1970). Ascaris produces less inflammation but gives the patient a feeling of irritation and movement in the nose.

Symptoms and signs

Mineral and vegetable foreign bodies

These generally give rise to a unilateral foetid discharge, usually mucopurulent and sometimes blood-stained. There is frequently unilateral nasal obstruction and there may be pain, epistaxis, and sneezing. A few foreign bodies are inert and cause either no symptoms, or solely a unilateral nasal obstruction if sufficiently large. The presence of a radiopaque foreign body may be identified on occasions as an incidental finding on a child's dental X-ray.

Examination of the nose shows reddened congested mucosa, mucopus, and sometimes granulations, ulceration, and necrosis. The foreign body may or may not be visible, depending on its size and nature, and on the degree of surrounding oedema.

Rhinoliths

As they increase in size slowly and are relatively inert, rhinoliths are initially symptomless and later cause nasal obstruction only if they become large enough. They may be discovered when a cause is sought for an unresolved sinus infection.

Examination of the nasal cavity shows a brown or greyish irregular mass, usually near the floor of the nose, which feels stony hard and gritty on probing. X-rays will reveal the extent of the rhinolith, which may attain a very large size, and may occasionally extend into the antrum.

Animate foreign bodies

The symptoms are often bilateral, and nasal obstruction, headaches and serosanguineous foetid discharge may occur within a few days of infestation. In the larval stage, pyrexia may occur. The patient has a constant feeling of formication in the nose. In poor communities the patients adapt surprisingly well to the condition, and instead of being driven to despair, have to be persuaded, on the grounds that complications may occur, to seek treatment.

Examination shows marked swelling of the mucosa, which is fragile and bleeds easily. In heavy infestations there is an appearance of constant motion, which on closer inspection is seen to be due to a mass of worms, which are firmly attached and are difficult to remove. In long-standing infestation there may be destruction of bone and cartilage.

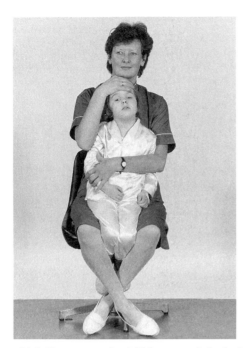

Figure 14.2 The position of a child for removal of a foreign body from the nose. Note that the child's head is slightly tilted back so that the floor of the nose is visible to the examiner

Owing to secondary infection and bone destruction complications are not rare, and patients may develop orbital infection or meningitis. In the rare case of ascaris in the nose, the worm is large (15–25cm) and easy to remove. There is minimal mucosal reaction.

Diagnosis

With inanimate foreign bodies, the suspicion usually arises because of a unilateral, foul-smelling, purulent nasal discharge, and in children this must be regarded as due to a foreign body until proved otherwise. Frequently the foreign body will be seen on anterior rhinoscopy (and sometimes on posterior rhinoscopy), but on occasions mucosal oedema or granulations will hide it. If such unilateral changes are seen, but no foreign body is evident, in cooperative older children the nose should be sprayed with a vasoconstrictor to shrink the mucosa and the fossa re-examined. Sometimes a foreign body will then be seen. If not, the nose should be X-rayed as many foreign bodies are radiopaque. In younger or very apprehensive children it may be necessary for the search to be carried out under a general anaesthetic.

Other conditions to be excluded are neoplasm (by biopsy of granulations), unilateral sinusitis (by X-ray), syphilis (by serology), diphtheria (by nasal swab) and unilateral choanal atresia (by passing a catheter through the nasal fossa or by X-ray after instilling a contrast medium).

The diagnosis of animate foreign bodies is usually all too apparent on inspection.

Management

Inanimate foreign bodies (except rhinoliths)

If the foreign body is easily seen, and the patient is a cooperative child, it is usually possible to remove the object through the anterior naris, either with no anaesthetic, or after spraying with a local anaesthetic solution such as (50:50) 4% lignocaine and 1/1000 adrenaline.

However, it cannot be too strongly emphasized that unskilled attempts to remove the foreign body in the accident and emergency department by personnel without appropriate training may result in disaster. The foreign body may be displaced backwards and may even reach the nasopharynx with risk of inhalation. Marked epistaxis may occur or a docile child may become terrified and require a general anaesthetic which might otherwise have been avoided.

The patient is placed in the usual upright position for routine otolaryngological examination (Figure 14.2), and the nasal fossa illuminated with a head mirror or headlight. It is important that the light source should be very bright. A suitable size speculum, probe, hook, forceps and suction should be available. The nasal speculum is inserted, and the hook passed beyond the object and the tip rotated to rest just posteriorly to the object. The object is then gently drawn forwards and removed completely, or brought almost to the nasal vestibule and then removed with forceps. This technique should be used whenever there is a risk of displacing the object backwards into the nasopharynx, as with spherical objects such as beads. Rough semi-impacted objects such as bits of paper, sponge and objects placed very near the vestibule, can be removed directly with forceps.

A general anaesthetic will be required in the following circumstances:

1 If the patient is uncooperative or very apprehensive
2 If there is likely to be troublesome bleeding, for instance if the foreign body is firmly embedded in granulation tissue
3 If the foreign body is posteriorly placed with a risk of pushing it back into the nasopharynx
4 If a foreign body is strongly suspected but cannot be found.

More extensive examination of the nose is required with the opportunity to deal with whatever is found. It must be emphasized that there is no need for haste on these occasions. The foreign body may have been in the nose for a considerable period and it is important to wait for ideal facilities, including an experienced anaesthetist. Unskilled manipulation in adverse conditions can lead to inhalation of the foreign body or blood.

The patient is anaesthetized and a cuffed oral endotracheal tube and a pharyngeal pack are inserted. With the patient in the usual position for nasal surgery, the nose is examined using a nasal speculum, headlight, and suction to remove secretions. To minimize bleeding, the affected nasal fossa may be sprayed with a local anaesthetic solution, in consultation with the anaesthetist. After waiting for this to take effect, the nose is then re-examined, and the foreign body is gently withdrawn.

If the object is wedged posteriorly and cannot be brought out through the anterior naris, it is occasionally necessary to push the foreign body backwards into the nasopharynx. Before doing so the patient is placed in the tonsil position, a Boyle-Davis gag is inserted, and the palate gently retracted with a soft catheter passed through the unaffected side of the nose and out through the mouth. The catheter is held while the foreign body is pushed back, at the same time watching the nasopharynx with a mirror. The foreign body cannot fall into the larynx because of the patient's position and the cuffed tube, and can readily be picked out of the nasopharynx with forceps.

Rhinoliths

These present a different problem as they are impacted and often large. It may be necessary to break up the rhinolith within the nasal fossa with forceps, and then to remove it piecemeal. This procedure should be carried out under a general anaesthetic. Rarely, a rhinolith is so large that it can only be removed through a lateral rhinotomy approach. Occasionally it may even extend into the antrum, in which case a Caldwell-Luc approach is required.

Animate foreign bodies

Infestations with maggots and screw worms are treated by instilling 25% chloroform solution into the nasal cavities. This is repeated two or three times a week for about 6 weeks until all larvae are killed. After each treatment the patient blows his nose to clear the dead worms and larvae. Sometimes treatment is given under general anaesthesia (with a cuffed endotracheal tube and throat pack), when repeated irrigation followed by suction can be carried out.

Ascaris is managed by removal of the worm with forceps, followed by treatment of the general condition with piperazine and magnesium sulphate purges to clear dead worms from the bowel.

References

FOSARELLI, P., FEIGELMAN, S., PEARSON, E. and CALIMANO-DIAZ, A. (1988) An unusual intranasal foreign body. *Pediatric Emergency Care*, **4**, 117–118

GUPTA, S. K. and NEMA, H. V. (1970) Rhino-orbital-myiasis. *Journal of Laryngology and Otology*, **84**, 453–455

MCRAE, D., PREMACHANDRA, D. J. and GATLAND, D. J. (1989) Button batteries in the ear, nose and cervical oesophagus: a destructive foreign body. *Journal of Otolaryngology*, **18**, 317–319

MUNTZ, H. R., PA-C, D. J. and ASHER, B. F. (1990) Embedded earrings: a complication of the ear-piercing gun. *International Journal of Paediatric Otorhinolaryngology*, **19**, 73–76

PELTOLA, T. J. and SAARENTO, R. (1992) Water used to visualize and remove hidden foreign bodies from the external ear canal. *Journal of Laryngology and Otology*, **106**, 157–158

PRIDE, H. and SCHWAB, R. (1989) A new technique for removing foreign bodies of the external auditory canal. *Pediatric Emergency Care*, **5**, 135–136

SCHIMANSKI, G. (1992) Silicone foreign body in the middle ear caused by auditory canal impression in hearing aid fitting. *HNO*, **40**, 67–68

15

Congenital anomalies of the nose

Michael J. Cinnamond

The nose has been called, for both literal and figurative reasons, 'the outstanding feature of the face'. Many parents will observe and comment on minor abnormalities of the nose, even when these are barely visible and are causing no functional disability. More major aberrations of the external nose may induce considerable parental dismay and may even, occasionally, give rise to rejection of the child.

It is fortunate, therefore, that despite its complicated embryological development most significant anomalies of the nose are rare. While a precise explanation for this is lacking, it may well be that, owing to the intimate association between development of the face and brain, severe structural abnormalities of this region are largely incompatible with continued fetal existence.

There is much to be said for entrusting the long-term management of children with congenital nasal defects to a few large centres where the necessary radiological, maxillofacial, neurosurgical and other skills are readily available. Few otolaryngologists will gain significant experience during their working lifetime in the care of such children and, moreover, many of these patients have additional congenital abnormalities, especially of the face and central nervous system.

Development of the nose

In order that the reader may understand more fully the teratogenesis of those anomalies which do occur, a brief summary of the embryology of the nose will be given here.

At about the third week of fetal life paired thickenings (the olfactory or nasal placodes) appear in the cranial ectoderm near the embryonic anterior neuropore.

Invagination of the placodes, consequent on growth of the surrounding mesoderm, results in the formation of the nasal pits which, as they deepen, serve to delineate medial and lateral prominences of the frontonasal process. The medial prominences fuse to form the central portion of the upper lip, the premaxilla and the primitive nasal septum (Figure 15.1).

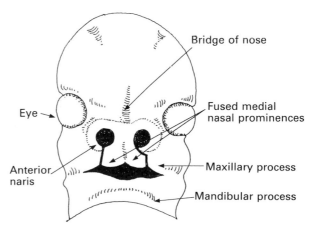

Figure 15.1 Development of the face and nasal pyramid

The floor of the nose is, at first, formed by medial growth of the maxillary processes of the mandibular arch. As the nasal pits deepen they become slit-like. Progressive thinning of the mesoderm, dorsally and caudally, results in the formation of the bucconasal membrane, separating the lumen of the nose from the buccal cavity.

The bucconasal membrane eventually breaks down, forming the primitive posterior nasal apertures which lie horizontally in the roof of the buccal cavity or stomatodaeum (Figure 15.2). At this stage, the lower free border of the developing nasal septum lies in contact with the dorsum of the tongue.

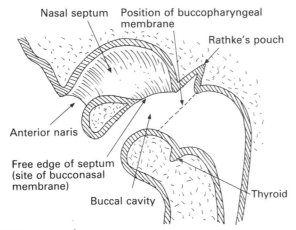

Figure 15.2 Early development of the nasal cavity and mouth

Meanwhile, paired lateral palatal processes are formed, one on each side of the tongue (Figure 15.3). Fusion of these with each other, with an unpaired, ventrally sited, median process and with the caudal border of the septum, gives rise to the definitive palate, finally separating the nasal and nasopharyngeal cavities from the mouth (Figure 15.4).

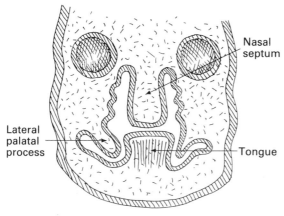

Figure 15.3 Lateral palatal processes

Choanal atresia

Choana is derived from a Greek word, χοανη, meaning a funnel. The choanae are, by definition, the posterior apertures of the nose (Friel, 1974). The use of the term 'posterior choanae' is, therefore, tautology.

Atresia of the choanae was first described by Roederer

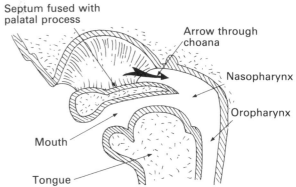

Figure 15.4 Formation of the definitive choana

in 1775 (Devgan and Harkins, 1977). It is one of the more commonly observed congenital abnormalities of the nose, although its true incidence is uncertain. The most consistently quoted figure is one per 8000 live births, but this is probably an underestimate. Bilateral choanal atresia is likely to have been, and may still be, a frequently unrecognized cause of death in the neonatal period. Females appear to be affected about twice as often as males and the condition may be unilateral or bilateral in the proportion 3:2 (Kaplan, 1985).

Choanal atresia has been associated with chromosomal abnormalities (Hurst, Meinecke and Baraitser, 1991; Katafuchi *et al.*, 1992; Shashi, Golden and Fryburg, 1994). It has been reported that non-syndromal choanal atresia can be transmitted as an autosomal recessive trait (Gershoni–Baruch, 1992).

Embryology

Much confusion exists about which embryological structure is actually involved in choanal atresia. Some authors (Sprinkle and Sporck, 1983; Kaplan, 1985) subscribed to the theory that the anomaly may arise as a result of persistence of the buccopharyngeal membrane. It is difficult to reconcile this view with the embryology of the region, however, as the buccopharyngeal membrane in the developing fetus lies posterior to the site of Rathke's pouch, which in turn lies posterior to the nasal septum (see Figure 15.2).

It has also been suggested that the aberration is due to a failure of the bucconasal membrane to undergo involution (Sprinkle and Sporck, 1983). The primitive posterior nasal apertures, produced by breakdown of the bucconasal membrane are, however, considerably more anteriorly placed than the definitive choanae. While this mechanism may explain some instances of choanal atresia, it is the author's view that the majority of cases are due to persistence of the epithelial cells which proliferate within the nasal cavities during the sixth to eighth weeks of intrauterine development.

Pathology

Choanal atresia may be bony (90%) or membranous (10%) and is generally sited just in front of the posterior end of the nasal septum. In most instances where the atretic plate is of the bony type, it is thin and easily perforated. Occasionally, a much more substantial atresia occurs, a considerable proportion of the posterior nasal cavity being obliterated by dense bone. In this latter form the nasal cavity is frequently funnel shaped (Pracy, 1979; Pirsig, 1986).

Asymmetry of the facial skeleton is common, especially in those with unilateral atresia, and most patients will have a high arched palate. Other orthodontic abnormalities such as transverse maxillary compression have been described and there may be deformed or absent teeth, especially those of the second dentition. Pirsig (1986) is of the opinion that congenital choanal atresia should not be considered as an isolated plate of bone but as one component of a skull base anomaly developing between the fourth and twelfth weeks of gestation.

Computerized tomography (CT) has demonstrated thickening of the vomer, bowing of the lateral wall of the nasal cavity and fusion of bony elements in the choanal region (Wetmore and Mahboubi, 1986). Maurizi *et al.* (1985) have observed various changes in the cell morphology of the nasal ciliated columnar mucous membrane. They described unevenness of the mucosal surface, thickening of the basal membrane and the presence of ciliary abnormalities including compound cilia, cilia with excessive cytoplasm and ciliary structures with loss of the peripheral membrane.

Incomplete obstruction of the posterior nasal aperture may also occur, usually taking the form of bony stenosis. If severe this may mimic true atresia necessitating similar management. Severe nasal mucosal congestion and inflammation will often present an identical clinical picture (Derkay and Grundfast, 1990).

Congenital nasal pyriform aperture stenosis has also been described (Arlis and Ward, 1992). This rare midfacial developmental anomaly is associated with a single, prominent central maxillary incisor, which is related to holoprosencephaly. Holoprosencephaly is a specific malformation complex associated with central nervous system abnormalities and endocrine defects involving the hypothalamic–pituitary–thyroid–adrenal axis.

Clinical features

Unilateral choanal atresia usually presents somewhat later than bilateral atresia (commonly 18 months) but may not become apparent until later childhood or even adulthood. Feeding difficulties may occur, especially during breast feeding when the non-affected side of the nose is occluded by contact with the breast. More commonly, however, it presents as a unilateral nasal discharge.

Bilateral atresia, on the other hand, almost always presents as a respiratory emergency, and is apparent at birth. Newborn infants are, by instinct, nose breathers. The reflexes, which in the older child or adult will result in breathing through the mouth in response to nasal obstruction, do not develop until some weeks or months after birth. If, however, the mouth is held open, either by insertion of an artificial airway or during crying, then mouth breathing will occur. Thus, neonates with bilateral choanal atresia or other cause of severe nasal obstruction will sometimes demonstrate a cyclical change in oxygenation, becoming cyanosed during quiet periods, normal colour returning when the child cries.

While choanal atresia may be found as an isolated anomaly about 60–70% of cases are associated with one or more other congenital defect (Kaplan, 1985; Morgan and Bailey, 1990). In addition to random affiliations, however, choanal atresia has been linked to a limited number of specific defects – the so-called CHARGE association (Pagon *et al.*, 1981):

C colobomatous blindness
H heart disease
A atresia of the choanae
R retarded growth or development, including the central nervous system
G genital hypoplasia in males
E ear deformities, including deafness.

Diagnosis

The time-honoured method of determining patency of the nose in the newborn infant is the ability to pass a soft red-rubber catheter through each side of the nose into the oropharynx. Failure to pass the catheter, however, is not conclusive evidence for the presence of atresia of the posterior nares. The tip may become impacted in the adenoid or may be deflected by minor abnormalities of the turbinates causing the catheter to curl up inside the nasal cavity. In consequence, the author prefers to use a stethoscope from which the bell has been removed, the open end of the tube being held over each nostril in turn and the presence or absence of an air-blast noted.

There are, however, causes of total nasal obstruction in the neonate other than choanal atresia. These include massive congenital hypertrophy of the turbinates or adenoid. Radiographic demonstration that contrast medium is held up at the choanae (choanography) has been the traditional method of confirming the diagnosis of atresia. The current investigation of choice, however, is computerized tomography. This gives rather more information, especially with regard to whether the obstruction is membranous or bony and, in the latter case, the actual structures involved and their thickness (Brown *et al.*, 1986). Kearns *et al.* (1988) have drawn attention to the potentially misleading effects of mucus within the nasal cavities. They stressed the need for careful preparation, including the use of vasoconstrictive drops and nasal suction, if high-quality images are to be obtained.

Management

The essential aim of treatment of choanal atresia is the creation of patent nasal airways. In the case of unilateral atresia, there is seldom any urgency in the presentation and surgery can be undertaken as a planned or 'cold' procedure. Bilateral atresia, however, always presents as a respiratory emergency and management must, therefore, be considered under two headings:

1 Primary, or emergency treatment
2 Secondary, or definitive surgery.

Emergency management

In most cases and especially where it is planned to proceed to definitive surgery within 24 hours or so, it will suffice to insert a standard neonatal Waters airway, taping it securely into position. The child may, if necessary, be fed through an indwelling naso-gastric tube. In a few cases, where the child's general condition is precarious, perhaps because of additional pathology, it is found necessary to delay surgery. In these circumstances, it is probably wiser to intubate the larynx or, if this is not possible, to perform a tracheotomy.

Definitive management

This is best carried out as soon as possible. Four approaches to the posterior end of the nasal cavity have been described:

1 Transnasal
2 Transpalatal
3 Trans-septal
4 Transantral.

Of these, only the first two are in common use. In all surgery of this region use of the operating microscope not only provides much better illumination but makes the operation easier and safer. Some authors consider that endoscopic transnasal repair provides better visualization and the ability to perform more exact surgery (Stankiewicz, 1990; El-Guindy *et al.*, 1992). General anaesthesia with orotracheal intubation is employed.

The transnasal route is valid only for membranous atresia or where the bony plate is thin. The simplest procedure is perforation of the atretic lamina followed by dilatation. Although Lichtwitz's trocar and cannula is often used to achieve the primary puncture,

there is an inherent risk in this method of causing serious damage to the cervical spine and spinal cord. Instead, the author recommends the use of female urethral dilators which, being curved, direct the perforating force safely downwards, into the lumen of the nasopharynx.

The atretic plate is almost always thinnest and weakest at the junction of the floor of the nose and posterior end of the septum. It is, therefore, towards this point that the tip of the instrument should be directed. If gentle pressure does not succeed in perforating the atresia, it is probably too thick and some other method should be employed instead. Once puncture has been achieved, the opening may be widened, using progressively larger dilators, up to about 5 mm (14–16 FG).

Many surgeons recommend the insertion of Portex or Silastic tubes to prevent re-stenosis of the choanae, but the author feels that these do not help and prefers instead to dilate the choanae once a week for 4–6 weeks. Other transnasal methods which have been advocated are drilling out the bony atresia with diamond paste burrs (Evans and Maclachlan, 1971) or vapourizing the obstruction using the CO_2 laser. In either case, it is imperative that an aural speculum is used to protect the skin of the nasal vestibule as it is very easy to cause circumferential damage, resulting in stenosis of the anterior naris.

Where the atresia is thick, it is preferable to employ the transpalatal approach. The most comfortable operating approach is similar to that used in cleft palate surgery, the child's head overhanging the end of the table and resting on the surgeon's lap. The Kilner-Dott mouth gag gives rather better exposure of the hard palate and is to be preferred to the more usual Boyle–Davis instrument.

An incision is made around the summit of the alveolar ridge or at the gingivopalatal margin if teeth are present. The mucous membrane of the hard palate is elevated, using a McKenty or Cottle septal elevator and the flap is developed posteriorly until the edge of the hard palate is reached. Care must be taken to avoid damage to the greater and lesser palatine vessels and nerves as they traverse the bony palate on either side close to its posterior edge. The nasopharynx is entered by separation of muscle fibres from the posterior edge of the hard palate and incision of the superior mucosal layer of the soft palate.

Using diamond paste or cutting burrs of suitable size, the posterior end of the hard palate is removed to expose the bony atresia. Much has been written about preservation of mucosal flaps intended to re-line the new choanae but, in the author's experience, this is almost always impossible to achieve. Continuity of the nasal cavity can now be restored by drilling away the obstructing bone, the posterior end of the vomer being removed at the same time. Care is needed at this stage to avoid damage to the vessels and nerves which run in the lateral nasal wall.

Before replacing and suturing the palatal flap, soft Silastic tubes may be inserted and anchored in position with an anterior septal transfixion suture. The tubes should be removed 4–6 weeks later. As in the transnasal approach the author does not believe that such tubes are necessary.

Pirsig (1986), in a very comprehensive review of the surgery of choanal atresia, has drawn attention to the possibility of subsequent maldevelopment of the upper dental arch in patients who have undergone the transpalatal operation. There is also a risk of palatal perforation if the palatal flap is too short.

Koltai, Hoehn and Bailey (1992) recommended the use of the external rhinoplasty approach in children. They have utilized this method for the correction of a wide range of rhinological problems, including septal deviation, unilateral choanal atresia, nasal dermoid and problems involving the sphenoidal sinus. In cases of unilateral atresia they considered that this technique provides as good exposure of the posterior vomer as the transpalatal approach but without the risk to palatal growth.

Septal deviation

Some degree of nasal septal deviation is found in 58% of all newborn babies, and in 4% of births there is also an associated external nasal deformity (Gray, 1985). Two mechanisms have been proposed to explain how such deformities may arise:

1 Differences in the rate of growth of the septum as compared to other midfacial structures, resulting in a septum which is too big for the space it has to occupy
2 Trauma to the nose, either as the result of prolonged contact with the uterine wall or during parturition, especially when this is protracted.

It should be noted that septal deviation is a frequent concomitant of cleft lip and palate.

The resulting nasal obstruction, which may affect one or both sides, usually presents in the neonate as difficult or slow feeding, often accompanied by colic due to air swallowing. If, as frequently happens, nasal infection supervenes, the child will become snuffly and in some cases the nasal blockage is so severe as to mimic choanal atresia.

Inspection of the nose may reveal displacement of the quadrilateral cartilage, but more posteriorly sited deformities of the perpendicular plate of the ethmoid or vomer are not always visible. Gray (1985) described specially shaped nasal struts which he used to determine the septal configuration. A good estimate of nasal patency may be made by comparing the air-blast heard over each nostril, as described in the section on choanal atresia.

Both external pyramidal and internal septal deformities may be corrected, within the first few days of life using specially designed neonatal nasal septum

forceps (Gray, 1985; Alpini *et al.*, 1986). By about 6 years of age the nose is large enough to allow septoplasty to be performed, but it is recommended that tissue removal be kept to an absolute minimum, otherwise subsequent growth and development of the nose may be jeopardized. The external rhinoplasty approach provides excellent access to the nasal septum (Koltai, Hoehn and Bailey, 1992).

Congenital nasal masses

Congenital nasal masses are rare, occurring once in every 20 000–40 000 live births. All intranasal masses in children, and especially if unilateral, should be treated with the gravest suspicion and circumspection. Failure to differentiate between a simple nasal polyp and a communicating meningoencephalocoele may lead to cerebrospinal fluid rhinorrhoea with the resultant risk of meningitis. The differential diagnosis of nasal swellings in a child is given in Table 15.1.

Table 15.1 Causes of nasal swellings in childhood

Cystic	Solid
Congenital	Congenital
meningoencephalocoele	glioma
meningocoele	haemangioma
dermoid cyst	lymphangioma
epidermoid cyst	congenital angiofibroma
nasolacrimal duct	neurofibroma
mucocoele	teratoma
	hamartoma
Acquired	hairy polyp
sebaceous cyst	neuroblastoma
lacrimal duct cyst	rhabdomyosarcoma
mucocoele	chordoma
	craniopharyngioma
	Acquired
	lipoma
	papilloma
	lymphoma
	nasopharyngeal carcinoma
	angiofibroma
	ethmoidal polyp
	antrochoanal polyp
	abscess

Nasal dermoids

These are solid tumours, cysts or sinuses, occurring anywhere in the midline of the nose from the glabella to the columella, whose walls contain skin adnexae (Bradley, 1981). Solid dermoids may also occur in the nasopharynx, where they take the form of 'hairy polyps' – the dermoid mass is covered with hair-bearing skin (Haddad *et al.*, 1990). Dermoids are formed as the result of sequestration of epithelial elements during fusion of the median nasal processes. The diagnosis is often delayed until adolescence or adulthood and may only become manifest if infection ensues (Figure 15.5). Multiple midline nasal dermoid cysts have been described (Posnick, Bortoluzzi and Armstrong, 1994).

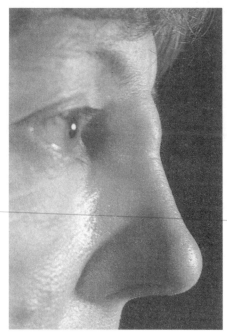

Figure 15.5 Nasal dermoid

Dermoid sinuses, recognized by a dimple or minute opening, sometimes containing a single hair, may extend deeply into the nasal septum, occasionally reaching as far as the cribriform plate. Contrast sinography will assist in determining both the extent and configuration of the sinus tract. Complete excision is usually difficult to achieve, but may be facilitated by prior cannulation of the external punctum and instillation of methylene blue. Intracranial extension can occur and this may necessitate a combined intracranial and extracranial approach if resection is to be effective (Brydon, 1992; Rouland *et al.*, 1993; Posnick *et al.*, 1994).

The external rhinoplasty approach can offer wider exposure with a better view of the operation field (Morrissey and Bailey, 1991; Koltai, Hoehn and Bailey, 1992).

Nasal gliomas

These account for approximately 5% of all congenital nasal swellings. They are said to be more common in males and may occur entirely outside the nasal cavity (60%), entirely within the nasal cavity (30%) or in a combination of both sites (10%).

Although the exact embryological details are uncertain, it seems likely that gliomas and meningo-encephalocoeles share a common origin, resulting from faulty closure of the anterior neuropore. However, while meningoencephalocoeles retain their communication with the subarachnoid space, gliomas become detached from the intracranial cavity by closure of the skull sutures, although in some cases a fibrous tract may remain connecting the glioma to the skull base (Figure 15.6).

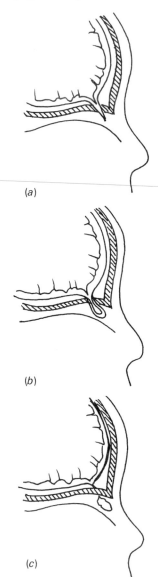

(a)

(b)

(c)

Figure 15.6 Embryogenesis of meningoencephalocoeles and gliomas. (*a*) Normal development – dura projecting into prenasal space; (*b*) meningoencephalocoele – herniation of intracranial tissue; (*c*) nasal glioma – neural tissue trapped by skull closure. (Modified from Swift and Singh, 1985, courtesy of the authors and publisher)

Macroscopically, gliomas are smooth and rubbery with a grey, yellow or purple surface. On histological examination there are aggregates of mature glial cells, predominantly astrocytes, interspersed with fibrous tissue (Swift and Singh, 1985).

Most cases are diagnosed at or soon after birth, presenting as either a subcutaneous lump to one side of the nasal bridge or as an obstructing intranasal mass. Unlike a meningoencephalocoele, a glioma does not increase in size with straining or crying. Tomography or CT scanning of the anterior skull base is usually carried out, though it should be noted that absence of a bony defect does not rule out an intracranial communication. Generally, the diagnosis is not in doubt but should always be confirmed by biopsy, having first checked for the presence of cerebrospinal fluid by needle aspiration.

Nasal gliomas tend to enlarge slowly with age though, occasionally, rapid expansion may occur. Treatment is by excision. Intranasal masses may require a lateral rhinotomy approach though laser excision is also effective. Incomplete removal may lead to recurrence. In those few cases where a dural connection can be demonstrated, anterior craniotomy will be necessary to prevent cerebrospinal fluid leak.

Nasal meningoencephalocoeles

Meningoencephalocoeles, sometimes incorrectly referred to as encephalocoeles, are local herniations of glial tissue and meninges through a defect in the skull. While these may occur at any site, they are commonly classified into five main groups depending upon the size and site of herniation (Table 15.2). Cranioschisis, it should be noted, refers to very large bony defects in the skull. Most of the meningoencephalocoeles seen by otorhinolaryngologists are of the frontoethmoidal or basal types.

Frontoethmoidal meningoencephalocoeles probably share a common origin with nasal gliomas as described in the previous section. The origin of other groups will depend upon local developmental abnormalities. The sac-like protrusion of meninges contains brain tissue and the subarachnoid space, which is filled with cerebrospinal fluid, communicates freely with the cranial cavity. Injury to a meningoencephalocoele is, therefore, likely to cause cerebrospinal fluid rhinorrhoea and meningitis.

A meningoencephalocoele usually presents as either a soft cystic mass overlying the root of the nose (frontoethmoidal type) or as a pedunculated intranasal swelling (basal type). Crying or straining is said to increase the size and tension of the mass though, in the case of intranasal swellings, this may not be easy to detect. All such swellings must be subject to rigorous radiological examination, including plain films, tomography and computerized tomography, to determine the exact site and size of the cranial defect. Magnetic resonance imaging has recently been shown to be superior to computerized tomography in distinguishing between brain parenchyma and inflamed nasal mucosa (Zinreich *et al.*, 1992).

In those few cases where the skull defect is small and readily accessible local external excision with careful plugging of the cranial opening may suffice. Most cases, however, will require the assistance of a neurosurgeon. Craniotomy is performed, with removal of the herniated brain tissue, followed by closure of the bony defect using tantalum mesh and repair of the meninges with fascia.

Other congenital nasal masses

Congenital nasolacrimal duct mucocoeles may prolapse or expand into the nose causing respiratory distress and feeding difficulties. Endoscopic marsupialization of the mucocoele, with lacrimal duct probing and insertion of lacrimal duct drainage tubes has been advocated (Yee *et al.*, 1994).

Nasal hamartomas may present with nasal obstruction, epistaxis and chronic rhinorrhoea. Local excision is the treatment of choice and may be done using standard functional endoscopic sinus surgery techniques (Terris, Billman and Pransky, 1993).

Nasopharyngeal angiofibromas, occurring in late childhood or early adult life, are a well recognized clinical entity. Manjalay *et al.* (1992), however, have described an angiofibroma occurring in the right maxillary sinus of a newborn child. Teratomas of the nasopharynx have also been reported (Rybak *et al.*, 1991). These may be associated with abnormalities of the central nervous system.

Other malformations
Haemangioma

Haemangiomas, which most authorities regard as vascular hamartomas rather than true neoplasms,

Table 15.2 Classification of meningoencephalocoeles

Occipital	Basal
Cranial vault	transethmoidal
interfrontal	sphenoethmoidal
anterior fontanelle	trans-sphenoidal
interparietal	frontosphenoidal or
posterior fontanelle	spheno-orbital
temporal	Cranioschisis
Frontoethmoid	cranial upper facial cleft
nasofrontal	basal lower facial cleft
nasoethmoidal	occipitocervical cleft
naso-orbital	acrania and
	anencephaly

Modified from Sprinkle and Sporck (1983) by courtesy of the authors and publisher

are common in childhood (Walter and Israel, 1970). Although the majority of these tumours are found in the head and neck region, primary involvement of the nose is relatively rare. Histologically haemangiomas have been identified as capillary, cavernous, mixed or hypertrophic, though the usefulness of this classification for either prognosis or typing has been questioned (Batsakis, 1974).

Despite being unsightly and disfiguring almost all of these lesions will regress spontaneously with little or no residual deformity (Thomson and Lanigan, 1979). Those few tumours which do not involute are said to be associated with increasing numbers of arteriovenous fistulae, the development of which can be monitored by serial Doppler examinations. In the majority of cases, therefore, masterly inactivity is the treatment of choice, active intervention being restricted to those instances where tumour growth continues.

Agenesis of the nose

Total agenesis of the nose is an exceptionally rare abnormality with fewer than a dozen cases having been reported in the literature (Sprinkle and Sporck, 1983). In two cases reported by Gifford and MacCollum (1972), there was an associated absence of the nasopharynx and no evidence of any nasal development. The child may learn to mouth breathe or surgery may be undertaken in a bid to establish a nasal airway. A nasal prosthesis is probably more cosmetically acceptable than the results of surgical reconstruction.

Partial agenesis with failed development of one nasal cavity has also been reported.

Cleft nose

This deformity is also very rare. The actual degree of cleft which occurs varies considerably from minor notching of the nasal tip to total midline division of the nose into widely separated nasal cavities. There may be an associated median cleft of the upper lip and palate or notching of the alar margins (Figure 15.7). Most cases exhibit hypertelorism and it has been suggested that there are strong associations between separation of the eyes, cephalic anomalies and the probability of mental deficiency (DeMyer, Zeman and Palmer, 1963).

Surgical repair of these anomalies is likely to require the assistance of a maxillofacial surgeon and perhaps a neurosurgeon. In the more severe cases multiple procedures will be necessary and, where bony elements are involved, it may be advantageous to delay repair until growth of the nose and face has ceased.

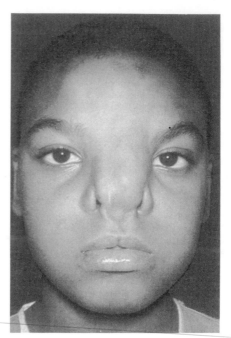

Figure 15.7 Bifid nose

Proboscis lateralis

This unusual deformity consists of a tube of skin and soft tissue, arising at the inner canthus of the eye. The nasal cavity on the affected side may be completely normal or there may be maldevelopment of varying degree up to and including total agenesis.

The embryological defect would appear to result from imperfect fusion of the lateral nasal and maxillary processes. As a consequence, there is also failure of development of the nasolacrimal duct. Proboscis lateralis has also been described in association with other congenital nasal defects, such as supernumerary nostrils (Coessens, De Mey and Lejour, 1992).

Where there is maldevelopment of the nasal cavity repair will be facilitated by incorporation of some of the extraneous tissue of the tube in reconstruction of the nose. Some form of dacryocystorhinostomy will also be required.

References

ALPINI, D., CORTI, A., BRUSA, E. and BINI, A. (1986) Septal deviation in newborn infants. *International Journal of Pediatric Otorhinolaryngology*, **11**, 103–107

ARLIS, H. and WARD, R. F. (1992) Congenital nasal pyriform aperture stenosis. *Archives of Otolaryngology – Head and Neck Surgery*, **118**, 989–991

BATSAKIS, J. (1974) *Tumours of the Head and Neck*. Baltimore: Williams and Wilkins, Co. p. 250.

BRADLEY, P. J. (1981) Nasal dermoids in children. *International Journal of Pediatric Otorhinolaryngology*, **3**, 63–70

BROWN, O. E., SMITH, T., ARMSTRONG, E. and GRUNDFAST, K. (1986) The evaluation of choanal atresia by computed tomography. *International Journal of Pediatric Otorhinolaryngology*, **12**, 85–98

BRYDON, H. L. (1992) Intracranial dermoid cysts with nasal dermal sinuses. *Acta Neurochirurgica*, **118**, 185–188

COESSENS, B., DE MEY, A. and LEJOUR, M. (1992) Correction of supernumerary nostrils *International Journal of Pediatric Otorhinolaryngology*, **23**, 275–280

DEMYER, W., ZEMAN, W. and PALMER, C. G. (1963) Familial alobar holoprosencephaly (arhinencephaly) with median cleft lip and palate. *Neurology*, **13**, 913–918

DERKAY, C. S. and GRUNDFAST, K. M. (1990) Airway compromise from nasal obstruction in neonates and infants. *International Journal of Pediatric Otorhinolaryngology*, **19**, 241–249

DEVGAN, B. K. and HARKINS, W. B. (1977) Congenital choanal atresia. Twenty years experience. *International Surgery*, **62**, 397–399

EL-GUINDY, A., EL-SHERIFF, S., HAGRASS, M. and GAMEA, A. (1992) Endoscopic endonasal surgery of posterior choanal atresia. *Journal of Laryngology and Otology*, **106**, 528–529

EVANS, J. N. G. and MACLACHLAN, R. F. (1971) Choanal atresia. *Journal of Laryngology and Otology*, **85**, 903–929

FRIEL, J. P. (ed) (1974) *Dorland's Illustrated Medical Dictionary*, 25th edn. Philadelphia: W. B. Saunders. p. 305

GERSHONI-BARUCH, R. (1992) Choanal atresia: evidence for autosomal recessive inheritance. *American Journal of Medical Genetics*, **44**, 754–756

GIFFORD, G. H. JR and MACCOLLUM, D. W. (1972) Congenital malformations. In: *Pediatric Otolaryngology*, edited by C. F. Ferguson and E. L. Kendig Jr. Philadelphia: W. B. Saunders. pp. 932–943

GRAY, L. (1985) Septal manipulation in the neonate: method and results. *International Journal of Pediatric Otorhinolaryngology*, **8**, 195–209

HADDAD, J. JR, SENDERS, C. W., LEACH, C. S. and STOOL, S. E. (1990) Congenital hairy polyp of the nasopharynx associated with cleft palate: report of two cases. *International Journal of Pediatric Otorhinolaryngology*, **20**, 127–135

HURST, J. A., MEINECKE, P. and BARAITSER, M. (1991) Balanced t(6;8)(6p8p;6q8q) and the CHARGE association. *Journal of Medical Genetics*, **28**, 54–55

KAPLAN, L. C. (1985) Choanal atresia and its associated anomalies. Further support for the CHARGE association. *International Journal of Pediatric Otorhinolaryngology*, **8**, 237–242

KATAFUCHI, Y., FUKUDA, T., MARUOKA, T., TOKUNAGA, Y., YAMASHITA, Y. and MATSUISHI, T. (1992) Partial trisomy 6p with agenesis of the corpus callosum and choanal atresia. *Journal of Child Neurology*, **7**, 114–116

KEARNS, D. B., WICKSTEAD, M., CHOA, D. I., LEITCH, R. N., BAILEY, C. M. and EVANS, J. N. G. (1988) Computed tomography in choanal atresia. *Journal of Laryngology and Otology*, **102**, 414–418

KOLTAI, P. J., HOEHN, J. and BAILEY, C. M. (1992) The external rhinoplasty approach for rhinologic surgery in children. *Archives of Otolaryngology – Head and Neck Surgery*, **118**, 401–405

MANJALAY, G., HOARE, T. J., PEARMAN, K. and GREEN, N. J. (1992) A case of congenital angiofibroma. *International Journal of Pediatric Otorhinolaryngology*, **24**, 275–278

MAURIZI, M., OTTAVIANI, F., PALUDETTI, G., SPRECA, A. and ALMADORI, G. (1985) Choanal atresia: a surface and ultrastructural study of the nasal mucous membranes. *International Journal of Pediatric Otorhinolaryngology*, **10**, 53–66

MORGAN, D. W. and BAILEY, C. M. (1990) Current management of choanal atresia. *International Journal of Pediatric Otorhinolaryngology*, **19**, 1–13

MORRISSEY, M. S. and BAILEY, C. M. (1991) External rhinoplasty, approach for nasal dermoids in children. *Ear, Nose and Throat Journal*, **10**, 445–449

PAGON, R. A., GRAHAM, J. M. JR, ZONANA, J. and YONG, S. L. (1981) Coloboma, congenital heart disease, and choanal atresia with multiple anomalies: CHARGE association. *Journal of Pediatrics*, **99**, 223–227

PIRSIG, W. (1986) Surgery of choanal atresia in infants and children: historical notes and updated review. *International Journal of Pediatric Otorhinolaryngology*, **11**, 153–170

POSNICK, J. C., BORTOLUZZI, P. and ARMSTRONG, D. C. (1994) Nasal dermoid sinus cysts: an unusual presentation, computed tomographic scan findings, and surgical results. *Annals of Plastic Surgery*, **32**, 519–523

POSNICK, J. C., BORTOLUZZI, P., ARMSTRONG, D. C. and DRAKE, J. M. (1994) Intracranial nasal dermoid sinus cysts: computed tomographic scan findings and surgical results. *Plastic and Reconstructive Surgery*, **93**, 745–754

PRACY, R. (1979) Congenital diseases of the nose. In: *Scott-Brown's Diseases of the Ear, Nose and Throat*, 4th edn. edited by J. Ballantyne and J. Groves. London: Butterworths. pp. 73–81

ROULAND, J. F., CHEVALIER, D., PIOUET, J. J., CONSTANTINIDES, G. and FRANÇOIS, P. (1993) Les fistules congénitales médianes du dos du nez. *Journal Francais D'Ophtalmologie*, **16**, 264–266

RYBAK, L. P., RAPP, M. F., MCGRADY, M. D., SCHWARTZ, M. R., MYERS, P. W. and ORVIDAS, L. (1991) Obstructing nasopharyngeal teratoma in the neonate. *Archives of Otolaryngology – Head and Neck Surgery*, **117**, 1411–1415

SHASHI, V., GOLDEN, W. L. and FRYBURG, J. S. (1994) Choanal atresia in a patient with the deletion (9p) syndrome. *American Journal of Medical Genetics*, **49**, 88–90

SPRINKLE, P. M. and SPORCK, F. T. (1983) Congenital malformations of the nose and paranasal sinuses. In: *Pediatric Otolaryngology*, edited by C. H. Bluestone and S. E. Stool. Philadelphia: W. B. Saunders. pp. 769–780

STANKIEWICZ, J. A. (1990) The endoscopic repair of choanal atresia. *Otolaryngology – Head and Neck Surgery*, **103**, 931–937

SWIFT, A. C. and SINGH, S. D. (1985) The presentation and management of the nasal glioma. *International Journal of Pediatric Otorhinolaryngology*, **10**, 253–261

TERRIS, M. H., BILLMAN, G. F. and PRANSKY, S. M. (1993) Nasal hamartoma: case report and review of the literature. *International Journal of Pediatric Otorhinolaryngology*, **28**, 83–88

THOMSON, H. G. and LANIGAN, M. (1979) The Cyrano nose: a clinical review of hemangiomas of the nasal tip. *Plastic and Reconstructive Surgery*, **63**, 155–160

WALTER, J. B. and ISRAEL, M. S. (1970) *General Pathology*, 3rd edn. London: J. & A. Churchill. pp. 578–582.

WETMORE, R. F. and MAHBOUBI, S. (1986) Computed tomography in the evaluation of choanal atresia. *International Journal of Pediatric Otorhinolaryngology*, **11**, 265–274

YEE, S. W., SEIBERT, R. W., BOWER, C. M. and GLASIER, C. M.

(1994) Congenital nasolacrimal duct mucocele: a cause of respiratory distress. *International Journal of Pediatric Otorhinolaryngology*, **29**, 151–158

ZINREICH, S. J., BORDERS, J. C., EISELE, D. W., MATTOX, D. E.,

LONG, D. M. and KENNEDY, D. W. (1992) The utility of magnetic resonance imaging in the diagnosis of intranasal meningoencephaloceles. *Archives of Otolaryngology – Head and Neck Surgery*, **118**, 1253–1256

16

Craniofacial anomalies

David R. James and Peter Ramsay-Baggs

The term *craniofacial anomalies* literally encompasses all congenital deformities of the cranium and face. More specifically, however, the term has come to imply congenital deformities of the head that interfere with physical and mental well-being (Marsh and Vannier, 1985). There are practically no epidemiological studies of craniofacial malformations. Myrianthopoulos (1982) reviewed data gleaned from epidemiological studies that were selected because of their careful design, large number of observations and high degree of 'ascertainment'. On this basis, there appear to be of the order of 175 major craniofacial malformations per 10 000 births, and the proportion of craniofacial malformations to all malformations is about 21%. For an authoritative overview of the spectrum of craniofacial abnormalities the reader is referred to Gorlin, Cohen and Levin (1990).

The initial attempts at surgical correction of facial deformity were directed at the mandible. Osteotomies of every part of the mandible have been described in order to achieve forward, backward, or rotational repositioning of the constituent parts. These techniques have been comprehensively reviewed by Rowe (1960). The most universally useful technique has proved to be the sagittal splitting osteotomy introduced by Trauner and Obwegeser (1957), with later modifications by Dal Pont (1961) and Hunsuck (1968).

The first maxillary osteotomies used to correct facial deformity were at the Le Fort I level, and the development of this procedure has recently been reviewed by Drommer (1986). Gillies performed the first craniofacial dysjunction at the Le Fort III level in 1942 (Gillies and Harrison, 1950). Obwegeser explored the techniques of subcranial facial osteotomy during the 1950s and 1960s laying the foundations for the routine surgical correction of the great majority of cases of facial deformity (Obwegeser, 1969).

During the 1960s, Tessier devised advanced techniques for the surgical correction of the craniofacial deformity which afflicted patients suffering from the craniosynostoses (Tessier, 1967). These patients, while comparatively few in number, suffer particularly severe forms of craniofacial deformity. Both Obwegeser and Tessier used subcranial osteotomies, but Tessier also addressed the problem of orbital hypertelorism. Segmental orbital movements had been used by a number of surgeons, but the results were unsatisfactory. Tessier reasoned that successful surgical correction required mobilization of the orbit posterior to the equator of the globe of the eye, and that this required a combined intracranial and extracranial approach. Tessier and his neurosurgical colleague Guiot were the first surgeons to reposition the bony orbits by a courageous craniofacial approach (Tessier *et al.*, 1967). Surgeons from all parts of the world subsequently journeyed to Paris to learn from Tessier before returning home to help develop the discipline of craniofacial surgery, of which he is the undisputed father.

Classification of craniofacial anomalies

Developments in craniofacial surgery in turn stimulated interest in the classification of craniofacial anomalies. Hitherto, descriptions of patients with such deformities were reported as individual cases, as groups of patients having similar collections of clinical signs (malformation syndromes), and in voluminous textbooks containing extensive lists of various types of facial dysmorphology.

More recently, an increasing understanding of the underlying genetic defects in many craniofacial anomalies has begun to offer new insights into diagnosis and treatment. Craniofacial anomalies can be broadly divided into three main subgroups:

The craniosynostoses
Craniofacial clefts
Miscellaneous craniofacial anomalies.

The craniosynostoses

At birth the cranial sutures are non-ossified zones between the bony plates of the cranial vault and the various small bones of the cranial base which appear as radiolucencies on routine skull radiographs. The sutures were originally considered to be the primary site of growth of the bony cranium, but they are now thought to be tension-responsive zones that deposit bone in response to intracranial expansion. The sutures remain biologically active for variable periods of time postnatally before fusing on a predictable schedule. *Craniosynostosis* is the term used to describe premature fusion of one or more cranial sutures *in utero*.

The incidence of craniosynostosis is not precisely known. In a World Health Organization study, several participating centres reported this condition with an incidence ranging from one in 4500 to one in 30 000 births; yet another study quoted an incidence of one in 2000 births (Myrianthopoulos, 1982).

Three types of craniosynostosis are described.

Primary craniosynostosis

This may be found as an idiopathic developmental error occurring in otherwise normal individuals. It also occurs as part of complex syndromes involving other developmental aberrations; such syndromes often show mendelian inheritance. It should be noted, however, that there is no familial incidence in the large majority of cases of primary craniosynostosis.

The inherited forms of craniostenosis can be subdivided into four groups:

1 Isolated craniostenosis
2 Craniostenosis with syndactyly
3 Craniostenosis with syndactyly and polydactyly
4 Craniostenosis with other abnormalities.

Secondary craniosynostosis

A failure of brain growth as in microcephaly or an encephaloclastic process occurring during the first years of life will result in premature fusion of the cranial sutures. A similar process may also be seen when severe hydrocephalus has been treated with a low pressure shunt.

Metabolic craniosynostosis

Metabolic craniosynostosis results from premature sutural fusion determined by obvious biochemical disorders such as the mucopolysaccharidoses, rickets, hypophosphatasia or hypercalcaemia.

Pathology of craniosynostosis

From a pathologist's point of view, craniosynostosis can be regarded as a normal developmental process occurring at an abnormally young age. Until recently there was little evidence of anything in the suture pathology to suggest that the process differs fundamentally from normal suture closure, but Pensler *et al.* (1994) have shown that osteoblasts cultured from sutures involved in stenosis differ from those in non-involved sutures in the same individual.

Histological studies of the sutures have concentrated mainly on those of the cranial vault, but it has become increasingly evident that, in many cases of craniosynostosis, the basal sutures are also involved.

The cranial deformities which are seen in the craniosynostoses represent the secondary pathology of the condition. Cranial vault bones that are prematurely fused act as a single bone plate with decreased growth potential.

The volumetric capacity of the skull is unlikely to be reduced by the premature fusion of one or two sutures. When multiple sutures are involved the cranial volume is affected. In this latter case the skull shows pathological changes indicative of raised intracranial pressure. These include convolutional impressions (circular or oval areas of thinning of the cranial vault seen on skull radiographs as 'hammer- or copper-beating'), and the formation of small cerebral herniae in areas of even more defective cranial development. The variations in skull shape consequent upon the premature fusion of specific sutures will be discussed below.

Changes in the brain, the organs of special sense and the facial viscera may be regarded as the tertiary pathology of craniosynostosis. Much concern over the condition relates to possible detrimental effects on the brain. There are few convincing reports of cerebral damage directly related to the distorted shape of the cranium, but minor degrees of cerebral damage would escape detection at post mortem. Serious cerebral anomalies are most often found in association with the genetically determined craniosynostoses. A neuropathological complication is hydrocephalus which may be severe enough to demand treatment. There is no direct relationship between intracranial volume and intracranial pressure (Gault *et al.*, 1992) and raised intracranial pressure is often seen in craniostenotic patients who do not have decreased intracranial volume (Fok *et al.*, 1992). Vision may be affected and perhaps mentality. When the cranial capacity is reduced, the term *craniostenosis* is applied.

Clinical presentations

Where medical and nursing scrutiny is routine and effective in the neonatal period, the majority of cases of craniosynostosis are diagnosed early. In a minority of patients, usually where the deformities are mild, the diagnosis may be delayed. A variety of signs and symptoms are associated with craniosynostosis.

Raised intracranial pressure

This is an important but relatively uncommon feature of craniosynostosis, with the associated symptoms of headache, fading vision and mental deterioration. Papilloedema is a very serious clinical finding, and is most likely to develop early in life, when there is maximum disproportion between the volume of the growing brain and the capacity of the stenosed skull. Mental changes occur in less than 20% of cases, and there is poor correlation between mental status and the severity of the craniosynostosis.

Exorbitism and orbitostenosis

Exorbitism or the protrusion of the orbital contents anterior to the bony orbit, is a feature of some cases of the complex craniosynostosis syndromes (Figure 16.1). The magnitude of the exorbitism varies between specific diagnoses as well as between individuals with the same syndrome. The orbital volume is reduced by encroachment of the roof, lateral and medial walls, reflecting disturbed bony development within the anterior and middle cranial fossae secondary to craniosynostosis. This reduction in orbital capacity is sometimes termed orbitostenosis. In addition, the orbital floor is hypoplastic as a result of the

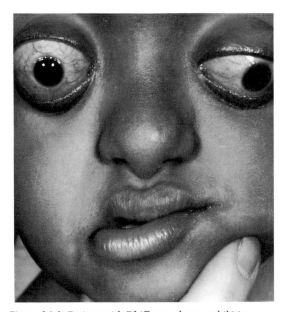

Figure 16.1 Patient with Pfeiffer syndrome exhibiting severe exorbitism and a divergent squint. He experienced occasional dislocation of the globes with retraction of the eyelids behind them

severe maxillary retrusion often seen in these syndromes. Exorbitism, apart from being unsightly, may interfere with function. The extrinsic ocular muscles, especially the medial recti, work at a disadvantage. There is a strong tendency to divergent squinting (see Figure 16.1) and binocular vision is frequently impossible. Exorbitism may be sufficiently marked to prevent lid closure during sleep, leading to keratitis and the danger of blindness (Figure 16.2). Thus sight may be in danger from both corneal damage and optic atrophy secondary to raised intracranial pressure. In some patients the globe is so proptosed that it may become dislocated through the palpebral fissure, when manual reduction may be necessary.

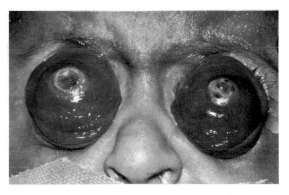

Figure 16.2 Extreme exorbitism in a neonate with Kleeblattschadel (clover-leaf skull) resulting in gross keratitis and loss of vision. (Courtesy of Mr Richard Hayward, FRCS)

Orbital hypertelorism

Greig (1924) coined the term *hypertelorism* to describe what he thought was a discrete syndrome consisting of excessive separation between the eyes. Greig's nomenclature of ocular hypertelorism has now been replaced by the term orbital hypertelorism in order to exclude excessive interpupillary distances secondary to exotropias. It should be distinguished from telecanthus, an increased distance between the medial canthi, which is frequently encountered in severe nasoethmoidal trauma. Orbital hypertelorism is not a primary anomaly *per se*, but is found in a number and variety of diseases and malformation syndromes, most notably the craniosynostoses and craniofacial clefting syndromes (see Figure 16.23). There is some evidence to suggest that the severity of hypertelorism progresses in craniosynostosis, whereas it remains constant with growth in patients with clefting. Not only is orbital hypertelorism unsightly, but there may be functional impairment of binocular vision and convergence.

The diagnosis depends on declining deviation from normality, usually two or three standard deviations from the mean. Various measurements such as inter-canthal distance and interpupillary distance, standardized for age and sex, are used to measure such deviation. The distribution of these differs in various ethnic groups. For example, intercanthal and interpupillary values for Negroes significantly exceed those for Caucasians. On this basis, Myrianthopoulos (1982) suggested an incidence of one per 1000 births.

Hypertelorism has been classified according to the degree of separation of the medial orbital walls measured at the anterior lacrimal crests on standard radiographic projections. In first degree hypertelorism the interorbital distance is 30–34 mm which is clinically insignificant. In second degree hypertelorism the interorbital distance is 34–40 mm which is clinically obvious, while a distance of greater than 40 mm signifies third degree hypertelorism which is unusual in craniosynostosis, but is seen in association with frontonasal dysplasia (see below). In this extreme state the orbits may appear to face laterally as well as forward, in which case the ocular movements are impaired.

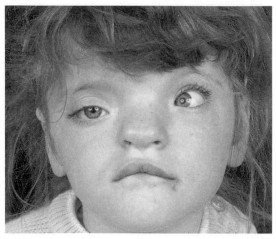

Figure 16.3 Orbital dystopia. The left orbit is displaced in all three planes of space, and demonstrates a degree of rotation

Orbital hypotelorism

An interorbital distance below the normal range (22–30 mm in the adult) is likely to give the eyes a close-set appearance known as *hypotelorism* (see Figure 16.25). It results from excessive medial migration of the orbits due to inadequate development of the frontal cribriform area as a result of either metopic craniosynostosis or neural hypoplasia. Vision is not affected.

Orbital dystopia

The term *dystopia* literally refers to an aberrant position of the globe. Orbital dystopia implies a displacement of the bony orbit in one or a combination of the axial (transverse), corneal (mediolateral) and sagittal (anteroposterior) planes. The malposition is usually associated with a degree of rotation (Figure 16.3). Dystopia may be a feature of the craniosynostoses or of the clefting syndromes such as Treacher Collins syndrome and craniofacial microsomia.

Midface hypoplasia

Craniosynostosis and midface retrusion are common features of a number of specific syndromes, most of which also include deformities of the hands and feet (see Figures 16.12 and 16.14). The membranous components of the facial skeleton fail to grow normally, while the cartilaginous components are largely unaffected. Consequently, relative overgrowth of the nasal septum may produce a prominent, often deviated nose with obstruction of the nasal airway. Delaire *et al.* (1963) have applied the term *faciosteno-*

sis to describe these states of midface hypoplasia. While it is not yet certain that this hypoplasia results from premature fusion of the facial sutures, the concept of faciostenosis is useful, as it emphasizes that affected patients suffer from disorders of visceral function analogous to those seen in craniostenosis and *orbitostenosis*.

Airway restriction

Maxillary hypoplasia is a three-dimensional phenomenon. The maxilla is narrow transversely, resulting in a narrow and frequently high-arched palate. The retruded position of the maxilla reduces the postnasal space, while diminished vertical height lowers the capacity of the nasal cavity and paranasal air sinuses. In addition, choanal atresia may occur in cases of Crouzon's syndrome. Some of the severely affected children may experience sleep apnoea, while older patients are often mouth breathers who snore unduly. It is possible that respiratory distress may cause some infant deaths, especially in Apert's syndrome, which carries a high infant mortality rate.

Speech

Severe midface retrusion can have marked effects on speech. Adequate accommodation of the tongue is precluded by the narrow palate, especially if there is an accompanying palatal cleft – a not uncommon association. Velopharyngeal incompetence is not usually a feature, but may occur in association with a cleft or after large surgical advancements of the maxilla. Crowding of the nasopharyngeal airway and varying degrees of nasal obstruction are common in

Crouzon's syndrome and this can result in hyponasal speech.

Hypoplastic paranasal sinuses may reduce vocal resonance, while severe dental malocclusions add to the articulation problems caused by the abnormal tongue position. Impaired hearing is a common finding in Apert's and Crouzon's syndromes and this can adversely affect the acquisition of normal speech, as may mental retardation.

Mastication

The skeletal disproportion between maxilla and mandible, and the accompanying dental malocclusion, can seriously impair normal mastication (see Figure 16.7). It should be noted that, although there is an apparent mandibular prognathism, the mandible is usually abnormally small in patients with craniosynostosis syndromes. This has important implications for surgical reconstruction, as it is frequently necessary to advance both maxilla and mandible to produce a satisfactory facial harmony (see Figure 16.21).

Simple calvarial deformities

There is considerable variation in the shape and size of heads, and when these variations are extreme, they are considered to be deformities. Such a judgement is essentially intuitive, and obviously varies in different ethnic groups and in different cultures. The *cephalic index* (more strictly the horizontal cephalic index), defined as (maximum breadth/maximum length) × 100 offers a useful means of quantitating a visual impression. The dimensions may be measured clinically or from skull radiographs. It will be obvious that it is very difficult to quantitate cranial asymmetry. All cranial vault sutures and fontanelles are patent in the normal neonatal skull. They ossify and become radiopaque in an orderly, but variable sequence, as follows:

Sutures – metopic (childhood); sagittal, coronal and lambdoid (adulthood); squamosal, occipitomastoid and sphenotemporal (may be patent in the elderly)
Fontanelles – posterior and anterolateral (infancy); posterolateral (during first year of life); anterior (during second year of life).

The shape of the skull may be significantly deformed by premature fusion of the cranial sutures. One must be careful to exclude cranial moulding which usually improves with time, while craniosynostosis becomes progressively more obvious.

The various types of calvarial deformity are summarized in Table 16.1. Sagittal synostosis is the most common (Figure 16.4), representing about 55–60%, with coronal synostosis being the next most common (20–30%). Metopic, lambdoidal and combinations of premature sutural fusions are far less frequent. While these cranial deformities are found in isolation, they frequently form part of one of the craniosynostosis syndromes described below.

Craniosynostosis syndromes

Cohen (1979) listed 57 craniosynostosis syndromes, as well as 22 combinations with secondary or occasional craniosynostosis. Simple calvarial deformities may be accompanied by unusual facial appearances, but they are primarily dysplasias of the cranium. Cases of identifiable craniofacial syndrome may present with deformities of the skull vault and minimal facial disturbance.

The commonest of the craniofacial syndromes is Crouzon's syndrome which primarily affects the craniofacial region. There is a number of craniofacial syndromes in which craniosynostosis occurs together with syndactyly, the most important of these being Apert's syndrome. A significant proportion of the cases of craniofacial syndromes are familial, usually exhibiting autosomal dominant transmission.

Table 16.1 The various types of calvarial deformity

Affected suture	Traditional name	Literal translation	Skull length	Skull width	Skull height
Sagittal	Scaphocephaly	Boat skull	Increased	Decreased	Normal or increased
Metopic	Trigonocephaly	Triangle skull	Normal or increased	Increased	Normal
Unicoronal	Plagiocephaly	Oblique skull	Decreased or normal	Increased	Normal or increased
Bicoronal	Brachycephaly	Short skull	Decreased	Increased	Increased
Multiple sutures	Turricephaly (acrocephaly)	Tower skull	Decreased	Increased	Increased
	Oxycephaly	Sharp skull	Decreased	Increased	Increased
	Kleeblattschädel	Clover-leaf skull	Decreased	Increased	Increased

Note: plagiocephaly is not necessarily synonymous with unilateral coronal synostosis

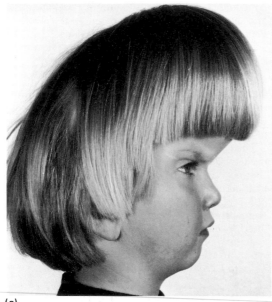

(a)

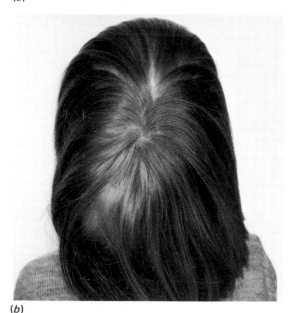

(b)

Figure 16.4 Scaphocephaly. In this child the sagittal suture is completely fused, while the remaining sutures of the cranial vault are normal

Only the commoner syndromes will be described. For an overall perspective of the various craniosynostosis syndromes the reader is referred to the excellent review article by Cohen (1979). A fuller account of the craniosynostoses is provided by David, Poswillo and Simpson (1982) and Cohen (1986).

Crouzon's syndrome

Although Friedenwald reported a case of steeple head with prominent eyes in 1893, Crouzon, in 1912, was the first to delineate the triad of calvarial deformity, midface hypoplasia and exorbitism. Crouzon's syndrome, also called *craniofacial dysostosis*, has autosomal dominant transmission, which maps to a locus on the long arm of chromosome 10. Up to 50% of cases occur sporadically, representing fresh mutations. The cause of the syndrome is thought to be mutation in the fibroblast growth factor receptor 2 gene (FGFR2) (Reardon *et al.*, 1994). This mutation has also been shown to be responsible for both Apert's and Pfeiffer syndromes (Wilkie *et al.*, 1995; Rutland *et al.*, 1995). The incidence is said to be 1/25 000 of the general population.

Clinical features

Cranium

Patients may exhibit any of the forms of calvarial deformity, depending on which sutures are involved, the chronological order in which they fuse and the extent of their involvement. The brachycephalic deformities predominate, but it is important to remember that many cases of the syndrome show no obvious calvarial deformity, even when there are marked radiological abnormalities.

Premature and progressive craniosynostosis is variable in onset, but frequently commences during the first year of life and is usually complete by 2–3 years of age. Radiographically, the coronal and sagittal sutures are nearly always involved, while the lambdoidal suture is affected in 80% of cases. Other findings include digital markings (90%), basilar kyphosis and widening of the pituitary fossa (Figure 16.5). The basal sutures may also fuse prematurely. While this is hard to demonstrate radiographically, post-mortem studies have revealed premature fusion of the sphenofrontal sutures (Kreiborg and Bjork, 1982), a finding which has been confirmed during surgery. Such sphenofrontal craniosynostosis is an important feature of orbitostenosis, since failure of growth across this suture results in reduced anteroposterior depth of the orbit. Cephalometric studies frequently indicate short calvaria, a steep forehead and flattened occiput. Often there is protrusion in the area of the anterior fontanelle (the clown's cap deformity) which exaggerates the oxycephalic head shape. The cranial base is commonly short and narrow with the clivus especially shortened. The patterns of dysmorphology in Crouzon's syndrome were well described by Kolar, Munro and Farkas (1988) in their study of 61 patients.

The signs of raised intracranial pressure may be evident, with headaches noted in 30% and epilepsy in 10%. While some cases of mental impair-

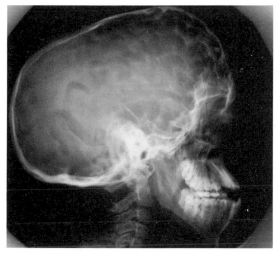

Figure 16.5 Crouzon's syndrome. Lateral skull radiograph which demonstrates scaphocephaly due to premature fusion of the sagittal suture, obvious digital markings, basilar kyphosis and widening of the pituitary fossa

ment result from this increased pressure, the extent to which mental deficiency exists *de novo* is uncertain.

Face

Midface hypoplasia with relative mandibular prognathism, drooping lower lip and short upper lip are typical features (Figure 16.6). The nasal bridge is often flattened, and the tip of the nose may appear beak like. There is deviation of the nasal septum in 35% and obstruction of the nasopharynx in 30% of cases.

Eyes

Proptosis is a constant finding, being secondary to the shallow orbits. Divergent strabismus, nystagmus and hypertelorism are frequently found. Exposure conjunctivitis (50%), keratitis (10%), poor vision (45%) and optic atrophy (25%) are reported; rarely there is luxation of the globes.

Oral findings

These include a narrow high-arched palate, crowding of the dental arches and an anterior open bite (Figure 16.7). Ectopic eruption of the maxillary first molar teeth occurs in about half of the patients and 35% are obligate mouth breathers. Lateral palatal swellings are present in 50% of cases, but are rarely large enough to give rise to the pseudo-cleft palate commonly seen in Apert's syndrome. Only some 3% of patients exhibit a cleft palate and 10% have a bifid uvula.

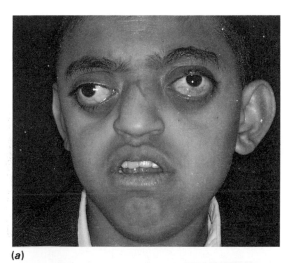

(a)

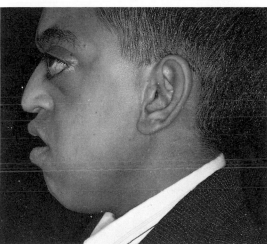

(b)

Figure 16.6 Crouzon's syndrome. This 13-year-old boy exhibits the classical features of maxillary hypoplasia with relative mandibular prognathism, exorbitism, short upper lip and drooping lower lip. He also has a divergent strabismus, flattened nasal bridge and beak-like nasal tip

Ears

More than 50% of patients have a conductive hearing loss associated with ossicular deformity and some 15% patients have atresia of the auditory canals.

Other anomalies

Stiffness of the joints, especially the elbows, has been reported. Cervical spine anomalies occur in 30–40% of patients, these being mostly intervertebral fusions and 85% exhibit calcification of the stylohyoid ligament. Acanthosis nigricans has been reported in the syndrome.

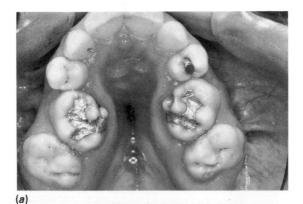

(a)

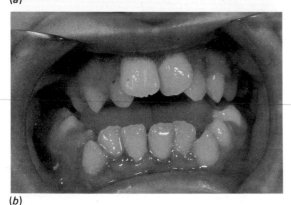

(b)

Figure 16.7 Crouzon's syndrome. (*a*) Typical narrow high-arched palate; (*b*) a degree of dental crowding and anterior open bite is also very common

Differential diagnosis

Having no abnormalities of the hands or feet, Crouzon's syndrome is easily distinguished from Apert's, Pfeiffer or Jackson-Weiss syndromes. It may be confused with Saethre-Chotzen syndrome in which the hand and feet anomalies may be minimal or absent. It should also be distinguished from simple craniosynostosis.

Apert's syndrome

In 1896 Apert observed an infant with a very brachycephalic head and severe syndactyly affecting all four limbs. Two similar cases had previously been described by Wheaton in 1894. By the time he described the case 10 years later (Apert, 1906), eight similar cases had been reported. Apert called the condition *acrocéphalosyndactylie*. The anglicized form *acrocephalosyndactyly* is now usually used to embrace all those syndromes which have the common features of craniosynostosis and digital anomalies. Apert's syndrome is distinguished from other acrocephalosyndactylies by the severity of the syndactyly, which involves fusion of the phalanges of at least the index,

middle and ring fingers. A birth prevalence of between 13.7 and 15.5 (Cohen and Krieborg, 1992; Cohen *et al.*, 1992) per 1 000 000 has been suggested, but due to high infant mortality, there is probably a significantly lower incidence in the general population. The syndrome represents around 4% of all cases of craniostenosis.

By 1991 only five familial instances were published in the world literature, the remaining cases being sporadic. Despite this, autosomal dominant inheritance is strongly suggested by the familial cases, the sex ratio of 1 : 1 and increased paternal age at the time of conception. Cohen and Krieborg (1991) felt that the high incidence of mental deficiency and the high level of severe deformity reduces the number of people with the syndrome who have children. Prenatal diagnosis has been made by ultrasound and fetoscopy, when hand and foot anomalies have been noted. It has now been shown that the syndrome is caused by the same mutation in fibroblast growth factor receptor 2 gene (FGFR2) that is responsible for both Crouzon's and Pfeiffer syndromes (Wilkie *et al.*, 1995; Lajeunie *et al.*, 1995).

Clinical features

Cranium

In typical cases the head is turribrachycephalic, with a high forehead and flattened occiput; the apex of the cranium is located near or anterior to the bregma (Figure 16.8). There is usually a congenital bone

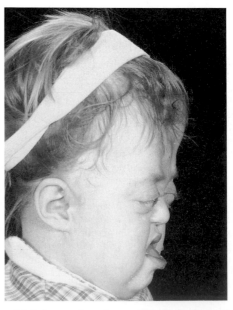

Figure 16.8 Crouzon's syndrome. This young patient has a turribrachycephalic skull with a high forehead; she also has a severe midface hypoplasia and exorbitism. A similar appearance is frequently seen in Apert's syndrome

defect in the metopic region, and consequently there may be a soft tissue bulge extending from the fontanelle to the roof of the nose (Figure 16.9). This defect is patent during infancy, closure usually commencing in the third year of life. There is invariably premature synostosis of the coronal sutures, and there may be additional premature fusion of the squamosal and sagittal sutures, but these are less obvious and usually appear later. The clivus is disproportionately small, and there is an associated shortening of the posterior

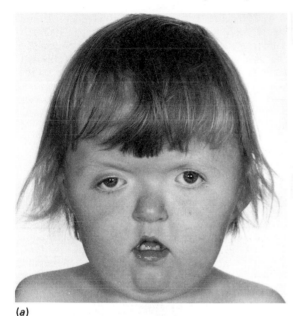

(a)

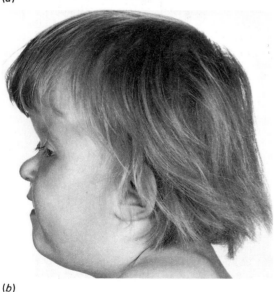

(b)

Figure 16.9 Apert's syndrome. Often a congenital bone defect in the metopic region permits bulging from the fontanelle to the root of the nose

fossa, but this may become less evident with growth. The mean head circumference is normal but the head length is significantly increased, leading to an increased intracranial volume. Post-mortem studies appear to indicate that the cranial malformation is determined before the sutures begin to fuse, and there are various patterns of synostosis in the chondrocranial components of the skull base. David, Poswillo and Simpson (1982) have suggested that, in Apert's syndrome, there is some more fundamental perversion of skull growth than is seen in other forms of craniosynostosis, perhaps due to an underlying biochemical defect in chondrogenesis. More recently, Kreiborg and Cohen (1990), in a study of the radiographs of 16 infant patients and measurements from two dried skulls, came to the conclusion that growth inhibition in the sphenofrontal and coronal suture area has its onset very early in fetal life.

Central nervous system

Some degree of mental retardation is found in most patients, although normal intelligence has been observed in some cases. It appears doubtful that cerebral damage results purely as a result of compression by the unyielding skull, and the basis of the mental retardation in Apert's syndrome remains unclear.

It may be related to malformations of the central nervous system. Cohen and Krieborg (1990), in their review of the literature and by analysis of their own clinical material, came to the conclusion that defects in the corpus callosum, and/or limbic systems may be responsible. Surgery seems to have no effect on intelligence (Patton *et al.*, 1988).

Face

The facial dysplasia is severe, especially in older patients. The maxilla is grossly hypoplastic, while the nose and mandible are relatively prominent, although the mandibular body length is actually short compared to the population norm. The ramal height, by comparison, is usually normal or increased (Costaras-Volarich and Pruzansky, 1984). Facial asymmetry is sometimes present, and can be very pronounced.

Oral findings

The palate is usually highly arched, constricted and may have a median furrow. The soft palate is cleft in about one-third of cases (Figure 16.10*a*), and a bifid uvula is occasionally seen. The maxillary dental arch may be V-shaped, with severe dental crowding and bulging alveolar ridges (Figure 16.10*b*). Lateral palatal swellings are common, caused by bulging of the alveolar ridges (Figure 16.10*b*). This can give rise to

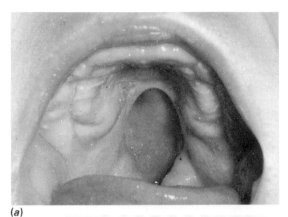

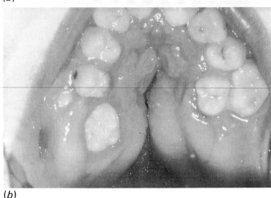

(a)

(b)

Figure 16.10 Apert's syndrome. (*a*) Cleft of the secondary palate; (*b*) maxillary dental arch exhibiting dental crowding, bulging alveolar ridges and a tendency towards a gothic shape

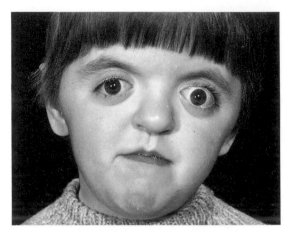

Figure 16.11 Apert's syndrome. Mild orbital hypertelorism with an antimongoloid slant of the palpebral fissures and some proptosis

a 'pseudo' cleft of the hard palate. A skeletal class III malocclusion is almost invariable, and an anterior open bite is often seen. Retarded dental eruption is common. All these deformities, together with mental impairment, frequently combine to impair speech.

Eyes

Hypertelorism is common, and there is usually some degree of proptosis. All degrees of orbitostenosis are seen in Apert's syndrome, but it is not generally as severe as in Crouzon's syndrome. The palpebral fissures may show an antimongoloid slant (Figure 16.11). Buncic (1991) reviewed the spectrum of ocular abnormalities.

Otolaryngological problems

Otitis media is common. Middle ear problems are related to the high incidence of cleft palate. Fixation

of the foot of the stapes is seen frequently. Sleep apnoea is common and can give rise to management problems (McGill, 1991).

Skeletal system

Deformities of the hands and feet are symmetrical. A mid-digital hand mass with bony and soft-tissue syndactyly of digits two, three and four is always found (Figure 16.12*a*); in addition, digits one and five may be joined to digits two and four respectively (Figure 16.12*b*). If free, the thumb is broad and deviates radially. The interphalangeal joints of the fingers are stiff, while the fingernails of the mid-digital hand mass may be continuous or partly continuous. In the feet, toes two, three and four are joined by soft-tissue syndactyly; toes one and five may be joined by soft-tissue syndactyly to the second and fourth toes respectively (Figure 16.12*c*). The great toes are broad and hallux varus is common. Toenails may be partially continuous with some segmentation.

The upper extremities are shortened, and there may be aplasia or ankylosis of several joints, especially the elbow, shoulder and hip. Progressive synostosis of the bones of the hands, feet and cervical spine has been reported. The epiphyses of the long bones are frequently dysplastic.

Other findings

An acneiform eruption, similar to acne vulgaris, commonly occurs, with extension to the forearm. A wide variety of cardiovascular and other internal anomalies has been reported (Cohen and Krieborg, 1993).

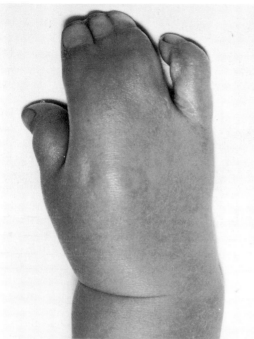

(a)

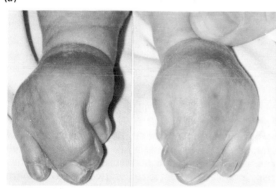

(b)

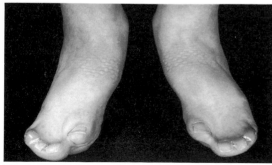

(c)

Figure 16.12 Apert's syndrome. Deformities of the hands and feet; (*a*) typical mid-digital hand mass with bony and soft tissue syndactyly of digits two, three and four; (*b*) fusion of all five digits; (*c*) syndactyly of all five digits of the feet

Differential diagnosis

The syndactyly of Apert's syndrome is much more severe and consistent than in other craniosynostosis-syndactyly syndromes such as Pfeiffer, Saethre-Chotzen and Carpenter's syndromes. The hands and feet are normal in Crouzon's syndrome.

Pfeiffer syndrome

In 1964, Pfeiffer described a syndrome consisting of craniosynostosis with turribrachycephaly, broad thumbs and great toes, and partial soft-tissue syndactyly of the hands and feet as a variable feature. Pfeiffer's report described eight affected individuals in three generations, with two instances of male-to-male transmission.

It has now been shown that the syndrome is caused by the same mutation in fibroblast growth factor receptor 2 gene (FGFR2) that is responsible for both Crouzon's and Apert's syndromes. In addition, there is also a mutation of FGFR1 (Rutland *et al.*, 1995; Lajeunie *et al.*, 1995; Schell *et al.*, 1995; Muenke *et al.*, 1995.

The syndrome as originally described by Pfeiffer is designated type 1. Type 2 consists of clover-leaf skull, Pfeiffer hands and feet plus elbow ankylosis. All cases have been sporadic to date. Type 3 is similar to type 2, without the clover-leaf skull but with severe ocular proptosis and marked shortening of the cranial base. Type 1 cases usually have normal intelligence (Cohen 1986, 1993).

Clinical features

Cranium

Turricephaly is the commonest deformity, being associated with premature fusion of the coronal sutures (Figure 16.13*a*). Other sutures may be involved, and cases with trigonocephaly and clover-leaf skull have been recorded.

Intelligence is usually normal, but mental retardation does occur, being most severe in those cases associated with clover-leaf skull.

Face

Maxillary hypoplasia with relative mandibular prognathism is common, and the ears are frequently low-set (Figure 16.13*b*). Facial asymmetry, orbital hypertelorism, antimongoloid palpebral fissures, proptosis and strabismus (see Figure 16.1) have all been reported.

Oral findings include a high-arched palate, dental malocclusion and, rarely, a bifid uvula. Supernumerary teeth and gingival hyperplasia are occasionally seen.

Hands and feet

The thumbs and great toes are broad, and usually show varus deformity (Figure 16.14). In some patients the

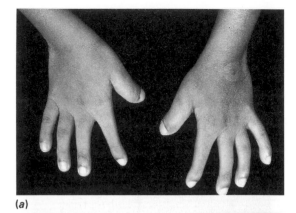

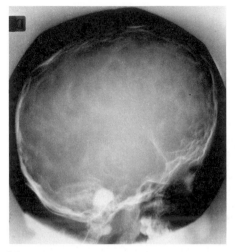

(a)

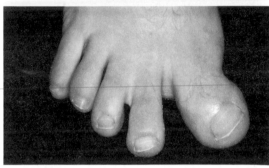

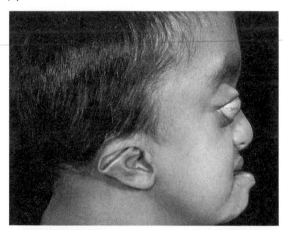

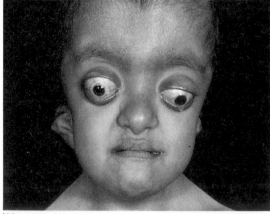

(b)

Figure 16.13 Pfeiffer syndrome. (*a*) Radiograph of the skull of a 9-year-old child demonstrating turricephaly due to premature fusion of the coronal sutures; (*b*) facial photographs of the same patient revealing severe maxillary hypoplasia with relative mandibular prognathism, low set ears, exorbitism and strabismus

Figure 16.14 Pfeiffer syndrome. Hands and feet displaying a varus deformity

great toes may be shortened, but without varus deformity. Cutaneous syndactyly is usually present, involving digits two and three, and at times three and four, of both hands and feet. Clinodactyly and symphalangism of both hands and feet have been reported. Other skeletal anomalies described include fused cervical vertebrae, radiohumeral and radioulnar synostoses (Figure 16.15).

Other anomalies

Other features occasionally seen are pyloric stenosis, bicuspid aortic valve, hypoplasia of the gallbladder, single umbilical artery, umbilical hernia, preauricular tags, choanal atresia and hearing loss.

Differential diagnosis

Pfeiffer syndrome should be distinguished from other craniosynostosis–syndactyly syndromes, notably Apert's and Saethre-Chotzen syndromes. Facially it is similar to Apert's syndrome, but in the latter, the degree of syndactyly is extreme and characteristic. The facial findings of asymmetry, low hairline and beaking of the nose in the Saethre-Chotzen syndrome are not typical of Pfeiffer syndrome. In Crouzon's syndrome the hands are normal, while in Pfeiffer syndrome the thumbs and great toes are typical.

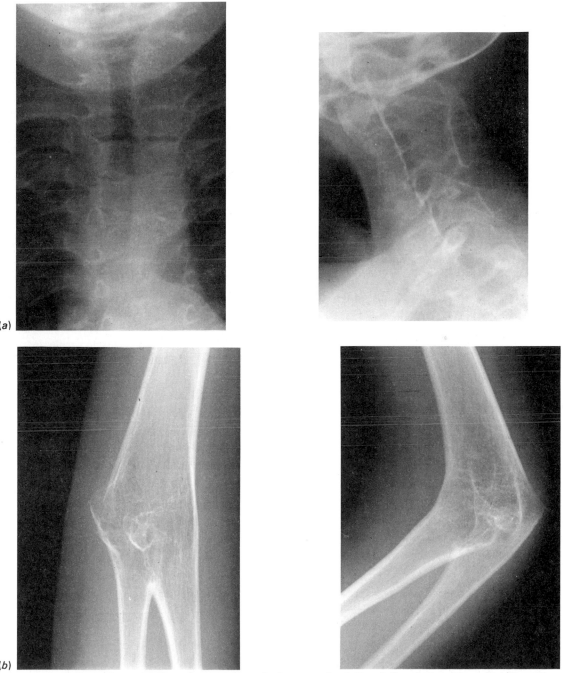

Figure 16.15 Pfeiffer syndrome. (*a*) Cervical spine radiographs demonstrating fusion of all cervical vertebrae; (*b*) radiographs of the elbows demonstrating radiohumeral and radioulnar synostosis with the left arm fully extended

Clover-leaf skull (Kleeblattschadel)

Although Vrolik described a case of clover-leaf skull in 1849 the condition was first identified in 1960 by Holtmuller and Weidman. This anomaly can be seen in many of the craniostenoses, although it may occur in isolation. Synostosis may involve the coronal, lambdoidal and metopic sutures with bulging of the cerebrum through the open sagittal suture or of the sagittal and squamosal sutures with cerebral bulging via a wide patent anterior fontanelle. Occasionally all the sutures may be stenosed.

The trilobular appearance is striking, and the degree of deformity depends on the underlying stenoses. In severe forms the ears may be displaced downwards. Antimongoloid slant of the palpebral fissures is common. Hypertelorism and exorbitism are frequently seen, and may be so severe that the eyelids fail to close leading to ocular damage. Midface hypoplasia is the rule. Hydrocephaly is common. Life expectancy is short (Cohen, 1986, 1987).

Treatment of the craniosynostoses

The most contentious debate in craniofacial surgery remains that concerning the timing of the various forms of surgery available. Regrettably, despite the fact that such surgery has now been practised for more than 30 years, there are no good objective and scientific studies indicating the long-term results in respect of the obvious parameters of brain and cranial growth, facial growth, eyesight and mental ability. Surgery has been performed at all ages from the neonatal period to adulthood, and the results presented have been largely anecdotal.

There is general agreement that the two conditions which make early surgery mandatory are raised intracranial pressure and the danger of visual impairment due to gross exorbitism. The aims of early craniofacial surgery for craniosynostosis are:

1 To allow the brain to expand normally
2 To provide a normal shape to the forehead and skull
3 To provide eye protection by reducing the exorbitism
4 To prevent or minimize the problem of impaired facial growth in faciostenosis.

Marchac and Renier (1981) reported the results of early surgery (preferably within the first 6 months of life), claiming good morphological and functional results that appeared to be maintained over periods up to 8 years (their longest follow-up period). Surgery involved frontal bone advancement by their 'floating forehead' technique and reshaping of the cranium. The photographs appear impressive, but no objective measurement of either morphology or function was made. They also claimed that 'there is a definite improvement in affected facial structures when early surgery has been performed', but no evidence is produced.

The severe midface retrusion seen in the craniosynostosis syndromes is almost certainly due to involvement of the sutures of the cranial base, and it is difficult to see how surgery which corrects the cranial vault can have any effect on the growth of the midface.

In 1989 Marchac and Renier published a further follow up and noted that in Crouzon's and Apert's syndromes early frontal advancement did not prevent midface retrusion. In 1994 the same authors, with Broumand, published a 20-year follow up of 983 operated patients. They still advocated early surgery for non-syndromic craniostenosis, but for syndromic craniostenosis they advocated a two-stage procedure, with forehead advancement first and midface advancement later unless there is severe exorbitism, in which case they advocated the frontofacial monobloc procedure.

Fearon and Whitaker (1993) compared the monobloc and Le Forte III osteotomy and concluded that aesthetically there was no difference between the two procedures, but that the monobloc procedure had a significantly higher rate of infection. The older the patients were when operated on the better the aesthetics were judged to be. Most younger patients required a repeat of the facial advancement. On the basis of their findings they recommended staging of the forehead and midface advancements.

Posnick (1991) emphasized the need for a team approach to the treatment of patients with craniostenosis. In addition, he suggested the following rationale for the timing of craniofacial surgery:

Infancy   cranial vault surgery to relieve intracranial pressure and papilloedema
Childhood   to increase intracranial volume further, improve nasal airflow, dental occlusion and body image
Adolescence to improve occlusion, speech and aesthetics.

This will avoid unproductive surgery and maximize long-term functional and aesthetic results. Examples of early craniofacial surgery are shown in Figures 16.16 and 16.17. Patients with hypertelorism lack stereoscopic vision. Tessier (1967) originally suggested that, if the hypertelorism could be corrected by early surgery, this may result in the acquisition of stereoscopic vision. Unfortunately, this does not appear to be the case. Seventy per cent of the adult interorbital distance is reached by the age of 2 years in the normal person, and it is thus assumed that surgical correction of hypertelorism is best delayed until after this age. The results of surgery for hypertelorism depend on the anatomy of the specific deformity and the skill of the surgeon (Figure 16.18).

Faciostenosis or midface retrusion, apart from producing severe facial deformity, may result in the functional problems of corneal exposure, impairment of breathing and poor mastication. There are obvious advantages to correcting the deformity early, both from a cosmetic and functional point of view. However this presents some technical problems, and it is almost certain that further correction will be necessary at a later date. Provided that everybody involved in the decision is aware of these constraints, it appears reasonable to agree to early surgery in

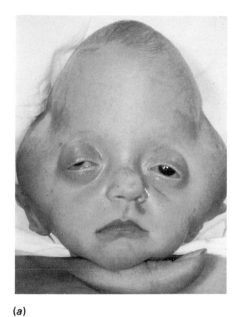

(a)

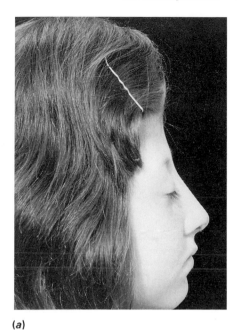

(a)

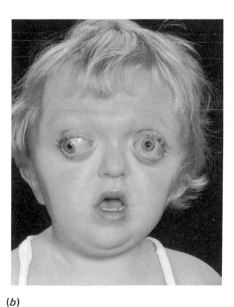

(b)

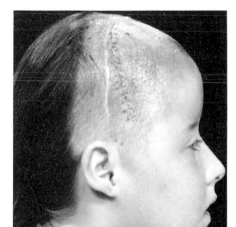

(b)

Figure 16.16 (a) Clover-leaf skull deformity in an infant with Apert's syndrome; (b) the patient at 3 years following surgical correction by means of frontal advancement and reshaping of the cranial vault. (Courtesy of Mr Richard Hayward, FRCS)

Figure 16.17 (a) An 8-year-old patient with Crouzon's syndrome exhibiting turricephaly and recession of the frontal bone; (b) appearance following frontal advancement and reshaping of the cranial vault. (Courtesy of Mr Richard Hayward, FRCS)

appropriate cases (Figure 16.19). Undoubtedly better results are obtained in those patients in whom surgery is delayed until after puberty (Figures 16.20 and 16.21).

Details of surgical technique are outside the scope of this chapter, and have therefore not been included.

Readers are directed to some of the texts included in the list of references at the end of the chapter. Henderson (1985) comprehensively covered the subcranial osteotomies and Caronni (1985) is a good source for information about cranial and orbital techniques.

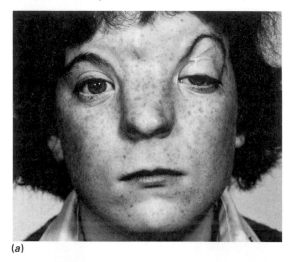

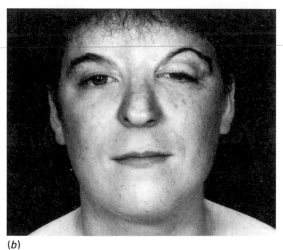

Figure 16.18 (*a*) A 13-year-old girl with hypertelorism; (*b*) the same patient at the age of 17, 4 years after transcranial correction of her hypertelorism and subsequent soft-tissue adjustment of the left upper eyelid

Craniofacial clefts

Cleft is a useful word for conveying the mechanism of a malformation, or the resultant features of the deformity. While clefts of the lip and palate are relatively common, there is a number of other clefts occurring in the craniofacial region which are rare. For many years the terminology for these conditions was confusing and often misleading. Terms such as nasomaxillary hypoplasia and frontonasal dysplasia were used, and adjectives such as orofacial, oronasal and otomandibular employed. Some malformations may bear many names, while others are subjected to eponymous terminology such as Treacher Collins and Goldenhar syndromes.

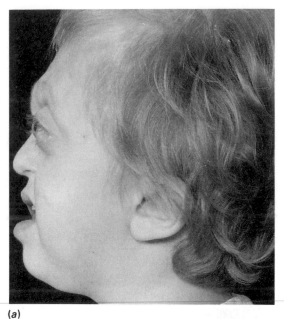

(*a*)

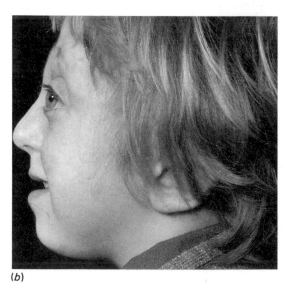

(*b*)

Figure 16.19 (*a*) A 3-year-old child with Apert's syndrome who has had previous cranial vault surgery; (*b*) appearance after a Le Fort III subcranial advancement

Numerous attempts have been made to classify craniofacial defects, but none has proved entirely satisfactory. Tessier (1976) devised a descriptive, clinical classification that is unrelated to the embryology of the malformation. It is based on his personal observation of 336 cases of craniofacial clefts. His analysis of this vast and unique collection of rare conditions included clinical and radiographic examination. In 254 cases he carried out an anatomical

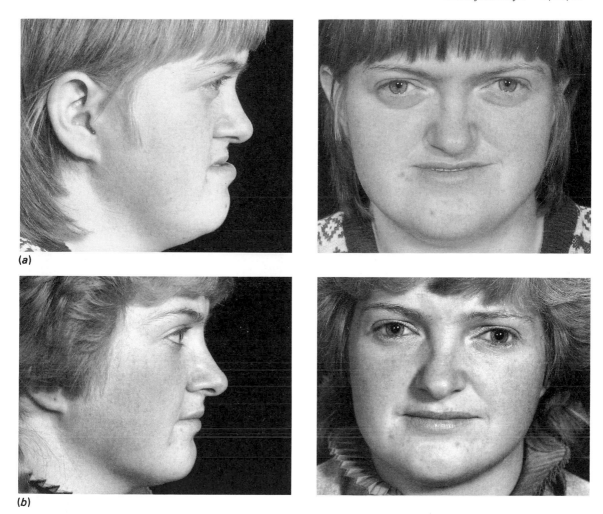

Figure 16.20 (*a*) Crouzon's syndrome in a 16-year-old girl; (*b*) appearance 4 years after a subcranial Le Fort III advancement

dissection at the time of surgery. As a result of this work Tessier found that true bony clefts were present where 'hypoplasia' had previously been described, this being the case in both Treacher Collins syndrome and craniofacial microsomia. Bone and soft tissues were rarely involved to the same extent. Between the midline and infraorbital foramen soft tissue defects were the more destructive, while lateral to this (with the notable exception of the auricle) bony defects were more severe. Clefts were located along some very definite axes; due to the constancy of most skeletal points, clefts are more easily described with reference to the skeleton than to the soft tissues.

Tessier classification

Tessier utilized the eyelids and orbits as a reference when describing clefts, as this enables both cranium and face to be included. His original diagrams present a graphic representation of the classification (Figure 16.22).

For the purpose of orientation the orbit is divided into two hemispheres. The lower lid with the cheek and lip constitutes the southern hemisphere, and clefts through it are facial. The upper lid is in the northern hemisphere, and clefts through it are cranial. Using the number zero as the mid-sagittal plane, each site of malformation has been assigned a respective number determined by its axis in relationship to the zero line. Fifteen locations for clefts (0–14) have been described, using the orbit as the point of reference. They are distributed according to eight 'time zones', cleft number seven being the most lateral. Cleft lip is not specifically described, but is encountered in most instances of clefts 1, 2 or 3. For specific details of the classification, readers are referred to Tessier's original paper. David, Moore and Cooter

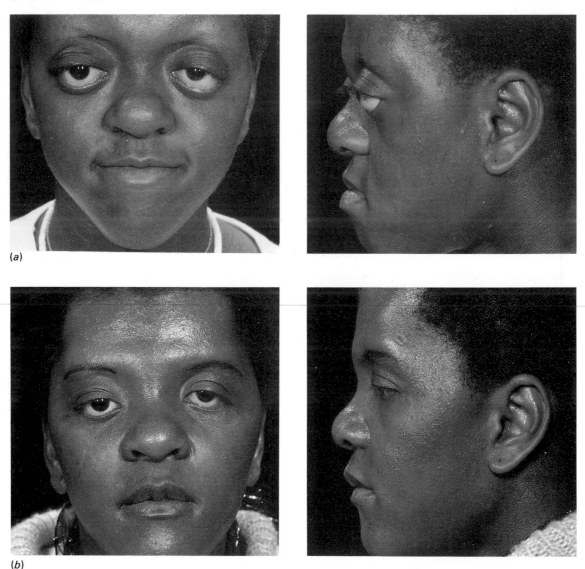

(a)

(b)

Figure 16.21 (*a*) A 15-year-old girl with Apert's syndrome; (*b*) same patient 2 years after simultaneous transcranial frontal advancement, Le Fort III maxillary advancement, mandibular advancement and genioplasty

(1989) illustrated each type and added a three-dimensional reconstruction.

It should be remembered that the spectrum of prevalence of the anomalies encompassed within the above classification varies from very uncommon to extremely rare. Selection has therefore been exercised, and only the 'commoner' conditions seen in a craniofacial unit have been included. Cleft lip and palate, along with the more common associated abnormalities, are covered in Chapter 19.

Frontonasal dysplasia

This condition, also known as *median cleft face* syn-drome, is an ill-defined syndrome. First described by Hoppe in 1859, it is a non-specific developmental alteration in which the defect occurs with a host of low-frequency anomalies (Goodman and Gorlin, 1983). Frontonasal dysplasia corresponds to clefts 0 and 14 in Tessier's classification. The main features are orbital hypertelorism, broad nasal root, lack of formation of the nasal tip, widow's peak hair anomaly and anterior cranium bifidum occultum. Sedano *et al.* (1970) published a comprehensive review of the condition and applied the term *frontonasal dysplasia*.

The basic defect is unknown. Embryologically, if the nasal capsule fails to develop, the primitive brain vesicle fills the space normally occupied by the

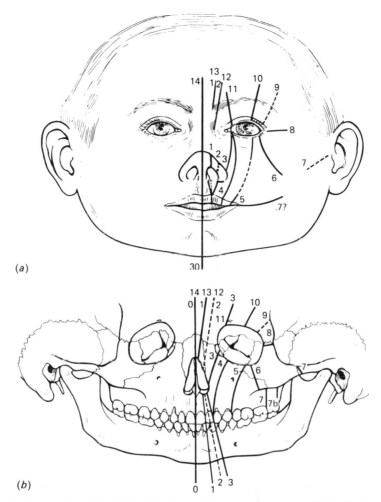

(a)

(b)

Figure 16.22 Tessier classification of craniofacial clefts. (*a*) Localization of soft-tissue clefts; (*b*) localization of skeletal (bony) clefts. Dotted lines represent either uncertain sites or uncertain clefts

capsule; this produces anterior cranium bifidum occultum, a morphokinetic arrest in the positioning of the eyes and lack of formation of the nasal tip. Most cases of this condition are sporadic.

Both autosomal inheritance and multifactorial transmission have been proposed, but the genetic mode of inheritance remains unclear. Fryburg, Persing and Lin (1993) and Kapusta, Brunner and Hamel (1992) presented series of patients with the condition consistent with an X-linked dominant inheritance. It is not known why twinning is commoner in families with frontonasal dysplasia than in the general population.

Clinical features

The facial malformation presents variable clinical combinations, and varies from mild (type A) to severe (type D). Orbital hypertelorism is a constant finding, and secondary telecanthus or narrowing of the palpe-

bral fissures occurs in severe cases (Figure 16.23). The anterior hairline may extend in a V shape onto the centre of the forehead (widow's peak).

Epibulbar dermoids are common, while anophthalmia, optic nerve hypoplasia, microphthalmia, upper eyelid colobomas and congenital cataracts occur rarely. Strabismus and anisometropia may lead to amblyopia.

Nasal deformities vary from colobomas of the nostrils to nasal flattening, with widely spaced nares and a broad nasal root (Figure 16.24).

Other findings include median cleft of the upper lip (cleft palate is rare), preauricular tags, low set ears, absent tragus and conductive deafness.

Mental deficiency is present in some cases, being more likely when the hypertelorism is severe or when extracephalic anomalies are present. Anterior cranium bifidum may be seen radiographically. A large anterior meningoencephalocoele, and rarely lipoma

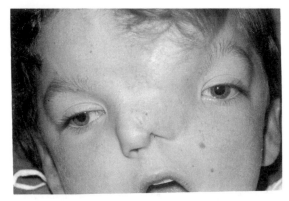

Figure 16.23 Frontonasal dysplasia. Gross orbital hypertelorism with secondary narrowing of the palpebral fissures and a widow's peak hair anomaly

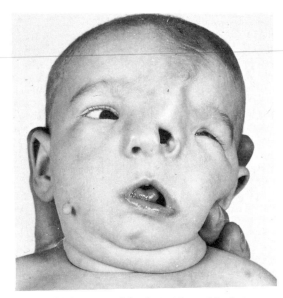

Figure 16.24 Frontonasal dysplasia. Many of the features of this condition are demonstrated; hypertelorism, broad nasal root with coloboma of the nostril, widow's peak hair anomaly, and a preauricular skin tag. This infant also has microphthalmia on the left side

or teratoma, is sometimes associated with frontonasal dysplasia. Craniosynostosis and brachycephaly have been reported, together with a variety of cerebral anomalies. Outside the craniofacial region occasional findings include preaxial polydactyly (with or without tibial hypoplasia – only seen in type D), syndactyly, clinodactyly, umbilical hernia and cryptorchidism.

Differential diagnosis

Orbital hypertelorism should be regarded as a non-specific malformation that may occur in a variety of different syndromes. Peterson *et al.* (1971) listed a variety of disorders in which orbital hypertelorism is

a feature. Bifid nose can occur with hypertelorism, several familial cases having been reported. When epibulbar dermoids, eyelid colobomas and preauricular tags are present, frontonasal dysplasia should be distinguished from craniofacial microsomia.

Treatment

Seventy per cent of the adult interorbital distance is reached by the age of 2 years in the normal person. It is thus generally assumed that surgical correction of hypertelorism should be delayed until after this age. In the majority of cases the optic canals are the normal distance apart. Occasionally they are wider apart, and this is usually associated with an increase in width of the cribriform plate. Before any surgery is contemplated, it is thus important that a precise assessment of the orbital anatomy is made. For a resumé of imaging techniques the reader should consult Marsh and Vannier (1985). The place of magnetic resonance imaging has not yet been fully determined.

For details of the surgical technique for the correction of orbital hypertelorism the reader is directed to a text on craniofacial surgery, e.g. Caronni (1985).

Median cleft lip with orbital hypotelorism

This rare syndrome is also known as *holoprosencephaly, arhinencephaly* and *median facial dysgenesis*. It results from impaired sagittal cleavage of the forebrain into cerebral hemispheres. There exists a whole spectrum of midline facebrain anomalies ranging from the extreme *cyclopia* (one central eye), through *cebocephaly* (orbital hypotelorism and a single blind-ended nostril nose) and *premaxillary agenesis* (hypotelorism, a flat boneless nose and a medial cleft lip) to the less severe forms of *midline facial dysmorphia*. In all forms the incidence is about one in 8000 births, and the frequency may be as high as one in 250 conceptuses from spontaneous abortion. The reader is referred to the extensive review of the subject by Cohen (1989).

Chromosomal anomalies are common in this group of disorders, and the majority of cases are sporadic. Some mild examples have exhibited mendelian inheritance. Gurrieri *et al.* (1993) and Hatziioannou *et al.* (1991) have shown that there is a locus on chromosome 7 which seems to be associated with the syndrome. The more severe forms do not survive long enough to reproduce.

Clinical features

It should be remembered that holoprosencephaly encompasses various gradations of facial dysmorphism, from cyclopia at one end of the spectrum to quite mild facial abnormalities, such as hypotelorism, at the other.

The characteristic features of the syndrome likely to be encountered by clinicians are:

1 Complete median cleft lip with absent premaxilla and prolabium
2 Flat nose with absent columella, septal cartilage and nasal bones
3 Orbital hypotelorism
4 Mongoloid slant of the eyes
5 Fusion of eyebrows in midline, and sparse frontal hair
6 Forebrain formed by a single large ventricle with little cerebral cortex
7 A cleft palate may be present.

Almost all these features are illustrated in Figure

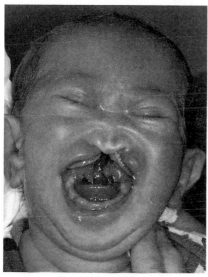

(a)

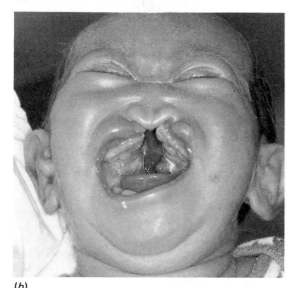

(b)

Figure 16.25 Median cleft lip with orbital hypotelorism. This baby exhibits virtually all the features of this syndrome

Treatment

Severe cases do not survive infancy, and many do not live past childhood. Most exhibit a moderate to severe degree of mental retardation. The degree of facial involvement usually, but not always, predicts the extent of brain malformation. It will thus be obvious that extensive treatment is unrealistic. Where appropriate, lip closure may be helpful.

Lateral and oblique facial clefts

Lateral facial cleft

This relatively rare cleft runs from the angle of the mouth towards the tragus of the ear, although its course is variable. The incidence is estimated to be between 1 : 50 000 and 1 : 175 000 live births. It results from failure of fusion of the maxillary and mandibular processes of the first branchial arch. It may be present as a shallow furrow throughout, or extend as a complete cleft into the oral cavity as far as the anterior border of the masseter muscle. There may be hypoplasia of the muscles of mastication, as well as of the maxilla, zygoma and auricle. Both Treacher Collins syndrome and craniofacial microsomia are forms of lateral facial clefting (Tessier no. 7); the macrostomia seen in the Goldenhar variant of craniofacial microsomia is an obvious manifestation of this cleft (Figure 16.26).

Some of the reported associated anomalies are syndactyly, absence of digits, micrognathia and bifid uvula.

Oblique facial cleft

Boo-Chai (1970), following Morian (1887), has subdivided these extremely rare clefts into:

1 *Naso-ocular cleft*, extending from the nostril to the lower eyelid border with possible extension to the temporal region (along the line of closure of the nasolacrimal groove) (40%)
2 *Oro-ocular cleft*, extending from eye to lip. There may be a further subdivision into medial and lateral types, depending on the relationship to the infraorbital foramen (60%).

Gorlin, Cohen and Levin (1990) believed that many of these clefts can be explained as the result of damage to the ectomesenchyme of the developing face caused by amniotic bands. About 25% of these rare clefts are bilateral, an example being illustrated in Figure 16.27.

Hernia, talipes, hydrocephalus, encephalocoele, genitourinary abnormalities and spinal abnormalities have been described in association with oblique facial clefts.

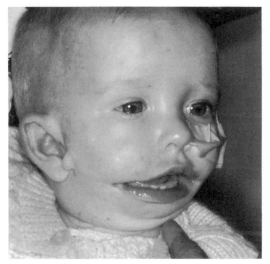

(a)

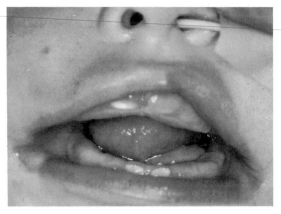

(b)

Figure 16.26 Macrostomia in craniofacial microsomia, an example of cleft no. 7 in the Tessier classification

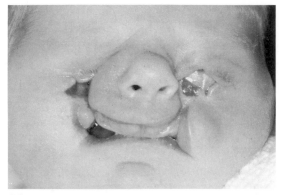

(a)

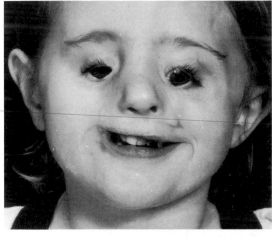

(b)

Figure 16.27 Bilateral oblique facial clefts. These oro-ocular clefts represent the medial variety above (Tessier no. 4) and the lateral variety below (Tessier no. 5). Such clefts present extremely difficult reconstructive problems. (Courtesy of Mr Eric Gustavson, FRCS)

Treatment

Treatment usually consists of one or more Z-plasties to bring tissue into the cleft. Eyelid colobomas are treated in the usual way by excision of the edges and closure of the defect.

Amniotic band disruption complex

The amniotic band disruption complex occurs in various forms. The most common involves the limbs only, but the complex embraces a spectrum ranging from a ring constriction of the finger to major craniofacial and visceral defects. The most severe combination of anomalies in this disorder includes limb and craniofacial abnormalities acronymically termed the

ADAM (amniotic deformity, adhesions, mutilations) complex. The incidence is estimated between one in 5000 and one in 10 000 for all forms of the complex, and craniofacial examples are obviously much rarer. There is no evidence that a genetic factor is involved.

The most common hypothesis concerning the complex is that the fetal deformities result from primary amnion rupture without chorionic sac damage at various stages of gestation. The placenta and membranes are often abnormal. Fibrous strands attached to the amnion or chorion have been observed, and rarely, a band is attached to the infant (Figure 16.28). The earlier the amniotic rupture, the more severe the anomalies.

Facial anomalies include cleft lip (usually bilateral), bizarre midfacial clefts (Figure 16.29), hydrocephalus, microcephalus, multiple anterior encephalocoeles and meningocoeles. It is postulated that an amniotic

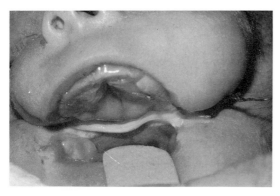

Figure 16.28 Amniotic band disruption complex. Amniotic band producing a most unusual cleft transversely across the palate

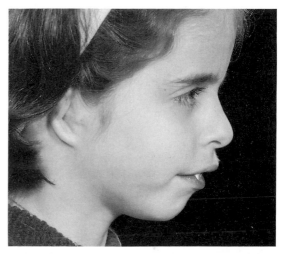

(a)

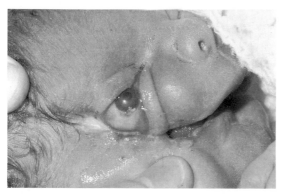

Figure 16.29 Amniotic band complex. Another view of the patient shown in Figure 16.28. The facial part of the cleft appears to mimic a Tessier no. 5 oblique facial cleft

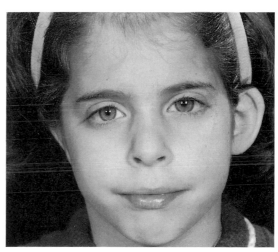

(b)

Figure 16.30 Craniofacial microsomia. Very mild example, with minimal facial asymmetry, but with deformity of the right auricle

strand is swallowed, becomes attached to the pharynx and slices the ectomesenchyme of the facial processes. Ocular findings include distorted or colobomatous palpebral fissures, microphthalmia, anophthalmia and corneal opacity. There may be complex nasal malformations, and major visceral anomalies comprise omphalocoele and gastroschisis (Gorlin, Cohen and Levin, 1990).

Treatment

The prognosis depends on the severity of the deformities. Many of those with the ADAM complex die, and mental retardation is common with central nervous system involvement. Due to the wide variety of clinical features, treatment plans have to be applied on an individual basis.

Craniofacial microsomia (Figures 16.30–16.34)

This condition is also known as hemifacial microsomia, first arch syndrome, first and second branchial arch syndrome, otomandibular dysostosis, oculo-auriculovertebral dysplasia, Goldenhar syndrome and lateral facial dysplasia. Most of these terms convey the erroneous impression that involvement is limited to facial structures, whereas cardiac, renal and skeletal anomalies may occur in addition. The condition was first reported by Arlt in 1881. Gorlin *et al.* (1963) used the term hemifacial microsomia to refer to patients with unilateral microtia, macrostomia and failure of formation of the mandibular ramus and condyle. They suggested that oculoauriculovertebral dysplasia (Goldenhar syndrome) was a variant, characterized by vertebral anomalies and epibulbar dermoids. From a craniofacial viewpoint, the most recent appellation of craniofacial microsomia proposed by Converse *et al.* (1977) has the merit of

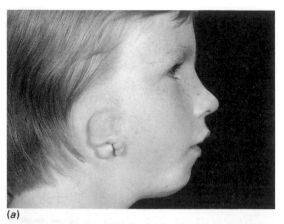
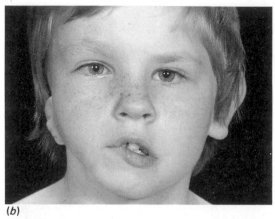

Figure 16.31 Craniofacial microsomia. Obvious facial asymmetry, with right auricular deformity

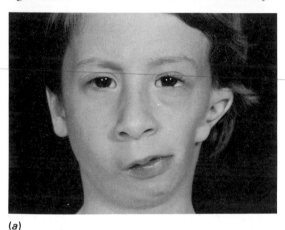
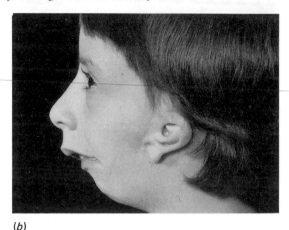

Figure 16.32 Craniofacial microsomia. Fairly severe example, with marked facial asymmetry due to mandibular, maxillary and zygomatic hypoplasia. Although abnormal, the left auricle is far less affected than the less severe cases shown in Figures 16.31 and 16.32

avoiding the implication that the condition is unilateral (it is frequently bilateral), and it emphasizes that the cranium may be involved.

The disorder may vary from mild to severe and several classification systems have been devised to aid in diagnosis, treatment planning and for predicting the outcome of treatment. David, Mahatumarat and Cooter (1987) proposed the SAT (combining *s*keletal, *a*uricular and soft *t*issue categories) and in 1991 Vento Labrie and Mulliken introduced the OMENS classification (*o*rbit, *m*andible, *e*ar, *n*erve and *s*oft tissue categories). The latter classification is quite sensitive to the wide phenotypic heterogenicity found in hemifacial microsomia.

Although craniofacial microsomia is usually sporadic, familial cases are known with a variety of transmission patterns. The incidence is reported as between 1:5000 and 1:5600 live births (Gorlin, Cohen and Levin, 1990) with a 1:1 sex ratio. In about 70% of cases the anomaly is unilateral. When

it is bilateral it is always asymmetrical, a notable difference from Treacher Collins syndrome.

Poswillo (1973, 1974), using an animal model, demonstrated that destruction of differentiating tissues in the region of the developing ear and jaws by a teratogenically induced, expanding haematoma produced a branchial arch dysplasia. The severity of the dysplasia was related to the degree of local destruction. This is supported by the clinical findings of Robinson *et al.* (1987). Thus craniofacial microsomia should probably be regarded as a non-specific symptom complex, the pathogenesis of which has several different aetiologies. When cardiac, renal or skeletal anomalies coexist, there appears to be an increased chance of genetic involvement.

Clinical features

Not uncommonly the infants are small-for-dates, and there may be feeding difficulties which, on occasions,

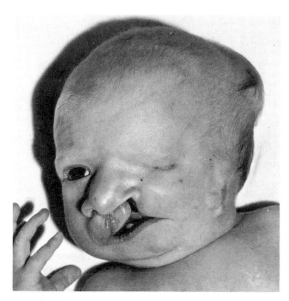

Figure 16.33 Craniofacial microsomia. Severe case of this syndrome, accompanied by a cleft of the lip and palate on the ipsilateral side. The microphthalmia resulted in enucleation of the affected eye

can necessitate tube feeding. In rare cases, nocturnal sleep apnoea may be severe enough to require tracheostomy (see Figure 16.38).

Facies

The facies may be striking because of the asymmetry. This may be partly due to hypoplasia and or displacement of the pinna, but the degree of involvement varies markedly. The maxilla, zygoma and temporal bones on the affected side are reduced and flattened (Figure 16.35). Frontal bossing is common and the ipsilateral eye may be set lower than its neighbour. The chin point is frequently deviated to the affected side due to mandibular hypoplasia, and the asymmetry can be further enhanced by hypoplasia of the parotid gland. Macrostomia, when it occurs, is usually mild (see Figure 16.26). Some 30% of patients with craniofacial microsomia have bilateral involvement, but the disorder is always more severe on one side (see Figure 16.36e).

Oral findings

Patients may exhibit all degrees of hypoplasia of the mandible, from a minimal decrease in size to complete agenesis of the ascending ramus and portion of the body on the affected side (Figure 16.36). When the condyle is absent, there is concomitant absence of the glenoid fossa. The gonial angle is often flattened, and this is a reflection of the decreased activity of the masticatory muscles. Moss and James (1984) have

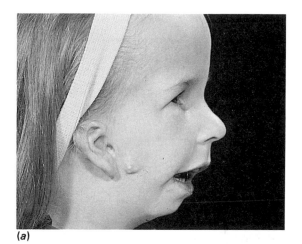

(a)

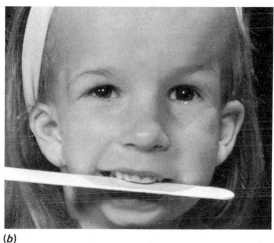

(b)

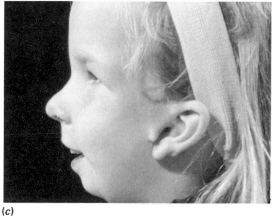

(c)

Figure 16.34 Craniofacial microsomia. Bilateral involvement; although there is reasonable symmetry with an absence of cant of the occlusal plane, the external ears are affected to varying degrees. The normal obliquity of the palpebral fissures and lack of zygomatic hypoplasia excludes a diagnosis of Treacher Collins syndrome

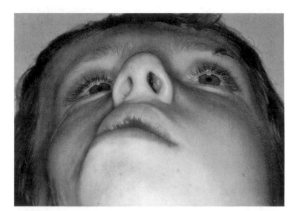

Figure 16.35 Craniofacial microsomia. This view of the face reveals hypoplasia of the mandible, maxilla, zygoma and temporal bones

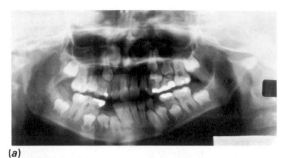

(a)

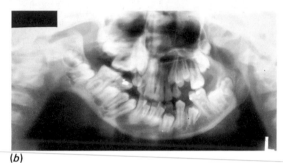

(b)

shown that there is a significant correlation between muscle activity and the morphology of the ascending ramus. The dental occlusal plane is frequently canted (Figure 16.37), and the degree of cant is a direct reflection of the severity of the mandibular and maxillary hypoplasia. Moss and James also found that the angle of the occlusal plane was negatively correlated with muscle activity and that, in unilateral cases, the deficiency of growth on the affected side was compensated by overgrowth of the other side. In bilateral cases, the occlusal plane is usually normal or only mildly canted, but in such cases the chin is often severely retruded (see Figure 16.34). In infants, when severe micrognathia is present, there is a risk of obstructive sleep apnoea (Figure 16.38). This risk is enhanced when the pharynx is hypoplastic. As well as hypoplasia and/or paresis of the palatal muscles, the tongue may be similarly affected, resulting in some degree of collapse of the dental arches. The incidence of cleft lip and palate is usually quoted as less than 10%, but at the Hospital for Sick Children, Great Ormond Street, London the incidence is 18% in a group of some 60 patients. Velopharyngeal insufficiency is seen in around 35% of cases.

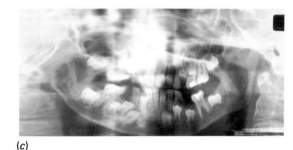

(c)

Figure 16.36 Craniofacial microsomia. Orthopantograms demonstrating varying degrees of mandibular involvement. (a) Mild left-sided mandibular hypoplasia; the lack of a well-defined angle reflects reduced activity of the medial pterygoid and masseter muscles; (b) mild right-sided hypoplasia; the pronounced antegonial notch indicates good pterygomasseteric activity, and hence a good prognosis for successful bony reconstruction; (c) more severe right-sided mandibular hypoplasia with a trivial ascending ramus and right temporomandibular joint; (d) complete agenesis of the left ascending ramus; this is the radiograph of the patient shown in Figure 16.45; (e) bilateral case with coincident right unilateral complete cleft of lip and palate; the right ascending ramus is absent, and the left condyle is hypoplastic

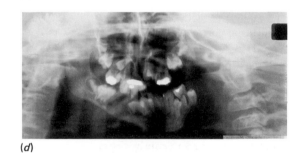

(d)

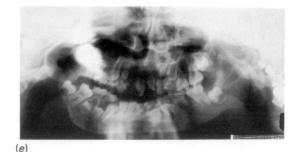

(e)

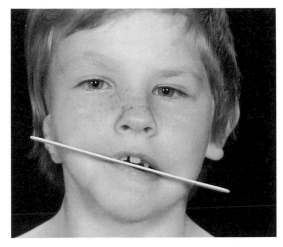

Figure 16.37 Craniofacial microsomia. A wooden spatula placed between the teeth reveals a marked cant of the occlusion. This is a reflection of the degree of mandibular and maxillary hypoplasia

Neuromuscular system

Hypoplasia of the masticatory muscles is present in all but the mildest cases, the masseter, temporalis and medial pterygoid being the most frequently involved, though to a variable degree.

A wide range of central nervous system defects may be associated with the condition. Encephalocoele is more common in the occipital region but may be seen anteriorly in hemifacial microsomia. When this occurs with ear tags and epibulbar dermoids it may give rise to a misdiagnosis as a frontonasal malformation. Facial weakness, usually affecting the lower face (Figure 16.39), occurs in 10% of patients; palatal and tongue musculature are less commonly affected. The incidence of mental retardation is reported as 10%, and occasional cases of occipital encephalocoele are recorded.

Ear

Malformations of the external ear may vary from complete aplasia to a crumpled, distorted pinna displaced anteriorly and inferiorly. Supernumerary ear tags can be found anywhere from the tragus to the angle of the mouth; ear tags may be bilateral, especially when epibulbar dermoids are present. Conductive hearing loss due to middle ear abnormalities and/or absence or deficiency of the external auditory meatus is found in some 40% of patients.

Eye

The palpebral fissure is often somewhat lowered on the affected side. Epibulbar dermoid and/or lipodermoid is a variable finding. It is milky-white to yellow

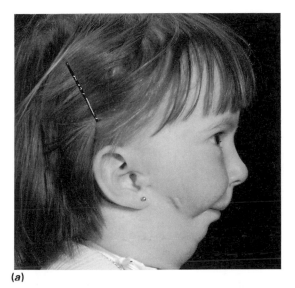

(*a*)

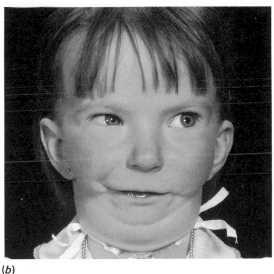

(*b*)

Figure 16.38 Craniofacial microsomia. This little girl with bilateral involvement has severe mandibular hypoplasia; this resulted in nocturnal sleep apnoea, severe enough to warrant a tracheostomy

in colour, flattened, ellipsoidal and usually solid rather than cystic. The dermoid is frequently located at the limbus or corneal margin in the *lower* and outer quadrant (Figure 16.40); by contrast, the lipodermoid is usually located in the *upper* and outer quadrant. In some patients both lesions are seen in the same eye. Unilateral coloboma of the upper lid is common in patients with epibulbar dermoids (it will be remembered that in Treacher Collins syndrome colobomas occur in the *lower* lid). Choroidal or iridial coloboma and congenital cystic eye can occur in this

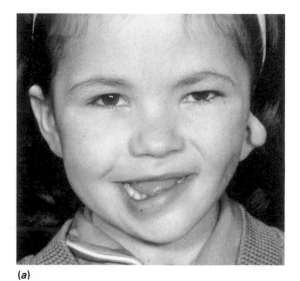

(a)

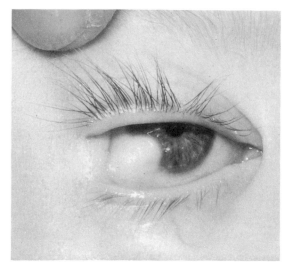

Figure 16.40 Craniofacial microsomia. Epibulbar dermoid affecting the lower and outer quadrant of the right eye

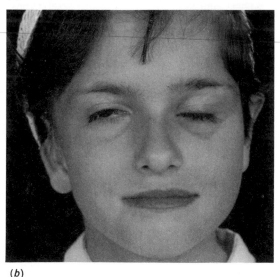

(b)

Figure 16.39 Craniofacial microsomia. (a) When facial weakness occurs in this syndrome, it more frequently affects the lower face as in this child with left-sided involvement; (b) upper facial weakness is occasionally a feature; this girl has trivial involvement of the hard and soft tissues of the face, but nevertheless has a right-sided weakness of the upper branches of the facial nerve

disorder. Microphthalmia (see Figure 16.33) and anophthalmia are associated with severely affected individuals in whom mental retardation is more common.

Skeletal anomalies

Vertebral anomalies are found in about half the patients, and include occipitalization of the atlas, cuneiform vertebrae, complete or partial synostosis of two or more vertebrae, supernumerary vertebrae, hemivertebrae and spina bifida. Anomalous ribs, talipes equinovarus, radial limb anomalies (e.g. hypoplasia of the radius and/or thumb) and other skeletal defects have been reported.

Other anomalies

Some 50% of affected patients have various forms of congenital heart disease (Gorlin, Pindborg and Cohen, 1976). This can be severe enough to preclude corrective facial surgery. Pulmonary agenesis or hypoplasia has been noted, usually on the affected side. A variety of renal abnormalities can be associated with the condition, including absent or ectopic kidney, double ureter and anomalous blood supply. Imperforate anus has been reported.

Differential diagnosis

This disorder should be distinguished from Pierre Robin anomaly and Moebius syndrome. Bilateral cases of craniofacial microsomia are frequently confused with Treacher Collins syndrome. Such confusion may be avoided if it is remembered that the former condition is asymmetrical, while the latter is symmetrical. Colobomas occur in the upper eyelid in craniofacial microsomia and the lower lid in Treacher Collins syndrome. Epibulbar dermoids may also be observed in frontonasal dysplasia.

Treatment

Three main problems have to be faced when considering surgical correction of craniofacial microsomia:

1 No general agreement exists regarding the best time to carry out reconstructive surgery. At one extreme are those who maintain that all treatment for these patients should be deferred until growth is complete, the argument being that the shortage of investing soft tissues will inevitably cause relapse during the growing stages. Others maintain that enlargement of the deficient mandibular ramus during growth (usually by serial bone grafting) will help stimulate any growth potential that may be present in the soft tissue

2 The hypoplasia seen in craniofacial microsomia affects all tissues, both hard and soft. Thus any bony reconstruction has to be planned within the constraints of limited soft tissue (functional) matrix

3 Facial asymmetries in general are more difficult to correct than horizontal or vertical disproportions. The fact that the hypoplasia of craniofacial microsomia affects all tissues presents one of the most difficult problems facing the maxillofacial surgeon.

The following observations reflect the authors' view about the management of this difficult problem.

1 In moderate to severe unilateral cases, complete symmetry can never be achieved

2 Early surgery is indicated in those patients who demonstrate activity in the masticatory muscles. Ideally, electromyography should be carried out. If this investigation is not available, the presence of certain indicators favours early surgery. These indicators are the presence of a condyle (however rudimentary), a reasonably sized coronoid process, a masseteric process at the angle of the mandible and a degree of antegonial notching, however slight (Towers, 1976). Very early surgery to the midface is better delayed due to the danger of damage to the developing tooth buds filling the maxilla, and the lack of patient cooperation for postoperative orthodontics. Mandibular surgery, however, can be performed at any time, but is better delayed until cooperation for functional orthodontic treatment is possible. If possible, the start of a 'growth spurt' is a useful time for surgical intervention

3 In unilateral cases of craniofacial microsomia the unaffected side is not 'normal'. It undergoes hyperplasia in order to compensate for underdevelopment of the affected side (Moss and James, 1984). In reconstruction it is important not to try to make the involved side the same length as the 'normal' side; some reduction in height of the longer side is advisable

4 The constraints of the restrictive soft tissue envelope may be managed by redistributing the bones within it, and not trying to introduce too much increase in bony volume. The reduction in lower face height referred to above will assist this process.

If the above is not possible, it will be mandatory to introduce soft tissue into the area

5 The bulk of a bone graft, whether it is vascularized or not, will only survive if subjected to the stimulus of muscle activity. Thus the quality of the masticatory muscles on the affected side is an important index of the prognosis for bone graft survival. When onlay bone grafts are used, cranial bone survives better than either rib or iliac crest – the two usual sources of bone for reconstruction (Zins and Whitaker, 1983)

6 The concept of the transfer of vascularized composite flaps containing both bone and soft tissue has received much attention recently. Vascularization of a bone graft in the absence of muscle activity will not ensure its survival. Similarly, muscles will atrophy and become fibrotic when they lack a nerve supply. The definitive assessment of these flaps is awaited with interest, but the optimism of some enthusiasts appears to ignore proven physiological concepts. Despite the above reservations, the microvascular transfer of soft tissue appears to offer definite advantages over other techniques when surface cover or soft-tissue bulk is required

7 In the past much time and effort was devoted to ear reconstruction. In the authors' experience the results were usually disappointing and sometimes frankly mutilating (Figure 16.41). When the time came for correction of the major part of the deformity, both parents and child were sometimes disillusioned and resentful. With the introduction of osseointegrated implants by Branemark in the 1960s a realistic alternative to surgery was provided (Branemark *et al.*, 1989). Fixtures and abutments were developed to support artificial ears constructed by a maxillofacial technician (Tjellstrom, 1990). The excellent results that can be obtained have made surgery virtually obsolete (Figure 16.42). In hemifacial microsomia great care is needed in placement of the fixtures as the quality and quantity of the temporal bone is often suboptimal.

For details of the surgical techniques currently employed in the treatment of craniofacial microsomia, the reader is referred to texts by Caronni (1985) and Henderson (1985). The results of such surgery are shown in Figures 16.43–16.46. Details of the techniques for prosthetic ear replacement can be found in Worthington and Branemark (1992).

Treacher Collins syndrome

Synonyms for this condition include *mandibulofacial dysostosis*, *Berry syndrome*, *Franceschetti-Zwahlen-Klein syndrome* and *bilateral facial agenesis*. Although the syndrome was probably first described by Thomson in 1846 (Gorlin, Pindborg and Cohen, 1976), credit for its discovery is usually given to Berry or, more commonly, to Treacher Collins, who described the

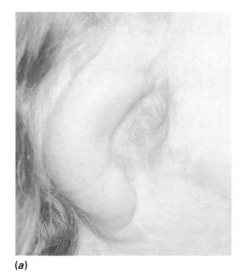

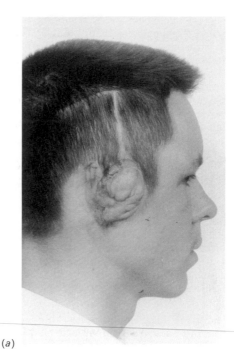

(a)

(a)

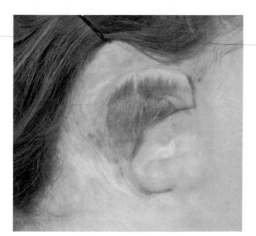

(b)

Figure 16.41 Craniofacial microsomia. Two examples of ear reconstruction which hardly justify the inconvenience and discomfort to the patient and the use of expensive resources

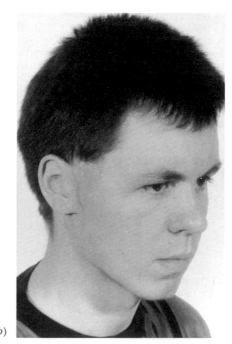

(b)

Figure 16.42 (a) Ear after multiple failed surgical procedures attempting to correct cosmetic deformity. (b) After excision of deformed auricle and fitting of prosthesis. (Courtesy of Mr. D. W. Proops)

essential features of the syndrome in 1900. Frances-chetti and Klein (1949) coined the term *mandibulo-facial dysostosis*.

The syndrome is inherited as an autosomal dominant trait with high penetrance and marked variability in expressivity. More than half the cases arise as fresh mutations, but before being so assigned, careful examination of family members should be performed, looking for minimal signs of the syndrome. Recent studies have shown the responsible gene to be located on the long arm of chromosome 5 (Dixon *et al.*, 1991). The abnormal gene may have a lethal effect, since miscarriage or early postnatal death is common. Poswillo (1975) used an experimental animal model to formulate an explanation for the causal mecha-

nism of Treacher Collins syndrome. He found that there was early destruction of the neural crest cells of the facial and auditory primordia which migrate to

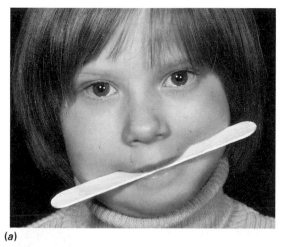

(a)

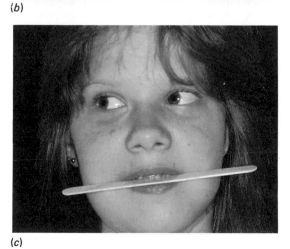

(b)

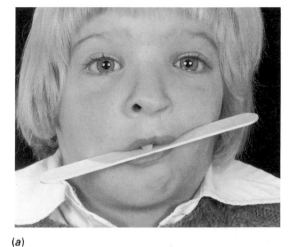

(a)

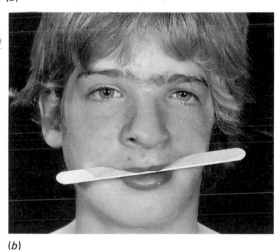

(b)

Figure 16.44 Craniofacial microsomia. (*a*) A more severe case, complicated by a complete left unilateral cleft of lip and palate. This 13-year-old boy underwent a two-stage reconstruction; a left malar osteotomy and temporal fossa reconstruction was followed by maxillary and mandibular osteotomies (*b*). Further surgery, including a rhinoplasty and soft-tissue augmentation will be necessary

(c)

Figure 16.43 Craniofacial microsomia. Two-stage correction of a moderately affected patient. (*a*) Prior to surgery; (*b*) appearance 4 years after mandibular osteotomy and bone grafting at 11 years of age; (*c*) patient aged 15 years following maxillary and mandibular osteotomies

the first and second branchial arches. This destruction, before migration is well under way, leads to the formation of a 'vacuum' in the area of the otic cup into which the surrounding tissues flow. The developing otic pit thus moves upwards into the first arch region and relocates over the angle of the mandible. Additionally, there is a symmetrical, overall hypoplasia of many of the derivatives of the first and second branchial arch mesenchyme.

Clinical features

Facies

The facial appearance is characteristic (Figure 16.47). The obliquely slanting palpebral fissures, depressed

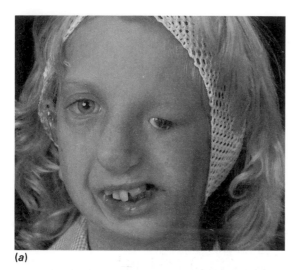
(a)

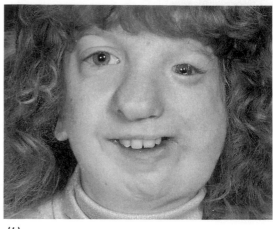
(b)

Figure 16.45 Craniofacial microsomia. (*a*) Patient very severely affected with gross soft-tissue and bony hypoplasia of the left side of the face, including microphthalmia; (*b*) multistaged reconstruction including a microvascular osteocutaneous groin flap has produced only a modest result in this girl at 19 years of age

cheekbones, deformed pinnas, receding chin and large, fish-like mouth present an unforgettable picture. The levator muscles of the mouth are absent, giving rise to the characteristic appearance. One-quarter of affected patients have a tongue-shaped process of hair that extends towards the cheek (Figure 16.48). The body of the malar bones may be totally absent, but more often is grossly and symmetrically underdeveloped, with discontinuity of the zygomatic arches (Figure 16.49). The paranasal air sinuses are usually small, and may be absent. The lower orbital rim is sometimes defective, giving support to Tessier's assertion that Treacher Collins syndrome is a clefting syndrome. The nasofrontal angle is usually obliterated, with a high nasal bridgeline. The nose appears large due to the lack of malar development, while the nares may be narrow and the alar cartilages hypoplastic.

Oral manifestations

The mandible is almost always hypoplastic, with the deficiency mainly in the ascending ramus; the gonial angle is high, and antegonial notching is seen. There is a downward curve in the body of the mandible and, together with the short ramus this results in gross retrusion of the chin (Figure 16.50). The articular eminence is rudimentary or absent. There is usually a high-arched palate, 30% of which are cleft. Macrostomia, seen in 15% of cases, may be unilateral or bilateral. Dental malocclusion is common, the teeth may be widely separated, hypoplastic, displaced or associated with an anterior open bite.

Eyes

There is an antimongoloid obliquity of the palpebral fissures, and a coloboma is present in the outer third of the lower lid in 75% of patients, half of whom also have a deficiency of eyelashes medial to the coloboma. Iridial coloboma may also occur. The lower lacrimal points, Meibomian glands and intermarginal strip may be absent. Microphthalmia has been reported.

Ears

Extra ear tags and blind pits may be found anywhere between the tragus and angle of the mouth. The external ear is frequently deformed, crumpled forward or misplaced toward the angle of the mandible. Some patients exhibit an absence or stenosis of the external auditory canal. Conductive deafness is common due to middle ear abnormalities. In many patients the middle ear cavity is bilaterally hypoplastic and dysmorphic, in severe cases there may be complete absence of the middle ear and epitympanic space. Anomalies of the ossicles include a fixed malleus, fusion of malformed malleus and incus, monopodal stapes, absence of stapes and oval window. The inner ear structures are normal.

Other anomalies

Those other abnormalities reported include absence of the parotid gland, congenital heart disease, malformed cervical vertebrae, defects of the extremities, cryptorchidism and renal abnormalities. Mental retardation does occur.

Differential diagnosis

The most important distinction is from bilateral craniofacial microsomia. Treacher Collins syndrome is usually a symmetrical facial deformity, although very occasionally a tendency towards asymmetry is

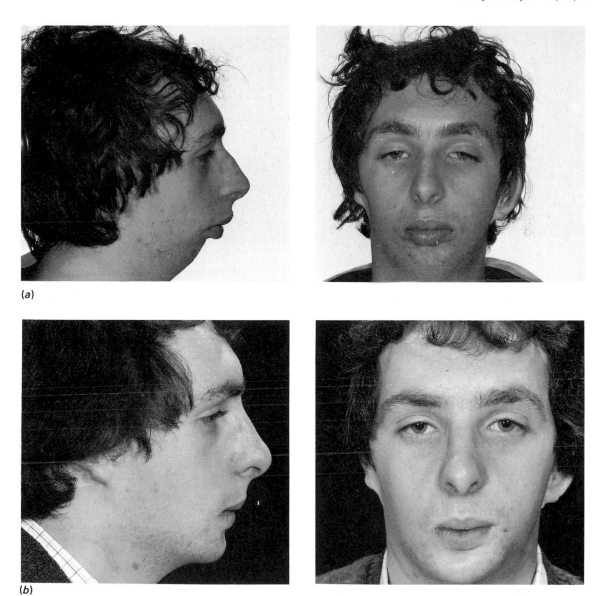

(a)

(b)

Figure 16.46 Craniofacial microsmia. (*a*) This patient with bilateral involvement exhibits very little asymmetry but gross micrognathia; (*b*) the appearance at the age of 18 years following a two-staged correction involving bilateral mandibular osteotomies with bone-grafting followed by genioplasty and rhinoplasty

seen. Craniofacial microsomia, however, is never symmetrical. Other isolated and rare syndromes may exhibit some of the facial features seen in Treacher Collins syndrome, and the 'commonest' of these is acrofacial dysostosis (Nager syndrome).

Treatment

Poswillo (1974) argued persuasively that the early reconstruction of the hypoplastic facial skeleton in Treacher Collins syndrome will permit expansion of the modified functional matrix. While the skeletal structures of the mid and lower face are morphologically deficient, their design is such that in the presence of a system of masticatory muscles there exists a reasonable functional matrix capable of growth and development after surgical reconstruction. Occasionally very early surgery is mandatory when obstructive sleep apnoea is precipitated by the severe micrognathia (Figure 16.51).

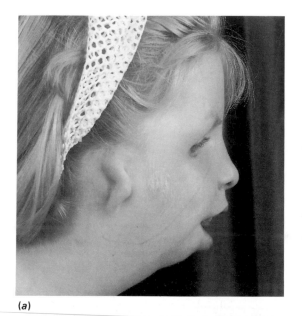

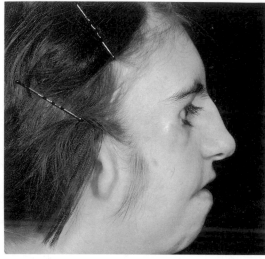

Figure 16.48 Treacher Collins syndrome. Tongue-shaped process of hair present in one-quarter of affected individuals

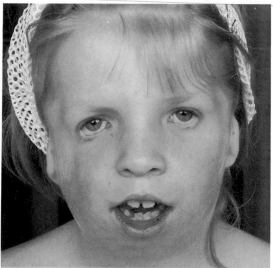

(b)

Figure 16.47 Treacher Collins syndrome. Characteristic facies of an 8-year-old patient with the condition

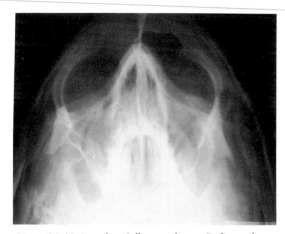

Figure 16.49 Treacher Collins syndrome. Radiograph demonstrating hypoplasia of the malar bones with absence of both zygomatic arches

Surgery is directed at three main areas:

1 The eyes, with antimongoloid slant of the palpebral fissures and lower lid colobomas
2 The malar hypoplasia
3 The mandibular hypoplasia with the marked retrognathia and anterior open bite.

For details of the techniques involved, readers should consult an appropriate craniofacial text such as that by Caronni (1985).

Miscellaneous conditions

Dysplasias of bone

The most interesting and extensive of these conditions are *fibrous dysplasia* and *cherubism*.

Fibrous dysplasia

Fibrous dysplasia of bone may affect the bones of the cranium and face in three ways:

1 As a monostotic lesion
2 As one or more of the lesions of polyostotic disease

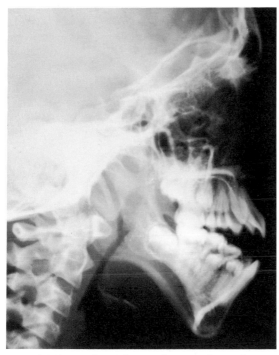

Figure 16.50 Treacher Collins syndrome. Radiograph showing the short ascending ramus of the mandible resulting in marked retrusion of the chin and anterior open bite

3 As one or more of the lesions of *Albright's syndrome*, in which the polyostotic lesions are accompanied by manifestations such as cutaneous pigmentation, endocrine disorders with precocious puberty and premature skull maturation.

The nature and aetiology of fibrous dysplasia are unknown, but the consensus of opinion at present regards it as a developmental defect. There is no evidence to suggest that the lesions are neoplastic, and they tend to become inactive or stabilized after the normal period of skeletal growth has come to an end. Fibrous dysplasia is not inherited, but there is a definite sex predilection, two to three times as many females being affected.

Distribution of lesions

In monostotic cases, practically any bone may be involved, but limb bones, ribs, jaws and cranial bones are those most frequently affected. The skull and facial bones are involved in 10–25% of cases. In polyostotic fibrous dysplasia the skull is involved in about half the cases in which there is a moderate degree of skeletal involvement, while in severe cases the skull is constantly involved. While almost any combination of lesions may occur, there is a well

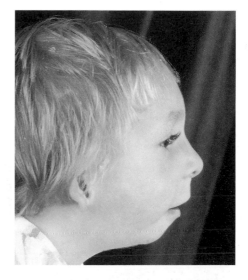

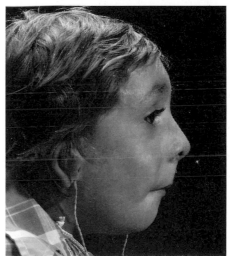

Figure 16.51 Treacher Collins syndrome. This 4-year-old boy experienced obstructive sleep apnoea which was relieved by mandibular advancement and bone-grafting

marked tendency for the lesions to occur segmentally, with localization in one limb or on one side of the body. When the jaws are involved, the lesion is usually solitary, occurring more often in the maxilla than the mandible. Multiple jaw lesions are less frequent, but when they occur may be accompanied by lesions in the facial and cranial bones (Figure 16.52).

Clinical features

Patients with polyostotic disease that is at all extensive practically always present as children, usually with deformity or pathological fracture (Figure 16.53). When solitary or relatively few lesions exist,

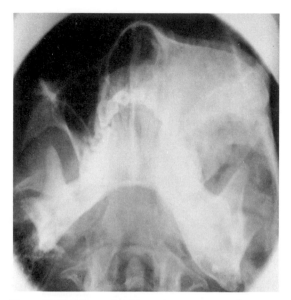
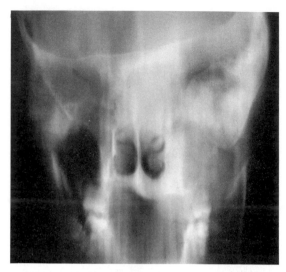

Figure 16.52 Fibrous dysplasia. Two radiographs of a patient showing extensive involvement of both facial bones and skull

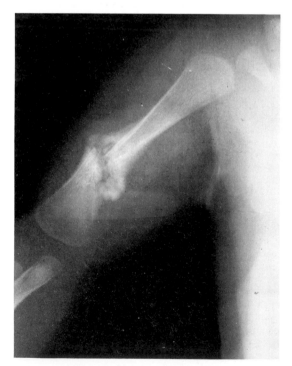

Figure 16.53 Fibrous dysplasia. Radiograph of a child with polyostotic disease demonstrating a pathological fracture of the humerus

presentation is usually in childhood or adolescence, but occasionally this is delayed until adult life. Jaw lesions occur as bony hard, non-tender swellings that expand the jaw, producing a gradually increasing facial asymmetry that may be first noticed by the parents. Often the deformity is slight, even when the lesion has ceased to be active. However, in some cases growth is more rapid and extensive, and in a comparatively short time there may develop a large mandibular swelling or a maxillary lesion that causes marked swelling of the cheek, exophthalmos or nasal obstruction. Such a case is shown in Figure 16.56. It is probable that many of the cases previously termed *leontiasis ossea* were examples of fibrous dysplasia.

Fibrous dysplasia is normally a slowly progressive and benign disease that develops over several years. It can also present as a rapidly growing 'aggressive' form, mimicking a malignancy.

Although rare, malignancies in fibrous dysplasia do occur. Ruggieri *et al.* (1994) found 28 cases of sarcoma in 1122 cases of fibrous dysplasia in a review of cases from the Mayo clinic. Thirteen of the sarcomas occurred in the craniofacial bones. The prognosis was poor.

Radiology

Radiographic appearances in the jaws (Figure 16.54) are generally similar to those seen in other bones. Both radiolucent and ground glass appearances are seen. On intraoral films a characteristic orange peel picture is seen in those areas that appear as a ground glass appearance in extraoral films. Diffuse lesions in the maxilla and facial bones may extend up to, and distort, the suture lines, but do not cross them. Skull radiographs in jaw cases frequently show that there is an increased density at the base of the skull (Figure 16.55).

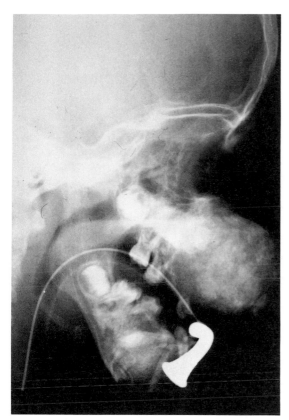

Figure 16.54 Fibrous dysplasia. Extraoral radiograph revealing a gross lesion in the maxilla and a smaller lesion in the mandible; both radiolucent and radiodense areas are seen

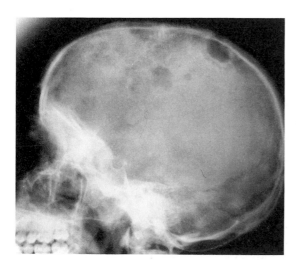

Figure 16.55 Fibrous dysplasia. Lateral skull radiograph of a young adult patient showing radiolucent lesions in the skull vault and increased density of the base of the skull

Computed tomography (CT scanning) will demonstrate the classic heterogeneous 'ground glass' appearance with calcifications. Sometimes areas of low enhancement and cystic areas can be seen. This can help to differentiate the lesion from a malignancy.

Magnetic resonance imaging (MRI) of fibrous dysplasia lesions are usually characterized by a decreased signal on T1- and T2-weighted images. The borders are usually well demarcated. Lesions enhance with gadolinium, but the degree of enhancement is variable. High clinical and pathological activity correlates with high signal intensity on both spin-echo sequences.

Pathology

The lesions are yellowish or greyish-white, and impart a gritty sensation to the knife when cut. Microscopically they consist of fibrous tissue that replaces normal bone and gives rise to osseous trabeculae. The proportion of fibrous to bony tissue varies from case to case and in different areas of the same lesion. It has been suggested that the proportion of fibrous tissue diminishes with the increasing age of a lesion, while calcification increases. This is no more than a trend, and is not necessarily a regular occurrence.

Differential diagnosis

This condition is sometimes confused with cherubism, but a careful family history and clinical examination of the jaws augmented by radiographic examination should clarify the situation. Fibrous dysplasia occurs in a totally different age group from Paget's disease, and the serum chemistry is within normal limits. Examination of biopsy material by an experienced oral pathologist should clinch the diagnosis.

Treatment

In the craniofacial region treatment is usually instituted for cosmetic reasons rather than for functional disability. Whenever possible, treatment should be deferred until after puberty when the progressive enlargement of the affected areas usually ceases. In some cases, due to the rapid progress of disease, it is necessary to intervene before maturation of the lesions (Figure 16.56). In this situation it may be necessary to repeat the surgery, sometimes several times, and at varying intervals.

Contouring of the affected areas is the treatment of choice. The consistency of lesions varies widely, some being amenable to paring with a scalpel, while others are hard enough to require shaping with osteotomes or mechanical instruments. Resection is both mutilating and unnecessary. On rare occasions, orbital and frontal bone involvement may necessitate a transcranial surgical approach (Figure 16.57).

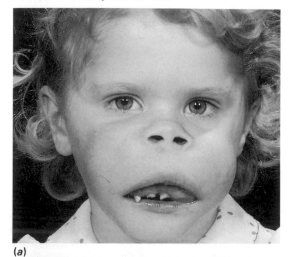

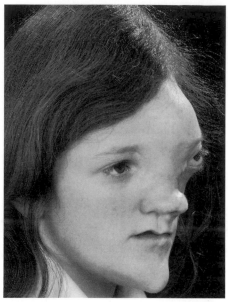

Figure 16.57 Fibrous dysplasia. Gross craniofacial involvement in an 11-year-old girl which will require a transcranial surgical approach for correction

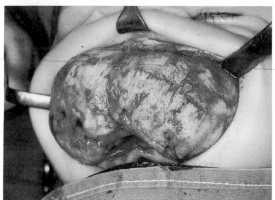

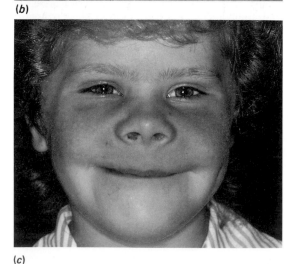

Figure 16.56 Fibrous dysplasia. (*a*) A 3-year-old girl with polyostotic disease, including gross involvement of the maxilla; (*b*) intraoperative photograph revealing the gross appearance of the affected bone; (*c*) early postoperative appearance. Further enlargement of the maxilla may be anticipated as facial growth proceeds

Cherubism

This condition was first described by Jones in 1933 as familial multilocular cystic disease of the jaws, but the term *cherubism*, coined by the same author, has gained wider acceptance. Lucas (1984) provided a good review of the condition. The familial incidence of cherubism is one of its characteristic features, probably being inherited as a dominant trait with variable expressivity. Males are affected twice as frequently as females. Children with cherubism appear normal at birth, but swellings appear in the jaws between 1 and 4 years of age; the mandible is always affected, and very often the maxilla. The lesions rapidly increase in size up to the age of about 7 years, then enter a static phase or progress slowly up to puberty. The facial appearance is then said to improve, despite abnormal radiological appearances.

Clinical features

Facial deformity is the chief complaint (Figure 16.58). There is a characteristic fullness of the cheeks and jaws, and there is often a slightly upturned appearance to the eyes, with a rim of sclera visible beneath the iris. This latter sign is due to involvement of the orbital floor causing upward displacement of the eyeball and loss of support for the lower eyelid. The upturned eyes and full cheeks produce a cherubic

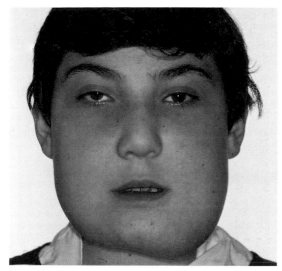

Figure 16.58 Cherubism. A 13-year-old child with asymmetrical cherubism

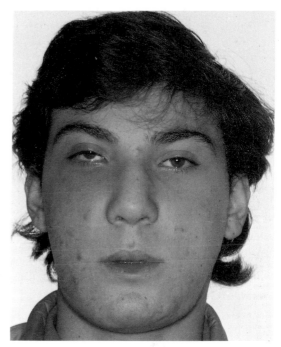

(a)

appearance. The submandibular lymph nodes are generally enlarged, and the cervical nodes are also sometimes involved. There is fibrous enlargement of large areas of the jaws, resulting in gross expansion and irregularity. The resulting irregular bulges are painless and not tender. Expansion of the mandible may elevate the tongue and cause a degree of speech impairment. The maxillary involvement is variable, sometimes being sufficiently extensive to produce nasal obstruction or ocular proptosis (Figure 16.59). The dentition is almost always abnormal.

Radiology

Radiographic appearances in the jaws are characteristic (Figure 16.60). Multiloculated radiolucencies produce considerable expansion of the bone; the loculi are sharply defined, and crossed by bony septa. The thinned and expanded cortex may be deficient in some areas without periosteal new bone formation.

Pathology

The tissue that replaces normal bone is soft, fibrous or friable, and mottled reddish-brown or greyish-brown. The main constituent of the lesion is fibrous tissue arranged in a whorled pattern. Giant cells are concentrated around the numerous thin-walled blood vessels that permeate this vascular lesion. The enlarged lymph nodes show reactive changes only.

Differential diagnosis

The main distinction is from fibrous dysplasia. Cherubism is almost always familial, and the lesions are

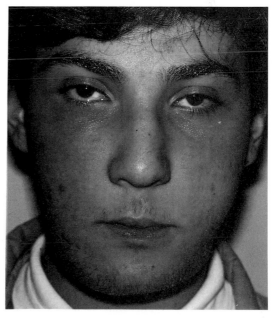

(b)

Figure 16.59 Cherubism. (*a*) The patient shown in Figure 16.58 underwent surgical correction of the facial deformity, but subsequently developed proptosis and elevation of the right globe due to involvement of the orbital floor; (*b*) same patient following surgical reduction of the enlarged orbital floor

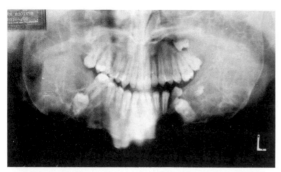

Figure 16.60 Cherubism. Orthopantogram showing the typical radiographic appearance of cherubism

bilateral. As in fibrous dysplasia, it is important that any biopsy material is examined by an experienced oral pathologist.

Treatment

Management is essentially the same as that described for fibrous dysplasia. Surgery should be conservative, and only performed before puberty when absolutely necessary.

Angiomatous malformations

Haemangioma

The appellation *haemangioma*, although generally accepted, is taxonomically erroneous, as the anomaly is a hamartoma rather than a true neoplasm. Haemangiomas are usually classified as capillary and cavernous, although mixed types are common. It is beyond the scope of this chapter to deal with them in a systematic way; rather, the discussion will be limited to those large, cavernous or mixed haemangiomas that occupy a substantial area in the craniofacial region and produce a significant deformity.

Clinical features

Facial cavernous and mixed haemangiomas may present as a very superficial, comparatively flat tumour at birth. They may enlarge slowly, but 60–70% of the lesions will regress completely by the age of 8 years if the parents will be patient and permit this approach. The occasional overwhelming lesion that has microarteriovenous fistulae demonstrates no regression, but continues to grow and expand. It rapidly develops a deeper cavernous element until the whole, or a large part, of the face becomes involved (Figure 16.61a).

The distended tissues may bulge out in the eyelids and around the mouth, so that the eye is completely hidden and the mouth may be partially obstructed.

The skin and musculature of the face are greatly stretched and feeding may become very difficult.

Differential diagnosis

The condition may be confused with lymphangioma, neurofibroma and congenital hemihypertrophy of the face. In young children it is important to exclude rhabdomyosarcoma. Fifty per cent occur before the age of 5 years, and 25% are in the head and neck region. If any doubt exists a biopsy is justified.

Investigations

MRI and CT scanning with contrast are useful, and can identify the limits, the major feeding vessels and the bony components of the lesion. Pooling of blood can occur in large lesions, which may not show on angiography or CT. The use of labelled red cells to demonstrate these areas can be helpful. Ultrasound can give information not only of the size of the lesion, but also about flow within it.

Treatment

Treatment of large facial haemangiomas should be embarked upon with considerable circumspection. The help of a neuroradiologist can be invaluable both in terms of defining the extent and nature of the lesion, and also carrying out microembolization with muscle or microspheres. This latter procedure is seldom anything other than transitory in its effect but it permits surgery under much more favourable conditions, thus reducing the operative risk. The results of surgery in such large lesions are usually disappointing. Occasionally, however, favourable results are obtained (Figure 16.61). For cavernous lesions that are not excessively large, Matthews (1968) advocated the use of saturated saline as a sclerosing fluid. An alternative is 50% dextrose. The use of radiotherapy in children is to be condemned.

Klippel-Trenaunay-Weber syndrome

The aetiology of this syndrome, also called vascular gigantism, is unknown, and almost all cases are sporadic. The original description defined the Klippel-Trenaunay-Weber syndrome as consisting of unilateral extremity enlargement with cutaneous and subcutaneous haemangiomas, varicosities, phlebectasia and occasionally arteriovenous fistulae. The syndrome has since been expanded to include almost every body area. Many additional abnormalities have been recognized, including lymphangiomatous anomalies, macrodactyly, syndactyly, polydactyly, oligodactyly and abdominal haemangiomas (Gorlin, Cohen and Levin, 1990).

Craniofacial involvement (Figure 16.62) is rare, but when present is similar to that seen in Sturge-

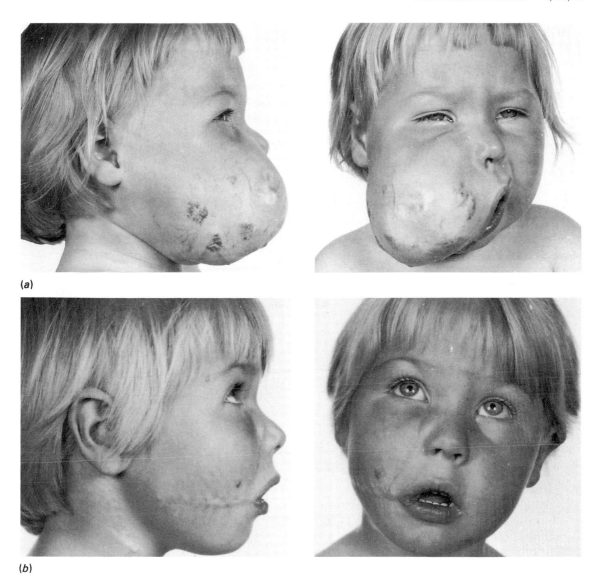

Figure 16.61 Haemangioma. (*a*) Expanding lesion of the right side of the face in a 16-month-old child; (*b*) appearance 9 months after surgical excision (*see* (*c*) *and* (*d*) *overleaf*)

Weber syndrome, both in distribution and the degree of variability. Patients may exhibit mental retardation when cutaneous involvement is present. Occasionally there may be bony enlargement of the jaws.

Differential diagnosis

Neurofibroma must be excluded, since limb hypertrophy and cutaneous haemangiomas may be associated with it. Café-au-lait spots do not occur in Klippel-Trenaunay-Weber syndrome. Hemihypertrophy and cutaneous haemangiomas occur in both Beckwith-

Weidemann syndrome and Maffucci syndrome. Vascular anomalies of the skin have also been reported in true congenital hypertrophy.

Treatment

Most patients do reasonably well. Some form of soft-tissue reduction such as filletting may be necessary. Care should be exercised, as wound healing is usually delayed and skin infarction is common. For this reason, considerable circumspection is necessary when dealing with facial lesions. In cases with se-

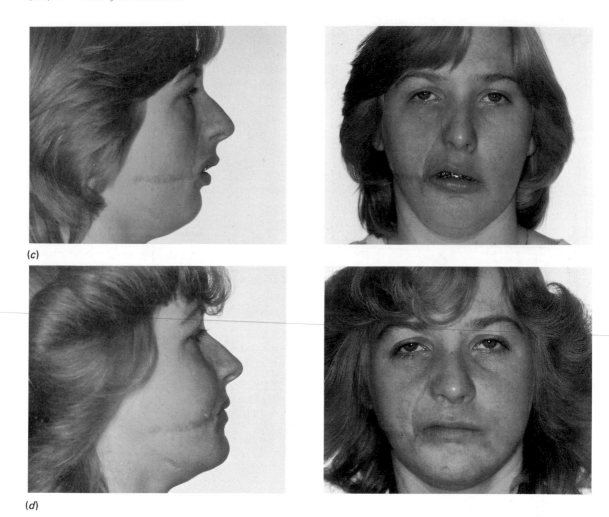

Figure 16.61 (*c*) same patient at the age of 20 years; (*d*) following orthognathic surgical correction of the facial disproportion

verely disproportionate growth in a limb, epiphyseal fusion or removal of a gigantic digit may be necessary. When gigantic extremities are gross enough to produce disseminated intravascular coagulation or evidence of high-output cardiac failure, amputation may be essential (Thomson, 1979).

Sturge-Weber syndrome

This syndrome is a non-hereditary condition that has neither sex nor ethnic predilection. It is characterized by:

1 Unilateral venous angiomatosis of the lepto-meninges
2 Ipsilateral facial angiomatosis
3 Ipsilateral gyriform calcifications of the cerebral cortex
4 Seizures, hemiplegia and mental retardation
5 Ocular defects.

A port-wine stain on the ipsilateral side of the face (Figure 16.63) occurs in 90% of individuals and this may extend onto the neck, chest and back. The colour varies from pink to purplish-red and rarely decreases in intensity with age. Occasionally there is an arteriovenous component.

Seizures, usually focal and rarely generalized, have been observed in 90% of patients. The symptoms appear during infancy on the side contralateral to the angiomatosis. Hemiparesis is less frequent. Mental impairment affects at least 30% of patients, being more severe with widespread cerebral involvement. Ophthalmic complications, including choroidal, conjunctival and episcleral haemangioma, are quite

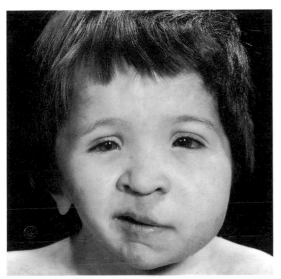

Figure 16.62 Klippel-Trenaunay-Weber syndrome. A 6-year-old boy with the rare craniofacial involvement

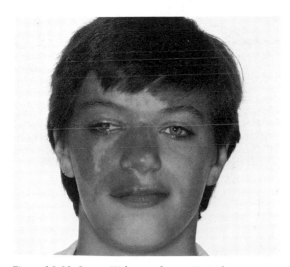

Figure 16.63 Sturge-Weber syndrome. Typical port-wine stain of the ipsilateral side of the face which affects 90% of affected individuals

common. Glaucoma may be seen in up to 70% of cases, with the onset occurring before the age of 2 years in 50%.

The diagnosis is usually clinical, but imaging can help to define the extent and severity of the leptomeningeal involvement. Marti-Bonmati *et al.* (1992) have shown that MRI imaging with contrast is probably the method of choice in the diagnosis of the syndrome, although CT scanning was better at showing the presence and extent of cortical calcification.

Differential diagnosis

The relationship between Sturge-Weber and Klippel-Trenaunay-Weber syndromes is not usually a problem, but the two may coexist, and could represent the same basic disorder in a different site (Goodman and Gorlin, 1983). Transitory port-wine stains are very common in the neonatal period, but dark supra-orbital involvement should arouse suspicion. The association of macrocephaly and angiomatosis may occur in disseminated haemangiomatosis, neurofibromatosis, Beckwith–Wiedemann syndrome, Klippel–Trenaunay–Weber syndrome and cutis marmorata telengiectatica congenita.

Treatment

Until recently satisfactory treatment of the patient with a port-wine stain had escaped all investigators (Thomson, 1979). Various modalities of treatment had been tried, but all have failed the patients' needs. These treatments included radiotherapy, cryotherapy and surgical tattooing.

The introduction of the tuneable pulse dye laser has overcome the previous problems associated with the argon laser, which proved disappointing because of scarring of the overlying tissues. Coherent light at 585 nm is applied with a 0.5 ms pulse over a 5 mm spot. This delivers 5–10 J/cm². The light passes through the overlying skin with no absorption, no thermal damage and thus no scarring. The energy is absorbed by the capillaries to a depth in excess of 1 mm causing disruption and scarring. The results are generally very good, and it is possible to adjust the amount of energy delivered to the tissues and thus match the final skin colour to the normal side. General anaesthesia is occasionally required for small children, but in most cases the treatment can be carried out without recourse to anaesthesia.

Cosmetic camouflage is now only used for treatment of cases unsuitable for laser therapy. Surgical tattooing may enable the patient to use a lighter cosmetic camouflage coverage, but fading or leaking out of the pigment is the major drawback; such fading appears less common in adult patients.

Lymphangioma

About 75% of cases of lymphangioma are found in the head and neck region. Like haemangiomas, these hamartomas are almost always evident by the age of 3 years. They may be present as unilocular or multi-locular (more commonly) masses, with thin, often transparent walls enclosing a straw-coloured fluid. Such lesions are known as *cystic hygromas* (Figure 16.64).

Cystic hygromas are usually slow-growing, unless there is an associated internal venous haemorrhage or infective lymphangitis. Most lesions appear in the posterior triangle of the neck, often occupying the

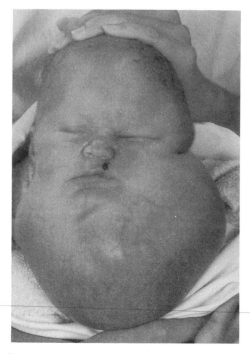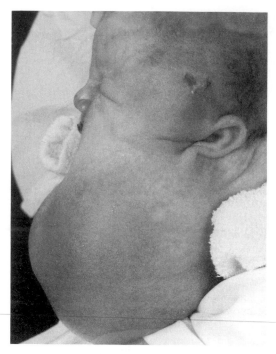

Figure 16.64 Cystic hygroma. Bilateral involvement in a neonate; any signs of respiratory distress will necessitate emergency surgical treatment. (Courtesy of Mr Ivor Broomhead, FRCS)

supraclavicular fossa. When they occur in the submandibular region or in the cervical prevertebral region, there may be severe respiratory distress in the neonatal period, especially if the disease is bilateral.

On rare occasions there is a rapid increase in growth. This can result in a grotesque enlargement of the affected side of the face, with the eye becoming obscured and gross distortion of the mouth. Hypertrophy of the maxilla and mandible may develop, but not to any marked extent.

There appears to be considerable disagreement about whether or not these lesions undergo spontaneous regression.

Treatment

This condition responds poorly to both radiotherapy and cryotherapy. Apart from the long-term danger of irradiating the neck in a child, radiotherapy produces extensive fibrosis, and this renders subsequent surgical dissection extremely difficult. Similar difficulty is experienced following the injection of sclerosing fluids. Ogita *et al.* (1994) reported encouraging results with intralesional injection of OK-432, an immunomodulatory agent prepared from an attenuated strain of *Streptococcus pyogenes*. This acts much like a sclerosing agent, but with significantly less inflamma-

tory response. It is at present too early to say whether this new agent will prove to be better than traditional sclerosants. It seems that radiotherapy, cryotherapy and sclerosing fluids should be avoided in the management of lymphangiomas.

Surgery remains the mainstay of treatment. Lymphangiomas of the neck and upper mediastinum which produce neonatal respiratory distress require to be treated as acute surgical emergencies. A preoperative chest radiograph is mandatory in order to exclude mediastinal extension. A tracheostomy and wide surgical excision is the treatment of choice. Cystic hygroma has an apparent disregard for anatomical planes, making total excision very difficult and sometimes impossible. For this reason, some surgeons prefer less radical means of surgical decompression, employing vacuum drains or marsupialization of the cysts (Thomson, 1979).

In gross cases, a radical approach should be made without regard for the facial nerve (Mustardé, 1979). Not only is it extremely difficult to dissect out the functioning branches of the nerve, but more importantly, gross involvement and stretching of the facial muscles renders their preservation pointless and usually impossible. A series of planned resections is necessary, and subsequent reconstruction involves the standard techniques for dealing with facial palsy. Readers are directed to Mustardé's account for information regarding management of grossly involved eyelids.

Benign neoplasms

Neurofibroma

This benign tumour of the nerve sheath is an important, if rare, cause of gross facial deformity. It occurs only rarely as a solitary tumour. Much more often there are multiple tumours (neurofibromatosis) occurring in connection with the nerves of the skin and subcutaneous tissues and also those of internal organs. Neurofibromatosis is an hereditary disorder transmitted as an autosomal dominant trait. The gene for type 1 neurofibromatosis has been located near the centromere of chromosome 17. It has the highest mutation rate known to man, 50% of cases representing a fresh mutation. The classification and clinical features of the nine currently recognized types are well described by Gorlin, Cohen and Levin (1990). The commonest presentation of this disease to the surgeon is that of facial deformity, and on rare occasions this may result in a gigantic overgrowth of one side of the face (Figure 16.65). While café-au-lait skin pigmentation may have been present since birth

or early childhood, tumour formation becomes evident during childhood, and is usually most aggressive at the time of puberty. The condition is progressive, not subject to spontaneous regression, and the pathology is that of plexiform neuroma. Both the Vth and VIIth cranial nerves are involved, and it is impossible to dissect them out from the mass of tumour tissue. In gross facial lesions the facial bones are involved and may show considerable enlargement and deformity. The skin is grossly expanded and may hang down in tumour-filled folds over the eye or cheek, the eyelids may be considerably elongated.

As in other areas of neuroimaging, MRI has taken over as the investigation of choice in the diagnosis of the condition. It is especially helpful in identifying acoustic neuroma (vestibular schwannoma) in type 2 neurofibromatosis and in detecting optic glioma and astrocytoma which can occur in any type of the condition.

Differential diagnosis

A gigantic plexiform neurofibroma of the face bears a resemblance to gross haemangiomas and lymphangiomas but is usually distinguished by the simultaneous presence of café-au-lait spots. Polyostotic fibrous

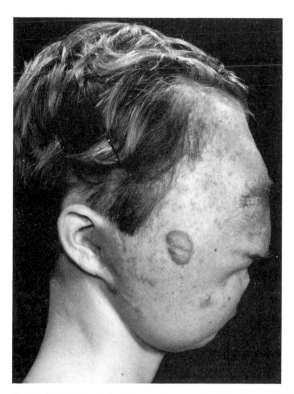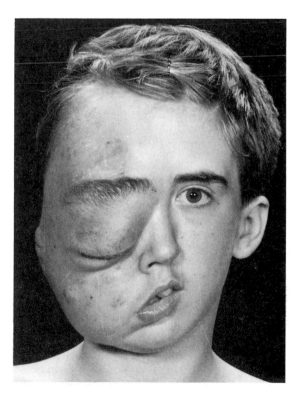

Figure 16.65 Craniofacial neurofibroma resulting in gross facial deformity with displacement of the right eye; the skin pigmentation is evident on the affected side of the face

dysplasia with grossly enlarged facial bones may also
have café-au-lait patches, but the enlargement is
bony rather than soft tissue. Hemifacial hypertrophy
is an enlargement of all the elements of the face, and
this should make it easy to distinguish from
neurofibroma.

Treatment

Treatment is directed at serial resection, access being
gained via an extended parotidectomy incision, with
secondary incisions in the nasolabial folds and eyelid
margins. No attempt is made to preserve neurological
function, and excess skin should be excised. The
neurofibromatous tissue is extremely vascular, but
preliminary carotid ligation does not usually result in
a significant reduction in peroperative bleeding. Complete removal of all the involved tissue is virtually
impossible. Resection of grossly involved parts of the
maxilla and mandible may be necessary. There is
considerable skeletal deformity in the orbital region.
Surgery is, of necessity, crude, and enucleation of the
globe may be required.

Prodigious efforts are usually expended over a
number of years to effect an improvement in appearance, but this is seldom acceptable to the patient or
his relatives. The prognosis is poor, as growth of the
incompletely excised tumour tissue is unavoidable.
In addition, there is the risk of malignant
transformation.

Miscellaneous malformations

Congenital hemihypertrophy of the face (facial gigantism)

Asymmetrical growth or development of the body or
any of its parts is not too unusual; this may be trivial
or very obvious. It may result from localized overgrowth of a single tissue or of all the tissues within a
part. In any case the condition is best regarded as a
hyperplasia, rather than a hypertrophy.

Marked asymmetry caused by localized overgrowth
of all the tissues within a part is rare. It is probably
due to faulty cell division of the zygote which results
in two daughter cells of unequal size, and has been
considered a form of incomplete twinning (Norman,
1983).

Congenital hemihypertrophy may be of several
types, and these have been classified by Rowe
(1962):

1 Complex hemihypertrophy involving an entire
half of the body, or at least an arm and a leg. Enlarged parts may be all on the same side of the
body (complex ipsilateral hemihypertrophy) or
crossed, in which case enlarged parts may be
found on both sides (complex contralateral
hemihypertrophy)

2 Simple hemihypertrophy, involving part or the
whole of a limb
3 Hemifacial hypertrophy, involving one side of the
face (Figure 16.66).

The criteria for the hemifacial type of congenital
hypertrophy are as follows:

1 Unilateral enlargement of the viscerocranium
bounded superiorly by the frontal bone (not including the eye), inferiorly by the inferior border
of the mandible, medially by the facial midline
and laterally by the ear, the pinna being
involved
2 Enlargement of *all* tissues – bone, teeth and soft
tissue – within this area.

Almost all instances of this condition are sporadic,
but a few familial cases have been reported. The
incidence is about one per 15000 births. Rowe
(1962) recorded that the enlargement results from
an increased number of cells rather than increase in
cell size. Asymmetry is usually evident at birth, but
may become accentuated with age, especially at puberty. Occasionally there is unilateral enlargement of
a cerebral hemisphere, and mental retardation is
reported in 15–20% of cases. When the hemihypertrophy is restricted to the face, there is usually macroglossia. The lips, palate, maxilla and dentition (especially
the permanent teeth) are all enlarged. Unlike both
hard and soft tissues, the teeth are unique in that
their form and size are determined early and thereafter are not modified. A consideration of the size of
the teeth on the affected side, therefore, is significant
in this condition as it establishes it as being congenital. Of special interest is the association with various
neoplasms such as adrenocortical carcinoma, nephro-
blastoma, hepatoblastoma, adrenal adenoma, adrenal
neuroblastoma and undifferentiated sarcoma of the
lung. Neoplasia and renal dysplasia may be the cause
of a reduced life span.

Differential diagnosis

Congenital facial hemihypertrophy may be confused
with lymphangioma, haemangioma, neurofibroma
and lipoma. It is usually distinctive due to involvement of all the tissues in the region, and it is the only
condition where the teeth are enlarged. There is
overlap with the rare Beckwith-Wiedman syndrome.
It is possible to mistake the condition with hemifacial
atrophy (Romberg's disease) of the contralateral side,
although this is usually progressive.

Treatment

Due to the involvement of all facial tissues, surgical
correction can be difficult, and as a result of the
extreme paucity of cases, few surgeons gain much
experience in treating such patients.

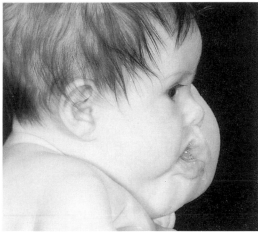

(a)

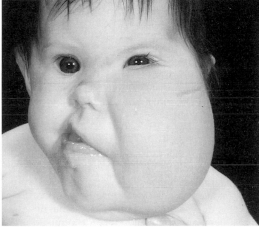

(b)

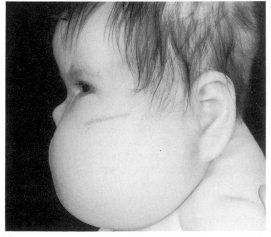

(c)

Figure 16.66 Congenital hemihypertrophy of the face in a 3-month-old girl

Progressive hemifacial atrophy

This disorder is also called Romberg's disease, Parry-Romberg syndrome and progressive facial hemiatrophy. Although it was mentioned by Parry in 1825 (Gorlin, Pindborg and Cohen, 1976), credit for its description is usually given to Romberg (1846). The condition consists of:

1 Slowly progressive atrophy of the soft tissues of essentially half the face, accompanied most often by
2 Contralateral Jacksonian epilepsy
3 Trigeminal neuralgia
4 Changes in the eyes and hair
5 Associated atrophy of half the body.

Nearly all cases are sporadic, but a few familial cases have been noted. There is no proven cause for progressive hemifacial atrophy. After a review of the various hypotheses, Rogers (1977) concluded that a sympathetic nervous system cause is the most likely. It is postulated that sympathetic tracts are affected centrally, perhaps directly in their centres in the diencephalon. There is a long-standing debate about the relationship between progressive and hemifacial atrophy and scleroderma, some authors asserting that the coup-de-sabre form of scleroderma is a special type of progressive hemifacial atrophy.

Clinical features

Progressive hemifacial atrophy usually commences in late childhood or adolescence, and 75% of cases appear before the twentieth year. It is usually limited to one side of the face, although bilateral disease has been reported. The 'active' period of the disease progression lasts for 2 to 10 years, but may stop at any time, leaving minimal deformity. Some cases of progressive hemifacial atrophy continue beyond a period of 10 years. The disease is slowly progressive, with atrophy of the subcutaneous fat in the paramedian area of the face (Figure 16.67). The process slowly spreads, so that atrophy of the underlying muscle, bone and cartilage becomes apparent. From the initial site, frequently in the area covered by temporalis and buccinator muscles, involvement extends to include the brow, angle of the mouth, neck or even half the body. There is a marked predilection for left-sided involvement, and the overlying skin often becomes darkly pigmented. Changes in the hair may precede those in the skin. The scalp on the affected side may exhibit complete alopecia limited to the paramedian area, eyelashes and medial part of the eyebrow. Poliosis (blanching of the hair) has been observed.

Loss of periorbital fat produces enophthalmos and the outer canthus may be displayed due to loss of the underlying bone. Muscular paresis, lagophthalmos and ptosis have all been reported, as well as a variety of inflammatory intraocular conditions.

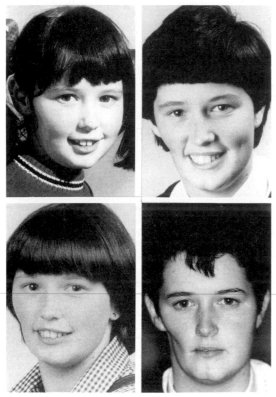

Figure 16.67 Progressive hemifacial atrophy seen in serial photographs at ages 8, 12, 17 and 24 years. (Courtesy of Mr. R. C. Boyd)

The bone and cartilage of the face are underdeveloped to a degree directly related to the age of onset of progressive hemifacial atrophy. The bony involvement is thus most severe when the disorder commences in early childhood. When the mandible is involved both ramus and body are shorter than the contralateral side, and teeth on the involved side may be retarded in eruption or may have atrophic roots. Resorption of the roots of teeth has been reported. Atrophy of half the tongue and upper lip is common, sometimes resulting in exposure of the teeth.

The commonest neurological abnormality is epilepsy, usually of the Jacksonian variety, which often appears late. Conversely, trigeminal neuralgia and/or facial paraesthesia appear early, and may precede the rest of the changes. Migraine is a common finding.

Differential diagnosis

The main conditions with which progressive hemifacial atrophy may be confused are scleroderma and craniofacial microsomia.

Treatment

Little information is published about the treatment of this condition, and the results are frequently disappointing. The main problem is that the same unknown factors which cause the initial atrophy frequently act against the success of the various forms of graft that have been used in reconstructive surgery. This is clearly a major problem when surgical procedures are undertaken during the 'active' phase of the disease. If at all possible, treatment is better delayed until the atrophy is no longer progressive.

Dimethylpolysiloxane fluid injections

This liquid form of silicone has been widely used in the USA, and is advocated by Grabb (1979) as the best treatment for progressive hemifacial atrophy. Plastic surgeons in the UK, however, have found this method of treatment less satisfactory. Inflammatory reactions, excessive fibrosis and migration of the fluid have all caused problems, and the technique has largely been abandoned.

Grafts

Dermo-fat grafts are still widely used. When they are inserted in areas not affected by progressive hemifacial atrophy, the resorption rate is unpredictable, and 50% or more of the original bulk is often lost. The resorption rate of dermo-fat grafts in tissues affected by the atrophy is even greater, and patients with severe forms of the disease have to be regrafted many times.

Flaps

Pedicled flaps of omentum have been used, but if this tissue is chosen, it is now more frequently used as a 'free' microvascular transfer. Temporalis muscle has been transferred on its pedicle in cases where the upper face has been largely spared, but this technique is clearly unsatisfactory in patients with extensive and severe involvement of the face.

The development of microvascular techniques has offered the best chance for reconstruction in progressive hemifacial atrophy. Each microvascular surgeon has his own preference in selecting the donor site. The main problems are the maintenance of an even distribution of soft tissue so transferred (it frequently 'sags') and variation in the bulk of the flap with changes in the weight of the patient due to its content of adipose tissue.

Moebius syndrome

This condition, while rare, is one of the commoner disorders of oromandibular limb hypogenesis. Moebius (1888), in attempting to classify multiple congenital cranial nerve palsies, created a group in which palsies of the VIth and VIIth cranial nerves were combined. Subsequently the concept of Moebius syndrome has been expanded to include:

VIth and VIIth cranial nerve palsies, usually bilateral
Occasionally other cranial nerve involvement (IIIrd, Vth, IXth and XIIth)
Reductive limb anomalies (30%)
Poland anomaly (15%), i.e. abnormality of pectoralis major muscle and ipsilateral syndactyly
Mild mental retardation (10–15%).

The aetiology of Moebius syndrome is unknown, and all cases are sporadic. Recent studies have suggested there may be an abnormality in chromosome 13. Post-mortem studies have demonstrated nuclear agenesis.

Clinical features

The mask-like facies is characteristic (Figure 16.68). Bilateral facial palsies usually impart a symmetrical appearance, but variation in the degree of involvement of each side of the face can cause significant asymmetry (Figure 16.69). Occasionally the facial palsy is unilateral.

Most patients cannot abduct either eye beyond the midline, but unilateral VIth nerve palsy does occur. Ptosis, nystagmus or strabismus may accompany the above features, and epicanthal folds are common (Figure 16.70). Some patients are unable to close their eyelids, resulting in conjunctivitis or corneal ulceration. The nasal bridge is often high and broad, especially during infancy and childhood. The broadness of the bridge extends downwards in a parallel fashion to include the nasal tip, thus providing midfacial prominence which is accentuated by the retruded mandible (see Figure 16.68).

The angles of the mouth droop, allowing saliva to escape. The mouth aperture is small, and mandibular opening may be restricted; this tends to improve spontaneously as the child develops. Unilateral or bilateral tongue hypoplasia is seen, and when combined with poor palatal mobility, can result in impaired feeding or speech. The mandible is frequently hypoplastic, adding to these problems. The pinnae may be hypoplastic, normal or large, and frequently protrude laterally.

Unilateral, bilateral or asymmetrical hypoplasia or aplasia of pectoralis major muscle or complete Poland anomaly occurs in 15% of cases. Limb defects occur in 50% of affected individuals, 30% constituting talipes deformities and the other 20% include hypoplasia of digits, syndactyly or more severe reductive deformities (Figure 16.71). Mental retardation, usually of a mild nature, occurs in 10–15% of patients with Moebius syndrome.

Differential diagnosis

There are variable degrees of overlap between the oromandibular limb hypogenesis syndromes. Thus Moebius syndrome must be distinguished from Charlie M. syndrome, glossopalatine ankylosis syndrome,

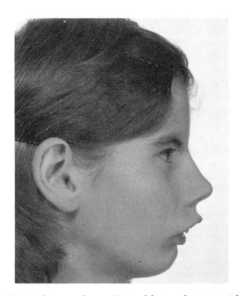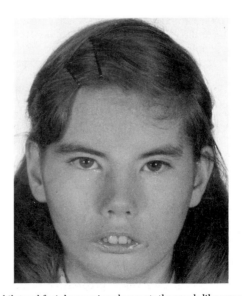

Figure 16.68 Moebius syndrome. Typical facies of patient with bilateral facial nerve involvement; the mask-like appearance is accompanied by mandibular retrusion, accentuated by the midfacial prominence

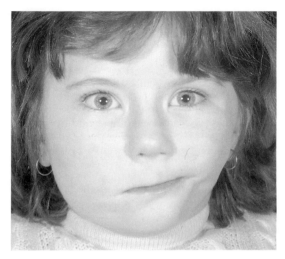

Figure 16.69 Moebius syndrome. Appearance of a child with asymmetrical facial nerve involvement

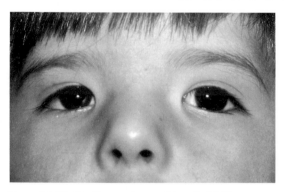

Figure 16.70 Moebius syndrome. Epicanthal folds

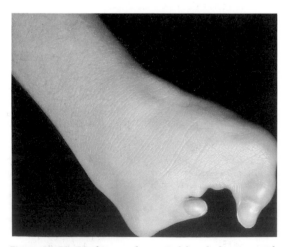

Figure 16.71 Moebius syndrome. Left hand of patient with severe reductive deformity

Hanhart syndrome and hypoglossia-hypodactylia syndrome. All these are much rarer than Moebius syndrome. Similar limb defects are seen in the Poland anomaly, amniotic band syndrome and other reductive limb anomalies.

Superficially, Moebius syndrome may be confused with craniofacial microsomia, Treacher Collins syndrome and Pierre Robin syndrome. Isolated facial palsy may occur as an inherited disorder, or may result from birth trauma.

Treatment

The treatment of Moebius syndrome has received scant attention. Much has, however, been written about the management of facial palsy. It is outside the scope of this chapter to cover this challenging field of reconstructive surgery. Static sling procedures and reanimation techniques each have their advocates. It is the authors' experience that results of reanimation are inconsistent and often disappointing, although satisfactory results are occasionally presented. Electromyographic feedback may have a role to play if surgery is not considered advisable or is to be delayed until after orthognathic surgery (Gallegos *et al.*, 1992). If advances in this field are to continue, it is essential that patients with facial palsy are referred to those surgeons with an interest in and experience of these problems.

If static slings are employed, it is preferable that they are delayed until after any orthognathic surgery has been performed, as they usually severely restrict access to the oral cavity. The same principle applies to orthodontic treatment which is usually necessary.

The upper lip is short and immobile. The only satisfactory way of managing this problem is by means of a Le Fort I osteotomy to intrude the maxilla. This will have to be accompanied by an osteotomy of the mandible which usually needs advancement. Surgical details of the various orthognathic techniques are well described by Henderson (1985). Repositioning of the jaws may have a beneficial effect on feeding and speech, although the results are frequently disappointing in this respect. The facial appearance can be further improved by correcting the wide nasal bridge and epicanthal folds when present.

References

APERT, E. (1906) De l'acrocephalosyndactylie. *Bulletin de la Societe Medicine du Hopital de Paris*, **23**, 1310–1330

ARLT, F. von (1881) *Klinische Darstellung der Krankheiten des Auges*. Vienna: W. Braunmuller.

BOO-CHAI, K. (1970) The oblique facial cleft: a report of 2 cases and a review of 41 cases. *British Journal of Plastic Surgery*, **23**, 352–359

BRANEMARK, P. I., BREINE, V., LINDSTROM, J., ADELL, R., HANSSON, B. O. and OHLSSON, A. (1989) Intraosseous anchorage of dental prostheses: 1. experimental studies. *Scandinavian Journal of Plastic and Reconstructive Surgery*, **3**, 81–100

BUNCIC, J. R. (1991) Ocular aspects of Apert syndrome. *Clinics in Plastic Surgery*, **18**, 315–319

CARONNI, E. P. (ed.) (1985) *Craniofacial Surgery*. Boston: Little, Brown and Company

COHEN, M. M. (1979) Craniosynostosis and syndromes with craniosynostosis: incidence, genetics, penetrance, variability and new syndrome updating. *Birth Defects*, **XV**, 13–63

COHEN, M. M. JR (1986) *Craniostenosis: Diagnosis, Evaluation, and Management*. New York: Raven Press

COHEN, M. M. JR (1987) Cloverleaf skull update. *Proceedings of the Greenwood Genetic Center* **6**, 186–187

COHEN, M. M. JR (1989) Perspectives on holoprosencephaly Part 1. Epidemiology, genetics and syndromology. *Teratology*, **40**, 211–236

COHEN, M. M. JR (1993) Pfeiffer syndrome update, clinical subtypes, and guidelines for differential diagnosis. *American Journal of Medical Genetics*, **45**, 300–307

COHEN, M. M. JR and KRIEBORG, S. (1990) The central nervous system in Apert' syndrome. *American Journal of Genetics*, **35**, 36–45

COHEN, M. M. JR and KRIEBORG, S. (1991) Genetic and family study of the Apert syndrome. *Journal of Craniofacial Genetics and Developmental Biology*, **11**, 7–17

COHEN, M. M. JR and KRIEBORG, S. (1992) New indirect method for estimating the birth prevalence of the Apert syndrome. *International Journal of Oral and Maxillofacial Surgery*, **21**, 107–109

COHEN, M. M. JR and KRIEBORG, S. (1993) Visceral anomalies in the Apert syndrome. (Review). *American Journal of Medical Genetics*, **45**, 758–760

COHEN, M. M. JR, KRIEBORG, S. LAMMER, E. J., CORDERO, J. F., MASTROIACOVO, P., ERICKSON, J. D. *et al.* (1992) Birth prevalence study of the Apert syndrome. *American Journal of Medical Genetics*, **42**, 655–659

COLLINS, E. T. (1900) Cases with symmetrical congenital notches in the outer part of each lid and defective development of the malar bones. *Transactions of the Ophthalmological Society of the United Kingdom*, **20**, 190–192

CONVERSE, J. M., MCCARTHY, J. G., WOOD-SMITH, D. and COCCARO, P. J. (1977) Craniofacial microsomia. In: *Reconstructive Plastic Surgery*, 2nd edn, edited by J. M. Converse. Philadelphia: W. B. Saunders. pp. 2359–2400

COSTARAS-VOLARICH, M. and PRUZANSKY, S. (1984) Is the mandible intrinsically different in Apert and Crouzon syndromes? *American Journal of Orthodontics*, **85**, 475–487

CROUZON, O. (1912) Dyostose craniofociale hereditaire. *Bulletin de la Societe Medicine du Hopital de Paris*, **33**, 545–555

DAL PONT, G. (1961) Retromolar osteotomy for the correction of prognathism. *Journal of Oral Surgery, Anaesthesia and Hospital Dental Services*, **19**, 42–47

DAVID, D. J., MAHATUMARAT, C. and COOTER, R. D. (1987) Hemifacial microsomia: a multisystem classification. *Plastic and Reconstructive Surgery*, **80**, 525

DAVID, D. J., MOORE, M. H and COOTER, R. D. (1989) Tessier clefts revisited with a 3rd dimension. *Cleft Palate Journal*, **26**, 163–185

DAVID, D. J., POSWILLO, D. and SIMPSON, D. (1982) *The Craniosynostoses – Causes, Natural History and Management*. Berlin: Springer-Verlag

DELAIRE, J., GAILLARD, A., BILLET, J., LANDAIS, H. and RENAUD, Y. (1963) Considerations sur les synostoses prematurées et leur consequences au crane et à la face. *Revue de Stomatologie*, **64**, 97–106

DIXON, M. J., READ, A. P., DONNAI, D., COLLEY, A., DIXON, J. and WILLIAMSON, R. (1991) The gene for Treacher Collins syndrome maps to the long arm of chromosome 5. *American Journal of Human Genetics*, **49**, 17–22

DROMMER, R. B. (1986) The history of the Le Fort I osteotomy. *Journal of Maxillofacial Surgery*, **14**, 119–122

FEARON, J. A. and WHITAKER, L. A. (1993) Complications with facial advancement: a comparison between the Le Fort III and monobloc advancements. *Plastic and Reconstructive Surgery*, **91**, 990–995

FOK, H., JONES, B. M., GAULT, D. G., ANDAR, U. and HAYWARD, R. (1992) Relationship between intracranial pressure and intracranial volume in craniosynostosis. *British Journal of Plastic Surgery*, **45**, 394–397

FRANCESCHETTI, A. and KLEIN, D. (1949) The mandibulofacial dysostosis: new hereditary syndrome. *Acta Ophthalmologica*, **27**, 143–224

FRIEDENWALD, H. (1893) Cranial deformity and optic nerve atrophy. *American Journal of Medical Science*, **105**, 529–535

FRYBURG, J. S., PERSING, J. A. and LIN, K. Y. (1993) Frontonasal dysplasia in two successive generations. *American Journal of Medical Genetics*, **46**, 712–714

GALLEGOS, X., MEDINA, R., SPINOSA, E. and BOUSTAMANANTE, A. (1992) Electromyographic feedback in the treatment of bilateral facial paralysis. *Journal of Behavioural Medicine*, **15**, 533–539

GAULT, D. T., RENIER, D., MARCHAC, D. and JONES, B. M. (1992) Intracranial pressure and intracranial volume in children with craniosynostosis. *Plastic and Reconstructive Surgery*, **90**, 377–381

GILLIES, H. D. and HARRISON, S. H. (1950) Operative correction by osteotomy of recessed malar maxillary compound in a case of oxycephaly. *British Journal of Plastic Surgery*, **2**, 123–127

GOODMAN, R. M. and GORLIN, R. J. (1983) *The Malformed Infant and Child*. New York: Oxford University Press

GORLIN, R. J., COHEN, M. M. JR and LEVIN, L. S. (1990) *Syndromes of the Head and Neck*, 3rd edn. Oxford: Oxford University Press

GORLIN, R. J., PINDBORG, J. J. and COHEN, M. M. (1976) *Syndromes of the Head and Neck*, 2nd edn. New York: McGraw-Hill

GORLIN, R. J., JUE, K. L., JACOBSEN, U. and GOLDSCHMIDT, E. (1963) Oculoauriculovertebral dysplasia. *Journal of Paediatrics*, **63**, 991–999

GRABB, W. C. (1979) Some anomalies of the head and neck. In: *Plastic Surgery*, 3rd edn, edited by W C. Grabb and J. W. Smith. Boston: Little, Brown and Company. pp. 115–130

GREIG, D. M. (1924) A hitherto undifferentiated congenital cranio-facial deformity. *Edinburgh Medical Journal*, **31**, 560–593

GURRIERI, F., TRASK, B. J., VAN DEN ENGH, G., KRAUSS, C. M., SCHINZEL, A., PETTENATI, M. J. *et al.* (1993) Physical mapping of the holoprosencephaly critical region on chromosome 7q36. *Nature Genetics*, **3**, 247–251

HATZIIOANNOU, A. G., KRAUSS, C. M., LEWIS, M. B. and HALAZONETIS, T. D. (1991) Familial holoprosencephaly associated with a translocation breakpoint at chromosomal position 7q36. *American Journal of Medical Genetics*, **40**, 201–205

HENDERSON, D. (1985) *A Colour Atlas and Textbook of Ortho-*

gnathic Surgery – The Surgery of Facial Skeletal Deformity. London: Wolfe Medical Publications

HOLTMULLER, K. and WEIDMAN, H.-R. (1960) Kleeblattschadel syndrome. *Medizinische Monatschrift,* **14,** 439–446

HOPPE, I. (1859) Eine angeboren Spaltung der Nase. *Preuss Medizinische-Zeitung Berlin,* **2,** 164–165

HUNSUCK, E. E. (1968) A modified intraoral sagittal splitting technique for correction of mandibular prognathism. *Journal of Oral Surgery,* **26,** 249–252

JONES, W. A. (1933) Familial multilocular cystic disease of the jaws. *American Journal of Cancer,* **17,** 946–950

KAPUSTA, L., BRUNNER, H. G. and HAMEL, B. C. (1992) Craniofrontonasal dysplasia. *European Journal of Pediatrics,* **151,** 837–841

KOLAR, J. C., MUNRO, I. R. and FARKAS, L. G. (1988) Patterns of dysmorphology in Crouzon syndrome: An anthropometric study. *Cleft Palate Journal,* **25,** 235–244

KREIBORG, S. and BJORK, A. (1982) Decription of a dry skull with Crouzon syndrome. *Scandinavian Journal of Plastic and Reconstructive Surgery,* **16,** 245–253

KREIBORG, S. and COHEN, M. M. JR (1990) Characteristics of the infant Apert skull and its subsequent development. *Journal of Craniofacial Genetic and Developmental Biology,* **10,** 399–410

LAJEUNIE, E., MA, H. W., BONAVENTURE, J., MUNNICH, A. and LE MERRER, M. (1995) FGFR2 mutations in Pfeiffer syndrome. *Nature Genetics,* **9,** 108

LUCAS, R. B. (1984) *Pathology of Tumours of the Oral Tissues,* 4th edn. Edinburgh: Churchill Livingstone. pp. 408–412

MCGILL, T. (1991) Otolaryngologic aspects of Apert syndrome. *Clinics in Plastic Surgery,* **18,** 309–313

MARCHAC, D. and RENIER, D. (1981) Cranio-facial surgery for craniosynostosis *Scandinavian Journal of Plastic and Reconstructive Surgery,* **15,** 235–243

MARCHAC, D. and RENIER, D. (1989) Craniosynostosis. *World Journal of Surgery,* **13,** 358–365

MARCHAC, D., RENIER, D. and BROUMAND, S. (1994) Timing of treatment for craniosynostosis and facio-craniosynostosis: a 20-year experience. *British Journal of Plastic Surgery,* **47,** 211–222

MARSH, J. L. and VANNIER, M. W. (eds) (1985) *Comprehensive Care of Craniofacial Deformities.* St Louis: C. V. Mosby Co

MARTI-BONMATI, L., MENOR, F., POYATOS, C. and CORTINA, II. (1992) Diagnosis of Sturge-Weber syndrome: comparison of the efficiency of CT and MRI imaging. *American Journal of Roentgenology,* **158,** 867–871

MATTHEWS, D. N. (1968) Haemangiomata. *Plastic and Reconstructive Surgery,* **41,** 528–535

MOEBIUS, P. J. (1888) Uber angeborene doppelseitige abducens-focialis lahmung. *Munchene Medizinische Wochenschrift,* **35,** 91–94 and 108–111

MORIAN, R. (1887) Uber die schrage Gisichtsspalte. *Arch. Clin. Chir.,* **35,** 245–288

MOSS, J. P. and JAMES, D. R. (1984) An investigation of a group of 35 consecutive patients with a first arch syndrome. *British Journal of Oral and Maxillofacial Surgery,* **22,** 157–169

MUENKE, M., SCHELL, U., HEHR, A., ROBIN, N. H., LOSKEN, H. W., SCHINZEL, A. *et al.* (1994) A common mutation in the fibroblast growth factor receptor 1 gene in Pfeiffer syndrome. *Nature Genetics,* **8,** 269–274

MUSTARDÉ, J. C. (ed.) (1979) Acquired hemifacial hypertrophy (hemifacial gigantism). In: *Plastic Surgery in Infancy and Childhood,* 2nd edn. Edinburgh: Churchill Livingstone. pp. 372–379

MYRIANTHOPOULOS, N. C. (1982) Epidemiology of craniofacial malformations. In: *Clinical Dysmorphology of Oral-Facial Structures,* edited by M. Melnick, E. D. Shields and N. J. Burzynski. Bristol: Wright. pp. 1–27

NORMAN, M. E. (1983) The bones and joints. In: *Nelsons Textbook of Pediatrics,* edited by R. E. Behrman and V. C. Vaughan. Philadelphia: W. S. Saunders. pp. 1614–1662

OBWEGESER, H. L. (1969) Surgical correction of small or retrodisplaced maxillae. *Plastic and Reconstructive Surgery,* **43,** 351–365

OGITA, S., TSUTO, T., NAKAMURA, K., DEGUCHI, E. and IWAI, N. (1994) OK-432 therapy in 64 patients with lymphangioma. *Journal of Pediatric Surgery,* **29,** 784–758

PATTON, M. A., GOODSHIP, J., HAWARD, R. and LANDSDOWN, R. (1988) Intellectual development in Apert syndrome: A long term follow up of 29 patients. *Journal of Medical Genetics,* **25,** 164–167

PENSLER, J. M., LEDESMA, D. F., HIJJAWI, J. and RADOSEVICH, J. A. (1994) Plagiocephaly: premature unilateral closure of the coronal suture: a potentially localized disorder of cellular metabolism. *Annals of Plastic Surgery,* **32,** 160–165

PETERSON, M. Q., COHEN, M. M., SEDANO, H. O. and FRERICHS, C. T. (1971) Comments on frontonasal dysplasia, ocular hypertelorism and dysplopia canthorum. *Birth Defects,* **VII,** 120–124

PFEIFFER, R. A. (1964) Dominant erbliche akrocephalosyndaktylie. *Zeitschrift für Kinderheilkunde,* **90,** 301–320

POSNICK, J. C. (1991) Craniofacial dysostosis. Staging of reconstruction and management of the midface deformity. *Neurosurgical Clinics of North America,* **2,** 683–702

POSWILLO, D. (1973) The pathogenesis of the first and second branchial arch syndrome. *Oral Surgery, Oral Medicine, Oral Pathology,* **3,** 302–328

POSWILLO, D. (1974) Otomandibular deformity: pathogenesis as a guide to reconstruction. *Journal of Maxillofacial Surgery,* **2,** 64–72

POSWILLO, D. (1975) The pathogenesis of the Treacher Collins syndrome. *British Journal of Oral Surgery,* **13,** 1–26

REARDON, W., WINTER, R. M., RUTLAND, P., PULLEYN, L. J., JONES, B. M. and MALCOLM, S. (1994) Mutations in the fibroblast growth factor receptor 2 gene cause Crouzon syndrome. *Nature Genetics,* **8,** 98–103

ROBINSON, L. K., HOYME, H. E., EDWARDS, D. K. and JONES, K. L. (1987) Vascular pathogenesis of unilateral craniofacial defects. *Journal of Pediatrics,* **111,** 236–239

ROMBERG, M. H. (1846) Trophoneurosen. In: *Klinische Ergebnisse.* Berlin: A. Forstner. pp. 75–81

ROGERS, B. O. (1977) Embryology of the face and introduction to craniofacial anomalies. In: *Reconstructive Plastic Surgery,* 2nd edn, edited by J. M. Converse. Philadelphia: W. B. Saunders. pp. 2296–2358

ROWE, N. H. (1962) Hemifacial hypertrophy: a review of the literature and addition of four cases. *Oral Surgery, Oral Medicine, Oral Pathology,* **15,** 572–587

ROWE, N. L. (1960) The aetiology, clinical features and treatment of mandibular deformities. *British Dental Journal,* **108,** 45–64 and 97–115

RUGGIERI, P., SIM, F. H., BOND, J. R. and UNNI, K. K. (1994) Malignancies in fibrous dysplasia. *Cancer,* **73,** 1411–1424

RUTLAND, P., PULLEYN, L. J., REARDON, W., BARAITSER, M., HAYWARD, R., JONES, B. *et al.,* (1995) Identical mutations in the FGFR2 gene cause both Pfeiffer and Crouzon syndrome phenotypes. *Nature Genetics,* **9,** 173–176.

SCHELL, U., HEHR, A., FELDMAN, G. J., ROBIN, N. H., ZACKAI, E. H., DE DIESMULDERS, C. *et al.*, (1995) Mutations in FGFR1 and FGFR2 cause familial and sporadic Pfeiffer syndrome. *Human Molecular Genetics*, **4**, 323–328

SEDANO, H. C., COHEN, M. M., JIRASEK, J. and GORLIN, R. J. (1970) Frontonasal dysplasia. *Journal of Paediatrics*, **76**, 906–913

TESSIER, P. (1967) Osteotomies totales de la face; syndrome de Crouzon; syndrome d'Apert: oxycephalies, scaphocephalies, turricephalies. *Annales de Chirurgie Plastique*, **12**, 273–286

TESSIER, P. (1976) Anatomical classification of facial craniofacial and lateral-facial clefts. *Journal of Maxillofacial Surgery*, **4**, 69–92

TESSIER, P., GUIOT, G., ROUGERIE, J., DELBERT, J. P. and PASTORIZA, J. (1967) Osteotomies cranio-naso-orbitofaciales – hypertelorisme. *Annales de Chirurgie Plastique*, **12**, 103–118

THOMSON, H. G. (1979) Hemangioma, lymphangioma, and arteriovenous fistula. In: *Plastic Surgery*, 3rd edn, edited by W. C. Grabb and J. W. Smith. Boston: Little, Brown and Company. pp. 518–529

TJELLSTROM, A. (1990) Osseointegrated implants for the replacement of absent or defective ears. *Clinics in Plastic Surgery*, **17**, 355–366

TOWERS, J. F. (1976) The management of congenital and acquired deformity of the mandibular condyle in children. *Cartwright Prize Essay*. London: Royal College of Surgeons of England

TRAUNER, R. and OBWEGESER, H. L. (1957) Surgical correction of mandibular prognathism and retrogenia with consideration of genioplasty. *Oral Surgery, Oral Medicine, Oral Pathology*, **10**, 677–689

VENTO, A. R., LABRIE, R. A. and MULLIKEN, J. B. (1991) The OMENS classification of hemifacial microsomia. *Cleft Palate and Craniofacial Journal*, **28**, 68–76; discussion 77

VROLIK, W. (1849) *Tabulae ad illustrandam embryogenesin Hominis et mamalium*. London: GMP

WHEATON, S. W. (1894) Two cases of congenital facial deformity in infants with fusion of the fingers and toes. *Transactions of the Pathological Society of London*, **45**, 238–241

WILKIE, A. O. M., SLANEY, S. F., OLDRIDGE, M., POOLE, M. D., ASHWORTH, G. J., HOCKLEY, A. D. *et al.* (1995) Apert syndrome results from localized mutations of FGFR2 and is allelic with Crouzon syndrome. *Nature Genetics*, **9**, 165–172

WORTHINGTON, P. and BRANEMARK, P.-I. (1992) *Advanced Osseointegration Surgery, Applications in the Maxillofacial Region*. Chicago: Quintessence Publishing Co

ZINS, J. E. and WHITAKER, L. A. (1983) Membranous versus endochondral bone: implications for craniofacial reconstruction. *Plastic and Reconstructive Surgery*, **72**, 778–784

17

Nasal obstruction and rhinorrhoea in infants and children

David Albert

The sight of a snuffly baby or a child with a blocked runny nose is sufficiently commonplace to engender a feeling of complacency in parents and doctors alike (Figure 17.1). In some patients the airway obstruction will be sufficiently severe to warrant urgent attention. In a few patients the benign nature of the symptoms will mask more sinister pathology. In most the symptoms are not that serious and can easily be disregarded but, if investigated appropriately and treated judiciously, these young patients can enjoy a significantly improved quality of life.

At the same time, otolaryngological surgeons who treat children must always remember that many symptoms will improve with age and that therefore the indications for any treatment, especially surgery, need to be very carefully considered. It is the balance between watchful waiting and appropriate intervention that is at the heart of successful treatment of paediatric otolaryngological conditions.

An *infant* with bilateral choanal atresia will obstruct and desaturate without making any attempt to open the mouth and use a perfectly good alternative oral airway. Infants thus rely on a patent nasal airway to survive; they are obligate nasal breathers. If an alternative airway is provided, such as a nasal stent or tracheostomy, they develop normally without the other nasal functions of humidification and smell. For the infant, nasal discharge is only relevant in that it obstructs an already small airway.

Older children are seldom, if ever, at risk merely through nasal obstruction, though severe sleep apnoea will occur if nasal obstruction is combined with significant oropharyngeal obstruction. More often children complain of the annoyance of nasal obstruction and resultant mouth breathing with only occasional complaints of hyposmia. Nasal discharge is more of a

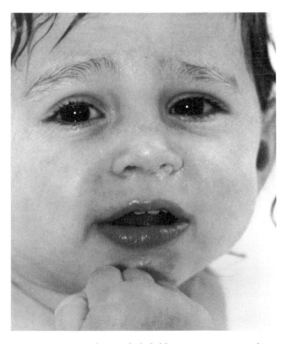

Figure 17.1 Typical catarrhal child – so common as to be considered normal?

problem for parents than for children. This is particularly true in the USA where access to child care facilities can be denied to children with nasal discharge and this will have a major impact on working mothers.

As aetiology and management differ between infants and children, this chapter first covers history, examination and investigation together but then separates the management of conditions found in infancy from those in childhood (Table 17.1).

Table 17.1 The causes of nasal obstruction and rhinorrhoea in infants and older children

	Infants	Older children
Congenital		
Skeletal abnormalities		
choanal atresia/stenosis	+	
nasal agenesis/stenosis	+	
cleft palate nose	+	+
Aperts/Crouzons syndromes	+	+
Down's syndrome	+	+
Nasal masses		
dermoid cysts	+	
mucous cysts	+	
meningo-/encephalocoeles	+	
nasal glioma	+	
nasopharyngeal teratomas	+	
haemangiomas	+	+
angiofibroma		+ (boys)
rhabdomyosarcoma		+
Acquired		
Septal deviation/haematoma	+	+
Infective		
viral 'cold'	+	+
snuffles (AIDS, syphilis)	+	
rhinosinusitis		+
Allergic		
allergic rhinitis	+	+ + +
allergic polyps		+
Non-allergic rhinitis		+
Adenoid hypertrophy	Seldom	+ + +
Foreign bodies		+ (unilateral)
Idiopathic		
Neonatal rhinitis	+ +	
Pubertal rhinitis		+
Associated with general paediatric disease		
Specific diseases		
cystic fibrosis		+
sickle cell		+
immotile cilia syndrome		+
immune deficiency	?	+

Most snuffly babies have idiopathic neonatal rhinitis, while most catarrhal children have a mixture of allergic rhinitis and adenoid hypertrophy. It is important however to exclude other causes.

History

To obtain the maximum useful information from a paediatric consultation, it is imperative that the parents and child feel at ease. This involves reducing waiting times, making waiting and consultation rooms child friendly and allowing the child to become used to the doctor. The clinic nurse, who can amuse patients and siblings, is invaluable in allowing time to obtain an accurate history from the parent. In younger children examination should be incorporated into play and may have to be performed as opportunities arise rather than to a set rote (Table 17.2).

Table 17.2 The symptoms associated with nasal obstruction and rhinorrhoea in infants and older children

	Infants	Older children
Sleep disturbance	+	+ *
waking	+	
recession	+	
struggling	+	
inability to settle	+	
apnoeas	+	
stertor	+	
snoring	+	+ *
Feeding difficulties	+	
Poor growth	+	
Nasal discharge	+	+
Mouth breathing	+	+
Inability to blow nose		+

* Sleep disturbance and snoring in older children are often due to a combination of nasal, nasopharyngeal and oropharyngeal obstruction.

In *infancy* the severity of airway obstruction is judged by the degree of disturbance of sleep, feeding and growth. These parameters distinguish infants with significant nasal obstruction from the many snuffly babies whose nasal obstruction and rhinorrhoea is benign. Parents can often accurately describe waking, struggling to breathe and an inability to settle, apnoeas, soft tissue recession or stertor. A useful question to ask the parent is if they are worried by the infant's sleep pattern. You may find that many parents insist on their baby sleeping in the same room for fear of cot death. It is often difficult to distinguish stridor and stertor on history and one may often have to resort to a quick impersonation of each!

Infants have disturbed feeding for many reasons but if the infant keeps 'coming up for air' during feeds, this implies nasal obstruction. Feeding at a time of airway obstruction may be associated with air swallowing and 'colic'. It is important to be aware that severe airway obstruction can result in failure to thrive, though there are many other causes. Where airway obstruction appears to be the sole cause in the first year of life, the mechanism is more likely to be due to increased energy expenditure rather than any disturbance of growth hormone secretion as growth in this age group is relatively independent of growth hormone.

In *older children* the symptoms are often less dramatic. While sleep disturbance can occur, it is often due to a combination of nasopharyngeal and oropharyngeal obstruction. The intensity of snoring is irrelevant in assessing airway obstruction, it is the periodicity and pauses which imply significant sleep disturbance. Audio tapes (Potsic, 1987) can be computer analysed to provide objective evidence of sleep disturbance without admitting the child. Ask about sleep during colds as nasal secretions will make all forms of upper airway obstruction worse.

Fixed unilateral nasal obstruction suggests a deviated nasal septum, possibly following an injury. During the day, mouth breathing due to nasal obstruction may concern parents and teachers more than the child. Rhinorrhoea similarly may be of little concern to children, though they tend to be teased about this more than mouth breathing. Thin, clear discharge is usually from a viral cold or due to allergic or perennial rhinitis while thick discoloured secretions do not necessarily imply bacterial infection. A foul smelling unilateral discharge strongly suggests a foreign body. With children aged 4–5 years, it is important to ask if they can effectively blow their nose. A family or patient history of asthma or eczema may suggest atopy. Ask about family pets in a way that does not suggest to the child that their favourite guinea-pig is about to 'disappear'. Many children will have been started on medication by their general practitioners prior to referral but it is important to determine if the patient was compliant before deciding that a particular treatment has been ineffective.

Examination

Infants should initially be observed without interference to assess the respiratory pattern, soft tissue recession, use of accessory muscles and the timing and character of any stertor. Even an infant with bilateral choanal atresia can breathe well if it is crying enthusiastically.

Auscultation with a stethoscope bell, observing misting patterns on a cold surface (Figure 17.2) and watching wisps of cotton wool move in the airstream are three complementary methods of assessing air flow. Gentle suction of nasal secretions is very helpful prior to examination using a modern halogen bulb fibreoptic otoscope. Misting can be reduced by cleaning the lens with soapy water or using a demisting agent. If there is no obvious mass causing nasal obstruction and secretions have been cleared, a soft catheter should be passed to determine choanal patency. In a child with recession, this test should only be performed with support available as the airway may be further compromised. Inability to pass catheters does not prove that the obstruction is at the choanae.

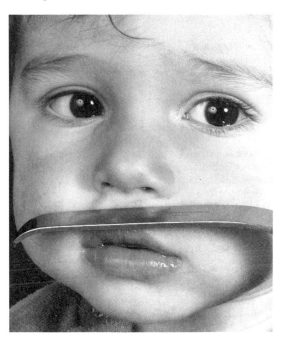

Figure 17.2 Observing misting patterns on a cold surface

Infants are often reluctant to open their mouths unless crying which tends to distort the view of the oropharynx and in particular the relative size of the tongue and the postnasal space. Occasionally a nasopharyngeal polyp may be seen hanging behind the palate.

In *children*, elevation of the nasal tip combined with headmirror illumination is preferable to using a nasal speculum. This can be supplemented by the use of the otoscope to obtain a magnified view of the anterior nares. A video-otoscope can also be used to examine the anterior nares and has the advantage that the child's cooperation is improved and abnormalities can be demonstrated to the parent. The video-otoscope (Jedmed instrument company, England) is described in the chapter on examination (see Chapter 1).

Investigations

Invasive investigations should always be used sparingly in children in order to retain a good child/doctor relationship. Fortunately a provisional diagnosis can often be arrived at from the history and examination without recourse to investigations and treatment started on the basis of this. If investigations are undertaken, they must be interpreted cautiously. X-rays of the sinuses and of the adenoids, for example, have a relatively low clinical correlation.

Radiology and ultrasound

The problem with X-raying children's sinuses is that a child with primarily allergic rhinitis can be labelled as having bacterial sinusitis on the basis of an abnormal X-ray. A clear Water's view will provide reassurance for parent and doctor alike that no intervention is required. Mucosal thickening is interpreted by most as part of allergic rhinosinusitis. An opaque antrum however, does not necessarily mean that bacterial infection is present and in one study bacterial infection was only found in 70% of patients with opaque sinus radiographs (Arruda *et al.*, 1990).

Computerized tomography (CT) provides much more information and is essential if functional endoscopic sinus surgery is being considered. The very sensitivity of the technique requires care in interpretation as CT abnormalities are often identified as an incidental finding in asymptomatic children. In one study, 41% of scans of asymptomatic children showed some mucosal thickening or opacification in at least one sinus (Lesserson, Kieserman and Finn, 1994). As a single Water's view detects maxillary sinus opacification or fluid level in 76% of cases when compared with CT (Garcia *et al.*, 1994), plain X-ray is more appropriate than a CT scan in the initial assessment of the chronic rhinitic who does not respond to simple medical treatment.

Ultrasound examination of the sinuses has the advantage not only of avoiding ionizing radiation, but also patient cooperation is easier as the child does not have to sit as still as for a conventional radiograph. Interpretation, however, does require considerable experience.

X-ray examination of the postnasal space (Figure 17.3) to determine adenoid size and postnasal airway correlates poorly with the size of adenoids at operation (Cohen, Koltai and Scott, 1992; Wormald and Prescott, 1992). In one study a better correlation was obtained with obstructive symptomatology (Wormald and Prescott, 1992).

Nasal swabs and nasal smears

While copious mucus can be obtained relatively easily, *bacteriology* is not usually useful in diagnosis or treatment. A smear from the turbinate can be processed to demonstrate *eosinophilia*, but the slide needs to be stained immediately and even the presence of a heavy eosinophilia does not confirm allergy, e.g. non-allergic eosinophilic rhinitis.

Cilial function

Brushings for cilial motility are easier to manage in an outpatient setting than biopsies because of the risk of haemorrhage. Children over the age of 6 years will usually cooperate with saccharine transport tests.

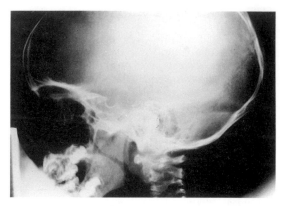

Figure 17.3 Clinical observation is better than postnasal X-ray in assessing the effect of adenoid size

Blood tests

A full blood count, even if it demonstrates eosinophilia, is seldom helpful in changing management of rhinitic children. A *radioallergosorbent test* (RAST) is less sensitive than skin testing and is expensive. As with skin testing, it may merely confirm the suspected allergen for which avoidance may be impractical or impossible. Immunoglobulin assay and in particular, *immunoglobulin subclass* estimation is, however, very valuable in children who have medically recalcitrant bacterial sinusitis. Demonstration of a degree of immune deficiency can prompt successful treatment with prophylactic antibiotics and also provides an explanation for the parents as to why their child has repeated infection.

Skin tests

Skin testing which is quick, easy and effective in adults is not popular in children, though they do appear to be safe with no deaths reported in a 4-year period in the USA (Reid *et al.*, 1993).

Rhinomanometry

Unlike lateral radiographs, *anterior rhinomanometry* correlates well with the size of adenoids at operation (Fielder, 1985; Kohli Dang and Crysdale, 1986), as does *acoustic rhinometry* (Elbrond *et al.*, 1991; Fisher *et al.*, 1995). This experimental technique (Figure 17.4) is less accurate in the nasopharynx with errors of 17% compared with errors of 3% in the nasal cavity (Lenders, Scholl and Brunner, 1992). If suitable portable hardwear could be developed, this non-invasive technique could have a place in the assessment of the paediatric nasal airway. Anterior rhinomanometry however, is probably not of clinical use in children as it is difficult and time consuming (Parker, Maw and Powell, 1989).

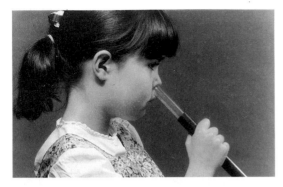

Figure 17.4 Acoustic rhinometry would be easier to use in clinical practice if the equipment could be made more compact

Sleep studies

Polysomnography is routinely used to detect periods of apnoea and oxygen desaturation while *sleep nasendoscopy* is useful for revealing the site of an obstruction (Croft *et al.*, 1990).

Management of neonatal conditions

While most children will have idiopathic neonatal rhinitis, some will have obvious congenital abnormalities and, in a few, investigation will reveal unexpected abnormalities.

Congenital syndromes

In the many craniofacial syndromes, patients will have nasal obstruction and even choanal atresia as part of the syndrome and initial management may require insertion of an *oral airway* (Handler, 1985). Subsequent treatment may be with the placement of a *nasopharyngeal airway* (see Figure 17.4) or even *long nasal stents* (Figure 17.5) which provide a more secure alternative. A large number of syndromes have, as either a frequent or occasional component, abnormalities that are significant in terms of nasal obstruction such as hypoplastic nares, choanal atresia and maxillary or malar hypoplasia with micrognathia (Smith, 1982).

Congenital masses

Morgan and Evans (1990) reviewed a 10-year series of congenital nasal anomalies other than choanal atresia. Of the 50 cases that underwent surgery there were two nasopharyngeal cysts, four hairy polyps, two meningoencephalocoeles, seven gliomas (Figures 17.6 and 17.7), 20 dermoids (Figure 17.8), two capillary haemangiomas, four fibromas, one fibromyxoma, one mucocoele, one granuloma, one

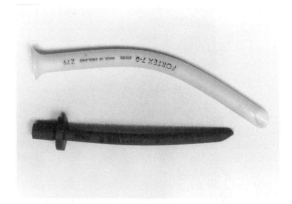

(*a*)

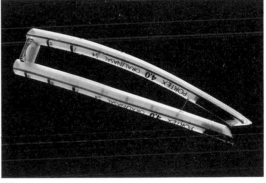

(*b*)

Figure 17.5 (*a*), (*b*) Nasopharyngeal airways and long nasal stents for nasopharyngeal obstruction. Note that the retaining suture exits through a hole in the stent to pass around the vomer

lipoma, two nasal aplasias, two nasal clefts and one nasal web. CT or MRI investigation is mandatory prior to surgery to assess *intracranial connection*. Midline nasal dermoids should be removed with an incision other than a simple midline incision as this leaves a very poor scar (MacGregor and Geddes, 1993). Haemangiomas, if detected preoperatively, can usually be left to resolve spontaneously by the time the child is 5 years of age with the occasional use of steroids if indicated.

Nasal septum

A severely deviated nasal septum can occasionally cause significant nasal obstruction in neonates. The reported prevalence varies from 1.9% (Sorri *et al.*, 1990), 6% (Alpini *et al.*, 1986) to 58% (Gray, 1978). The wide variation reflects the subjective nature of assessment of septal deviation. Controversy exists, however, as to whether these abnormalities will correct spontaneously with growth and moulding (Sorri

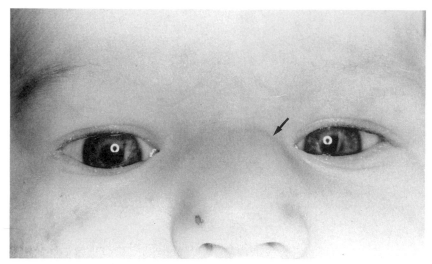

Figure 17.6 Nasal glioma displacing left nasal bone

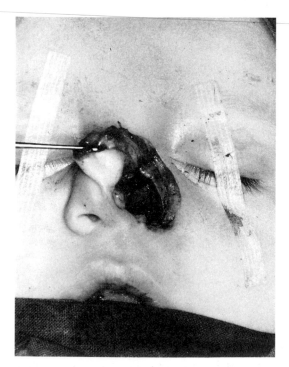

Figure 17.7 Glioma being excised via a lateral rhinotomy

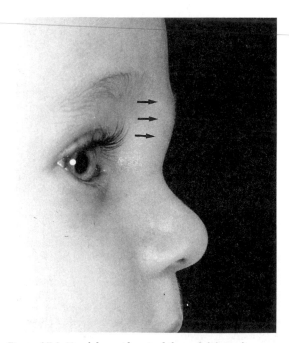

Figure 17.8 Nasal dermoid excised through bilateral
Howarth's incisions

et al., 1990) or whether more active treatment is
required. Sorri *et al.* (1990) found no difference between a group of neonates whose septa were straight-
ened after birth and a group who were left alone.
Gray (1978, 1983) recommended simple replacement
of the septum in the midline without anaesthetic
while for more severe abnormalities, Healey (1986)
suggested a sublabial approach. Other than in exceptional circumstances, neonatal septal deviations
should be observed (Figure 17.9).

Choanal atresia

Patients with bilateral choanal atresia require an
oral airway prior to definitive surgery. A CT scan

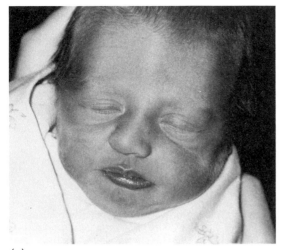

(a)

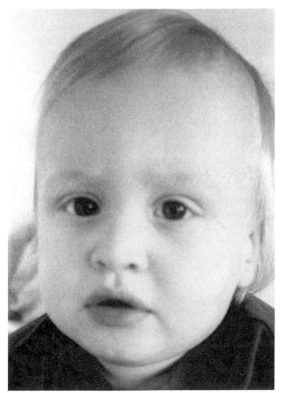

(b)

Figure 17.9 (a) Nasal septal deviation at birth and (b) at 16 months after *no* treatment

after nasal suction and vasoconstriction is helpful but not mandatory in experienced hands. Transnasal drilling of the choanae under video control, using a 120° telescope provides the best chances of success.

Drilling should be undertaken even if the stenosis appears membranous and stents should be left in place for at least 6 weeks to prevent restenosis.

Nasal stenosis

Recently, congenital nasal *pyriform aperture stenosis* (Bignault and Castillo, 1994) has been recognized; this is a CT diagnosis usually discovered in a child being assessed for choanal atresia. *Congenital nasal stenosis* has similarly only been reported recently with a reduced transverse width of the bony nasal passage, again seen on CT (Koga *et al.*, 1993).

Syphilitic neonatal rhinitis

Thin discharge starts in the third week and then becomes purulent with crusting around the nares. As this can also occur with non-specific infections, access to the mother's prenatal screening (with permission) will usually rule out this rare cause of snuffly babies.

Chlamydial rhinitis

One of the few occasions when nasal bacteriology will be helpful is if it demonstrates the intracellular parasite *Chlamydia trachomatis* acquired during vaginal delivery.

Idiopathic neonatal rhinitis

A number of neonates will have significant nasal obstruction and discharge for no obvious cause. Some may have a bacterial or allergic basis (Tolley, Ford and Commins, 1992), while other authors have suggested that there may be a deficiency in autonomic control (Teoh, Fox and Matthews, 1992). There is also an association with gastro-oesophageal reflux (Wang *et al.*, 1993) though it is always difficult to determine which is the primary phenomenon as low negative intrathoracic pressures from upper airway obstruction may predispose to gastro-oesophageal reflux. Many of these patients will benefit from simple extraction of nasal mucus using a *nasal mucus sucker* (Figure 17.10) and the administration of beclomethasone nose drops sometimes combined with neomycin. Very occasionally turbinate oedema and excess secretions are sufficiently severe that nasal stents need to be placed to provide an airway.

Management of general childhood conditions

General paediatric disease can affect the nose and sinuses, and once diagnosed may require close collaboration with the relevant paediatric specialist.

Immune deficiency in children, if severe, may present

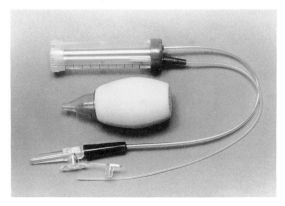

Figure 17.10 Nasal mucus suckers; trap specimen type and bulb syringe type

with rhinitis/rhinosinusitis as part of a spectrum of other infections but if less severe, the sinonasal lining may be the only area affected. Lack of history of generalized infections does not rule out immune deficiency and is not a reason for failing to test for immunoglobulins and immunoglobulin subclasses in a child with recalcitrant rhinitis. Many of these less severely deficient children can be helped with prophylactic antibiotics (Barlan, Geha and Schneider, 1993; Gandhi, Brodsley and Ballow, 1993) though the safety of co-trimoxazole, which is very effective, has recently been questioned. Very rarely treatment will be required with replacement gamma globulin.

Cystic fibrosis

This generalized condition primarily affects the lungs but also affects the sinuses and to a lesser extent the ears. Polyps are present in 45% of children over 5 years of age and there is CT evidence of sinusitis in 12% of children between 3 months and 8 years of age (Brihaye *et al.*, 1994). Taking a slightly older age group Triglia *et al.* (1993) demonstrated CT abnormalities in all patients. There is quite a variation in how severe an effect the general disease has on the nose and some patients do not develop polyps until quite late. There is no genetic difference between the mild and severe cases (Bautsch *et al.*, 1988), nor is there a difference in antral washout cultures or in atopy (Drake Lee and Morgan, 1989). Medical treatment with a topical nasal steroid such as beclomethasone or fluticasone should be used in mild cases of polyposis (Donaldson and Gillespie, 1988) though some authors feel that medical treatment is universally ineffective (Triglia *et al.*, 1993). Simple nasal polypectomy combined with external or internal ethmoidectomy and the Caldwell-Luc operation has been the mainstay of treatment for many years (Cepero *et al.*, 1987; Crockett *et al.*, 1987; Triglia *et al.*, 1993)

though many would now see cystic fibrosis as one of the key indications for functional endoscopic sinus surgery in children (Cuyler and Monaghan, 1989; Jones, Parsons and Cuyler, 1993). These cases can prove challenging for extensive endoscopic functional surgery because of the grossly disordered nasal anatomy. An 'endoscopic polypectomy' appears to last longer than conventional polypectomy.

Immotile cilia syndrome

The inability of cilia to transport mucus affects the lungs causing bronchiectasis in 29% of patients as well as causing sinusitis and otitis in 100% and nasal polyps in 29% (Turner *et al.*, 1981). Situs inversus, which is a feature of Kartagener's syndrome, occurs in 49% of patients with immotile cilia syndrome. While isotopes can be used to measure nasal mucociliary transport (Escribano *et al.*, 1993), saccharine transport times are easy to perform in the clinic. Although many would advocate medical treatment for ciliary dyskinesia, Parsons and Greene (1993) reported good results from functional endoscopic sinus surgery.

Sickle cell disease

Obstructive sleep apnoea secondary to adenotonsillar hypertrophy in these patients is particularly important as it may predispose to vasculo-occlusive episodes. The adenotonsillar hypertrophy is part of the body's response to the disease rather than to infection. While it is important to relieve obstruction with adenotonsillectomy, this must be done safely with preoperative transfusion to decrease the body's own erythropoiesis and decrease the concentration of HbS to less than 30% (Derkay *et al.*, 1991). Given these precautions, adenotonsillectomy is safe and effective in the patient with sickle cell disease (Sidman and Fry, 1988; Maddern *et al.*, 1989).

Down's syndrome

Abnormalities during sleep studies have been demonstrated in 100% of children with Down's syndrome with true obstructive sleep apnoea present in 45% (Marcus *et al.*, 1991.) Adenotonsillectomy helped all of the patients in this study though Strome (1986) suggested that the obstruction is due more to the craniofacial make up and a small postnasal space than to the size of the tonsils.

Pubertal rhinitis

Intermittent nasal obstruction and even rhinorrhoea can occur during puberty (Taylor, 1973). Reassurance is usually all that is required but ipratropium bromide will help the rhinorrhea though not the obstruction.

Management of specific childhood conditions of the nose and sinuses

Adenoids

The concept of *adenoiditis* is not as well accepted or as widely discussed as tonsillitis. However, most adenoids removed at operation are infected (Brodsky and Koch, 1993; Forsgren *et al.*, 1993). Interestingly the predominant flora is *Haemophilus influenzae*, irrespective of whether the adenoids were thought to be infected or merely hypertrophic. This hypertrophic response of adenoids to chronic bacterial infection in some children probably therefore represents an excessive local immune response.

As with obstructing tonsils, it is not the absolute size of the adenoid which is important, but the size relative to the postnasal space and the airway that is remaining. Objective assessment is difficult because of the limitations of radiology, anterior rhinometry and acoustic rhinometry. A clear parental history of obstruction, mouth breathing and perhaps nocturnal apnoea is anyway more important than pseudo-precise cephalometry. The site of airway obstruction can be placed in the postnasal space if the child is mouth breathing with an obstructed airway despite clear anterior nares. Postnasal mirror examination of the adenoids can be achieved in most children over the age of 6 years but the view is distorted and only a gross assessment of the impact of the adenoids on the airway can be achieved. Sleep nasendoscopy most closely correlates with the clinical situation (Croft *et al.*, 1990).

Few surgeons would perform adenoidectomy on a child whose only symptom was snoring without nasal obstruction and, similarly, almost all would recommend adenoidectomy in a child whose adenoids were contributing to significant obstructive sleep apnoea. The vast majority of patients however fall somewhere between these two extremes and, as always, a balance has to be struck between surgical risks and the benefit to the child. The risk of haemorrhage can be almost eliminated by using a technique of *suction diathermy* (Figure 17.11) and this is very important in a day case setting (Yardley, 1992). The risk of *hypernasality* following surgery is estimated at 1 in 15 000 (Donnelly, 1994). Surgery should be avoided not only if there is an obvious submucous cleft palate or bifid uvula, but also if there is a significant history of nasal regurgitation as an infant. Overall, adenoidectomy is effective (Khalifa *et al.*, 1991) but blind adenoidectomy has the risk of leaving some obstructive tissue behind particularly in the choanae; so-called *choanal adenoids* (Phillips *et al.*, 1989; Donnelly, 1994). The morbidity and mortality are very low though extra care should be taken with cases of obstructive sleep apnoea and these are not suitable to be undertaken as day cases (Price, Hawkins and Kahlstrom, 1993).

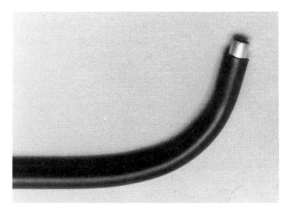

Figure 17.11 Suction diathermy used to remove adenoids under vision and without haemorrhage

Adenoidectomy is also effective in controlling rhinorrhoea though if chronic rhinitis is present as well, medical treatment for this may be necessary before the discharge finally ceases. Overall parents are usually more impressed with the improvement in obstruction than with cessation of rhinorrhoea.

Rhinitis

The response of the nasal lining to inhaled *allergens* and *pollutants* is the commonest cause of chronic rhinitis in children. About 15% will have no obvious allergy but will have eosinophils present on nasal smear. This condition of *eosinophilic non-allergic rhinitis* corresponds to that of intrinsic asthma. In a few children the rhinitis will be a response to drugs or general disease while in others no obvious cause may be found.

Allergic rhinitis

House dust mite faeces have long been considered an important factor in allergic rhinitis though interestingly the number of mites found in the mattresses of rhinitics was no higher than in controls (Pauli *et al.*, 1993). It would seem that it is the body's response to the allergen which is abnormal rather than increased allergen load. With increased environmental awareness there has recently been a lot of interest in the possibility that pollution (Koltai, 1994) acts as an adjuvant in allergic rhinitis. In London in 1994 a temperature inversion retained pollutants and allergens alike in the atmosphere and provoked increased rhinitis and asthma. Traffic density has been shown to correlate with allergic rhinitis (Weiland *et al.*, 1994) but, interestingly, rhinitis was no more common in urban than rural locations (Ross and Fleming, 1994). Ten per cent of school children are thought to have rhinitis (Saval *et al.*, 1993). Weeke (1992) stated that 90% of children with rhinitis are allergic with pollen being the commonest of a number of factors. Linna, Kokkonen and Lukin (1992) showed that the prognosis for rhinitis in children was quite poor with some symptoms present in 90% of patients 10 years later. Fifty per cent were managing without medication though this may represent poor compliance rather than a change in the disease. Perennial rhinitis became seasonal and vice versa.

Infective rhinosinusitis

As the nasal lining is continuous with that of the sinus, the distinction between rhinitis and sinusitis is difficult and somewhat artificial. No clear difference between rhinitis and sinusitis was demonstrated on history, examination, X-ray, ultrasound or sinus washings in one study (Van Buchem, Peeters and Knottnerus, 1992).

Acute viral rhinitis is common, while bacterial infections are sited primarily in the sinuses or ad-enoids. The common cold is usually caused by a rhinovirus but may also be caused by adenovirus or coxsackievirus A or B. Specific nasal infections such as diphtheria and tuberculosis are now seen very rarely.

Eosinophilic non-allergic rhinitis

In these patients the nasal symptoms of congestion, rhinorrhoea, itching and sneezing may well suggest allergy but the symptoms do not fluctuate with allergen exposure and skin tests are negative. Eosinophils will be seen on a nasal smear but the serum IgE will be normal or low. There is an increased incidence of nasal polyps as well as of intrinsic asthma.

Medical treatment of childhood rhinitis
(Table 17.3)

The vast majority of rhinitic children are allergic. Much has been done in the past to identify the

Table 17.3 Treatment of nasal obstruction and rhinorrhoea in infants and children

Medical		*Surgical*	
Allergen avoidance/reduction		Adenoidectomy	Effective
Plastic covers for mattress			
Damp dusting		Turbinate surgery	
Ascarides (chemicals that kill house dust mite)	Often *less* effective than one would hope	Submucous surgery	Short lived
Freeze duvets, pillows and toys for 6–24 hours		Antroconchopexy	
		Turbinate trim	Significant haemorrhage possible
Keep pets out of bedroom		Total turbinectomy	
Hyposensitization		Polypectomy	
		Endoscopic	Probably superior to conventional removal
Nasal suction			
Portable electric sucker		With headlight illumination	
Trap type nasal sucker			
Bulb syringe	Very useful for snuffly infants	Sinus surgery	
Maternal oral suction (popular in Nigeria)		Antral washouts	Overused
		Inferior antrostomy	Non-physiological drainage
Saline nasal drops			Requires training – rarely needed
		Functional endoscopic surgery	
Vasoconstrictors			Minimal interference until growth has stopped
Topical		Septal surgery	
oxymetazoline	Limit use to 1 week because of rebound	Septoplasty	
ephedrine		Submucous resection	
Systemic: pseudoephedrine			
Cromoglycate	q.d.s. dosage – ?compliance		
Steroid nasal drops/spray	?Concerns re growth		
Non-sedating antihistamines	Helps drip more than blockage		
Short courses of antibiotics	Discharge recurs		
Prophylactic antibiotics	Diarrhoea/thrush/? safety		
Immunoglobulin replacement	Rarely necessary		
Homeopathic medicine	Some parents are keen		

allergens from history and skin tests and then to recommend allergy avoidance and a course of hyposensitization. While skin testing is essentially safe, there were 17 deaths in the USA between 1985 and 1989 associated with this technique. This relates to a total of 1–2 million doses (Reid *et al.*, 1993). Appreciation of the risks and disillusionment with the results other than perhaps with house dust mite and pollen desensitization have steered many practitioners away from hyposensitization. Oral hyposensitization which is thought to have less risk, has been shown to be successful though prolonged courses are necessary (Giovane *et al.*, 1994; Ukai *et al.*, 1994). Other than avoiding contact with animals, reducing allergen contact with house dust mite and pollen has proved much more difficult and less successful. Using chemicals to kill the house dust mite may reduce the live mite population but will be ineffective if the quantity of mite faeces left in bedding remains (Brown and Merrett, 1991; Mezei, Cserhati and Pusztai, 1994).

The new non-sedating antihistamines (terfenadine, astemizole, loratadine) have certainly found a place in the treatment of childhood as well as adult allergic rhinitis (Wood, 1992; Simons *et al.*, 1994). The topical antihistamine azelastine, which has created a lot of interest in the adult literature is yet to be licensed for use in children (Grossman *et al.*, 1994; Storms *et al.*, 1994). Levocabastine is an H1 receptor antagonist which can be used topically and which may become available for use in paediatric allergic rhinitis (Janssens, 1992).

Topical vasoconstrictors cause rebound vasodilatation and are thought to be associated with rhinitis medicamentosa, although a true cause and effect has never been proven. Systemic pseudoephedrine is popular and effective.

An array of competing topical nasal steroids provides the back bone of therapy for adult allergic rhinitis but have always been treated with some caution in children because of conflicting reports as to their potential for affecting axial growth (Balfour Lynn, 1986; Bisgaard *et al.*, 1988; Wolthers and Pedersen, 1993). Children who are also taking inhaled steroids for asthma are at particular risk, but in the correct dosage children taking once a day preparations such as fluticasone are probably not at risk.

Inhaled cromoglycate, though effective, needs to be taken four times a day which is unrealistic for the long-term treatment of most school children.

If nasal obstruction and rhinorrhoea are a problem, initial therapy with once a day topical nasal steroid is appropriate, while if rhinorrhoea is the presenting complaint antihistamines or systemic pseudoephedrine can be tried. If parents have great reluctance to use steroid preparations or if the patient is already on inhaled steroids for asthma, cromoglycate can be tried but encouragement towards effective compliance is essential. Table 17.4 summarizes the doses of the more commonly used drugs.

Surgical treatment of childhood rhinitis
(Table 17.3)

In medically recalcitrant nasal obstruction due to allergic and non-allergic rhinitis with significant *turbinate hypertrophy*, surgery to the turbinates can have a dramatic and long lasting beneficial effect on the nasal airway. Turbinate surgery remains controversial because of the possible complications. The concerns of rhinitis sicca are unfounded but even simple submucous diathermy can occasionally result in significant haemorrhage (von Haacke and Hardcastle, 1985; Ophir *et al.*, 1992). Over zealous diathermy can result in a two-stage turbinectomy (Williams, Fisher and Golding Wood, 1991). Total turbinectomy (Ophir, Shapira and Marshak, 1985) not only carries a significant risk of haemorrhage but also the postoperative course is complicated by crusting and bleeding for some time. Cryosurgery to the turbinates (Scheeren *et al.*, 1993), especially with a smaller instrument (Williamson, Timms and Canty, 1988) seems to be as effective as conventional turbinectomy but without the risk of haemorrhage. Similar claims are made for laser turbinectomy (Fukutake *et al.*, 1986). The almost historical operation of antroconchopexy (Figure 17.12), in which the turbinate is swung into an inferior antrostomy has similarly swung out of fashion though the risk of haemorrhage was small and the airway much improved.

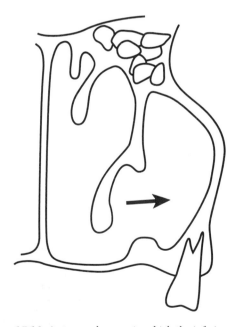

Figure 17.12 Antroconchopexy, in which the inferior turbinate is fractured laterally into an inferior antrostomy

Table 17.4 Paediatric doses and age limits

	Drug	Dose	Age
Antihistamines *(Non-sedating)*	Astemizole	10 mg daily 5 mg daily	Over 12 years 6–12 years
	Loratadine	10 mg daily 5 mg daily	Over 12 years or over 30 kg Over 2 years but under 30 kg
	Terfenadine	60 mg b.d. 30 mg b.d. 15 mg b.d.	Over 12 years 6–12 years 3–6 years
(Sedating)	Brompheniramine	4 mg at bedtime 2 mg	6–12 years 3–6 years
(Topical)	Azelastine	1 spray b.d.	Not yet recommended in children
Systemic antibiotics	Amoxycillin	250 mg t.d.s. 125 mg t.d.s. 10–20 mg/kg/dose t.d.s.	Over 10 years Children up to 10 years Accurate dose helps avoid diarrhoea
	Co-amoxiclav	250/125 mg tabs t.d.s. 250/62 (5 ml) t.d.s. 125/31 (5 ml) t.d.s. 125/31 0.8 ml/kg/day	Over 12 years 6–12 years 1–6 years Under 1 year
	Erythromycin	250–500 mg q.d.s. 250 mg q.d.s. 125 mg q.d.s.	Over 8 years 2–8 years Up to 2 years
Topical nasal steroids + topical cromoglycate	Beclomethasone Betamethasone drops	2 sprays b.d. 2 drops b.d./t.d.s.	Children over 6 years Avoid prolonged use especially in small children
	Budesonide Flunisolide	2 sprays b.d. 2 sprays b.d./t.d.s. 1 spray b.d./t.d.s.	Children over 12 years Children over 12 years Children over 5 years
	Fluticasone	1–2 sprays o.d. 1 spray o.d.	Children over 12 years Children 5–12 years
	Cromoglycate 4%	1 spray q.d.s.	Adults and children
Topical nasal decongestants	Ephedrine 0.5% Oxymetazoline 0.05% Xylometazoline 0.1% Xylometazoline 0.05%	1–2 drops t.d.s. 1 spray t.d.s. 2–3 drops t.d.s. 1–2 drops b.d.	Caution in infants under 3 months Adults and children over 5 years Not under 12 years Not under 3 months
Systemic nasal decongestants	Pseudoephedrine elixir	10 ml t.d.s. 5 ml t.d.s. 2.5 ml t.d.s.	Over 12 years 6–12 years 2–5 years

From: British National Formulary. Lower age limits are recommendations which are sometimes 'stretched'. o.d., once daily; b.d., twice daily; t.d.s., three times a day; q.d.s., four times a day.

Sinusitis

Acute bacterial sinusitis is relatively common and responds to decongestants and antibiotics in almost all cases without recourse to antral lavage.

Chronic sinusitis refers to a spectrum of disease. There are many children who have long-term radiological sinus abnormalities, either on plain X-ray or CT, associated with rhinorrhoea and minor degrees of pain and headache. Most of these patients will respond to prolonged antibiotics (Wald, 1992; Gandhi, Brodsky and Ballow, 1993; Lund, 1994) and topical nasal steroids as well as simple antral lavage (Manning, 1992).

The controversy that exists at present is what to do with the small proportion of children whose symptoms and radiological abnormalities persist despite maximal medical therapy. Historically, very few children underwent either intranasal or external ethmoidectomy but with the rapid expansion in functional endoscopic sinus surgery it was only a matter of time before some of the experts in the field used these new instruments and techniques in the paediatric population. Certainly their results demonstrate efficacy and safety in skilled hands (Stammberger, 1986a,b; Kennedy *et al.*, 1987; Lusk, 1992; Poole, 1994). The problem as always with paediatric conditions is to know to what extent the condition will be self-limiting. This clearly tips the balance away from invasive surgery especially if the potential risks are serious. At present the vogue for paediatric functional endoscopic sinus surgery in the USA seems to be diminishing (Poole, 1992, 1994; Cotton *et al.*, 1993; Proffitt, 1993). There will always be a place for this surgery in cystic fibrosis and in a few cases of medically resistant symptomatic sinusitis.

Nasal polyps

Nasal polyps (Figure 17.13) can occur in children who do not have cystic fibrosis and normally this occurs in the presence of non-allergenic eosinophilic rhinitis (Yamashita *et al.*, 1989). Most of these polyps respond well to nasal steroids (Drake Lee, 1994) but a proportion of these will be larger antrochoanal polyps (Figures 17.14 and 17.15), perhaps more commonly in children than in adults (Chen, Schloss and Azouz, 1989). These cannot be expected to shrink with even long-term steroid therapy and therefore require surgery.

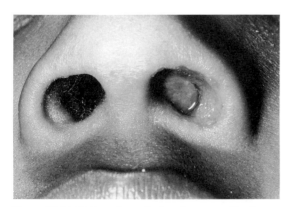

Figure 17.13 Unilateral nasal polyp shown on CT to be antrochoanal

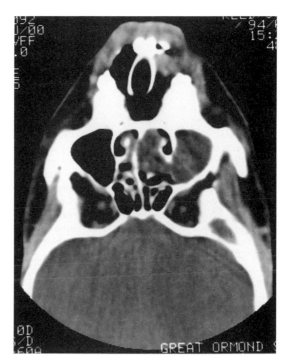

Figure 17.14 Coronal CT demonstrating polyp

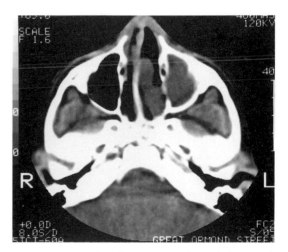

Figure 17.15 Axial CT demonstrating choanal element of polyp

Nasal septal deformities

In neonates the question is whether or not the septum will correct spontaneously. In children there has long been a taboo on early corrective septoplasty because of possible damage to the growth centres. In severe nasal obstruction or where the appearance is such as to create social and psychological difficulties, limited surgery is acceptable after 5 years of age.

Care must be taken to preserve cartilage and in particular to retain support. Even external septorhinoplasty has been shown to be safe and this approach can also be used to access nasal masses in infants as well as children.

Summary

Dealing with children does require a different approach and ideally a different setting from adults. In paediatric nasal obstruction and rhinorrhoea the history and examination are all important so that invasive investigations are required only occasionally.

Much can be done for the snuffly infant even if it is only using a nasal sucker. In older children allergy is the commonest cause of catarrh. While most children can be effectively treated medically, compliance over a long period can be a real problem. Simple surgery such as adenoidectomy is very effective but complex surgery such as functional endoscopic sinus surgery should be reserved for exceptional cases. Never forget that most children will literally 'grow out' of their nasal misbehaviour.

References

ALPINI, D., CORTI, A., BRUSA, E. and BINI, A. (1986) Septal deviation in newborn infants. *International Journal of Pediatric Otorhinolaryngology* 11, 103–107

ARRUDA, L. K., MIMICA, I. M., SOLE, D., WECKX, L. L., SCHOETTLER, J., HEINER, D. C. *et al.* (1990) Abnormal maxillary sinus radiographs in children: do they represent bacterial infection? *Pediatrics*, 85, 553–558

BALFOUR LYNN, L. (1986) Growth and childhood asthma. *Archives of Disease in Childhood*, 61, 1049–1055

BARLAN, I. B., GEHA, R. S and SCHNEIDER, L. C. (1993) Therapy for patients with recurrent infections and low serum IgG3 levels. *Journal of Allergy and Clinical Immunology*, 92, 353–355

BAUTSCH, W., PONELIES, N., DARNEDDE, T., FRYBURG, K., GROTHUES, D. HUNDRIESER, J. *et al.* (1988) The nasal polyps as a tool for basic research in cystic fibrosis. *Scandinavian Journal of Gastroenterology*, 143, (suppl.), 5–8

BIGNAULT, A. and CASTILLO, M. (1994) Congenital nasal piriform aperture stenosis. *American Journal of Neuroradiology*, 15, 877–878

BISGAARD, H., DAMKJAER NIELSEN, M., ANDERSEN, B., ANDERSEN, P., FOGED, N., FUGLSANG, G. *et al.* (1988) Adrenal function in children with bronchial asthma treated with beclomethasone dipropionate or budesonide. *Journal of Allergy and Clinical Immunology*, 81, 1088–1095

BRIHAYE, P., CLEMENT, P. A., DAB, I. and DESPRECHIN, B. (1994) Pathological changes of the lateral nasal wall in patients with cystic fibrosis (mucoviscidosis). *International Journal of Pediatric Otorhinolaryngology*, 28, 141–147

BRODSKY, L. and KOCH, R. J. (1993) Bacteriology and immunology of normal and diseased adenoids in children. *Archives of Otolaryngology – Head and Neck Surgery*, 119, 821–829

BROWN, H. M. and MERRETT, T. G. (1991) Effectiveness of an acaricide in management of house dust mite allergy. *Annals of Allergy*, 67, 25–31

CEPERO, R., SMITH, R. J., CATLIN, F. I., BRESSLER, K. L., FURUTA, G. T. and SHANDERA, K. C. (1987) Cystic fibrosis – an otolaryngologic perspective. *Otolaryngology – Head and Neck Surgery*, 97, 356–360

CHEN, J. M., SCHLOSS, M. D. and AZOUZ, M. E. (1989) Antrochoanal polyp: a 10-year retrospective study in the pediatric population with a review of the literature. *Journal of Otolaryngology*, 18, 168–172

COHEN, L. M., KOLTAI, P. J. and SCOTT, J. R. (1992) Lateral cervical radiographs and adenoid size: do they correlate? *Ear, Nose and Throat Journal*, 71, 638–642

COTTON, R. T., MYER, C. M., SHOTT, S. R. and WILLGING, J. P. (1993) Pediatric sinusitis is not a surgical disease (letter; comment). *Ear, Nose and Throat Journal*, 72, 306

CROCKETT, D. M., MCGILL, T. J., HEALY, G. B., FRIEDMAN, E. M. and SALKELD, L. J. (1987) Nasal and paranasal sinus surgery in children with cystic fibrosis. *Annals of Otology, Rhinology and Laryngology*, 96, 367–372

CROFT, C. B., THOMSON, H. G., SAMUELS, M. P. and SOUTHALL, D. P. (1990) Endoscopic evaluation and treatment of sleep-associated upper airway obstruction in infants and young children. *Clinical Otolaryngology*, 15, 209–216

CUYLER, J. P. and MONAGHAN, A. J. (1989) Cystic fibrosis and sinusitis. *Journal of Otolaryngology*, 18, 173–175

DERKAY, C. S., BRAY, G., MILMOE, G. J. and GRUNDFAST, K. M. (1991) Adenotonsillectomy in children with sickle cell disease. *Southern Medical Journal*, 84, 205–208

DONALDSON, J. D. and GILLESPIE, C. T. (1988) Observations on the efficacy of intranasal beclomethasone dipropionate in cystic fibrosis patients. *Journal of Otolaryngology*, 17, 43–45

DONNELLY, M. J. (1994) Hypernasality following adenoid removal. *Irish Journal of Medical Science*, 163, 225–227

DRAKE LEE, A. B. (1994) Medical treatment of nasal polyps. *Rhinology*, 32, 1–4

DRAKE LEE, A. B. and MORGAN, D. W. (1989) Nasal polyps and sinusitis in children with cystic fibrosis. *Journal of Laryngology and Otology*, 103, 753–755

ELBROND, O., HILBERG, O., FELDING, J. U. and BLEGVAD ANDERSEN, O. (1991) Acoustic rhinometry, used as a method to demonstrate changes in the volume of the nasopharynx after adenoidectomy. *Clinical Otolaryngology*, 16, 84–86

ESCRIBANO, A., ARMENGOT, M., MARCO, V., BASTERRA, J. and BRINES, J. (1993) An isotopic study of nasal mucociliary transport in newborns: preliminary investigation. *Pediatric Pulmonology*, 16, 167–169

FIELDER, C. P. (1985) The effect of adenoidectomy on nasal resistance to airflow. *Acta Otolaryngologica*, 100, 444–449

FISHER, E. W., PALMER, C. R., DALY, N. J. and LUND, V. J. (1995) Acoustic rhinometry in the pre-operative assessment of adenoidectomy candidates. *Journal of Laryngology and Otology*, 109, 503–508.

FORSGREN, J., SAMUELSON, A., LINDBERG, A. and RYNNEL DAGOO, B. (1993) Quantitative bacterial culture from adenoid lymphatic tissue with special reference to *Haemophilus influenzae* age-associated changes. *Acta Otolaryngologica*, 113, 668–672

FUKUTAKE, T., YAMASHITA, T., TOMODA, K. and KUMAZAWA, T. (1986) Laser surgery for allergic rhinitis. *Archives of Otolaryngology – Head and Neck Surgery*, 112, 1280–1282

GANDHI, A., BRODSKY, L. and BALLOW, M. (1993) Benefits of antibiotic prophylaxis in children with chronic sinusitis: assessment of outcome predictors. *Allergy Proceedings*, 14, 37–43

GARCIA, D. P., CORBETT, M. L., EBERLY, S. M., JOYCE, M. R., LE, H. T., KARIBO, J. M. *et al.* (1994) Radiographic imaging studies in pediatric chronic sinusitis. *Journal of Allergy and Clinical Immunology*, **94**, 523–530

GIOVANE, A. L., BARDARE, M., PASSALACQUA, G., RUFFONI, S., SCORDAMAGLIA, A., GHEZZI, E. *et al.* (1994) A three-year double-blind placebo-controlled study with specific, oral immunotherapy to Dermatophagoides: evidence of safety and efficacy in paediatric patients. *Clinical and Experimental Allergy*, **24**, 53–59

GRAY, L. P. (1978) Deviated nasal septum, incidence and etiology. *Annals of Otology, Rhinology and Laryngology*, **87**, 3–20

GRAY, L. P. (1983) The development and significance of septal and dental deformity from birth to eight years. *International Journal of Pediatric Otorhinolaryngology*, **6**, 265–277

GROSSMAN, J., HALVERSON, P. C., MELTZER, E. O., SHOENWETTER, W. F., VAN BAVEL, J. H., WOEHLER, T. R. *et al.* (1994) Double-blind assessment of azelastine in the treatment of perennial allergic rhinitis. *Annals of Allergy*, **73**, 141–146

HANDLER, S. D. (1985) Upper airway obstruction in craniofacial anomalies: diagnosis and management. *Birth Defects*, **21**, 15–31

HEALEY, G. B. (1986) An approach to the nasal septum in children. *Laryngoscopy*, **96**, 1239–1242

JANSSENS, M. M. (1992) Levocabastine: a new topical approach for the treatment of pediatric allergic rhinoconjunctivitis. *Rhinology*, **13** (suppl.), 39–49

JONES, J. W., PARSONS, D. S. and CUYLER, J. P. (1993) The results of functional endoscopic sinus (FES) surgery on the symptoms of patients with cystic fibrosis. *International Journal of Pediatric Otorhinolaryngology*, **28**, 25–32

KENNEDY, D. W., ZINREICH, S. J., SHAALAN, H., KUHN, F., NACLERIO, R. and LOCH, E. (1987) Endoscopic middle meatal antrostomy: theory, technique, and patency. *Laryngoscope*, **97**, 1–9

KHALIFA, M. S., KAMEL, R. H., ZIRKY, M. A. and KANDIL, T. M. (1991) Effect of enlarged adenoids on arterial blood gases in children. *Journal of Laryngology and Otology*, **105**, 436–438

KOGA, K., KAWASHIRO, N., TSUCHIHASHI, N. and ARAKI, A. (1993) Congenital nasal stenosis – new concept and its cases. *Nippon Jibiinkoka Gakkai Kaiho*, **96**, 1869–1877

KOHLI DANG, N. and CRYSDALE, W. S. (1986) Cephalometric radiographs and nasal resistance. *Journal of Otolaryngology*, **15**, 112–115

KOLTAI, P. J. (1994) Effects of air pollution on the upper respiratory tract of children. *Otolaryngology – Head and Neck Surgery*, **111**, 9–11

LENDERS, H., SCHOLL, R. and BRUNNER, M. (1992) Acoustic rhinometry: the bat principle of the nose. *HNO*, **40**, 239–247

LESSERSON, J. A., KIESERMAN, S. P. and FINN, D. G. (1994) The radiographic incidence of chronic sinus disease in the pediatric population. *Laryngoscope*, **104**, 159–166

LINNA, O., KOKKONEN, J. and LUKIN, M. (1992) A 10-year prognosis for childhood allergic rhinitis. *Acta Pediatrica*, **81**, 100–102

LUND, V. J. (1994) Bacterial sinusitis: etiology and surgical management. *Pediatric Infectious Diseases Journal*, **13**, 58–63

LUSK, R. P. (1992) Endoscopic approach to sinus disease. *Journal of Allergy and Clinical Immunology*, **90**, 496–505

MACGREGOR, F. B. and GEDDES, N. K. (1993) Nasal dermoids:

the significance of a midline punctum. *Archives of Disease in Childhood*, **68**, 418–419

MADDERN, B. R., REED, H. T., OHENE FREMPONG, K. and BECKERMAN, R. C. (1989) Obstructive sleep apnea syndrome in sickle cell disease. *Annals of Otology, Rhinology and Laryngology*, **98**, 174–178

MANNING, S. C. (1992) Surgical management of sinus disease in children. *Annals of Otology, Rhinology and Laryngology*, **155** (suppl.), 42–45

MARCUS, C. L., KEENS, T. G., BAUTISTA, D. B., VON PECHMANN, W. S. and WARD, S. L. (1991) Obstructive sleep apnea in children with Down syndrome. *Pediatrics*, **88**, 132–139

MEZEI, G., CSERHATI, E. and PUSZTAI, A. (1994) Effect of a mite-killing agent on house dust and on symptoms of house dust allergy. *Orvosi Hetilap*, **135**, 969–972

MORGAN, D. W. and EVANS, J. N. (1990) Developmental nasal anomalies. *Journal of Laryngology and Otology*, **104**, 394–403

OPHIR, D., SHAPIRA, A. and MARSHAK, G. (1985) Total inferior turbinectomy for nasal airway obstruction. *Archives of Otolaryngology*, **111**, 93–95

OPHIR, D., SCHINDEL, D., HALPERIN, D. and MARSHAK, G. (1992) Long-term follow-up of the effectiveness and safety of inferior turbinectomy. *Plastic and Reconstructive Surgery*, **90**, 980–984

PARKER, A. J., MAW, A. R. and POWELL, J. E. (1989) Rhinomanometry in the selection for adenoidectomy and its relation to preoperative radiology. *International Journal of Pediatric Otolaryngology*, **17**, 155–161

PARSONS, D. S. and GREENE, B. A. (1993) A treatment for primary ciliary dyskinesia: efficacy of functional endoscopic sinus surgery. *Laryngoscope*, **103**, 1269–1272

PAULI, G., QUOIX, E., HEDELIN, G., BESSOT, J. C., OTT, M. and DIETEMANN, A. (1993) Mite allergen content in mattress dust of Dermatophagoides – allergic asthmatics/rhinitics and matched controls. *Clinical and Experimental Allergy*, **23**, 606–611

PHILLIPS, D. E., BATES, G. J., PARKER, A. J., GRIFFITHS, M. V. and GREEN, J. (1989) Digital and mirror assessment of the adenoids at operation. *Clinical Otolaryngology*, **14**, 131–133

POOLE, M. D. (1992) Pediatric sinusitis is not a surgical disease (see comments). *Ear, Nose and Throat Journal*, **71**, 622–623

POOLE, M. D. (1994) Pediatric endoscopic sinus surgery: the conservative view. *Ear, Nose and Throat Journal*, **73**, 221–227

POTSIC, W. P. (1987) Comparison of polysomnography and sonography for assessing regularity of respiration during sleep in adenotonsillar hypertrophy. *Laryngoscope*, **97**, 1430–1437

PRICE, S. D., HAWKINS, D. B. and KAHLSTROM, E. J. (1993) Tonsil and adenoid surgery for airway obstruction: perioperative respiratory morbidity. *Ear, Nose and Throat Journal*, **72**, 526–531

PROFFITT, S. D. (1993) Pediatric sinusitis is not a surgical disease (letter; comment). *Ear, Nose and Throat Journal*, **72**, 306–307

REID, M. J., LOCKEY, R. F., TURKELTAUB, P. C. and PLATTS MILLS, T. A. (1993) Survey of fatalities from skin testing and immunotherapy 1985–1989. *Journal of Allergy and Clinical Immunology*, **92**, 6–15

ROSS, A. M. and FLEMING, D. M. (1994) Incidence of allergic rhinitis in general practice, 1981–92. *British Medical Journal*, **308**, 897–900

SAVAL, P., FUGLSANG, G., MADSEN, C. and OSTERBALLE, O. (1993) Prevalence of atopic disease among Danish school children. *Pediatric Allergy and Immunology*, **4**, 117–122

SCHEEREN, R. A., KEEHNEN, R. M., MEIJER, C. J. and VAN DER BAAN, S. (1993) Defects in cellular immunity in chronic upper airway infections are associated with immunosuppressive retroviral p15E-like proteins. *Archives of Otolaryngology – Head and Neck Surgery*, **119**, 439–443

SIDMAN, J. D. and FRY, T. L. (1988) Exacerbation of sickle cell disease by obstructive sleep apnea. *Archives of Otolaryngology – Head and Neck Surgery*, **114**, 916–917

SIMONS, F. E., REGGIN, J. D., ROBERTS, J. R. and SIMONS, K. J. (1994) Benefit/risk ratio of the antihistamines (H1-receptor antagonists) terfenadine and chlorpheniramine in children. *Journal of Pediatrics*, **124**, 979–983

SMITH, D. W. (1982) Recognizable patterns of human malformation: genetic embryologic and clinical aspects. *Major Problems in Paediatrics*, 3rd edn, edited by K. Lyons Jones. Philadelphia: W. B. Saunders. pp. 723–725

SORRI, M., LAITAKARI, K., VAINIO MATTILA, J. and HARTIKAINEN SORRI, A. L. (1990) Immediate correction of congenital nasal deformities; follow-up of 8 years. *International Journal of Pediatric Otorhinolaryngology*, **19**, 277–283

STAMMBERGER, H. (1986a) Endoscopic endonasal surgery – concepts in treatment of recurring rhinosinusitis. Part I. Anatomic and pathophysiologic considerations. *Otolaryngology – Head and Neck Surgery*, **94**, 143–147

STAMMBERGER, H. (1986b) Endoscopic endonasal surgery – concepts in treatment of recurring rhinosinusitis. Part II. Surgical technique. *Otolaryngology – Head and Neck Surgery*, **94**, 147–156

STORMS, W. W., PEARLMAN, D. S., CHERVINSKY, P., GROSSMAN, J., HALVERSON, P. C., FRIETAG, G. G. et al. (1994) Effectiveness of azelastine nasal solution in seasonal allergic rhinitis. *Ear, Nose and Throat Journal*, **73**, 382–386, 390–394

STROME, M. (1986) Obstructive sleep apnea in Down syndrome children: a surgical approach. *Laryngoscope*, **96**, 1340–1342

TAYLOR, M. (1973) The vasomotor reaction. *Otolaryngologic Clinics of North America*, **6**, 645

TEOH, T. G., FOX, G. P. and MATTHEWS, T. G. (1992) Snuffles in infants – infection or autonomic dysfunction. *Irish Journal of Medical Science*, **161**, 44–45

TOLLEY, N. S., FORD, G. and COMMINS, D. (1992) The management of neonatal rhinitis. *International Journal of Pediatric Otorhinolaryngology*, **24**, 253–260

TRIGLIA, J. M., BELUS, J. F., DESSI, P., NOIRCLERC, M. and CANNONI, M. (1993) Rhinosinusal manifestations of cystic fibrosis. *Annales d'Otolaryngologie et de Chirurgie cirvico faciale*, **110**, 98–102

TURNER, P. J., CORKEY, C. W., LEE, J. Y., LEVISON, H. and STURGESS, J. (1981) Clinical expression of immotile cilia syndrome. *Pediatrics*, **67**, 805–810

UKAI, K., AMESARA, R., MASUDA, S., NAKAMOTO, S., OHKAWA, C., OKAMOTO, K. et al. (1994) The evaluation of hyposensitization with house dust in patients with nasal allergy to house dust-mite. *Arerugi*, **43**, 16–21

VAN BUCHEM, F. L., PEETERS, M. F. and KNOTTNERUS, J. A. (1992) Maxillary sinusitis in children. *Clinical Otolaryngology*, **17**, 49–53

VON HAACKE, N. P. and HARDCASTLE, P. F. (1985) Submucosal diathermy of the inferior turbinate and the congested nose. *Journal of Otorhinolaryngology and Related Specialties*, **47**, 189–193

WALD, E. R. (1992) Antimicrobial therapy of pediatric patients with sinusitis. *Journal of Allergy and Clinical Immunology*, **90**, 469–473

WANG, W., TOVAR, J. A., EIZAGUIRRE, I. and ALDAZABAL, P. (1993) Airway obstruction and gastroesophageal reflux: an experimental study on the pathogenesis of this association. *Journal of Pediatric Surgery*, **28**, 995–998

WEEKE, E. R. (1992) Epidemiology of allergic diseases in children. *Rhinology*, **13** (suppl.), 5–12

WEILAND, S. K., MUNDT, K. A., RUCKMANN, A. and KEIL, U. (1994) Self-reported wheezing and allergic rhinitis in children and traffic density on street of residence. *Annals of Epidemiology*, **4**, 243–271

WILLIAMS, H. O., FISHER, E. W. and GOLDING WOOD, D. G. (1991) 'Two-stage turbinectomy': sequestration of the inferior turbinate following submucosal diathermy. *Journal of Laryngology and Otology*, **105**, 14–16

WILLIAMSON, I. G., TIMMS, M. and CANTY, P. (1988) A new cryoprobe with advantages in turbinate freezing. *Journal of Laryngology and Otology*, **102**, 503–505

WOLTHERS, O. D. and PEDERSEN, S. (1993) Short-term growth in children with allergic rhinitis treated with oral antihistamine, depot and intranasal glucocorticosteroids (see comments). *Acta Paediatrica*, **82**, 635–640

WOOD, S. F. (1992) Clinical experience with non-sedating antihistamines in paediatric allergic rhinitis. *Rhinology*, **13** (suppl.), 27–37

WORMALD, P. J. and PRESCOTT, C. A. (1992) Adenoids: comparison of radiological assessment methods with clinical and endoscopic findings. *Journal of Laryngology and Otology*, **106**, 342–344

YAMASHITA, T., TSUJI, H., MAEDA, N., TOMODA, K. and KUMAZAWA, T. (1989) Etiology of nasal polyps associated with aspirin-sensitive asthma. *Rhinology*, **8** (suppl.), 15–24

YARDLEY, M. P. (1992) Tonsillectomy, adenoidectomy and adenotonsillectomy: are they safe day case procedures? *Journal of Laryngology and Otology*, **106**, 299–300

18

Tonsils and adenoids

David L. Cowan and John Hibbert

Acute tonsillitis

This is a common disorder in children and it is unusual for a child not to have at least one or two episodes of tonsillitis. These attacks are particularly liable to occur when the child is exposed to large numbers of other children for the first time, that is on entering nursery school or primary school.

The bacteriology of acute tonsillitis and the normal flora of the throat in children is interesting and somewhat puzzling. Several studies (Box, Cleveland and Willard, 1961; Reilly *et al.*, 1981; Toner *et al.* 1986) have shown that the culture of throat swabs taken from children with a history of acute tonsillitis does not differ, in terms of organisms cultured, from those taken from normal children. Box, Cleveland and Willard (1961), in a study of normal children and those with recurrent tonsillitis, showed that a high proportion of normal children grow pathogenic organisms from throat swabs. In this series of normal children, 96% of swabs grew *Streptococcus pneumoniae* (pneumococcus), 50% grew *Staphylococcus aureus*, 30% grew *Haemophilus influenzae* and 5% grew a β-haemolytic streptococcus. Similarly, a fair proportion of normal children (10% in a series from Moffett, Siegle and Doyle, 1968) will have viruses present in their throats and also anaerobic organisms (25% in the series of Reilly *et al.*, 1981).

Doubt remains regarding the most common causative organisms in acute tonsillitis in children. It has been stated that a virus infection initiates an attack of tonsillitis and predisposes to a bacterial infection (Everett, 1979). On the other hand, a virus may be the sole agent responsible and adenoviruses, Epstein-Barr virus and herpes simplex virus have been implicated (Sprinkle and Veltri, 1976). Of the bacteria causing acute tonsillitis, β-haemolytic streptococci, *Streptococcus pnemoniae* and *Haemophilus influenzae* are

the most numerous. Stjernquist–Desatnik, Prellner and Schalen (1991) cultured the organisms in the tonsil core of 126 patients with acute tonsillitis and found *Haemophilus influenzae* in 20% and group A streptococci in 17%. Anaerobes have been found to be present in moderate to heavy amounts in about 32% of superficial swabs but their significance is not fully known.

Clinical features

The clinical features of true acute tonsillitis are fairly classical. The onset is abrupt and may be ushered in by a nightmare or shivering attack, followed by pyrexia up to 39°C and pain in the throat. Swallowing is acutely sore and solid food is refused at the height of the inflammation although fluids are usually accepted and must be encouraged. Occasionally febrile convulsions occur. The glands in the neck are usually enlarged and painful. Although this is the classical presentation the problem may present in different ways. The child may often be generally unwell and present with abdominal pain and vomiting. Unless the tonsils are examined the diagnosis may be missed. Otalgia, either referred from the tonsils or as a result of acute otitis media, may on occasions be the presenting feature. Examination of the tonsils will always show a generalized erythematous reaction which may or may not be associated with the appearance of white/yellow beads of purulent exudate in the tonsillar crypts.

Treatment

There is dispute about the appropriate treatment for acute tonsillitis as many physicians will say that due to the possibility of a viral aetiology, antibiotics should be withheld until a swab result is available. In reality a child with acute tonsillitis is ill and requires fluids by mouth, paracetamol in a dose of 10 mg/kg 4–6 hourly, and penicillin. The administration of the penicillin may be intravenous, intramuscular or oral. In seriously ill children the best route is intravenous (10–20 mg/kg daily). In hospital, parenteral administration is easy. At home it is much more difficult and perhaps treatment is best initiated by intramuscular penicillin followed by oral dosage. If the patient is allergic to penicillin, erythromycin (25 mg/kg daily) should be used.

Differential diagnosis

The following alternatives may be seen only rarely but should be borne in mind.

Diphtheria

The Western World has controlled the spread of this disease by vaccination. Diphtheria, however, does still occur and affects principally the 2–3-year-old age group. The onset is insidious and local pain is less of a feature than general prostration from toxaemia. A tough false membrane appears on the tonsils and this may spread to the pharyngeal wall or the larynx. Treatment is by antitoxin, in doses of 10 000–80 000 units depending upon the severity of the disease, and combined with a full course of penicillin or erythromycin.

Infectious mononucleosis

Infectious mononucleosis or glandular fever is due to the Epstein–Barr (EB) virus. Examination of the peripheral blood shows an increase in atypical lymphocytes in a leukocytosis. A positive monospot test will confirm the diagnosis, although it is sometimes negative at the first visit. If clinical suspicion remains it can be repeated a week later. There is no specific treatment apart from rest, analgesics and adequate fluid intake and the disease can run a protracted course. Antibiotics are of little use and ampicillin is directly contraindicated as it causes an extensive skin rash. It is much commoner in older teenage children than in the younger child.

Other blood disorders

Acute lymphatic leukaemia may have an onset in the pharynx. Ulcerative lesions may be found with pur-purpic haemorrhages in the tonsils or buccal and pharyngeal mucosa. The blood picture will usually be diagnostic. Hodgkin's disease may of course affect the lymphoid tissue of the pharynx and show characteristic enlargement of the cervical lymph glands.

Complications of acute tonsillitis

The local complications of acute tonsillitis are discussed in Volume 5 and include respiratory obstruction, peritonsillar and parapharyngeal abscess. In addition, in children, acute otitis media may occur at the same time or be a complication of acute tonsillitis, as may an acute retropharyngeal abscess (see below).

The systemic or general complications of acute tonsillitis are rare and almost confined to childhood. They are discussed below.

Septicaemia

Untreated acute tonsillitis can result in septicaemia with septic abscesses, septic arthritis and meningitis.

Acute rheumatic fever and glomerulonephritis

These are diseases of unknown aetiology and follow infection with a β-haemolytic streptococcus of Lancefield group A. The current belief as to aetiology is that antibodies produced against the streptococcus may, in some instances, cross-react with the patient's own tissues. Thus the effect on the tissue may be an arthritis, an endocarditis or myocarditis, or a dermatitis, and in rheumatic chorea there is inflammation of the cerebral cortex and basal ganglia. In acute glomerulonephritis there is damage to the glomeruli, possibly caused by immune complexes.

The incidence of acute rheumatic fever following streptococcal tonsillitis is variable but in 1950 was of the order of 2% if the tonsillitis was not treated and 0.3% if the tonsillitis had been treated with penicillin (Denny, Wannamaker and Brink, 1950). The incidence of a second attack of rheumatic fever is approximately 60% and this is reduced to 4% if the patient is on long-term prophylactic penicillin (sulphonamides if the patient is allergic to penicillin). Tonsillectomy does not influence the recurrence rate of rheumatic fever in patients who are given adequate prophylactic penicillin and has no place in the management of this condition.

Tonsillectomy has sometimes been advised for children who are not prepared to take antibiotic prophylaxis (Feinstein and Levitt, 1970) but this certainly does not eliminate streptococcal infections. Acute glomerulonephritis does not recur after a single attack although the effects of the attack may be long-standing. Again, tonsillectomy has no place in the management of this condition.

Peritonsillar abscess in children

As stated above this is a rare condition in childhood. In 1981, Holt and Tinsley reported a series of 41 children seen over a 10-year period in San Antonio, Texas. The interesting facts to emerge from this series are that only 15% of the children had a previous history of recurrent tonsillitis and this is the experience in adults with a quinsy. Of the 41 children, 11 had tonsillectomy and of the remaining children only two had a further quinsy. Here again it seems that the chances of having a second quinsy are not very high and certainly do not justify routine tonsillectomy.

Acute retropharyngeal abscess

A collection of pus in the retropharyngeal space occurs in three situations. First, and most commonly in children, it occurs as suppuration in a retropharyngeal lymph node. This is most likely to occur after an upper respiratory tract infection. The other two causes of retropharyngeal abscess are a perforating foreign body (Figure 18.1) or following tuberculous disease of the cervical spine (this produces a chronic retropharyngeal abscess and is discussed in Volume 5).

Clinical features

Acute retropharyngeal abscess is most common in infancy and in young children (up to the age of 5 years) (Figure 18.2). There may have been a previous upper respiratory tract infection and the child with an abscess is pyrexial and ill. There is dysphagia with marked pain on swallowing and the patient may drool saliva. Respiration is somewhat noisy, in part as a result of accumulated secretions, but also because the abscess obstructs the airway and causes oedema of the larynx. The patient often holds the neck rigid and resists attempts to move it. There may be cervical lymphadenopathy or a very large abscess may be palpable in the neck. Examination of the child's throat is difficult, but if the posterior pharyngeal wall can be seen this is erythematous and bulging. A lateral radiography to show the soft tissues of the neck will demonstrate an abscess, initially as an increase in the prevertebral soft tissue shadow but, later, may show an abscess with a fluid level. The dangers of a retropharyngeal abscess are airway obstruction and spread of the infective process to involve the carotid sheath laterally or the mediastinum inferiorly.

Treatment should not be delayed. The child should be started on intravenous penicillin and arrangements made to drain the abscess under general anaesthesia. This is a hazardous general anaesthetic because intubation may be difficult and rupture of the abscess may result in inhalation of infected material into the bronchial tree. Because of these dangers, facilities should be available for emergency laryngotomy or tracheostomy. Tracheostomy may be necessary anyway to safeguard the airway postoperatively if the abscess is large. When the airway has been established the abscess should be drained. This is usually carried out by incising the posterior pharyngeal wall at the point where the abscess seems to be most prominent and breaking down all loculi with artery forceps. In a very large abscess which has extended into the neck, incision of the posterior pharyngeal wall may be insufficient and the abscess may need to be drained through the neck by a cervical incision and dissection medial to the anterior border of the sternomastoid muscle.

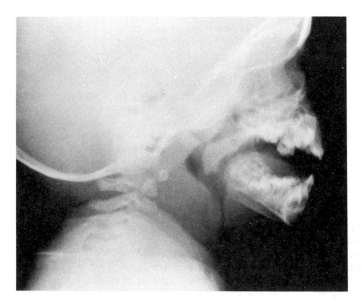

Figure 18.1 Acute retropharyngeal abscess in an infant

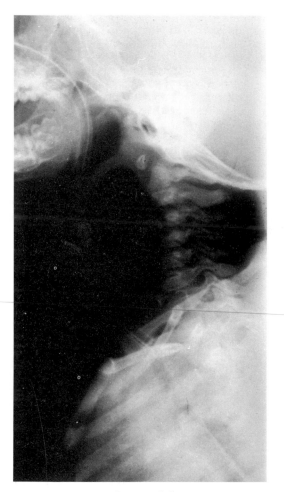

Figure 18.2 Acute retropharyngeal abscess containing gas. The patient has a nasotracheal tube

Diseases of the adenoids

When considering diseases of the adenoids it is as well to remember that the mass of lymphoid tissue in the nasopharynx generally referred to as the adenoids is a normal structure with a definite function, namely the production of antibodies (IgA locally, and IgG and IgM systemically). Many consider it pedantic to insist on the singular expression, the adenoid, so the more common term, adenoids, will be used here.

The size of the adenoids varies from child to child and also in the same individual as she grows. In general, the normal adenoids attain their maximum size between the ages of 3 and 7 years and then regress. What may be important in considering the harmful effects of the adenoids is not the absolute size, but more the size in relation to that of the nasopharynx. The disease processes which affect the adenoids and cause problems are infective. An acute upper respiratory tract infection affects the adenoids and results in hyperplasia with enlargement and multiplication of the lymphoid follicles. It is certainly possible that recurrent acute infections are the sole cause of abnormally large adenoids, although it has been suggested that allergic episodes also result in adenoidal enlargement. It is likely that most of the harmful effects caused by adenoids are related to size, although it is often accepted that they may become chronically infected. There is very little evidence that this occurs and histological studies of adenoidal tissue very rarely show septic foci or microabscesses. They simply show hyperplasia of lymphoid follicles. Chronic adenoiditis is therefore not a proven entity and there is even less evidence for its existence as a clinical condition than for chronic tonsillitis. It is safest when considering diseases of the adenoids to limit discussion to acute infection and to chronic enlargement.

Acute infection

It is only relatively recently that the term acute adenotonsillitis has been used with any frequency, but logically it is inconceivable that the adenoids or tonsils can be acutely infected independently of each other. It is easier to see the tonsils during acute infection which is probably why the term acute tonsillitis is most commonly used, but it is almost certain that the adenoids are infected at the same time. Bacteriological culture of tonsils and adenoids removed from the same patient are very similar indeed (Polvogt and Crowe, 1929). Viral cultures of tonsils and adenoids yield similar results, namely adenoviruses, Epstein-Barr virus and herpes simplex virus (Sprinkle and Veltri, 1976).

Enlargement of the adenoids

As stated above it is the size of the adenoids relative to the nasopharynx that may be important, rather than the actual size. The effects of such enlargement produce impairment of nasal respiration and possible obstruction of the eustachian tube openings.

Nasal obstruction

There is no doubt that large adenoids can partially or totally obstruct nasal respiration causing snoring, hyponasal speech and forcing the child to breathe through the mouth. This is well documented and certainly the experience of all otolaryngologists. Unfortunately there are other causes of nasal obstruction and mouth breathing, and adenoidectomy in these circumstances will be of no benefit. One of the sources of confusion is that a child with an open lip posture, that is with his lips apart at rest, is automatically assumed to be a mouth breather. In fact a number of studies have shown that this is not the case and that an open lip posture may be totally unrelated to respiration. In 1969, Rasmus and Jacobs showed that children clinically assessed as being mouth breathers by virtue of an open lip posture had identical air flow studies to normal children.

Clinical examination of children with nasal obstruction is notoriously unreliable. Examination of the nasal cavities by anterior rhinoscopy may be normal or may show increased secretion, hypertrophy or congestion (hyperaemia or blueness) of the inferior turbinates. Murray (1972) showed a positive statistical correlation between enlarged adenoids and nasal congestion on anterior rhinoscopy, and while this association may be true in some children, these are precisely the appearances on anterior rhinoscopy of children with allergic rhinitis. In some children examination of the nasopharynx with a postnasal mirror will identify large adenoids. Unfortunately in many children it is impossible to assess the adenoids in this way.

The most reliable way of assessing the size of the adenoids is to take a lateral radiograph. This will give a measure of the absolute size of the adenoids and also an assessment of the relation to the size of the airway (Hibbert and Whitehouse, 1978; Maw, Jeans and Fernando 1981; Cohen and Konak, 1985). In an individual child with nasal obstruction, this is the best method of assessing whether adenoidectomy will improve the symptoms (Figures 18.3, 18.4 and 18.5).

Adenoid facies

It is generally stated that a child with enlarged adenoids has a characteristic facial appearance but it is not the authors' view that this is a reliable fact.

The so-called classical appearances include:

1 An open lip posture with prominent upper teeth and a short upper lip. It is not our experience that children with this facial appearance necessarily have enlarged adenoids and in fact persistent thumb sucking or the use of a dummy may be more likely causes.
2 A thin nose with a hypoplastic maxilla, narrow upper alveolus and a high arched palate. There is indeed a group of children who fall into this category but again there is no reliable evidence that enlarged adenoids would on their own cause these changes. Tulley (1964) suggested that these are merely inherited variations of the normal. It is certainly possible that normal sized adenoids in an inherited hypoplastic maxilla may give rise to symptoms whereas this might not occur in a normal maxilla.

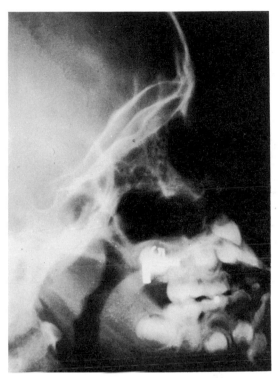

Figure 18.3 Lateral soft tissue radiograph with a normal airway and normal nasopharynx

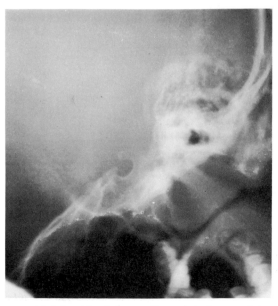

Figure 18.4 Lateral soft tissue radiograph to show partial encroachment of the adenoids on the airway

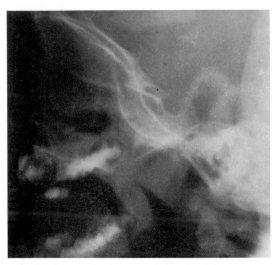

Figure 18.5 Lateral soft tissue radiograph to show apparent total occlusion of the nasopharyngeal airway by the adenoids. There almost certainly is an airway to either side of the main prominence of the adenoids but this, of course, does not show on the radiograph

Effects of adenoids on the ear

This has long been and remains a controversial subject. The classical concept is that enlargement of the adenoids or repeated recurrent infections of the adenoids results in recurrent acute otitis media and of otitis media with effusion (glue ear). It has been demonstrated both by radiological techniques (Bluestone 1971) and by pressure studies (Bluestone, 1975a,b) that adenoids can and do obstruct the eustachian tube and that adenoidectomy relieves the obstruction. As children who have had their adenoids removed still do suffer from acute otitis media and recurrent glue ear they are obviously not the sole cause of the problem.

It is difficult to carry out controlled preoperative trials in children but two studies (Maw, 1983; Bulman, Brook and Berry, 1984) have shown a definite reduction in the recurrence rate of glue ear in children who have had an adenoidectomy. There are, however, other studies (Rynnel-Dagloo, Ahlbom and Schiratzki, 1978; Fiellau-Nicholajsen, Falbe-Hansen and Knudstrup, 1980; Roydhouse, 1980; Widemar *et al.*, 1986) which have suggested that adenoidectomy has no part to play in the treatment of childhood ear problems. It is the authors' experience that, although obviously not the sole cause, removal of the adenoids does help to prevent or reduce the frequency of attacks of otitis media and the incidence of glue ear. Further discussion of the aetiology of glue ear is presented in Chapter 7.

Sleep apnoea

The condition known as sleep apnoea was first described by Gastaut, Tassinari and Duron in 1966, and is characterized by apnoeic episodes during sleep associated with hypersomnolence during the day. In normal children brief episodes of apnoea occur during sleep and definition of the abnormal is difficult. This has been arbitrarily chosen as at least 30 episodes of apnoea lasting 10 seconds or more during 6 hours of sleep. Pathological episodes are associated with hypoxaemia and bradycardia which do not occur in normal children (Tilkian *et al.*, 1976).

Apnoeic episodes may be obstructive, central or mixed. Obstructive apnoea occurs when increasing respiratory effort produces no airflow; central apnoea occurs when respiratory effort ceases and the defect is in the central control mechanism, either in the brain stem, chemoreceptors, or connections of these. The otolaryngologist is concerned with obstructive apnoea and the role that enlargement of the tonsils and adenoids plays in its aetiology. Luke *et al.* (1966) reported a series of children who had developed right ventricular failure and pulmonary oedema. These complications were felt to be related to upper airway obstruction and were completely relieved by tonsillectomy and adenoidectomy in three children and by adenoidectomy in one. Since then a number of reports have confirmed that adenoidectomy alone or combined with tonsillectomy will reverse upper airway obstruction which has caused pulmonary hypertension and right-sided heart failure. In 1977, Mangat, Orr and Smith showed that obstructive apnoea during sleep could be cured by adenoidectomy. Similarly it has been shown and documented by polysomnography that tonsillectomy and adenoidectomy will improve obstructive apnoea and oxygen desaturation in children (Eliaschar *et al.*, 1980; Mauer, Staats and Olsen, 1983).

The current theory regarding obstructive sleep apnoea is that if untreated, apart from the problems of daytime sleepiness, a proportion of these children will go on to develop pulmonary hypertension and cor pulmonale. The prevalence of pathological sleep apnoea is unknown and the risks of development of cor pulmonale as a result are also unknown and remain to be investigated. These risks must be very small because the number of children who develop cor pulmonale with otherwise normal hearts and respiratory systems is low.

The recognition of sleep apnoea clinically and its treatment are difficult problems. It is surprising how many parents, when questioned about snoring in children, will volunteer the information that as well as snoring their children have apnoeic episodes which, quite naturally, alarm the parents considerably. Clinical examination may confirm noisy respiration even when the child is awake and examination of the throat may show very large tonsils. However, in most children the diagnosis is not nearly so easy to make. Radiology with a soft tissue lateral view may show totally obstructive adenoids and observation in hospital may confirm or refute the diagnosis of sleep apnoea.

Ideally these children should be monitored during sleep with electrocardiography, strain gauges for chest movement and ear lobe oximetry for oxygen saturation recording. As Croft *et al.* (1990) pointed out sleep screening is a very effective and inexpensive method of making a definite diagnosis and if the child is thought to be suffering from sleep apnoea overnight observation with oximetry is a very reliable technique and can be undertaken in most paediatric wards. Oximetry is increasingly being used in routine anaesthesia and equipment is therefore often available -for use in sleep screening and requires little additional expense. Such observation, however, is essential to avoid unnecessary and wholesale surgery. Once it has been demonstrated that a child has significant obstructive sleep apnoea and that other conditions such as micrognathia or Treacher Collins syndrome are not responsible, the question still remains as to whether the child should have adenoidectomy alone or whether the tonsils should also be removed. Some advocate that the size of the adenoids should be assessed radiologically and if they appear to be obstructing the nasopharynx significantly, then they alone should be removed. It is the authors' opinion that radiology offers very little help and that decisions have to be made on clinical grounds with the help of the observations during sleep that have already been mentioned. On most occasions it is the tonsils and the adenoids that are involved and both should be removed.

Tonsillectomy and adenoidectomy

The fact that removal of tonsils and adenoids is frequently undertaken at a single operation while indications for the removal of each differ considerably has not helped the popularity of the surgical procedure among paediatricians. In the past it has been called 'a prophylactic ritual carried out for no particular reason with no particular result'. It is beholden on the surgeon to be certain that each of these operations is performed only when there is a valid indication. No doctor has any right to promise more from the removal of tonsils other than that the child will have no further attacks of acute tonsillitis. The idea that one was removing a source of focal sepsis and hence treating a nephritic or rheumatic condition has long since become outdated.

The general feeling among the profession is that the operation is being performed less frequently than it used to be. However, Scottish Health Statistics from the library of the Scottish Office reveal that in 1977 the operation was performed on 12 447 occasions

and in fact this figure remains almost the same over the years, e.g. in 1990, 12 652 procedures were performed. There is no reason to believe that the figures for other parts of the UK are any different.

However, in the USA the perceived trend of decreasing operations is borne out in the statistics with the number of tonsil and adenoid procedures having fallen from 1019×10^3 in 1971 to 259×10^3 in 1987 (National Center for Health Statistic: National Hospital Discharge Survey, 1988).

The indications for performing this operation, both in general and on every occasion it is done, need to be rigorously examined. The morbidity and mortality associated with such surgery in childhood are not to be taken lightly. Some of the reasons advocated for tonsillectomy and adenoidectomy in the past were plainly ridiculous and it is embarrassing to read them in medical literature. Ideally, an objective way of evaluating the problem is needed before advising any surgical procedure. The more that a surgical procedure relies upon subjectivity either in the patient or the doctor, the less likely is the efficacy of that procedure. In fact, tonsillectomy in particular is the prime example of a surgical procedure the performance of which depends upon the subjective assessment by the parents of the child and, to a lesser extent, by the general practitioner.

Clinical examination is unlikely to be a decisive factor in the assessment of a child for tonsillectomy. Certainly clinical assessment of the size of the tonsils is not particularly reliable and the size is not related to the severity of previous infection (Weir, 1972). Cervical lymphadenopathy is probably related to recurrent tonsillitis and it has been shown that children with a history of tonsillitis are more likely to have large palpable glands in the neck than normal children (Mills and Hibbert, 1983). However, this is a very imprecise method of assessment and 75% of normal children have palpable cervical lymph nodes.

It is most unlikely that bacteriological examination of throat swabs will be helpful in assessing children with recurrent tonsillitis. Serological tests have been explored as a possible indicator of recurrent or chronic infection and a report by Veltri *et al.* (1972) seemed to be encouraging. In this study, elevated levels of IgG and IgA were found in a small group of children with recurrent tonsillitis or recurrent otitis media. After tonsillectomy and adenoidectomy these levels returned to normal. However, Kerr, Basuttil and Mandell (1977) could not substantiate these findings and found no differences in IgM, IgA or IgG levels in children undergoing tonsillectomy compared with normal individuals. Even if there are changes in immunoglobulins produced by recurrent tonsillitis, these are almost certainly fairly non-specific and unlikely to be a major contribution to the decision of whether or not to remove the tonsils.

We are therefore left with a history of recurrent tonsillitis as the main method of assessing children for tonsillectomy. Based on this history a number of clinical trials have been designed to evaluate tonsillectomy. At the present time five such controlled trials have been published (Kaiser, 1930; McKee, 1963; Mawson, Adlington and Evans, 1968; Roydhouse, 1970; Paradise *et al.*, 1984). The control patients in these trials are those who, although thought to need operation, have not had surgery and so they are compared with the operated children. Unfortunately the assessment of the children after surgery is necessarily subjective and therefore the bias introduced by the placebo effect of surgery is not eliminated. This fundamental drawback in such trials is inevitable, the only way round this problem being unethical and not possible, namely the performance of sham operations (that is, the child is anaesthetized but no surgery is performed), and even this would not be blind because it would be obvious which children had had surgery and which had not. Despite this limitation, these trials are of value and, particularly in the case of the Pittsburgh Children's Hospital study, some interesting and relevant facts have been produced.

From the Pittsburgh study it became obvious that a history of recurrent sore throats did not mean that these continued. In fact, of children with a history of recurrent episodes of tonsillitis, only 17% continued to have such episodes when supervised and examined at regular intervals by a team of doctors and nurses (Paradise *et al.*, 1978). Since the history of recurrent episodes were quite rigorous (five to seven a year for 2 years) most of these children, if seen by an otolaryngologist, would have been advised to have surgery. If these figures are representative it means that, based on history, 80% of tonsillectomies are unnecessary and that we are performing five times as many as are needed. The second fact which has so far emerged from this study is that tonsillectomy did significantly reduce the incidence of sore throats when compared with control children with a similar history of repeated episodes of acute tonsillitis. However, the problems encountered by the control children (that is non-operated children) were not excessive and many of the sore throats which they suffered were classified as mild. This implies that the benefits bestowed by tonsillectomy were not necessarily great, even if it did mean tonsillitis was eliminated. Paradise *et al.* (1984) did, however, conclude that tonsillectomy was warranted for children meeting strict criteria.

Having said this, the results of the surgery, at least to the parents of the children, are commonly good. A Scottish National Audit on 5923 children (age under 14 years) operated on between February 1992 and February 1993 gave interesting results in a follow-up questionnaire. Over 60% said their child's appetite was better and 80% said the operation had helped their child 'greatly'. In response to the question, 'Are you glad your child had the op-

eration?', 98% said they were (Scottish Otolaryngological Society National Audit Office, 1994). Questionnaires are notoriously unreliable and these of course are subjective responses. It is extremely difficult to identify satisfactory objective criteria that are readily measurable.

Indications for tonsillectomy

Recurrent episodes of acute tonsillitis

All children will have one or more episodes of acute tonsillitis and this is not abnormal. A series of many attacks in childhood is unusual and there is no doubt that these can be avoided by tonsillectomy. This has advantages in that if it is possible to prevent these attacks education may not be harmed and if a child can be saved these illnesses it is an advantage. It is unlikely that there are any long-term sequelae from recurrent tonsillitis and serious complications of tonsillitis are unusual (see above) in the present day because of antibiotics. There is no evidence that recurrent tonsillitis affects growth (Mills and Hibbert, 1983).

When an otolaryngologist sees a child with a history of recurrent acute tonsillitis – a diagnosis possibly supported by examination during acute episodes by the general practitioner and defined as severe illness, pyrexia, dysphagia, lasting at least 5 days – he is asked to predict whether these attacks are going to continue or whether they will cease spontaneously. If it is felt that they are likely to continue then tonsillectomy is reasonable. It is this prediction which is so difficult. However, it is assumed that if a child has had six attacks of genuine tonsillitis per year for at least 2 years then they are likely to continue. This, therefore, is our prime indication for tonsillectomy and doubt is cast even on this by the Pittsburgh Children's Hospital study. It is important to determine that the attacks of sore throat are those of tonsillitis and not an upper respiratory tract virus infection – the latter possibly associated with coryza and usually a shorter-lived illness. If there is doubt the patient can be seen during an acute episode. If the history is questionable then the patient should be reassessed 6 months later. It is surprising how this will reduce parental anxiety and very often avoid the need for surgery.

Tonsillectomy should never be used as a means of placating anxious parents when the indications are not present. On the other hand, parental anxiety is to be respected and can be allayed by careful and sympathetic history taking and examination of the child.

Peritonsillar abscess

This is rare in childhood. Wolf *et al.* (1988) reviewed 38 children seen with peritonsillar abscess between

1976 and 1986; 20% of these had a previous history of recurrent tonsillitis while 74% had had no previous trouble. These results are in keeping with most people's findings and their conclusion, that one episode of peritonsillar abscess does not constitute an absolute indication for tonsillectomy, is now generally accepted.

Sleep apnoea

As has already been discussed, there is no doubt that in a small number of children who have been properly evaluated, the removal of tonsils and adenoids is indicated for this disorder.

In the Scottish Audit the indications for operation were recurrent acute tonsillitis in 80% of the 5923 children; 10% of the operations were performed for sleep apnoea specifically or for 'obstructive symptoms'. The remaining 10% were for more vague and hence possibly inappropriate reasons.

Contraindications to tonsillectomy

Recent upper respiratory tract infection

A recent upper respiratory tract infection is an absolute contraindication to tonsillectomy and the operation should be postponed for 3 weeks unless there are urgent obstructive symptoms. Primary and secondary haemorrhage are considered to be more likely if an acutely inflamed tonsil is removed. Pulmonary complications of anaesthesia are more likely when the child has an upper respiratory tract infection.

Haematological problems

Anaemia is a contraindication to surgery unless the haemoglobin is more than 10 g/dl. Surgery should be deferred until the anaemia is corrected. It is essential when considering a child for tonsillectomy that a history of bleeding in the patient or family is ascertained. If there is any such history the child must be fully investigated and if a bleeding disorder is discovered the indications for surgery must be reviewed though minor coagulation defects can be corrected or may not cause any difficulty.

The operation of tonsillectomy (Figures 18.6–18.10)

The important points about the surgical techniques of tonsillectomy are discussed in the adult in Volume 5 and will not be repeated here. The essential difference in the technique is that, in the child, an oral endotracheal tube is used. This must be positioned

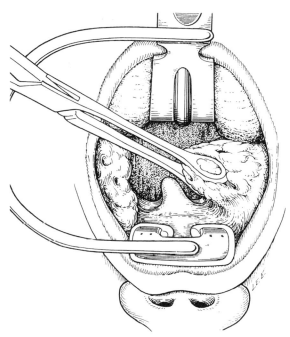

Figure 18.6 The tonsil is grasped and pulled medially. As in all surgery dissection of tissues under tension is the easiest and least traumatic

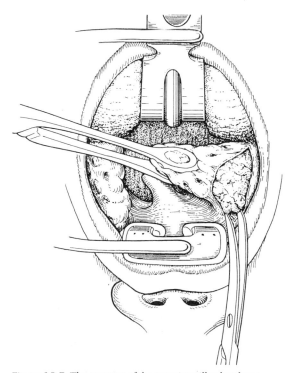

Figure 18.7 The mucosa of the anterior pillar has been incised, the upper pole of the tonsil is being dissected prior to incision of the posterior pillar

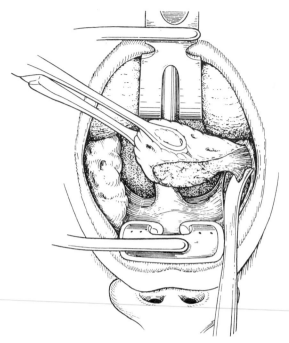

Figure 18.8 The areolar tissue between the tonsillar capsule and the superior constrictor muscle is being dissected. Sufficient tension must be exerted on the tonsil

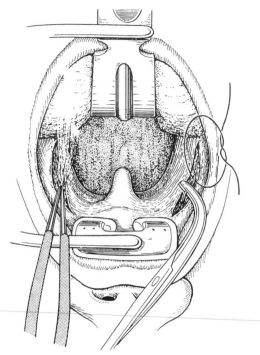

Figure 18.10 Absolute haemostasis must be achieved, either using ligatures or diathermy

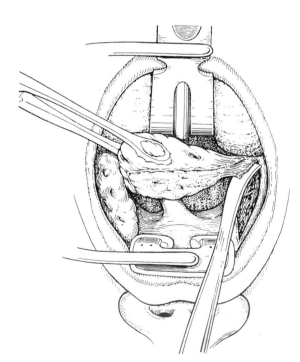

Figure 18.9 The dissection is almost complete but should be continued just onto the base of the tongue

centrally on the dorsum of the tongue and fixed in this position in the slot of the Doughty blade of a Boyle–Davies gag. Unless the tongue is carefully positioned before surgery access to one tonsil will be totally inadequate. It is essential to choose the correct size of Doughty blade. In the average child aged 6 or 7 years a 9 cm (3.5 inch) blade will be found to be appropriate. The cross bar at the tip of a blade which is too small will compress and obstruct the orotracheal anaesthetic tube. A small blade will also allow the base of the tongue to obstruct the view of the lower parts of the tonsillar fossae and make adequate tonsillectomy impossible.

It goes without saying that the blood volume of a child is less than that of an adult and this is an important consideration when performing surgery in children. The average blood loss during a routine tonsillectomy and adenoidectomy is between 100 and 130 ml (Shalom, 1964; Holden and Maher, 1965). If the blood volume of a child is calculated as 75 ml/kg this means that a child weighing 13 kg or less will lose nearly 14% of the blood volume in an uncomplicated procedure; 14% is the point of blood loss in a child at which transfusion is felt to be necessary (British Medical Journal, 1965). Excessive bleeding, postoperative bleeding or preoperative anaemia thus assume great importance in the child, particularly the young child. The blood loss during tonsillectomy can be measured so that excessive loss can be documented and corrected, though this is rarely done in clinical practice.

The postoperative care of a child undergoing tonsillectomy is of critical importance. The position immediately following extubation should be such that if any bleeding does occur the blood will run out of the mouth and nose and not into an unprotected larynx. Thus the child should lie on the side with the head below the level of the shoulders.

The postoperative observations include regular recording of the pulse rate (every 15 minutes for the first 2 hours, every 30 minutes for the next 2 hours and hourly thereafter) and close observation of the child's breathing pattern. A semiconscious child with blood in the pharynx will always make an audible noise on respiration and this should also be an indication to examine the child's pharynx for haemorrhage. Excessive swallowing or vomiting of blood is a sign that bleeding has occurred and here again the pharynx should be examined. A rapidly rising pulse rate with a child looking increasingly grey in colour is also an indication that haemorrhage is occurring.

Control of postoperative pain is always difficult. The postoperative administration of diamorphine is popular in some centres while in others rectal nonsteroidal anti-inflammatory preparations are now used. For ongoing analgesia paracetamol (250–500 mg) as an oral suspension is usually sufficient. Aspirin should be avoided as it increases the risk of primary haemorrhage (Carrick, 1984) by reducing the platelet adhesiveness and prolonging the bleeding time. The administration of aspirin has been incriminated in the causation of Reye's syndrome and its use is contraindicated in children under 12 years of age. The vast majority of children can be discharged home 24 hours after tonsillectomy without increasing the risk of haemorrhage (Siodlak, Gleeson and Wengraf, 1985).

Laser tonsillectomy

There have been several reported series of laser tonsillectomy using the KTP-532 laser in the past number of years. Strunk and Nichols (1990) stated that the only advantage was a reduction in blood loss during the procedure, which they judged would only be of significance in the very young or those with coagulopathies. The disadvantages cited included an increase in total operative time (due mostly to increased anaesthetic time), delayed healing and increased cost. Other authors have reported similar findings. Laser tonsillectomy might be expected to result in a reduction in pain postoperatively, however, Das and Bartels (1990) found that although the pain was reduced initially it became worse in the later phases of healing than with standard dissection techniques.

Complications of tonsillectomy

These are fully discussed in Volume 5 and will not be restated in detail here. Clearly the most important factor and the cause of most of the deaths associated with tonsillectomy is haemorrhage and the delay in treating it. Tate (1963) investigated the cause of death in 93 children over a 5-year period and stated that this delay was the primary cause of death following tonsillectomy. The death rate was approximately one child per 10 000 operations. The factors which make the operation more serious in a child than an adult are the relative blood volumes, the difficulty in recognition of haemorrhage in children and the problems in coping with it in an uncooperative child. If there is thought to be haemorrhage in a child following tonsillectomy, venous access should be established, blood taken for cross matching and base-line haemoglobin, and the child prepared for anaesthesia. A minor bleed may occur which ceases after a few minutes and, in this situation, a child should be observed very closely with regular inspection of the tonsillar fossae. Any child bleeding significantly after tonsillectomy should be re-anaesthetized and the bleeding point dealt with. This second anaesthetic is hazardous (Davies, 1964) and should only be administered by a very experienced anaesthetist.

Incidence of complications

Chowdhury, Tewfik and Schloss (1988) carried out a retrospective review of 6842 tonsillectomies and adenoidectomies performed over a 7-year period at the Montreal Children's Hospital. The total incidence of postoperative bleeding was 2.5%. The incidence of primary or reactionary haemorrhage was 1% with 78% of these bleeds within 12 hours of surgery. Only one-third of these haemorrhages required a second anaesthetic to control the bleeding. The overall incidence of secondary post-tonsillectomy haemorrhage was 1.2% with 24% of these requiring blood transfusion.

Day-patient tonsillectomy

With increasing demand on surgeons to reduce the length of stay in hospital there is increasing pressure to perform day-patient tonsillectomy. In papers describing the experience of 6998 patients undergoing such surgery in the USA and UK the conclusion was that the procedure may be performed safely as a day case (Maniglia, Kushner and Cozzi, 1989; Helmus, Grin and Westfall, 1990; Reiner *et al.*, 1990; Yardley, 1992).

Colcalasure and Graham (1990) found a major complication rate of 1.4% in 3340 day-case tonsillectomy and adenoidectomy operations. These included primary haemorrhage, anaesthetic complications, severe nausea and dehydration. It is the authors' opinion that day-case tonsillectomy and adenoidectomy should only be considered under the most rigid guidelines. The social circumstances and access to both telephone and private transport are important considerations in assessing patient suitability. Close cooperation with anaesthetic colleagues is vital to achieve the degree of pain control required to allow successful implementation of a day-care policy. Willingness of parents to agree to the discharge of their children depends significantly on the effectiveness of postoperative pain control. The degree of reliance on opiates with their associated side effects, particularly nausea, is also important. In a recent survey at one local hospital only a very small percentage of parents showed any wish to take their children home on the same day of the operation.

There is a clear need to develop guidelines to influence the increasing trend to day-case tonsillectomy. The impact of such an increase on complication rates and on primary care services also needs to be monitored.

Indications for adenoidectomy

Nasal obstruction

Children who have an obstructed nasal airway should be evaluated by clinical examination and by radiography. If the latter shows the airway to be obstructed by the adenoids then adenoidectomy is indicated.

Otitis media with effusion

The evidence that the adenoids are a causative factor in otitis media with effusion is equivocal and was discussed previously. Some surgeons advocate adenoidectomy as primary treatment for otitis media with effusion either alone or combined with insertion of ventilation tubes. Other surgeons advise the insertion of ventilation tubes possibly reserving adenoidectomy for children whose effusion recurs after extrusion of the tubes. A third approach is to advise insertion of ventilation tubes as primary treatment, only removing the adenoids if they are large.

Recurrent acute otitis media

Although historically adenoidectomy has been advised to prevent recurrent attacks of acute otitis media these is no evidence that it is effective.

Sleep apnoea

As discussed above either adenoidectomy alone or combined with tonsillectomy is valuable in the treatment of obstructive sleep apnoea.

Contraindications to adenoidectomy

Recent upper respiratory tract infection

A recent upper respiratory tract infection is an absolute contraindication to adenoidectomy.

Bleeding

As with tonsillectomy, a suspected bleeding disorder must be investigated before adenoidectomy.

Cleft palate

As discussed in the complications, in certain instances the adenoids assist the soft palate in closure of the nasopharynx from the oropharynx during speech and deglutition, and removal of the adenoids may impair speech. The adenoids should never be removed in a child who has had a cleft palate repair, one who has a congenitally short palate or in one who has a submucous cleft of the palate.

The operation of adenoidectomy

This operation is by no means a minor procedure. Far from being an afterthought following tonsillectomy it should be regarded as a major surgical procedure with significant risks and complications. For example 60–70% of the blood loss during tonsillectomy and adenoidectomy is due to the adenoidectomy and control of excessive bleeding following adenoidectomy is more difficult than after tonsillectomy.

The preoperative considerations and preparation of a child for adenoidectomy are identical to those for tonsillectomy. The anaesthesia is also the same using an orotracheal tube which is stabilized in a Doughty blade using a Boyle-Davies gag.

When performing tonsillectomy and adenoidectomy it is usual to extend the neck of the patient using a sandbag under the shoulders of the child. This accentuates the curvature of the cervical spine and probably makes a complete adenoidectomy more difficult. A more neutral position of the neck, neither flexed nor extended may be preferable.

The adenoids are palpated with an index finger and it is important that the soft palate is relaxed during this manoeuvre or it will be torn. It is usual to dissect, using the finger, the lateral extension of the adenoids towards the midline. A St Clair Thomson curette is then inserted into the nasopharynx, gently positioned against the posterior surface of the nasal septum and swept downwards (Figures 18.11 and 18.12). It is important to select a curette of the correct size. Too large a curette will damage the eustachian cushions and one which is too small will mean that the adenoidectomy is incomplete. As the main mass of adenoids is curetted, the blade of the curette is brought forwards to avoid running it down

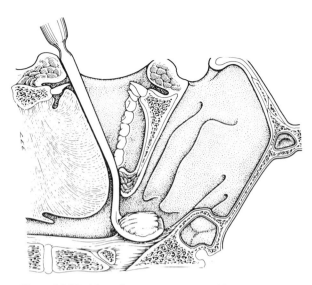

Figure 18.11 Adenoidectomy – insertion of the curette

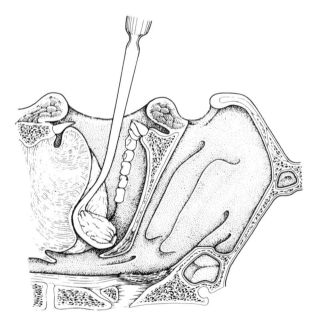

Figure 18.12 Adenoidectomy – curettage of adenoids. The adenoids are shaved away with a firm sweeping movement of the wrist until the curette emerges from behind the soft palate

the posterior pharyngeal wall and stripping the mucosa. On occasions the adenoid mass remains attached by mucosal strands inferiorly. These should be avulsed using Luc's forceps, but the direction of avulsion should be cranial, otherwise the mucosa of the posterior pharyngeal wall will be stripped. The nasopharynx is palpated and any adenoidal remnants

are curetted. A pack is then placed in the nasopharynx to help haemostasis. Modifications of this adenoidectomy technique are numerous. Inspection of the nasopharynx with a mirror and removal of remnants of lymphoid tissue have been advocated (Sheridan, 1951). A fundamentally different approach is direct adenoidectomy in which the soft palate is retracted and the adenoids removed under direct vision using punches forceps and scissors (Guggenheim, 1957).

If bleeding continues after removal of the pack a second pack should be inserted and left for a further 5 minutes. If bleeding still continues mirror examination of the nasopharynx may reveal a bleeding point which can be cauterized or an adenoid tag which can be removed. If at this point bleeding continues some surgeons will resort to the use of topical adrenalin (1:1000) on a swab and others will insert a postnasal pack to remain for 24 hours. There must be absolutely no bleeding from the nasopharynx before anaesthesia is terminated.

Complications of adenoidectomy

The possible complications of adenoidectomy are basically the same as for tonsillectomy and will not be considered here in detail. However, there are certain other considerations associated with adenoidectomy.

Excessive haemorrhage

Occasionally there will be excessive haemorrhage at adenoidectomy. Aberrant vessels have been described (Grant, 1944; Duncan, 1963) and occasionally an aberrant internal carotid artery has been damaged at surgery (Harmer, 1914; McKenzie and Woolf, 1959). In general, excessive haemorrhage should be investigated by coagulation studies, blood should be replaced and the haemorrhage corrected by diathermy if possible or with a postnasal pack. Postoperative bleeding from the adenoidal bed is serious and the child should be returned to theatre immediately and a postnasal pack inserted (Figure 18.13).

Surgical trauma

The soft palate, particularly if it is not relaxed, can be damaged during adenoidectomy. The eustachian cushions can be injured and stenosis can occur (see below). Dislocation of the cervical spine has been described (Gibb, 1969) but usually this is caused by infection affecting the anterior ligaments of the spine and resulting in subluxation of the atlanto-occipital joint about 10 days after surgery.

Effect of adenoidectomy on speech

Children with large obstructive adenoids may have hyponasal speech, that is the speech of nasal obstruc-

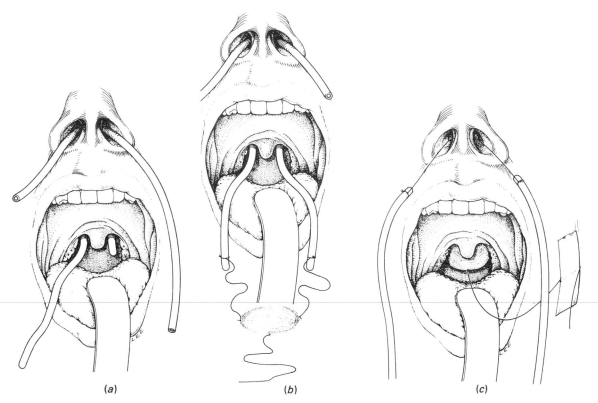

(a)   (b)   (c)

Figure 18.13 Insertion of a postnasal pack. The illustrations here depict insertion of a pack under local anaesthesia. It is necessary in a child to perform the same manoeuvres under general anaesthesia. (*a*) A small soft rubber or plastic catheter is passed through each nostril via the nasopharynx into the oropharynx. The catheters are drawn out through the mouth; (*b*) a piece of strong thread attached to each side of the pack is tied to the distal end of each catheter; (*c*) the catheters are then withdrawn through the anterior nares and the pack firmly settled into the postnasal space. The threads are tied across the columella and a third piece of thread, previously sutured to the centre of the lower edge of the pack is loosely secured on the cheek with adhesive tape. The pack is removed 24 hours later through the open mouth

tion, and one would expect this to be improved following adenoidectomy. Hypernasal speech following adenoidectomy has been estimated to occur once every 1450 operations (Gibb, 1958). This is almost certainly a lower figure than the actual incidence because less severe cases may be overlooked or may be only temporary. The reason for hypernasality (nasal escape speech like that with cleft palate) following adenoidectomy is that the adenoids assist the soft palate in closing the nasopharynx during speech. Hypernasality is therefore more likely to occur postoperatively in those children with an abnormal soft palate. This may be congenitally short or its musculature may be defective in a patient with a submucosal cleft. The latter is associated with a bifid uvula and a notch in the hard palate, and adenoidectomy should be avoided in this situation. If the above obvious examples of palatal abnormality are excluded only a small number of children should develop hypernasality following surgery and one would expect this to be only temporary and to respond to speech therapy.

Scarring following surgery

It is not unusual to see fibrous bands or adhesions in the nasopharynx following adenoidectomy and normally this will cause no harm. Trauma to the eustachian openings may well produce stenosis and may impair eustachian tube opening and this has been suggested as one of the causes of failure of adenoidectomy to cure ear symptoms. Rarely, adenoidectomy results in total obliteration of the nasopharynx by scar tissue.

Persistence of symptoms following surgery

It is not unusual for symptoms to persist following adenoidectomy. Dawes (1970) has stated that 70% of children in his series with otitis media with effusion had previously had an adenoidectomy. There are three possible explanations for this:

1 The adenoid was not responsible for the symptoms in the first place
2 Postoperative scarring, particularly of the eustachian openings nullifies any benefit of surgery
3 Lymphoid tissue left in the nasopharynx following incomplete adenoidectomy results in symptoms. Much has been made of adenoid remnants causing symptoms and the proponents of direct adenoidectomy use it to justify their approach. There is no doubt that some lymphoid tissue must remain in the nasopharynx following adenoidectomy and on occasions this tissue can undergo hypertrophy and cause symptoms. This is probably rare and may be more likely to happen in the very young child.

References

BLUESTONE, C. D. (1971) Eustachian tube in cleft palate. *Annals of Otology, Rhinology and Laryngology*, **80**, (suppl. 2), 1–25

BLUESTONE, C. D. (1975a) Obstructive adenoids in relation to otitis media. *Annals of Otology, Rhinology and Laryngology*, **84**, (suppl. 19), 44–48

BLUESTONE, C. D. (1975b) Certain effects of adenoidectomy on eustachian tube ventilatory function. *Laryngoscope*, **85**, 113–127

BOX, Q. T., CLEVELAND, R. T. and WILLARD, C. Y. (1961) Bacterial flora of the upper respiratory tract. *American Journal of Diseases of Children*, **102**, 293–330

British Medical Journal (1965) Editorial. Bleeding after adenotonsillectomy. **2**, 1321–1322

BULMAN, C. H., BROOK, S. J. and BERRY, M. G. (1984) A prospective randomised trial of adenoidectomy vs. grommet insertion in the treatment of glue ear. *Clinical Otolaryngology*, **9**, 67–75

CARRICK, D. G. (1984) Salicylates and post-tonsillectomy haemorrhage. *Journal of Laryngology and Otology*, **98**, 803–805

CHOWDHURY, K., TEWFIK, T. L. and SCHLOSS, M. D. (1988) Post tonsillectomy and adenoidectomy hemorrhage. *Journal of Otolaryngology*, **17**, 46–49

COHEN, D. and KONAK, S. (1985) The evaluation of radiographs of the nasopharynx. *Clinical Otolaryngology*, **10**, 73–78

COLCALASURE, J. B. and GRAHAM, S. S. (1990) Complications of outpatient tonsillectomy and adenoidectomy: a review of 3,340 cases. *Ear, Nose and Throat Journal*, **69**, 155–160

CROFT, C. B., BROCKBANK, M. J., WRIGHT, A. and SWANSTON, A. R. (1990) Obstructive sleep apnoea in children undergoing routine tonsillectomy and adenoidectomy. *Clinical Otolaryngology*, **15**, 307–314

DAS, R. E. and BARTELS, J. P. (1990) KTP/532 laser tonsillectomy: a comparison with standard technique. *Laryngoscope*, **100**, 385–388

DAVIES, D. D. (1964) Re-anaesthetising cases of tonsillectomy and adenoidectomy because of persistent post-operative haemorrhage. *British Journal of Anaesthesia*, **36**, 244–249

DAWES, J. D. K. (1970) The aetiology and sequelae of exudative otitis media. *Journal of Laryngology and Otology*, **84**, 563–610

DENNY, F. W., WANNAMAKER, L. W. and BRINK, W. R. (1950) Prevention of rheumatic fever. *Journal of the American Medical Association*, **143**, 151–153

DUNCAN, R. B. (1963) New concept of adenoidectomy haemorrhage. *Archives of Otolaryngology*, **76**, 721–728

ELIASCHAR, I., LAVIE, P., HALPERIN, E., GORDON, G. and ALROY, G. (1980) Sleep apnoeic episodes as indications for adenotonsillectomy. *Archives of Otolaryngology*, **106**, 492–496

EVERETT, M. T. (1979) The cause of tonsillitis. *Practitioner*, **223**, 253–259

FEINSTEIN, A. R. and LEVITT, M. (1970) The role of tonsils in predisposing to streptococcal infections and recurrences of rheumatic fever. *New England Journal of Medicine*, **282**, 285–291

FIELLAU–NICHOLAJSEN, M., FABLE–HANSEN, J. and KNUDSTRUP, P. (1980) Adenoidectomy for middle ear disorders: a randomised controlled trial. *Clinical Otolaryngology*, **5**, 323–327

GASTAUT, H., TASSINARI, C. and DURON, B. (1966) Polygraphic study of the diurnal and noctural (hypnic and respiratory) manifestations of the Pickwickian syndrome. *Brain Research*, **2**, 167–186

GIBB, A. G. (1958) Hypernasality following tonsil and adenoidal removal. *Journal of Laryngology and Otology*, **83**, 1159–1174

GIBB, A. G. (1969) Unusual complications of tonsil and adenoid removal. *Journal of Laryngology and Otology*, **83**, 1159–1174

GRANT, H. (1944) Hydrostatic pressure in adenoid haemorrhage. *Annals of Otology, Rhinology and Laryngology*, **53**, 576–577

GUGGENHEIM, P. (1957) Direct adenoidectomy. *Archives of Otolaryngology*, **66**, 26–32

HARMER, D. (1914) Large pulsating vessel in the right portion of the posterior pharyngeal wall partly concealed behind the right tonsil in a boy aged five. *Proceedings of the Royal Society of Medicine*, **7**, 26

HELMUS, C., GRIN, M. and WESTFALL, R. (1990) Same-day-stay adenotonsillectomy. *Laryngoscope*, **100**, 593–596

HIBBERT, J. and WHITEHOUSE, G. H. (1978) The assessment of adenoidal size by radiological means. *Clinical Otolaryngology*, **3**, 43–47

HOLDEN, H. B. and MAHER, J. J. (1965) Some aspects of blood loss and fluid balance in paediatric adenotonsillectomy. *British Medical Journal*, **2**, 1349–1351

HOLT, C. R. and TINSLEY, P. P. (1981) Peritonsillar abscesses in children. *Laryngoscope*, **91**, 1226–1230

KAISER, A. D. (1930) A comparative study of twenty-two hundred tonsillectomised children with an equal number of controls three and ten years after operation. *Journal of the American Medical Association*, **95**, 837–841

KERR, A. I. G., BASUTTIL, A. A. and MANDELL, C. M. (1977) A study of serum IgA levels in children undergoing tonsillectomy. *Clinical Otolaryngology*, **1**, 85–91

LUKE, M. J., MEHRIZI, A., FOLGER, G. M. and ROWE, R. D. (1966) Chronic nasopharyngeal obstruction as a cause of cardiomegaly; cor pulmonale and pulmonary oedema *Paediatrics*, **37**, 762–768

MCKEE, W. J. E. (1963) A controlled study of the effects of tonsillectomy and adenoidectomy in children. *British Journal of Preventative and Social Medicine*, **17**, 133–140

MCKENZIE, W. S. and WOOLF, C. J. (1959) Carotid abnormalities and adenoid surgery. *Journal of Laryngology and Otology*, **73**, 596–602

MANGAT, D., ORR, C. W. and SMITH, R. C. (1977) Sleep apnoea, hypersomnolence and upper airway obstruction secondary to adenotonsillar enlargement. *Archives of Otolaryngology*, **103**, 383–386

MANIGLIA, A. J., KUSHNER, H. and COZZI, L. (1989) Adenotonsillectomy. A safe outpatient procedure. *Archives of Otolaryngology – Head and Neck Surgery*, **115**, 92–94

MAUER, K. W., STAATS, B. A. and OLSEN, K. D. (1983) Upper airway obstruction and disordered nocturnal breathing in children. *Mayo Clinic Proceedings*, **58**, 349–353

MAW, A. R. (1983) Chronic otitis media with effusion and adenotonsillectomy; prospective randomised controlled study. *British Medical Journal*, **287**, 1586–1588

MAW, A. R., JEANS, W. D. and FERNANDO, D. J. J. (1981) Interobserver variability in the clinical and radiological assessment of adenoid size and the correlation with adenoid volume. *Clinical Otolaryngology*, **6**, 317–322

MAWSON, S. E., ADLINGTON, P. and EVANS, M. (1968) A controlled study evaluation of adenotonsillectomy in children. *Journal of Laryngology and Otology*, **82**, 963–979

MILLS, R. P. and HIBBERT, J. (1983) The effects of recurrent tonsillitis on growth and cervical lymphadenopathy in children. *International Journal of Paediatric Otolaryngology*, **1**, 77–82

MOFFETT, H. L., SIEGLE, A. C. and DOYLE H. K. (1968) Non-streptococcal pharyngitis. *Journal of Paediatrics*, **73**, 51–60

MURRAY, A. R. (1972) The appearance of the turbinates and nasal allergy in children. *Annals of Allergy*, **30**, 245–249

NATIONAL CENTER FOR STATISTICS: National hospital discharge summary (1988)

NATIONAL HEALTH SERVICE IN SCOTLAND Edinburgh: Information and Statistics Division

PARADISE, J. L., BLUESTONE, C. D., BACHMAN, R. Z., KARANTONIS, G., SMITH, I. H., SAEY, C. A. *et al.* (1978) History of recurrent sore throats as an indication for tonsillectomy. *New England Journal of Medicine*, **298**, 409–413

PARADISE, J. L., BLUESTONE, C. D., BACHMAN, R. Z., COLBURN, B. S., BERNARD, B. S., TAYLOR, F. H. *et al.* (1984) Efficacy of tonsillectomy for recurrent throat infections in severely affected children. Results of a parallel randomised and non-randomised study. *New England Journal of Medicine*, **310**, 674–683

POLVOGT, L. M. and CROWE, S. J. (1929) Predominating organisms found in cultures from tonsils and adenoids. *Journal of the American Medical Association*, **92**, 962–964

RASMUS, R. L. and JACOBS, R. M. (1969) Mouth breathing and malocclusion: quantitative technique for measurement of oral and nasal air flow velocities. *Angle Orthodontist*, **39**, 269–299

REILLY, S., TIMMIS, P., BEEDEN, A. G. and WILLIS A. T. (1981) Possible role of the anaerobe in tonsilliis. *Journal of Clinical Pathology*, **34**, 532–547

REINER, S. A., SAWYER, W. P., CLARK, K. F. and WOOD, M. W. (1990) Safety of outpatient tonsillectomy and adenoidectomy. *Otolaryngology – Head and Neck Surgery*, **102**, 161–168

ROYDHOUSE, N. (1970) A controlled study of adenotonsillectomy. *Archives of Otolaryngology*, **92**, 611–616

ROYDHOUSE, N. (1980) Adenoidectomy for otitis media with mucoid effusion. *Annals of Otology, Rhinology and Laryngology*, **89**, (suppl. 68), 312–315

RYNNEL–DAGLOO, B., AHLBOM, A. and SCHIRATZKI, H. (1978) Effects of adenoidectomy. *Annals of Otology, Rhinology and Laryngology*, **87**, 107

SCOTTISH OTOLARYNGOLOGICAL SOCIETY NATIONAL AUDIT OFFICE (1994) Ninewells Hospital, Dundee, Scotland

SHALOM, A. S. (1964) Blood loss in ear, nose and throat operations. *Journal of Laryngology and Otology*, **78**, 734–756

SHERIDAN, M. R. (1951) Observations on the nasopharynx and removal of adenoids. *Journal of Laryngology and Otology*, **65**, 609–613

SIODLAK, M. Z., GLEESON, M. J. and WENGRAF, C. L. (1985) Post-tonsillectomy secondary haemorrhage. *Annals of the Royal College of Surgeons of England*, **67**, 167–168

SPRINKLE, P. M. and VELTRI, R. W. (1976) The tonsils and adenoids. *Clinical Otolaryngology*, **2**, 153–167

STJERNQUIST–DESATNIK, A., PRELLNER, K. and SCHALEN, C. (1991) High recovery of *Haemophilus influenzae* and group A streptococci in recurrent tonsillar infection or hypertrophy as compared with normal tonsils. *Journal of Laryngology and Otololgy*, **105**, 439–441

STRUNK, C. L. and NICHOLS, M. L. (1990) A comparison of KTP/532 laser tonsillectomy vs. traditional dissection/ snare tonsillectomy. *Otolaryngology – Head and Neck Surgery*, **103**, 966–971

TATE, N. (1963) Deaths from tonsillectomy. *Lancet*, ii, 1090–1091

TILKIAN, A. C., GUILLEMINAULT, C., SCHRODER, J. S., LOHRMAN, K. L., SIMMONS, F. B. and DEMENT, W. C. (1976) Sleep wakefulness and sleep. *Annals of Internal Medicine*, **85**, 714–719

TONER, J. G., STEWART, T. J., CAMPBELL, J. B. and HUNTER, J. (1986) Tonsil flora in the very young tonsillectomy patient. *Clinical Otolaryngology*, **11**, 171–174

TULLEY, W. J. (1964) Malformation of the jaws and teeth in relation to upper repiratory symptoms and certain speech disorders. *Guy's Hospital Reports*, **113**, 261–272

VELTRI, R. W., SPRINKLE, P. M., KELLER, S. A. and CHICKLO, J. M. (1972) Immunoglobulin changes in a paediatric otolaryngologic patient sample subsequent to T and A. *Journal of Laryngology and Otology*, **86**, 905–916

WEIR, N. F. (1972) Clinical interpretation of tonsillar size. *Journal of Laryngology and Otology*, **86**, 1137–1144

WIDEMAR, L., SVENSON, C., RYNNEL–DAGLOO, B. and SCHIRATZKI, H. (1985) The effect of adenoidectomy on secretory otitis media; a two year controlled prospecive study. *Clinical Otolaryngology*, **10**, 345–350

WOLF, M., KRONENBERG, J., KESSLER, A., MODAN, M. and LEVENTON, G. (1988) Peritonsillar abscess in children and its indication for tonsillectomy. *International Journal of Paediatric Otolaryngology*, **16**, 113–117

YARDLEY, M. P. (1992) Tonsillectomy and adenoidectomy and adenotonsillectomy procedures: are they safe for day case procedures. *Journal of Laryngology and Otology*, **106**, 299–300

19

Dental development, orthodontics, cleft lip and palate

Terry Gregg and Andrew Richardson

Orthodontics has been defined as the study of growth and development of the masticatory apparatus and the prevention and correction of anomalies of this development. Many orthodontic patients treated in general or specialist practice present with anomalies of the teeth and facial shape which are not in themselves pathological but are cosmetically detrimental, make the teeth difficult to clean and may be associated with painful disturbances of the temporomandibular joint and masticatory musculature. These may simulate migraine or conditions of the ear, nose or throat.

Hospital orthodontists also provide orthodontic treatment for patients needing alveolar or maxillo facial surgery and are involved in the treatment of syndromal conditions such as first arch anomalies, cleft palate, Treacher Collins and Pierre Robin's syndromes, and hemifacial microsomia in which they share an interest with the otolaryngologist.

Since the basic science of orthodontics is the growth and development of the dentition and face, orthodontists prepare serial study casts of the mouth (Figure 19.1) and have devised equipment called a cephalostat (Broadbent, Broadbent and Golden, 1975) to take serial cephalometric radiographs of the head in a reproducible position (Figure 19.2).

The casts are used to make measurements such as the size of teeth, the amount of crowding or spacing of the teeth, dental arch breadths, palate depth, the overjet (the horizontal protrusion of the upper incisors relative to the lower incisors) and the overbite (the vertical overlap of the upper incisors over the lowers). Cephalometric radiographs can be used to measure the shape of the face, facial growth and the size of the tongue, airway and adenoids in two dimensions. A simple cephalometric analysis is shown in Figure 19.3.

The bones of the jaws and face

The relationship of the jaw bones is influenced by the size and shape of the cranial base because the maxilla is attached to the anterior part and the glenoid fossa to the posterior part. Thus, malocclusion is common in such conditions as achondroplasia and cleidocranial dysostosis where the cranial base is abnormal.

Growth of the facial bones is both transformative – in which the shape of a bone is changed – and translatory – a process by which a bone moves in space. The mechanisms involved are subperiosteal apposition and resorption, sutural growth and interstitial growth of cartilage. Surface apposition and sutural growth are involved in transformative growth. Growth of cartilage is involved in translatory growth of the cranial base at the spheno-occipital synchondrosis and of the maxilla at the nasal septum. The factors controlling these growth mechanisms are unclear, although there is an obvious genetic influence. The primary factor in translatory growth of the calvaria is growth of the brain. Sutural growth in this area is a secondary mechanism to maintain bony continuity. The functional matrix theory (Moss, 1968; Moss and Salantijn, 1969) proposes that growth of the functioning spaces of the mouth, pharynx, larynx and nasal cavities acts in a similar manner to the brain and promotes translatory growth of the jawbones.

Early work using cephalometric radiographs showed that the average face grows downwards and forwards in a straight line. This tends to mask the growth spurt which more or less coincides with the growth spurt in stature at about the time of puberty and to minimize important interindividual variations. Some faces grow predominantly downward and others grow predominantly forward and it is these variations which are important in orthodontics (Greenberg and Johnston, 1975). By superimposing

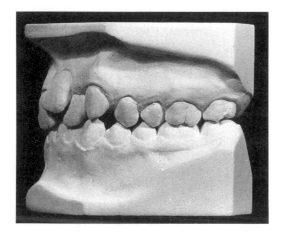

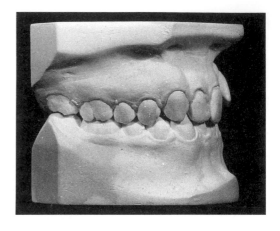

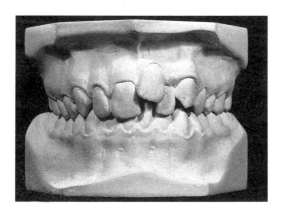

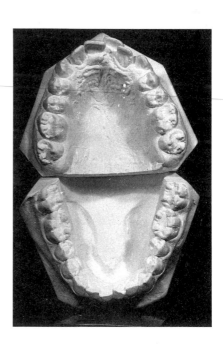

Figure 19.1 Orthodontic study casts

cephalometric films on titanium implants placed in the bone, it has been found that both the maxilla and mandible rotate as they translate during growth (Björk and Skeiller, 1972). Viewed from the right side most mandibles rotate counterclockwise as they grow but much of the rotation is masked by surface apposition going on at the same time.

As age advances the profile tends to straighten, the dentition becomes less prominent and the external nose gets bigger. Between the ages of 6 and 18 years the soft tissue of the nose grows 16–17 mm in length and 12–13 mm in height. During the adolescent growth spurt, growth of the soft tissue of the nose greatly exceeds growth of the maxilla.

Large adenoids may lead to mouth breathing, an altered posture of the head with the neck extended, and development of a long face. Removal of adenoidal tissue reverses the process to a certain extent (Linder-Aronson, 1970; Linder-Aronson *et al.*, 1993).

The 'soft tissues'

In orthodontic terminology, the 'soft tissues' include the lips, tongue and cheeks, the floor of mouth, the soft palate and throat and associated musculature.

Lips

At birth, the shape of the vermilion borders of the lips is almost round. During the first 2 years of life

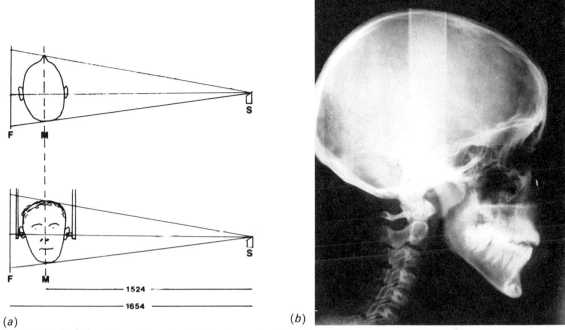

(a)   (b)

Figure 19.2 Cephalometric radiography. (a) Superior and anterior views of the arrangements for cephalometric radiography. The central ray of the X-ray beam passes from the source (S), through the ear rods and impinges on the film at right angles. Typical distances from the source to the midsagittal plane and film holder are shown. The enlargement of a midline structure is approximately 8%. (b) A cephalometric radiograph. The exposure of the lips and nose is reduced by an aluminium wedge. The nasopharyngeal airway is clearly demonstrated. F: Film; M: mid sagittal plane

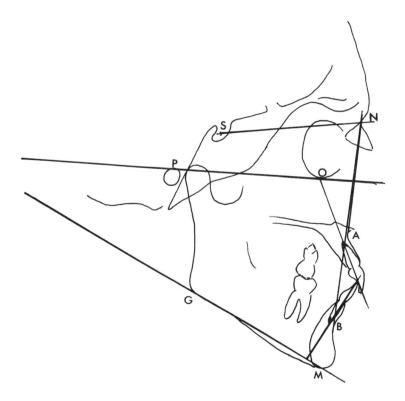

Figure 19.3 A simple cephalometric analysis. S = Sella, the centre of the sella turcica; N = nasion, the junction of the frontal and nasal bones in the midline; P = porion, the highest point on the external auditory meatus; O = orbitale, the lowest point on the rim of the orbit; G = gonion, the lowest, most posterior point at the angle of the mandible; M = menton, the lowest point on the symphyseal outline; A = the most posterior point on the concave outline of the maxilla anterior to the upper incisors; B = the most posterior point on the concave outline of the mandible anterior to the lower incisors. Ideal data would be as follows: ANB angle = 2–4 degrees, OP/MG angle = 27 degrees, upper incisor/OP = 109 degrees, lower incisor/MG = 90 degrees

the width of the mouth doubles while the height diminishes, thus converting a sphincter suitable for suckling into a slit. Subsequent lip growth is greater than growth of the lower face. Lips tend to become more competent with the lower lip covering more of the upper incisors (Burke, 1980; Vig and Cohen, 1979). Competent lips are defined as the condition in which the lips form an anterior oral seal without contraction of the perioral musculature when the mandible is in the rest position. Incompetent lips are those which do not meet under the same conditions. Patients with incompetent lips which are normally separated at rest may be mistakenly diagnosed as mouth breathers. This may not necessarily be so as a posterior oral seal is frequently produced between the dorsum of the tongue and soft palate.

The habitual position of the lower lip in relation to the upper incisors is very important in orthodontics. Normally, the lower lip covers the lower one third of the upper incisors. In patients whose lower lip lies below or behind the upper incisors, the overjet is usually increased.

Tongue

The interesting features of the tongue are the size, the resting position and function in swallowing and speech. Large tongue areas measured on cephalometric films are associated with proclination of the incisor teeth and small tongue areas with retroclination. After the age of 13 years, the area of the tongue increases more than the area of the intermaxillary space. Where there is nasal obstruction and mouth-breathing the tongue has a low resting position, the upper arch is narrow and the lower incisors are retroclined. The lower incisors procline spontaneously following adenoidectomy and the consequent altered mode of breathing. Patients with long faces have a large angle between the ramus and body of the mandible, narrow mandibular rami and poorly developed muscles of mastication. Patients with shorter faces have smaller angles between the ramus and body of the mandible, broader mandibular rami and high muscular activity.

The suckling behaviour in an infant is with the jaws widely separated and the tongue protruded. The normal swallowing behaviour in an adult is with the teeth together, the tongue contained within the dental arches and little or no contraction of the circumoral musculature. Children usually change from the infantile to the adult behaviour sometime between 2 and 5 years of age. An anterior resting position of the tongue with tongue-thrusting behaviour is associated with an anterior open bite where there is a vertical space between the anterior teeth when the posterior teeth are brought together. Providing the abnormality of tongue behaviour is not very vigorous, an open bite in young children is likely to close of its own accord. Rarely, the tongue thrust is

endogenous and is present throughout life. This may impose serious limitations on the possibilities for orthodontic treatment.

So far as speech is concerned, most children seem to cope with the changing environment of the mouth cavity as teeth erupt and are shed without undue difficulty, but an interdental sigmatism or lisp is quite a common developmental feature.

In the vast majority of children the pattern of soft tissue behaviour matures but the combination of a vigorous tongue thrust on swallowing and a lisp is a traditional warning sign to the orthodontist that tooth positions will not improve spontaneously and that treatment results are likely to relapse.

Dental development

Development of the dentition and the occlusion of teeth (the bite) occurs in five stages (Richardson, 1995).

Edentulous stage (Figure 19.4)

At birth, the infant has no teeth. He has instead two tough, firm edentulous arches known as gum pads. The upper gum pad is usually in the shape of a horseshoe whereas the lower is more flattened anteriorly. The gum pads are segmented – each segment corresponding to a developing deciduous tooth. The sulcus demarcating the posterior edge of the developing deciduous canine runs over onto the buccal side of the pad, where it is called the lateral sulcus. The relationship of the upper lateral sulcus to the lower is used to measure the anteroposterior gum pad relationship. At birth, the lower gum pad is usually posterior to the upper and there is a vertical space anteriorly into which the tongue protrudes. Both of these features would be regarded as malocclusions if teeth were present. They are usually transitory and facilitate simultaneous suckling and nasal breathing. The postnormality is usually corrected by forward growth of the mandible during the first few months of life,

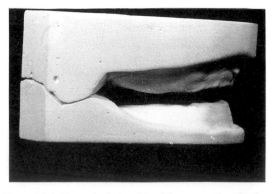

Figure 19.4 Normal relationship of the gum pads at birth

and the vertical space has been considered by some authorities as a favourable feature which may prevent an excessive overbite when the teeth erupt.

Eruption of deciduous teeth

The deciduous teeth normally erupt between the ages of 6 months and 2.5 years. The average ages of eruption in Caucasian children are shown in Table 19.1.

Table 19.1 Average age of eruption of deciduous teeth in Caucasian children

Tooth	Age of eruption (months)
Lower central incisor	7.28
Upper central incisor	9.18
Upper lateral incisor	10.55
Lower lateral incisor	11.55
Upper canine	18.17
Lower canine	18.27
Upper first molar	14.72
Lower first molar	14.83
Upper second molar	26.31
Lower second molar	25.72

The typical order of eruption is the central incisor followed by the lateral incisor, then the first deciduous molars and canine, with the second deciduous molar coming last. Normally, each lower tooth erupts before its upper counterpart, but variation in the order and timing of eruption is common and has little significance.

Functional deciduous dentition (Figure 19.5)

In the fully developed deciduous dentition seen after the age of 2.5 years, the incisor teeth are normally spaced from each other. Such spaces help to accommodate the larger permanent teeth. It is only when the total spacing between the deciduous teeth exceeds 6 mm that there is little chance of crowding of the permanent teeth. While an extremely large overbite or overjet in the completed deciduous dentition may indicate a similar arrangement of the permanent successors, lesser variations have a much diminished predictive value.

Between the ages of 2.5 and 6 years the deciduous teeth wear away and this may allow forward shift of the mandible and mandibular teeth in relation to the maxillary teeth which reduces the overbite and overjet and the incisor teeth may meet edge-to-edge before the age of 6 years.

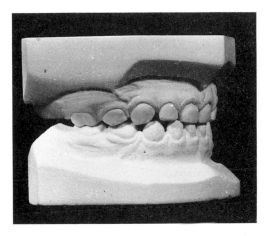

Figure 19.5 Normal relationship of the deciduous teeth

Eruption of permanent teeth (mixed dentition)

The permanent teeth usually erupt between the ages of 6 and 13 years, excepting the third molars (or wisdom teeth) which are frequently delayed in their eruption due to lack of space. Average ages of eruption of permanent teeth for Caucasian boys are shown in Table 19.2 and for girls in Table 19.3.

As a general rule, each lower tooth erupts before its counterpart in the upper arch. Usually, the earliest permanent teeth to erupt are the first permanent molars (commonly referred to as the sixes) followed by the central and lateral incisors. In the uncrowded lower arch these are usually followed by the canines, premolars and second molars. In the upper arch, by contrast, the eruption of premolars usually precedes eruption of the canines. The late-erupting upper canine is frequently displaced by crowding.

Table 19.2 Average age of eruption of permanent teeth in Caucasian boys

Tooth	Age of eruption (years)
Lower central incisor	6.2
Upper central incisor	7.2
Upper lateral incisor	8.2
Lower lateral incisor	7.4
Upper canine	11.5
Lower canine	10.6
Upper first premolar	10.6
Lower first premolar	10.7
Upper second premolar	11.4
Lower second premolar	11.5
Upper first molar	6.3
Lower first molar	6.2
Upper second molar	12.4
Lower second molar	11.9

Table 19.3 Average age of eruption of permanent teeth in Caucasian girls

Tooth	Age of eruption (years)
Lower central incisor	6.0
Upper central incisor	7.0
Upper lateral incisor	7.8
Lower lateral incisor	7.1
Upper canine	10.8
Lower canine	7.6
Upper first premolar	10.1
Lower first premolar	10.0
Upper second premolar	11.0
Lower second premolar	11.0
Upper first molar	6.1
Lower first molar	6.0
Upper second molar	11.9
Lower second molar	11.4

When the permanent incisors first erupt a transitional open bite may persist for some months as the teeth come under the influence of the lips, tongue and cheeks. This open bite is often associated with a habit of thumbsucking and is likely to close of its own accord providing the habit is abandoned. In the majority of Caucasian children, the permanent incisor teeth erupt in crowded positions. The upper and lower lateral incisors usually develop on the lingual side of the arch.

Another frequent abnormality is a midline space between the upper permanent central incisors when they first erupt. This may close on eruption of the lateral incisors or may be associated with the lateral fanning of the upper incisors called the 'ugly duckling stage'. As the name suggests, spontaneous correction is the rule in these cases.

Functional permanent dentition (Figure 19.6).

Following the attainment of occlusion, teeth continue

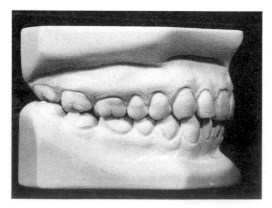

Figure 19.6 Normal relationship of the permanent teeth

to erupt and tend to drift in a forward direction. Incisor teeth tend to become more crowded between the ages of 13 and 18 years.

The interplay of aetiological factors

In the course of growth and development of the child, the rest position (or endogenous postural position) of the mandible precedes the eruption of teeth. It is said to be present by the third month of life and to be still present even if all the teeth are extracted. The inviolable nature of the rest position of the mandible, which is mediated through the length of ligaments and resting length of muscles, is derived from its importance in maintenance of the airway. The teeth and alveolar processes grow into the intermaxillary space dictated by the rest position and centric relation of the jaws and the occlusion of the teeth is established.

From the moment the first pair of upper and lower teeth make occlusal contact, two factors exist: the muscles and the teeth, influencing the mandible in its functional range of movement. Ideally, the range of mandibular movement imposed by the muscles should coincide with that dictated by the teeth. Unfortunately, this does not always occur. Where there is a discrepancy between muscular positioning and the jaw relationship determined by the teeth, the jaws are not in centric relation when the teeth are in occlusion and the patient will show a displacement or deflection of the mandible in closing from the rest position. These displacements may be anterior, lateral or posterior and are commonly associated with temporomandibular dysfunction later in life. The uninitiated must be very wary about diagnosing displacements because young children will frequently protrude the mandible when asked to bring their teeth together.

Temporomandibular disorders

Dynamic abnormalities of the masticatory apparatus may lead to disorders of the teeth, jaws, temporomandibular joints and associated muscles (Gray, Davies and Quayle, 1995). Patients present with one or more of the features of pain dysfunction syndrome comprising clicking, pain or locking of the joint, headache, pain on palpation of the muscles of mastication and a history of noisy grinding of the teeth during sleep or when concentrating. The juxtaposition of the joint and the ear invites misdiagnosis. There may have been an episode of acute trauma such as wide opening of the mouth during anaesthesia or dental procedures. Much more commonly the aetiology is multifactorial with stress an important feature in many cases. There is frequently a displacement of the mandible as the teeth are brought together. The classical group presenting for treatment is women of child-bearing age, but signs of temporo-mandibular disorders can be elicited in more than half of the population, including men and women in approximately equal proportions. Temporomandibular disorders are rare in young children. It is important to exclude general causes of joint pain before making a diagnosis of a temporomandibular disorder. Treatment depends on aetiology, but initial treatment in the form of physiotherapy or a bite raising appliance is effective in many cases.

Orthodontic treatment

The causes of malocclusion may be considered under the following headings:

The relationship of the jawbones
The effect of the soft tissues
Crowding or spacing of the teeth
Local factors.

Anteroposterior abnormalities of the skeletal pattern may be treated with functional appliances during the growing phase, by altering the positions of the incisor teeth (thus camouflaging the skeletal discrepancy), or by a combined orthodontic and surgical approach at the end of the growth period.

Functional appliances work best in children who wear the appliance assiduously and who have a favourable growth pattern. The extent of possible camouflaging with fixed or removable appliances is limited by the thickness of the alveolar processes and the fact that moving lower incisors forward very rarely produces a stable result. Patients who have a lip-apart habitual posture frequently seal the lips after correction of the overjet. Bringing the upper incisors within the control of the lower lip promotes stability of the treatment result.

Orthodontic treatment is more successful in treating horizontal as against vertical skeletal discrepancies.

The concensus of orthodontic opinion is that there is little scope for training lip and tongue function, but some orthodontists believe that exercises and appliances which stimulate or educate muscle behaviour can improve soft tissue function.

Crowding of the teeth is very common in Caucasians. Only a minority can accommodate a full complement of well-aligned teeth in stable positions. Crowding can be treated interceptively in the early stages of development by holding space open for erupting teeth or by extraction of other teeth. At a later stage crowding may be treated by fixed or removable appliances usually associated with extraction of teeth.

Malocclusions resulting from local factors, such as supernumerary teeth or absence of teeth can usually be treated by orthodontic appliances.

The vast majority of patients treated in orthodontic practice have crowding, one or more local factors or a moderate skeletal discrepancy or more than one of these in combination.

The combination of orthodontic and surgical treatment is usually done in the hospital environment. It is the most versatile treatment available, but has the greatest risk of iatrogenic effects.

Respiratory pattern in relation to the teeth and face

The long-standing interest of orthodontists in respiration stems partly from the proximity of the mouth and nose, and partly from the availability of cephalometric radiography which has fostered quantitative research work into the relationship between the mode of respiration and the teeth and face.

Although cephalometric measurement of the airway and the size of the adenoidal pad is two-dimensional, there is a good correlation between cephalometric measurements and the size of adenoids assessed by nasopharyngoscopy.

The classic 'adenoidal facies' comprises a long narrow face, a large angle between the ramus and body of the mandible, narrow mandibular rami and poorly developed muscles of mastication. The upper arch is narrow with protruding upper incisors, the overjet is large and the overbite is diminished. The lips are incompetent and held apart to facilitate mouth-breathing (Figure 19.7). This classical picture is somewhat undermined by the fact that many such patients do not breathe exclusively through the mouth and many subjects who do not have adenoidal facies breathe partially through the mouth under conditions of stress.

Whether the genetic contribution to the shape of the face subscribes to nasal obstruction does not seem to be known. While it is not unreasonable to suggest that it does, most of the limitation of air flow seems to occur at the nostrils. Children with long faces have a higher percentage of airflow through the mouth than control children. In adults with long faces, the nasal resistance is greater on average than in controls with normal faces and competent lips, but the range of variation is great and the differences insufficient to sustain a diagnosis of increased resistance from facial morphology alone.

The other question is whether chronic nasal obstruction has an effect on facial shape. If the nose is blocked experimentally there is an immediate extension of the neck with the head tilting upwards by about 5° on average. The extension strains the submandibular muscles and the mandible drops. It is hypothesized that chronic nasal obstruction produces a similar effect and that the tension in the submandibular muscles causes the mandible to grow downwards rather than forwards. There is an associa-

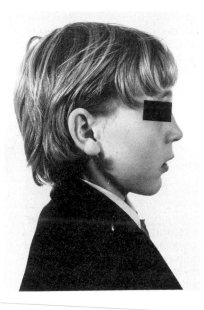

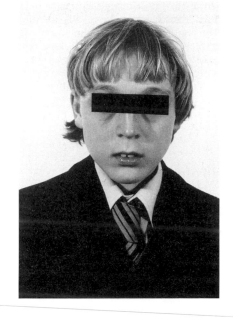

Figure 19.7 Adenoidal facies

tion between perennial allergic rhinitis and a long face, increased overjet and diminished overbite. Children scheduled for adenoidectomy have significantly longer faces than control children. In the first 5 years following adenoidectomy the abnormalities of facial shape diminish but are still characteristic. The lower incisor teeth move forward during the same period (Linder-Aronson, 1970).

It seems that the mode of breathing has an effect on facial shape and tooth positions which is statistically significant but quantitatively is not large. The effect is of the order of 3 mm in terms of facial height and of 2.5 mm in the position of the lower incisors (Linder-Aronson *et al.*, 1993).

Orthodontic appliances in relation to respiratory pattern

Some functional appliances and oral screens which are worn at night inhibit oral breathing and have been said to promote nasal breathing during the waking hours. There seems to be no scientific evidence supporting these claims, but both types of appliance reduce the overjet which makes an anterior oral seal more readily attainable.

Maxillary expansion

Simple upper removable appliances can be used to expand the upper arch. A typical appliance is shown in Figure 19.8. The expansion screw in the midline is opened one quarter turn once or twice each week by the patient. Each quarter turn opens the screw about 2 mm. The principal effect is lateral tipping of the teeth which is approximately equal in the molar and canine regions. A Coffin spring (Figure 19.9) may be used to produce differential dental expansion. Much

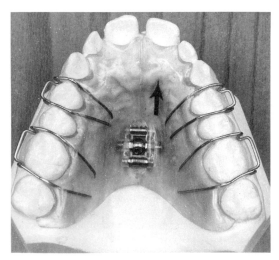

Figure 19.8 A removable screw appliance to expand the upper arch

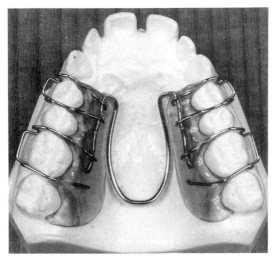

Figure 19.9 A removable Coffin spring appliance which can be adjusted to produce different degrees of expansion in the molar and premolar areas

higher forces can be exerted by the quadhelix (Figure 19.10) which is cemented to the teeth. It can be adjusted to produce differential expansion. Routine activation by the orthodontist is about 10 mm at monthly intervals. Quite high forces can be exerted by the quadhelix and some orthopaedic expansion of the basal bones is possible. In the technique of rapid maxillary expansion (Timms, 1980) cast silver splints are cemented to the teeth and expansion is produced by the patient turning the screw twice each day. The effect is largely orthopaedic. The mid-palatal suture

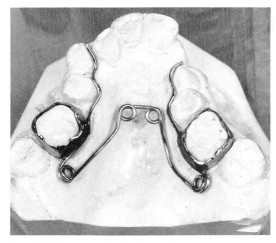

Figure 19.10 A fixed Quadhelix appliance. The bands are cemented to the molar teeth. Different degrees of expansion in the molar and premolar areas are possible

opens and a frighteningly large space appears between the central incisors. The palatal vault is lowered. The increase in size of the nasal airway is said to promote nasal breathing, improve respiratory physiology and improve conductive hearing loss due to alterations in tone of the levator and tensor palati and the effect on the eustachian tube (Hershley, Steward and Warren, 1976).

Scientific evidence for these claims is scant. Following removal of the appliance, the expansion may relapse by about 50%. Dehiscence or clefting of the alveolar process may occur on the buccal sides of the teeth as they are driven through the bone.

Snoring and sleep apnoea

The noise of snoring is caused by vibration of the soft palate or the walls of the oropharynx when they become relaxed during sleep. In sleep apnoea breathing ceases for 10 seconds or longer and there may be 30 or many more such episodes during a 7-hour period of sleep. The cause may be central in which there is disruption of the central nervous impulses initiating a breath or obstructive in which the walls of the oropharynx collapse as a result of reduced muscle tone. Sleep apnoea syndrome is the condition in which there is sleep apnoea associated with excessive drowsiness during the waking hours. Contributory factors are airway narrowing caused by tumours, adenotonsillar hypertrophy, macroglossia or the dentofacial morphology. This has been studied extensively using CT scans and cephalometric radiography (Lowe, Gionhaku and Takeuchi, 1986; Bacon, 1990). Characteristically the face is long with a steep jaw angle, clockwise rotation of the mandible, retropositioning of the maxilla and mandible, a large tongue and soft palate, proclined incisor teeth and open bite. Similarities with the adenoidal facies are striking.

Pierre Robin syndrome

Pierre Robin syndrome arises through a delay in extension of the neck which seriously interferes with mandibular growth and prevents descent of the tongue *in utero*, thus causing cleft palate. The tongue may obstruct the airway which calls for skilled nursing. Appliances have been devised to hold the tongue forward (Cookson and Hall, 1968) and cradles in which infants are nursed belly-down. Mandibular growth usually catches up quite well.

Hemifacial microsomia

In the typical hemifacial microsomia there are severe deficiencies of the ramus of the mandible and muscles of mastication; the mandible is markedly asymmetrical with deviation to the affected side. The occlusal plane of the teeth is canted up to the affected side.

The external ear is anomalous with accessory ear tags. Treatment is by costochondral grafting associated with a functional orthodontic appliance which centralizes the mandible and blocks the eruption of teeth on the unaffected side while allowing eruption of teeth on the affected side.

Treacher Collins syndrome

In Treacher Collins syndrome (mandibulofacial dysostosis) the face is bird-like with poor development of both maxilla and mandible. There are associated abnormalities of the eyes and ears with variable hearing loss. There is usually a severe anterior open bite. Since the origin of the problem is skeletal, the major role in treatment is in the hands of the maxillofacial surgeon. The orthodontist can correct crowding of the teeth and prepare the arches for surgery.

Cleft lip and palate

About one in 750 British Caucasian children is born with cleft lip and/or palate. Each type of cleft has different implications for the patient in terms of appearance, speech and treatment. The cosmetic detriment of cleft lip and the speech difficulties of cleft palate are significant and the psychological effect on the child and parents may be devastating. There are important implications for mastication, swallowing, hearing and speech. Chronic inflammation of the nasal and pharyngeal mucosa and middle ear infection are common. Malalignment of the teeth in the region of the cleft together with decreased growth of the maxilla following palatal surgery also affect appearance adversely. All of these deficiencies are treatable by a range of specialists including paediatric dentists, orthodontists, restorative dentists, plastic and maxillofacial surgeons, otolaryngologists, geneticists and speech therapists. Some are involved at decisive stages of treatment, others have a constant and less dramatic commitment throughout the first 16 or 17 years of life. Since a sound dentition, primary and secondary, is required to facilitate orthodontic treatment, alveolar bone grafting, and orthognathic surgery, all specialists must have an understanding of the tooth-bearing region. The reader is referred to the section on normal dental development and orthodontics at the beginning of this chapter.

A great deal of medical and dental effort is involved in the treatment of the cleft child. Perhaps more importantly, a great deal of commitment is required of the patient and parents. At some stages patients and parents cry out for treatment and may be disappointed when the perceived problem cannot be rectified immediately. At other times they may become disenchanted with long, slow treatment and frequent visits to hospital. It is incumbent on members of the

medical team to make visits to hospital meaningful and fruitful in order to maintain parental enthusiasm and patient compliance. If the outstanding possibilities for treatment are to be fully realized, orchestration of the medical team is essential to make the most of these important factors. Close support and encouragement is essential and each cleft palate team should have one member easily contactable by the family for advice in times of difficulty.

Assessment of the treatment modalities which have been used over the years is bedevilled by the involvement of many surgeons, many orthodontists and many techniques. Some treatments benefit one aspect of the problem to the detriment of others. It is therefore important that each operator has an adequate understanding of the aims and timing of treatment of the other specialists involved and the possible interaction of each treatment phase. This communication between specialists has improved greatly in recent years and an international pattern of treatment seems to be evolving. There is no question that the results of cleft treatment have vastly improved over the working lifetime of these authors.

Embryology of facial development

In order to understand the nature of the cleft defect a basic knowledge of normal facial development is essential. For more detailed information a specialist textbook should be consulted (Ferguson, 1988, 1991, 1993).

Initially the right and left facial processes are widely separated from each other. The central block of the face constitutes about 60% of the total face width at 7 weeks' gestation but, with differential growth, particularly the lateral to frontal migration of the developing eye fields, this central facial block occupies only 20% of the total face width by 9 weeks' gestation. This proportion remains relatively constant until birth and it is this central facial block which ultimately makes up the philtrum of the lip, columella, nose and interorbital distance. The right and left lateral maxillary processes grow medially and at about 8 weeks' gestation fusion occurs between these and the medial nasal process (Figure 19.11). Failure of fusion results in either unilateral or bilateral clefting, complete or incomplete, of the lip and/or primary palate as far back as the incisive foramen. Fusion of the developing palatal shelves occurs a little later, beginning anteriorly and finally forming the posterior soft palate. Females elevate their palatal shelves 1 week later than males (Figure 19.12). Cleft palate occurs when the shelves fail to fuse in the midline and can occur completely or incompletely involving all or part of the hard and soft palate as far forward as the incisive foramen. The disruption of development which results in isolated cleft palate is different from that in anterior

1 Hypoplasia of the facial processes
2 Altered facial geometry
3 Defective ability of the surface epithelia to participate in the fusion process
4 Excessive cell death in the fusing epithelial seams, mesenchymal deficiency and postfusion rupture.

A spectrum of malformations can occur ranging from simple grooving to complete clefting. Where weak fusion occurs the subsequent growth tractional forces can pull tissues apart, often incompletely, resulting in Simonart's bands.

Such events may occur unilaterally or bilaterally in which case the central portion of the lip contains little or no muscle as a result of deficient mesenchymal consolidation. Lip pits can occur without lip clefting and may represent a microform of the same process, but are more likely to be associated with partial persistence of the sulcus between the pars villosa and pars glabra. Complete persistence of this sulcus results in the so-called 'complete double lip' often seen in Ascher's syndrome.

Isolated cleft palate may be a result of disruption of one or more of a number of mechanisms:

1 Palatal shelves too small to meet – hypoplasia
2 Failure of palatal shelf elevation at the correct time either due to diminished intrinsic force, or due to increased resistance, principally by the tongue position remaining high and between the palatal shelves (see Figure 19.12). Defective growth of Meckel's cartilage also can inhibit tongue drop by an underdeveloped mandible which normally grows down and forward. Postural moulding defects also play a part, e.g. Pierre Robin syndrome. In this case the mandible becomes trapped behind the sternum and increases resistance to tongue dropping
3 Excessive head width causing failure of normal sized palatal shelves to meet
4 Failure of shelf fusion due to defective epitheliomesenchymal interactions. This may occur at different stages producing a spectrum of clinical presentations ranging from complete midline cleft, along the entire length of the palate, to cleft of the soft palate only. Sometimes the mucosa overlying the palate appears normal but fusion below has not occurred resulting in 'submucous' cleft palate.

Pierre Robin syndrome is a triad of small retrusive mandible, cleft palate and weak tongue. The palatal shelves are intrinsically normal and the cleft is usually extremely wide due to the tongue position preventing fusion (Figure 19.13). Unlike isolated cleft palate caused by defective shelf growth there is some catch up growth which decreases the size of the cleft after birth when tongue resistance is removed.

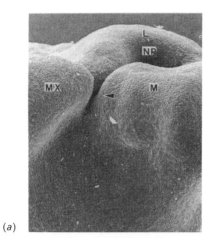
(a)

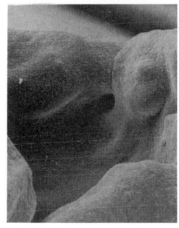
(b)

Figure 19.11 (a) Intraoral view of the closing medial nasal (M), lateral nasal (L) and maxillary (MX) processes to form the primary nasal choanae (arrowed). NP, nasal pit. (b) Illustrates the closure of these processes and the fusion of the epithelium at the base of the nasal pit with that of the oronasal cavity to form the primary nasal choanae. Note how the closure of the medial nasal, lateral nasal and maxillary processes also contributes to the formation of the primary nasal choanae. (Courtesy of M. Ferguson)

clefting and should be considered separately. When cleft of lip and palate occur together the cleft palate is almost always a secondary result of the lip cleft. In this case the tongue tip becomes trapped above the cleft premaxilla, increasing the resistance to palatal shelf elevation, which is accordingly delayed or prevented, resulting in cleft palate.

Cleft lip results from a failure of fusion of the medial nasal, lateral nasal and maxillary processes on either or both sides. It has been suggested that several interactive processes can lead to this failure:

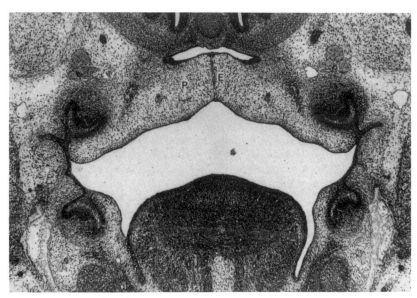

Figure 19.12 Coronal histological section illustrating horizontal fused palatal shelves (P). Note the epithelial seam (E) and the first molar tooth germs now at the bell stage of development. (Courtesy of M. Ferguson)

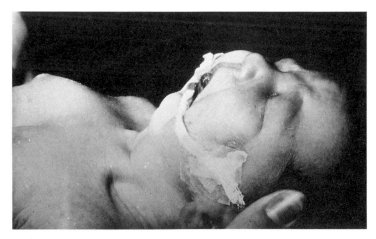

Figure 19.13 Pierre Robin syndrome. Note very retrusive chin and respiratory difficulty when lying on the back as tongue strength is poor and the tongue falls backward on the nasopharynx to occlude the airway

Clinical classification of cleft type

Since the time of Veau (1932, quoted by Kernahan and Stark, 1958) several attempts have been made to classify clefts diagrammatically. The Veau classification was improved by Kernahan and Stark (1958) but still had shortcomings when describing the degree of clefting of both primary and secondary palate. In recent years, a more detailed classification method has been developed in several centres in the UK which allowed the separate recording of whether a cleft is complete or incomplete in each anatomical region of lip, alveolus, hard and soft palates. Such

incoordinated efforts have been made in Scotland, Northern Ireland, and several centres in England and Wales. In 1994, the Faculty of Dental Surgery of the Royal College of Surgeons of England, through the Orthodontic Audit Committee, commissioned the development of a common Cleft Palate Database for the registration of births in the UK. In 1995 and in conjunction with the CARE committee of the Craniofacial Society the aim is to appoint a 'caretaker' in each region whose duty is to record standard details of every cleft birth and provide these to a central database which, in time, will allow accurate epidemiological studies to be performed for the whole of the

UK. In addition the family history of clefting together with possible environmental stimuli which could be implicated in the cause of the defect will also be recorded.

Relative incidence of cleft types

Retrospective epidemiological studies of cleft lip and/or palate have been unreliable for many years because the description of cleft type in clinical notes is often incomplete or inconsistent. The present authors have published a report of cleft births in Northern Ireland over a 10-year period, 1980– 1989 (Gregg, Boyd and Richardson, 1994). This probably represents the most recent and accurate study in a population within the UK. Cleft type was recorded according to the Kernahan and Stark classification (Figure 19.14). Fifty three per cent of clefts involved the secondary palate only, 16% the primary palate/lip only, 26% involved both primary and secondary palate and 5% were unconnected. More males than females were affected overall and there were more males than females in the group having complete

clefts. Unilateral clefts were more common on the left side.

Within the group showing complete unilateral cleft of the primary and secondary palate, left-sided clefts were more commonly male, right-sided clefts were more commonly female. There were no sex differences between sides in the unilateral primary palate cleft group. Separate clefts of lip and palate occurred almost exclusively in males. These findings suggest a strong sex-linked genetic background in clefts affecting the primary palate/lip but not in clefts affecting the secondary palate only. However, a specific gene has not yet been identified, nor has a specific environmental stimulus been implicated, although it has been shown that presence of receptors for teratogens (e.g. phenytoin) artificially induced in animals does cause failure of palatal shelf elevation and resultant cleft palate. This has not been shown in humans. It is known that when a close family history of clefting exists, either in a sibling or in either parent, the chance of a cleft occurrence increases to approximately 1:30 compared to 1:750 where no previous family history exists.

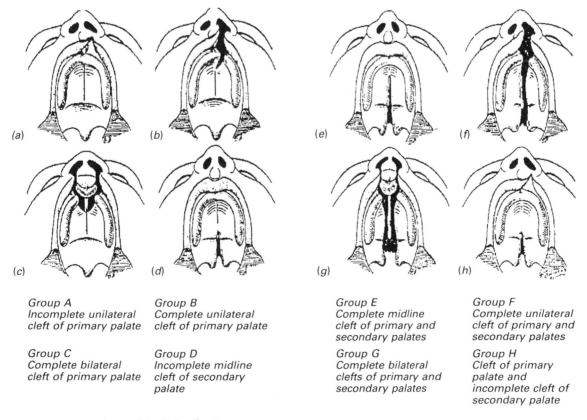

Group A
Incomplete unilateral
cleft of primary palate

Group B
Complete unilateral
cleft of primary palate

Group C
Complete bilateral
cleft of primary palate

Group D
Incomplete midline
cleft of secondary
palate

Group E
Complete midline
cleft of primary and
secondary palates

Group F
Complete unilateral
cleft of primary and
secondary palates

Group G
Complete bilateral
clefts of primary and
secondary palates

Group H
Cleft of primary
palate and
incomplete cleft of
secondary palate

Figure 19.14 Kernahan and Stark classification

Clinical management and coordination of treatment

This will be considered in the chronological order in which each aspect of treatment is usually undertaken. While no single child would have all of the treatments, and there are still variations between treatment centres, a list of possible decisive events in chronological order is shown in Table 19.4.

Table 19.4 Chronological list of possible treatment events

Birth	Parental counselling
	Presurgical orthopaedics
3 months	Lip repair
6–12 months	Palate repair
2–5 years	Speech therapy
4–5 years	Surgery for velopharyngeal incompetence
	Further speech therapy
7–9 years	Initial orthodontic treatment
	Arch expansion
9 years	Secondary alveolar grafting
	Elevation of nasal tip
12 years	Final orthodontic alignment
	Temporary prosthesis
17 years	Orthognathic surgery combined with orthodontic treatment
	Definitive prosthesis
	Revision of nose and lip

Parental counselling, presurgical orthopaedics and feeding aids

There is great variation in reaction between parents after a cleft baby is born. Some will cope very well and soon adopt a pragmatic approach when they realize that the problem is not life threatening and surgical repair is possible. An early visit from a member of the cleft palate team can relieve many fears and a demonstration of 'before and after' photographs of a repaired cleft lip is very reassuring. Similarly a full description of the extent of potential speech and hearing problems is always appreciated. Most centres also have a small booklet which can be given to parents for information. A short explanation of the cause and incidence of clefting is requested by some parents and it is important to explain this without attributing blame to either parent. Usually both parents and family very quickly recover from the initial shock and wish to deal with the most immediate problem of successful feeding to ensure that the baby is discharged from hospital as soon as possible.

Presurgical orthopaedics is the term used to describe orthodontic manipulation of the cleft alveolar segments in an effort to obtain better alignment prior to surgical repair. This is not carried out for isolated midline clefts of the palate only. Ideally the cleft alveolar segments should be positioned end to end, as in a butt joint. This in turn causes the soft tissues of the lip to be in better apposition which will facilitate surgical repair. This is usually performed at 3 months of age.

Presurgical orthopaedics is considered for any cleft involving the primary palate, unilateral or bilateral, where unrestrained growth has displaced the alveolar segments significantly (Figure 19.15). In a bilateral

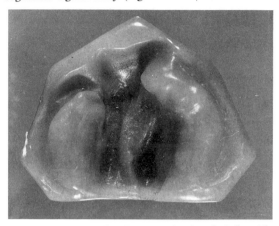

Figure 19.15 A model of the upper alveolus of a baby with a complete unilateral cleft of lip and palate. Note the displacement of the alveolar segments and resultant lateral position of the midline fraenum

cleft at birth the alveolar segments often collapse medially behind a premaxillary segment which is protruded by unrestrained growth of the nasal septum (Figure 19.16). Repositioning of the segments can be achieved with an intraoral plate to expand the lateral segments together with elastic strapping to retract the protrusive premaxilla. The method described by McNeill (1954) and Burston (1958) has been most commonly employed. The technique involves sectioning a model of the mouth, repositioning the lateral segments and making an acrylic plate to

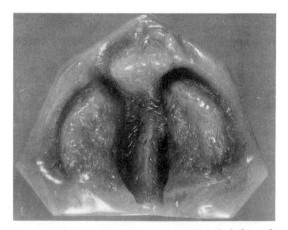

Figure 19.16 A model of the upper alveolus of a baby with a complete bilateral cleft of lip and palate. Note the unrestrained growth of the nasal septum pushes the premaxilla forward and upwards. Sometimes the lateral alveolar segments collapse medially behind the premaxilla

the new position. When the baby closes the mouth around a teat, the acrylic plate is gently pressed into the alveolar segments which are guided to the new position. This in turn allows the protruded premaxilla to be retracted using elastic strapping fixed in front of the ear on both sides (Figure 19.17). Huddart (1962)

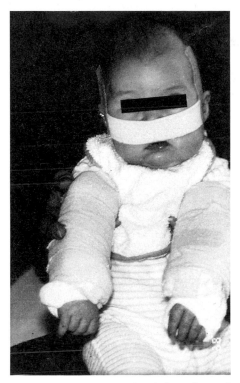

Figure 19.17 Burston strapping for a baby with complete unilateral cleft of lip and palate. In this case arm splints were used for a period to prevent the baby from disturbing the strapping

and later DiBiase and Hunter (1983) described a modification of the Burston method involving an active appliance which used springs and screws, as with an orthodontic appliance used in the dentate adolescent, in an effort to achieve even better alignment of the alveolus.

For unilateral complete clefts (involving both primary and secondary palate) Latham, Kusy and Georgiade (1976) modified a technique first developed by Georgiade, Nladick and Thorne (1968) which involves fitting a sectional plate pinned to the alveolar segments. A screw is turned by the parent each day resulting in the eventual active forcing together of the alveolar segments (Figure 19.18). They designed a similar appliance for bilateral complete clefts which involves additional intraoral elastic traction to reposition a protruded premaxilla, thus obviating the need for extraoral strapping as described earlier. These methods have been recommended by Millard (1994) to allow not only easier repair of the soft tissues but also, when the gap between the alveolar segments can be reduced to less than 4 mm, it may be possible to close the mucoperiosteum without relieving incisions. This may reduce the need for an alveolar bone graft at 9 years of age. This has yet to be proven conclusively as the technique is still relatively new. A further benefit of easing lip repair, it is hypothesized, is that when surgical repair requires less undermining in order to achieve closure of the lip there will be less scar tissue and less hindrance to future growth as a result. This also has not been proven satisfactorily as yet. The initial results seem encouraging but as the child matures the differences between children having and not having presurgical orthopaedics diminishes. A survey by Ascher-McDade and Shaw (1990) revealed that presurgical orthopaedics is used by 56.8% of clinicians in the UK for alignment of complete unilateral and bilateral clefts. Of these 53.9% use a

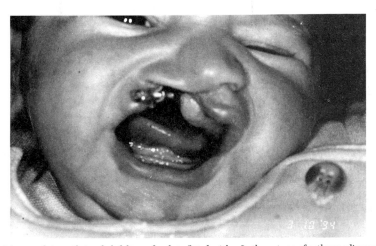

Figure 19.18 Baby with complete unilateral cleft lip and palate fitted with a Latham type of orthopaedic appliance. Note the screw which protrudes and is easily turned each day by the parents to draw gradually the alveolar segments into close apposition

Burston type appliance and a further 25.5% use an active appliance of some kind. As an alternative, some surgeons attempt to restrain the premaxillary segment by initial lip adhesion soon after birth followed by definitive lip closure a few months later. However, although this may ease lip repair a little, it does not achieve significant improvement of the position of the alveolar segments.

It is important to distinguish between premaxillary orthopaedics and the fitting of an inactive feeding plate from birth until lip repair on the grounds that it will normalize tongue position and function and eliminate the harmful false suckle and swallowing pattern. This is only of use in complete clefts for the short period before lip repair, usually at 3 months of age, and should not be used for long periods. It is suggested that the presence of a plate blocking off the cleft also facilitates feeding by providing a false alveolus and hard palate allowing an anterior seal in the absence of a complete lip closure. Saunders *et al.* 1988) described an acrylic plate lined with a soft material which provides a better fit and has the additional benefit of achieving adequate retention without the need for external straps (Figure 19.19). However feeding problems can also be met, albeit less well, with modified teats alone, which allow easier flow of milk as the baby tires. The Habermann bottle provides a useful alternative as flow can be altered through the teat by rotating the bottle to one of three positions (Figure 19.20). In contrast, it is important to realize that babies with isolated clefts of the secondary palate feed satisfactorily by using modified teats and variance of flow as described above and there is no significant benefit from a feeding plate. In any case, since palate repair is not carried out until 6–12 months of age, it is undesirable to fit an appliance for this length of time. In this case additional benefit for feeding is obtained by maintaining the baby in an upright position during feeding to maximize the effect of gravity and decrease the likelihood of milk passing

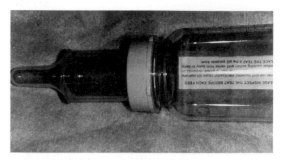

Figure 19.20 Habermann feeding bottle allows the flow speed to be varied by turning the bottle into one of three positions (denoted by a different length of line on the teat). The need for different teats with different sized holes is obviated

backwards and into the nose in the absence of a soft palate closure. It is also useful to encourage frequent winding as air through the nose will be swallowed during sucking.

Surgical repair of cleft lip

It is not proposed to describe the surgical procedures for repair of the cleft lip in detail in this chapter. Such procedural details can be found in a textbook of plastic surgery. Rather an overview of preparation, timing of surgery, and follow up will be described.

It is first important to realize that complete repair of cleft lip and palate is not carried out at the same time. Usually surgery to the lip is performed at around 3 months of age or when the baby reached 4.5 kg (10 lb) weight. This timing is the result of anaesthetic considerations rather than for any reason associated with the cleft lip. With the improvements in safety of anaesthesia for babies in recent years some surgeons have carried out surgery in the first week of life in an effort to achieve normal appearance as soon as possible and also to allow easier feeding in the presence of a lip seal. However, there has not been any other benefit claimed by such early intervention and the majority of surgeons still operate at 3 months. The technique described by Millard (1957) is almost universally used. Photographs of 'before and after' lip repair are shown in Plates 6/19/I and 6/19/II. Patients who have a cleft of lip only without involvement of the alveolus can reasonably expect complete success in one operation. When the alveolus is affected then soft tissue of the lip on either side of the cleft may be so far apart that surgery is extremely difficult and a secondary procedure is required in later years to tidy the vermilion border or raise the tethered prolabium. One can also expect some disturbance in the eruption and form of the teeth in the region and patients are enrolled in a joint cleft palate clinic with an orthodontist and paediatric dentist who will monitor development of the permanent

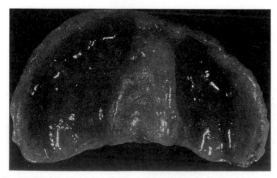

Figure 19.19 Saunders feeding plate with a soft lining of Visco Gel dental material which improves the fit and increases retention

dentition and prepare the dental arch for an alveolar bone graft around the age of 9 years as indicated.

In the case of very wide clefts, where closure will require much undermining of tissues, some surgeons like to perform a lip adhesion in the first few weeks as a preparation for definitive closure at 3 months. This method hopes to ease the tissue tension immediately postoperatively and promote better healing. It is also hypothesized that there is some narrowing of the cleft due to the tension produced by the 'tacking' of the soft tissue which acts in a similar way to presurgical orthopaedic strapping. In the case of bilateral clefts another approach is to carry out closure on one side only at the first operation, allow this to heal for a few weeks, and repair the second side separately. There is no universal agreement as to the indications for these variations, or to perform presurgical orthopaedics, and each method has very enthusiastic proponents. It remains the preference of different surgeons which determines the method used in most centres.

Palate repair and functional implications for speech

Successful treatment of congenital and acquired conditions affecting the palate depends on an understanding of its functions. As the floor of the nose, it provides part of the airway, isolating the nasal cavity from obstruction by food during mastication, and as the roof of the mouth, it provides a surface against which food may be broken up by the tongue and neatly passed back as manageable boluses for swallowing. In humans its smooth surface is also concerned with the production of distinguishably different sounds which can be combined together to produce intelligible speech. The soft palate has the additional ability to contribute to closure of the velopharyngeal isthmus to prevent food entering the nose in swallowing and also to conserve and direct respired air through the mouth under pressure for speech.

Timing of palate repair

During the normal development of speech patterns, the first phonemes that require velopharyngeal closure are used between 6 and 9 months of age suggesting that repair should precede this period. In 1927 Veau demonstrated that patients who underwent repair of the palate after 2 years of age had notably worse speech than those whose palates were repaired before that age. Pigott and McManamny (1987) suggested that there is a statistically significant higher rate of velopharyngeal insufficiency in those operated on before 1 year compared with those operated on between 1 and 2 years. An additional practical consideration is that at 1 year of age the bulk of muscle in the palate is much larger than at 3 months,

making tension-free repair easier. Many surgeons now compromise and aim to carry out palate repair around 6 months of age to facilitate speech development as early as possible.

Extent of repair

There has always been some controversy regarding how much of the palate should be repaired at the primary procedure. The most common approach in the UK is to repair the soft palate, and all of the hard palate in need of closure. An alternative is to repair the soft palate only at first operation and repair the mucoperiosteum of the hard palate in later years. The former method avoids the postoperative requirement of an obturator which needs to be worn continuously for several years if harmful tongue positions during speech are to be avoided. The permanent presence of a dental plate for long periods presents many problems including dental decay, mucosal irritation, frequent replacement as teeth erupt and fit is lost and, most importantly, lack of compliance from the child who quickly learns to eject the plate from the mouth. Hotz *et al.* (1978) and Schweckendiek (1978) favoured early repair of the soft palate and delayed repair of the hard palate, varying between 4 and 12 years. They pointed out that considerable narrowing of the cleft takes place so that extensive mucoperiosteal undermining and displacement are not required. This they claimed would have considerable benefits for long term growth of the maxilla and some surgeons persist with this approach in spite of the logistical difficulties of compliance.

Technique (Pigott and McManamny, 1987)

A modified von Langenbeck technique will be described. The use of this method depends on closure of the anterior palate at the same time as the lip is repaired in those cases of complete cleft of lip and palate. This is usually performed 3 months before palatal repair (Figure 19.21).

Longitudinal studies of facial growth (Ross, 1970) have shown a significantly greater proportion of midface retrusion in the patients who underwent the Veau procedure (Figure 19.22) compared with the von Langenbeck procedure (Figure 19.23). This has been attributed to the reduced amount of dissection of the hard palate in the von Langenbeck procedure. Veau's technique has, in the past, been considered to give superior speech results because it lengthened the palate. However, in 1959 and 1960, Calnan reported that the palatal lengthening achieved by the Veau V to Y pushback operation is not sustained. Reports of better speech results with the Veau operation compared to the Langenbeck's and vice versa abound but some authors find no real difference (Jolleys, 1954; Witzel *et al.*, 1979).

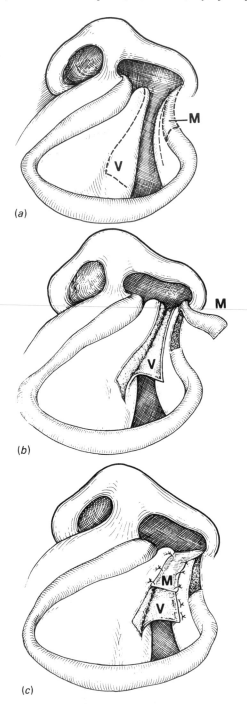

(a)

(b)

(c)

Figure 19.21 Repair of alveolus and anterior hard palate. (*a*) Lines of incision in palatal mucoperiosteum, of vomer and lesser segment for nasal layer closure and lines of incision in lateral labial mucosa for oral flap; (*b*) cleft is closed by approximating mucoperiosteal layers of alveolus and vomerine flap (V) of major segment beneath the mucoperiosteum of lesser flap; (*c*) a two-layer closure is achieved anteriorly by using the labial mucosa flap (M)

Preoperative preparation

Bacteriological swabs are taken from the nose and throat 3 days preoperatively. The operation is postponed if group A beta haemolytic streptococci are cultured, and treatment with penicillin is commenced. Staphylococci are treated with nasal chlorhexidene and flucloxacillin.

Operation (Pigott and McManamny, 1987)

Under endotracheal anaesthesia using a non-cuffed tube, gauze swabs soaked in 3% cocaine are placed along the margins of the cleft, and are inserted into the nostrils. Care is taken not to exceed a dose of 3 mg/kg bodyweight. An intravenous drip is inserted. The patient is positioned with a sandbag placed beneath the shoulders, and the head extended on the neck. Both headlight and magnification with 2.5 loupes are used by the surgeon. Suction apparatus is available with a paediatric measuring facility. A Dott mouth gag and a throat pack are inserted. The palate is infiltrated with a solution of 1% lignocaine hydrochloride with 1:250 000 adrenalin. Seven minutes are allowed for the vasoconstrictor to take effect. The initial incision is made in the oral mucosa down to bone just medial to the sulcus between alveolar and palatal mucosa from a point a little anterior to the forward limit of the cleft, back to the maxillary buttress, then laterally to the outer margin of the alveolus and then back again to the tip of the hamulus. A second incision is made on the oral side of the margin of the cleft, along a line between oral and nasal mucosa where a distinct colour change from the redder nasal to the whiter oral mucosa exists. A small periosteal elevator such as a Mitchell's timmer is used to separate the mucoperiosteum from the underlying bony palate starting from the lateral incision and working across to the cleft margin. Care must be taken to avoid damage to the greater palatine vessels. After exposure of the bony cleft margin, the nasal mucosa is mobilized blindly for a short distance laterally from the cleft margin.

With the posterior border of the hard palate in view, the soft palate musculature is gently mobilized at the line of attachment to the posterior margin of the hard palate using a combination of sharp and blunt dissection. Laterally, fibres of tensor palati can be seen passing around the hook of the hamulus. The tensor is preserved and the hamulus is not fractured. The lesser palatine nerve which supplies musculus uvulae is also preserved, if possible. The nasopharyngeal mucosa is mobilized from the medial surface of the pterygoid plate up to the base of skull. Both oral mucosa and mucous glands are separated from the muscular layer of the soft palate for about 1 cm to permit displacement of the musculus uvulae onto the palatal dorsum while uniting the levator and depressors beneath it. Oral and nasal flaps must

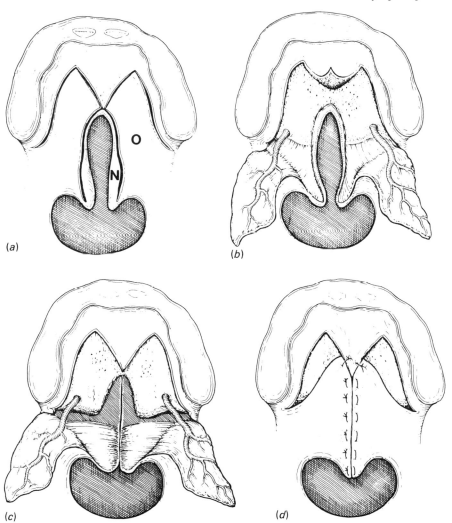

Figure 19.22 Veau technique of cleft palate repair with veloplasty. (*a*) Lines of incision in palatal mucosa; (*b*) flaps are elevated based on the greater palatine arteries; (*c*) musculature of the soft palate is approximated; (*d*) mucosal closure, with V–Y pushback. O: Oral mucosa; N: nasal mucosa

reach easily to the midline. A similar procedure is performed on the remaining side.

The nasal layer is closed first using interrupted absorbable sutures, beginning anteriorly and working back. Then a heavy (3.0 chromic) horizontal mattress suture is placed at the junction of the middle and posterior thirds of the soft palate. It passes through both muscle and nasal mucosa layers lateral to the musculus uvulae fibres, with the aim of bunching up the tissue on the dorsum midline of the palate to recreate the uvula muscle ridge (Figure 19.24). The oral layer is then closed with interrupted mattress sutures, one suture being placed between oral and nasal layers at the junction of the hard and soft palate to obliterate a potential dead space. Small

wedges of absorbable haemostatic agent (Oxycel) are placed in the lateral defects, which heal rapidly by secondary intention. Postoperatively thumb sucking may be prevented by armsplints for 2 weeks if required, although such methods of restraint do not have universal approval. The patient remains in hospital for 7–10 days after surgery. The use of a teat should also be avoided and it is useful to ask parents to accustom the child to feeding with fluids from a spoon for a period before admission.

A routine postoperative follow up is arranged for 6 months, and the first formal speech assessment is carried out at 18 months. By this time it is already possible to assess velopharyngeal competence in some children, but most children can be more reliably

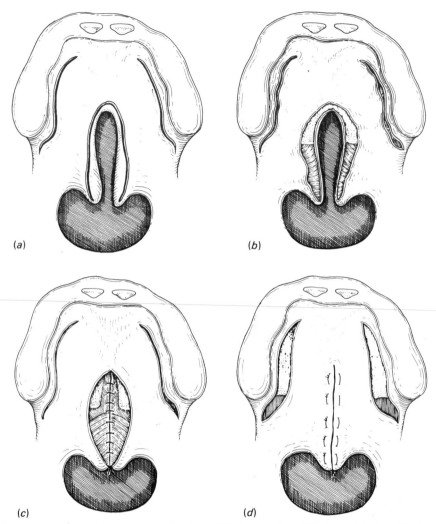

Figure 19.23 Von Langenbeck repair incorporating Pigott and McManamny's modifications. (*a*) Lines of incision in palatal mucosa; (*b*) flaps are elevated. Muscle layer of soft palate is defined but not dissected completely. Nasopharyngeal mucosa adherent to medial pterygoid plate is mobilized; (*c*) muscle layers are sutured in the midline and the nasal mucosa everted with a horizontal mattress suture; (*d*) oral mucosa closure. No pushback and minimal exposure of palatal bone occurs

assessed at 30 months (van Demark and van Demark, 1970).

Early complications

The majority of children recover quickly from cleft palate repair and the incidence of complications is low in experienced hands. Of the problems that can occur postoperatively, airway obstruction and bleeding are the two most dangerous.

Difficult intubation due to micrognathia, subglottic stenosis, cervical spine anomalies or incorrect tube selection may cause oedema of the glottis and tracheostomy may be required. More often, a tongue-stitch may be used to hold the tongue forward for a few hours in some micrognathic infants. It also facilitates pharyngeal suction. Humidification has been found useful in about 10% of infants and betamethasone has produced dramatic improvement on rare occasions. Usually bleeding can be controlled in the ward with direct pressure using a swab placed over the bleeding point and digital compression. Haemorrhage sufficient to require return to theatre occurs in approximately 5% of cases. Secondary haemorrhage is very uncommon, but if it occurs it can be life-threatening. Return to theatre and surgical control of the bleeding is necessary, as are antibiotics. The most common pathogen under these circum-

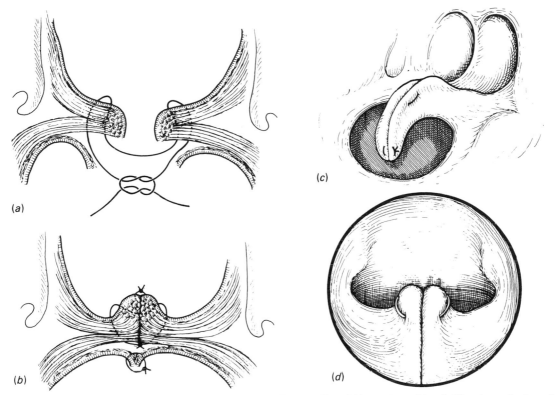

Figure 19.24 Musculus uvulae eversion suture. (*a*) Placement of suture; (*b*) and (*c*) eversion achieved; (*d*) endoscopic view of eversion achieved

stances is the group A beta-haemolytic streptococcus and penicillin is the drug of choice for treatment. Mixed infections are not uncommon and flucloxacillin should be added pending swab results. Group A streptococcal infection may also result in wound breakdown and fistula formation. Fistula repair should be deferred for a minimum of 6 months to allow scars to mature and the tissues to soften.

Late complications

Maxillary retrusion

The significant long-term problem following early total cleft palate repair is the effect that this surgery has on the growth of the midface. Some 80% of children with total clefts will require orthodontic correction for dental arch collapse and 10% will require surgery in the late teens for severe maxillary hypoplasia. Against this must be set evidence suggesting that early repair of the palate may reduce the incidence of ear infections and deafness and also reduce the incidence of severe articulatory disturbances leading to markedly impaired intelligibility.

Fistulae

While many fistulae remaining after cleft palate repair are small and asymptomatic, the following symptoms may be sufficient to merit surgery. Nasal dribbling, especially of ice cream or chocolate rubbed against the palate for taste, is a significant social disability and may occur with pinhole fistulae. Alteration of nasal resonance and loss of oral air pressure may occur. The tongue may naturally occlude the fistula for some sounds but trick movements to occlude it for other sounds distort articulation. Symptoms of rhinitis are not uncommon and ironically an enlarged turbinate may obturate a large fistula. Fistulae are described as being pre-, per- or postalveolar, hard palate, soft palate or a combination.

Treatment

Treatment may be by dental obturation or surgical closure. Dental obturation is particularly suitable if the patient must wear a partial denture due to loss of teeth. However, partial dentures frequently cause dental decay and mucosal inflammation. While some patients wish to avoid surgery if at all possible, others may find the need to wear a plate unacceptable. Surgical management to close the fistula requires tissue which may be available locally or may need to be imported. A surprisingly large flap of oral mucosa may be 'hinged' on the scar and turned up to line the nose. This is then reinforced, often as a double-breasting manoeuvre, with a flap transposed from the opposite side (Figure 19.25). Another local flap may be developed by advancing a segment of palatal mucoperiosteum on the greater palatine artery. After teasing out the vessel from the foramen, up to 2 cm of anterior displacement may be obtained. This opera-

tion described by Widmaier in 1973 has been christened, most aptly, the tadpole flap by Henderson (1982).

Where local tissue is considered to be too scarred or insufficient in area, distant flaps may be obtained from the buccal sulcus or tongue. Buccal sulcus mucosa may be transposed on a posterior base round behind the maxillary tuberosity, or anteriorly through the alveolar cleft. The tongue provides a major reservoir of tissue where previous surgery has rendered repair with local tissue impracticable. A flap of mucosa with a shaving of muscle is raised, usually on an anterior base which should be sited beneath the posterior margin of the fistula and rotated through 180° to be sutured to the freshened edges of the fistula. Detachment of the pedicle is usually possi-

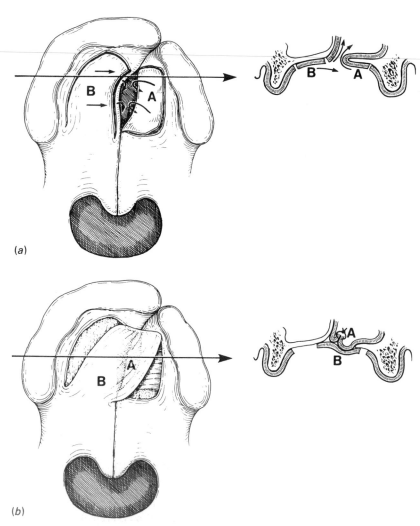

Figure 19.25 Local flap repair of hard palate fistula. The turnover flap is based on a scar at the edge of the fistula and must be elevated with great caution

ble at 10–14 days. The mucosa retains its papillae and if a very large flap is taken sensation of the tongue may be impaired (Pigott, Reiger and Frazer Moodie, 1984).

Velopharyngeal incompetence

The incidence of velopharyngeal incompetence or insufficiency after cleft palate repair varies from less than 10% (Morley, 1970) up to more than 50% in other series, but many authors accept a figure in the region of 20% for patients operated upon in the first 2 years of life.

Improved velopharyngeal function in speech can be achieved by modifying one or more of the walls of the velopharyngeal isthmus.

Anterior wall

The failed repaired cleft palate shares several stigmata with submucous cleft (see below). In particular, the points of lift seen on the oral side of the palate are more widely separated than normal, causing the palate to assume a square, rather than a Gothic pointed arch or the lift may be diffuse, producing a Norman or rounded arch. At the same time, ridges of muscle may be seen to build up towards the posterior nasal spine from the region of the eustachian tubes (Boorman and Sommerlad, 1985). The dorsal surface seen endoscopically has a V-shaped midline valley and this may be the site of failure to close as the palate shoulders reach the posterior wall. Alternatively, there may be a total failure of the palate to reach the posterior wall, a pharyngeal disproportion, indicating a degree of hypoplasia of the palate. Restoration of normal function may require some or all of the following (Figure 19.26):

1 Realignment of muscles by intravelar veloplasty (Kriens, 1975)
2 Reconstruction of the musculus uvulae ridge
3 Correction of the disproportion by lengthening the palate (Honig, 1967)
4 Augmentation of the palatal dorsum (Moore, 1960).

Posterior wall

The posterior wall may be advanced by insertion of materials such as cartilage, muscle, bone or synthetics such as Teflon and silastic. Alternatively the wall may be advanced by construction of a mucomuscular ridge on the posterior wall above the level of the arch of the atlas vertebra (Hynes, 1953; Orticochea, 1967). In order to perform this part of the operation the soft palate is retracted out of the way and a transverse incision is made across the posterior wall as far above the level of the arch of the atlas as

possible. Bilateral flaps of posterior tonsillar pillar are raised, with bases orientated superiorly, at the same level as the transverse pharyngeal incision. The posterior margins of the flaps are continuous with this transverse incision. The flaps must contain some palatopharyngeus fibres if they are to be dynamic, but some muscle must be left behind, otherwise active palatal depression is reduced, with subsequent hyponasality. The flaps are transposed through 90° and sutured end to end. The inferior border of this newly created horizontal bar is then attached to the inferior border of the transverse incision in the posterior pharyngeal wall.

The pharyngoplasty is given time to heal and, although it may initially be immobile, on reassessment some months later, it will be seen to contract during speech. There are two possible explanations for the delay in function of this muscle bar. One is that cortical representation of the muscle activity, which was originally concerned with palatal depression, must have time to reorganize to coordinate with palatal elevation and velopharyngeal closure. Another explanation is that during elevation and transposition of the muscle flaps, they become denervated, and they do not become active again until they have reinnervated with nerve fibres from the posterior pharynx. This muscle ridge will usually produce a static advancement of 5 mm, but in some cases it is dynamic, thus permitting sphincteric closure of the isthmus (Lendrum and Dhar, 1984).

Surgical obturation by pharyngeal flap

A superiorly or inferiorly based trapdoor of mucosa and muscle from the posterior wall (Schoenborn, 1876) is attached to the soft palate to obstruct the central part of the isthmus. These operations rely on adduction of the lateral pharyngeal walls to the flap to complete closure. The defect on each side of the bar is known as a port or gutter. The bridge of the mucosa is usually passive, although a few studies have suggested residual activity of the accompanying superior constrictor muscle. The width of the flap may be adjusted to take advantage of observed mobility of the lateral pharyngeal walls which provide the opening/closing element as they adduct against the bridge.

A method of employing several of these techniques dependent on the endoscopic and radiological findings is given in Table 19.5. Although good success has been reported with any one of the above operations, better results follow selection of the operation to fit the individual patient. Complications particular to these operations include hyponasality, due to overclosure of the isthmus or inability of the palate to descend rapidly between phonemes; pooling of mucus occurs and may be due to impaired nasal drainage or to importing oral mucosal glands onto

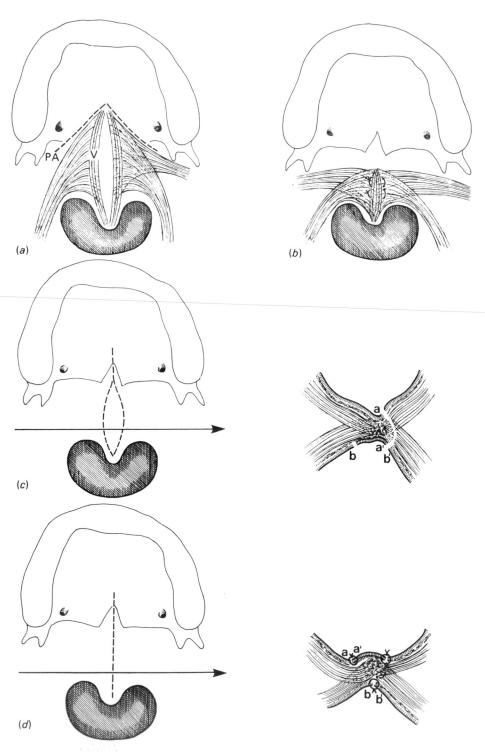

Figure 19.26 Techniques for restoring velopharyngeal competence. (*a*) Re-repair of the palate by intravelar veloplasty. Dotted line indicates incision through the palatine aponeurosis (PA) and Veau's muscle (V); (*b*) muscles retroposed and sutured in the midline; (*c*) oral mucosa island based on the muscles of one side; (*d*) after transposition to the nasal layer carrying fibres of the musculus uvulae onto the dorsum;

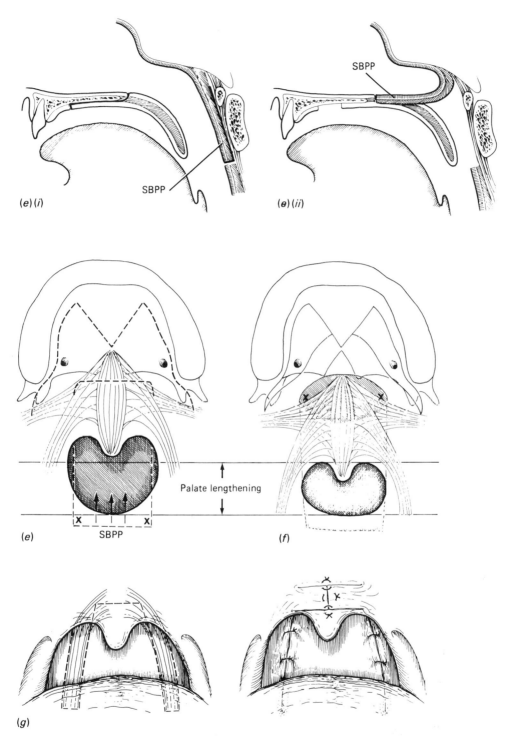

Figure 19.26 (*e*) palate lengthening by V–Y pushback (Veau) of oral layer combined with inset of tip of pharyngeal flap, with superior base (SBPP) into the nasal layer (Honig); (*f*) flap inset into nasal layer; (*g*) lateral wall flaps containing palatopharyngeus and salpingopharyngeus transposed into a horizontal incision above the level of the arch of the atlas (Hynes). Incisions outlined and flaps transposed

Table 19.5 Method of pharyngoplasty selection

Observation	Deduction	Operation
1 V-shaped upper surface of palate Anteroposterior gap less than 2 mm	Inadequate muscle union No disproportion Lateral wall movement irrelevant	Re-repair palate
2 V-shaped upper surface of palate Anterioposterior gap of 2–5 mm	Inadequate muscle union Moderate disproportion Lateral wall movement irrelevant	Re-repair palate plus Hynes pharyngoplasty
3 Anteroposterior gap greater than 5 mm	Severe disproportion Lateral wall movement irrelevant	Palate re-repair with lengthening by pharyngeal flap (Honig)
4 Lateral walls adduct to close lateral 1/6 isthmus each	Disproportion irrelevant	Wide pharyngeal flap
5 Lateral walls adduct to close lateral 1/3 isthmus each	Disproportion irrelevant	Narrow pharyngeal flap
6 Asymmetrical movement		Modification of one of above to close residual defect

the nasal surface of the palate; difficulty in eating may be experienced due to inability to inspire air with the mouth due to overclosure of the isthmus. While snoring may occur due to altered air flow and turbulence, some patients who snore before operation are cured by pharyngoplasty.

Prosthetic obturation

An alternative approach is the non-surgical obturation of the defect with an acrylic mould. A piece of softened gutta percha or other suitable dental impression material is introduced into the velopharyngeal isthmus on a bent wire attached to the back of the denture and the patient is asked to make a prolonged closure sound such as S-S-S, thus 'muscle trimming' the obturator. When the muscles relax there should be adequate space for nasal respiration and mucus drainage. Accurate addition and subtraction from the obturator is facilitated by nasal endoscopic control. Once a satisfactory shape has been achieved, the obturator is cast in acrylic.

Follow up and speech analysis

One of the main aims of the management of patients with cleft palate is the provision of an anatomical and physiological environment in which comprehensible speech can be produced. The speech of a patient with an unrepaired cleft palate is characterized by features which are instantly recognizable by most people, lay public and medical professionals alike. However, it is misleading to assume that the speech defects of patients with this problem are identical. The speech of any individual patient will alter, depending on such factors as the inability to bring the lips together, necessary to pronounce /p/ and /b/; the

configuration of the hard palate and alveolar arch and the integrity of the dental arcade which may affect sounds such as /s/ and /z/; the presence of fistulae at different points in the palate which can alter air escape affecting consonants such as /d/ /g/ and /k/ made against the hard or soft palate and, most importantly, the competence of the velopharyngeal isthmus which conserves the air stream and directs it past the articulators or allows it to escape through the nose to produce nasal consonants. In this light, speech analysis may seem a difficult and complicated task, but it becomes straightforward when an ordered approach is taken. As well as analysing the various components of speech, the degree to which the patient becomes breathless on talking is one of the first aspects to be noted. This can be assessed by asking the patient to count up to 20 rapidly. With velopharyngeal competence it should be unnecessary for the patient to take more than one breath to complete the task; with severe incompetence a breath may be taken for every few digits.

For the purposes of defining various speech defects with greater precision, and comparing different methods of treatment, articulation, velopharyngeal function and intelligibility are considered separately.

Diagnostic techniques for velopharyngeal incompetence

Oral examination

Direct observation of the oral cavity provides essential but limited information about the cleft palate patient. Unfortunately, the competence or otherwise of the velopharyngeal sphincter cannot be determined by looking into the mouth, since the point of closure lies above the soft palate, not directly behind it. Examination of the oral cavity must include a good view right back to the uvula and pharyngeal walls.

Videofluoroscopic lateral radiological examination while talking provides additional information as to whether the soft palate achieves contact with the posterior pharyngeal wall. However, this view does not reveal inadequate closure laterally and only direct viewing from above via an endoscope will allow full assessment. The rigid endoscope has the best optics for this purpose but the flexible endoscope is much kinder to the young patient and achieves greater compliance. Pigott and Makepeace (1982) reported 30% success with the rigid endoscope in 3 year olds compared to 100% success in 10 year olds providing gross nasal obstruction was not present.

Late presentation of unrepaired cleft or submucous cleft

The stimulus for late presentation of cleft palate is usually poor speech development. If there is an unrepaired cleft, the extent and the width of the defect should be noted. In patients where there is no obvious cleft the examiner should look for signs of a submucous cleft. Not all the signs are found in each patient. There is often a translucent stripe running down the centre of the soft palate. This represents an area devoid of muscle. The posterior border of the palate should be palpated for a notch in place of the nasal spine. Presence of a notch is pathognomonic of submucous cleft and probably represents the anterior insertion of the palate muscles exactly as seen in overt clefts. The levator lift dimples should be examined as the patient says 'ah'. Lateral placement also indicates muscle separation. The uvula is bifid in four out of five cases of submucous cleft, but this is not a reliable sign of a submucous cleft, as it occurs in more than 1% of the population. Irregularities of the dental arcade and collapse of the arch should be noted as they will make articulation more difficult.

Repaired cleft palate

In the case of a repaired palate, examination will reveal the quality of the resultant scar and apparent mobility, and the presence or absence of a fistula. Although nasopharyngeal closure cannot be confirmed by oral examination, a fair assessment of palate mobility can be achieved. The time-honoured sound the patient is asked to utter, /ah/, is not as effective in achieving maximum velar elevation as the vowel /ee/. Formation of this sound normally lifts the soft palate to a level well above the hard palate, and should be used instead. Both Calnan (1952) and Sommerlad (1981) pointed out that in the normal palate elevation is accompanied by the presence of dimples on the oral surface at points of the attach-

ment of the levator palati muscles to the soft palate. In the cleft palate, these dimples may be displaced laterally, or grooves running forward to the posterior edge of the hard palate may be seen instead. Large tonsils may be responsible for obstruction of either nasal or oral air flow which can lead to hyper- or hyponasality or to a 'hot potato' quality of the patient's speech.

Some idea can be gained of the relative sizes of the oral cavity, palate and pharynx. In a small group of patients with velopharyngeal incompetence no abnormality will be found other than a disproportionately large pharynx. Passavant's ridge is sometimes visible on saying /ah/, but even if the ridge itself cannot be seen, bunching of the mucosa may be visible below the palate. Mirror examination will confirm this. Although further investigations are required, a provisional diagnosis of pharyngeal disproportion can be made on oral examination.

Closure patterns of the velopharyngeal isthmus

From a few well documented direct observations following maxillectomy, but mainly from radiological and endoscopic studies, normal and abnormal patterns of closure of the velopharyngeal isthmus have been defined both for swallowing and for speech (Calnan, 1952; Astley, 1958; Massengill *et al.*, 1966; Pigott, 1969; Skolnick, McCall and Barnes, 1973). Further information has come from electromyography (Fritzell, 1969; Bell-Berti, 1976; Mulder, 1976). These patterns may be summarized as follows.

Swallowing

Swallowing is a relatively slowly developed, powerful sphincteric movement involving approximation of the posterior third of the palate to the pharyngeal wall. The action of swallowing is innervated by the IXth, Xth and XIth cranial nerves via the pharyngeal plexus and invariably functions normally in the group of patients whose behaviour is considered in this chapter. One principal muscle is the superior constrictor with assistance from palatopharyngeus and to a lesser extent levator palati. Closure is below the level of the area of the atlas.

Speaking

Closure for speech, by contrast, occurs rapidly (e.g. the palate must rise and fall eight times to produce the 13 syllables in counting from 15 to 20 at a normal speed (in 3 seconds). If the movements were equally distributed this would give a cycle open-closed-open of 0.36 seconds but very much higher speeds have been recorded. The role of the palate depressors is very important under these circum-

stances. The sacrifice of all the fibres of the palatopharyngeus muscle in certain pharyngoplasties may
lead to the palate remaining up for open nasal sounds
with resultant hyponasality; at least part of this
muscle should be conserved during surgery. The closure takes place above the level of the arch of the
atlas in adults, at the level of the basiocciput in
children, and at the level of the basisphenoid in
infants (Calnan, 1959). These changes are due to
descent of the maxilla, with the attached hard palate
and soft palate, with age and also to atrophy of the
adenoids against which they actually make contact
in infants and younger children. In these younger
groups the palate rotates up as a fixed length structure to touch the adenoid mass, but with increasing
age it also lengthens (velar stretch).

Muscular control

The principal muscle is the levator palati and when
this contracts alone the palate rises as a simple valve
(Figure 19.27). More often there is a contribution to
closure from the superior constrictor and/or the horizontal fibres of the palatopharyngeus which originate
in the soft palate and sweep around the pharynx as
the palatopharyngeal sphincter (Whillis, 1930;
Calnan, 1952). It is likely that velar stretch is due to
these horizontal fibres. Whatever muscle is responsible, the effect is advancement of the lateral and
posterior walls, each to a greater or lesser degree,
resulting in a final pattern of closure which may be
coronal, sagittal or sphincteric (Skolnick, McCall and
Barnes, 1973; Shprintzen *et al.*, 1979) and is as
idiosyncratic to that person as the movements of
their mouth (Figure 19.28).

The less the movement of the palate, the greater
the movement of the lateral and posterior walls,
which may be compensatory, since in cases of unrepaired or inadequately repaired palate clefts, a well-

defined semicircular shelf develops on the posterior
wall, known as Passavant's ridge. Evidence from
neurological syndromes (Sedlakova, Lastovka and
Scram, 1973), observations on patients with facial
palsy (Podvinec, 1952), from human observation
studies (Nickl, 1950), and from animal experiments
(Nishio *et al.*, 1976a, b) support the view that the
VIIth cranial nerve innervates the levator for speech,
possibly via the chorda tympani, or the greater superficial petrosal nerves, in addition to fibres from the
pharyngeal plexus.

The vertical fibres of the palatopharyngeus actively
depress the palate, assisted by elastic fibres in the
palatoglossus, the muscle fibres, like those of salpingopharyngeus, being small and inconstant (Kuehn
and Azzam, 1978).

The upper surface of the soft palate is convex at
the level of the levator eminence over its median
third, due to the bulk of the paired musculus uvulae
and the associated mass of mucosal glands (Pigott,
1969; Azzam and Kuehn, 1977). This allows it to fit
snugly into the concavity of the posterior pharyngeal
wall. Laterally, the inconstant ridges of salpingopharyngeus advance medially to fit against the sides
of the musculus uvulae ridge.

Submucous cleft palate

Submucous cleft palate, first described by Kelly
(1910), is an infrequently diagnosed condition and
anatomically is the least obvious form of cleft palate.
It can be the cause of infant feeding difficulty, otitis
media, deafness and velopharyngeal incompetence
and treatment is necessary in many cases. The precise
incidence of submucous cleft palate will probably never
be known as there are cases where there are no
significant symptoms and treatment is not required
and probably more cases which never present at all.

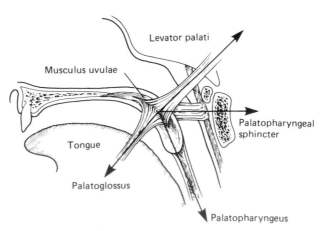

Figure 19.27 Muscle vectors. Palatoglossus and palatopharyngeus are seen to be antagonists to levator palati. The
palatopharyngeal sphincter aids closure by advancing the lateral and posterior walls and causing velar stretch

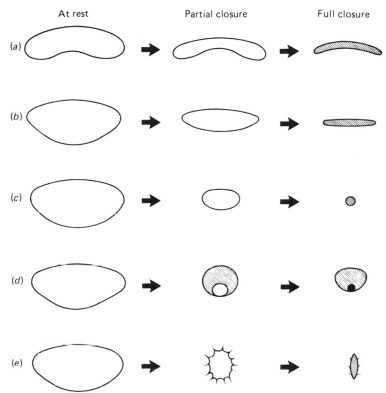

Figure 19.28 Patterns of velopharyngeal closure (Skolnick, 1973). Basal view. (*a*) Normal subject. Note musculus uvulae bulge; (*b*) coronal pattern; repaired cleft palate subject; (*c*) circular closure pattern, repaired cleft palate; (*d*) circular closure pattern with Passavant's ridge (shaded area); (*e*) sagittal closure pattern, repaired cleft palate

Classification

Submucous clefts may be considered overt or occult. They may also be associated with pharyngeal disproportion.

In 1954, Calnan described the classic triad of examination findings associated with this condition:

1 Bifid uvula
2 Palatal muscle diastisis giving a translucent zone
3 Bony notch in the hard palate.

Essentially the same abnormal muscle configuration as seen in overt clefts leads to inadequate soft palate movement. This produces, initially, difficulty in feeding in a small number of cases, and subsequently, nasal escape on speaking. In addition, the same abnormality results in poor eustachian tube function.

As Kaplan (1975) has pointed out, a spectrum of severity exists with regard to clefts of the secondary palate. This ranges from the complete overt cleft of both hard and soft palates, through to the classical submucous cleft and eventually to an entity termed the 'occult' submucous cleft in which velar function is abnormal, but there are no oral signs. The diagnosis is indicated by the symptomatology and must be confirmed by endoscopy, basal view X-rays and eventually by surgery. It is important to appreciate that submucous cleft may also be associated with pharyngeal disproportion, hypoplasia, etc.

Hypoplasia occurs in submucous cleft as it does in overt clefts and probably becomes worse with age (Skoog, 1965). Well developed adenoids may mask the disproportion. It is most important, therefore, to be aware of submucous cleft prior to adenoidectomy in order to warn the patient or family of the possibility of speech impairment. Furthermore, if adenoidectomy had been recommended for recurrent otitis media there is a real possibility that the deranged musculature is responsible and not the adenoidal cushion. It is best to avoid adenoidectomy in the presence of a submucous cleft.

Diagnosis

The diagnosis should be considered in all children with evidence of palatal incompetence, especially if there is a history of feeding difficulty in infancy, and it becomes almost certain if there is also a history of otitis media. The corollary is that it should always be excluded before treating cases of otitis media. An oral examination allows the diagnosis to be made on Calnan's criteria. In addition, on induction of a gag reflex, or if the patient is capable of saying 'ee-ee', the vault of the soft palate may be seen to rise and assume a box shape rather than the usual Gothic arch configuration, due to separation of the levator lift points (Figure 19.29). The soft palate itself may be seen to be short in comparison to the pharynx.

Kaplan (1975) has pointed out the association of the following facial features as characteristic of patients with classic submucous cleft, occult submucous cleft, and some overt clefts of the secondary palate. They are present to varying degrees.

1 Maxillary hypoplasia – 'dish face'
2 Lip contour deformity at vermilion border – 'gull wing'
3 Drooping of oral commissure
4 Hypodynamic facial muscles
5 External ear abnormality – flat arc of superior helix
6 Alveolar arch abnormality.

Submucous clefting has been associated with a number of conditions. These include cleft lip, Treacher Collins, Klippel-Feil and Fanconi syndromes, congenital rubella, albinism, choanal atresia, Moebius syndrome, ring 18 chromosome and mental retardation. If any of these conditions is diagnosed early in life and a submucous cleft is recognized as well, speech development can be monitored carefully and, at the first signs of ear symptoms or speech problems associated with velopharyngeal incompetence, appropriate measures can be taken.

Investigation

A speech assessment is undertaken, and if surgery is considered appropriate radiological and endoscopic assessments are made. The shape, size, and level of the incompetent velopharyngeal isthmus are recorded as for patients with an overt cleft.

Repair

Inevitably most submucous clefts are diagnosed late compared with overt clefts. The speech or ear problems with which they present will dictate correction as early as possible. Aberrant speech patterns may have become fixed, with grossly impaired intelligibility, and treatment can be quite difficult. Surgery should be combined with intensive speech therapy in a residential course if progress is slow. However, a child with a submucous cleft may have normal articulation and intelligibility where nasal escape has been masked by large adenoids. If adenoidectomy is performed with subsequent intractable nasal escape and hypernasal resonance, an excellent result can be achieved by repair of the submucous cleft with or without pharyngoplasty.

Technique

A number of options is available in the surgical management of these patients. The choice of procedure depends on the findings at investigation.

If a palate with good length and mobility has been demonstrated radiographically (reaching to within 3 mm of the posterior pharyngeal wall), a standard cleft palate repair is undertaken. The soft palate is split in the midline and the velar musculature mobilized. The muscles of the two halves of the palate are brought together in the midline. The nasal midline bulge is carefully reconstructed with judicious placement of a horizontal everting mattress suture and the palate closed. For a gap of 3–5 mm a Hynes-type pharyngoplasty is added to the procedures above. Palates so short that they fail to achieve closure by more than 5 mm are comparatively rare and may require a Honig pharyngoplasty.

Results

The results of surgery for submucous cleft palate are variable and in general are not as good as for cleft palate repair. The most important aetiological factor in this regard is that surgery is not undertaken until

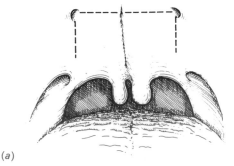   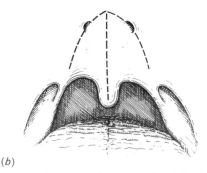

(a)   (b)

Figure 19.29 (a) Submucous cleft palate. Bifid uvulae and 'box-like' soft palate elevation with laterally placed dimples are demonstrated; (b) normal palate. 'Gothic arch' elevation is demonstrated

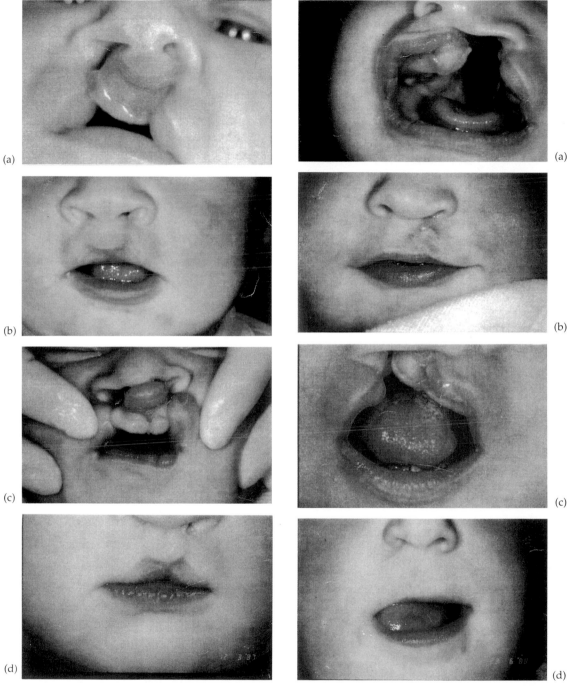

Plate 6/19/I Photographs of 'before and after' lip repair using the Millard technique. Such photographs provide great encouragement to parents if shown soon after the baby is born. (*a*) Bilateral cleft of lip and palate at 2 months old; (*b*) photographed at 9 months old after surgery at 3 months old; (*c*) bilateral cleft of lip and palate at 2 months old; (*d*) photographed at 12 months old after surgery at 3 months old

Plate 6/19/II Photographs of 'before and after' lip repair using the Millard technique. (*a*) Unilateral cleft of lip and palate at birth; (*b*) cleft lip repaired at 3 months old. The lip scar is quite red and raised; (*c*) unilateral cleft lip and palate at birth; (*d*) at 2 years and 6 months the old lip scar has flattened and paled becoming less obvious

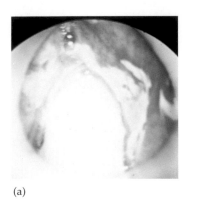

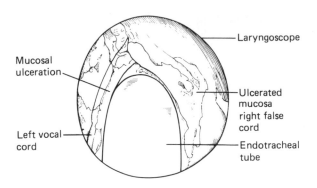

(a)

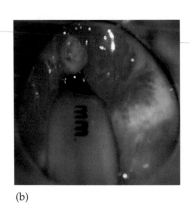

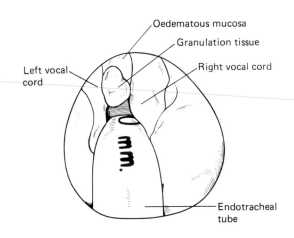

(b)

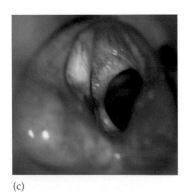

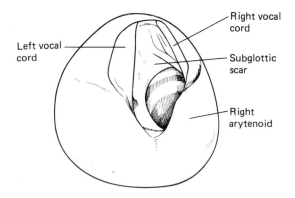

(c)

Plate 6/23/I Microlaryngoscopy showing (*a*) mucosal ulceration of the vocal cords and right false cord 24 hours after intubation for ventilatory support for respiratory distress; (*b*) granulation tissue filling the glottis in front of the endotracheal tube; (*c*) a fibrous subglottic stenosis

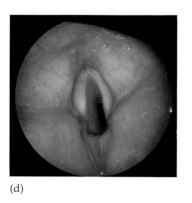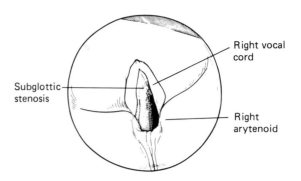

(d)

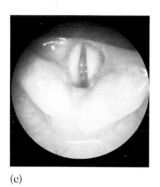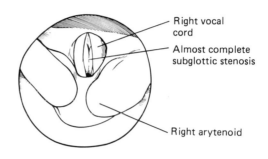

(e)

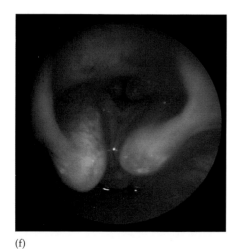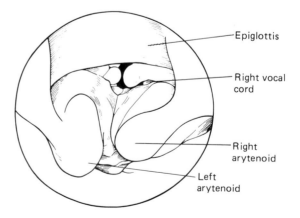

(f)

Plate 6/23/I (*continued*) Microlaryngoscopy showing (*d*) mild congenital subglottic stenosis; (*e*) severe congenital subglottic stenosis; (*f*) mucus retention cysts after intubation

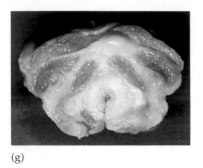

(g)

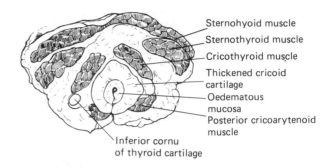

Sternohyoid muscle

Sternothyroid muscle

Cricothyroid muscle

Thickened cricoid
cartilage

Oedematous
mucosa

Posterior cricoarytenoid
muscle

Inferior cornu
of thyroid cartilage

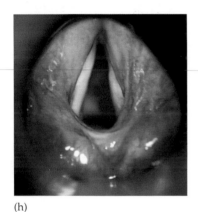

(h)

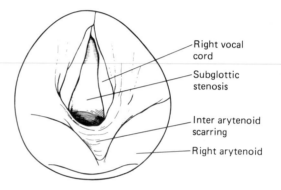

Right vocal
cord

Subglottic
stenosis

Inter arytenoid
scarring

Right arytenoid

Plate 6/23/I (*continued*) (*g*) post-mortem specimen showing an abnormally thick cricoid and hyperplasia of the submucosa (courtesy of Mr R. Pracy); (*h*) microlaryngoscopy showing interarytenoid fixation

significantly later compared with surgery for the overt cleft and the earlier a cleft is repaired, the more likely a satisfactory outcome will be achieved. Only one-third of patients over 2 years of age achieve palatal competence if no additional manoeuvre is undertaken. However, with intensive speech therapy, good hearing and intelligence and, perhaps most importantly, the incentive to relearn articulation patterns, dramatic improvements often follow quickly (within 6 months) of the provision of a competent velopharyngeal mechanism.

Orthodontic treatment of the cleft palate

Initial orthodontic treatment

Patients who have had an isolated midline cleft of the palate repaired may need expansion of the upper arch if it has collapsed as a result of the scar tissue following palatal surgery. A short period of orthodontic treatment, using either removable or fixed appliances, will generally be sufficient to expand the arch and correct the crossbite of the posterior teeth.

Initial orthodontic treatment for the patient who has had a cleft involving the alveolus and anterior palate is usually carried out at about 7 years of age when the permanent incisor teeth erupt. Similarly treatment begins at this age for complete unilateral or bilateral clefts. The abnormalities typically present at this age are as follows:

1 The upper incisors are often poorly formed (Figure 19.30). It seems likely that this results from manipulation of the alveolar process during lip closure before calcification of the tooth germs has occurred. Enamel hypoplasia can be masked at a later date by veneers. More severe dysplasia of the teeth involving bending of the roots may complicate orthodontic treatment.
2 The upper lateral incisor is frequently absent on the cleft side (Figure 19.31). At a superficial level, this may be interpreted as an interference with tooth development in the region of the cleft. The fact that the lateral incisor may be missing on the non-cleft side suggests a more complex explanation.

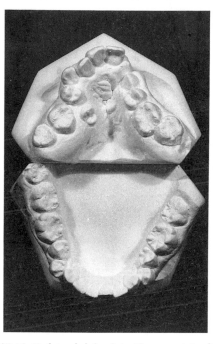

Figure 19.31 Unilateral cleft palate. The upper lateral incisor is absent

3 There is frequently a supernumerary tooth distal to the cleft (Figure 19.32). This is called a precanine tooth. There may be a precanine in both the deciduous and permanent series. When secondary alveolar grafting is carried out, the precanine is almost invariably removed to make way for eruption of the permanent canine.
4 There is, less frequently, a supernumerary tooth mesial to the cleft. These teeth are usually poorly-formed but may be retained.
5 The upper incisors bite behind the lower incisors (Figure 19.33). This may be corrected with a simple removable appliance providing the skeletal discrepancy is not severe.
6 There is usually medial rotation of the lesser segment or both posterior segments in bilateral cases with a unilateral or bilateral crossbite of the canine and premolar teeth. Examination of unoperated adult cleft palate patients where there are large clefts but few crossbites leaves little doubt that surgical palatal closure is a primary factor in causing this anomaly. Very significant improvements in surgical techniques have reduced crossbites in frequency and severity. Crossbites may be treated by arch expansion with removable or fixed appli-

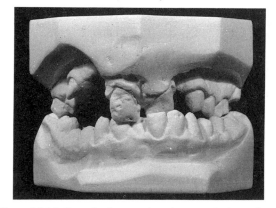

Figure 19.30 Hypoplastic enamel on the upper incisors of a cleft palate patient

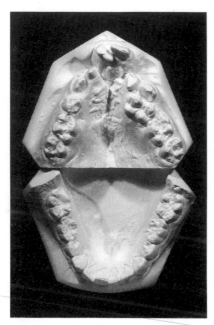

Figure 19.32 Bilateral cleft palate. Both upper lateral incisors are absent. On the right side there is a conical supernumerary tooth behind the cleft and anterior to the upper right canine tooth

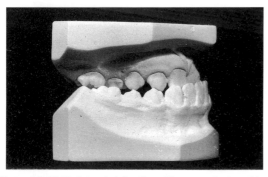

Figure 19.33 Unilateral cleft palate. The upper incisors bite behind the lower incisors and there is crossbite of the molar and premolar teeth

ances. The Quadhelix fixed appliance is preferred. Claims have been made that rapid maxillary expansion followed by bone grafting in cleft cases permanently improves the nasal airway. It seems clear that the advantages have been overstated. Grafted bone, or local bone replacing grafted bone, seems just as labile as any other bone and allows a variable degree of relapse. There is no scientific evidence that airway resistance is reduced by the procedure which does nothing for septal deviation or resistance at the nostrils.

7 There may be mandibular protrusion (Figure 19.34). The protrusion may be due to a true skeletal discrepancy or to overclosure of the mandible resulting from poor occlusion of the posterior teeth. Poor posterior occlusion allows the mandible to swing upwards but, since it is hinged at the temporomandibular joint, the movement is upwards and forwards thus producing a functional mandibular protrusion. This can be improved quite dramatically by expanding the upper arch, thus providing posterior occlusion which swings the mandible downwards and backwards. Overclosure of this kind is becoming much less common as a result of improved palatal surgery.

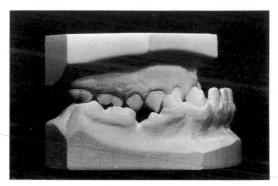

Figure 19.34 Mandibular protrusion

Secondary alveolar grafting

Following expansion of the arch, the deciduous canine is removed and the socket is allowed to heal. Precanine teeth are removed at the time of operation and the alveolar cleft packed with chips of cancellous bone taken from the hip.

Secondary grafting closes oronasal fistulae, provides support for the alar base and provides bone through which the upper canine will erupt in a mesial position. The significant dental advantage is that the patient does not have to wear a prosthesis in more than 90% of cases.

Definitive orthodontic treatment

Definitive orthodontic treatment with fixed appliances is carried out after eruption of the canine and premolar teeth at about 12 years of age. In many cases this is the final event in the dental programme. Some patients, however, need restorative treatment in the form of veneers or bridgework. Where there is a skeletal discrepancy, combined orthodontic and maxillofacial surgical treatment will be needed at the end of the growth period. If the need for maxillary surgery can be predicted, the lesser segment may be advanced and residual defects grafted at this operation.

Orthognathic surgery

In broad principle, the orthodontist produces two good arches of teeth which will fit together after surgery. The fixed orthodontic appliances are used for intermaxillary fixation and traction after surgery. The surgery usually takes the form of maxillary advancement at the Le Fort I level but care must be taken that the pharynx is not sufficiently enlarged to produce nasal speech. A compensatory mandibular osteotomy is sometimes required.

Conclusions

Most cleft patients need closure of lip and palate, production of velopharyngeal competence, production of two continuous dental arches of well-aligned teeth which occlude well, and correction of skeletal discrepancies.

Traditionally, lips and palates have been closed surgically with or without the aid of presurgical orthopaedics, incisors in lingual occlusion have been treated with removable appliances at the age of 7 years with a second course of orthodontic treatment after the age of 12 years to expand the arches and align the teeth. Since surgical closure of the palate produced gross contraction of the upper arch, large crossbites and postural protrusion of the mandible were frequent. Massive expansion of the upper arch was needed. This opened up spaces in the upper arch which were filled with a life-long removable prosthesis which also stabilized the expansion.

The most significant improvement in recent years has been the improvement in primary surgery. Crossbites and postural protrusions are now less frequent and greatly reduced in magnitude. Since the required expansions are smaller, the spaces produced in the upper arch are much diminished and this has brought about the possibility of closing the upper arch spaces. This in turn has led to the introduction of secondary alveolar grafting allowing mesial eruption of the maxillary canine to replace the lateral incisor and the possibility of producing an intact arch of natural teeth so that the need for long term prosthetic replacement is almost eliminated.

Bearing in mind possible difficulties with patient compliance, anything which can be done to reduce the length and number of interventions should be done. In terms of orthodontic treatment, patients may have preliminary orthodontic treatment at age 7–9 years, definitive orthodontic treatment after the age of 12 years and a third bout of treatment to prepare for maxillofacial surgery if required at the end of the growth period. The key issue is whether the patient will need maxillofacial surgery after facial growth has been completed. If this is predictable, there are many attractions in leaving orthodontic treatment until immediately before this procedure

and advancing the maxilla combined with a lesser segment osteotomy and grafting as one surgical intervention. This approach, pioneered by Bruce Ross and his team in Toronto has two difficulties (Ross, 1987). First, patients may not be prepared to accept crooked teeth until the age of 17 years and second, many cleft patients have a marked deterioration in skeletal relationships towards the end of the growth period so that the need for maxillary advancement is difficult to predict. The way ahead may lie in more precise prediction of facial growth.

References

ASHER-MCDADE, C. and SHAW, W. C. (1990) Current cleft lip and palate management in the United Kingdom. *British Journal of Plastic Surgery*, **43**, 318–321

ASTLEY, R. (1958) The movements of the lateral walls of the nasopharynx: a cineradiographic study. *Journal of Laryngoscopy*, **72**, 325-328

AZZAM, N. A. and KUEHN, D. P. (1977) The morphology of musculus uvulae. *Cleft Palate Journal*, **14**, 78–87

BACON, W. H. (1990) Cephalometric evaluation of pharyngeal obstructive factors in patients with sleep apnea syndrome. *Angle Orthodontist*, **60**, 115–122

BELL-BERTIE, F. (1976) An electromyographic study of velopharyngeal function in speech. *Cleft Palate Journal*, **19**, 225–240

BJÖRK, A. and SKIELLER, V. (1972) Facial development and tooth eruption. *American Journal of Orthodontics*, **62**, 339–383

BOORMAN, J. G. and SOMMERLAD, B. C. (1985) Levator palati and palatal dimples: their anatomy, relationship and clinical significance. *British Journal of Plastic Surgery*, **38**, 326–332

BROADBENT, B. H. SR, BROADBENT, B. H. JR and GOLDEN, W. H. (1975) *Bolton Standards of Dentofacial Developmental Growth*. St Louis: CV Mosby.

BURKE, P. H. (1980) Serial growth changes in the lips. *British Journal of Orthodontics*, **7**, 17–30

BURSTON, W. R. (1958) The early orthodontic treatment of cleft palate conditions. *Dental Practitioner*, **9**, 41–56

CALNAN, J. S. (1952) Movements of the soft palate. *British Journal of Plastic Surgery*, **5**, 286–296

CALNAN, J. S. (1954) Submucous cleft palate. *British Journal of Plastic Surgery*, **6**, 264–282

CALNAN, J. S. (1959) The surgical treatment of nasal speech disorders. *Annals of the Royal College of Surgeons England*, **25**, 119–141

CALNAN, J. S. (1960) Cleft palate: lengthening of the soft palate following the V-Y repair. *British Journal of Plastic Surgery*, **13**, 243–248

COOKSON, A. and HALL B. D. (1968) Use of obturators in the early management of a case of Pierre Robin syndrome. *Transactions of the British Society for the Study of Orthodontics*, 8–10

DIBIASE, D. D. and HUNTER, B. (1983) A method of pre-surgical oral orthopaedics. *British Journal Orthodontics*, **10**, 25–31

FERGUSON, M. W. I. (1988) Palatal development. *Development*, **1035**, 41–60

FERGUSON, M. W. I. (1991) The orofacial region. In: *Textbook of Fetal and Perinatal Pathology*, edited by J. S. Wigglesworth and D. B. Singer. Oxford: Blackwell. pp. 843–880

FERGUSON, M. W. I. (1993) Craniofacial morphogenesis and prenatal growth. In: *Orthodontics and Occlusal Management*, edited by W. C. Shaw. Oxford: Butterworth-Heinemann. pp. 1–25

FRITZELL, B. (1969) The velopharyngeal muscles in speech. *Acta Otolaryngologica Supplementum*, **250**, 48

GEORGIADE, N., NLADICK, R. and THORNE, F. (1968) Positioning of the premaxilla in bilateral cleft lips by oral pinning and traction. *Plastic and Reconstructive Surgery*, **41**, 240

GRAY, R. M., DAVIES, S. J. and QUAYLE, A. A. (1995) *Temporomandibular Disorders – a Clinical Approach*. London. British Medical Association

GREENBERG, L. Z. and JOHNSTON, L. E. (1975) Computerized prediction: the accuracy of a contemporary language forecast. *American Journal of Orthodontics*, **67**, 243–253

GREGG T. A., BOYD, D. H. and RICHARDSON, A. (1994) Incidence of cleft lip and palate in Northern Ireland 1980–1990. *British Journal of Orthodontics*, **21**, 387–392

HENDERSON, H. P. (1982) An advancement island flap for the closure of anterior palatal fistulae. *British Journal of Plastic Surgery*, **35**, 163–166

HERSHLEY, H. G., STEWARD, B. L. and WARREN, D. W. (1976) Changes in nasal airway resistance associated with rapid maxillary expansion. *American Journal of Orthodontics*, **70**, 274–284

HONIG, C. A. (1967) The treatment of velopharyngeal insufficiency after palatal repair. *Archivum Chirurgicum Neerlandicum*, **19**, 71–81

HOTZ, M. M., GNOINSKI, W. M., NUSSBAUMER, H. and KISTLER, E. (1978) Early maxillary orthopaedics in cleft lip and palate cases: guidelines for surgery. *Cleft Palate Journal*, **15**, 405–411

HUDDART, A. G. (1962) Pre-surgical dental orthopaedics. *Dental Practitioner*, **12**, 339–350

HYNES, W. (1953) The results of muscle transplantation in 'failed cleft palate' cases, with special reference to the influence of the pharynx on voice production. *Annals of the Royal College of Surgeons*, **13**, 17–35

JOLLEYS, A. (1954) A review of the results of operations on cleft palates with reference to maxillary growth and speech function. *British Journal of Plastic Surgery*, **7**, 229–241

KAPLAN, E. N. (1975) The occult submucous cleft palate. *Cleft Palate Journal*, **12**, 356–368

KELLY, A. B. (1910) Congenital insufficiency of the palate. *Journal of Laryngology, Rhinology and Otology*, **25**, 281–342

KERNAHAN, D. A. and STARK, R. B. (1958) A new classification for cleft lip and palate. *Plastic and Reconstructive Surgery*, **22**, 435–441

KRIENS, O. (1975) Anatomy of the velopharyngeal area in cleft palate. *Clinics in Plastic Surgery*, **2**, 261–283

KUEHN, D. P. and AZZAM, N. A. (1978) Anatomical characteristics of palatoglossus and the anterior faucial pillar. *Cleft Palate Journal*, **15**, 349–359

LATHAM, R. A., KUSY, R. P. and GEORGIADE, N. G. (1976) An extraorally activated expansion appliance for cleft palate infants. *Cleft Palate Journal*, **13**, 253–261

LENDRUM, J. and DHAR, B. K. (1984) The Orticochea dynamic pharyngoplasty. *British Journal of Plastic Surgery*, **37**, 160–168

LINDER-ARONSON, S. (1970) Adenoids, their effect on the mode of breathing and nasal air flow and their relationship to characteristics of the facial skeleton and the dentition. *Acta Otolaryngologica Supplementum*, **265**

LINDER-ARONSON, S., WOODSIDE, D. G., HELLSING, E. and EMERSON, W. (1993) Normalisation of incisor position after adenoidectomy. *American Journal of Orthodontics and Dentofacial Orthopedics*, **103**, 412–427

LOWE, A., GIONHAKU, N. and TAKEUCHI, K. (1986) Three-dimensional CT reconstructions of tongue and airway in adult subjects with obstructive sleep apnea. *American Journal of Orthodontics and Dentofacial Orthopedics*, **90**, 364–374

MCNEIL, C. K. (1954) *Oral and Facial Deformity*. London: Pitman

MASSENGALL, R., QUINN, G., BARRY, W. F. and PICKRELL, K. (1966) The development of rotational cinefluorography and its application to speech research. *Journal of Speech and Hearing Research*, **9**, 259–265

MILLARD, D. R. (1957) A primary camouflage of the unilateral harelip. *Transactions of the First International Congress of Plastic Surgeons*. Baltimore: Williams and Wilkins. pp. 160–165

MILLARD, D. R. (1994) Embryonic rationale for the primary correction of classical congenital clefts of the lip and palate. *Annals of the Royal College of Surgeons England*, **76**, 150–160

MOORE, F. T. (1960) A new operation to cure nasopharyngeal incompetence. *British Journal of Surgery*, **47**, 424–428

MORLEY, M. E. (1970) *Cleft Palate and Speech*, 7th edn. Edinburgh: Livingstone. pp. 124–127

MOSS, M. L. (1968) The primacy of functional matrices in orofacial growth. *Transactions of the British Society for the Study of Orthodontics*, 107–115

MOSS, M. L. and SALANTIJN, L. (1969) The primary role of functional matrices in facial growth. *American Journal of Orthodontics*, **55**, 566–577

MULDER, J. W. (1976) Velopharyngeal function and speech. *Doctoral thesis*. Amsterdam: Van Gorcum B. V. Assen

NICKL, A. (1950) Uber die Innervation des musculus levator veli palatini durch den N. facialis. *Archiv für Psychiatrie und Zeitschrift Neurologie*, **184**, 117–132

NISHIO, J., MATSUYA, T., MACHIDA, J. and MIYAZAKI, T. (1976a) The motor nerve supply of the velopharyngeal muscles. *Cleft Palate Journal*, **13**, 20–30

NISHIO, J., MATSUYA, T., IBUKI, K. and MIYAZAKI, T. (1976b) Roles of the facial, glossopharyngeal and vagus nerves in velopharyngeal movements. *Cleft Palate Journal*, **13**, 201–214

ORTICOCHEA, M. (1967) Construction of a dynamic muscle sphincter in cleft palates. *Plastic and Reconstructive Surgery*, **41**, 323–327

PIGOTT, R. W. (1969) The nasendoscopic appearance of the normal palato-pharyngeal valve. *Plastic and Reconstructive Surgery*, **43**, 19–24

PIGOTT, R. W. and MCMANAMNY D. S. (1987) The management of cleft palate. In: *Scott Brown's Otolaryngology*, 5th edn, edited by A. G. Kerr, Vol. 6. *Paediatric Otolaryngology*, edited by J. N. G. Evans. London: Butterworths. pp. 310–333

PIGOTT, R. W. and MAKEPEACE, A. P. (1982) Some characteristics of endoscopic and radiological systems used in elaboration of the diagnosis of velopharyngeal incompetence. *British Journal of Plastic Surgery*, **35**, 19–32

PIGOTT, R. W., REIGER, F. W. and FRAZER MOODIE, A. (1984) Tongue flap repair of cleft palate fistulae. *British Journal of Plastic Surgery*, **37**, 285–293

PODVINEC, S. (1952) The physiology and pathology of the soft palate. *Journal of Laryngology and Otology*, **66**, 452–461

RICHARDSON, A. (1995) *Interceptive Orthodontics*, 3rd edn. London: British Dental Association

ROSS, R. B. (1970) The clinical implications of facial growth in cleft lip and palate. *Cleft Palate Journal*, 7, 37–47

ROSS, R. B. (1987) Treatment variables affecting facial growth in complete unilateral cleft lip and palate. Part 2: Presurgical orthopaedics. *Cleft Palate Journal*, 24, 24–32

SAUNDERS, L. D. F., GEARY, L., FLEMING, P. and GREGG, T. A. (1989) A simplified feeding appliance for the infant with a cleft lip and palate. *Quintessence International*, 20, 907–910

SCHOENBORN, D. (1876) Uber eine neue methode der staphylorrhaphie. *Archiv für Klinische Chirurgie*, 9, 527

SCHWECKENDIECK, W. (1978) Primary veloplasty: long term results without maxillary deformity. *Cleft Palate Journal*, 15, 268–274

SEDLAKOVA, E., LASTOVKA, M. and SCRAM, F. (1973) Contribution to knowledge of soft palate innervation. *Folia Phoniatrica*, 25, 434–441

SHPRINTZEN, R. J., LEWIN, M. L., CROFT, C. B., DANILLER, A. I., ARGAMASO, R. V., SHIP, A. G. et al. (1979) A comprehensive study of pharyngeal flap surgery. Tailor made flaps. *Cleft Palate Journal*, 16, 46–55

SKOLNICK, M. L., MCCALL, G. N. and BARNES, R. T. (1973) The sphincteric mechanism of velopharyngeal closure. *Cleft Palate Journal*, 10, 286–305

SKOOG, T. (1965) The management of the bilateral cleft of the primary palate (lip and alveolus). *Plastic and Reconstructive Surgery*, 35, 35–44

SOMMERLAD, B. (1981) Nasendoscopy. In: *Recent Advances in Plastic Surgery*, vol. 2, edited by I. T. Jackson. Edinburgh: Churchill Livingstone. pp. 11–27

TIMMS, D. J. (1980) A study of basal movement with rapid maxillary expansion. *American Journal of Orthodontics*, 77, 500–507

VAN DEMARK, D. and VAN DEMARK, A. (1970) Speech and sociovocational aspects of individuals with cleft palate. *Cleft Palate Journal*, 7, 284–299

VEAU, V. (1927) The treatment of cleft palate by operation. *Proceedings of the Royal Society of Medicine*, 20, 1916–1926

VIG, P. S. and COHEN, A. M. (1979) Vertical growth of the lips: a serial cephalometric study. *American Journal of Orthodontics*, 75, 405–415

WHILLIS, J. (1930) A note on the muscles of the palate and the superior constrictor. *Journal of Anatomy*, 65, 92–95

WIDMAIER, W. (1973) Beitrag zum Verschluss schwieriger Restperforationen am Gaumen mit Insellappen und Lyodura. In: *Fortschritte der Kiefer- und Gesichts-Chirurgie*, edited by K. Schuchardt, G. Steinhardt and N. Schwenzer Stuttgart: Thieme. pp. 299–320

WITZEL, M. A., CLARKE, J. A., LINDSAY, W. K. and THOMSON, H. G. (1979) Comparison of results of pushback or Von Langenbeck repair of isolated cleft of the hard and soft palate. *Plastic and Reconstructive Surgery*, 64, 347–352

20

Sleep apnoea

C. M. Bailey and C. B. Croft

In 1889 Dr William Hill presented a paper to the autumn meeting of the Royal Society of Medicine in Leeds entitled 'On some cases of backwardness and stupidity in children relieved by adenoidal scarification'. In this paper Hill associated symptoms of snoring and restless sleep with mental dullness and lethargy which he presumed were due to the disturbed sleep pattern. The children Hill described benefited from adenoidectomy and the credit for first recognizing the association between partial upper airways obstruction and significant respiratory disturbances during sleep must go to him. The great increase in sleep research during the 1950s and 1960s has resulted in recognition of normal sleep patterns, i.e. rapid eye movement (REM) and non-rapid eye movement (non-REM) sleep with their characteristic EEG patterns. Most significantly, such sleep research has demonstrated the existence of a host of sleep-related disorders of breathing and clearly demonstrated the relationship between these disorders and significant disturbances of the cardiorespiratory and central nervous systems. During the past decade more than a dozen sleep clinics have been established in the UK and the increasing availability of non-invasive monitoring equipment has allowed other less specialized units to undertake screening of respiration during sleep in both the paediatric and adult populations.

Definitions

Snoring: a noise generated from the upper airway due to partial obstruction of the airway.

An apnoea: cessation of airflow at the nostrils and mouth for at least 10 seconds.

Apnoea index (AI): the number of apnoeas occurring per hour of sleep.

An hypopnoea: reduction in tidal volume.

Sleep apnoea syndrome is diagnosed when 30 or more apnoeic episodes occur during a 7-hour sleep period. This would give an apnoea index equal to or greater than 5. Recognition that partial airways obstruction results in reduced ventilation or hypopnoea has resulted in some sleep laboratories working on an apnoea/hypopnoea index where hypopnoea is defined as a decrease in airflow at the lips or nose associated with oxygen desaturation (Guilleminault *et al.*, 1984). Current thinking is that an apnoea/hypopnoea index of 15 should be present before diagnosing the sleep apnoea syndrome. The American Sleep Apnoea Association currently grades sleep apnoea as follows:

Mild   = 5–20 apnoeas per hour
Moderate = 20–40 apnoeas per hour
Severe   = > 40 apnoeas per hour.

Sleep apnoea is further complicated by the classification of pathological sleep apnoea as *central*, *obstructive* or *mixed*. In central sleep apnoea there is no airflow at the nose or mouth and this is associated with the cessation of all respiratory effort. Obstructive sleep apnoea occurs in the presence of continued and continuous respiratory effort – such obstructive apnoeas are accompanied by paradoxical movements of the chest and abdomen in an attempt to overcome the upper airway obstruction. Mixed apnoea begins as a central apnoea with no airflow and no respiratory effort, followed by increasingly forceful respiratory effort until airflow is re-established. It is important to note that normal individuals have occasional physiological central apnoeic episodes during REM sleep or at least at the onset of sleep. However, the mean apnoea index in control subjects is only 0.3 apnoea/hour (women) and one apnoea/hour (men) (Guilleminault, van den Hoed and Mitler, 1978).

Although the above definitions are reasonably

clear, there is a progression from natural and completely unobstructed respiration during sleep to the previously mentioned syndromes. Two conditions which are manifested by partial airway obstruction with secondary cardiorespiratory effects are:

1 *High upper airways resistance syndrome.* Patients with this disorder demonstrate episodes of marked partial upper airway obstruction but do not actually completely obstruct their airway. They are able to maintain oxygen saturation at a normal level (around 95 %) but the extra respiratory effort required to overcome partial obstruction of the airway induces frequent microarousals. These patients may develop significant cardiovascular strain because of the excessive and prolonged respiratory effort and are likely to suffer marked daytime sleepiness (Stoohs and Guilleminault, 1990).

2 *Nocturnal hypoventilation and hypoxia.* Hypoventilation occurring nocturnally in patients with pre-existing hypoxaemia from pulmonary or cardiac disorders may develop into significant arterial desaturation. Patients with pulmonary fibrosis, cystic fibrosis and respiratory muscle weakness due to myasthenia gravis, bulbar poliomyelitis or Guillain-Barré syndrome may develop this disorder.

Normal sleep

Mention should be made of the physiology of normal sleep, noting that respiration when a patient is awake is mainly under voluntary control, but during sleep automatic mechanisms assume greater importance.

Normal individuals pass through a cycle of REM and non-REM sleep stages 1–4 approximately every 120 minutes. At the onset of sleep respiration is often irregular with short apnoeic episodes but, as sleep becomes deeper, progressing into non-REM sleep, breathing becomes more regular. It is particularly important to note that during REM sleep there is a tendency to decreased muscle tone with diminished responsiveness to hypoxic or hypercapnic stimuli secondary to airway obstruction. There is a slight associated drop in oxygen saturation and a rise in $P_a\mathrm{CO_2}$, with a tendency to some irregularities of breathing and an occasional physiological apnoeic episode (Apps, 1983).

Obstructive apnoea

Obstructive sleep apnoea in children is caused by either physical or dysfunctional obstruction of the upper airway during sleep. It is this type of sleep apnoea which is most likely to present to the otolaryngologist. Physical obstruction of the upper airway is especially common in children. Causes of physical obstruction extend from the alar nasi to the glottis (Table 20.1).

Table 20.1 Causes of obstructive sleep apnoea

Nose
  Polyps
  Deviated nasal septum
  Rhinitis
  Nasal packing

Pharynx
  Nasopharyngeal tumour
  Enlarged adenoids
  Enlarged palatine tonsils
  Enlarged lingual tonsils
  Retropharyngeal mass
  Large tongue
    myxoedema
    acromegaly
  Micrognathia/retrognathia
  Obesity

Larynx
  Tumours
  Oedema
  Shy-Drager syndrome

Congenital conditions

Nasal obstruction

Total nasal obstruction, as for example caused by complete nasal agenesis or bilateral choanal atresia is immediately life-threatening as all neonates are obligate nose-breathers for the first 2–3 months of life (Stool and Houlihan, 1977). Presentation of these patients is usually dramatic with respiratory and feeding difficulties which are life-threatening. Such patients would certainly manifest obstructive sleep apnoea.

Causes of partial nasal obstruction (which present later with stertor and nocturnal snoring) include neonatal rhinitis and congenital cysts of the nasal cavity (i.e. dermoids, nasoalveolar cysts, dentigerous cysts and mucous cysts of the floor of the nose arising in Jacobson's organ). Partial nasal obstruction in the neonatal period may also be caused by a swelling of neural origin extending into the nose; this may be a meningocoele (meninges alone), meningoencephalo-coele (meninges plus brain tissue) or an encephalocoele (glial tissue with no remaining connection to the brain) (Furstenberg, 1936). Choanal stenosis may also produce partial nasal obstruction with stertorous respiration and snoring, but is extremely uncommon.

Facial skeletal anomalies

Children with craniofacial abnormalities may develop stertor as a result of obstruction of the nose, nasopharynx or oropharynx. Nasopharyngeal airway obstruction occurs in Apert's and Crouzon's syndromes as a result of severe posterior displacement of the midfacial skeletal structures with consequent narrowing of the nasopharyngeal airway. Oropharyngeal obstruction is a feature of glossoptosis in which micrognathia results in the tongue sitting in a posterior position and tending to fall back into the oropharynx. Treacher Collins syndrome is an example of micrognathia in which this may occur. Significantly, patients with Treacher Collins syndrome have been shown to have obstructive sleep apnoea and to be particularly difficult to manage during induction and recovery from anaesthesia. This latter finding is typical of children with obstructive sleep apnoea (Shprintzen *et al.*, 1979). Pierre Robin syndrome, in which the tongue is even more likely to fall posteriorly in the presence of a cleft palate, is also frequently associated with obstructive sleep apnoea.

Macroglossia

The tongue can produce significant respiratory obstruction if it is much enlarged even if the mandible is normal. This can occur in Down's syndrome and as part of the organomegaly of Beckwith's syndrome, or it may be an isolated and idiopathic finding. Enlargement of the tongue may also occur due to a cystic hygroma or haemangioma in the floor of the mouth, although it is rare for partial respiratory obstruction or embarrassment to ensue.

Pharyngeal swelling

A large lingual thyroid mass can produce respiratory obstruction, as may a lingual thyroglossal duct cyst or any of the rare congenital tumours of the pharynx which include Thornwald's bursa, branchial cleft cyst, teratoma, hairy polyp, chordoma or craniopharyngioma, cystic hygroma and haemangioma (Parkin and Thomas, 1974).

Acquired conditions

Traumatic

The authors have certainly seen obstructive sleep apnoea in a patient with a traumatic and completely obstructing nasal septal haematoma.

Inflammatory

Children with partial upper airways obstruction often deteriorate in the presence of upper respiratory tract inflammation such as the common cold. Parents commonly describe exacerbation of breathing difficulties with snoring progressing to definite sleep apnoea. This is presumably secondary to further reduction of an already minimal nasal and upper pharyngeal airway due to mucosal oedema and excessive secretions. Tonsillitis rarely causes respiratory embarrassment except in children with extremely large tonsils. Infectious mononucleosis can produce life-threatening airway obstruction as a result of massive inflammatory swelling of all the pharyngeal lymphoid tissues with grossly stertorous respiration and increased breathing difficulties and dangers when the patient is asleep. The most common cause of obstructive sleep apnoea in children is undoubtedly non-inflammatory enlargement of the adenoids and/or tonsils. It is relatively rare for secondary acute inflammation, such as a peritonsillar abscess, parapharyngeal or retropharyngeal abscess, to present with sleep-disordered breathing.

Neoplastic

The neoplasm most likely to produce nasal obstruction and nocturnal snoring with obstructive sleep apnoea in older children and adolescents is the postnasal angiofibroma which may enlarge to fill the nasopharynx completely. Other tumours such as neuroblastoma, lymphoma or rhabdomyosarcoma, may less commonly produce similar symptoms.

Iatrogenic

Nasal obstruction, snoring and sleep apnoea may result from stenosis of the nasopharyngeal isthmus. Rarely this can develop after tonsillectomy and/or adenoidectomy. It has been described after 'sandwich', wide-flap pharyngoplasty operations performed for velopharyngeal insufficiency. Surgical obstruction of the velopharyngeal port following pharyngoplasty has caused death and subsequent evaluation of other similarly-treated children has confirmed the presence of significant obstructive sleep apnoea (Kravath *et al.*, 1980). Insertion of a postnasal pack can have a similar effect.

Other conditions

Hypertrophic adenoids and tonsils have already been mentioned as the most common cause of partial upper airways obstruction in secondary sleep apnoea. Nasal polyps in children are usually associated with cystic fibrosis and there is often a concomitant chronic mucosal swelling and abnormally thick nasal mucus aggravating the obstruction. An antrochoanal polyp may rarely present in children with complete nasopharyngeal airway obstruction and sleep apnoea.

Pharyngeal airway dysfunction

In the past decade, the evaluation of children with obstructive sleep apnoea with no definite or obvious physical cause for upper airways obstruction has revealed evidence of dysfunction of the pharyngeal constrictor muscles which maintain upper airway patency during sleep. Fluoroscopic and fibreoptic nasendoscopic studies have demonstrated a small group of children with classical obstructive sleep apnoea in whom the episodes of obstruction are caused by collapse of the pharyngeal muscles during sleep (Southall *et al.*, 1988; Croft *et al.*, 1990). Diminished pharyngeal muscle tone, especially during REM sleep, precipitates collapse of an already partially narrowed pharyngeal airway as a result of the Venturi or negative pressure effect, caused by rapid air flow through a narrow pharynx. Subsequently, increasing airway obstruction results in oxygen desaturation and a rise in $P_a\text{co}_2$, producing increased muscle tone and arousal (often accompanied by awakening), which terminates the apnoea. These patients with pharyngeal airway dysfunction appear to show maturation of their respiratory control mechanisms during childhood with a diminishing tendency to pharyngeal airway collapse during sleep.

Finally, it is worth noting that children with obstructive sleep apnoea and snoring present as a continuum, from those patients who may tend to mouth-breathe and snore intermittently to the full-blown picture of obstructive sleep apnoea described above. It is very worthwhile directly questioning the parents of such children about the degree of snoring, sleep position and presence of apnoea. By no means all parents are aware of the potential significance of these symptoms.

Central apnoea

Central apnoea is caused by an instability of the automatic control of respiration by the respiratory centre in the medulla. This pattern of respiration can be induced in normal subjects when awake by a voluntary period of hyperventilation, when it is termed periodic breathing. When an individual hyperventilates for 2–3 minutes, and then stops and permits his respiration to continue without exerting any voluntary control over it, there is a period of apnoea. This is followed by a few shallow breaths, and then by another period of apnoea, followed again by a few breaths. The apnoea is the result of hypocapnia induced by the period of hyperventilation. During the apnoea the alveolar $P\text{o}_2$ falls and the $P\text{co}_2$ rises. Breathing resumes because of hypoxic stimulation of the peripheral (carotid and aortic body) chemoreceptors before the CO_2 level has returned to normal. A few breaths eliminate the hypoxic stimulus, and breathing stops until the alveolar $P\text{o}_2$ falls again. Gradually, however, the $P\text{co}_2$ returns to normal, the central (medullary) CO_2-driven chemoreceptors come back into play and normal breathing resumes (Ganong, 1973). Periodic breathing in disease states is called Cheyne-Stokes respiration.

This same imbalance of respiratory control between the central and peripheral chemoreceptors can occur during sleep in some normal individuals at high altitudes as a result of overbreathing induced by hypoxia. A similar sequence of events is induced by congestive cardiac failure (as a consequence of an imbalance between central and peripheral chemoreceptor responses caused by the prolonged circulation time) and myxoedema can cause central sleep apnoea by the same mechanism.

Neurological lesions in the brain stem or above may produce central apnoea. Some patients with brain-stem lesions (e.g. infarcts) lose automatic control of respiration altogether and stop breathing when they go to sleep. The congenital form of this central hypoventilation syndrome is termed Ondine's curse, after the mythical water nymph whose human suitor was cursed to stop breathing and die if ever he fell asleep. It is thought to be due to a brain-stem lesion in the area where chemoreceptor input is integrated (Marcus *et al.*, 1991a).

Other neurological causes in this category include brain-stem encephalitis, bulbar poliomyelitis and supratentorial space-occupying lesions. Some patients with central apnoea have no demonstrable neurological or cardiovascular cause, however, and often are found to have a diminished responsiveness to hypoxia and hypercapnia even when they are awake. Table 20.2 lists the causes of central sleep apnoea.

Table 20.2 Causes of central sleep apnoea

Ondine's curse
Altitude
Cheyne-Stokes respiration
Congestive heart failure
Myxoedema

Neurological lesions
    Brain-stem infarct
    Brain-stem encephalitis
    Bulbar poliomyelitis
    Supratentorial space-occupying lesions

Complications of sleep apnoea

The clinical features and complications associated with obstructive sleep apnoea result from two main factors. These are oxygen desaturation with associated hypercapnia and the generation of high negative intrathoracic pressure.

Oxygen desaturation

During an apnoeic episode no air flows into the lungs and as time elapses the patient becomes both hypoxic and hypercapnic. Very low levels of oxygen saturation can be reached during a long obstructive event. The degree of hypoxia will be determined by the duration of the apnoeic event, the lung volume (which is reduced in obesity) and any coexistent neuromuscular, cardiac or pulmonary disorder. Hypoxia is associated with a rise in sympathetic output (Hedner *et al.*, 1988) and the resulting peripheral vasoconstriction causes transient pulmonary and systemic hypertension. Particularly in children, long-standing sleep apnoea will result in irreversible pulmonary hypertension with subsequent development of cor pulmonale (Kravath, Pollak and Borowiecki, 1977). Those patients with some degree of daytime desaturation may also develop secondary polycythaemia. Systemic hypertension may ensue. Hypoxia can also cause a variety of cardiac dysrhythmias which range from bradycardia to ventricular ectopic beats. During an obstructive episode the effort of trying to inspire results in increased vagal activity with subsequent bradycardia. The presence of hypoxia significantly worsens this bradycardia (Shephard, 1984). There is some evidence that sleep apnoea may play a minor part in some cases labelled sudden infant death syndrome or 'cot death' (Guilleminault *et al.*, 1984). However, most experts on sudden infant death syndrome feel that obstructive sleep apnoea and sleep-related upper airways obstruction could be responsible only for a minority of cases.

Generation of high negative intrathoracic pressure

The efforts of the respiratory system to overcome upper airway obstruction results in the generation of high negative intrathoracic pressures. This results in arousal from sleep and the termination of the obstructive episode. It is now thought that termination of such episodes is heavily dependent upon arousal rather than hypoxia or hypercapnia (Phillipson and Sullivan, 1978). The patient is often unaware of these arousals which can occur many hundreds of times throughout the night. The effect of repeated arousals is a grossly disturbed sleep pattern which is reflected in the symptom of excessive daytime sleepiness, one of the commonest symptoms of obstructive sleep apnoea. Excessive daytime sleepiness also occurs in patients with partial upper airways obstruction and in some patients who snore loudly without any obstructive episodes. Presumably these patients are generating sufficiently high negative intrathoracic pressures from their partial obstruction to stimulate arousal on a frequent basis. It is well recognized that the threshold for arousal is elevated during REM sleep so that obstructive episodes are more prolonged and severe during this sleep stage.

There are some children who present with a combination of the complications outlined in association with obesity. Stool *et al.* (1977) described the 'chubby puffer' syndrome in three children with obesity and airway obstruction caused by enlarged tonsils and/or adenoids, associated with hypersomnolence and cardiopulmonary disturbance. This seems to be closely related to the classical Pickwickian syndrome (so-called after Joe, the fat boy, in 'The Pickwick Papers') of obesity, hypoventilation, daytime hypersomnolence, cor pulmonale and polycythaemia. The cause of the Pickwickian syndrome is considered to be multifactorial but some patients have obstructive sleep apnoea due to pharyngeal airway collapse (Sharp, Barroc and Chokroverty, 1980) as well as hypoventilation secondary to obesity.

Obesity affects nocturnal respiration in two significant ways. First, there is a direct compression of the pharyngeal airway by excess fat deposits in the soft tissues of the neck. CT scan studies of pharyngeal airway size in obese sufferers from obstructive sleep apnoea confirm gross and statistically significant reductions in the pharyngeal airway particularly at the level of the oropharynx and tongue base (Bohlman *et al.*, 1983). There does not appear to be direct fatty infiltration of the pharyngeal wall or pharyngeal constrictor muscles. The second effect of obesity is to cause reduction in lung volume and to derange the pulmonary-pharyngeal reflexes which allow phasic and appropriate dilatation of the pharyngeal airway during inspiration.

Clinical features

Symptoms of obstructive sleep apnoea

The cardinal and universal symptom of obstructive sleep apnoea is loud and persistent *snoring*. Snoring may be described as the 'stridor of the pharynx' and is produced by vibration of the nearly apposed walls of the pharynx and soft palate. The actual site of noise generation may vary from patient to patient and in children may vary from the level of the palatopharyngeal sphincter and adenoid pad through the oropharynx (with pharyngeal walls apposed to the palatine tonsils) and on down to the tongue-base level of obstruction which is characteristically seen in Down's syndrome (Croft *et al.*, 1990). Evaluation of the upper airway using fibreoptic flexible endoscopic techniques has revealed a spectrum of sites and causes of upper airway obstruction ranging from those described above to pharyngeal airway dysfunction and rarely even laryngomalacia (Croft *et al.*, 1990).

It is important to remember that snoring is a sign of partial airways obstruction and progression of the events leading to this obstruction will eventually lead to shut-down of the airway as increasing velocity of inspiratory airflow through the narrowed pharynx creates an irresistible collapsing force on the compliant pharyngeal walls (Venturi effect). This produces the classical obstructive apnoeic episode which is the second major hallmark symptom of the obstructive sleep apnoea syndrome. Any degree of intrinsic airway compromise is of considerable importance in generating these obstructive episodes. Clearly, patients with massive obstructing tonsils and adenoids or reduced pharyngeal airway dimensions, as in the Treacher Collins syndrome (Shprintzen *et al.*, 1979) or Crouzon's or Apert's syndromes will tend to obstruct with little provocation and the addition of sleep-induced relaxation of the pharyngeal walls completes the embarrassment and obstruction of the upper airway.

During periods of apnoea the high negative intrathoracic pressures and decrease in oxygen saturation interact to produce arousal. The airway is restored as the patient wakes but frequent wakening and disturbed sleep pattern are a direct consequence of these events. This may result in abnormal sleep movements and restlessness, with the child adopting abnormal positions during sleep and likely to wake frequently with sweating and cyanosis, accompanied by gasping or choking episodes. A major consequence of multiple arousals and disturbed sleep pattern is daytime hypersomnolence. In the child this may result in constant daytime sleepiness and a fall-off in school performance, as these patients tend to fall asleep as soon as their concentration lapses. There is some evidence that sleep deprivation in children with obstructive sleep apnoea may result in retarded growth and development (Richardson *et al.*, 1980). It is known that growth hormone secretion is maximal nocturnally with 'pulses' of growth hormone released during sleep. There is some evidence that in children with severe sleep disruption growth hormone secretion may be reduced. However, definitive research is still being undertaken into this interesting possibility. It is also thought that nocturnal enuresis may be exacerbated in children with sleep-related breathing disorders such as obstructive sleep apnoea (Richardson *et al.*, 1980).

In the adult, obesity is often present, although this finding is less usual in children. The child may be excessively sleepy and drowsy and have difficulty in concentrating and staying awake during the taking of a medical history.

Symptoms of central sleep apnoea

There may be few symptoms in patients with central apnoea as the events are essentially silent and hypersomnolence is unusual. The patient may be aware of stopping breathing at night with a tendency to wake in a 'panic or choking attack', or of being unable to breathe when going to sleep.

Signs of obstructive sleep apnoea

The great difficulty in diagnosing sleep apnoea on general examination is that there may be few, if any, daytime physical signs. However, in the child, a poor nasal airway with constant mouth-breathing is usual. The upper lip is often coated with nasal mucus and daytime respiration may be noisy with variable stertor present. Grossly hypertrophic tonsils may cause real physical difficulties in swallowing solids and the child may be underweight and undersized for his age as a result.

Examination of the chest may reveal signs of chronic inspiratory airway obstruction with a pectus excavatum deformity and a rib sulcus similar to the 'Harrison's sulcus' seen in rickets. Examination of the throat may show 'midline tonsils' which appear to occupy the oropharynx completely, and nasal airflow may be minimal on objective testing. Physical signs may dramatically increase when the child is asleep, with obvious signs of respiratory embarrassment, sweating, stertor and tracheal tug with intercostal recession. Asking the parents to record the child with a simple tape recorder or with their home videocamera is often useful in screening for the presence of real nocturnal respiratory difficulty.

Examination of the nasal airway should be carefully undertaken, usually with the help of fibreoptic endoscopic equipment. The association of obstructive sleep apnoea with reduced nasopharyngeal and hypopharyngeal dimensions in patients with skull base abnormalities and syndromes such as Treacher Collins have already been discussed.

Signs of central sleep apnoea

Central sleep apnoea is very much less common than sleep apnoea of the obstructive type. Patients may present with signs germane to the causal pathology in the central nervous system. Thus patients who have had encephalitis affecting the brain stem, or patients with lesions in the pons, midbrain or above would manifest signs of other neurological disorders. Alternatively, patients may present with signs relating to disruption of their sleep pattern. Hypersomnolence, irritability and, paradoxically, insomnia may be present. However, a proportion of patients with central sleep apnoea have little in the way of signs of neurological or cardiac disease and diagnosis will depend upon the history and subsequent positive identification with a sleep study.

Investigations
Sleep studies

Although the history and examination may be highly suggestive of sleep apnoea, observation of the patient during sleep is definitely required if the presence of sleep disordered breathing is to be recognized and quantified.

A *polysomnograph* or full sleep study is a detailed examination during sleep, with monitoring of sleep stage as active or quiet sleep (sometimes including EEG, EMG and eye movement recordings), chest and abdominal movements (for paradoxical movements during efforts to respire), and transcutaneous monitoring of oxygen saturation with measurement of nasal or oral airflow, end tidal CO_2 and continuous ECG recording (Figure 20.1). Video monitoring of sleep during the study is also helpful.

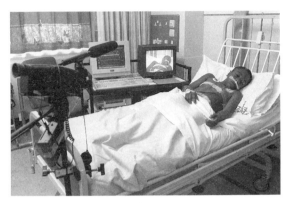

Figure 20.1 Polysomnography

Such a study is detailed and expensive and the authors believe an initial screening or 'mini-sleep study', with observation during sleep and transcutaneous oximeter monitoring of oxygen saturation, together with an ECG and rhythm strip and postnasal space and chest X-rays, is useful in identifying those patients who require a full study, and in most children it is sufficient to document the need for adenotonsillectomy without proceeding further. There is no doubt that if major surgery or tracheostomy is being contemplated a full sleep study is warranted, and as other appropriate treatments are developed for obstructive apnoea, such as uvulopalatopharyngoplasty, this will increasingly be the case. However, in most children a screening study is probably more appropriate unless there are doubts about the site of obstruction. Overnight studies can be reduced to 4 hours without loss of clinical significance (Smith *et al.*, 1992).

Sleep sonography has proved a reliable method for evaluating patients with upper airway obstruction due to adenotonsillar hypertrophy (Potsic, 1987). Agreement between polysomnography and sleep sonography is very high in scoring the respiratory pattern and detecting apnoea, and where it is available this technique could replace the need for nurse observation during a 'mini-sleep study'.

Polysomnographic results in the paediatric age group differ from those in adults, and recommendations for normal values are given by Marcus *et al.* (1992). In the context of a mini-sleep study, arterial oxygen saturations measured by pulse oximetry of below 90% represent significant hypoxia.

Radiology

A plain lateral X-ray of the postnasal space and upper airway is extremely useful in identifying and documenting adenoidal obstruction of the nasopharynx and tonsillar obstruction of the oropharynx (Figure 20.2). It also shows the position of the lower jaw and tongue base in addition to outlining the airway.

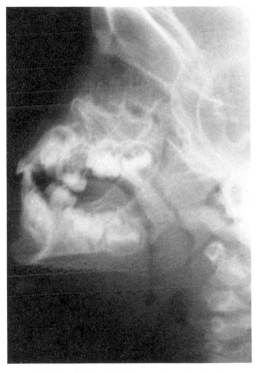

Figure 20.2 Lateral X-ray of the head and neck, showing a 3 year old with massive tonsils and adenoids obstructing the postnasal and oropharyngeal airway

Computerized tomographic scans of the pharyngeal airway in patients with obstructive sleep apnoea (Bohlman *et al.*, 1983) have shown significantly reduced dimensions of the airway at the naso- and oropharyngeal levels. This is really of research interest only and it is not appropriate to perform CT scanning routinely.

Chest radiography should be performed to exclude cardiomegaly and right heart failure.

Nasendoscopy

The use of the flexible fibreoptic endoscope to examine the physical state and dynamics of the upper airway is extremely valuable in documenting both physical and functional airway obstruction. The Olympus ENF P flexible laryngoscope (Figure 20.3) is ideal in having a 2.9 mm bundle which allows examination of the upper airway in the smallest infants. The nasal cavity, postnasal space, velopharyngeal sphincter and hypopharynx and larynx are examined in turn and, if no obvious physical obstruction is seen, a Muller (reverse Valsalva) manoeuvre can be performed by older patients to try to document areas of functional obstruction.

It may be necessary to perform this examination under light general anaesthesia without intubation (sleep nasendoscopy) to identify pharyngeal airway dysfunction in children (Southall *et al.*, 1988; Croft *et al.*, 1990). If adenotonsillar obstruction is confirmed, the child is then intubated and adenotonsillectomy can proceed immediately.

Intubation

In children with both congenital cyanotic heart disease and upper airway obstruction (e.g in Down's syndrome) it can be difficult to separate the effects of one from the other. Kasian *et al.* (1987) have shown that in this situation elective intubation can be useful, by demonstrating the result of relieving the airway obstruction on pulmonary artery pressure and systemic arterial oxygen saturation. In two of their three patients, the pulmonary pressures immediately decreased and systemic arterial oxygen saturations increased: both of these children showed dramatic improvement after tonsillectomy.

Treatment of obstructive sleep apnoea

Medical and conservative measures

Medication has little to offer, but in Hurler's syndrome, bone marrow transplantation can produce effective metabolic correction with resolution of obstructive sleep apnoea (Malone *et al.*, 1988).

Continuous positive airway pressure

Continuous positive airway pressure can be helpful in patients with a tendency to pharyngeal airway collapse (pharyngeal airway dysfunction) during sleep. This type of dysfunction can be minimized by increasing the pressure of the inspired air. This requires either a plastic pressure chamber to fit over the head for infants, or alternatively a face mask or nasal inserts for older children. There are problems in maintaining treatment in this way, particularly in children, but more major surgical intervention may be avoided (British Medical Journal, 1986).

Use of the nasopharyngeal airway ('nasal prong')

Pharyngeal airway obstruction may be dramatically relieved by employing a nasopharyngeal airway (Aubert, 1992). This technique is particularly useful in the Pierre Robin syndrome (Heaf *et al.*, 1982) and in Apert's syndrome where midface recession is accompanied by a very shallow nasopharynx.

A Portex endotracheal tube is employed; for a neonate a 3.0 or 3.5 mm diameter tube is appropriate, and the length required can be estimated from the crown/heel measurement (Heaf *et al.*, 1982). The tube is mounted on a Tunstall connector, passed through the nose and secured with a conventional head band and tapes across the cheeks (Figure 20.4). Alternatively, a Portex endotracheal tube holder can be fitted and its 'wings' taped to the cheeks ('Brompton prong'): this is a less secure method of fixing the tube, but it is aesthetically more acceptable for parents managing their child at home.

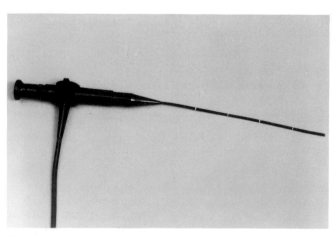

Figure 20.3 Olympus ENF P flexible nasolaryngoscope

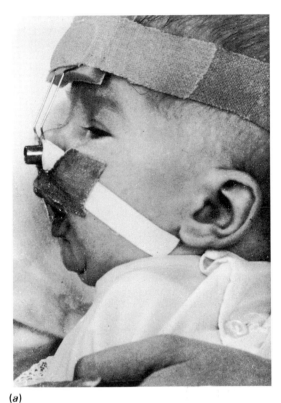 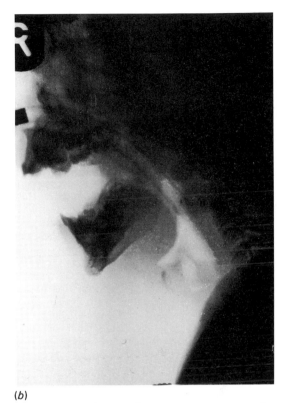

(a)   **(b)**

Figure 20.4 (*a*) A 5-month-old infant with Pierre Robin syndrome showing a nasopharyngeal airway in position, secured with a Tunstall connector, head band and cheek tapes. (*b*) Lateral neck X-ray of an infant with a nasopharyngeal airway in place, demonstrating the splinting effect of the tube on the tongue. The position of the anterior tube bevel is seen just above the epiglottis. (From Heaf *et al.*, 1982, by kind permission of the Editor and Publisher of the *Journal of Pediatrics*)

Lateral neck radiography is necessary to check the tube position. For the Pierre Robin syndrome, where the site of obstruction is at the tongue base, the tube tip should ideally be just above the epiglottis: if the tube is too long, choking and vomiting are induced; but if it is too short, relief of airway obstruction is not achieved. For Apert's syndrome, where the site of obstruction is the nasopharynx, the tube tip should lie at the level of the free edge of the soft palate.

To maintain tube patency, regular suction with a catheter is undertaken, preceded by instillation of 0.5 ml of isotonic saline; this is carried out routinely before feeds and at other times as required. If possible the tube is changed every week and the new tube passed through the opposite nostril.

Occasionally vestibulitis develops around the tube, requiring topical antibiotic therapy. Crusting and blockage may sometimes occur and necessitate a tube change. Parents can be trained to manage the tube at home, with weekly visits to the hospital.

A nasopharyngeal airway may be the only treatment required for some children. Those with the Pierre Robin syndrome, for example, often grow to develop an adequate airway by the age of about 3

months, and use of the 'prong' can then be discontinued. In other children, the nasopharyngeal airway is an invaluable temporary measure, allowing full assessment of their clinical condition to be made prior to more definitive treatment (e.g. adenotonsillectomy or tracheostomy).

In some children with severe pharyngeal airway obstruction, e.g. where there is pharyngeal collapse, a nasopharyngeal airway alone is insufficient, but the addition of continuous positive airway pressure overcomes the residual obstruction by distending the pharynx during inspiration. A ventilator is not required; continuous positive airway pressure may be applied via a special valve, or by underwater immersion of the exhalation arm of a T-piece system.

Surgical

The major complications of obstructive sleep apnoea are potentially reversible, although end-stage cor pulmonale is not; therefore identifiable obstructive lesions in the upper airway should be dealt with surgically as soon as possible. This usually involves simple adenotonsillectomy in children, but obstruction may occur at any site from the nasal cavity to the larynx and careful evaluation is required to reveal the site of obstruction (Kravath, Pollak and Borowiecki, 1977).

Adenotonsillectomy

Increased awareness has made upper airway obstruction an important indication for adenotonsillectomy. Indeed, in the USA, airway obstruction has become the indication for surgery in one-third of all children undergoing adenotonsillectomy (Derkay, 1993).

Clearly, the removal of enormously hypertrophic tonsils and adenoids will improve the airway. However, it is important to appreciate that some children with sleep apnoea caused by anatomical restriction of the upper airway (e.g. some of the craniofacial anomalies) may benefit from tonsillectomy and adenoidectomy even though hypertrophy of the tonsils and adenoids is not the primary cause of the problem. This is because the flow of air through a tube increases as a function of the fourth power of the radius of the tube in accordance with Poiseuille's formula, and so a small increase in radius is accompanied by a large increase in flow. It is therefore often beneficial to remove the tonsils and adenoids in such a situation even if they are not unduly large, as the consequent improvement in respiratory function may avoid the need for tracheostomy (Hultcrantz, Svanholm and Ahlqvist-Rastad, 1988).

Uncommonly, lingual tonsil hypertrophy may be responsible for upper airway obstruction in children and lingual tonsillectomy (using diathermy or the CO_2 laser) can be highly effective (Guarisco, Littlewood and Butcher, 1990).

Other surgical techniques

Surgical modification of the major site of pharyngeal airway shutdown is possible and interest has centred on surgical modification of the velopharyngeal sphincter by uvulopalatopharyngoplasty (UPPP) as described by Fujita *et al.* (1981). This operation has been performed on large numbers of adults and is successful in relieving obstructive sleep apnoea in between 50 and 70 % of cases, depending on the criteria involved in selecting the patients (Sher *et al.*, 1985). The operation has not been widely used in children where lymphoid obstruction of the upper airway is generally the rule, but it may have a place for some children such as those with Down's syndrome (Donaldson and Redmond, 1988; Seid *et al.*, 1990).

Tracheostomy

Some children with pharyngeal airway dysfunction experience major nocturnal arterial desaturation (to around 50% P_aO_2) and may show major cardiac dysrhythmias. These patients represent a high risk group and may well progress to cardiac failure or to life-threatening dysrhythmias (Southall *et al.*, 1988). Tracheostomy is indicated if adenotonsillectomy fails to help these unusually severe cases, and is rapidly effective in reversing the gross cardiorespiratory abnormalities described.

Premedication and postoperative care

Patients with the obstructive sleep apnoea syndrome are extremely sensitive to sedation. Heavy premedication prior to surgery may cause a marked deterioration in the patient's respiratory status and even produce a respiratory arrest. The same strictures apply to postoperative sedation and both should be avoided in patients with obstructive sleep apnoea. Anaesthetists involved in treating these patients should be alerted to the dangers of over-sedation.

Children with obstructive sleep apnoea are at risk of respiratory compromise immediately following adenotonsillectomy; young age and severe sleep-related upper airway obstruction significantly increase this risk. These children are *not* suitable for day case surgery, and postoperative pulse oximetry monitoring is recommended for children undergoing adenotonsillectomy for obstructive sleep apnoea (McColley *et al.*, 1992). It is sometimes wise to leave a nasal prong *in situ* for the first 12–24 hours postoperatively in high-risk children.

Treatment of central sleep apnoea
Medical therapy

Theophylline may be useful in improving respiratory function in mild cases, by providing central respiratory stimulation.

Ventilation and diaphragm pacing

Children with congenital central hypoventilation syndrome are traditionally managed with positive-pressure ventilation via a tracheostomy, and can be looked after at home with appropriate support. During the neonatal period complete ventilator-dependency is usual, but most then become able to sustain normal gas exchange when awake and only require ventilation when asleep (Oren, Kelly and Shannon, 1987).

Negative-pressure ventilation is also used successfully in a number of these patients, and may avoid the need for tracheostomy (Samuels and Southall, 1989).

Recently it has proved possible to manage a few of these children by diaphragm pacing using implanted bilateral phrenic nerve electrodes (Weese–Mayer *et al.*, 1989; Marcus *et al.*, 1991b). However, a tracheostomy is still necessary owing to impaired neuromuscular control of upper airway patency during pacing (Hunt *et al.*, 1988).

References

APPS, M. C. P. (1983) Sleep disordered breathing. *British Journal of Hospital Medicine*, 30, 339–347

AUBERT, G. (1992) Alternative therapeutic approaches in sleep apnea syndrome. *Sleep*, 15 (suppl.), 69–72

BOHLMAN, M. E., HAPONIK, E. F. and SMITH, P. L. (1983) CT demonstration of pharyngeal narrowing in adult obstructive sleep apnoea. *American Journal of Roentgenology*, 14, 543–548

BRITISH MEDICAL JOURNAL (1986) PEEP and CPAP. Editorial. 292, 643

CROFT, C. B., THOMSON, H. G., SAMUELS, M. P. and SOUTHALL, D. P. (1990) Endoscopic evaluation and treatment of sleep-associated upper airway obstruction in infants and young children. *Clinical Otolaryngology*, 15, 209–216

DERKAY, C. S. (1993) Pediatric otolaryngology procedures in the United States: 1977–1987. *International Journal of Pediatric Otorhinolaryngology*, 25, 1–12

DONALDSON, J. D. and REDMOND, W. M. (1988) Surgical management of obstructive sleep apnea in children with Down syndrome. *Journal of Otolaryngology*, 17, 393–403

FUJITA, S., CONWAY, W., ZORICK, F. and ROTH, T. (1981) Surgical correction of anatomic abnormalities in obstructive sleep apnoea syndrome: uvulopalatopharyngoplasty. *Otolaryngology – Head and Neck Surgery*, 89, 923–934

FURSTENBERG, A. C. (1936) *A Clinical and Pathological Study of Tumours and Cysts of the Nose, Pharynx, Mouth and Neck of Teratological Origin*. Ann Arbor: Edward Brothers

GANONG, W. F. (1973) *Review of Medical Physiology*, 6th edn. Los Altos: Lange. p. 507

GUARISCO, J. L., LITTLEWOOD, S. C. and BUTCHER, R. B. (1990) Severe upper airway obstruction in children secondary to lingual tonsil hypertrophy. *Annals of Otology, Rhinology and Laryngology*, 99, 621–624

GUILLEMINAULT, C., VAN DEN HOED, J. and MITLER, M. M. (1978) Clinical overview of the sleep apnea syndromes. In: *Sleep Apnea Syndromes*, edited by C. Guilleminault and W. C. Dement. New York: Alan R. Liss. pp. 1–2

GUILLEMINAULT, C., HILL, M. W., SIMMONS, F. B. and DEMENT, W. C. (1978) Obstructive sleep apnea: electromyographic and fiberoptic studies. *Experimental Neurology*, 62, 48–67

GUILLEMINAULT, C., SOUQUET, M., ARIAGNO, R. L., KOROBKIN, R. and SIMMONS, F. B. (1984) Five cases of near-miss sudden infant death syndrome and development of obstructive sleep apnea syndrome. *Pediatrics*, 73, 71–78

HEAF, D. P., HELMS, P. J., DINWIDDIE, R. and MATTHEW, D. J. (1982) Nasopharyngeal airways in Pierre Robin syndrome. *Journal of Pediatrics*, 100, 698–703

HEDNER, J. A., EJNELL, H. and SELLGREN, J. et al. (1988) Is high and fluctuating muscle nerve sympathetic activity in the sleep apnoea syndrome of pathogenic importance for the development of hypertension? *Journal of Hypertension*, 6, 529–531

HILL, W. (1889) On some cases of backwardness and stupidity in children relieved by adenoidal scarification. *British Medical Journal*, 2, 711–712

HULTCRANTZ, E., SVANHOLM, H. and AHLQVIST–RASTAD, J. (1988) Sleep apnea in children without hypertrophy of the tonsils. *Clinical Pediatrics*, 27, 350–352

HUNT, C. E., BROUILLETTE, R. T., WEESE–MAYER, D. E., MORROW, A. and ILBAWI, M. N. (1988) Diaphragm pacing in infants and children. *PACE (Pacing Clinical Electrophysiology)*, 11, 2135–2141

KASIAN, G. F., DUNCAN W. J., TYRRELL, M. J. and OMAN GANES, L. A. (1987) Elective oro-tracheal intubation to diagnose sleep apnea syndrome in children with Down's syndrome and ventricular septal defect. *Canadian Journal of Cardiology*, 3, 2–5

KRAVATH, R. E., POLLAK, C. P. and BOROWIECKI, B. (1977) Hypoventilation during sleep in children who have lymphoid airway obstruction by nasopharyngeal tube and T and A. *Pediatrics*, 59, 865–871

KRAVATH, R. E., POLLAK, C. P., BOROWIECKI, B. and WEITZMANN, E. (1980) Obstructive sleep apnea and death associated with surgical correction of velopharyngeal incompetence. *Journal of Pediatrics*, 96, 645–648

MCCOLLEY, S. A., APRIL, M. M., CARROLL, J. L., NACLERIO, R. M. and LOUGHLIN, G. M. (1992) Respiratory compromise after adenotonsillectomy in children with obstructive sleep apnea. *Archives of Otolaryngology – Head and Neck Surgery*, 118, 940–943

MALONE, B. N., WHITLEY, C. B., DUVALL, A. J., BELANI, K., SIBLEY, R. K., RAMSAY, N. K. et al. (1988) Resolution of obstructive sleep apnea in Hurler syndrome after bone marrow transplantation. *International Journal of Pediatric Otorhinolaryngology*, 15, 23–27

MARCUS, C. L., BAUTISTA, D. B., AMIHYIA, A., WARD, S. L. and KEENS, T. G. (1991a) Hypercapneic arousal responses in children with congenital central hypoventilation syndrome. *Pediatrics*, 88, 993–998

MARCUS, C. L., JANSEN, M. T., POULSEN, M. K., KEENS, S. E., NIELDS, T. A., LIPSKER, L. E. et al. (1991b) Medical and psychosocial outcome of children with congenital central hypoventilation syndrome. *Journal of Pediatrics*, 119, 888–895

MARCUS, C. L., OMLIN, K. J., BASINKI, D. J., BAILEY, S. L., RACHAL, A. B., VON PECHMANN, W. S. et al. (1992) Normal polysomnographic values for children and adolescents. *American Review of Respiratory Disease*, 146, 1235–1239

OREN, J., KELLY, D. H. and SHANNON, D. C. (1987) Long-term follow-up of children with congenital central hypoventilation syndrome. *Pediatrics*, 80, 375–380

PARKIN, J. L. and THOMAS, G. K. (1974) Benign masses of the pharynx. *Rocky Mountain Medical Journal*, 71, 34

PHILLIPSON, E. A. and SULLIVAN, C. E. (1978) Arousal: the forgotten response to respiratory stimuli. *American Review of Respiratory Diseases*, 118, 807–809

POTSIC, W. P. (1987) Comparison of polysomnography and sonography for assessing regularity of respiration during sleep in adenotonsillar hypertrophy. *Laryngoscope*, 97, 1430–1437

RICHARDSON, M. A., SEID, A. B., COTTON, R. T., BENTON, C. and KRAMER, M. (1980) Evaluation of tonsils and adenoids in the sleep apnea syndrome. *Laryngoscope*, 90, 1106–1110

SAMUELS, M. P. and SOUTHALL, D. P. (1989) Negative extrathoracic pressure in treatment of respiratory failure in infants and young children. *British Medical Journal*, 299, 1253–1257

SEID, A. B., MARTIN, P. J., PRANSKY, S. M. and KEARNS, D. B. (1990) Surgical therapy of obstructive sleep apnea in children with severe mental insufficiency. *Laryngoscope*, 100, 507–510

SHARP, J. T., BARROC, A. S. and CHOKROVERTY, S. (1980) The cardiorespiratory effects of obesity. In: *Clinics in Chest Medicine*, edited by M. H. Williams. Philadelphia: W. B. Saunders. p. 103–118

SHEPHARD, J. W. (1984) Pathophysiology and medical therapy of sleep apnea. *Ear, Nose and Throat Journal*, 63, 24–29

SHER, A. E., THORPY, M. J., SHPRINTZEN, R. J., SPIELMAN, A. J.,

BURASK, B. and MCGREGOR, P. A. (1985) Predictive value of Muller manoeuvre in selection of patients for uvulopalato-pharyngoplasty. *Laryngoscope*, **95**, 1483–1487

SHPRINTZEN, R. J., CROFT, C. B., BERKMAN, M. D. and RAKOFF, S. J. (1979) Pharyngeal hypoplasia in the Treacher Collins syndrome. *Archives of Otolaryngology*, **105**, 127–131

SMITH, T. C., PROOPS, D. W., PEARMAN, K. and HUTTON, P. (1992) Hypoxia in sleeping children: overnight studies can be reduced to 4 hours without loss of clinical significance. *Clinical Otolaryngology*, **17**, 243–245

SOUTHALL, D. P., CROFT, C. B., IBRAHIM, H., BUCHDALHL, R. and WARNER, J. (1988) Detection of sleep-associated, dysfunctional pharyngeal obstruction in infants. *European Journal of Paediatrics*, **302**, 353–359

STOOHS, R., and GUILLEMINAULT, C. (1990) Obstructive sleep apnoea syndrome or abnormal upper airways resistance during sleep. *Journal of Clinical Neurophysiology* **7**, 83–92

STOOL, S. E. and HOULIHAN, R. (1977) Otolaryngologic management of craniofacial anomalies. *Otolaryngologic Clinics of North America*, **10**, 41–44

STOOL, S. E., EAVEY, R. D., STEIN, N. L. and SHARRAR, W. G. (1977) The 'chubby puffer' syndrome. *Clinical Pediatrics*, **16**, 43–50

WEESE–MAYER, D. E., MORROW, A. S., BROUILLETTE, R. T., ILBAWI, M. N. and HUNT, C. E. (1989) Diaphragm pacing in infants and children. A life-table analysis of implanted components. *American Review of Respiratory Disease*, **139**, 974–979

21

Stertor and stridor

Michael J. Cinnamond

Definitions

Stertor and stridor are both auditory manifestations of disordered respiratory function, and as such merit investigation in every case. Not all sounds emanating from the respiratory tract, however, are stridorous or stertorous: voluntary or involuntary vocalizations, moist sounds, such as rattling or bubbling of secretions in the pharynx or larynx and rales or crepitations, arising in the distal portions of the bronchial tree or alveoli, should be excluded.

Stertor, from the Latin *stertere* meaning 'to snore', is caused by obstruction of the airway above the level of the larynx. It is a low-pitched snoring or snuffly sound produced by vibrations in the tissues of the nasopharynx, pharynx or soft palate.

Stridor is due to air-flow changes within the larynx, trachea or bronchi. Despite its derivation from the Latin, *stridere*, meaning a harsh, creaking or grating sound (Onions, 1978), stridor is not always discordant but is, in fact, more often musical or sibilant in character. The frequency of the sound produced also varies from low-pitched and sonorous to high-pitched squeaking or whistling.

Aerodynamic considerations

Stridor and stertor are due to turbulence of the airflow within a partially obstructed respiratory tract. In order to understand the mechanisms by which these sounds are produced it is necessary first to review a few of the basic physical principles pertaining to contained gases at rest and in motion. Pascal's principle states that: 'in a fluid (whether liquid or gaseous) at rest, a pressure change in one part is transmitted, without loss, to every portion of the fluid and to the walls of the container' (adapted from Encyclopaedia Britannica, 1981).

In other words, the pressure exerted by the gas is the same at every point on the containing walls. Steady gas flow, along a tube, is described by Bernoulli's equation which, in simple terms, relates velocity of the gas to the pressure which it exerts. If the tube is constricted or throttled, the gas velocity increases through the narrowed portion and, in order to preserve the law of conservation of energy, the local gas pressure falls.

Application of Bernoulli's equation to airflow through the respiratory tract, especially the flaccid, compressible airway of the child, demonstrates that an increased transmural pressure gradient will occur at sites of constriction, resulting in collapse of the airway and temporary cessation of airflow (Forgacs, 1978). Pascal's principle and the resilience of the cartilaginous support causes the airway to spring open again and the cycle is repeated.

The fluttering vibrations thus created are amplified by the resonators of the vocal tract and chest cavity, giving rise to the audible sounds which are known as stertor or stridor, depending on where they are generated. Both stertor and stridor can be described in terms of the component frequencies and tonal qualities of the noise. While stertor is always inspiratory in timing, stridor can also be categorized in relation to the phase of the respiratory cycle during which it occurs. To a certain extent some categories of stridor so defined can be assigned to specific causes of respiratory obstruction, although considerable overlap occurs and caution should be exercised in the application of such diagnostic criteria to individual patients.

The following points should be noted:

1 During inspiration, the relatively mobile, poorly supported structures of the infantile supraglottis tend to be drawn into the glottic aperture, as a result of the pressure differential between pharynx

and trachea; expiration, on the other hand, forces the prolapsing tissues out of the laryngeal inlet. The inspiratory stridor thus produced is often low-pitched and harsh in character

2 In the smaller bronchi and bronchioles, accentuation of the normal physiological contraction, which occurs during expiration, combined with high velocity gas flow, results in collapse of the airway; this type of stridor is exemplified by the expiratory wheeze of asthma but may also be caused by retained bronchial foreign bodies

3 The relatively rigid walls of the rima glottis, subglottis and trachea prevent collapse and stridor arising in these areas is presumably due to turbulence of the airflow alone. In severe obstruction, biphasic or to-and-fro stridor may result.

Associated signs and symptoms

A variety of other signs and symptoms may be found in association with stertor and stridor.

Dyspnoea

Dyspnoea, like stertor and stridor, is a manifestation of airway obstruction; severity of one tends to reflect severity of the other. Thus, loud raucous stertor or stridor, audible at a distance from the patient, generally occurs in the presence of other signs of respiratory embarrassment, such as flaring of the alae nasi, use of the accessory muscles of respiration or, in extreme cases, actual cyanosis. The high negative pleural pressures which develop during inspiration against an obstructed airway may cause indrawing of the soft tissues in the subcostal, intercostal, suprasternal and supraclavicular regions. Marked recession of the suprasternal notch gives rise to the phenomenon of 'tracheal tug' when the trachea appears to be pulled down into the chest with each inspiration.

There are, however, pitfalls for the unwary in relation to the detection of dyspnoea in the neonate and small infant. In many normal, non-airway-obstructed infants, the soft, compliant nature of the chest wall may give rise to a false impression of intercostal or sternal recession; this may become extreme with relatively minor degrees of obstruction. In contrast, cases of severe, chronic airway obstruction are seen in which signs of respiratory distress are minimal – the author has observed this in children with congenital subglottic stenosis in whom the airway was reduced to pinhole size. It is difficult to explain the exact mechanism by which this perplexing phenomenon occurs but it is presumably, in part, one of necessary adaptation. A rather similar picture, though for different reasons, occurs in acute epiglottitis: in the early stages of the disease, the child may learn that increased respiratory effort serves only to exacerbate 'corking' of the glottic aperture by the swollen supraglottic structures; at a later stage, simple exhaustion may account for the decreased respiratory effort.

The respiratory obstruction which produces stertor and stridor can lead to hypoxia, hypercapnia, pulmonary oedema, cor pulmonale, vomiting, aspiration pneumonia and occasionally death.

Cough

Cough is usually harsh and barking in nature and is particularly associated with subglottic inflammation and tracheal compression.

Hoarseness

Hoarseness, whether of speech or the cry, reflects changes in the structure and/or function of the vocal cords and suggests laryngeal inflammation, trauma, tumours or vocal cord immobility. In the stertorous child there will be no hoarseness but the cry is often muffled.

Deglutition and respiration

Deglutition and respiration share a common pathway, namely the oropharynx. It is not surprising, therefore, that disorders of swallowing may interfere with breathing and vice versa; thus stertor and stridor are often observed to increase during feeding. Conversely, and especially in the suckling infant, tachypnoea and prolongation of inspiration conspire to impede or even prevent normal swallowing activity. Infants with noisy breathing, even in the absence of overt respiratory distress, are frequently noted to be poor or slow feeders. In some cases this may lead to failure of growth, due both to lack of nutrition and to the increased expenditure of energy on respiration (Heaf *et al.*, 1982). Choking, caused by accidental inhalation of ingested liquids or solids, may further compound the difficulties.

General features

Noisy breathing in the form of stertor or stridor is always a symptom or a sign, never a diagnosis or a disease. Although it may often appear innocuous, fleeting and of little import, it is well to remember that stertor or stridor is *always* indicative of obstruction of the airway. This does not, of course, imply that every child with noisy respiration must be regarded as an emergency but, rather, that a search for the cause should always be made.

Although endoscopy will be the final arbiter in most instances of stridor, time spent on a careful history and a thorough physical examination is time well spent. This is particularly true for the inexperienced or occasional endoscopist, as the information thus obtained will often direct the attention to areas which might otherwise have been overlooked.

History

Character

Stertor and stridor are often described by the parents as 'noisy breathing'. Others, perhaps of a more perspicacious nature, will characterize the noise as wheezing, crowing, whistling, croaking, sighing, rattling or snoring. These latter terms may be useful in evoking a mental image of the sound when it is absent at the time of examination. Stridor may be continuous or intermittent; the former suggests a more serious cause than the latter.

Severity

The loudness of the stertor or stridor, as measured by the distance from the patient at which it can be heard, may provide information about its severity. The parents should also be asked specifically about features of obstructed respiration such as shortness of breath, difficult or laboured breathing, cyanosis and periods of apnoea.

Age at onset

It is a curious feature of congenital stridor that the symptom may not make an appearance for some considerable time after birth. This may reflect the increasing activity of the older infant or the stridor may not become manifest until the child suffers from his first upper respiratory tract infection. Congenital causes of stertor, on the other hand, usually present at or soon after birth. This is especially true of neonates with nasal obstruction in whom the onset will be immediate and dramatic owing to their obligatory nasal breathing.

Relationship to feeding, crying and exercise

Many patients with stertor or stridor will exhibit alteration in severity of the sound in relation to changes in position. This tends to be rather variable. Shallower, slower breathing during sleep will often result in diminution of the sound while increased respiration during crying, feeding or when the child is active, all tend to make it louder. In some children, the respiratory noise will only be noticeable during such activity.

Related diseases

Enquiry should also be made about other known congenital or acquired disorders particularly in relation to the respiratory, cardiovascular and neurological systems.

In stridorous children it is essential to ask about problems associated with previous endotracheal intubation and whether the child has undergone any prolonged periods of assisted ventilation.

Stertor of rapid onset may be associated with a history of preceding trauma or upper respiratory tract infection, indicating respectively the likelihood of faciomaxillary fractures or an inflammatory condition as the cause. Slowly progressive stertor suggests a neoplastic cause. The older child who mouth breathes during the day and snores at night may have obstructive sleep apnoea and specific enquiry should be made about sleep patterns.

Physical examination

General appearance

An alert, active, happy and well-fed infant is unlikely to have any serious pathology. In some children there may be pectus excavatum (Lane *et al.*, 1984), although the significance of this finding in relation to airway obstruction is not clear.

Marked head retraction is a feature of some types of upper respiratory obstruction; extension of the neck will often reduce the stridor in laryngomalacia (Cotton and Reilly, 1983). In babies with the Pierre Robin syndrome or other forms of macroglossia or micrognathia, the stertor is often markedly diminished by lying the patient prone with the head extended.

Signs of increased airways resistance to be looked for are flaring of the nostrils, intercostal, suprasternal or substernal recession, tachypnoea and cyanosis. In the acutely obstructed child, a rising pulse rate is the most reliable sign of increasing distress. The pattern of respiration is important. In neonates especially, the increased effort of breathing through an obstructed airway may lead to periods of apnoea, sometimes prolonged. Reflex apnoea, after coughing or during feeding, may indicate the presence of innominate artery compression of the trachea (Macdonald and Fearon, 1971).

Nose and oral cavity

Stertor is caused by congenital or acquired disorders of the nose, nasopharynx, mouth or pharynx. Examination of the nose may reveal septal deviation, haematoma or abscess, congenital cysts or swellings and choanal atresia. Inflammation of the nasal mucosa resulting from chronic infective rhinitis, allergic rhinitis or rhinitis medicamentosa should also be sought; these may be associated with hypertrophy of the inferior turbinates (Mugliston and Mitchell, 1984). Children with cystic fibrosis may develop nasal polyps or chronic maxillary sinusitis and, in the older child, stertor may be associated with an antrochoanal polyp.

Outpatient examination of the nasopharynx is difficult in the young child, but in older children it may be possible to obtain an adequate view of the postnasal space using a mirror or a Hopkins' rod nasopharyngoscope. Indirect evidence of nasopharyngeal obstruction includes nasal or postnasal discharge and the presence of diminished nasal airflow in the absence of an obvious intranasal cause. Adenoidal hypertrophy or tumours of the nasopharynx, such as angiofibroma, lymphoma, rhabdomyosarcoma and neuroblastoma, should also be sought.

Micrognathia and macroglossia are potent causes of stertor. Micrognathia or retrognathia is a feature of the Treacher Collins and Pierre Robin syndromes; the latter may be associated with cleft palate. Enlargement of the tongue is found in Down's syndrome or as part of the organomegaly of Beckwith's syndrome.

The most common pharyngeal disorders causing stertor are tonsillar hypertrophy, infectious mononucleosis or peritonsillar abscess. More rarely, hypertrophy of the lingular tonsils, a lingular thyroid or one of the rare congenital pharyngeal swellings including cystic hygroma, haemangioma, teratoma or branchial cleft cysts, may be found (Parkin and Thomas, 1974).

Nutritional status

Overweight children are more likely to develop croup or airway obstruction, perhaps due to increased effort of breathing and higher oxygen requirements. Poor nutrition, in infants with noisy respiration, may be ascribed to the slow, laboured feeding, marked by frequent, and often prolonged, pauses for breath and, perhaps also, to the higher energy expenditure consequent upon increased airways resistance. Anaemia, from deficient nutrition may further add to the child's respiratory difficulties.

Auscultation

The importance of listening to the respiratory noise cannot be overemphasized. Attention should be paid to the timing of the sound in relation to the respiratory cycle, its quality and pitch. Listening, with the child lying on his back, front and side and while sitting up, may yield valuable clues; if possible, the child should also be observed during feeding, sleeping and crying. Very quiet stertor or stridor is often audible only when listened to with a stethoscope held close to the child's nose or open mouth. When heard through a stethoscope placed over the trachea or upper chest, stridor is often 'purer' in pitch due to the filtering action of the chest cavity (Forgacs, 1978).

Tape recording

Magnetic recording of the sound can be a valuable method of detecting change in the quality of stertor or stridor over a period of time. On occasions, it may also be useful as a means of convincing worried parents that their child's condition is improving.

Palpation

In some low-pitched stridors, palpable vibrations are transmitted through the chest wall. Palpation of the neck may reveal congenital thyroid enlargement, thymic tumours or cysts extending upwards from the superior mediastinum or teratomas involving the anterior wall of the trachea.

Related organ systems

Congenital causes of stridor are frequently associated with other congenital disorders; special attention should be paid to the state of the lungs, heart and central nervous system. Bronchopneumonia often supervenes in the child with an obstructed airway and atelectasis may follow impaired coughing ability. In the acute phase of foreign body impaction in the bronchial tree there may be signs of air trapping while prolonged retention of a foreign body can lead to the development of bronchiectasis. In severe cases of chronic obstruction of the respiratory tract there may be evidence of right heart failure with pulmonary congestion.

Investigations

Physiological

Regular observations of temperature, pulse, respiratory rate and blood pressure must be charted. Normal values for neonates and older children are given in Table 21.1.

The resting respiratory rate is a sensitive index of pulmonary function. Tachypnoea and tachycardia are early and important compensatory mechanisms in children with respiratory distress. Bradycardia is a late sign that indicates terminal decompensation, and is accompanied by hypotension (although neonates often develop bradycardia as an immediate response to acute hypoxia).

The single most important laboratory test of respiratory efficiency in the critically ill child is measurement

Table 21.1 Normal physiological values for neonates and older children

	Neonate	Child
Resting respiratory rate	40/min	15/min
Resting heart rate	140/min	80/min
P_aO_2	9.3 kPa	11.97 kPa
P_aCO_2	3.99–4.66 kPa	4.66–5.99 kPa
pH	Range 7.30–7.45	

of arterial blood gas levels. The P_aO_2 indicates the level of oxygen being delivered to the tissues. Serious tissue hypoxia results when the P_aO_2 falls below 6.65 kPa (50 mmHg). The P_aCO_2 is the best indicator of alveolar ventilation, but it must be remembered that P_aCO_2 is inversely related to respiratory minute volume, and so if the alveolar minute volume doubles the P_aCO_2 is halved. The pH is a measure of respiratory and metabolic acidosis or alkalosis.

When serial measurements of arterial blood gases are needed, an indwelling arterial line is necessary. However, a transcutaneous oxygen sensor (ear lobe oximeter) can be invaluable for continuously monitoring tissue oxygenation. Similarly, continuous automatic monitoring of temperature, pulse, blood pressure and ECG can be undertaken if the child's condition is unstable, together with respiratory rate if the patient is intubated. In this situation an intravenous line is mandatory for administration of fluids and drugs.

Laboratory

Malnutrition, particularly in the neonate, is a frequent concomitant to respiratory difficulty. Blood chemistry analysis may reveal evidence of dehydration or depleted serum proteins, while haematological investigations will be of value in the detection and management of anaemia. Ampicillin-resistant strains of *Haemophilus influenzae* are being increasingly reported (Schwartz *et al.*, 1978); it is, therefore, imperative that all children with acute epiglottitis should have blood culture studies, to ensure that the correct antibiotic therapy is instituted. In the patient with an acutely obstructed airway, arterial blood gas estimation can give an accurate, dynamic analysis of the respiratory state. Incompetence of the immunological system is occasionally found in children with repeated episodes of viral croup and may be a factor in some cases of persistent laryngeal papillomatosis.

Radiology

Plain lateral soft-tissue X-rays of the head, neck and upper thorax will often reveal a surprising amount of detail of the functional anatomy of the airway, providing the films are of good quality (Dunbar, 1970). Even small degrees of rotation in either the sagittal or coronal planes, however, will obscure detail by superimposing other structures on the airway shadow; this is especially true in the infant. Owing to the laxity of the soft tissues and the flexible nature of the cartilaginous structures of the child's larynx, care must be taken in the interpretation of such X-rays (Valvassori *et al.*, 1984). Thus, during inspiration, the subglottic region may collapse, giving rise to the mistaken view that stenosis is present; a film taken during expiration will demonstrate the error. Similarly, films taken during expiration with the head

and neck flexed, especially if the child is crying, produce dramatic distortions of the pharyngeal tissues which can mimic the appearance of a retropharyngeal abscess or mass (Figure 21.1). Anteroposterior and lateral plain X-rays of the chest may show distortion of the tracheobronchial air shadow in cases of vascular anomaly or mediastinal cysts. The high-kV 'Cincinnati' posteroanterior view of the mediastinum enhances the air column in the trachea and bronchi by providing improved contrast between air and soft tissues. Lobar atelectasis and areas of consolidation, related to a foreign body or other causes of airway obstruction, may be demonstrated.

Xeroradiography gives enhanced soft tissue differentiation allowing detailed visualization of stenoses, granulomas and other lesions, but at the cost of greatly increased radiation exposure; the technique should, therefore, be used sparingly.

Hypocycloidal polytomography shows bone destruction well and is used when a neoplasm is suspected, e.g. a postnasal angiofibroma. For a vascular tumour such as this, angiography is employed in addition.

Although computerized tomographic scanning has dramatically enhanced the visualization of many parts of the body, it has proved to be something of a disappointment in the elucidation of upper airway disease in small children. There are two reasons for this: first, the avoidance of motion artefact, consequent upon the long scan times needed, is difficult to achieve in children (Valvassori *et al.*, 1984), and second, there is a lack of deep body fat in babies, an essential requirement in obtaining good differentiation between tissue layers. An important exception to this rule occurs in the case of bony abnormalities such as choanal atresia or stenosis. In general, magnetic resonance imaging has proved to be much more valuable.

Contrast studies, using barium or Gastrografin, with fluoroscopic screening, enable the surgeon to obtain valuable information about the dynamic relationships between the air and food passages; they may also demonstrate encroachment on the oesophageal lumen by aortic arch anomalies or distortion of the tracheo-oesophageal complex by mediastinal masses. Aortography with videotaping is an essential tool in the investigation of great vessel anomalies causing tracheal or bronchial compression. Where possible, the surgeon should attend contrast screening sessions in person, in order to obtain first hand knowledge of the altered anatomical and physiological relationships.

Future trends

A number of recent studies have suggested the possibility of characterization of stridor and other airway sounds using Fourier analysis (Hirschberg, 1980; Mori *et al.*, 1980) or electronic filtering (Malone *et*

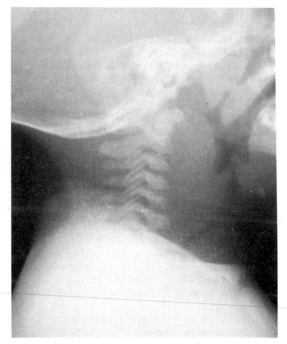

(a)

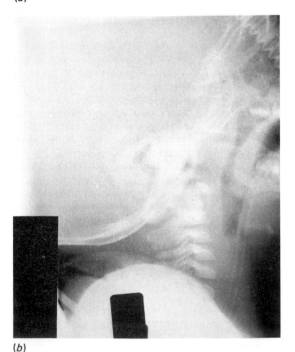

(b)

Figure 21.1 (*a*) Lateral soft-tissue X-ray of a child taken in slight flexion while crying, apparently showing a retropharyngeal mass. (*b*) X-ray of the same child taken shortly afterwards during an examination under anaesthesia. With the head extended and the child relaxed, the retropharyngeal pseudomass has disappeared. (Courtesy of C. M. Bailey and C. B. Croft)

al., 1992). The hope has been expressed that further development of the method could provide matching of specific spectral patterns with individual pathological causes for stridor, enabling diagnosis without the need for endoscopic examination (Gray *et al.*, 1985). Comparison of preoperative and postoperative spectral analyses could be useful in evaluating treatment. Should the early promise shown by such techniques be confirmed, the paediatric laryngologist might be provided with a tool equivalent to evoked response audiometry.

Endoscopy

Stertor

Endoscopic examination is often needed to confirm the diagnosis, especially in the neonate and small child. Under general anaesthesia, via an orotracheal tube, the nose, oral cavity, nasopharynx, oropharynx and hypopharynx are examined.

The nasal cavities are inspected using a headlight and the smallest Cottle's speculum. If available, examination should also be carried out with straight-ahead (0°) and angled (30° or 70°) Hopkins' rod telescopes or a small-bundle, flexible fibreoptic nasendoscope such as the 2.9 mm Olympus ENF 'P'. Inspection of the oral cavity and pharynx is facilitated by inserting a Boyle-Davis gag. Finally, examination of the postnasal space is accomplished with a mirror or a 120° retrograde telescope, passed behind the posterior edge of the soft palate.

At the end of the procedure the endotracheal tube should be removed to permit observation of the airway as the child awakens. This may reveal airway obstruction in the dynamic state (such as pharyngeal collapse) that was not apparent when the tube was in place.

Stridor

All children with stridor should be endoscoped. Where the onset has been recent or sudden this must be carried out as a matter of urgency; in well established cases, however, provided there is no respiratory distress, laryngoscopy and bronchoscopy may be delayed.

The larynx and tracheobronchial tree continue to grow throughout childhood. In order to allow for this, a minimum set of paediatric laryngoscopes, bronchoscopes, oesophagoscopes and endoscopic instruments, as outlined in Table 21.2, should be available. Refinements to the basic list of instruments might include additional sizes of bronchoscopes, a selection of Hopkins' rod telescopes, fibreoptic endoscopes or facilities for photographic or video recording.

The author has found the Stortz instruments to be the most satisfactory. Older, non-ventilating bronchoscopes such as the Negus instruments, make the task

Table 21.2 Instrumentation

Instruments	Diameter (mm)	Length (cm)
Intubating laryngoscopes		11
		9.5
		8.5
Anterior commissure laryngoscope		11
Ventilating bronchoscopes	2.5	20
	3	20
	3.5	20
	3.5	30
	4	30
	5	30
	6	30
Oesophagoscopes	3	20
	3.5	20
	4	30
	5	30
	6	30
Metal suction tubes		35
(with and without rubber tips)		25
Bronchoscopic instruments	2	35
	1.5	25
Forceps		
Alligator		
Sharp-pointed rotating		
Peanut		
Circular cup		
Retroangle cup		

not only more difficult but less safe; whenever possible these endoscopes should be replaced. A good light source and carefully maintained fibreoptic light cords are essential. For lesions affecting the larynx, and especially where biopsy or removal of tissues is contemplated, an operating microscope fitted with a 350 mm or 400 mm focal length objective lens, is essential.

Technique

Development of a good technique demands practice and patience. A well-performed endoscopy is characterized by skill, gentleness and thoroughness; it should be unhurried and safe. Particular care should be taken to avoid trauma to the subglottis, especially when there is pre-existing oedema or inflammation.

Laryngoscopy

The instrument is inserted into the right-hand corner of the mouth with the tip of the middle finger resting on the hard palate. The thumb is placed beneath the instrument and is used to protect the upper teeth by acting as a fulcrum. The tongue is displaced to the left hand side to minimize its tendency to flop over the laryngoscope, causing obstruction to the view. At the same time, the laryngoscope is pushed forwards against the base of the tongue, opening up the pharyngeal lumen and allowing the epiglottis to be visualized. Once this has been achieved, the beak of the instrument is moved to the midline and, by a combination of caudal displacement of the laryngoscope into the vallecula and anterior pressure on the base of the tongue, the epiglottis is persuaded to ride forwards away from the laryngeal inlet thus uncovering the vocal cords and rima glottis. This affords the best view of the larynx and allows thorough inspection of the supraglottic and glottic larynx, at the same time causing the least interference with vocal cord movement.

Where the larynx is difficult or impossible to visualize in this way, the tip of a standard laryngoscope can be placed posterior to the epiglottis allowing it to be held forwards more positively, or an anterior commissure laryngoscope may be used. In exceptional cases, and particularly in children with the Pierre Robin or Hunter-Hurler syndromes, it may prove to be completely impossible to gain any view of the larynx by these means. In such circumstances a tracheoscope or flexible laryngoscope, if available, can be very helpful; as an alternative, the forward view Hopkins' rod telescope may be used on its own.

Bronchoscopy

The correct size of bronchoscope to be used in any individual child is a function of that child's weight and maturity. A rough guide is given in Table 21.3. Where significant narrowing of the airway is suspected and, particularly if the subglottis is involved, a size smaller bronchoscope than that which would normally be employed, should be tried first. While intubation of the airway should be performed in as calm and unhurried a fashion as possible, access should be given back immediately to the anaesthetist if there is cause for alarm.

Intubation may be achieved either using the intubating laryngoscope or by direct insertion of the bronchoscope. Inexperienced or casual bronchoscopists are strongly advised to use the former method, especially in cases of acute obstruction; no

Table 21.3 Selection of bronchoscopes by age

Bronchoscope size External diameter (mm)	Length (cm)	Age of child
2.5 or 3	20	Preterm (< 2.5 kg)
3.5	20 or 30	0–6 months
3.5	30	6–18 months
4	30	18 months–3 years
5	30	3–12 years
6	30	> 12 years

credit is given for an apparently slick approach when the end result is a traumatized larynx or a dead child.

Before inserting the laryngoscope it is wise to ascertain that the chosen bronchoscope will pass easily through the lateral opening of the laryngoscope blade; if not, a straight bladed Magill's laryngoscope may be used instead. The bronchoscope is then inserted, through the laryngoscope, under direct visual control, until the tip lies at the level of the false cords. From this point onwards, passage of the instrument is achieved by looking through the bronchoscope itself.

The major problem that occurs at this stage is displacement of the tip of the bronchoscope posterior to the arytenoids with subsequent passage of the scope into the oesophagus; failure to identify any tracheal rings should alert the operator to the possibility that this has happened.

The bronchoscope should now be rotated through 90° so that the 'handle' points directly to the right. The tip is moved laterally until the right vocal cord can be identified and is then moved medially until the left cord appears. At this point, the tip of the scope should lie directly in line with the glottic aperture. The bronchoscope is advanced through the glottis and subglottis with a 'screwing' motion returning the 'handle' to its original straight ahead position. This manoeuvre ensures that the cords are gently separated and reduces the possibility of trauma to the vulnerable subglottic region. If the cords are in spasm, the tip of the scope may become accidentally displaced into the right laryngeal ventricle with the possibility of penetration into the neck. No advancement of the scope should be attempted unless the airway can be seen. The arytenoids are also at risk during this manoeuvre and care must be taken to avoid engaging the superior process of the arytenoid (especially the left one) with the bronchoscope, otherwise accidental dislocation at the cricoarytenoid joint may occur. The laryngoscope can now be removed.

Having achieved passage of the bronchoscope through the subglottis, it should be advanced to the carina and the anaesthetic gas supply connected to the side arm. The more experienced endoscopist will have taken the opportunity to form an impression of the state of the subglottis and trachea during this part of the procedure, but once the child's blood oxygen level has been replenished the scope should be gently and carefully withdrawn again to the subglottis to allow for a more detailed examination. Next, the bronchoscope is passed into each main bronchus in turn and the various segmental bronchial orifices identified and inspected. It should be noted that, unlike the situation in the adult, it is usually possible to obtain a direct and satisfactory view of the upper lobe bronchi in the small child by suitable positioning of the head and neck.

Particular care is required, when using rigid metal suckers, to avoid traumatizing the bronchial mucosa. Any bleeding which occurs may seriously impair the view obtained and, especially during attempted removal of a bronchial foreign body, this is likely to have profound consequences. Because of the small lumen of the paediatric bronchoscopes, only uniocular vision is possible; use of the bronchoscopic forceps is, therefore, difficult and success depends more on gentle touch and experience than on good eyesight. Practice in the use of the instruments is essential; clumsy, inexperienced snatching at an impacted peanut may turn a difficult problem into an impossible one.

Microlaryngoscopy

The small adult-sized operating laryngoscope may be used for older children, but for babies and small children a paediatric model is necessary (the Stortz or Holinger instruments are recommended). For preference, a suspension system such as Vaughan's modification of the Boston University holder should be used, rather than the more commonly available Loewy's jack. The former reduces the likelihood of damage to the upper teeth and helps also in stabilizing the head, especially in dolichocephalic patients.

The endoscope is inserted in the midline of the mouth, although when the larynx lies very anteriorly it is sometimes better to introduce the instrument from the right side. Unlike the beaked, intubating laryngoscope, the operating laryngoscope should be placed posterior to the epiglottis holding it forwards to expose the glottic aperture. The operating microscope must be fitted with either a 400 mm or 350 mm focal length objective lens; the latter is better with the paediatric scope as it brings the operator slightly closer to the patient, making the use of the long shanked instruments somewhat easier. A padded Mayo table or some similar support, placed between the surgeon and patient's head, upon which the operator may rest the forearms, makes prolonged endolaryngeal microsurgery somewhat less tiring. Placing the patient in a partial reverse Trendelenburg position will often result in a more comfortable operating stance.

Flexible endoscopy

In difficult cases, where a rigid endoscope cannot be passed or where a satisfactory view is not obtained, flexible laryngoscopes, bronchoscopes or oesophagoscopes may be invaluable. These instruments, however, are not only costly and easily damaged but are much less versatile than their rigid counterparts and are generally more difficult to use. The flexible bronchoscope, in particular, creates problems in the maintenance of a satisfactory airway in the infant.

Documentation

A simple line drawing of the larynx, trachea and bronchi, indicating the pathology, is always much more informative than a few terse sentences and should be used in every case. This is especially true where repeated endoscopic examination proves necessary, both in reminding the surgeon of the circumstances found on the previous occasion and how the situation has changed since. The shape, position and distribution of nodules, papillomas and similar lesions can be documented with considerable accuracy by this method.

Estimation of the size of the airway is often useful and is mandatory when subglottis stenosis is present. In its simplest form this may be merely a note to the effect that, for example, while a 3.0 mm bronchoscope could be inserted easily, a 3.5 mm one could not. For more accurate measurement, a graduated series of endotracheal tubes (Pracy, 1979) or gum elastic oesophageal dilators may be used.

Still photography, cine photography and video techniques are very useful for teaching purposes but are difficult to use routinely. The interested reader is advised to study the methods and equipment described by Benjamin (1981).

Classification

The causes of childhood stertor, stridor and upper airway obstruction may be classified according to aetiology, pathology, anatomical site of origin or individual characteristics of the respiratory noise, such as pitch or timing.

The subject is complex and several authors have produced extensive lists of possible causes (Kelemen, 1953; Cotton and Reilly, 1983). In practice, however, the actual number of different causes commonly met with is relatively small, as reference to Tables 21.4 and 21.5 will show. What the classification used here lacks in refinement, it makes up for in simplicity. For further details of diagnosis and management the reader is referred to the relevant chapters in this volume.

Table 21.4 Causes of stertor

Congenital	Acquired
Dysgenesis	Traumatic
agenesis	septal haematoma
hypoplasia	septal abscess
stenosis of the anterior	faciomaxillary fractures
nares	Inflammatory
choanal atresia or stenosis	common cold
median facial anomalies	chronic rhinitis
Cysts	sinusitis
dermoid	nasopharyngitis
nasoalveolar	acute and chronic
dentigerous	pharyngitis
mucous	tonsillitis
Neurological swellings	infectious mononucleosis
meningocoele	peritonsillar abscess
meningoencephalocoele	parapharyngeal abscess
glioma	retropharyngeal abscess
Facial skeletal abnormalities	Ludwig's angina
Apert's syndrome	Allergic rhinitis
Crouzon's syndrome	Neoplastic
Glossoptosis and	angiofibroma
micrognathia	neuroblastoma
Treacher Collins	lymphoma
syndrome	rhabdomyosarcoma
Pierre Robin syndrome	Other conditions
Macroglossia	rhinitis medicamentosa
Down's syndrome	hypertrophic tonsils or
Beckwith's syndrome	adenoid
cystic hygroma	nasal polyp
haemangioma	antrochoanal polyp
Pharyngeal swellings	idiopathic neonatal
lingual thyroid mass	mucosal swelling
congenital tumours	Iatrogenic

Table 21.5 Causes of stridor

Congenital	Acquired
Larynx	Trauma
supraglottis	thermal and chemical
laryngomalacia	external
web	intubation
saccular cyst	surgical
cystic hygroma	Foreign body
laryngocoele	laryngeal
glottis	tracheal
web	bronchial
cri-du-chat syndrome	oesophageal
vocal cord paralysis	Inflammatory
subglottis	acute laryngitis
web	laryngotracheobronchitis
stenosis	acute epiglottitis
haemangioma	diphtheria
Trachea and bronchi	Allergy
web	Neoplasms
stenosis	papilloma
tracheomalacia	
vascular compression	
tracheogenic cyst	
bronchogenic cyst	
Mediastinal tumours	

References

BENJAMIN, B. (1981) Documentation in paediatric laryngology. *Annals of Otology, Rhinology and Laryngology,* **90,** 478–482

COTTON, R. and REILLY, J. S. (1983) Stridor and airway obstruction. In: *Pediatric Otolaryngology*, edited by C. H. Bluestone and S. E. Stool. Philadelphia: W. B. Saunders. pp. 1190–1204

DUNBAR, J. S. (1970) Upper respiratory tract obstruction in infants and children. *American Journal of Roentgenology*, 109, 227–246

ENCYCLOPAEDIA BRITANNICA (1981) 15th edn. Pascal's principle, VII, 780. Chicago: Encyclopaedia Britannica Inc.

FORGACS, P. (1978) *Lung Sounds*. London: Baillière Tindall

GRAY, L., DENNENY, J. C., CARVAJAL, H. and JAHRSDOERFER, R. (1985) Fourier analysis of infantile stridor: preliminary data. *International Journal of Pediatric Otorhinolaryngology*, 10, 191–199

HEAF, D. P., HELMS, P. J., DINWIDDIE, R. and MATTHEW, D. J. (1982) Nasopharyngeal airways in Pierre Robin syndrome. *Journal of Paediatrics*, 100, 689–703

HIRSCHBERG, J. (1980) Acoustic analysis of pathological cries, stridors and coughing sounds in infancy. *International Journal of Pediatric Otorhinolaryngology*, 2, 287–300

KELEMEN, G. (1953) Congenital laryngeal stridor. *Archives of Otolaryngology*, 58, 245–268

LANE, R. W., WEIDER, D. J., STEINEM, C. and MARIN-PADILLA, M. (1984) Laryngomalacia. A review and case report of surgical treatment with resolution of pectus excavatum. *Archives of Otolaryngology*, 110, 546–555

MACDONALD, R. E. and FEARON, B. (1971) Innominate artery compression syndrome in children. *Annals of Otology, Rhinology and Laryngology*, 80, 535–540

MALONE, M., BLACK, N. D., LYDON, M. and CINNAMOND, M. J. (1992) Acoustic analysis of infantile stridor: a review. *Medical and Biological Engineering and Computing*, 31, 85–96

MORI, M., KINOSHITA, K., MORINARI, H., SHIRAISHI, T., KOIKE, S. and MURAO, S. (1980) Waveform and spectral analysis of crackles. *Thorax*, 35, 843–850

MUGLISTON, T. A. H. and MITCHELL, D. B. (1984) Nasal obstruction in healthy neonates. *British Medical Journal*, 289, 1659–1660

ONIONS, C. T. (ed.) (1978) *The Oxford Dictionary of English Etymology*. Oxford: Clarendon Press

PARKIN, J. L. and THOMAS, G. K. (1974) Benign masses of the pharynx. *Rocky Mountain Medical Journal*, 71, 34

PRACY, R. (1979) Congenital diseases of the larynx. In: *Scott–Brown's Diseases of the Ear, Nose and Throat*, vol. 4, 4th edn, edited by J. Ballantyne and J. Groves. London: Butterworths. pp. 309–328

SCHWARTZ, R., RODRIGUEZ, W., KHAN, W. and ROSS, S. (1978) The increasing incidence of ampicillin resistant *Haemophilus influenzae*. A cause of otitis media. *Journal of the American Medical Association*, 239, 320–323

VALVASSORI, G. E., POTTER, G. D., HANAFEE, W. N., CARTER, B. L. and BUCKINGHAM, R. A. (1984) *Radiography of the Ear, Nose and Throat*. Philadelphia: W. B. Saunders

22

Congenital disorders of the larynx, trachea and bronchi

Michael J. Cinnamond

The true incidence of congenital deformities of the upper airway is not known for certain, but van den Broek and Brinkman (1979) quoted an incidence for congenital laryngeal defects of between 1:10 000 and 1:50 000 births. Of 219 children with stridor who underwent endoscopic examination, Hollinger (1980) found 81% to have evidence of congenital abnormalities of the larynx, trachea or bronchi. Of the total, 60% had abnormalities of the larynx, 16% had tracheal abnormalities and 5% had congenital anomalies of the bronchi. Significantly, 45% of the patients had more than one congenital abnormality; it is thus mandatory that a full endoscopic examination be carried out in all children presenting with congenital stridor (Shugar and Healy, 1980).

Larynx

Supraglottis

Laryngomalacia

The term 'laryngomalacia' (malacia is derived from a Greek word, μαλακια, indicating morbid softening of a part) was introduced by Jackson and Jackson (1942), to describe a form of congenital laryngeal stridor characterized by flaccidity of the supraglottic structures.

Although the exact pathophysiological correlates of the condition are not known for certain, the following features have been noted (Sutherland and Lack, 1897; Kelemen, 1953):

1 Softness, flabbiness or lack of consistency of the laryngeal tissues
2 Thinning and hypocellularity of the laryngeal cartilages
3 Wrinkled, loose or redundant mucosa, especially over the arytenoid cartilages.

Laryngomalacia is by far the commonest cause of congenital stridor, accounting for 60–70% of all cases (Fearon and Ellis, 1971; Holinger, 1980). The male to female ratio is approximately equal (McSwiney, Cavanagh and Languth, 1977).

In the vast majority of patients, inspiratory stridor is the only symptom. Characteristically the stridor is high pitched, crowing and fluttering. It is usually first noticed within a few days of birth but, in some patients, it may not become obvious until the child begins to be more active or develops an acute upper respiratory tract infection. The stridor tends to increase in severity during the first 8 months of life, reaching a maximum between 9 and 12 months, thereafter beginning to resolve (Lane *et al.*, 1984). The stridor is often intermittent, appearing only while the child is feeding or crying and may be much more pronounced during sleep, especially if the child lies on its back. Hyperextension of the head sometimes results in significant lessening of the stridor.

The diagnosis can only be established for certain by direct observation of the appearance and movement of the laryngeal structures at endoscopy. Four significant findings are consistently noted, either separately or in combination:

1 A tall, tubular, in-rolled epiglottis, with a tendency to prolapse backwards and which is often likened to the Greek letter omega (Ω). It should be noted, however, that this is a common finding in otherwise normal neonates and, almost certainly, merely represents an exaggeration of the infantile form (Lane *et al.*, 1984)
2 Short, sometimes almost non-existent, flaccid, medially prolapsing aryepiglottic folds
3 Prominent, elongated arytenoid cartilages, often covered by loose, redundant mucosa and separated

by a deep interarytenoid cleft. On inspiration, the arytenoids will be seen to be sucked inwards, often crossing one over the other, obstructing the airway and giving rise to the typical stridor

4 The whole supraglottic larynx is deepened and narrowed with the result that the vocal cords are often quite difficult to see.

In order to observe these features properly, it is not only essential that the child is breathing spontaneously but that the respiratory efforts should be deep and vigorous. These conditions are perhaps best achieved during recovery from anaesthesia. It is likewise important to avoid splinting of the laryngeal inlet; the beak of the laryngoscope must be kept in the vallecula with as little disturbance as possible to the supraglottic structures. Insertion of the tip of the laryngoscope between the aryepiglottic folds will usually result in the cessation of the stridor.

One important feature of this condition is that the stridor will often become more noticeable during the early stages of anaesthesia, especially the phase of excitation; this might be explained perhaps by the supine position of the child under anaesthesia and the increased respiratory effort.

In most cases, laryngomalacia is otherwise asymptomatic. Occasionally, however, there may be associated feeding difficulties, sometimes severe enough to produce failure to thrive. Rarely, the child will have respiratory distress of such a degree as to require active treatment – this may take the form of tracheotomy, excision of redundant mucosa (Prescott, 1991) or division of the aryepiglottic folds (Seid *et al.*, 1985).

Although the stridor will, in most cases, have disappeared spontaneously by 18 months to 2 years, this is not invariably the case (Smith and Cooper, 1981). The author has seen children in whom both the stridor and the characteristic appearance of the larynx persisted into late childhood and adolescence.

Bifid epiglottis, an extremely rare laryngeal anomaly, has a very similar presentation and course. It is often associated with other congenital anomalies, especially abnormalities of the digits and hypothalamic–pituitary dysfunction (Prescott, 1994).

Laryngeal cyst

A laryngeal (saccular) cyst is a mucus-filled dilatation of the laryngeal saccule which may distort the aryepiglottic fold, the false cord or the laryngeal ventricle (Suhonen *et al.*, 1984). Saccular cysts may sometimes be confused with laryngocoeles. In the former, however, there is no communication with the airway and the contents are fluid rather than gaseous. Most laryngeal cysts are sited in the supraglottis but may, occasionally be found in the subglottis (Smith, Cotton and Meyer, 1990).

Generally, such cysts are asymptomatic and are only noted incidentally during endotracheal intubation. Occasionally, however, the cysts enlarge or become infected, resulting in a rather hoarse stridor and rapidly increasing airway obstruction. Endoscopic examination reveals a large bluish swelling in the region of the aryepiglottic fold (Ostfeld *et al.*, 1990), sometimes totally obscuring the vocal cords. Treatment is aimed at endolaryngeal excision of the cyst or, if this proves impossible, wide marsupialization. Very occasionally tracheotomy may be required if the respiratory distress becomes severe.

Extensive cystic hygromas (lymphangiomas) can involve the posterior part of the tongue, the vallecula and the epiglottis, resulting in airway obstruction. The most satisfactory method of dealing with this problem is wide excision of the cystic masses using the CO_2 laser, but recurrence is common and tracheotomy may prove necessary.

Congenital laryngocoele

A laryngocoele is an air-filled dilatation of the ventricular sinus of Morgagni. If the sac extends beyond the limits of the thyroid cartilage, piercing the thyrohyoid membrane, the laryngocoele is classified as being external, the internal variety remaining deep to the laryngeal cartilages. Clinically the condition is recognized by intermittent hoarseness or respiratory distress which increases on crying or straining. Rarely, the external variety may be diagnosed by palpation of a soft, fluctuant swelling in the neck presenting above the thyroid cartilage. Plain X-rays of the neck may demonstrate the air-filled sac.

Glottis

Laryngeal web

Formation of a normal laryngeal lumen depends upon complete canalization of the epithelial lamina between the vestibulotracheal canal above and the pharyngotracheal canal below, a process which begins at about the fifth week of intrauterine development. Total failure of this process will produce a complete laryngeal atresia but, more commonly, partial canalization occurs resulting in the formation of a laryngeal web. Such webs may involve the supraglottis, or subglottis, but by far the greatest number (over 75%) are sited in the glottis (McHugh and Loch, 1942).

Most glottic webs are located anteriorly, involving a variable length of the vocal cords. They may be thin and membranous or, rather more frequently, thick and fibrotic, often extending downwards to involve the subglottis. The symptoms produced depend, to a degree, upon the extent and thickness of the web but stridor, which may be biphasic in timing, hoarseness of the voice or cry and respiratory distress may all occur.

Thin webs can be divided endoscopically using scissors, knife or laser. Thick, fibrotic webs, however, are much more difficult to treat successfully. Some authors advocate the formation, as an initial stage, of an anteriorly sited, epithelial-lined tract (Lynch and LeJeune, 1960): others recommend insertion of a keel, either endoscopically or via a laryngofissure approach (van den Broek and Brinkman, 1979). In many cases, however, where the web is small and causing little in the way of symptoms, the best approach is to leave well alone.

Posterior (interarytenoid) webs are much less common and are often difficult to diagnose (Benjamin and Mair, 1991). Congenital interarytenoid webs may be associated with ankylosis of the cricoarytenoid joints or subglottic stenosis (Irving, Bailey and Evans, 1993).

Cri-du-chat syndrome

The most striking feature of this relatively uncommon condition is the characteristic high pitched 'mewing' stridor. At endoscopy, the rima glottis is observed to be diamond shaped, the vocal cords are narrow and the supraglottis is curved and elongated. Respiratory distress is uncommon and tracheotomy rarely required (Ward, Engel and Nance, 1968). Chromosomal investigation confirms the diagnosis, showing partial deletion of the short arm of the fifth chromosome in group B (Cotton and Reilly, 1983).

Vocal cord paralysis

Congenital paralysis of the vocal cord is the third most common cause of congenital stridor, accounting for between 6% and 13% of all cases (Fearon and Ellis, 1971; Holinger, 1980). It may be unilateral or bilateral, the former occurring four times more frequently than the latter (Emery and Fearon, 1984).

In unilateral paralysis the cry is often breathy or weak, stridor is uncommon and there is little tendency to airway obstruction. In contrast, bilateral paresis is associated with a normal cry and stridor and significant respiratory distress are almost invariable, though these may not appear until the child becomes more active.

The diagnosis is confirmed at laryngoscopy with direct observation of vocal cord movement but this can be difficult, particularly in the small child and undoubtedly many cases are missed. Problems may arise from incorrectly placing the tip of the laryngoscope posterior to the epiglottis causing distortion of the glottis or from too deep an anaesthetic causing inhibition of laryngeal reflexes. The best opportunity to observe vocal cord movement is during recovery from anaesthesia. Care must also be taken to distinguish between true paresis of the vocal cord and fixation of the cricoarytenoid joint – this may be achieved by gentle palpation of the arytenoid cartilage.

Many of these infants exhibit other congenital defects involving the central or peripheral nervous systems, the heart and great vessels or the respiratory tract. Thus neonates with hydrocephalus, meningo-encephalocoele, meningocoele, meningomyelocoele, or the Arnold–Chiari malformation, who present with stridor or abnormality of the cry should have their vocal cords inspected. Congenital myasthenia gravis, which is characterized in the child by drooping of the eyelids (ptosis), inability to suck or intermittent facial paralysis, may present with progressive weakness of the cry and stridor (Winter and Koopmann, 1990). Cardiomegaly or abnormalities of the great vessels may result in stretching of the left recurrent laryngeal nerve. Either recurrent laryngeal nerve may be involved in abnormalities of the tracheobronchial tree or oesophagus.

Benign congenital hypotonia, Werdnig–Hoffmann disease, leucodystrophy, Charcot–Marie–Tooth disease and other progressive congenital muscular disorders may demonstrate paralysis of the vocal cords (Dedo and Dedo, 1983).

Most cases of unilateral vocal cord paralysis can be treated expectantly. In the author's opinion there is no justification for the use of Teflon paste injection in the management of this condition in childhood. Bilateral paralysis will almost always necessitate tracheotomy to protect the airway, at least initially. Late recovery of one or both vocal cords has been noted – in one case this occurred at the age of 9 years (Emery and Fearon, 1984). Attempts at improving the airway by lateralization of the vocal cord should, therefore, be postponed. Reduction of one cord using the laser, with or without arytenoidectomy, may be an effective alternative.

Subglottis

Subglottic stenosis

It is often difficult to distinguish between the congenital and acquired varieties of this condition, indeed the two frequently coexist. Stenosis may be considered to be present if the diameter of the subglottic space is less than 3.5 mm as measured by failure to achieve the unforced passage of a bronchoscope of this size (Fearon and Cotton, 1972). The abnormality lies in the cricoid cartilage which is thickened and oval in shape. There is also a concomitant increase in the thickness of the submucosa giving rise to the characteristic crescentic narrowing of the anterior subglottic space, maximal 2–3 mm below the true vocal cords. Occasionally this submucosal thickening extends upwards to involve the cords at the anterior commissure.

Congenital subglottic stenosis demonstrates a wide variation, both in severity and in symptomatology. Airways resistance changes as the fourth power of the radius (Poiseuille's law); as a consequence even minor degrees of subglottic oedema will produce a disproportionately large increase in airways resistance. Thus, in mild cases of subglottic stenosis, there may be no stridor until the child develops an upper respiratory tract infection or the subglottis is traumatized by endotracheal intubation. In such patients the stridor is usually inspiratory in nature whereas, in the more severe case it is often biphasic. Every once in a while a child will present with such severe stenosis that the subglottic airway is reduced to pinhole dimensions. Remarkably, a few of these children, while noted to be stridorous, do not appear to get into respiratory difficulty until infancy has passed and the ambulatory phase of childhood has begun.

Demonstration of the characteristic endoscopic findings referred to above and the absence of a history of previous prolonged endotracheal intubation provide the mainstays of diagnosis. Plain X-rays of the neck and thoracic inlet are notoriously unreliable with many instances of both false-positive and false-negative findings reported. Considerable care and gentleness must be employed during bronchoscopy in these patients in order to avoid damage to the subglottic area otherwise the airway may be further compromised, precipitating the need for tracheotomy. It is the author's practice to record the diagnosis clearly on the front of the patient's chart to warn anaesthetic personnel should the child require endotracheal intubation in the future.

There is a tendency towards spontaneous improvement in congenital subglottic stenosis and in mild cases it is often sufficient to advise the parents that problems are only likely to arise during upper respiratory infections or following intubation for anaesthesia. In more severe cases tracheotomy may be required and should be performed earlier rather than later. Treatment consists of either serial dilatation or laryngotracheoplasty, though the former method is of much less value in congenital stenosis than in the acquired form of the disease. In the acquired form of subglottic stenosis it has been suggested that there may be an autoimmune response to type II collagen. This may explain the different outcomes with prolonged intubation where most infants do not acquire stenosis, but others, with comparable birthweights, gestational ages and duration of intubation go on to develop stenosis (Stolovitzky and Todd, 1990). In general congenital stenosis responds rather better to treatment than does acquired stenosis (Narcy *et al.*, 1990). For further details on management, the reader is referred to Chapter 23.

Subglottic haemangioma

Congenital haemangiomas are hamartomas of blood-vessel origin. The association between skin haemangiomas and vascular tumours affecting internal organs is well recognized (Garfinkel and Handler, 1980). The best known of these symptom complexes is the Sturge-Weber syndrome in which 'port wine stains' in the area of distribution of one trigeminal nerve are coupled with angiomas of the cerebral cortex. Other locations which may be affected include the abdomen, skeleton and eyes.

Similarly, laryngeal haemangiomas, almost always affecting the subglottis, may appear in conjunction with capillary naevi of the face or neck. Symptomatically the affected child presents with inspiratory or biphasic stridor, dyspnoea and a rather harsh cry. Haemoptysis may occur (Premachandra and Milton, 1991). On direct laryngoscopy, the distinctive appearance of the subglottis is almost diagnostic. There is a bluish, pear-shaped swelling arising from the lateral wall of the subglottic space often extending upwards to involve the undersurface of the vocal cord. In most cases the subglottis is affected on one side only, but occasionally there are bilateral tumours. Although often associated with facial lesions, subglottic haemangiomas may also be present in isolation. The tumours are soft and compressible and can be easily bypassed with the bronchoscope. In the author's experience the angiomas are always of the capillary type, do not bleed and may, therefore, be safely biopsied to provide a tissue diagnosis.

Like the facial haemangiomas, the subglottic lesions often rapidly increase in size during the first few years, thereafter spontaneously regressing. A tracheotomy is usually necessary, at least initially, though some authors have claimed that this can be avoided by using steroid therapy (Cohen and Wang, 1972; Sadan, Sade and Grunebaum, 1982); others, however, disagree (Leikensohn, Benton and Cotton, 1976). Laser excision is probably the treatment of choice in most centres (Wenig and Abramson, 1988).

Laryngotracheal cleft

The respiratory primordium is derived from the foregut at about day 20 of embryonic life by the development of the median pharyngeal groove. Subsequently, the groove deepens to form the pharyngotracheal canal, becoming separated from the oesophagus by development of a tracheo-oesophageal septum which starts caudally and grows in a cephalad direction. Failure in the formation of this septum, or arrest of its rostral advancement, will result in open communication between the laryngotracheal airway and the oesophageal lumen (van den Broek and Brinkman, 1979).

Pettersson (1955) has classified these clefts into three types:

1 Laryngotracheal cleft
2 Partial laryngotracheo-oesophageal cleft
3 Total laryngotracheo-oesophageal cleft.

The hallmark of this condition is persistent aspiration, sometimes accompanied by stridor, respiratory distress and a toneless cry. Diagnosis is difficult and is frequently missed (Garel *et al.*, 1992); in one series 42% were diagnosed at autopsy (Burroughs and Leape, 1974). Screening of the swallow using Gastrografin or dilute barium will demonstrate aspiration, although the precise site of occurrence may be difficult to determine and is, of course, found in other conditions, such as H-type tracheo-oesophageal fistula. More recently, magnetic resonance imaging has been advocated (Garel *et al.*, 1992). Any patient in whom the possibility of a cleft is considered should be examined, using the laryngeal microscope, and the interarytenoid cleft palpated using a blunt hook or similar instrument. The defect between the larynx and oesophagus may be repaired via a lateral pharyngotomy (Kauten, Konrad and Wichterman, 1984). Supraglottic interarytenoid clefts may be repaired endoscopically (Koltai, Morgan and Evans, 1991).

Laryngotracheal clefts occur in isolation, but may also be associated with other congenital abnormalities as in the 'G' or Opitz-Frias syndrome (Opitz *et al.*, 1969). This is an autosomally dominant disease with male predominance, characterized by craniofacial, aerodigestive and urogenital anomalies. The head and neck manifestations are related to midline defects, including cleft lip and palate, laryngotracheal cleft and neuromuscular dysfunction of the pharynx and oesophagus (Kimmelman and Denneny, 1982).

Anterior clefts of the larynx, due to failure of fusion of the laminae of the thyroid cartilage, creating an anterior midline defect, have also been described (Montgomery and Smith, 1976). It should be noted, however, that these are glottic rather than subglottic.

Trachea and bronchi

Abnormalities of the tracheobronchial tree account for about 26% of congenital causes of stridor (Holinger, 1980).

Agenesis

Complete or partial agenesis of the trachea is incompatible with life. Short-term survival may be possible, however, if there is a fistulous connection between the oesophagus and bronchus, but utilization of the oesophagus as a tracheal replacement has proved unsuccessful (Peison, Levitsky and Sprowls, 1970). Agenesis of one main bronchus and its associated lung is, however, survivable, although most affected infants are weak and tend to succumb to chest infections. In the majority of cases there are other severe, associated congenital abnormalities which further diminish the chances of survival of these patients beyond the neonatal period.

Anterior vertical fusion of tracheal cartilages may

be found in association with craniosynostosis or with Goldenhar's syndrome (Inglis *et al.*, 1992).

Stenosis

Congenital narrowing of the tracheal or bronchial lumen may take the form of membranous webs, segmental or whole organ stenosis. Where the obstruction is sited in the lower trachea or main bronchi, treatment is confined to attempts at gentle dilatation using bronchoscopes of increasing diameter. Rather surprisingly, such management is often successful and should certainly be tried. Stenosis of the upper trachea may be managed in the same way or recourse may be had to tracheoplasty where the lumen is increased by making a vertical incision in the anterior tracheal wall and inserting an elliptical wedge of costal cartilage. Where the stenosis affects a long segment of the trachea an attempt may be made to increase the lumen by separation of one side of the trachea from the oesophagus and reattachment more laterally.

Tracheal narrowing due to mucopolysaccharide infiltration of the tracheal connective tissue has been described in Hurler's syndrome (Adachi and Chole, 1990).

Tracheomalacia

Tracheomalacia exists in both generalized and localized forms, of which the latter is much more common. Although there are some pathological correlates between tracheomalacia and laryngomalacia and, occasionally, they may coexist, there is no proven relationship between the two. The characteristic stridor, which is high pitched and expiratory is said to resemble the expiratory wheeze of asthma (Baxter and Dunbar, 1963). In the localized form, cough is a frequently associated symptom and is harsh and barking in quality, rather like that of viral croup. At bronchoscopy, the trachea is seen to be compressed in its anteroposterior diameter due to a flattening of the anterior aspect of the cartilaginous rings (Morehead and Parsons, 1993). This abnormal appearance is accentuated by expiration and even more so by coughing, when the anterior and posterior walls may come in contact. Care must be taken, however, to distinguish between this anomaly and that produced by laxity of the trachealis muscle with forward ballooning of the posterior wall – an almost universal finding in the neonate.

As with laryngomalacia, complete spontaneous recovery is the rule. In a few cases, however, where approximation of the anterior and posterior walls is marked, severe obstruction to the airway may be present and a tracheotomy found to be necessary. In these circumstances, it is often imperative to use a longer than usual tracheotomy tube, one which will reach to just above the carina, otherwise the infalling anterior wall may block the end of the tube (Cinnamond, 1977). Suspension of the anterior tracheal wall from the inner surface of the sternum has also been recommended.

In a high proportion of cases of the generalized type, the malacic process will be found to be also affecting the main bronchi. In about 10% of cases, additional abnormalities of the trachea will be present, especially tracheo-oesophageal fistulae, which are considered in Chapter 26. In every case, a careful search should be made for the tracheal opening of an H-type tracheo-oesophageal fistula as this condition may otherwise be missed.

The localized form of the disease is almost always due to compression of the affected portion of the anterior tracheal wall from without. The most probable causes are vascular rings or abnormal vessels, congenital mediastinal or cervical tumours or bronchogenic cysts.

Long-standing tracheotomies can give rise to severe peristomal tracheomalacia which may be helped by anterior cricoid/tracheal suspension after excising and closing the tracheocutaneous fistula. The fibromuscular tissue overlying the cricoid and peristomal trachea is sutured to the musculofascia of the strap muscles adjacent to the sternum (Azizkhan, Lacey and Wood, 1993).

Severe tracheomalacia may require segmental resection and possibly reconstruction with rib cartilage graft (deLorimer *et al.*, 1990). Animal experiments have been performed using expandable stents (Mair *et al.*, 1991) and artificial grafts (Hanawa *et al.*, 1990; Shaha *et al.*, 1991).

Vascular compression

The primary cause of anomalies of the great vessels of the neck and thorax is faulty embryonic development and the only adequate way to classify them is embryologically. Desnos *et al.* (1980) have suggested a simplified but satisfactory classification based on endoscopic findings.

Vascular ring

1 Double aortic arch, in which the ascending aorta divides into two arches, one passing to the right of the trachea and the other to the left, rejoining posterior to the oesophagus to form the descending aorta. The trachea and oesophagus are thus confined within a compressing ring of vascular structures. There is considerable variation in the morphology of these rings, the arches may be of equal or unequal size and different configurations of the main branches may occur.
2 Neuhauser's anomaly, where the aorta is single

but passes to the *right* of the trachea. In this case the ring is only partly vascular, the component to the left of the trachea being formed by the ligamentum arteriosum, the remnant of the ductus arteriosus which, in the fetus, connects the pulmonary artery to the descending aorta.

Vascular sling

Here, the left pulmonary artery, instead of passing anterior to the trachea, passes between it and the oesophagus compressing the trachea from behind and the oesophagus from in front. Tracheal stenosis or tracheobronchial branching abnormalities are sometimes found in association with this condition (Sailer *et al.*, 1992).

Anterior compression

1 Compression of the anterior tracheal wall by an anomalous innominate artery, the origin of which from the aortic arch is more posteriorly sited and more to the left than normal. This produces a characteristic sloping compression of the lower trachea 1–2 cm above the carina, more marked on the right anterolateral aspect. Further confirmation is afforded by noting diminution or absence of the patient's right radial or right carotid pulses, using the tip of the bronchoscope to collapse the vessel against the sternum. On rare occasions, the anomalous innominate artery may be associated with an aberrant right subclavian artery, which passes posterior to the oesophagus (Macdonald and Fearon, 1971).
2 A larger than normal pulmonary artery may compress the trachea and bronchi at or just below the carina.
3 Anterior compression of the left main bronchus may occur as a result of left atrial enlargement (Dailey, O'Loughlin and Smith, 1990).

Posterior compression

This is usually due to an aberrant right or, more rarely, left subclavian artery passing posterior to the oesophagus. The oesophagus alone is compressed in this case.

In those instances where both trachea and oesophagus are involved the patient may present with symptoms which can be referred to either. In practice, however, the tracheal symptoms of stridor, dyspnoea and a harsh, brassy cough tend to dominate the picture. Similar symptoms are found where the trachea alone is affected. In about one-third of those children in whom there is significant airway obstruction due to innominate artery compression, stimulation of the area of compression with the tip of the bronchoscope may initiate reflex apnoea (Moes, Izukawa and Trusler, 1975). It has been suggested that activation of this reflex may explain some cases of sudden infant death syndrome.

Barium swallow may show indentation of the oesophagus – this will be bilateral when the abnormality is a double aortic arch or Neuhauser's anomaly, anteriorly in vascular sling or posteriorly with an aberrant subclavian artery. High-resolution ultrasound scanning is often helpful and computerized tomography or magnetic resonance imaging may give additional information (Myer *et al.*, 1990), but the conclusive investigation, in all cases, is aortography.

In those patients in whom the symptoms are severe and, especially, when the tracheal airway is judged to be inadequate as demonstrated by an inability to see the carina from a position proximal to the compression, surgical decompression should be undertaken. In almost all cases of vascular ring surgery will be necessary, the definitive management being division of the lesser component of the ring. Where the compression is due to an anomalous innominate artery, the vessel may be slung anteriorly away from the trachea by suturing the adventitia to the undersurface of the sternum (Gross and Neuhauser, 1948; Mustard *et al.*, 1969). This, however, is seldom necessary and indeed, in the neonate, some degree of innominate artery compression of the trachea is so common as to be the rule rather than the exception.

In all types of vascular compression, tracheotomy should be avoided as bypassing the obstruction may result in intubation of the right main bronchus and, in addition, there is significant, and usually fatal, risk of erosion of the vessel by the tip of the tracheotomy tube. In all cases where surgical correction of the deformity has been undertaken, it should be borne in mind that the localized area of tracheomalacia, which invariably accompanies compression, may remain for many months or even years postoperatively (Van Son *et al.*, 1993).

Anomalous bronchial bifurcations

A right upper lobe bronchus originating from the right lateral wall of the trachea above the carina is relatively common. In almost every case this is an incidental finding and is entirely asymptomatic. Bronchography may be required to delineate the exact morphology. Other minor variations in the bronchial tree also occur and are, likewise, symptom free.

Congenital cysts and tumours

These cause non-pulsatile compression of the trachea and main bronchi but their presentation and appearance on endoscopy are otherwise similar to vascular compression.

Tracheogenic and bronchogenic cysts are thought to originate from evaginations of the primitive tracheal bud. They are lined with respiratory epithelium and may contain thick, inspissated mucus. In contrast to bronchogenic cysts, those arising from the trachea do not usually communicate with the lumen. Infection may occur with resulting increased compression of surrounding structures. Thoracotomy and excision of the cyst will often be required.

Cervical and mediastinal cysts or tumours, including thymomas, teratomas and branchial arch anomalies may compress the trachea or bronchi from without (Mills and Hussain, 1984; Morrish and Manning, 1991). Teratomas affecting the anterior neck present particular difficulties as the tumour may intimately involve the anterior wall of the trachea. Complete excision of the mass is likely to entail removal of part of the tracheal wall with the possibility of long-term airway stenosis.

References

ADACHI, K. and CHOLE, R. A. (1990) Management of tracheal lesions in Hurler syndrome. *Archives of Otolaryngology – Head and Neck Surgery*, **116**, 1205–1207

AZIZKHAN, R. G., LACEY, S. R. and WOOD, R. E. (1993) Anterior cricoid suspension and tracheal stomal closure for children with cricoid collapse and peristomal tracheomalacia following tracheostomy. *Journal of Paediatric Surgery*, **28**, 169–171

BAXTER, J. D. and DUNBAR, J. S. (1963) Tracheomalacia. *Annals of Otology, Rhinology and Laryngology*, **72**, 1013–1023

BENJAMIN, B. and MAIR, E. A. (1991) Congenital interarytenoid web. *Archives of Otolaryngology – Head and Neck Surgery*, **117**, 1118–1122

BURROUGHS, N. and LEAPE, L. L. (1974) Laryngotracheoesophageal cleft: report of a case successfully treated and review of the literature. *Pediatrics*, **53**, 516–522

CINNAMOND, M. J. (1977) Tracheomalacia – or is it? *Proceedings of the Irish Otolaryngological Society*, **18**, 33–35

COHEN, S. R. and WANG, C. (1972) Steroid treatment of hemangiomas of the head and neck in children. *Annals of Otology, Rhinology and Laryngology*, **81**, 584–590

COTTON, R. and REILLY, J. S. (1983) Stridor and airway obstruction. In: *Pediatric Otolaryngology*, edited by C. H. Bluestone and S. E. Stool. Philadelphia: W. B. Saunders. pp. 1190–1204

DAILEY, M. E., O'LOUGHLIN, M. P. and SMITH, R. J. H. (1990) Airway compression secondary to left atrial enlargement and increased pulmonary artery pressure. *International Journal of Pediatric Otorhinolaryngology*, **19**, 33–44

DEDO, D. D. and DEDO, H. H. (1983) Neurogenic diseases of the larynx. In: *Pediatric Otolaryngology*, edited by C. H. Bluestone and S. E. Stool. Philadelphia: W. B. Saunders. pp. 1278–1284

DELORIMER, A. A., HARRISON, M. R., HARDY, K., HOWELL, L. J. and ADZICK, N. S. (1990) Tracheobronchial obstructions in infants and children. Experience with 45 cases. *Annals of Surgery*, **212**, 277–289

DESNOS, J., ANDRIEU-GUITRANCOURT, J., DEHESDIN, D. and DUBIN, J. (1980) Vascular strictures of the respiratory tract in children. *International Journal of Pediatric Otorhinolaryngology*, **2**, 269–285

EMERY, P. J. and FEARON, B. (1984) Vocal cord palsy in pediatric practice: a review of 71 cases. *International Journal of Pediatric Otorhinolaryngology*, **8**, 147–154

FEARON, B. and COTTON, R. B. (1972) Subglottic stenosis in infants and children. The clinical problem and experimental surgical correction. *Canadian Journal of Otolaryngology*, **1**, 281–289

FEARON, B. and ELLIS, D. (1971) The management of long term airway problems in infants and children. *Annals of Otology, Rhinology and Laryngology*, **80**, 669–677

GAREL, C., HASSAN, M., HERTZ-PANNIER, L., FRANÇOIS, M., CONTENCIN, P. and NARCY, P. (1992) Contribution of MR in the diagnosis of 'occult' posterior laryngeal cleft. *International Journal of Pediatric Otorhinolaryngology*, **24**, 177–181

GARFINKEL, T. J. and HANDLER, S. D. (1980) Hemangioma of the head and neck. *Journal of Otolaryngology*, **9**, 435–450

GROSS, R. E. and NEUHAUSER, E. D. B. (1948) Compression of the trachea by an anomalous innominate artery. An operation for its relief. *American Journal of Diseases of Childhood*, **75**, 570–574

HANAWA, T., IKEDA, S., FUNATASU, T., MATSUBARA, Y., HATAKENAKA, R., MITSUOKA, A. *et al.* (1990) Development of a new surgical procedure for repairing tracheobronchomalacia. *Journal of Thoracic and Cardiovascular Surgery*, **100**, 587–594

HOLINGER, L. D. (1980) Etiology of stridor in the neonate, infant and child. *Annals of Otology, Rhinology and Laryngology*, **89**, 397–400

INGLIS, A. F., KOKESH, J., SIEBERT, J. and RICHARDSON, M. A. (1992) Vertically fused tracheal cartilage. *Archives of Otolaryngology – Head and Neck Surgery*, **118**, 436–438

IRVING, R. M., BAILEY, C. M. and EVANS, J. N. G. (1993) Posterior glottic stenosis in children. *International Journal of Pediatric Otorhinolaryngology*, **28**, 11–23

JACKSON, C. and JACKSON, C. (1942) *Diseases and Injuries of the Larynx*. New York: McMillan Publishing Co. Inc. pp. 63–68

KAUTEN, J. R., KONRAD, H. R. and WICHTERMAN, K. A. (1984) Laryngotracheoesophageal cleft in a newborn. *International Journal of Pediatric Otorhinolaryngology*, **8**, 61–71

KELEMEN, G. (1953) Congenital laryngeal stridor. *Archives of Otolaryngology*, **58**, 245–268

KIMMELMAN, C. P. and DENNENY, J. C. III (1982) Opitz (G) syndrome. *International Journal of Pediatric Otorhinolaryngology*, **4**, 343–347

KOLTAI, P. J., MORGAN, D. and EVANS, J. N. G. (1991) Endoscopic repair of supraglottic laryngeal clefts. *Archives of Otolaryngology – Head and Neck Surgery*, **117**, 273–278

LANE, R. W., WEIDER, D. J., STEINEM, C. and MARIN-PADILLA, M. (1984) Laryngomalacia. A review and case report of surgical treatment with resolution of pectus excavatum. *Archives of Otolaryngology*, **110**, 546–555

LEIKENSOHN, J. R., BENTON, C. and COTTON, R. (1976) Subglottic hemangioma. *Journal of Otolaryngology*, **5**, 487–492

LYNCH, M. G. and LEJEUNE, F. E. (1960) Laryngeal stenosis. *Laryngoscope*, **70**, 315–317

MACDONALD, R. E. and FEARON, B. (1971) Innominate artery compression syndrome in children. *Annals of Otology, Rhinology and Laryngology*, **80**, 535–540

MCHUGH, H. E. and LOCH, W. E. (1942) Congenital web of the larynx. *Laryngoscope*, **52**, 43–65

MCSWINEY, P. F., CAVANAGH, N. P. C. and LANGUTH, P. (1977)

Outcome in congenital stridor. *Archives of Disease in Childhood*, **52**, 215–218

MAIR, E. A., PARSONS, D. S., LALLY, K. P. and VAN DELLEN, A. F. (1991) Comparison of expandable endotracheal stents in the treatment of surgically induced piglet tracheomalacia. *Laryngoscope*, **101**, 1002–1008

MILLS, R. P. and HUSSAIN, S. S. M. (1984) Teratomas of the head and neck in infancy and childhood. *International Journal of Pediatric Otorhinolaryngology*, **8**, 177–180

MOES, C. A. F., IZUKAWA, T. and TRUSLER, G. A. (1975) Innominate artery compression of the trachea. *Archives of Otolaryngology*, **101**, 733–738

MONTGOMERY, W. W. and SMITH, S. A. (1976) Congenital laryngeal defect in the adult. *Annals of Otology, Rhinology and Laryngology*, **85**, 491–497

MOREHEAD, J. M. and PARSONS, D. S. (1993) Tracheobronchomalacia in Hunter's syndrome. *International Journal of Pediatric Otorhinolaryngology*, **26**, 255–261

MORRISH, T. N. and MANNING, S. C. (1991) Branchial anomaly in a newborn presenting as stridor. *International Journal of Pediatric Otorhinolaryngology*, **21**, 259–262

MUSTARD, W. T., BAYLISS, C. E., FEARON, B., PELTON, D. and TRUSLER, G. A. (1969) Tracheal compression by the innominate artery in children. *Annals of Thoracic Surgery*, **8**, 312–319

MYER, C. M. III, AURINGER, S. T., WIATRAK, B. J. and BISSET, G. (1990) Magnetic resonance imaging in the diagnosis of innominate artery compression of the trachea. *Archives of Otolaryngology – Head and Neck Surgery*, **116**, 314–316

NARCY, P., CONTENCIN, P., FLIGNY, I. and FRANÇOIS, M. (1990) Surgical treatment for laryngotracheal stenosis in the pediatric patient. *Archives of Otolaryngology – Head and Neck Surgery*, **116**, 1047–1050

OPITZ, J. M., FRIAS, J. L., GUTENBERGER, J. E. and PELLETT, J. R. (1969) The G syndrome of multiple congenital anomalies. In: *Malformation Syndromes, Birth Defects: Original Article Series*, edited by D. Bergsma. White Plains: The National Foundation – March of Dimes. pp. 95–101

OSTFELD, E., HAZAN, Z., RABINSON, S. and AUSLANDER, L. (1990) Surgical management of congenital supraglottic lateral saccular cyst. *International Journal of Pediatric Otorhinolaryngology*, **19**, 289–294

PEISON, B., LEVITSKY, E. and SPROWLS, J. J. (1970) Tracheoesophageal fistula associated with tracheal atresia and malformation of the larynx. *Journal of Pediatric Surgery*, **5**, 464–467

PETTERSSON, G. (1955) Inhibited separation of the larynx and upper part of the trachea from the esophagus in the newborn: report of a case successfully operated on. *Acta Chirurgica Scandinavica*, **110**, 250–254

PREMACHANDRA, D. J. and MILTON, C. M. (1991) Childhood haemangiomas of the head and neck. *Clinical Otolaryngology*, **16**, 117–123

PRESCOTT, C. A. J. (1991) The current status of corrective surgery for laryngomalacia. *American Journal of Otolaryngology*, **12**, 230–235

PRESCOTT, C. A. J. (1994) Bifid epiglottis: a case report. *International Journal of Pediatric Otorhinolaryngology*, **30**, 167–170

SADAN, N., SADÉ, J. and GRUNEBAUM, M. (1982) The treatment of subglottic hemangiomas of infants with prednisone. *International Journal of Pediatric Otorhinolaryngology*, **4**, 7–14

SAILER, R., ZIMMERMANN, T., BÖWING, B., SCHARF, J., ZEILINGER, G. and STEHR, K. (1992) Pulmonary artery sling associated with tracheobronchial malformations. *Archives of Otolaryngology – Head and Neck Surgery*, **118**, 864–867

SEID, A. B., PARK, S. M., KEARNS, M. J. and GUGENHEIM, S. (1985) Laser division of the aryepiglottic folds for severe laryngomalacia. *International Journal of Pediatric Otorhinolaryngology*, **10**, 153–158

SHAHA, A. R., BURNETT, C., DIMAIO, T. and JAFFE, B. M. (1991) An experimental model for the surgical correction of tracheomalacia. *American Journal of Surgery*, **162**, 417–420

SHUGAR, M. A. and HEALY, G. B. (1980) Coexistent lesions of the pediatric airway. *International Journal of Pediatric Otorhinolaryngology*, **2**, 323–327

SMITH, J. D., COTTON, R. and MEYER, C. M. III (1990) Subglottic cysts in the premature infant. *Archives of Otolaryngology – Head and Neck Surgery*, **116**, 479–485

SMITH, G. J. and COOPER, D. M. (1981) Laryngomalacia and inspiratory obstruction in late childhood. *Archives of Disease in Childhood*, **56**, 345–349

STOLOVITZKY, J. P. and TODD, N. W. (1990) Autoimmune hypothesis of acquired subglottic stenosis in premature infants. *Laryngoscope*, **100**, 227–230

SUHONEN, H., KERO, P. O., PUHAKKA, H. and VILKKI, P. (1984) Saccular cyst of the larynx in infants. *International Journal of Pediatric Otorhinolaryngology*, **8**, 73–78

SUTHERLAND, G. A. and LACK, H. L. (1897) Congenital laryngeal obstruction. *Lancet*, ii, 653–655

VAN DEN BROEK, P. and BRINKMAN, W. F. B. (1979) Congenital laryngeal defects. *International Journal of Pediatric Otorhinolaryngology*, **1**, 71–78

VAN SON, J. A., JULSRUD, P. R., HAGLER, D. J., SIM, E. K., PAIROLERO, P. C., PUGA, F. J. *et al.* (1993) Surgical treatment of vascular rings: the Mayo clinic experience. *Mayo Clinic Proceedings*, **68**, 1056–1063

WARD, P. H., ENGEL, E. and NANCE, W. E. (1968) The larynx in the cri-du-chat syndrome. *Laryngoscope*, **78**, 1716–1733

WENIG, B. L. and ABRAMSON, A. L. (1988) Congenital subglottic haemangiomas: a treatment update. *Laryngoscope*, **98**, 190–192

WINTER, P. H. and KOOPMANN, C. F. JR (1990) Juvenile myasthenia gravis: an unusual presentation. *International Journal of Pediatric Otorhinolaryngology*, **19**, 273–276

23

Stenosis of the larynx

J. N. G. Evans

Stenosis of the larynx is more frequent than tracheal stenosis; in a review of 752 cases of stridor seen at The Hospital for Sick Children, Great Ormond Street, London, laryngeal pathology accounted for 88% of the cases (Evans, 1986). The major cause of airway obstruction was as a result of congenital anomalies of the larynx and trachea. Holinger (1980), in his review of 219 patients with stridor, noted that it was caused by a congenital anomaly of the larynx or trachea in 87.2% of the patients. Congenital laryngeal anomalies are discussed in Chapter 22.

The incidence of acquired subglottic stenosis is increasing, resulting from the increased survival rate of preterm infants ventilated for bronchopulmonary dysplasia and hyaline membrane disease. The precise incidence of subglottic stenosis following intubation is difficult to establish. It is certainly less than the high figure of up to 20% reported in the late 1960s and early 1970s, the true incidence probably lying between 1 and 8% (Parkin, Stevens and Jung, 1976; Strong and Passy, 1977; Papsidero and Pashley, 1980; Ratner and Whitfield, 1983). This figure almost certainly underestimates the true incidence since, sadly, many low-birthweight infants do not survive, and minor degrees of subglottic stenosis may go undetected. Some are recognized only later as a result of persistent stridor following an upper respiratory tract infection, or as an incidental finding on intubation for general anaesthesia.

Aetiology and pathology

Many factors are involved in the creation of subglottic stenosis due to intubation; these include the material from which the tube is made, the shape and size of the tube (Marshak and Grundfast, 1981; Gould and Howard, 1985), its method of fixation and, above all, the skill and care which the intubated patient re-

ceives. Increased awareness of all these factors is extremely important if the incidence of subglottic stenosis is to be reduced further (Nicklaus et al., 1990).

There are two varieties of acquired laryngeal stenosis related to intubation: *soft* and *hard* stenosis. In soft stenosis, acute inflammatory oedema of the mucosa and submucosal connective tissue occurs (Rasche and Kuhns, 1972; Hawkins, 1978; Quiney and Gould, 1985). Mucosal ulceration (see Plate 6/23/Ia) will then supervene, because of mucosal abrasion resulting from poor fixation of the endotracheal tube, or because of pressure if the endotracheal tube is too large. The process of ulceration will be accelerated by infection; good aseptic technique and strict hygiene will, therefore, minimize the infective complications of intubation. Chemical irritation from rubber or plasticizers used to soften plastic tubes may further aggravate the process of mucosal ulceration, as will any residue of chemicals used in the sterilization of the tubes, e.g. ethylene oxide (Guess and Stetson, 1970). The process of ulceration eventually exposes the perichondrium of the cricoid cartilage causing perichondritis and chondritis. This is usually associated with the production of granulation tissue and fibrosis (see Plate 6/23/Ib). The stenosis associated with infection of the cricoid cartilage is of the hard variety. Hard stenosis may be further subdivided into two categories: fibrous and cartilaginous (Holinger, 1982). The fibrous stenoses can be dilated but tend to re-stenose (see Plate 6/23/Ic), whereas the cartilaginous stenoses cannot be dilated.

Subglottic stenoses may also occur as a result of acute infection of the larynx (see Chapter 24) and of blunt trauma to the neck in hanging injuries. The incidence of direct laryngeal trauma as a result of road traffic accidents has declined as a consequence of legislation prohibiting the transport of children under the age of 5 years in the front passenger seat of cars, and the compulsory wearing of seat belts by older children. Iatrogenic stenosis of the larynx may also occur as a result of prolonged treatment of juvenile laryngeal papillomas and the injudicious use of the CO_2 laser. Whatever the aetiological factor, the end result is a scarred contracted laryngeal opening. Although the number of cases of acquired subglottic stenosis is increasing due to increased survival rates of preterm infants of low birthweight, the actual incidence of subglottic stenosis is falling due to the improved care of preterm babies who are intubated endotracheally. The histological nature of the cricoid cartilage of preterm babies has been noted by Hawkins (1978) to be hypercellular with a scant gel-like matrix, and it may be that it is more distensible; this would account for the fact that these tiny babies may tolerate endotracheal intubation for several weeks without gross damage to the subglottic larynx.

There is certainly no point in laying down arbitrary time scales for endotracheal intubation before a tracheostomy becomes necessary. In general, it is essential to use an endotracheal tube that is as small as possible and which allows a leak of air during positive pressure ventilation. If the air leak disappears and a smaller endotracheal tube cannot be used, then a cricoid split procedure as advocated by Cotton and Seid (1980) and Frankel *et al.* (1984) may allow a further period of between 10 and 14 days' intubation before tracheostomy is necessary due to developing perichondritis or chondritis of the cricoid. A single laryngotracheal reconstruction using a cartilage graft at this early age, in order to try to avoid a tracheostomy with all its potential problems, has been advocated by Cotton, Myer and O'Connor (1992), Lusk, Gray and Muntz (1991) and Albert (personal communication). It has been suggested by Quiney *et al.* (1986) that, even if chondritis of the cricoid is present, epithelialization of the laryngeal mucosa may occur around the endotracheal tube – an argument for prolonged undisturbed intubation!

The investigation of the patient with acquired laryngeal stenosis is similar to that required for congenital laryngeal anomalies and is dealt with in Chapter 22.

Treatment of laryngeal stenosis

The treatment of laryngeal stenosis is one of the most controversial topics in paediatric otolaryngology. Therapeutic procedures range from repeated dilatation, prolonged laryngeal stenting with or without the use of steroids, the use of the CO_2 laser to create an airway with or without tracheostomy, to early tracheostomy and open surgical operation on the child's larynx.

Congenital subglottic stenosis

Congenital subglottic stenosis is on the whole less severe than acquired stenosis and, in some cases,

mild congenital subglottic stenosis can be treated without performing a tracheostomy (see Plate 6/23/Id). Holinger (1982) reported a series of 24 infants with severe subglottic stenosis, six of whom were treated with the CO_2 laser, so avoiding tracheostomy.

Almost half of the patients with congenital subglottic stenosis will require a tracheostomy (Cotton and Myer, 1984). Most of these patients will be decannulated within 2–5 years without requiring any operative procedure on the larynx. The process of natural resolution makes the effect of treatment difficult to assess. This difficulty is compounded by the fact that there are two basic types of congenital subglottic stenosis, the first being the result of soft tissue abnormality, the second of abnormalities of the cricoid cartilage (see Plate 6/23/Ie).

Soft tissue abnormalities

Submucosal fibrosis, hyperplasia of the submucous glandular tissue and frank granulation tissue usually occur as a result of intubation (Holinger, 1982; Quiney *et al.*, 1986). The hyperplasia of the submucous glandular tissue may be so exuberant as to present as submucous retention cysts (Mitchell *et al.*, 1987) (see Plate 6/23/If) and these cysts respond well to deroofing with the CO_2 laser, cup forceps or diathermy.

Abnormalities of the cricoid

In the review by Morimitsu *et al.* (1981) of congenital cricoid stenosis, 12 cases had a large anterior lamina with a very small posteriorly sited airway having an average diameter of 1.9 mm. In one case, there was a thickened posterior lamina (see Plate 6/23/Ig), and in another, the cricoid cartilage itself was oval. Tucker *et al.* (1979) also described a trapped first tracheal ring as an abnormality associated with subglottic stenosis. Thickening of the cricoid with a small posterior lumen is certainly the author's experience. The clinical importance of identifying thickening of the cricoid is fundamental, since these cases do not respond to dilatation, and treatment with the CO_2 laser is also likely to be unsuccessful. After a period of observation of approximately 1 year, in the case of neonates, or until the child's weight exceeds 10 kg, an open procedure on the larynx should be considered.

An open procedure on the larynx is also necessary in acquired stenosis were there is a hard cicatrix which has formed as a result of cricoid perichondritis.

Dilatation

The soft tissue stenoses may respond to simple dilatation, whereas dilatation is contraindicated, and may indeed be harmful, in patients with abnormalities of the cricoid cartilage.

Steroids

The use of steroids as an adjunct to dilatation and simple excision of scar tissue either by CO_2 laser or cup forceps might be accepted, on theoretical grounds, to aid decannulation. Baker and Whitaker (1950) demonstrated that the administration of corticosteroids during wound healing stopped fibroplasia and the growth of granulation tissue. Successful decannulation after the intralesional injection of steroids was reported by Waggoner, Belenky and Clark (1973). Peerless, Pillsbury and Peerless (1981) showed that the inhalation of beclomethasone dipropionate was an excellent adjunct therapy for the treatment of laryngeal stenosis. Birck (1970) reported seven patients with subglottic stenosis who were successfully decannulated within 2 months of treatment which involved dilatation and systemic administration of steroids. In spite of occasional reports of successful treatment with steroids, most practitioners have not found them to be helpful in the management of subglottic stenosis because the delayed healing process increases the patient's susceptibility to infection and thereby delays epithelial healing. It is the practice of the author to use systemic steroids in a dose of 0.5 mg/kg to reduce oedema after bronchoscopy in a difficult case, e.g. after the removal of a foreign body from the trachea of a young child.

Endoscopic resection

Various endoscopic methods of resection have been employed and include infant urethral resectoscopes (Downing and Johnson, 1979) and cryogenic probes (Rodgers and Talbert, 1978). It is probably true to say that the majority of paediatric otolaryngologists who specialize in the management of laryngeal stenosis would favour the use of the CO_2 laser for endoscopic resection (Strong *et al.*, 1979, Friedman, Healy and McGill, 1983; Carruth *et al.*, 1986). The successful endoscopic management of laryngeal stenosis depends upon careful patient selection. Simpson *et al.* (1982) reviewed 60 cases of laryngeal stenosis, 31 of whom had subglottic stenosis, and they were able to identify factors which indicated where endoscopic treatment was likely to be unsuccessful. These included cases of combined laryngeal and tracheal stenosis, particularly if the stenotic areas were wide or circumferential or if they were accompanied by significant loss of cricoid or tracheal cartilage.

If abundant scar tissue was present involving at least 1 cm of larynx or trachea vertically, the scar tissue was circumferential or the posterior commissure was involved and the arytenoids were fixed, then an unsuccessful outcome was likely.

If bacterial infection of the trachea associated with perichondritis occurred prior to treatment, an unsuccessful outcome was noted in 87.5% of the cases.

If these adverse factors are noted then an open operation upon the larynx is advised and, if there has been evidence of perichondritis with significant cartilage loss, it is essential to wait for at least 6 months to 1 year before attempting an open operation. This interval allows the active inflammatory process to resolve and increases the chance of a successful outcome of a procedure which may involve free grafts of cartilage where infection is likely to prejudice the success of the operation.

Open operations

Many surgical procedures for the correction of subglottic stenosis have been described; in the main they involve the use of autogenous grafts, hyoid bone (Abedi and Frable, 1983), sternohyoid myo-osseous flaps (Close, Lozano and Schaeffer, 1983) and nasal septal cartilage (Toohill, Martinelli and Janowak, 1976). The techniques of laryngotracheoplasty (Evans and Todd, 1974) and laryngotracheal reconstruction using free costal cartilage grafts (Cotton, 1978) are the most popular and will be discussed in some detail (Cotton and Evans, 1981; Ochi, Evans and Bailey, 1992a, b).

Laryngotracheoplasty

This technique is used in congenital subglottic stenosis where the cricoid cartilage is abnormally thick; it may also be used in cases of laryngeal webs where there is often an associated anomaly of the cricoid cartilage. In this procedure, a midline incision is made through the thyroid cartilage and cricothyroid membrane, a castellated incision (Figure 23.1) then

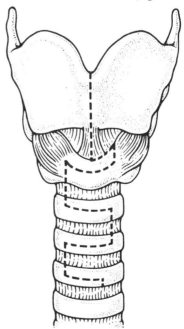

Figure 23.1 Castellated incision

being fashioned through the cricoid cartilage and involved tracheal rings. The larynx is opened from above and the vocal cords separated at the anterior commissure under direct vision. Once the larynx is opened, a submucosal dissection and removal of the scar tissue is made using scissors designed for microscopic surgery. As much laryngeal mucosa as possible is saved to line the stenotic segment. If the cricoid is abnormally thick, cartilage may be pared or cored from its internal surface to increase the lumen (Figure 23.2). An internal stent consisting of a 'swiss-roll' of Silastic sheeting (Figure 23.3) is inserted and the cartilaginous laryngeal and tracheal pegs are sutured in their displaced position. The Silastic roll is secured by a transfixion suture (Figure 23.4) which is brought out over the strap muscles and buried subcutaneously. The Silastic roll is removed endoscopically 6 weeks later.

Laryngotracheal reconstruction

This procedure is indicated where there has been loss of cartilage due to perichondritis and chondritis in acquired stenosis. If the stenosis is confined to the anterior part of the larynx and upper trachea, then it is only necessary to insert the cartilage graft anteriorly (Figure 23.5). A standard laryngofissure incision is made and a free graft of costal cartilage is inserted. The cartilage graft is taken from the costal margin and trimmed until it exactly fits the defect, the perichondrial surface is placed internally and the graft is sutured in position using 5/0 polypropylene sutures.

If the scarring involves the posterior part of the glottis with interarytenoid fixation (see Plate 6/23/Ih), the posterior lamina of the cricoid is divided and a smaller graft of costal cartilage inserted, as described by Rethi (1956) (Figure 23.6). If combined anterior and posterior stenoses are present or if the stenosis is complete, combined anterior and posterior grafts may be used (Cotton, 1991).

Stenting

The author prefers to stent the larynx and upper trachea in most cases, the best material probably being a Silastic swiss roll because it has the advantage of being self-adjusting. Rigid stents, such as the Montgomery Silastic laryngeal stent, the Montgomery T tube or the Aboulker Teflon stent (Aboulker *et al.*, 1966), do not have this advantage and, if the selected stent is too big, it may cause further damage to the laryngeal and tracheal mucosa. The Silastic stent is usually retained for 6 weeks, but in severe cases it may be retained for 6 months and in one of the author's cases the stent was retained for 2 years before successful decannulation (Evans, Batch and Leitch, 1986).

The management of laryngeal stenosis in infants and young children should be conservative, since in the majority of cases the stenosis will improve with laryngeal growth. The utmost gentleness must be employed in the inspection and endoscopic treatment of the infant larynx. Open surgical procedures are only to be recommended when it has been established

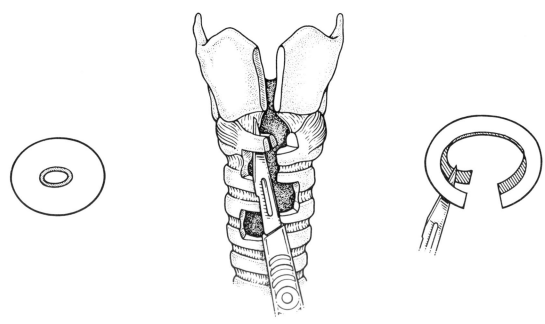

Figure 23.2 The coring out of the abnormally thick cricoid

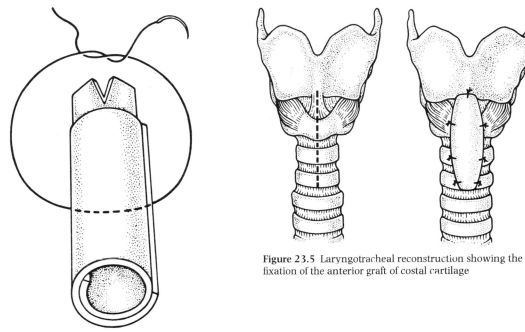

Figure 23.5 Laryngotracheal reconstruction showing the fixation of the anterior graft of costal cartilage

Figure 23.3 Internal stent of rolled Silastic (swiss roll)

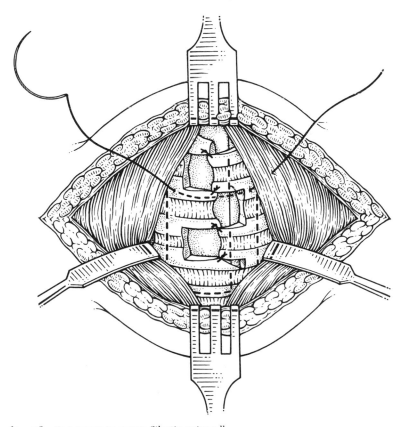

Figure 23.4 Insertion of transfixation suture to secure Silastic swiss roll

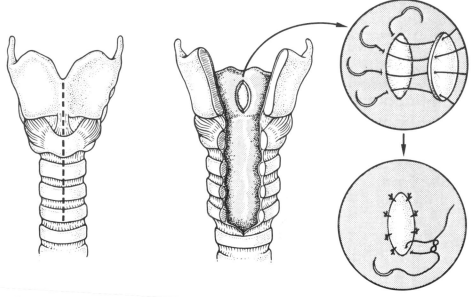

Figure 23.6 The technique of insertion of a graft in the posterior lamina of the cricoid

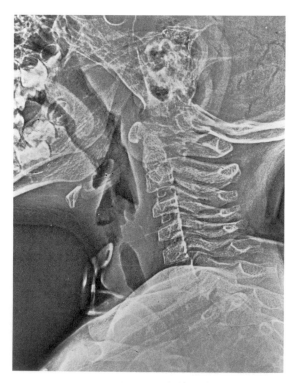

Figure 23.7 Xerogram showing subglottic stenosis, after intubation following cardiac surgery

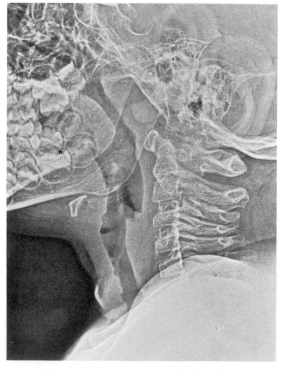

Figure 23.8 Xerogram showing normal subglottic airway after laryngotracheoplasty

by careful endoscopic assessment that the laryngeal lumen has not increased in size. The surgeon should be prepared to graft the larynx or to perform laryngotracheoplasty and often the appropriate procedure can only be determined when the cricoid cartilage is exposed at operation (Figures 23.7 and 23.8). Currently, the efficacy of operations on the larynx has been established and it has been shown that there is a reasonable prospect of achieving decannulation in the majority of cases. One can at least give the parents of these children a reasonably accurate prognosis, and the hope that their child can be restored to normality and to a state that is no longer dependent on tracheostomy (Ochi, Evans and Bailey, 1992a, b).

References

ABEDI, E. and FRAMBLE, M. A. S. (1983) Conjoint hyoid bone segment for the repair of severe laryngeal stenosis. *Archives of Otolaryngology*, **109**, 482–484

ABOULKER, P., STERKERS, J. M., DEMALDENT, J. E. and SAUTON, P. (1966) Modifications apportees a l'intervention de Rethi. *Annals of Otology and Laryngology*, **83**, 98–106

BAKER, B. L. and WHITAKER, W. I. (1950) Interference with wound healing by the local action of adrenocortical steroids. *Endocrinology*, **46**, 544–551

BIRCK, H. B. (1970) Endoscopic repair of laryngeal stenosis. *Transactions of the American Academy of Ophthalmology and Otolaryngology*, **74**, 140–143

CARRUTH, J. A. S., MORGAN, N. J., NIELSEN, M. S., PHILLIPPS, J. J. and WAINWRIGHT, A. C. (1986) The treatment of laryngeal stenosis using the CO_2 laser. *Clinical Otolaryngology*, **11**, 145–148

CLOSE, L. G., LOZANO, A. J. and SCHAEFFER, S. D. (1983) Sternohyoid myo-osseous flap for acquired subglottic stenosis in children. *Laryngoscope*, **93**, 433–439

COTTON, R. T. (1978) Management of subglottic stenosis in infancy and childhood: review of a consecutive series of cases managed by surgical reconstruction. *Annals of Otology, Rhinology and Laryngology*, **87**, 649–657

COTTON, R. T. (1991) The problem of pediatric laryngotracheal stenosis: a clinical and experimental study on the efficacy of autogenous cartilaginous grafts placed between the vertically divided halves of the posterior lamina of the cricoid cartilage. *Laryngoscope*, **101** (suppl. 56), 1–34

COTTON, R. T. and EVANS, J. N. G. (1981) Laryngotracheal reconstruction in children. Five-year follow up. *Annals of Otology, Rhinology and Laryngology*, **90**, 516–520

COTTON, R. T. and MYER, C. M. (1984) Contemporary surgical management of laryngeal stenosis in children. *American Journal of Otolaryngology*, **5**, 360–368

COTTON, R. T. and SEID, A. B. (1980) Management of the extubation problem in the premature child: anterior cricoid split as an alternative to tracheostomy. *Annals of Otology, Rhinology and Laryngology* **89**, 508–511

COTTON, R. T., MYER, C. M. and O'CONNOR, D. M. (1992) Innovations in pediatric laryngotracheal reconstruction. *Journal of Pediatric Surgery*, **27**, 196–200

DOWNING, T. P. and JOHNSON, D. G. (1979) Excision of subglottic stenosis with the urethral resectoscope. *Journal of Pediatric Surgery*, **14**, 252–257

EVANS, J. N. G. (1986) Laryngeal and upper tracheal stenosis in children. *Proceedings of the Fourth International Congress of Paediatric Otorhinolaryngology*, edited by J. Hirschberg and Z. Labas. Kultura Budapest

EVANS, J. N. G. and TODD, G. B. (1974) Laryngotracheoplasty. *Journal of Laryngology and Otology*, **88**, 589–597

EVANS, J. N. G., BATCH, A. J. G. and LEITCH, R. N. (1986) Tracheal problems in children. *Proceedings of the Fifth World Congress for Bronchology, 5th World Congress on Bronchoesophagology*, edited by F. Aprigliano and L. Fernando P. de Mello. Rio de Janeiro. pp. 147–150

FRANKEL, L. R., ANAS, N. G., PERKIN, R. M., SEID, A. B., PETERSON, B. and PARK, S. M. (1984) Use of anterior cricoid split operation in infants with acquired subglottic stenosis. *Critical Care Medicine*, **12**, 395–398

FRIEDMAN, E. M., HEALY, G. B. and MCGILL, T. J. I. (1983) Carbon dioxide laser management of subglottic and tracheal stenosis. *Otolaryngologic Clinics of North America*, **16**, 871–877

GOULD, S. J. and HOWARD, S. (1985) Histopathology of the larynx in the neonate following endotracheal intubation. *Journal of Pathology*, **146**, 301–311

GUESS, W. I. and STEISON, J. B. (1970) Tissue toxicity of rubber endotracheal tubes. *International Anaesthesiology Clinics*, **8**, 823–828

HAWKINS, D. B. (1978) Hyaline membrane disease of the neonate prolonged intubation in management: effect on the larynx. *Laryngoscope*, **88**, 201–224

HOLINGER, L. D. (1980) Etiology of stridor in the neonate infant and child. *Annals of Otology, Rhinology and Laryngology*, **89**, 397–400

HOLINGER, L. D. (1982) Treatment of severe subglottic stenosis without tracheostomy: a preliminary report. *Annals of Otology, Rhinology and Laryngology*, **91**, 407–412

LUSK, R. P., GRAY, S. and MUNTZ, H. R. (1991) Single stage laryngotracheal reconstruction. *Archives of Otolaryngology – Head and Neck Surgery*, **117**, 171–173

MARSHAK, G. and GRUNDFAST, K. M. (1981) Subglottic stenosis. *Pediatric Clinics of North America*, **28**, 941–948

MITCHELL, D. B., IRWIN, B. C., BAILEY, C. M. and EVANS, J. N. G. (1987) Cysts of the infant larynx. *Journal of Laryngology and Otology*, **101**, 833–837

MORIMITSU, T., MATSUMOTO, I., OKADA, S., TAKAHASHI, M. and KOSUGI, T. (1981) Congenital cricoid stenosis. *Laryngoscope*, **91**, 1356–1364

NICKLAUS, P. J., CRYSDALE, W. S., CONLEY, S., WHITE, A. K., SENDI, K. and FORTE, V. (1990) Acquired neonatal subglottic stenosis. *Archives of Otolaryngology – Head and Neck Surgery*, **116**, 902

OCHI, J. W., EVANS, J. N. G. and BAILEY, C. M. (1992a) Paediatric airway reconstruction at Great Ormond Street: a ten year review. I Laryngotracheoplasty and laryngotracheal reconstruction. *Annals of Otology, Rhinology and Laryngology*, **101**, 465–468

OCHI, J. W., EVANS, J. N. G. and BAILEY, C. M. (1992b) Paediatric airway reconstruction at Great Ormond Street: a ten year review. II Revisional airway reconstruction *Annals of Otology, Rhinology and Laryngology*, **101**, 595–597

PAPSIDERO, M. J. and PASHLEY, N. R. T. (1980) Acquired stenosis of the upper airway in neonates. *Annals of Otology, Rhinology and Laryngology*, **89**, 512–514

PARKIN, J. L., STEVENS, M. H. and JUNG, A. L. (1976) Acquired and congenital subglottic stenosis in the infant. *Annals of Otology, Rhinology and Laryngology*, **85**, 573–581

PEERLESS, S. A., PILLSBURY, H. R. and PEERLESS, A. G. (1981) Treatment of laryngeal stenosis a conservative new approach. *Annals of Otology, Rhinology and Laryngology*, **90**, 512–515

QUINEY, R. E. and GOULD, S. J. (1985) Subglottic stenosis: a clinico-pathological study. *Clinical Otolaryngology*, **10**, 315–327

QUINEY, R. E., SPENCER, M. G., BAILEY, C. M., EVANS, J. N. G. and GRAHAM, J. M. (1986) Management of subglottic stenosis: experience from two centres. *Archives of Disease in Childhood*, **61**, 686–690

RASCHE, R. F. H. and KUHNS, L. R. (1972) Histopathologic changes in airway mucosa of infants after endotracheal intubation. *Pediatrics*, **50**, 632–637

RATNER, I. and WHITFIELD, J. (1983) Acquired subglottic stenosis in the very low birth weight infant. *American Journal of Diseases of Children*, **137**, 40–43

RETHI, A. (1956) An operation for cicatricial stenosis of the larynx. *Journal of Laryngology and Otology*, **70**, 283–293

RODGERS, B. M. and TALBERT, J. L. (1978) Clinical application of endotracheal cryotherapy. *Journal of Pediatric Surgery*, **13**, 662–668

SIMPSON, G. T., STRONG, M. S., HEALY, G. B., SHAPSHAY, S. M. and VAUGHAN, C. W. (1982) Predictive factors of success or failure in the endoscopic management of laryngeal and tracheal stenosis. *Annals of Otology, Rhinology and Laryngology*, **91**, 384–388

STRONG, R. M. and PASSY, V. (1977) Endotracheal intubation complications in neonates. *Archives of Otolaryngology*, **103**, 329–335

STRONG, M. S., HEALY, G. B., VAUGHAN, C. W., FRIED, M. P. and SHAPSHAY, S. (1979) Endoscopic management of laryngeal stenosis. *Otolaryngologic Clinics of North America*, **12**, 797–806

TOOHILL, R., MARTINELLI, D. and JANOWAK, M. (1976) Repair of laryngeal stenosis with nasal septal graft. *Annals of Otology, Rhinology and Laryngology*, **85**, 601–608

TUCKER, G. F., OSSOFF, R. H., NEWMAN, A. N. and HOLINGER, L. D. (1979) Histopathology of congenital subglottic stenosis. *Laryngoscope*, **89**, 866–876

WAGGONER, L. G., BELENKY, W. M. and CLARK, C. E. (1973) Treatment of acquired subglottic stenosis. *Annals of Otology, Rhinology and Laryngology*, **82**, 822–826

24

Acute laryngeal infections

Andrew P. Freeland

Laryngeal infections in childhood may result in airway obstruction, the prime symptom of which is stridor. This chapter discusses the various causes of laryngeal infection and their management so that a safe course of action is followed, resulting in a favourable outcome.

The first aim in management is to establish a diagnosis rapidly and this is dependent on a good knowledge of the various possibilities. From a practical point of view it is vital to distinguish inflammation *above the glottis* (epiglottitis or supraglottitis) from inflammation *at* or *below the glottis* (laryngotracheobronchitis). A variety of organisms, both bacterial and viral, has replaced *Corynebacterium diphtheriae* as the commonest cause of acute laryngeal infection. Diphtheria, however, still needs to be considered, as do conditions which may mimic laryngeal infections such as acute retropharyngeal abscess and foreign bodies.

Stridor is the noise caused by obstruction of airflow due to narrowing in the respiratory tract. It may be inspiratory, biphasic or expiratory, but in most cases of acute laryngeal infection inspiratory stridor dominates. An expiratory phase is very common when the tracheal lumen is also narrowed by oedema or inflammation. Inspiratory stridor alone usually indicates that the lesion is at vocal cord level or above. Tucker (1979) pointed out that in a full-term baby's larynx measuring 7×4 mm, 1 mm of oedema reduces the lumen to 35% of normal. It is therefore not surprising that the child with laryngeal infection develops airway obstruction, whereas the adult with similar disease does not.

Croup, as defined by the Shorter Oxford English Dictionary is 'an inflammatory disease of the larynx and trachea of children marked by a peculiar, sharp, ringing cough'. An alternative definition is to 'cry hoarsely, or to make the hoarse, ringing cough of croup'. There is a tremendous variation in the diseases included in the literature under the term 'croup'. It appears to be more of a lay term rather than a pathological entity and parents seem to adhere more to the dictionary definition by referring to their children as having 'croupy' coughs than do the medical profession who usually mean airway obstruction. Since it is an imprecise term, it would seem more acceptable to classify all children as having acute inflammatory stridor until a more specific diagnosis can be established. Margolis (1980) pointed out that there is a major problem in deciding whether drug therapy is effective if the definition of the disease is inaccurate in the first place. There is even confusion as to whether croup includes epiglottitis. Since there is no generally agreed classification of this group of diseases, the present author feels that epiglottitis is a separate entity and that 'croup' includes acute viral laryngotracheobronchitis, bacterial laryngotracheobronchitis (pseudomembranous croup), spasmodic croup and diphtheria.

Anatomy of the larynx

The larynx is relatively and absolutely smaller than in the adult (Pracy, 1979) and is higher in the neck and more difficult to see. The coronal (Figure 24.1) and sagittal (Figure 24.2) whole organ laryngeal sections show two important points in relation to childhood infections. The epiglottis is surrounded by loose connective tissue – the pre-epiglottic and paraglottic spaces – and inflammation may spread quickly from the epiglottis within these spaces. Rough instrumentation or even tongue depression, may encourage inflammatory oedema to surround the laryngeal inlet completely. This is a hazard referred to in the section on management of epiglottitis. Secondly, the mucosa

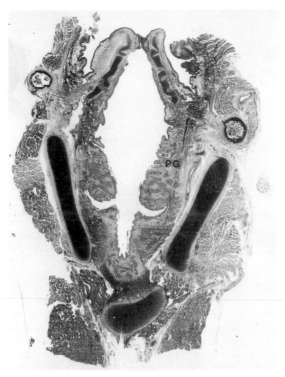

Figure 24.1 Coronal section through an infant larynx. Note the loose connective tissue in the paraglottic space (PG) into which inflammation from the epiglottis may quickly spread

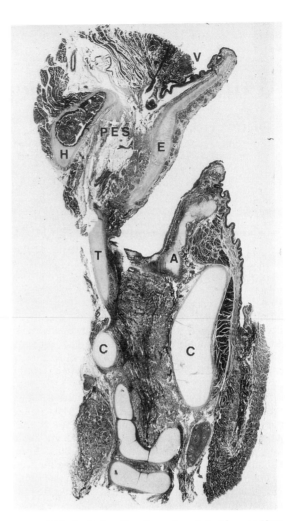

Figure 24.2 Sagittal section through an infant larynx. Note the pre-epiglottic space (PES) bounded by the hyoid (H) anteriorly, the vallecular (V) superiorly and the epiglottis (E) posteriorly into which epiglottitis can quickly spread. This space is continuous with the paraglottic space shown in Figure 24.1. T = thyroid; A = arytenoid cartilage; C = cricoid cartilage

in the subglottis (within the cricoid ring) is lax, full of mucous glands and easily becomes oedematous. If it does so, a biphasic stridor occurs since this is the only part of the laryngotracheobronchial tree that is completely surrounded by cartilage; it is therefore rigid and the airflow is restricted in both inspiratory and expiratory phases. It is also worth noting that laryngeal spasm occurs more easily in the child than in the adult. The childhood larynx seems to be physiologically more brittle.

Causes of laryngeal infection in childhood

The causes of acute laryngeal infection in childhood will be considered first in isolation. Their management, however, will be discussed together since in most cases the child will present in the casualty department as an acute infective airway obstruction of unknown cause. The correct management depends on an accurate diagnosis for a successful outcome for each condition.

Acute epiglottitis (acute supraglottic laryngitis, acute supraglottitis)

Acute epiglottitis is the most frightening of paediatric emergencies. If unrecognized it can kill and all medical practitioners should be aware of its existence and significance. It is rare, occurring 43 times less frequently than laryngotracheobronchitis, but the mortality, even in experienced hands, is 3–4% (Fearon, 1975). *Haemophilus influenzae* type B is, in the vast majority of cases, the causative organism. The β-haemolytic streptococcus, pneumococcus and staphylococcus have also been reported as causal agents

(Schwartz *et al.*, 1982). *H. influenzae* type B epiglottitis may present at any time during the year, although it is more common in the winter months (Walker and Crysdale, 1992). Drake-Lee, Broughton and Grace (1984) found no cases in the months of July, August or September over a 7-year period. There is considerable evidence that the introduction of Hib vaccine has reduced the incidence of acute epiglottitis. Kessler, Wetmore and Marsh (1993) described a series in which 27% of affected children had been vaccinated, though these all occurred before 1990. Since then there have been no affected vaccinated children in their series, probably due to the introduction of a more effective vaccine.

The disease is concentrated maximally on the epiglottis, but it is common to find inflammation involving the whole supraglottic compartment of the larynx. The infection spreads in the loose connective tissue anterior and posterolateral to the epiglottis (see Figures 24.1 and 24.2). The laryngeal surface of the epiglottis is largely spared.

Most cases are seen in children between the ages of 1 and 6 years with the peak incidence occurring between the ages of 3 and 4 years. This is in contrast with laryngotracheobronchitis which usually affects younger children, the peak incidence being 18 months of age. Recently several authors have described an age shift towards younger children (Singer and McCabe, 1988; Emmerson, Richman and Spahn, 1991; Kessler, Wetmore and Marsh, 1993). In the latter's series the mean age, as compared to a previous study, had not changed, though there was higher incidence of the disease in younger children. Epiglottitis is occasionally seen in adults, but most children over the age of 6 years have protective antibodies against *H. influenzae* type B and it also seems that some immunity exists below the age of 2 years. However, in this younger age group, haemophilus meningitis is more common. Why the organism spares the epiglottis in preference to the meninges is not clear. It has been suggested that previous contact with *H. influenzae* in early childhood may later be followed by a type III Arthus hypersensitivity reaction which would account for the rapid onset of epiglottitis (Broniatowski, 1985).

Clinical features

The most striking feature of this disease is the transformation of a fit child into one who is desperately ill, often within a period of only a few hours. However, not all cases present in this classical manner and Welch and Price (1983) found that one-third of their patients with epiglottitis had a history of an upper respiratory tract infection during the previous 24 hours and some had a surprisingly long history of stridor prior to admission. The classical presentation is described below.

A fit child, aged about 3 years, complains of a sore throat which intensifies and within half an hour dysphagia is reported. Rapidly worsening inspiratory stridor then develops and within 2 hours a critically ill child presents to the casualty department. The child will be sitting up and leaning forward, partly because if he lies back, suffocation may occur as a result of the epiglottis occluding the laryngeal inlet and partly because he is using his arms to fix the chest wall in order to use the accessory muscles of respiration (Figure 24.3). Dribbling of saliva will be profuse since dysphagia is total. His voice, if he is strong enough to speak, will not be hoarse but muffled. Inspiratory stridor is usually present but, as time goes by, the child will become quiet and floppy and the respiratory distress seems to lessen. This is an ominous sign caused by extreme fatigue and indicates that respiratory and cardiac arrest are imminent.

Unlike laryngotracheobronchitis where children are restless and pink, most children with epiglottitis are quiet, pale and look terrified. This is a systemic infection and the bacteraemia causes shock which gives rise to the pallor. Pyrexia is always present, although the degree is variable. Some authors feel

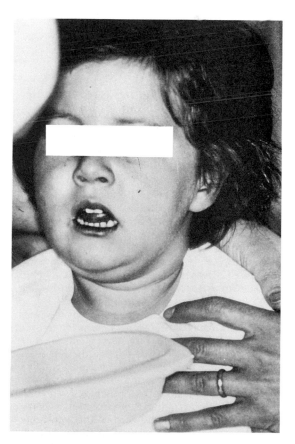

Figure 24.3 Epiglottitis illustrating a frightened child, sitting up, dribbling with cervical lymphadenopathy

that marked cervical lymphadenopathy is always present and in the casualty department this is the only physical sign, other than observation from a distance, that it is safe to elicit. On no account should the pharynx be examined since immediate asphyxia may ensue. Walker and Crysdale (1992) reported that 90% of the children in their series presented with odynophagia and stridor, with drooling present in 64%.

Radiology of this condition is discussed in the section on management, but it is the author's view that, although X-rays of the epiglottis in this condition are frequently found in articles and textbooks, the taking of an X-ray may be a dangerous practice. This is due to the delay and distress caused by aligning the child for an X-ray which is usually quite unnecessary for the diagnosis to be made.

The above picture is enough to raise suspicion that the child has epiglottitis and no further investigations should be carried out until an alternative airway has been established. Throat swabs, taking of blood cultures, and sampling for blood gases are liable to agitate the child, increase the likelihood of airway obstruction and waste valuable time.

The only time to confirm the diagnosis is as the child is being provided with an alternative airway. The further management of epiglottitis is considered later.

Laryngotracheobronchitis (croup, acute subglottic laryngitis, non-diphtheritic croup, acute laryngotracheitis)

This is the commonest infective cause of upper respiratory tract obstruction in children (Walker and Crysdale, 1992). As the name implies, laryngotracheobronchitis involves a larger proportion of the respiratory tract than epiglottitis but the maximum effect is in the subglottic area. In most cases the causative organism is parainfluenza virus type I, but parainfluenza virus types II and III, influenza virus type A, respiratory syncytial virus and rhinoviruses may also be responsible. Laryngotracheobronchitis may follow measles. It is not uncommon for secondary bacterial infection to supervene.

The vocal cords are inflamed and may be ulcerated, but it is the subglottis that seems to bear the brunt of the disease. Here there is gross oedema and occasionally ulceration. As the name implies, the rest of the tracheobronchial tree may also be affected.

As mentioned previously the incidence of hospital admissions for laryngotracheobronchitis is about 40 times more frequent than for epiglottitis (Fearon, 1975). Figures 24.4 and 24.5 show that experience in Oxford with age and seasonal incidence is very much the same as in other reports. The mean age is about 18 months and boys are more frequently

affected than girls. Denny *et al.* (1983) reported that boys are affected 1.43 times as commonly as girls and also stated that November is the peak month for the disease in North Carolina. Walker and Crysdale (1992) reported a male predominance of 2:1 in Canada, again with most children presenting in the winter months. It is certainly more common in the winter months in temperate climates, particularly in October, November and December, and there is often another peak in early spring (see Figure 24.5).

Clinical features

Unlike epiglottitis, laryngotracheobronchitis is always preceded by an upper respiratory tract infection, usually of at least 48 hours' duration. It is not uncommon for the child to have had a previous history of inflammatory stridor. The initial symptom is hoarseness and this is followed by a 'croupy' cough which is sometimes described as a 'musical cough of crowing quality', or the 'bark of a seal'. In the series reported by Walker and Crysdale (1992) the commonest presenting feature was cough, with stridor second. Signs

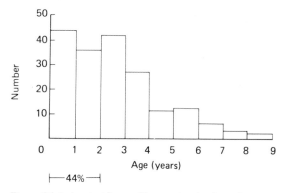

Figure 24.4 Age incidence of laryngotracheobronchitis

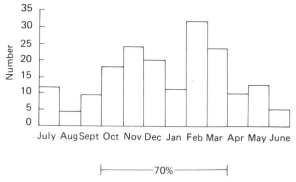

Figure 24.5 Seasonal incidence of laryngotracheobronchitis. Total = 183; 128 male (70%), 55 female (30%)

of respiratory distress then appear, often at night. There is usually a slight pyrexia. Although stridor is initially inspiratory, it soon becomes biphasic as subglottic oedema develops. Flaring of the ala nasae and suprasternal and intercostal recession develop as respiratory distress increases. At this stage, the child becomes very restless and prefers to lie down. Crying and coughing occur, which make the stridor worse and give rise to the physician's natural inclination to sedate the child. The safety of this will be discussed later. Careful assessment is needed as the child's stridor and chest retraction diminish; it may mean there is a genuine improvement, but occasionally it represents exhaustion with imminent respiratory failure.

It is unknown how many children are managed at home, usually with some form of moist inhalation administered by their parents and family doctors, and how many are admitted to hospital. It is therefore difficult to know what the true incidence of this disease is. According to Mitchell and Thomas (1980), only 5–10% of all croup cases need hospital admission and, in the USA, an overall incidence of 5–10/1000 preschool children is quoted (Hall and Hall, 1975). A rough estimate from 10 Oxford general practitioners suggests that they request hospital admission for one in every six cases they are called to see. The management in hospital will be discussed later, approximately one of 20 of these admissions needs an alternative airway. Milner (1984) quoted an even lower incidence of 1% requiring intubation. This is in contrast to epiglottitis where nearly all patients need an alternative airway.

Bacterial laryngotracheobronchitis (*pseudomembranous croup*)

This condition may be a separate disease or be caused by a secondary bacterial infection of viral laryngotracheobronchitis. Some authors call this disease bacterial tracheitis (Broniatowski, 1985) since it seems to involve the trachea predominantly. It is a much more severe illness than laryngotracheobronchitis, but very much less common (Walker and Crysdale, 1992). Henry (1983), over a 2-year period, reported seven children who had this condition and exhibited sloughing of the respiratory epithelium. The children were older than is normally associated with laryngotracheobronchitis and they had more severe obstruction. An artificial airway is often needed but this may easily obstruct with crusts of sloughed epithelium. The causative organism in most cases is *Staphylococcus aureus*. A similar experience with this condition was reported by Friedman *et al.* (1985), who described 10 patients ranging in age from 3 months to 12 years, three of whom required intubation and seven needed bronchoscopy for diagnosis and treatment.

Clinical features

Bacterial laryngotracheobronchitis begins in a fairly insidious way with a history of an upper respiratory infection. It progresses, however, and is accompanied by a brassy cough and high fever. The child becomes toxic and the white blood count is greatly elevated. It is likely on admission that the child will be diagnosed as having severe laryngotracheobronchitis and, because of respiratory distress, an alternative airway will be considered. If a bronchoscopy is performed the trachea will be seen to be ulcerated and sloughed epithelium will be aspirated. This should be sent for bacterial culture since, if bacterial laryngotracheobronchitis is suspected, appropriate antibiotic therapy is essential.

The condition poses major problems for intensive care nurses because of the marked tendency to endotracheal tube obstruction. Very efficient humidity and expert nursing care are necessary to manage these patients successfully. A tracheostomy may be safer since there is less risk of obstruction of the tube from inspissated secretions.

Spasmodic laryngitis (*spasmodic croup, acute subglottic oedema, laryngismus stridulus*)

This condition is not universally recognized in all classifications but has the following characteristics. Recurrent attacks are common. The bouts usually begin very suddenly at night without any prodromal features and disappear just as rapidly, often in the morning. The attacks respond to mist therapy and may stop after vomiting (Davis *et al.*, 1981). If the child is bronchoscoped for any reason, subglottic oedema is the abnormal finding. Most cases, however, do not require an alternative airway.

Zach (1983) studied immunoglobulin levels in recurrent croup and demonstrated low IgA levels in spasmodic laryngitis and showed that an association existed between the disease activity and the IgA levels. Some children seem to grow out of these attacks only to develop asthma or other allergic states.

There may be a place for treating spasmodic laryngitis with anti-asthma inhalants such as topical steroids or sodium cromoglycate. Systemic corticosteroids also relieve this condition (Koren *et al.*, 1983). These authors found that dexamethasone 0.6 mg/kg as a single dose was useful in spasmodic laryngitis but had no effect in laryngotracheobronchitis.

Diphtheria

Diphtheria is extremely rare in countries where routine immunization is the rule. In 1984 there were only 70 cases in the USA (Broniatowski, 1985), but it is still an important differential diagnosis of airway obstruction in children, especially in immigrants who may not have been immunized. Laryngeal diphtheria nearly always follows pharyngeal infection.

The causative organism is *Corynebacterium diphtheriae* and of the three strains – gravis, intermedius and mitis – it is nearly always the gravis strain that has been responsible for the major epidemics and high mortality rates. Clinical variants are reported as causing membranous pharyngitis. It is rare to see diphtheria in children over the age of 10 years.

It is not only the laryngeal obstruction that causes mortality in this condition, but also the production of an endotoxin with the risk of myocarditis and peripheral neuritis. The initial lesion is usually in the region of the tonsil where necrosis is seen and the characteristic grey membrane is formed – a mixture of necrotic tissue, a rich fibrinous exudate and a large number of bacteria. Attempts to remove the membrane often produce bleeding. The membrane appears to become thicker later in the disease process and is easier to separate from underlying mucosa. The characteristic bull neck appearance is due to cellulitis and regional lymphadenopathy.

Clinical features

The onset is insidious and begins with a barking cough, followed by inspiratory stridor with chest wall recession as the disease spreads from the pharynx to the larynx. General symptoms of malaise, pyrexia and sore throat are often present early in the disease but, occasionally, a membrane over the faucial pillars is the only sign during the early stages. General signs of toxaemia then occur, and dysphagia increases prior to laryngeal involvement which is evidenced by a barking cough, and stridor. The cough comes in paroxysms and exhaustion from coughing and toxaemia soon occurs unless an alternative airway is provided. Many children die, however, from acute toxic myocarditis occurring during the second week of the illness. Palatal paralysis is the most common of the peripheral neuropathies to occur, and presents with nasal regurgitation of food and 'nasal escape' to the voice.

Management

The main problem nowadays is to remember that laryngeal diphtheria still exists. *Corynebacterium diphtheriae* is penicillin sensitive and penicillin therapy is therefore the mainstay in treatment but, because of the danger of diphtheritic toxins, antitoxin treatment is also essential and both should be used early in the management. Intravenous benzyl penicillin, 600 mg 6-hourly, should be used and the dose of antitoxin, which may also be given intravenously, varies from 10 000 to 100 000 units, dependent on the severity of the infection.

It may also be necessary to remove the membrane from the larynx and insert an endotracheal tube for airway support. The decision to do this will depend entirely on the clinical situation and will probably be reserved for failed conservative treatment which should include humidification and oxygen therapy. Extubation (if intubation has been necessary) can be commenced early since the disease responds very well to medical therapy. Once the airway obstruction has been successfully managed, the child will need careful assessment and possibly total bed rest for 2–4 weeks until the danger of myocarditis is past.

Conditions which mimic laryngeal infections in childhood

Conditions that must be eliminated as mimics of acute laryngeal infections are foreign bodies, infectious mononucleosis (glandular fever), peritonsillar abscess, retropharyngeal abscess and paraquat poisoning.

Foreign bodies

This subject is beyond the scope of this chapter since it appears elsewhere in this volume (see Chapter 25) but a history of a child who is apyrexial who has been playing with small objects and who then begins to have paroxysms of coughing, suggests the inhalation of a foreign body. Removal via endoscopy is obviously essential. Absence of pyrexia is the most obvious way to distinguish foreign body impaction from acute inflammatory disease in the childhood larynx.

Infectious mononucleosis (glandular fever)

A full description will be found elsewhere in this volume (see Chapter 18), but mention is appropriate here since airway obstruction may occasionally occur. The membrane in glandular fever is less adherent than in diphtheria, but tonsillar hypertrophy may be massive and may result in inspiratory stridor. Glandular fever is more common in young adults, but is not infrequently found in children. If the airway becomes embarrassed and the stridor increases, large doses of intravenous dexamethasone often alleviate the need for an alternative airway. Ampicillin and amoxycillin should be avoided.

Peritonsillar abscess (quinsy)

Peritonsillar abscess occurs more commonly in adolescence than retropharyngeal abscess, but the reverse is true in infancy (White, 1985). The clinical features are of trismus, dribbling and airway obstruction which occurs as a result of the tonsils being displaced medially to threaten the oropharyngeal airway. There may be a history of antecedent recurrent tonsillitis.

It can be difficult to decide whether frank pus is present or whether the disease is in the cellulitic stage. If the airway is in jeopardy, it is recommended that surgical drainage of the abscess be carried out. The usual site of the incision, or needle aspiration, for the evacuation of pus is at a point which is transected by a line drawn horizontally from the base of the uvula with one drawn vertically from the anterior pillar of the tonsil. Release of pus by open drainage results in rapid improvement of the symptoms and of the child's well-being.

Retropharyngeal abscess

Retropharyngeal abscess is the commonest of the deep neck space infections occurring in infancy and may well mimic laryngotracheobronchitis by presenting with airway embarrassment. Young children have many retropharyngeal lymph nodes and these may become infected via lymphatics from the tonsils, teeth, nasopharynx or paranasal sinuses (Walker and Crysdale, 1992). Most children will have a history of a previous upper airway tract infection. Unsuspected foreign bodies are another important cause. Syphilis and tuberculosis affecting the cervical spine may also present with a retropharyngeal abscess. Children over the age of 4 years have far fewer nodes in the retropharyngeal space, hence this infection is more common in very young children (Brodinski and Holyoke, 1938; Walker and Crysdale, 1992).

Once necrosis of the retropharyngeal lymph node takes place or there is direct extension from tuberculosis of the cervical spine, an abscess is formed which bulges anteriorly into the pharynx. The child becomes toxic, has dysphagia and may dribble. His head is held stiffly and is eventually hyperextended. Prominent cervical glands are present. Inspiratory stridor may occur from associated laryngeal oedema or forward displacement of the laryngopharynx.

Examination is difficult, for apart from the signs referred to above, the oropharynx is not easy to see in an infant, especially with unswallowed secretions pooling in the throat. The retropharyngeal space is in direct continuity with the posterior mediastinum and palpation of the pharynx may well strip the abscess inferiorly or else cause it to be inadvertently ruptured with the consequent risk of inhalation of pus.

The management of this condition is considered later, but by far the most reliable way of diagnosing a retropharyngeal abscess is with a lateral soft tissue neck X-ray (Figure 24.6).

Paraquat poisoning

Paraquat (1,1'-dimethyl 4,4'-bipyridyldiyliumdichloride) is a herbicide which is occasionally ingested and gives rise to a pseudodiphtheritic picture (Broniatowski, 1985). It causes a marked pharyngeal membrane which is less adherent to underlying tissues than that associated with diphtheria. The tongue, characteristically, is more heavily involved with membrane than are the tonsils (Stevens, Walker and Schaffner, 1981). Systemic signs of shock and sepsis are also present.

The management of acute laryngeal infections in childhood

The two aims in management are to arrive swiftly at the correct diagnosis and to treat safely the child's airway obstruction. In order that this may be achieved, there must be an admissions policy laid down in each district which all family doctors are aware of and adhere to. The ambulance crew must also know of the arrangements and the hospital staff from different specialties must cooperate smoothly. There is a necessity for frequent reminders in the form of postgraduate seminars to all grades of staff to keep those who may have only just joined a general practice or hospital department informed as to local procedures.

It is only by adhering to a rigid protocol that safety in the management of airway obstruction in the

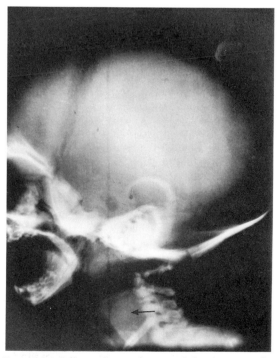

Figure 24.6 Infant with retropharyngeal abscess (arrowed). Note the width of the cervical spine, compared with the width of the retropharyngeal space. The trachea is displaced anteriorly

child will be maintained. Each hospital receiving such children should work out their own arrangements, but cooperation between anaesthetists, otolaryngologists and paediatricians (alphabetical order only!) is essential. Ideally, there should be a special resuscitation room near an operating theatre suite where children may be managed. Personnel involved in the management should be as senior as possible. It is not the situation for the newly appointed anaesthetist or inexperienced otolaryngologist.

The equipment in the resuscitation rooms needs to be checked daily to make sure it is complete and in working order – particularly bulbs, fibre light cables and suction equipment. The room must have enough space to house the mother and child, an anaesthetist, nurse, otolaryngologist and a paediatrician. In practice, other personnel frequently swell the numbers. The resuscitation trolley requirements include a full range of naso- and orotracheal tubes ranging from 2.5 mm upwards. Introducers for the endotracheal tubes are essential. Two laryngoscopes with straight blades should be available in case one fails. A complete anaesthetic machine is needed with all the necessary anaesthetic drugs and intravenous equipment. There will also need to be bronchoscopy equipment and the Storz rigid fibre light bronchoscopes are a personal preference, six sizes being available ranging from 2.5 mm to 5 mm. These need to be equipped with side arms for anaesthetic ventilation. A Venturi system may be used with a bronchoscope provided the bronchoscope is quite clear to allow air to escape back up it; its use is not advisable when a bronchoscope telescope is in place. Pneumothorax is the common complication of Venturi bronchoscopy. Various foreign body forceps for use down the bronchoscope need to be at hand, as do the correct lengths of suction cannulae. A paediatric tracheostomy set must also be available, although is rarely needed in the author's practice.

One of the most important pieces of equipment is the suction apparatus. There need to be two separate units; one being a large pharyngeal sucker, such as a Yankauer, for pharyngeal secretions and occasional sudden vomits, and the other for fine catheters or fine rigid metal suction tubes required for the bronchoscope. A Magill sucker is also well worth having on the trolley, since it can also be used to intubate the patient and provide a temporary airway.

The first stage of management is to arrive at a sensible diagnosis in a short space of time. Unnecessary questioning of parents for irrelevant information is a waste of precious time. The most important consideration is to distinguish epiglottitis and laryngeal foreign body from laryngotracheobronchitis and its mimics, since the former need immediate attention, whereas the latter can usually be managed in a more leisurely fashion. Although not all cases are typical, the boundary between the supraglottic compartment, the rest of the larynx and the tracheobronchial tree is crossed in both directions by both groups of infections. Table 24.1 may help to summarize the usual distinguishing features.

If all cases were typical, as in Table 24.1, there would be no difficulty distinguishing one disease from another. The signs of retropharyngeal abscess and epiglottitis appear to be much the same, except that the former is usually accompanied by a history of a previous upper respiratory tract infection and is of much slower onset. A laryngeal foreign body can be distinguished from epiglottitis, despite the equally rapid onset of symptoms, by the absence of pyrexia and the history of a foreign body being inhaled. The most important decision to be made in the emergency department is whether the child has epiglottitis or if his airway is immediately threatened by one of the other causes. In either event, an alternative airway must be secured without delay and no further investigation or radiology should be carried out.

Management of epiglottitis

If the child is thought to have epiglottitis, the following protocol should be adopted. The terrified child is comforted and his mother allowed to hold him upright (see Figure 24.3). No attempt should be made to restrain or undress him, carry out venepuncture, X-ray or examine him further since all these procedures may cause crying and precipitate immediate respiratory arrest (Goel, 1984; Tarnow-Mordi *et al.*, 1985; Williams *et al.*, 1985). Radiology is not advised though lateral neck X-ray may show the classical 'thumb' sign of the swollen epiglottis (Figure 24.7). Unless radiological services are present in the emergency room and the child's condition is so stable as to throw some doubt on the diagnosis of epiglottitis, there is no point in confirming it with what might turn out to be a fatal X-ray.

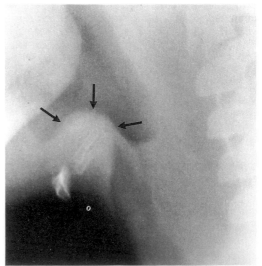

Figure 24.7 'Thumb sign' in epiglottitis

Table 24.1 Summary of differential diagnosis

	Epiglottitis	Laryngotracheobronchitis	Laryngeal foreign body	Retropharyngeal abscess
Pathology	Bacterial, usually *Haemophilus influenzae* type B	Viral, Parainfluenza virus type I		Bacterial, *Staphylococcus aureus*
Age	2–6 years	Under 3 years	Any	1–4 years
History				
onset	Rapid – less than 6 hours	Slow – usually 48 hours	Rapid	Slow – usually history of tonsillitis or upper respiratory tract infection
previous attacks	Not reported	Quite often	Occasional	Not reported
Symptoms				
cough	Absent	Barking cough	Paroxysms of coughing	Absent
dysphagia	Severe	None	Occasional	Severe
stridor	Inspiratory	Biphasic	Inspiratory	Inspiratory
Signs				
temperature	Elevated	Elevated	Apyrexial	Elevated
posture	Sitting, leaning forward	Lying on back	Variable	Sitting, stiff neck
drooling	Marked	None	Occasional	Marked
cervical glands	Large	Small	None	Large
behaviour	Quiet and terrified	Struggling	Variable	Restless
colour	Pale or grey	Pink – cyanotic in late stages	Usually normal	Flushed
voice	Muffled	Hoarse	Hoarse	Hoarse
X-ray	'Thumb sign' dangerous to perform	'Steeple sign'	Foreign body is visible if opaque	Marked widening of retropharyngeal space

Examination of the throat using a tongue depressor is particularly dangerous and should *not* be carried out since respiratory obstruction may occur suddenly, possibly from increase and spread of the swelling in the pre-epiglottic space or from vagal stimulation.

The child is carried by his mother to the resuscitation room, described above, where experienced anaesthetic, otolaryngological and paediatric staff will prepare to secure an alternative airway. Since the airway may obstruct completely if the child is supine, anaesthesia should be induced in the upright position. Occasionally, the child collapses prior to anaesthesia, in which case, intubation or bronchoscopy is required without delay and without induction of anaesthesia.

The otolaryngologist is present in case intubation fails, in which case rigid bronchoscopy is necessary, followed possibly by tracheostomy onto the bronchoscope through which anaesthesia is maintained. How-

ever, in most cases, the anaesthetist will successfully perform the intubation.

If the anaesthetic mask frightens the child, the gases are applied as near to the child's face as possible using the anaesthetist's cupped hand as a mask. Muscle relaxants are not used as there is risk of producing an apnoeic patient with a mechanically obstructed airway. Intravenous induction is generally avoided since obstruction may occur if the child cries as the needle is inserted and apnoea may result.

As soon as the child is asleep, the mother is shown from the room and the child laid on his back ready to be intubated. Anaesthesia is then deepened as much as possible using a partially closed system to allow the application of continuous positive airway pressure (CPAP) which tends to prevent complete obstruction by producing a 'pneumatic splint' for the airway. The airway may be more easily maintained with the patient in the lateral semiprone position at this stage, as the epiglottis will tend to fall back across the laryngeal inlet in the supine position. However, most anaesthetists will prefer to turn the patient supine for intubation. The cardinal error is to attempt intubation too early and provoke laryngospasm. A laryngoscope is inserted and the diagnosis of epiglottitis is confirmed. The usual description is of a cherry red, swollen epiglottis, but very often the aryepiglottic folds are grossly oedematous and the picture is more one of *supraglottitis* rather than inflammation being confined to the epiglottis alone. It is at this stage that a powerful pharyngeal sucker may be necessary to clear all the secretions.

The anterior nature of the oedema of epiglottitis closes the natural inverted 'V' of the epiglottis and obliterates a view of the laryngeal inlet. It is necessary therefore to attempt intubation at the anterior point of the closed 'V' and to displace the epiglottis anteriorly. If the tube is inserted centrally or posteriorly it will deflect off the posterior larynx into the pharynx. This requirement for anterior displacement of the epiglottis makes essential the use of a semi-rigid introducer or stylet such as the Portex (Portex, UK) intubating stylet within the endotracheal tube. If the entrance to the laryngeal inlet is not apparent, sudden compression of the child's chest will often produce a bubble of air in the mucus to indicate the position of the glottis. An appropriately sized orotracheal tube is inserted and hopefully the airway is fully and suddenly restored.

If the first attempt at intubation fails, further manipulation may increase soft tissue oedema and obscure the airway as well as causing marked vagal stimulation resulting in severe bradycardia or cardiac arrest. Further attempts at intubation with floppy plastic tubes will probably also fail and at this stage the patient should be handed over to the otolaryngologist who should be able to insert a rigid bronchoscope behind the epiglottis and into the trachea. Experience has shown that if a bronchoscope is not available, intubation can often be achieved using a Magill sucker which has the advantage of being rigid, hollow and readily available. Once the airway is secured, by whichever method, the immediate danger is over and at this stage an intravenous cannula is inserted to allow the anaesthetist better control.

Andreassen *et al.* (1992) described the use of the rigid bronchoscope in cases of difficult intubation. A suction catheter could then be inserted through the bronchoscope and used as a guidewire for an oral endotracheal tube.

The decision now has to be made about the type of airway to stay in place for the next 24–48 hours. The present author prefers nasotracheal intubation, as do Andreassen *et al.* (1992) and Kessler, Wetmore and Marsh (1993). If the orotracheal tube was only inserted with great difficulty, then it would seem unwise to remove it, unless the degree of swelling was relatively slight and intubation was easy. If this was the case a nasotracheal tube can be inserted via

the nose to a position adjacent to the oral tube, behind the epiglottis, and the latter removed with immediate placement of the former. If bronchoscopy has been necessary, it is probably safer to perform a tracheostomy onto the bronchoscope, although personal recent experience has not required this, the bronchoscope being replaced with a nasotracheal tube as described above.

At this stage culture swabs from the epiglottis and a blood culture sample are taken. A good intravenous infusion line is inserted for fluid replacement and for antibiotic therapy. Because epiglottitis is a short-lived illness, nasogastric feeding is usually unnecessary, but a nasogastric tube should be passed to decompress the stomach which may have been inflated from ventilation during 'bagging' in anaesthesia. Sedation should be used to avoid swallowing movements and struggling against the endotracheal tube, which would otherwise abrade the inflamed epiglottis. One advantage of a tracheostomy is that it allows the child to be ambulant and swallow normally. Cantrell, Bell and Morioka (1978) reviewed 19 series, totalling 738 cases of epiglottitis, and found that the mortality rate if tracheostomy was performed was 0.86% compared with 0.92% if endotracheal intubation had been utilized. However, this rate rose to 6.1% if an artificial airway of some sort was not used in the treatment of epiglottitis. It seems clear, therefore, that whether a tracheostomy or an endotracheal tube is used, there is little change in the outcome, but there is a significant difference if the child is treated without an alternative airway. The morbidity of tracheostomy and endotracheal intubation will be considered later.

Secure fixation of the endotracheal tube is extremely important prior to transfer, as disastrous accidental extubation at this stage is possible. Every anaesthetist has his own method, but painting the face with Compound Benzoin Tincture BP helps secure the Elastoplast strapping around the tube to the face. The child is now transferred from the emergency room to a paediatric intensive care unit. If he has been intubated, sedation is necessary prior to transfer to avoid the risk of extubation during transfer, with the addition of an opiate such as morphine to control the pain of epiglottitis, and intravenous midazolam 0.1 mg/kg as a bolus followed by continuous infusion of approximately 0.1 mg/kg per hour. The choice of antibiotic is difficult since the emergence of ampicillin-resistant and occasionally chloramphenicol-resistant strains of *Haemophilus influenzae* type B have been reported (Philpott-Howard and Williams, 1982). It has been suggested that one of the newer cephalosporins – cefotaxime (Claforan) – is highly effective against both ampicillin-resistant and chloramphenicol-resistant strains (Drake-Lee, Broughton and Grace, 1984). Other organisms, such as the β-haemolytic streptococcus, pneumococcus and staphylococcus, require appropriate treatment once blood cultures and epiglottic swabs are available. The author's current choice of antibiotic is chloramphenicol, 100 mg/kg of body weight/24 hours, although some would favour cefotaxime 200 mg/kg per day in divided 6-hourly doses, or cefuroxime (Walker and Crysdale, 1992).

Steroids are not indicated for the treatment of epiglottitis, although Cantrell, Bell and Morioka (1978) reported their widespread use. However, a single dose of 1 mg/kg of dexamethasone seems to allow earlier extubation and this is sometimes possible as little as 6 hours after the original intubation.

The most important feature about the care of endotracheal tubes is the personnel who look after the airway. It requires highly trained nurses, and enough of them, to care for these patients and it is only in an intensive care situation that these criteria are likely to be met. If an alternative airway has had to be secured in a hospital without intensive care facilities, then a tracheostomy is likely to be safest, since it requires less intense nursing skills in the immediate postoperative period.

Intravenous fluids are necessary to keep the child hydrated. The nasogastric tube is used more for aspiration of the stomach contents to prevent vomiting than for feeding.

Extubation is usually possible within 48 hours, but opinions on the criteria for extubation vary. Most practitioners first look for a leak around the tube with an airway pressure of some 20/30 cm of water. If a leak is present, extubation may be performed immediately if the sedation level is not too great. Corticosteroids may be given half an hour before extubation, to help reduce subglottic oedema caused by the irritant nature of the endotracheal tube. If there is doubt about whether a child can be extubated, then it is sensible to inspect the epiglottis. This can either be done by spraying the nose with lignocaine and using a flexible fibreoptic laryngoscope, or else a single dose of 2–3 mg/kg of propofol allows an atraumatic direct laryngoscopy, with rapid recovery of consciousness, to be carried out. Caution needs to be used since propofol has no product licence for children under the age of 3 years. It is obviously important to plan extubation for a time of day when staffing levels are highest.

One of the most rewarding features about managing this most frightening of paediatric emergencies is that, if cared for correctly, most children with epiglottitis are extubated within 48 hours, having been transformed from a moribund to a fully active, apparently healthy child within that time.

Complications are rare once an airway has been established, accidental extubation perhaps being the most common, but occasionally pulmonary oedema may become apparent after relief of the obstructed airway. A combination of hypoxia and negative intrathoracic pressure during acute obstruction may lead to an increase in pulmonary arterial pressure, damage to alveolar capillaries and to transudation of fluid into the alveoli. Mechanical ventilation of the lungs with a small amount of positive end-expiratory pressure (PEEP) and appropriate added oxygen is the treatment of choice, the oedema usually resolving rapidly (Soliman and Richer, 1978).

Deaths still occur (Welch and Price, 1983) but with a protocol such as suggested above the outcome should be favourable. Since it is the observed cases that die, it is essential that every practitioner is aware of this condition. If there is the slightest suspicion that a child might have epiglottitis, then immediate transferral to hospital is mandatory, if necessary in the practitioner's car, so that an alternative airway can be secured as soon as possible.

In certain circumstances epiglottitis probably can be managed without intubation. Butt *et al.* (1988) described a series in which 13% of children with epiglottitis were not intubated. The diagnosis of epiglottitis in this group was, in most cases, confirmed by a lateral neck X-ray. These patients were treated with antibiotics and were closely managed in an intensive care unit with experienced medical staff present at all times. If the first level of care is not available, intubation would seem mandatory.

It is important to remember that *Haemophilus influenza* type B infection is contagious, and that prophylactic antibiotics should be given to siblings. The North American policy of using rifampicin has generally been followed in Britain (Dale and Court, 1990), although this may not be the most appropriate antibiotic. The advent of Hib vaccine is likely to render this approach redundant and it is probable that epiglottitis will be a very rare disease in childhood in years to come. At the moment, Hib vaccine is in routine use as a public health measure in the UK, USA and Finland, but is not yet fully adopted in other countries. It is at least 90% effective (Moxon, 1994, personal communication).

Management of laryngotracheobronchitis

Some children with acute laryngotracheobronchitis will need an alternative airway on admission, especially if the diagnosis is bacterial laryngotracheobronchitis (pseudomembranous croup), in which case the preceding protocol for epiglottitis will serve to describe appropriate management. However, since only approximately 1% of patients with laryngotracheobronchitis will need intubation (Milner, 1984), a different approach is usually adopted.

Provided epiglottitis is unlikely, then conservative management with careful observation is usually all that is required as the disease settles. There are many controversial aspects of the management of laryngotracheobronchitis and these will be discussed.

Radiology

While in the emergency department lateral and anteroposterior neck, and chest X-rays are performed. The lateral neck X-ray is the only reliable way to exclude a retropharyngeal abscess (see Figure 24.6) and hopefully will not demonstrate a swollen epiglottis which should have been excluded clinically. Foreign bodies may also be seen. The neck X-ray may show a narrowed subglottis (Figure 24.8), with the so-called 'steeple' sign typical of laryngotracheobronchitis and may also show 'ballooning' of the hypopharynx. The chest X-ray is a helpful baseline to exclude collapsed lobes, mediastinal shift or obstructive emphysema as may occur with bronchial foreign bodies. Pulmonary oedema and pneumonia are also occasionally seen.

Once the X-ray has been taken, the child is admitted to the appropriate ward for observation.

Observation

Croup scoring systems are used in some hospitals (Davis *et al.*, 1981), but a numerical score has been found not to influence the clinical management of patients. It is to be hoped that clinical observations will show the stridor lessening, the restlessness settling, the colour remaining pink and the respiration and cardiac rates reducing. These parameters will not improve readily if the child is frightened, and removing him from his mother, placing him in a cold fog in a dripping plastic tent where he cannot see his surroundings, subjecting him to frequent pulse readings and painful blood gas estimations, does not help the situation (Henry, 1983; Walker and Crysdale, 1992).

Reassurance

Most of the treatments suggested for laryngotracheobronchitis are controversial, but the one aspect on which all authors agree is that the child needs strong reassurance, as do the parents (Walker and Crysdale, 1992). It is recommended practice not to separate parents and child and once in a calm, confident, reassuring atmosphere all seem to relax. Sedation is rarely necessary and there are serious dangers in suppressing the central drive to respiration with some drugs. If sedation seems essential, then chloral hydrate 30 mg/kg is the safest choice.

Humidification

Most authors agree that warm, moist air does little harm (Henry, 1983) and others suggest it should be delivered via a head box in very young children or in

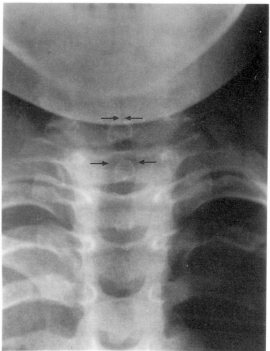

(a)

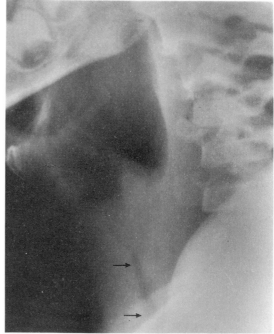

(b)

Figure 24.8 (*a*) Anteroposterior neck X-ray of laryngotracheobronchitis showing 'steeple sign'. (*b*) Lateral X-ray of laryngotracheobronchitis showing 'steeple sign' and 'ballooning of hypopharynx'. Lower arrows show normal trachea and upper arrows narrowed area ('steeple')

a tent with those who are older (Davis *et al.*, 1981). Most parents whose children have had recurrent problems will report the beneficial effects of a steam kettle at home, or a shower, but there has been no controlled trial providing evidence that humidity is efficacious in laryngotracheobronchitis, although there seems to be evidence that spasmodic laryngitis responds to mist therapy (Fogel *et al.*, 1982). However, since it does no harm and probably helps prevent drying of secretions in the respiratory tract, some form of humidity should be given but there is no place for cold mist. Jet nebulizers do not humidify the larynx and ultrasonically generated mist increases airway obstruction in children with abnormally labile airways (Henry, 1983).

The-ideal situation is to have a 'croup room' where the relative humidity of the atmosphere in the whole room can be kept high. Placing the child in a plastic humidified tent, which may increase the anxiety of the child and make careful observation more difficult through the fog, is not recommended, nor is a nebulizer blowing warm, wet air as near as possible to the face of the child. Hydration of the child is essential, with oral fluids if possible. If the child is not willing to drink, then intravenous fluids are necessary.

Oxygen

Oxygen therapy is also controversial. If a decision is made that the child needs an alternative airway, then obviously oxygen is used until the new airway is secured. In less severe cases, there is a view (Welch and Price, 1983) that its use may mask early signs of hypoxia but, on the other hand, Broniatowski (1985) feels that oxygen is mandatory since hypoxia is the most important blood gas abnormality. It is also suggested that supplemental humidified oxygen in the presence of diffuse bronchial involvement will help to prevent reflex bronchoconstriction, sputum retention and pulmonary oedema (Levison, Tabachnik and Newth, 1982). If oxygen is not used for fear of missing cyanosis, it should be pointed out that this is a late clinical sign, when arterial oxygen saturation is less than 40%. The problem with oxygen therapy is in its mode of application. Unless it is given via a face mask, the inspired percentage is variable and certainly the concentration of oxygen in an average plastic tent when 100% is delivered is only 35%. Unless there is evidence of severe bronchial involvement, or a decision has been made to intubate, the routine use of oxygen is not advised because of the fear induced by a face mask. Pulse oximetry should be mandatory and oxygen should be administered based on oxygen saturation.

Steroids

The place of steroids is not agreed, probably because response has not been related to the cause of the airway obstruction. One double-blind trial (Koren *et al.*, 1983), using dexamethasone 0.6 mg/kg as a single dose against placebo, found the steroid to be helpful in spasmodic laryngitis, but not in laryngotracheobronchitis. Severe cases of laryngotracheobronchitis were not accepted into this study and the difficulty in clinically distinguishing spasmodic laryngitis from laryngotracheobronchitis was pointed out. A totally opposite opinion was expressed in another report (Asher and Beaudry, 1981), where steroids were found to have a dramatic effect on laryngotracheobronchitis but not on spasmodic laryngitis. A previous study showed no significant benefit from steroid usage (Eden, Kaufman and Yu, 1967). On the other hand, Walker and Crysdale (1992) stated that there is evidence that they are of benefit in laryngotracheobronchitis, particularly if used earlier in the course of the disease.

Since there is confusion the author feels, therefore that the routine use of steroids is not recommended except possibly as a last resort to resuscitate a child in the hope of avoiding intubation, and occasionally to reduce oedema prior to extubation if this has previously failed or to reduce the duration of, and thus the complications of intubation.

Antibiotics

There is no evidence that antibiotics are of benefit in viral laryngotracheobronchitis except when secondary bacterial bronchitis supervenes. Bacterial laryngotracheitis (pseudomembranous croup) is probably a separate disease and since *Staphylococcus aureus* is normally the causative organism, flucloxacillin is given.

In practice, most children who are intubated for laryngotracheobronchitis receive antibiotics which are changed depending on the culture sensitivities from aspirates.

Racemic adrenalin (epinephrine)

There has been enthusiasm for this form of treatment in the USA, Canada, Australia and more recently the UK (Walker and Crysdale, 1992). According to Fogel *et al.* (1982) racemic adrenalin, nebulized and delivered by intermittent positive pressure breathing (IPPB) seems effective in uncontrolled studies, but in controlled studies it has been shown to be no more effective than nebulized saline. Fogel *et al.* (1982) designed a randomized trial whereby nebulized racemic adrenalin was compared with its delivery via intemittent positive pressure breathing. They included only patients who failed to respond to nebulized saline. The results show that a delivery via intemittent positive pressure breathing was not necessary for the effect and that it did reduce obstruction for up to 30 minutes in laryngotracheobronchitis. Spasmodic laryngitis responded to normal saline mist alone. These authors used 0.25 ml of 2.25% racemic adrenalin diluted with isotonic saline, nebulized and given via a tight-fitting face mask. Continuous ECG monitoring is necessary and there are dangers of a rebound effect. It is therefore only appropriate as a hospital management. The use of a tight fitting mask is controversial and because of its uncertain value the use of this treatment as a routine form of therapy is not recommended. However, in severe croup, adrenalin inhalation may buy a little time while intubation is undertaken and may render induction of anaesthesia less fraught.

Summary of management of laryngotracheobronchitis

Since only 1% of children with laryngotracheobronchitis fail to respond to conservative management, however controversial, the main reason for admission to hospital is to observe and secure an airway should that be necessary. Recommended management includes effective reassurance and possibly efficient humidification. It does not include routine use of oxygen, steroids, antibiotics or racemic adrenalin. Careful monitoring of the progress of the child is the most important aspect.

Monitoring of laryngotracheobronchitis

As mentioned previously, croup scoring systems have been suggested. They are useful as an initial baseline measurement but need to be continuously updated by the same nurses and the same medical staff, since they are very subjective. Objective methods of monitoring include pulse and respiration rates and blood gas estimation. Blood gas analysis is only used on rare occasions because it is a disturbing and painful procedure. It is necessary when there is significant bronchial involvement. Unfortunately, transcutaneous oxygen and carbon dioxide probes are not easy to use in restless children as the transducers move and their readings are unreliable, and pulse oximetry may be more valuable.

A quarter-hourly pulse rate charted from a monitor is of most value. Respiration rates can also be used and, according to Newth, Levison and Brown (1972), they correlate best with arterial oxygen tension. In practice, it is often a combination of a falling pulse rate, relaxation of a restless child, quietening of stridor and maintenance of a good colour that suggests favourable progress. There is no substitute for experience in assessing this condition and a good deal can be learnt by trainee doctors and nurses sitting for 2 or 3 hours with the child and observing progress. If a decision is made that a child needs an alternative airway, the same anaesthetic care is required as was described for epiglottitis.

Management of retropharyngeal abscess

As mentioned in the description of the clinical features of this infection, a lateral neck X-ray (see Figure 24.6) is the most reliable method of establishing the diagnosis. CT scanning has also been shown to be of value, especially in assessing the extent of the abscess cavity (White, 1985). This makes it easier to decide which route to use for drainage. X-rays, however, must be interpreted correctly and a true lateral X-ray is necessary (Seid, Dunbar and Cotton, 1979).

Normal variance must not be confused with disease, for instance neck flexion causes a widening of the retropharyngeal space and a reversed lordosis of the cervical spine can be caused by any condition that gives rise to muscle spasm and not just by infection. A useful rule is that the anteroposterior diameter of the prevertebral soft tissues should not exceed the diameter of the vertebral bodies. Pathological lesions of the vertebral bodies and discs must also be excluded. A chest X-ray needs to be performed to exclude spread from the neck into the posterior mediastinum. Providing that the child is not in immediate danger of serious airway embarrassment and if the X-rays suggest a retropharyngeal abscess, intravenous antibiotics should be the first line of treatment. *Staphylococcus aureus*, *Staphylococcus pyogenes* and anaerobic bacteria are the most common organisms in deep neck space infections (White, 1985). It is personal practice to use a combination of penicillin, flucloxacillin and metronidazole in appropriate doses for the weight of the child. Walker and Crysdale (1992) use clindamycin because of the increased incidence of infection due to Gram-negative rods and β-lactamase-producing organisms.

If the airway is compromised, or if there is no response to antibiotic therapy, drainage will be necessary. The safety of modern anaesthesia is such that, with an experienced anaesthetist, intubation is possible without trauma. A danger exists, however, of rupturing the abscess before the airway is secured or stripping the abscess into the posterior mediastinum.

Once the child is safely intubated, the posterior pharyngeal wall can be examined using a standard tonsillectomy gag. The abscess can then be aspirated or incised through the pharynx. External approaches, either anterior or posterior to the sternomastoid muscle have been suggested (Levitt, 1976) and are appropriate if extension of the abscess has occurred into the parapharyngeal space or posterior mediastinum. Cultures of the pus can now be obtained and the antibiotic therapy adjusted depending on the bacteria found.

It is recommended that intubation is continued for at least 24 hours after aspiration or incision of the abscess, or until there is an obvious clinical improvement in the child's condition as judged by radiology and settling of the pyrexia.

Choice and care of an alternative airway in inflammatory laryngeal obstruction

Tracheostomy is discussed in Chapter 26 and only brief comments relevant to the infected airway will be made here.

The choice as to whether endotracheal intubation or tracheostomy is performed may be a personal one or may be dependent upon local nursing services. There is no doubt that specialized intensive care facilities are necessary for the management of endotracheal tubes, whereas tracheostomy care, although intensive in the first few hours, needs less specialist facilities. Therefore, individual hospitals will have different criteria depending on local circumstances. The mortality rates between the two modalities of intubation and tracheostomy for epiglottitis are said to be very similar at 0.92% and 0.86% respectively. However, Friedberg and Morrison (1974) demonstrated a 3% mortality rate due to childhood tracheostomy from pneumothoraces and displacement or obstruction of the tube.

The differences in morbidity rates are more striking. Mitchell and Thomas (1980) reporting a series of 2567 patients with laryngotracheobronchitis admitted to the Hospital for Sick Children, Toronto, stated that 2% required airway support. With tracheostomy the tubes were placed for a mean time of 11 days, whereas endotracheal tubes stayed *in situ* for only 6 days. There were no deaths in the tracheostomy group, but there was one fatality caused by airway obstruction in the children treated with endotracheal tubes. Despite this, their preferred management has changed from tracheostomy tubes to endotracheal tubes, but they do emphasize the need for experienced nursing care in the management of the intubated patient.

Endotracheal intubation

Whether intubation is via naso- or oroendotracheal routes, the major complications are tube obstruction and accidental extubation. Occasionally multiple intubations are necessary to replace blocked tubes or because of failed trials of extubation. Mitchell and Thomas (1980) found that there were no cases of subglottic stenosis from intubation, but it did occur four times in 30 tracheostomies.

It must be emphasized that an endotracheal tube used in an inflammatory disease of the larynx will pass through the affected site. It is therefore essential that good fixation of the tube is achieved and that the child is sedated enough to avoid struggling which might cause movements of the tube and further damage the inflamed larynx. The vocal cords are, of course, splinted apart by the tube and this prevents the child from being able to cough or talk. A nasogastric tube is also necessary for feeding. Expert nursing care is obviously required, not only to manage the above problems, but also to provide adequate humidity and regular aspiration of the tube to prevent obstruction.

The type of the tube is a matter of personal preference. Most units use polyvinyl chloride (PVC) endotracheal tubes. It may be sensible to spray these with a silicone compound to increase lubrication of the tube. Silastic tubes are available but are expensive and have a thicker wall which tends to increase the size of the tube necessary to maintain adequate ventilation. The size of the tube is extremely important. It should be as small as possible to prevent traumatizing already damaged tissue. A rough guide to the size of the tube needed in normal patients without inflammatory airway disease can be worked out by the formula of dividing the child's age by four and adding 4.5 mm. It is recommended that a tube one size smaller than would be required for the normal child is selected for the inflamed larynx. Epiglottitis is often managed by applying a continuous positive airway pressure circuit to the endotracheal tube as there is usually no lower airway involvement. In laryngotracheobronchitis, however, mechanical ventilation may be required as secretions lead to lower airway occlusion and lobar collapse or pneumonia.

Fixation of a nasotracheal tube is easier than an orotracheal tube and requires a brace onto the forehead. Regular aspiration with suction catheters is necessary to prevent accumulation of secretions. Humidification is vital to prevent the secretions becoming too tenacious. This may take the form of a warm nebulizer attached by a T-tube to the endotracheal tube with or without added oxygen depending on the child's blood gases. Humidification may be supplemented by the installation of 2 ml of normal saline immediately prior to aspiration. The suction catheters used should be graduated and measured against the known length of the endotracheal tube. It is important that the catheter tube goes beyond the endotracheal tube to clear it, but not so far that it continually abrades the carina of the trachea, thereby causing a granuloma. Regular physiotherapy is essential to prevent bronchopneumonia. Extubation is usually possible within 48 hours with epiglottitis but, as mentioned previously, 6 days seems an average length of time in laryngotracheobronchitis (Mitchell and Thomas, 1980). Every child will be different but it would seem reasonable to attempt extubation when there is no evidence of any chest infection and the secretions are less tenacious. There should be an obvious leak around the tube indicating that the oedema has lessened. It may be worth using corticosteroids for 6 hours prior to extubation to reduce any postintubation oedema. Racemic adrenalin can also be used via a nebulizer prior to extubation for similar purposes. Once the child has been extubated, then efficient humidification is necessary as is very careful observation for the first few hours. Within an hour or two it is usually obvious whether the child will be able to cope without re-intubation. The parents will need to be reassured about the very weak, husky voice that often follows prolonged intubation, but this is usually nearly back to normal within 24 hours.

Tracheostomy

The main advantages of tracheostomy are that the disease process is bypassed, the child does not need sedating and normal feeding is usually possible. Occlusion of the tube with a finger on expiration or with the use of a valve allows talking and coughing to occur. However, tracheostomy has its disadvantages. The mortality rate and increased length of time before extubation is possible have already been mentioned. The operation of tracheostomy leaves a scar which, in some instances, can be quite unsightly. Although tracheostomy on the whole requires less skilled nursing care, there is a risk of accidental extubation, especially on return from the operating theatre. It may be extremely difficult to replace the tube, with disastrous consequences.

A less serious complication, but nevertheless, a well-recognized one, is pneumothorax and air tracking in the neck. It is recommended that immediately after a tracheostomy has been performed a chest X-ray is carried out to make sure there is no pneumothorax present. It is also recommended that on the first postoperative day a lateral neck X-ray is taken to ensure that the tracheostomy tube is in line with the trachea and not causing backward displacement of the anterior wall of the trachea immediately above the tracheostomy site. If this complication is seen on X-ray it is worth changing the tracheostomy tube for one with a different shape which will not produce this deformity. If it is unrecognized, then there may be permanent tracheal stenosis which will cause difficulty in extubation.

A personal preference in design of tracheostomy tube is the Great Ormond Street pattern which is usually made from polyvinyl chloride (PVC). Silastic may be a preferable material. Although this does not have the advantage of an inner tube or a fenestra and valve to aid in extubation, it becomes soft at body temperature and moulds itself well to the correct shape of the trachea.

In ideal situations, it would seem that endotracheal intubation is preferable to tracheostomy as an alternative airway in acute laryngeal inflammatory obstruction in childhood.

References

ANDREASSEN, U. K., BEAR, S., NIELSEN, T. G., DHAM, S. L. and ARNDAL, H. (1992) Acute epiglottitis – 25 year experience with nasotracheal intubation, current management policy and future trends. *Journal of Laryngology and Otology*, **106**, 1072–1075

ASHER, M. I. and BEAUDRY, P. H. (1981) Croup and corticosteroid therapy. *Journal of Pediatrics*, **97**, 506–507

BRODINSKI, M. and HOLYOKE, E. A. (1938) The fascia and fascial spaces of the head, neck and adjacent regions. *American Journal of Anatomy*, **63**, 367–408

BRONIATOWSKI, M. (1985) Epiglottitis. *Ear, Nose and Throat Journal*, **64**, 22–27

BUTT, W., SHANN, E., WALKER, D., WILLIAMS, J., DUNCAN, A. and PHELAN, P. (1988) Acute epiglottitis: a different approach to management. *Critical Care Medicine*, **16**, 43–47

CANTRELL, R. W., BELL, R. A. and MORIOKA, W. T. (1978) Acute epiglottitis: intubation versus tracheostomy. *Laryngoscope*, **88**, 994–1005

DALE, A. and COURT, S. (1990) *Haemophilus influenzae* infections in siblings: the need for prophylaxis. *Archives of Disease in Childhood*, **65**, 489–490

DAVIS, H. W., GARTNER, J. C., GALVIS, A. G., MICHAELS, R. H. and MESTAD, P. H. (1981) Acute upper airway obstruction: croup and epiglottitis. *Pediatric Clinics of North America*, **28**, 859–880

DENNY, F. W., MURPHY, T. F., CLYDE, W. A. COLLIER, A. M. and HENDERSON, F. W., (1983) Croup: an 11 year study in pediatric practice. *Pediatrics*, **71**, 871–876

DRAKE-LEE, A. B., BROUGHTON, S. J. and GRACE, A. (1984) Children with epiglottitis. *British Journal of Clinical Practice*, **38**, 218–220

EDEN, A. N., KAUFMAN, A. and YU, R. (1967) Corticosteroids and croup. *Journal of the American Medical Association*, **200**, 133

EMMERSON, S. G. P., RICHMAN, B. and SPAHN, T. (1991) Changing patterns of epiglottis in children. *Otolaryngology, Head and Neck Surgery*, **104**, 287–292

FEARON, B. (1975) Acute epiglottitis: a potential killer. *Canadian Medical Association Journal*, **112**, 760

FOGEL, J. M., BERG, I. J., GERBER, M. A. and SCHERTER, C. B. (1982) Racemic epinephrine in the treatment of croup: nebulization alone versus nebulization with intermittent positive pressure breathing. *Journal of Pediatrics*, **101**, 1028–1031

FRIEDBERG, J. and MORRISON, M. D. (1974) Paediatric tracheotomy. *Canadian Journal of Otolaryngology*, **3**, 147–155

FRIEDMAN, E. M., JORGENSEN, K., HEALY, G. B. and MAGILL, T. J. I. (1985) Bacterial tracheitis – 2 year experience. *Laryngoscope*, **95**, 9–11

GOEL, K. M. (1984) Are neck radiographs necessary in the management of croup syndrome? *Archives of Diseases of Childhood*, **59**, 980

HALL, C. B. and HALL, W. J. (1975) Viral croup: acute laryngotracheobronchitis. *Update*, **10**, 561

HENRY, R. (1983) Moist air in the treatment of laryngotracheitis. *Archives of Diseases of Childhood*, **59**, 577

KESSLER, A., WETMORE, R. F. and MARSH, R.R. (1993) Childhood epiglottitis in recent years. *International Journal of Pediatric Otorhinolaryngology*, **25**, 155–162

KOREN, G., FRAND, M., BARZILAY, Z and MACLEOD, S. M. (1983) Corticosteroid treatment of laryngotracheitis v spasmodic croup in children. *American Journal of Diseases of Children*, **137**, 941–944

LEVISON, H., TABACHNIK, E. and NEWTH, C. J. L. (1982) Wheezing in infancy, croup and epiglottitis. *Current Problems in Paediatrics*, **12**, 38–60

LEVITT, G. W. (1976) Cervical fascia and deep neck infections. *Otolaryngologic Clinics of North America*, **9**, 703–716

MARGOLIS, C. Z. (1980) Definition of croup. *Journal of Pediatrics*, **96**, 1123–1124

MILNER, A. D. (1984) Acute stridor in the pre-school child. *British Medical Journal*, **28**, 811–812

MITCHELL, D. P. and THOMAS, R. L. (1980) Secondary airway support in the management of croup. *Journal of Otolaryngology*, **9**, 419–422

NEWTH, C. J. L., LEVISON, H. and BROWN, A. C. (1972) The respiratory status of children with croup. *Journal of Pediatrics*, **84**, 1068

PHILPOTT-HOWARD, J. and WILLIAMS, J. D. (1982) Increase in antibiotic resistance in *Haemophilus influenzae* in the UK since 1977: report of a study group. *British Medical Journal*, **284**, 1597–1599

PRACY, R. (1979) Congenital diseases of the larynx. In: *Scott-Brown's Diseases of the Ear, Nose and Throat*, 4th edn, vol. 4, edited by J. Ballantyne and J. Groves. London: Butterworths. pp. 308–328

SCHWARTZ, R. H., KNERR, R. J., HERMANSEN, K. and WIENTZEN, R. L. (1982) Acute epiglottitis caused by beta-hemolytic group C streptococci. *American Journal of Diseases of Children*, **136**, 558–559

SEID, A. B., DUNBAR, J. S. and COTTON, R. T. (1979) Retropharyngeal abscesses in children revisited. *Laryngoscope*, **89**, 1717–1724

SINGER, J. I. and MCCABE, J. B. (1988) Epiglottitis at the extremes of age. *Journal of Emergency Medicine*, **6**, 228–231

SOLIMAN, M. G. and RICHER, P. (1978) Epiglottitis and pulmonary oedema in children *Canadian Anaesthetic Society*, **20**, 270–275

STEVENS, D. L., WALKER, D. H. and SCHAFFNER, W. (1981) Pseudodiphtheria: prominent pharyngeal membrane associated with fatal paraquat ingestion. *Annals of Internal Medicine*, **94**, 202–204

TARNOW-MORDI, W. D. BERRILL, A. M., DARBY, C. W., DAVIS, P. and POOK, J. (1985) Precipitation of laryngeal obstruction in acute epiglottitis. *British Medical Journal*, **290**, 629

TUCKER, J. A. (1979) Obstruction of the major pediatric airway. *Otolaryngologic Clinics of North America*, **12**, 329–341

WALKER, P. and CRYSDALE, W. S. (1992) Croup, epiglottitis, retropharyngeal abscess and bacterial tracheitis: evolving patterns of occurrence and care. *International Anaesthesiology Clinics*, **30**, 57–70

WELCH, D. B. and PRICE, D. G. (1983) Acute epiglottitis and severe croup. Experience in two English regions. *Anaesthesia*, **38**, 754–759

WHITE, B. (1985) Deep neck infections and respiratory distress in children. *Ear, Nose and Throat Journal*, **64**, 30–38

WILLIAMS, P. A., ARMITAGE, E. N., FISHER, N. G. and HATCHER, G. W. (1985) Precipitation of laryngeal obstruction in acute epiglottitis. *British Medical Journal*, **290**, 1007

ZACH, M. S. (1983) Airway reactivity in recurrent croup. *European Journal of Respiratory Disease*, **128** (Suppl.), 81–88

25

Foreign bodies in the larynx and trachea

J. N. G. Evans

Even the most experienced of endoscopists would agree that the prospect of having to deal with a very young child with a history of possible inhalation of a foreign body fills them with some trepidation – not only because of the demands that the removal of a foreign body makes on their skill as an endoscopist, but also because of the unpredictability in the degree of difficulty of the procedure. The degree of difficulty will depend on a number of factors: the age of the patient, the type of foreign body inhaled, the interval between inhalation and removal, the skill of the anaesthetist and the equipment available.

A strong case can be made for every 6-month-old child with a suspected peanut in the bronchus being referred to a specialist centre for its removal.

Modern techniques of endoscopic removal of bronchial foreign bodies stem from the advances made in the early part of the century by Chevalier Jackson, who reduced the mortality of removal of foreign bodies from over 20% to approximately 2%. He achieved a 98% success rate of bronchoscopic removal of foreign bodies, all the procedures being performed under local anaesthesia.

Since then improvement in the illumination provided by the Hopkins rod lens system and the advent of the ventilating bronchoscope (Hopkins, 1976), coupled with the advances in anaesthesia, have further reduced the mortality and greatly facilitated the task of the endoscopist (Tucker, 1985). Most paediatric endoscopists use these instruments and perform the removal of the foreign body under general anaesthesia (Gans and Berci, 1971).

Other techniques such as postural drainage (Burrington and Cotton, 1972; Campbell, Cotton and Lilly, 1982), the Heimlich (1975) manoeuvre and the introduction of fingers into the pharynx in an attempt to remove the foreign body, are to be deprecated, since these manipulations may dislodge the foreign body

and cause total respiratory obstruction and hypoxic cardiac arrest.

Incidence

The maximum incidence of inhalation of foreign bodies occurs between the age of 1 and 3 years: 74% of 115 patients (Brown and Clark, 1983) and 77% of 225 patients (Rothman and Boeckman, 1980); 74% in a much larger series (Jackson and Jackson, 1936). Holinger (1962) found that children under 4 years old constituted 55% of their series of foreign bodies, but their cases included adults.

The most common cause of accidental death in the home in children under 6 years of age is the inhalation of a foreign body (National Safety Council of America, 1980). It is estimated that almost 600 children under 15 years old die each year in the USA from asphyxia following the aspiration or ingestion of large foreign bodies. The peak incidence of inhalation of foreign bodies in early childhood is of course related to the fact that children have a habit of putting objects into their mouths to determine their texture and taste, and to chew on when teething. It is extremely important, therefore, where possible to keep objects which might be inhaled out of the reach of small children. Table 25.1 shows the types of foreign body removed in Rothman's series (Rothman and Boeckman, 1980). Boys are more likely to inhale foreign bodies than girls by almost 2:1 (Rothman and Boeckman, 1980; Brown and Clark, 1983; O'Neill, Holcomb and Neblett, 1983; Schloss, Pham–Dang and Rosales, 1983). The reasons for this are not clear!

A minority of these objects impact in the larynx; 4% in Cohen's series (Cohen *et al.*, 1980) were removed from the larynx. Foreign bodies lodge in the

Table 25.1 Type of foreign body

Type	Number
Portion of nut	86
Food	32
Carrot	18
Popcorn	8
Fruit (stem/seed)	5
Bone	8
Plastic	27
Metal	19
Tooth	4
Stone	4
Timothy hay	4
Bead	2
Mucus	2
Balloon	1
Crayon	1
Wood	1
Paper	1
Acorn	1
Pine needle	1

From Rothmann and Boeckman (1980).

Table 25.2 Duration of enlodgement

Duration	Number
2–8 hours	24
8–24 hours	35
1–5 days	14
5–10 days	14
10–30 days	19
1–6 months	9
6 months–1 year	2
Longer	1

From Cohen *et al.* (1980).

larynx if they are too large to pass through or if they are of an irregular shape or have sharp edges which can catch on the laryngeal mucosa. Egg shells and fragments of glass or plastic are not infrequent offenders.

History

In most cases of inhaled foreign body, there is a definite history of choking followed by paroxysmal coughing which then subsides. In 85% of the patients in Rothman's series (Rothman and Boeckman, 1980) a positive history of aspiration was obtained but in some patients this positive history was only obtained retrospectively, after removal of the foreign body (Cohen, 1981).

After the initial paroxysm of coughing the tracheo-bronchial mucosa becomes tolerant of the foreign body and coughing ceases. This feature is often responsible for delays in diagnosis – 18% of cases of foreign body were diagnosed one week and 8% one month after the event (Rothman and Boeckman, 1980). In Cohen's series, 50% of the cases were recognized and treated within 24 hours and, by 10 days, 74% of the cases had been treated, 26% of the cases being diagnosed between 10 days and one month (Cohen *et al.*, 1980) (Table 25.2). In a series of 51 cases of foreign body reported by Ross and McCormick (1980) there was no history of aspiration in 8%. One symptom of the triad – coughing, choking and wheeze – was present in 91% of patients with foreign body aspiration (Black *et al.*, 1984).

A history of wheeze, often diagnosed and treated as asthma, is the next most common symptom. Sudden onset of a wheeze in a child not previously known to have asthma, should alert one to the possibility of a foreign body being the cause – especially if the wheeze is predominantly unilateral. Unexplained persistent fever, a fever associated with persistent respiratory symptoms which continues in spite of treatment, and persistent or recurrent lobar pneumonia demand a diagnostic bronchoscopy to exclude a foreign body (Hoeve, Rombout and Pot, 1993).

Most endoscopists have, on some occasion, found an unsuspected foreign body at routine endoscopy for other reasons. The author has removed the horizontal limb of a Montgomery 'T' tube from the trachea of a child with laryngeal stenosis. There was no history of any previous treatment of his stenosis and the plastic tube was found quite by chance at routine endoscopy.

Acute respiratory distress is, fortunately, an uncommon but most alarming presentation of an inhaled foreign body. Fourteen or 6% of the patients in Rothman's series (Rothman and Boeckman, 1980) presented with respiratory distress, five of these patients having had a laryngeal foreign body. Pain at the root of the neck or over the larynx also suggests the presence of a laryngeal foreign body. Large oesophageal foreign bodies may compress the trachea and cause symptoms of respiratory obstruction. Sharp and long-standing oesophageal foreign bodies may produce a fistula between the oesophagus and trachea and cause respiratory symptoms (Yee, Schild and Holinger, 1975).

Clinical examination

A general examination of the child is essential. Respiratory distress or cyanosis demands immediate action; special care should be taken during the induction of anaesthesia in these patients since the foreign body may change position and completely obstruct the airway.

Inhaled foreign bodies are more common in children with upper respiratory tract infections, caused presumably by mouth breathing and the presence of a cough – inhalation of food particles may easily occur with the sharp intake of breath which follows a cough.

If there is a change in the child's cry or if the cry becomes hoarse or stridulous, a laryngeal foreign body should be suspected. Excessive salivation may also occur.

In the first few hours after aspiration the signs in the chest are due to changes in air flow through the tracheobronchial tree. These changes may be detected with a stethoscope on auscultation of the chest. An audible click may be heard due to movement of the foreign body up and down the trachea; a fluttering noise may also be detected due to rapid oscillation of the object in the air stream in the trachea or main bronchi. A unilateral expiratory wheeze and reduced air entry may indicate a foreign body in the bronchus.

Obstructive emphysema may be detected by mediastinal shifts, but is most easily detected radiologically and will be discussed more fully later in the chapter.

If the foreign body is not removed within 24 hours pneumonic signs supervene. The severity of these signs will depend on the reaction of the bronchial mucosa and the size of the foreign body (Strome, 1977). If the foreign body is of vegetable origin an intense inflammatory reaction of the bronchial mucosa occurs, ultimately with the production of granulation tissue. The mucosal swelling and inflammatory exudate may then obstruct the bronchial lumen, causing atelectasis of the distal lung. A lung abscess may supervene but this takes several months. An unusual complication of a foreign body in the bronchus, namely a brain abscess, was reported by Spencer et al. (1981) – a child inhaled a grass head which entered the bronchus, stem first. This enabled the grass head to migrate peripherally, causing pneumonia and a lung abscess, which in turn caused a cerebral abscess. The time interval between inhalation and development of the brain abscess was 3 months.

Dry vegetable foreign bodies, e.g. a bean, cause very rapid obstructive changes due to a combination of mucosal irritation and swelling of the bean itself by hygroscopic action. Atelectasis of the occluded segment of lung occurs with the utmost rapidity in this type of foreign body.

The presence of florid granulation tissue around the inhaled foreign body may also cause haemoptysis. It occurred in 6% of cases in a series reported by Ross and McCormick (1980). Haemoptysis itself is a rather uncommon symptom in children. Tom, Weisman and Handler (1980) investigated 40 patients who presented with this symptom and found 15% of the cases were due to a foreign body.

If the foreign body is made of ferrous metal or it has a particularly rough surface, some bronchial

irritation will occur, but the process of bronchial occlusion will take much longer.

If the foreign body is inert and has a smooth surface, very little mucosal reaction takes place and pneumonic changes may never supervene.

Radiological findings

X-ray examination of the patient must be performed and should include all the structures from the nasopharynx to the tuberosities of the ischia, otherwise a foreign body may be overlooked (Jackson and Jackson, 1936). X-rays should be taken with the neck extended with anteroposterior and lateral views. Anteroposterior views in expiration and inspiration should be taken, although these views are sometimes difficult to obtain in very young children. A lateral chest X-ray completes the examination.

Screening may also help, but standard X-rays are usually sufficient (Gaafar et al., 1982). Computerized tomographic studies may help to show a foreign body not seen with conventional studies (Berger, Kuhn and Kuhns, 1980). Isotope scans will demonstrate changes in ventilation and perfusion of lung tissues. These more sophisticated radiographic techniques are rarely necessary in obvious cases of inhaled foreign bodies. They should not be ordered if they delay the definitive endoscopic assessment of the patient.

Obstructive emphysema

Obstructive emphysema is produced by a valvular obstruction to the expiratory air stream due to the presence of a foreign body in the lumen of the air passage. It also occurs in endogenous extrinsic compression of the intrathoracic air passages. The action of the valve is due to the fact that the air passages dilate on inspiration and contract on expiration. Thus, on each respiration, a small volume of air is trapped beyond the obstruction and the lung is literally pumped up with air during each phase of the respiratory cycle (Figure 25.1). There is mediastinal shift during expiration to the unobstructed side of the chest; in inspiration the mediastinum may be in the midline (Figures 25.2 and 25.3). In atelectasis of the lung, mediastinal shift occurs towards the obstructed side of the chest, the mediastinum remaining deviated during inspiration and expiration. Tables 25.3 and 25.4 show the relative incidence of radiological findings in the Rothman (Rothman and Boeckman, 1980) and Black series (Black et al., 1984).

Positive plain X-ray evidence suggestive of a foreign body was obtained in 81% of patients in a review by Black et al. (1984), who also reported 88% of radiographic screenings to be positive. Normal radiographs were noted in approximately 10% of the patients in

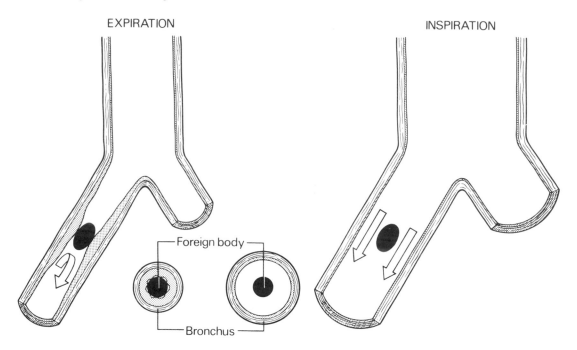

Figure 25.1 Demonstrating the mechanism by which obstructive emphysema occurs with a foreign body in the right main bronchus

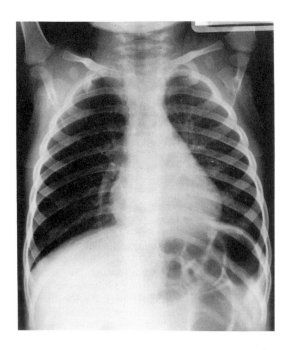

Figure 25.2 X-ray showing obstructive emphysema of the right lung due to the presence of a cashew nut in the right main bronchus, which had been present for one month. Note the radiolucency of the right lung compared with the left

Table 25.3 X-ray findings

Radiographic signs	Patient nos.
Obstructive emphysema	135
Foreign body visualized	31
Atelectasis	27
Pneumonia	18
Normal	17
Mediastinal emphysema	4

From Rothmann and Boeckman (1980).

whom foreign bodies were found at bronchoscopy. The time interval between inhalation and abnormal radiological findings was noted by Baraka (1974) and he found no X-ray evidence of a foreign body within 24 hours of inhalation in his paediatric patients; this figure altered dramatically after 24 hours when abnormal X-rays were noted in 90% of the patients.

Site of foreign body

The majority of foreign bodies come to rest in the right bronchial tree, since the right main bronchus is wider than the left and the interbronchial septum projects to the left. The effect of the inspiratory air currents also determines the site of final impaction

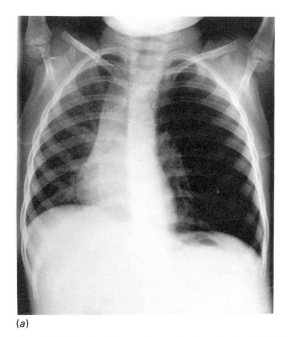
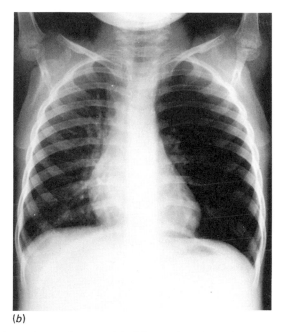

(a)   (b)

Figure 25.3 The two X-rays demonstrate mediastinal shift due to obstructive emphysema of the left main bronchus. The mediastinal shift is to the right and is maximal on expiration (*a*), since the unobstructed right lung can empty more easily. On inspiration (*b*) the mediastinum moves back towards the midline

Table 25.4 Radiographic findings in patients with airway foreign bodies

Radiographic signs	Patients	
	No.	%
Air trapping	91	41
Atelectasis	27	12
Perihilar infiltrates	24	11
Opaque foreign body	24	11
Lobar collapse	4	2
Other	9	4
Normal radiograph	29	13
Radiography not obtained	31	14

From Black *et al.* (1984).

and the anatomical differences between the right and left bronchial septum are of less significance than might be supposed (Moazamn, Talbert and Rodgers, 1983). In Jackson's series (Jackson and Jackson, 1936), 588 foreign bodies were on the right and 322 on the left, a ratio of 1.82:1.

In young children, where the difference is less pronounced, there is a more equal distribution of foreign bodies between the right and left bronchial tree. In Svensson's (1985) series of children only, there were 59 foreign bodies in the right bronchial tree and 46 in the left, a ratio of 1.28:1.

Management

If a foreign body in the respiratory tract is suspected or diagnosed radiologically, endoscopic examination and removal under general anaesthesia is the method of choice. In the case of laryngeal or large tracheal foreign bodies this should be performed as an emergency procedure. If the airway is compromised the endoscopy must be performed immediately with the facilities for performing an emergency tracheostomy. Large tracheal foreign bodies may have to be delivered through a tracheostomy (Swensson *et al.*, 1985). Bowdler and Emery (1985) recorded two cases of unusual foreign bodies in the trachea. In both cases silver tracheostomy tubes became detached from their neck plates – due to failure of the braising material. The tubes had been in use for a number of years, and the inhaled tubes were removed from the tracheostome with some difficulty! If the airway is not compromised the procedure should be performed within hours, allowing suitable time to elapse for the stomach to empty.

Laryngeal foreign bodies are removed by direct laryngoscopy. In the majority of cases this is accomplished without difficulty, often indeed in the anaesthetic room much to the delight of anaesthetic colleagues. Rarely, large foreign bodies may cause total respiratory obstruction during induction of anaesthesia and an emergency tracheostomy will then be necessary. A commonly encountered difficulty in cases of laryngeal foreign body is delay in diagnosis (Moskowitz, Gardiner and Sasaki, 1982).

Tracheal and bronchial foreign bodies are best removed using a rigid bronchoscope. In the absence of respiratory distress the operation should be performed as an elective procedure, by the 'surgical team' that are used to working together in their accustomed operating theatre. Under these 'ideal' circumstances, a 99% success rate for removal of foreign bodies should be achieved. There is no place for endoscopy for a foreign body being performed in an infant by inexperienced personnel in unfamiliar surroundings (Bush and Vivori, 1981).

In the author's opinion the efficiency and safety of rigid bronchoscopy completely supersedes any form of conservative approach using bronchodilators, thoracic percussion and postural drainage (Burrington and Cotton, 1972). Indeed this technique of inhalation and postural drainage may be the cause of severe respiratory obstruction and even hypoxic cardiac arrest if the foreign body is moved and impacts in the subglottis (Kosloske, 1980). Preoperative physiotherapy, together with the administration of antibiotics is, however, useful in patients with a peripherally situated, usually organic, foreign body of long standing, in which there is considerable atelectasis of the lung with pneumonia or a lung abscess. Postoperative physiotherapy is also helpful in expanding areas of atelectatic lung.

In cases where there is granulation tissue present the application of a 10% solution of adrenalin will shrink the granulation and reduce bleeding to a minimum (Harries and Albert, 1993).

In the rare event of being unable to remove a foreign body endoscopically, in spite of satisfactory operating conditions, it must be removed by thoracotomy and bronchotomy. In practice this generally has to be organized as a separate procedure, since the decision to abandon the bronchoscopic attempt at removal is only made after an already prolonged struggle. The author recalls having to abandon a bronchoscopy in a 2-year-old child who had choked on a pebble, after his father, in attempting to remove it with his finger, had pushed it through the laryngeal inlet. The pebble was oval in shape and almost exactly fitted the glottis. Once in the trachea sufficient air was able to pass around it to maintain respiration, but the author was unable to exert sufficient traction with a pair of forceps to pull it back through the larynx. It was successfully removed at thoracotomy the following day.

Technique of removal

In most cases removal of the foreign body is undertaken as an elective procedure – in this instance the surgical, anaesthetic and nursing personnel know

each other and the 'team' are able to perform their allotted tasks efficiently and peacefully. These factors increase the chances of a successful removal of the foreign body and reduce the operative morbidity.

Instruments

A complete set of ventilating bronchoscopes with a Hopkins rod lens system, such as that manufactured by Karl Storz (Figure 25.4) is used by many paediatric endoscopists (Table 25.5). These instruments, by virtue of their superior illumination and optics, which magnify the image nine times, improve the visualization of the foreign body in the infant and young child. The bronchoscopes are equipped with two side channels, one for ventilation and the other for instrumentation and suction.

Table 25.5 Recommended set of Storz bronchoscopes

Diameter (mm)	Length (cm)
2.5 3.0	20
3.0 3.5	25
4.0 5.0 6.0	30

In children where the Storz bronchoscope 3.5 or larger can be used then the combined bronchoscope and grasping forceps (Figures 25.5 and 25.6) are especially helpful in dealing with peanuts and other softer foreign bodies. The endoscopist must make a careful assessment of the forceps space between the foreign body and the bronchial wall so the best position for the insertion of the jaws of the instrument can be determined. The irregular shape of most foreign bodies will allow the forceps to be inserted in the gap between the foreign body and the bronchial wall, thus reducing the risk of pushing it distally and jamming it in the bronchus.

In neonates and infants where the combined bronchoscope and grasping forceps cannot be used then a set of open tube bronchoscopes of the Negus pattern suckling and infant sizes with a swing-arm magnifier (Figure 25.7) should be available and provides a magnification of × 4. The foreign body may need to be removed with Chevalier Jackson foreign body forceps.

In some centres (Kosloske, 1980), Fogarty balloon catheters designed for arterial embolectomy are used particularly in the removal of peanuts (Stein, 1970). The catheter size 3 or 4 is passed down the side-arm of the Storz bronchoscope. The tip of the catheter is passed beyond the foreign body and the balloon is

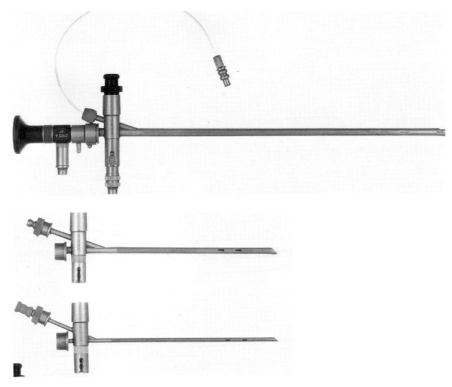

Figure 25.4 Storz ventilating brochoscope

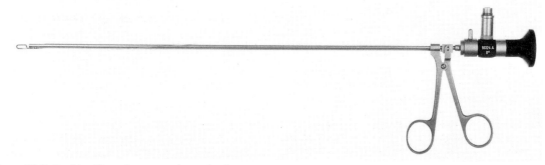

Figure 25.5 Combined bronchoscope and grasping forceps

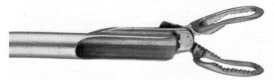

Figure 25.6 Enlarged view of forceps of combined bronchoscope and grasping forceps

inflated with saline (Wiesel *et al.*, 1982; Bannerjee, Khanna and Narayanan, 1984). The telescope is withdrawn approximately 1 cm to allow space for the presenting part of the peanut to be accommodated within the lumen of the bronchoscope as traction is exerted on the Fogarty catheter. The catheter, bronchoscope and foreign body are removed together (Figure 25.8).

The Fogarty catheter is also useful for removing foreign bodies with holes, e.g. beads: the catheter can be threaded through the hole, inflated and the foreign body removed. A Dormia basket used by urologists to remove ureteric calculi may also be used in a similar manner (Dajani, 1971) (Figure 25.9).

Before commencing endoscopy the surgeon must be satisfied that all the equipment is in working order. This applies particularly to the jaws of the

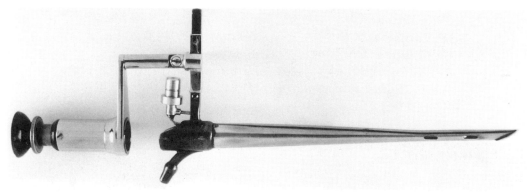

Figure 25.7 Swing-arm magnifier for Negus bronchoscope

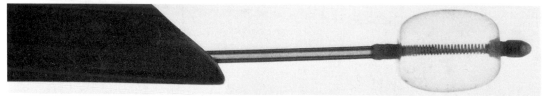

Figure 25.8 Fogarty balloon catheter

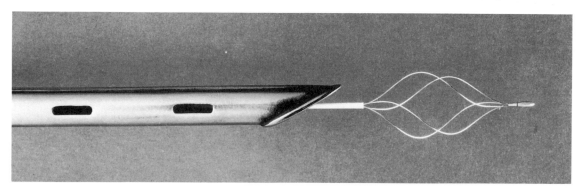

Figure 25.9 Dormia basket

Jackson forceps – these are made of spring steel which tends to rust and, therefore, may jam in the outer casing of the forceps. Suckers must be checked for patency and also that they are long enough to protrude beyond the end of the bronchoscope.

Bronchoscopes and forceps, suitable in size and shape for the case in hand, are selected (Figures 25.10–25.13). Practice passes of the forceps through the chosen bronchoscope are made, the blades of the forceps are inserted into the bronchoscope and then opened. The emergence of the opened forceps beyond the tip of the bronchoscope is felt rather than seen, because of the lack of stereoscopic vision down the bronchoscope. This manoeuvre is practised, while the patient is being anaesthetized, until the surgeon is confident that he will know when the tip of the forceps is just protruding beyond the end of the bronchoscope. This is the correct position for grasping the foreign body (Figure 25.14).

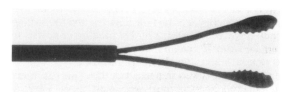

Figure 25.10 Typical Chevalier Jackson grasping forceps

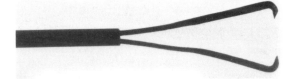

Figure 25.11 Rotation forceps

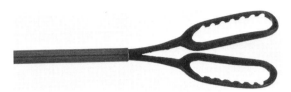

Figure 25.12 Fenestrated forceps – useful for removing peanuts

Figure 25.13 Ball forceps for removal of small hard round objects such as ball-bearings

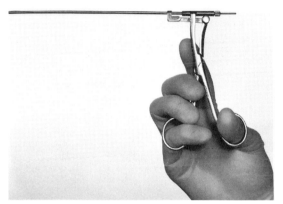

Figure 25.14 Demonstrates the correct method of holding the Chevalier Jackson forceps – traction is made with the index finger in the deviation of the long axis of the forceps

In cases where a particular difficulty is likely to be encountered, e.g. open safety pins or other sharp foreign bodies (Figures 25.15 and 25.16), the use of a dummy tracheobronchial tree and a duplicate foreign body (Figure 25.17) will enable the surgeon to practise the manoeuvre necessary to remove the foreign body safely. Time spent in practice will be amply rewarded by reducing the time spent during the actual endoscopy.

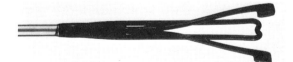

Figure 25.15 Clerf-Arrowsmith safety-pin closing forceps

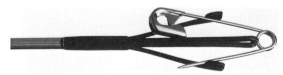

Figure 25.16 Clerf-Arrowsmith safety-pin closing forceps, closing safety pin

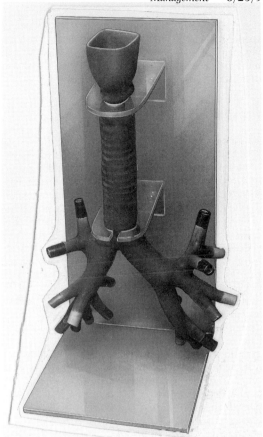

Figure 25.17 Bronchial tree – Manikin (Richard Wolf UK Ltd)

The actual technique of bronchoscopy is described in Volume 5. Special care must be taken in young children to keep the bronchoscope in line with the trachea to ensure adequate ventilation of the patient. Ventilation may be difficult when the bronchoscope is passed deeply into the obstructed bronchus; adequate ventilation will be maintained if the holes in the side of the bronchoscope remain unobstructed, and directed towards the normal main bronchus.

When the precautions mentioned above are taken a successful removal of a foreign body can be achieved in the majority of cases.

Following removal

It is very important after removal of the foreign body, while the child is still anaesthetized, that a *second look* is taken to ensure that a second foreign body has not been overlooked, and to remove any remaining small fragments particularly in the case of peanuts. Pus and mucus can be aspirated from the distal bronchus – speeding the resolution of atelectasis or pneumonia. It is also important to make sure that all major bronchopulmonary segments including the upper lobe orifices are inspected.

If the bronchoscopy is prolonged, or if the broncho-scope was noted to be a tight fit in the subglottic larynx, the use of a systemic corticosteroid, dexamethasone 0.5 mg/kg, is advised to reduce the incidence of laryngeal oedema postoperatively.

Prevention

The vast majority of cases of inhaled or ingested foreign bodies occur as a result of carelessness either in the preparation or ingestion of food or drinks, or as a result of placing inedible or unsuitable objects in the mouth. The accidental inhalation or ingestion of foreign bodies is therefore almost entirely preventable. Infants and children under the age of 2 years should not be allowed to eat peanuts, and their play areas should be cleared of small objects that could be inhaled. Adults should set a good example by never placing pins or tacks in their mouths. The long-term deleterious effects of a foreign body on the lung parenchyma, such as lung abscesses or bronchiectasis, are also preventable provided that the medical attendant of the child always considers the possibility that a foreign body may be present (Clerf, 1952), even in a case where a good history of inhalation has not been obtained, in a patient who develops a wheeze where asthma has not been previously diagnosed, or when pneumonic signs persist for a longer period than one would expect. In such cases a bronchoscopy should always be performed.

References

BANERJEE, A., KHANNA, S. K. and NARAYANAN, P. S. (1984) Use of Fogarty catheters for removal of tracheobronchial foreign bodies (letter). *Chest*, **85**, 452

BARAKA, A. (1974) Bronchoscopic removal of inhaled foreign bodies in children. *British Journal of Anaesthesia*, **46**, 125–126

BERGER, P. E., KUHN, J. P. and KUHNS, L. R. (1980) Computed tomography and the occult tracheobronchial foreign body. *Radiology*, **134**, 133–135

BLACK, R. E., CHOI, K. J., SYME, W. C., JOHNSON, D. G. and MATLAK, M. E. (1984) Bronchoscopic removal of aspirated foreign bodies in children. *American Journal of Surgery*, **148**, 778–781

BOWDLER, D. A. and EMERY, P. J. (1985) Tracheostomy tube fatigue. An unusual cause of inhaled foreign body. *Journal of Laryngology and Otology*, **99**, 517–521

BROWN, T. C. and CLARK, C. M. (1983) Inhaled foreign bodies in children. *Medical Journal of Australia*, **2**, 322–326

BURRINGTON, J. D. and COTTON, E. K. (1972) Removal of foreign bodies from the tracheobronchial tree. *Journal of Pediatric Surgery*, **7**, 119–122

BUSH, G. H. and VIVORI, E. (1981) How to remove a foreign body from the trachea and bronchial tree (letter). *British Journal of Hospital Medicine*, **26**, 102

CAMPBELL, D. N., COTTON, E. K. and LILLY, J. R. (1982) A dual approach to tracheobronchial foreign bodies in children. *Surgery*, **91**, 178–182

CLERF, L. H. (1952) Historical aspects of foreign bodies in the air and food passages. *Annals of Otology, Rhinology and Laryngology*, **61**, 5–17

COHEN, S. R. (1981) Unusual presentations and problems created by mismanagement of foreign bodies in the aerodigestive tract of the pediatric patient. *Annals of Otology, Rhinology and Laryngology*, **90**, 316–322

COHEN, S. R., HERBERT, W. I., LEWIS, G. B. JR and GELLER, K. A. (1980) Foreign bodies in the airway. Five-year retrospective study with special reference to management. *Annals of Otology, Rhinology and Laryngology*, **89**, 437–442

DAJANI, A. M. (1971) 'Bronchial foreign body' removed with a Dormia basket. *Lancet*, i, 1076–1077

GAAFAR, H., ABDEL–DAYEM, M., TALAAT, M. and MANDOUR, M. (1982) The value of X-ray examination in the diagnosis of tracheobronchial foreign bodies in infants and children. *Journal of Otorhinolaryngology and its Related Specialties*, **44**, 340–348

GANS, S. L. and BERCI, G. (1971) Advances in endoscopy of infants and children. *Journal of Pediatric Surgery*, **6**, 199–234

HARRIES, M. L. and ALBERT, D. M. (1993) Bronchoscopic foreign bodies: overcoming granulation tissue, *Journal of Otolaryngology*, **22**, 134

HEIMLICH, H. J. (1975) A life saving manoeuvre to prevent food choking. *Journal of the American Medical Association*, **234**, 398–401

HOEVE, L. J., ROMBOUT, J. and POT, D. J. (1993) Foreign body aspiration in children. The diagnostic value of signs, symptoms and pre-operative examination. *Clinical Otolaryngology*, **18**, 55–57

HOLINGER, P. H. (1962) Foreign bodies in the food and air passages. *Transactions of the American Academy of Ophthalmology and Otolaryngology*, **66**, 193–210

HOPKINS, H. H. (1976) *Endoscopy*. New York: Appleton Century Crofts. p. 17

JACKSON, C. and JACKSON, C. L. (1936) *Diseases of the Air and Food Passages of Foreign Body Origin*. Philadelphia: W. B. Saunders

KOSLOSKE, A. M. (1980) Tracheobronchial foreign bodies in children: back to the bronchoscope and a balloon. *Pediatrics*, **66**, 321–323

KOSLOSKE, A. M. (1982) Bronchoscopic extraction of aspirated foreign bodies in children. *American Journal of Diseases of Children*, **136**, 924–927

MOAZAMN, F., TALBERT, J. L. and RODGERS, B. M. (1983) Foreign bodies in the pediatric tracheobronchial tree. *Clinical Pediatrics*, **22**, 148–150

MOSKOWITZ, D., GARDINER, L. J. and SASAKI, C. T. (1982) Foreign-body aspiration. Potential misdiagnosis. *Archives of Otolaryngology*, **108**, 806–807

NATIONAL SAFETY COUNCIL OF AMERICA (1980) *Accident Facts*, 7

O'NEILL, J. A. JR, HOLCOMB, G. W. JR and NEBLETT, W. W. (1983) Management of tracheobronchial and esophageal foreign bodies in childhood. *Journal of Pediatric Surgery*, **18**, 475–479

ROSS, A. H. and MCCORMICK, R. J. (1980) Foreign body inhalation. *Journal of the Royal College of Surgeons of Edinburgh*, **25**, 104–109

ROTHMANN, B. F. and BOECKMAN, C. R. (1980) Foreign bodies in the larynx and tracheobronchial tree in children. A review of 225 cases. *Annals of Otology, Rhinology and Laryngology*, **89**, 434–436

SCHLOSS, M. D., PHAM-DANG, H. and ROSALES, J. K. (1983) Foreign bodies in the tracheobronchial tree – a retrospective study of 217 cases. *Journal of Otolaryngology*, **12**, 212–216

SPENCER, M. J., MILLET, V. E., DUDLEY, J. P., SHERROD, J. L. and BRYSON, Y. J. (1981) Grassheads in the tracheobronchial tree: two different outcomes. *Annals of Otology, Rhinology and Laryngology*, **90**, 406–408

STEIN, L. (1970) Foreign bodies of the tracheobronchial tree and oesophagus – a new approach to therapy. *Annals of Thoracic Surgery*, **9**, 382–383

STROME, M. (1977) Tracheobronchial foreign bodies: an updated approach. *Annals of Otology, Rhinology and Laryngology*, **86**, 649–654

SVENSSON, G. (1985) Foreign bodies in the tracheobronchial tree. Special reference to experience in 97 children. *International Journal of Pediatric Otorhinolaryngology*, **61**, 5–17

SWENSSON, E. E., RAH, K. H., KIM, M. C., BROOKS, J. W. and

SALZBERG, A. M. (1985) Extraction of large tracheal foreign bodies through a tracheostoma under bronchoscopic control. *Annals of Thoracic Surgery*, **39**, 251–253

TOM, L. W. C., WEISMAN, R. A. and HANDLER, S. D. (1980) Haemoptysis in children. *Annals of Otology, Rhinology and Laryngology*, **89**, 419–424

TUCKER, G. JR (1985) Instrumentarium for foreign body removal. *New Dimensions in Otorhinolaryngology – Head and Neck Surgery*, **1**, 585–588

WIESEL, J. M., CHISIN, R., FEINMESSER, R. and GAY, I. (1982) Use of a Fogarty catheter for bronchoscopic removal of a foreign body (letter). *Chest*, **81**, 524

YEE, K. F., SCHILD, J. A. and HOLINGER, P. H. (1975) Extraluminal foreign bodies (coins) in the food and air passages. *Annals of Otology, Rhinology and Laryngology*, **84**, 619–623

26

Tracheostomy and decannulation

J. H. Rogers

A tracheostomy involves the construction of an opening between the trachea and the skin surface of the neck in the midline. With time, this opening may acquire an epithelial lining and may then qualify in pathological parlance as a 'fistula'. The alternative spelling of 'tracheotomy' is often employed but etymological discussion is best avoided and in this chapter the more traditional 'tracheostomy' is preferred. The operation is performed at all ages but there are significant differences between children and adults because of the smaller structures involved and the degree of immaturity which may be present in children. With medical progress, the emphasis on these differences becomes greater as the operation is performed on the infant, the neonate and now the preterm neonate.

History

Historical accounts of this operation vie with each other in plumbing the depths of antiquity for plausible evidence (Goodall, 1934; Salmon, 1957; Nelson, 1958; Frost, 1976). The operation has been attributed to various oriental potentates who employed the sword as scalpel and hazy descriptions have been given by certain medicophilosophers. No doubt some fossil-find, decorated potsherd or deciphered hieroglyphic will eventually push its origins even further into prehistory.

Since the Renaissance, this life-saving operation has been better described and certain trends become apparent. Initially it was performed for choking, caused either by an inhaled foreign body, drowning or trauma to the upper respiratory tract. Indeed, the first successful tracheostomy in a child was reported in 1766 by Caron, a French surgeon who removed an inhaled bean from a 7-year-old boy. Later a common indication was 'croup', a label given by a

Scottish physician, Francis Home (Home, 1765) to the combination of sore throat and stridor. Some of these patients would probably have suffered from laryngotracheobronchitis, but more probably from 'diphtheria', a term coined later by a French physician, Pierre Bretonneau. Indeed, the term 'croup' is still reserved exclusively for diphtheria in many parts of western Europe. In the nineteenth century, tracheostomy became widely used in the treatment of diphtheria in children and, by 1887, some 20 000 such operations had been reported in western Europe and the USA. About this time, intubation became a feasible alternative with the appearance of the O'Dwyer tube and the discovery of diphtheria antitoxin in 1895 hastened the demise of diphtheria as the preeminent indication for childhood tracheostomy. However, the operation continued to be carried out for various forms of upper respiratory obstruction, although the notoriety resulting from a 30% survival rate caused many parents to refuse the operation.

The employment of tracheostomy for the removal of bronchial secretions is a relatively recent innovation and it was first described by Galloway in patients with bulbar poliomyelitis. Subsequently a similar approach was taken for chronic chest disease. The poliomyelitis epidemics of the early 1950s stimulated the use of tracheostomy for positive pressure respiration and this opened the doors for similar treatment in tetanus, cardiac surgery, severe burns and, most recently, the care of the preterm infant. The introduction of active immunization against diphtheria in 1940 and poliomyelitis in 1956 almost eliminated these diseases and left epiglottitis and laryngotracheobronchitis as the principal indications for tracheostomy in children. Over the last 20 years, intubation has taken over as the treatment of choice in these conditions and the frequency of tracheostomy has, therefore, decreased dramatically in the developed world. In the last decade, the increased skills of the neonatologists have permitted the increased survival of the very preterm infant with its concomitant multiple problems. These infants require prolonged ventilation and the resulting subglottic stenosis and failure of extubation necessitates tracheostomy. However, even in these infants, the need has again decreased as the neonatologists have become more adept in avoiding subglottic trauma.

The historical vista of tracheostomy depicts a lifesaving operation which becomes superseded as less traumatic treatment becomes available. It remains a life-saving operation, but with the associated improvements in anaesthesia, antibiotics and surgical technique, the morbidity and mortality of the operation have been greatly reduced.

Anatomy and physiology

In the child, the air passages are both absolutely and relatively smaller than in the adult (Tucker and Tucker, 1979). The cervical trachea usually lies in the midline of the neck and its length varies with body build and the degree of extension. The distance from the cricoid to the suprasternal notch varies from 2.5 cm in neonates to 6.0 cm in the 10-year-old child, but in short, heavy individuals the cricoid cartilage may be sited almost within the suprasternal notch. The larynx is higher in the child and the cricoid cartilage lies at the level of the third cervical vertebra in the infant and descends to the sixth cervical vertebra at puberty. Since the thyroid cartilage does not take on its adult configuration until adolescence, the larynx is not easily palpable in the infant and the cricoid may be the easiest landmark to identify. The trachea is softer and lies nearest the skin at the cricoid, but it becomes deeper as it approaches the thoracic inlet. The thyroid isthmus varies in size but crosses the trachea at the second, third and fourth tracheal rings (Figure 26.1). The recurrent laryngeal nerves lie laterally and a pretracheal pad of fat is generally present in the suprasternal notch in infants. In extension, the mediastinal contents may enter the neck so that the surgeon may encounter a high pleural dome, large vessels crossing the midline and, rarely the thymus. The articulation between the head and neck is considerably more mobile in infants and the chin may easily deviate from the midline during surgery.

The trachea provides an air passage between the larynx and the lungs. Since it needs to maintain its lumen and to remain flexible, it is constructed of incomplete cartilaginous rings. It is lined by respiratory mucosa which continues the process of warming and humidifying the inspired air, and the cilia waft the mucous blanket upwards to the larynx. The larynx is a valvular mechanism which allows the passage of air but normally denies access to solids

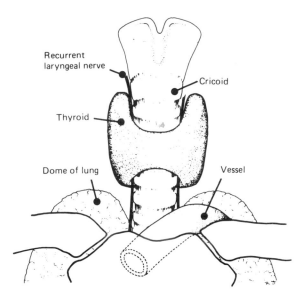

Figure 26.1 The essential anatomy of the cervical trachea

and fluids. It also provides a defence mechanism in the form of the cough reflex and it has been adapted to a sophisticated degree for the production of sound.

Indications for tracheostomy

The indications for tracheostomy in the past have been largely usurped by the indications for intubation and a tracheostomy may only become necessary when intubation is no longer feasible. In general, the indications are conveniently placed in three groups, as in the adult, although the specific details are different in the child.

Airway obstruction

Obstruction or the threat of obstruction to the upper respiratory tract is an indication for tracheostomy. Apart from laryngeal and subglottic lesions, indications include physical trauma to the face, jaws, oral and pharyngeal cavities as well as burns by corrosive chemicals or the inhalation of smoke or gases.

Dead space and secretions

Tracheostomy is indicated for improved respiration where a reduction in dead space or the removal of bronchial secretions is considered to be advantageous. This situation is found in chronic lung disease and in certain neonatal chest conditions.

Ventilation

The provision of prolonged positive pressure ventilation where voluntary or spontaneous respiration is not possible is an indication for tracheostomy. The patient with poliomyelitis, tetanus or brain damage may require such assistance, as also will the child with a damaged chest wall. Positive pressure ventilation is also employed as an adjunct to cardiac surgery, in patients with severe burns and the preterm neonate.

In the first and last groups, intubation may be employed in the short term but, for prolonged treatment, the tracheostomy is easier to manage. Until recently, intubation was only employed for periods of up to 3 weeks, but improvements in technique now permit intubation for periods of several months. A tracheostomy, therefore, becomes a necessity whenever prolonged endotracheal intubation poses the threat of laryngotracheal injury.

Several authors have reviewed their indications for tracheostomy over the last 15–20 years (Cohen *et al.*, 1977; Rodgers, Brooks and Talbert, 1979; Tepas *et al.*, 1981; Gerson and Tucker, 1982; Wetmore, Handler and Potsic, 1982; Carter and Benjamin, 1983; Line *et al.*, 1986; Swift and Rogers, 1987). There is no purpose in quoting the statistics from these reviews because they reflect the different patterns of referral to the centres concerned. Rapid changes have occurred over the last 15 years and the indications will vary with the precise period under review. The specific indications are, therefore, described below in general terms and in order of decreasing frequency.

Congenital laryngeal abnormalities

Although there are variations as described above, this group now accounts for the largest proportion of tracheostomies. In one series (Carter and Benjamin, 1983), laryngeal webs and subglottic haemangiomas accounted for most cases within this group, but this is unusual and the unit in question attracts these cases from a large area. Bilateral vocal cord paralysis is generally found to be the most common single indication, while congenital subglottic stenosis and cysts come next in frequency. Laryngomalacia or supraglottic floppiness is by far the most common laryngeal abnormality, but tracheostomy is very rarely required for its treatment.

Prolonged ventilation

Trauma to the head or chest continues to be common and is even increasing. Eventually it may, therefore, be the most common indication for tracheostomy. Tetanus occurs intermittently and is still very common in some large rural areas (Mukherjee, 1979). Poliomyelitis has largely been eliminated in the developed world, but continues to be a threat elsewhere.

Supralaryngeal obstruction

This may be present or threatened and is commonly seen in conditions such as the Pierre Robin syndrome, severe sleep apnoea and craniofacial surgery. Advances in the surgical treatment of congenital facial abnormalities are making tracheostomy more common in this latter group.

Severe spinal deformities can prevent easy access to the larynx and make the administration of general anaesthesia difficult. Although initial intubation may be possible, rapid re-intubation could be difficult and dangerous if the tube were dislodged and a temporary tracheostomy is helpful.

Acquired laryngeal abnormalities

Ten years ago, acquired subglottic stenosis would have been one of the most common indications for tracheostomy because of the increased resuscitative skills of the neonatologist. Although it is still a very significant problem in those units which attract the worst problems of this nature (Black, Baldwin and Johns, 1984; Quincy *et al.*, 1986), improved intubation skills have in general reduced the necessity for tracheostomy. Indeed, in one series (Carter and Benjamin, 1983), no tracheostomies were performed for acquired subglottic stenosis over a period of 10 years, although some 300 infants were intubated annually in the associated neonatal and intensive care units. Those authors attributed this remarkable success to the use of small-diameter (2.5 or even 2.0 mm) polyvinylchloride (PVC) nasotracheal tubes. Other centres receive patients from areas where such expertise may not be available.

Laryngeal papillomatosis as an indication for tracheostomy is also on the decline. The need in this condition is dictated not only by the virulence of the causative agent but by the degree of oedema and scarring following treatment. The use of the laser has reduced the postoperative oedema and the frequency of removal and has consequently obviated the need for an alternative airway.

Acute infections

Twenty years ago, infections of the respiratory tract were the most common indication for tracheostomy, but oro- and nasotracheal intubation has changed that (Crysdale and Sendi, 1988). Intubation is now widely used for acute epiglottitis and laryngotracheobronchitis, although it makes great demands on medical and nursing facilities and is, therefore, not so available in less developing countries (Mukherjee, 1979; Okafor, 1983; Soni, Chatterji and Thind, 1984), where tracheostomy is still widely employed (Prescott and Vanlierde, 1989).

Miscellaneous

This review is necessarily based on trends in the developed world but indications differ elsewhere. Diphtheria is an important acute infection and inhaled foreign bodies are a common indication, particularly where patients may take several days to reach hospital and, if still alive, will therefore have considerable oedema around the impacted object.

The operation of tracheostomy

The operation is more common in males because of their increased susceptibility to congenital and acquired disorders. The aim of the operation is to construct an airway into the trachea as safely as possible.

Since the emphasis is on safety, the operation should be carried out in an environment where there is complete control of the airway at all times. There are rare occasions when an emergency tracheostomy is life saving but, in the hospital environment, intubation or cricothyroidotomy is preferable when that urgent need arises. The technique of emergency tracheostomy will not be described here since, by definition, the facilities available are unknown, but the aim is to provide an airway as rapidly as possible by whatever means possible.

Since more than half of all paediatric tracheostomies are performed on children under the age of 1 year, it is essential that the operation is carried out in a paediatric unit or hospital where the nursing and medical staff are accustomed to the care of infants and neonates. Details of the anaesthetic and general care of a neonate will not be included here, although these are obviously of the greatest importance.

The operation should be performed electively in a sterile environment under a general anaesthetic administered through an endotracheal tube. The anaesthetic should be given by an experienced paediatric anaesthetist and the operation should be performed by, or supervised by, an experienced paediatric otolaryngologist. Some surgeons prefer to use a bronchoscope to establish the airway. It also makes identification of the airway easier and obviously allows preoperative inspection.

Preparation

Antibiotics are not needed prophylactically but they should be given if there is some medical reason to do so. A sample of sputum should be taken for culture and antibiotic sensitivity in readiness for a possible postoperative infection. Blood loss is minimal during the operation but, since the blood volume of a neonate may be very small, it is wise for a sample of blood to be grouped and kept for cross-matching.

The infant, suitably warmed, is laid supine on the operating table. The head is extended to increase the distance between the chin and sternal notch, to smooth out the redundant folds of skin in the neck and to bring the trachea and larynx closer to the skin surface (Figure 26.2). This is achieved by placing a suitable roll of soft material under the neck and the head is prevented from lolling by using a small head ring. When extension is difficult, it can be assisted by passing

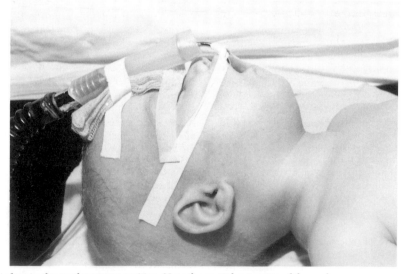

Figure 26.2 An infant in the tracheostomy position. Note the partial extension of the neck

a long piece of strapping beneath the chin and attaching both ends to the top of the operating table. It is important not to overdo the extension as this draws the lower trachea and mediastinal contents into the neck. Not only does this place the lung apices and mediastinal vessels at risk but it may tempt a low tracheal incision, which retreats into the chest on flexion.

The skin of the chin, neck and upper chest is cleaned with a suitable disinfectant and the surrounding area is draped with sterile towels. The chin is left uncovered in order that the surgeon can check the midline and some anaesthetists like to keep the face uncovered. Before the towels are positioned a little adrenalin (1:80 000 or 1:200 000 if halothane is being used) and local anaesthetic are infiltrated subcutaneously between the cricoid and the sternal notch. This allows the adrenalin to disperse and to exert its vasoconstrictive effect before the incision is made a few minutes later. The local anaesthetic reduces postoperative discomfort. At this stage it is also wise to check that the intended tracheostomy tube is available and that the proper connections are at hand.

Surgical technique

Either a vertical or a horizontal skin incision may be used, but there are theoretical and practical reasons for preferring the vertical incision. The horizontal skin crease incision has its supporters in the adult because of the better cosmetic result, but in the infant both incisions are so small that they produce similar scars. The main advantage of the vertical incision is that it runs in the line of the trachea. This is important in the infant since it is often difficult to judge the precise level of the proposed tracheostomy externally and the improved access gives a greater freedom of choice. The midline is also less vascular and for both these reasons the vertical incision is best used.

The cricoid cartilage is palpated, often with some difficulty, and a vertical midline skin incision of 1.5 cm is made with the upper end at the level of the cricoid. If a horizontal incision is to be employed, it should be of similar length and sited in a skin crease midway between the cricoid and the suprasternal notch. It is important that the chin and sternal notch are in line when the skin is incised. The bleeding is usually minimal but diathermy should be employed if necessary. An assistant retracts the edges of the incision with a skin hook or small retractor and blunt dissection is carried out in the midline with artery forceps or small scissors. It is important not to open up tissue planes unnecessarily as this encourages surgical emphysema later. As the dissection probes deeper, the assistant repositions the retractors and in this way the strap muscles are separated and the trachea approached. If the surgeon stays in the midline this procedure can usually be completed without any bleeding, but the degree of difficulty in exposing the trachea varies greatly. Even in the more difficult cases persistence is rewarded as long as the midline is sought and the level of the cricoid checked.

It is difficult to mistake the trachea when it is reached although the tracheal rings are softer and less obvious then in the adult. It is, however, sometimes a problem to identify an individual tracheal ring and this may be facilitated by exposing the cricoid cartilage and its attached cricothyroid muscle and numbering the rings from that level. The identification of the thyroid isthmus also provides a landmark for the tracheal rings. Although the isthmus varies in width from a tenuous sliver of connective tissue to a more substantial mass, it consistently overlies the second, third and fourth tracheal rings (see Figure 26.1). Some authorities feel that the isthmus should always be cut and sutured (Gerson and Tucker, 1982) in order to facilitate recannulation later, but this is rarely necessary. It is usually simple to free the isthmus from the underlying trachea and to retract it superiorly or inferiorly for the exposure of the relevant tracheal rings. Good access to the trachea is obtained by clearing the fascia from its anterior surface, although care must be taken not to disturb the recurrent laryngeal nerves which lie posterolaterally. The trachea should now be exposed in a small but bloodless field and, after rechecking the tracheostomy tube and its attachments, the anaesthetist is alerted to the imminent incision of the trachea itself.

The tracheal incision

In the adult, there has always been considerable discussion about the best form of tracheal incision but in the infant it is generally agreed that the vertical incision is simplest and best. This is given support by an attempt to evaluate the relative merits of the vertical slit, the inferiorly based trapdoor and the horizontal H (Fry *et al.*, 1985). Using young ferrets as a paediatric model the authors assessed the tracheal airway after decannulation and healing and demonstrated that the vertical slit resulted in less stenosis and less airway resistance.

It is important that the vertical incision is made at the correct level. If it is too near to the cricoid, it will predispose to subglottic stenosis and the surgeon should, therefore, aim at keeping the upper tracheal ring intact. Conversely, if the incision is made too low, the tip of the tracheostomy tube may enter the right main bronchus and the tube is more likely to come out accidentally. The tracheal rings are identified again and a vertical incision is made through the second, third and fourth rings. A larger incision should be extended to include the fifth ring. The slit is made from below upwards to avoid damage to the mediastinal contents and it should be made in a controlled manner because a slip will extend the incision into the cricoid. Even in the infant, the tracheal wall is rather thicker than one would suspect but care must be taken not to damage the posterior wall of the trachea with the point of the scalpel. In practice this is most unlikely since the anaesthetist's endotracheal tube lies in the tracheal lumen, unless it has become displaced superiorly. There is sometimes a little bleeding from the tracheal mucosa and the perichondrium of the ring, but this is rarely significant.

Some surgeons feel that the procedure is assisted by the insertion of a silk suture, to either side of the midline. Before the vertical incision is made, a black silk suture is introduced to circle the third and fourth tracheal rings on either side. These are left long and initially are held laterally in artery forceps. After the vertical incision has been made between them these sutures are retracted to assist cannulation. Later they are taped to the chest wall for up to one week and may be used for recannulation if necessary. In the author's experience, these sutures are not mandatory since there is rarely any problem in introducing the tracheostomy tube at operation and decannulation is prevented by other means described below. In addition, there is a possibility that the sutures will weaken the anterior tracheal wall and the threads become sodden and something of an obstacle during subsequent care of the tracheostomy.

The anaesthetist now withdraws the endotracheal tube just proximal to the upper end of the incision under the guidance of the surgeon. The trachea is sucked out and a tracheostomy tube of suitable design and size is inserted under direct vision. This is done in a calm, unhurried way since the anaesthetist still has full control of the airway. If any difficulty is experienced in introducing the tube the following points may be helpful. The incision may need to be lengthened and stay sutures should be retracted if they are available. If the tube is a metal one then the introducer should be properly in place while, if it is plastic, the ends can be compressed in an artery forceps and inserted through the incision (Pracy, 1979) (Figure 26.3). The tracheostomy tube can also be 'railroaded' down a fine catheter which has been passed through the tube and the tracheal incision.

Unless there is good reason, a synthetic plastic or silicone tube should be used for the initial intubation. The standard tube used by the author is the Great Ormond Street pattern of the Aberdeen tube made by Franklin, but other models are available and are described below. The standard size used for a 3-month-old baby is the 3.5 mm (internal diameter), but the tube should obviously be measured for the patient in terms of its lumen and length.

The correct position of the tube in the tracheal lumen is checked and the anaesthetist makes the attachments for continued ventilation. Once the anaesthetist is satisfied that both lungs are being ventilated, the endotracheal tube is fully withdrawn. No sutures are placed in the edges of the skin incision

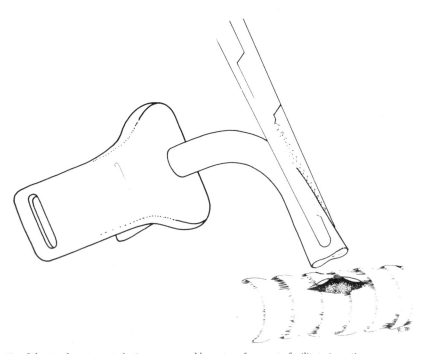

Figure 26.3 The tip of the tracheostomy tube is compressed by artery forceps to facilitate insertion

which usually fits comfortably around the tube and in any case a tight fit is to be avoided since it predisposes to surgical emphysema.

The tube is now held in place by suturing the flange to the neck skin and by tying tapes around the neck (Figure 26.4). The importance of securing the tube cannot be overestimated since accidental decannulation is avoided if it is done properly. Silk sutures are placed through the upper border of the flange and adjacent skin just lateral to the opening of the tube. This positioning prevents the substantial tube movement which can occur if the sutures are placed towards the tip of the flange or through the lower border of the flange. Another technique of fixation

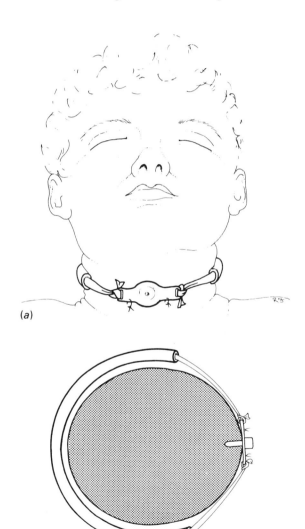

(a)

(b)

Figure 26.4 (a) The flanges are secured to the neck skin by a tape and by sutures adjacent to the collar of the tube. (b) A cross-section of the neck demonstrating the tape passing through protective tubing

has been described (Black, Fernandes and Carr, 1988). A silk suture is placed through each wing of the tracheostomy tube, close to the cannula and tied over the wing. A tape is then tied from one side of the flange to the other around the back of the neck. One end of the tape is knotted to one side of the flange while the other is passed through a piece of tubing of suitable length. This tubing conforms to the convexity of the baby's neck and protects the skin from the rubbing of the tape. The free end of the tape is then knotted to the other end of the flange and is adjusted so that the tube is held firmly, but not tightly, in place. It is most important that these adjustments to the tape are carried out while the neck is in slight flexion. If they are done while the neck is extended, the tube will loosen on subsequent flexion and accidental decannulation may occur. It is, therefore, important that the tape adjustments are made by the surgeon or the anaesthetist and the task should not be delegated to an inexperienced member of the team. Children over the age of 6 months are given sedation, but younger babies are best left without to discourage apnoeic attacks. The child is now moved from the operating table and care is taken to avoid traction on the tube while this is being carried out.

Postoperative care

For the first few days the child should be in an intensive care unit where there are adequate trained nursing and medical staff on duty for 24 hours of the day. As soon as the infant arrives on the ward, an X-ray of the chest and neck is taken to confirm that the tip of the tracheostomy tube is not so low that it impinges on the carina or enters the right main bronchus. The X-ray may also demonstrate surgical emphysema in the superficial tissues or in the mediastinum. Initially feeding is via the intravenous drip which is established during the operation, but within a few hours, the baby is able to feed by mouth. The maintenance of adequate hydration is important since it contributes to the prevention of tracheal crusting.

If the baby has previously suffered from chronic airway obstruction, the sudden relief may produce apnoea and it may be wise initially to increase the dead space by a suitable attachment. In the preterm baby, positive end expiration pressure may be necessary to maintain lung stability. The chin may also obstruct the stomal opening in the small baby, but this can be avoided by choosing a suitable tube (as described below), or by inserting a segment of plastic tubing into the opening of the tracheostomy.

Since the tracheostomy has bypassed the nose it is essential that humidified air is supplied to the infant, but care must be taken to avoid over-humidification. Particle size is not as important as was previously thought but cold humidity is probably best and an ultrasonic humidifier may be necessary to provide a sufficient volume. The glottis is also bypassed by the operation and the cough reflex is therefore lost. The trachea and bronchi respond to the surgical insult by an increase in mucus secretion and, because the cough reflex is lost, suction is essential. Regular aseptic suction is required but the frequency varies and must be assessed by the experienced attendant staff. The catheter is inserted without suction and the negative pressure is exerted as the catheter is withdrawn. The size of the catheter is most important. The external diameter of the catheter should be less than half the internal diameter of the tracheostomy tube because, if not, hypoxia or, at worst, lung collapse may occur.

At first a careful watch must be kept for surgical emphysema or pneumothorax, but these are unlikely to occur after 12 hours. It is not usually necessary to place a dressing between the peristomal skin and the tubal flanges, but a barrier cream is helpful if skin excoriation threatens.

The parents of the child are encouraged to take an active role in the routine care from the outset. In the neonate, this is important for bonding, but it is particularly important in the older child because speech will now be impossible and a parent must be immediately available for reassurance and communication. Both parents should initially observe the routine procedures of tracheostomy care and should then be supervised in doing it themselves to overcome their natural fear. At this stage they should also be introduced to the idea of contacting one of the relevant parental organizations such as 'Aid for children with tracheostomies'.

One week after the tracheostomy the track will be well formed. The tube can now be changed, although this is not mandatory and it can be left longer if it is clean and well positioned. The first change is best done in the intensive care unit or in the operating theatre where emergency facilities are available. An endotracheal tube, spare tracheostomy tube and tracheal dilators are essential and the change is done after cutting the flange sutures by an experienced doctor, whether surgeon or anaesthetist. The tapes are again tied with great care and the position of the tube is checked. The baby can now be returned to a normal ward but only if the staff are accustomed to dealing with a patient with a tracheostomy and are capable of continuing with the training of the parents. Regular aseptic suction and humidification are continued and the necessary equipment is ordered for the home care of the child. Before a return home is contemplated, both parents should be able to change the tracheostomy tube and the surgeon must be happy that they are confident about the routine daily care.

Later, if decannulation has not been achieved, questions will arise concerning the development of speech and the proposed nature of future education. The problem of speech is linked to the type of tracheostomy tube used and this is discussed in a separate section below. It is imperative to seek the aid of an experienced speech therapist and every effort must be made to enrol the otherwise normal child in a normal school, although this may prove to be difficult.

Complications

Since the tracheostomy is now the main route for respiration, any complication which interferes with this route may be fatal. The mortality and morbidity following the tracheostomy itself (as opposed to the associated disease) is now much less than it was 20 years ago (Fearon and Cotton, 1974), although results still vary from different centres. The improvement is attributed to the avoidance of emergency tracheostomies where possible and to the emphasis on basic surgical technique as described above. If these guidelines are followed, complications are infrequent, although the vulnerability of the tracheostomized child must never be forgotten. Complications are conveniently considered as being early or late, the dividing line being about 1 week into the postoperative period. Some problems such as crusting and granulation formation are so common that they may be regarded as the normal consequences of the operation, but if these are exaggerated, they qualify as complications.

Early complications

Apnoea

Apnoeic attacks are more likely to occur in the small infant with chronic airway obstruction. Such a child should not be given postoperative sedation and the dead space can be increased temporarily by a suitable attachment to the tracheostomy tube.

Air in the tissues

A little surgical emphysema is commonly seen immediately after the operation and it may only be recognized on the postoperative X-ray. Usually the emphysema resolves without any treatment but the position of the tube and the tightness of the skin around the stoma should be checked. *Pneumomediastinum* presents in a similar manner and should be treated in the same way but a *pneumothorax* is more serious and is treated on its merits. A low tracheostomy predisposes to a pneumothorax and a tight stoma aggravates the situation. Prevention is therefore the best form of treatment. The neck should not be overextended during the operation and blunt dissection in the midline will avoid the opening up of lateral tissue planes.

Accidental decannulation

This can be a serious complication in the first 2 or 3 days after surgery because the fistula track will not have formed and the slit incision in the trachea will make recannulation difficult. If the tracheostomy has been performed at the right level and the tube has been sutured and taped accurately, it should not occur. In this situation stay sutures come into their own but, even in their absence, the experienced staff of an intensive care unit should be able to recannulate or pass an endotracheal tube and the necessary instruments should always be immediately available.

Creation of a false passage

The changing of the tube or its reinsertion following accidental decannulation may lead to the creation of a false passage. It is particularly likely to occur before the track is well formed and the tube should not normally be changed until this has occurred. The false passage may lead to obstruction or to a pneumothorax and the position of the tube should always be carefully checked after recannulation.

Obstruction

This is obviously a potentially fatal complication. If the tube is the correct length and is positioned correctly, the most common cause is the accumulation of mucus and crusts in the tube or the tracheal lumen and it is best prevented by adequate humidification and suction. Intermittent obstruction by the baby's chin is prevented by a suitable restraining attachment to the tube and this is discussed below.

Haemorrhage

Blunt dissection in the midline during the operation will often result in a bloodless field but a little bleeding may occur from the skin edges, the tracheal perichondrium and the tracheal mucosa. Such bleeding is usually trivial and will stop after an hour or two. Serious haemorrhage from the erosion of a large vessel is often fatal but rarely occurs in the first week since the most common cause is secondary infection.

Chest infections

Even with strict attention to aseptic technique during suction, pulmonary infections occur, particularly in the infant with previous lung problems. In this latter group, prophylactic antibiotics should be given preoperatively and in all cases the appropriate medical treatment is commenced. The choice of antibiotic is aided by taking a sample of sputum or tracheal aspirate at operation and sending it for culture and sensitivity.

Late complications

All the complications mentioned above may occur later but their importance varies. The most common and, therefore, the most important fatal complications, are accidental decannulation and obstruction and these are particularly likely to happen at home.

Accidental decannulation

Accidental decannulation at a later stage is less dangerous because the tube can be easily replaced into the established track within a few minutes of decannulation. However, the track can stenose rapidly and tracheal dilators may be required even within 10 minutes of the decannulation. The avoidance of decannulation at home is most important and the parents must be instructed to tie the securing tapes firmly. To counteract the efforts of an active child, it may be necessary to have tapes which are tight enough to mark the neck, but a marked neck is preferable to a decannulated child.

Obstruction

This may be caused by a granuloma or by a mucus plug. Granulations almost always appear at the site of the stoma, particularly within the tracheal lumen above the stoma (Figure 26.5). They may obstruct the tracheal lumen following elective or accidental decannulation, but may also block the tube or cause

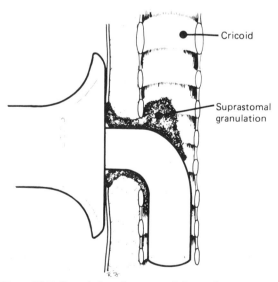

Figure 26.5 Granulations form around the tracheostomy tube. The suprastomal granulation is seen above the tube on the anterior wall

bleeding during recannulation. Granulations are very likely to occur when a metal tube is used. The characteristics of the various tubes and the management of granulations are discussed below. Obstruction of the tube or the tracheal lumen by a mucus plug is best prevented by adequate humidification and suction. Such humidification is provided by a plastic humidifier in the home but also by a heat-moisture exchanger, of which there are several models, which is easily connected to the tube. This device allows freedom in the open air without the encumbrance of a standard humidifier and may even permit the child to play in sand under supervision. An attempt has been made to detect obstruction in the tracheostomy tube by electronic means and this may indicate the direction of future progress. Accumulated mucus activates electrodes inserted into the wall of the tube and this produces an audible signal (Rao *et al.*, 1989).

Haemorrhage due to the erosion of a large vessel is usually fatal and can only be prevented by the proper positioning of the tracheostomy, by attention to operative technique, and the prompt treatment of infection. Haemorrhage and mediastinitis have also been caused by erosion of the tracheal wall by the tip of a badly positioned tube. Chest infections continue to be more frequent than in the normal child and are treated symptomatically.

Tracheostomy tubes

Every otolaryngologist must have wished many times that an available tracheostomy tube could be modified to suit the problem of the patient in hand. The perfect tube does not exist but successive modifications have occurred with advances in medical knowledge and in the science of materials (Pracy, 1976).

The early tracheostomy tubes were made of bone, rubber or metal and the paediatric tube was a smaller version of the adult model. The tubes were of varying curvature with a flange around the external opening for the attachment of stabilizing tapes. Latterly, these tubes were made of silver and incorporated an inner tube, which was longer than the outer and could be easily removed when blockage occurred. Later a valve was fitted to the tube by Negus to allow inspiration through the tube and expiration through the glottis for phonation. Forty years ago, Wilson introduced a silver tube for children with a funnel-shaped projection, which could be easily attached to a respirator. This tube also had a window in the shoulder of the outer tube to allow transglottic breathing prior to decannulation. The addition of a window and a valve to the inner tube produced the Alder Hey tube, which has been widely used in the UK for many years.

A great advance was made with the discovery of flexible plastics such as polyvinylchloride and silicone rubber. Since several of these are thermoplastic, the initial curvature of the tube is not so important because the shaft conforms to the shape of the track as the material warms. Unfortunately, the wall of these tubes needs to be thicker in order to preserve sufficient rigidity. This reduces the size of the lumen and makes the use of an inner tube impracticable in the smaller paediatric models. The theoretical characteristics of an ideal tube are discussed in detail elsewhere (Pracy, 1976), but a few factors are summarized here. The design of the tube should permit an optimum flow of air, a situation which is favoured by a shorter shaft, a greater radius of curvature and a smooth inner surface (Yung and Snowdon, 1984). The material should be non-toxic and should possess minimal tissue reactivity as demonstrated by implantation tests. It is probable that various chemicals are leached out from these plastic tubes while they are in use and that their tissue reactivity changes. However, it is not known if, or how rapidly, this occurs and, therefore, how long to leave a tube in place before disposing of it (Bush, 1986, personal communication).

There are also desirable practical considerations. The tube should be comfortable, easy to clean and easy to change. It must be easily connected to ventilation equipment and attachments should fulfil standard international requirements. At present it is agreed that the external opening of the tube, known as the collar, should have an internal diameter of 15 mm. In babies and small children it is helpful to have a projection from the opening of the tube, a chin restrainer, which will prevent the chubby chin of the baby occluding the tube. It would also be most desirable if the measurements of the tubes were easily accessible and expressed clearly. The choice of an ideal tube would be facilitated by a knowledge of the internal and external diameters of the tube and the length of the shaft. Unfortunately, there is a confusing lack of uniformity in the description of various tubes and this problem has recently been well described (Irving *et al.*, 1991). There is therefore a tendency for practitioners to persevere with those tubes they know and whose measurements they understand. In practice there are two groups of tubes, the metal tubes and the synthetic tubes. The characteristics of those in common use are described.

Metal tubes

The Alder Hey tube is typical of this group and is described above. It has an inner tube which is easily cleaned and it inspires confidence in the inexperienced parent who, initially, does not need to change the complete tube. It has a large radius of curvature and its smooth surface encourages laminar air flow (Yung and Snowdon, 1984). Both the inner and outer tubes are fenestrated and a valve is available to allow transglottic expiration and speech. Similar, but not identical, paediatric metal tubes are those of Jackson and Holinger, but all are durable and may last for several years.

There are also disadvantages. They are said to be less comfortable than the synthetic tubes and cosmetically they are less satisfying. The edges of the fenestra and the shaft-tip are sharp and it is the impression of the author and others (Quiney *et al.*, 1986) that granulations are more likely to occur in the trachea and around the stomal skin. The tracheal granulations are sited above the stoma, at the level of the tube tip and at the level of the fenestra on the posterior wall. The fenestrated tube was designed for transglottic air flow. This was thought to be of major importance for the continued development of the child's larynx, as a prelude to decannulation (Pracy, 1976) and in the production of speech. This theory of laryngeal development is no longer thought to be true and it is now known that an adequate air flow through the glottis can be achieved by employing a smaller tube. In addition, it has proved difficult to site the fenestra at a suitable point on the curvature. The tube sits differently in different patients and in spite of the adjustable plates, the opening of the fenestra often impinges on the posterior tracheal wall.

A death has occurred due to a fracture caused by corrosion between the plate and the tube of a silver tracheostomy tube (Brockhurst and Feltoe, 1991). This was believed to be due to the effect of body fluids or the disinfecting solutions and it is recommended that the junction should be checked from time to time.

In spite of these defects, metal tubes have their place and the recently introduced Sheffield tube has its admirers. Its winged flange is less traumatic, an extra inner tube facilitates cleaning and the full length obturator prevents crusting during decannulation.

Synthetic tubes

Those commonly used in the UK are the Franklin tube of Great Ormond Street pattern, the Portex paediatric tube and the Shiley paediatric or neonatal tube. The Great Ormond Street tube is a winged tube which sits comfortably on the infant neck. Its external opening does not project and lies flush with the winged flanges. The outer section of the lumen expands to an opening of constant size and this is convenient for the attachment of anaesthetic or ventilation equipment. A version with a fixed extension and side holes is now available and the extension doubles as a chin restrainer. If the extended tube is not available, there is an attachment which can be used and a suitable length of tubing can achieve the same effect. A De Santi speaking valve can be attached, but these are poorly tolerated and block easily.

The Portex tube is not winged but it has square-ended flanges and a projecting collar connector of international standard dimensions. This connector is sometimes found to be rather bulky. Unlike the Great Ormond Street tube it does not have a bevelled tip and it is, therefore, a little more difficult to introduce through a vertical slit in the trachea. The quoted size of this and the Great Ormond Street tube refers to their internal diameter.

The Shiley tube comes in a paediatric or neonatal size. It has a large winged flange with a standard projecting connector and both structures make an effective chin restrainer. An investigation (Yung and Snowdon, 1984) into the respiratory resistance of these tubes showed that resistance to air flow was greater in the Shiley tube owing to the rougher inner surface. However, it is doubtful whether this is of practical importance (Figure 26.6). The shortened length of the neonatal grades prevents occlusion of the bronchus in the smallest babies.

A range of silicone paediatric and neonatal tubes

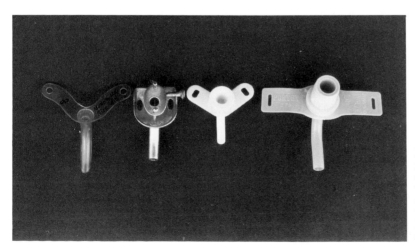

Figure 26.6 A selection of paediatric tracheostomy tubes in common use. From left to right: the Great Ormond Street tube (Franklin): the silver Alder Hey tube; the Shiley tube; and the Portex tube. Note the standardized collars on the latter two tubes

has recently become available from Kapitex. Both the tube and the flange are very flexible although the tube shaft is reinforced to prevent kinking. The tip is soft and tapered. The author has limited experience of this tube but it has proved very useful in one difficult case.

Although the metal tubes still have their use, many practitoners (Line *et al.*, 1986; Quiney *et al.*, 1986) including the author have virtually ceased to use them routinely. The synthetic tubes are cosmetically better and parents seem to have little trouble in cleaning and changing them.

Obstruction of the tube at home is the most common fatal complication but it does not appear to be more common with the use of synthetic tubes. Indeed, the standard connectors now available for the synthetic tubes allow the attachment of a heat-moisture exchanger with consequent avoidance of dry mucoid plugs. Until recently the metal tubes were valuable in the provision of speech by means of the fenestra and the valved inner tube. However, an effective phonation valve as made by Rusch is available and can be simply attached to a standard connector (Figure 26.7). The use of a tube of lesser diameter provides an adequate expiratory flow through the cords.

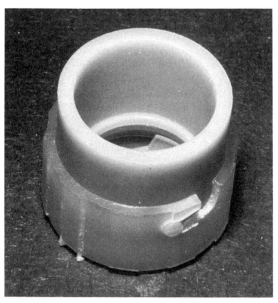

Figure 26.7 Phonation valve (Rusch) which can be attached to any tube with a standardized collar

Decannulation

It is always hoped that any child with a tracheostomy will eventually be decannulated. The outcome obviously depends upon the original lesion, but fortunately many resolve either spontaneously or with medical or surgical treatment. The time comes when the airway appears to be adequate and it is felt that the patient will manage without the tracheostomy. However, it is well established that the removal of the tracheostomy tube in these circumstances may still result in problems and it is these which are discussed below.

Assessment before decannulation

Children with tracheostomies may be in hospital or at home, but in both situations they are seen at regular intervals and assessed clinically. The child should appear to be well and show no sign of aspiration during eating and drinking. It should be noted that he has a good voice or cry in the absence of a valved tube and the temporary occlusion of the tube with the finger permits respiration to continue adequately through the glottis. Radiography and particularly CT scanning or MRI of the larynx and trachea will demonstrate any narrowing of the airway and a picture taken during temporary extubation may be particularly helpful. A method for physiological assessment has been described (Mallory *et al.*, 1985) whereby the peak inspiratory flow through the tracheostomy tube is compared with that through the mouth. Lastly, endoscopy is carried out and the larynx, trachea and bronchi are examined with special attention to the sites of the original lesion and the tracheal stoma. The lumen of the subglottis is also measured by the passage of an endotracheal tube of known diameter and the vocal cords are observed for normal movement towards the end of the anaesthetic.

It is advisable to carry out such endoscopic examinations at least every 6 months (Tom *et al.*, 1993) because a tracheostomy carries a morbidity and mortality rate which justifies decannulation as soon as it is feasible.

In most cases this assessment will lead to a definite decision with regard to decannulation but there will be some where considerable doubt will remain. The child may suffer from recurrent chest infections or the lumen of the subglottis may be smaller than was expected. There are occasions when the presence of a tracheostomy predisposes to chest infections and to adjacent subglottic oedema. This latter finding is more significant when there is a mild congenital subglottic narrowing which has not previously been diagnosed. In these borderline cases a trial of decannulation may be necessary.

When the endoscopy is carried out a suprastomal granulation of varying size is nearly always seen on the anterior tracheal wall. Indeed, this finding is so common that it should be regarded as a normal consequence of tracheostomy rather than as a complication. The suprastomal granulation, which may be mixed with fibrous tissue, is more likely to be present with a long-standing tracheostomy but a substantial granulation can be present after only 1 week. It has been suggested (Prescott, 1992) that a formal skin-to-trachea stoma reduces granulation formation and should be constructed if a long-term tracheostomy is anticipated. In the infant even a small granulation causes a significant blockage of the lumen and it should be removed endoscopically or surgically through the stoma. Endoscopically, the granulation is removed with microscopic cup forceps, diathermy, cryosurgery or the laser (Maddern, Weskhaven and Stool, 1989). The granulation is removed through the stoma at the time of the endoscopy (Reilly and Myer, 1985) or during surgical decannulation as described below. Varying degrees of anterior tracheal wall collapse may also be noted above the stoma at endoscopy.

The decannulation procedure

Broadly speaking decannulation may be performed in two ways. The most common method is to remove the tube and to allow the track to close down and heal. The alternative is to excise the track and allow it to heal by first intention. In both methods the final decannulation is preceded by various manoeuvres which constitute a trial decannulation and are aimed at ensuring the safety of a final extubation.

The child is brought into hospital for a period of observation which need not exceed 2 or 3 days. If there is any choice in the timing then it is preferable to do it in the early summer when there is a low incidence of respiratory infection. The general health is checked, chest physiotherapy is arranged and a sample of sputum is taken for culture and sensitivity. Although the tube may already have been blocked for a trial period, this period should be repeated and the child should be watched carefully by the ward staff while he carries out normal physical activities. Some advocate the use of a fenestrated metal tube such as the Alder Hey tube (Black, Baldwin and Johns, 1984) for this procedure, but a small plastic tube allows an adequate airway around it. Indeed, this latter method is preferable, since the partial blockage of the tracheal lumen by the tube makes the trial more stringent and, if it is well tolerated, then the final decannulation is even more likely to be successful. If blocking is well tolerated during the day, then it should be continued at night as long as there are enough qualified nursing staff to provide a constant watch. If there are still no problems, the tube is removed and the stoma is covered by a sterile dressing. The child is then kept under observation as an inpatient for at least 1 week before being allowed home. Various other pre-decannulation procedures are practised but they are all variations on a theme of progressive tube blockage with an increase in the dead space.

During the whole of the decannulation and pre-decannulation period essential emergency equipment must be at the bedside and humidification must be continued. The equipment should include a tracheostomy tube, an endotracheal tube, a laryngoscope, suitable retractors or skin hooks and tracheal dilators. Antibiotics are only given if there is a medical reason for doing so and there is no indication for routine mucolytics or steroids.

Decannulation problems

Although the airway is deemed to be adequate or near adequate before the decannulation trial is commenced, significant numbers of children still have problems. In one report (Black, Baldwin and Johns, 1984), 30% had an initial problem with chest infections and respiratory distress but this large percentage is unusual and can be attributed to the large numbers of problem patients with subglottic stenosis who are referred to that centre. Others (Carter and Benjamin, 1983; Line *et al.*, 1986) reported very few problems and the present author shares this experience. When respiratory distress does occur the causative factors are thought to be as described below.

Dead space

An increase in the dead space occurs when the tracheostomy is closed. In addition, the infant's air passages are absolutely and relatively smaller than those of an adult and the airway resistance will, therefore, be relatively increased. An increased oxygen requirement in children will emphasize any airway resistance and further compromise previously diseased lungs. However, these factors should have manifested their effects in the early assessment prior to decannulation and it is doubtful whether they would be very significant after decannulation.

Tracheal narrowing above the stoma

This is the most probable cause of decannulation problems and there is more than one aetiology. First, a significant granuloma may have been misjudged at the endoscopic assessment, or it may have increased in size or reappeared in the interval between assessment and decannulation. A failed decannulation should, therefore, be followed by a repeated endoscopic assessment and a removal of the granulation if necessary. Second, there may be a flap of fibrous tissue or a displaced anterior tracheal wall above the stoma which may not be immediately obvious to the uninitiated. In the author's experience a flap of fibrous tissue is much more common. It has been claimed that the flap can be repositioned by inserting a nasotracheal tube for 72 hours (Carter and Benjamin, 1983), but it can also be sutured forwards (Benjamin and Curley, 1990; Azizkhan, Lacey and Wood, 1993) or removed surgically through the stoma (Rogers, 1980). Third, the trachea may be weakened in the vicinity of the stoma by a low-grade chondritis and this may cause collapse of the trachea during inspiration. Lastly, the repeated interference with the larynx, which occurs during the period of assessment and decannulation, may cause oedema in the subglottis where the lumen is critical for decannulation. This is particularly likely to occur where there was previously some congenital narrowing or where the original problem was one of acquired subglottic stenosis.

Reduced movement of vocal cords

It has been reported that the reflex abduction of the vocal cords with inspiration is dependent on airway resistance and that this reflex disappears in the presence of a long-standing tracheostomy (Sasaki, Fukuda and Kirchner, 1973). Although this had been demonstrated electromyographically and is a possible source of trouble, practical experience shows that it has no real clinical significance.

All the above may combine to cause trouble but the most likely problems are those of *suprastomal granulations* and *tracheal narrowing* due to tracheal weakness or a displaced anterior tracheal wall. Both these common problems are well treated by surgical decannulation.

Surgical decannulation

In this operation, the tracheostomy track is excised and the tracheal stoma is examined under direct vision. A pre-decannulation assessment is carried out as described above and endoscopy is performed immediately prior to the operation to confirm the presence or otherwise of granulations or a displaced anterior tracheal wall flap. A suitable orotracheal tube is introduced for general anaesthesia.

A horizontal elliptical skin incision is made around the external stoma and the resulting island of skin is grasped in an Allis forceps. The track with its surrounding cuff of fibrous tissue is freed down to the trachea with cutting diathermy. It is important not to pull too hard on the fibrous track as the weakened trachea may be tented upwards and damaged when the track is incised horizontally at the tracheal stoma. The tracheal opening and the intraluminal orotracheal tube can now be clearly seen and any visible granulations or excessive fibrous tissue are excised. A small triangular piece of anterior tracheal wall tissue, about 2 mm long, is now excised from the superior border of the tracheal stoma. This piece of tracheal wall is made up of fibrous tissue which may have been displaced posteriorly into the tracheal lumen and it often carries on its internal surface the suprastomal granuloma (Figure 26.8). One horizontal Vicryl suture is now placed in the stoma to recon-

struct the tubular structure of the trachea at this level and a repeat endoscopy is performed to ensure that there is no residual granuloma or displaced anterior wall flap. There must be no excessive narrowing of the tracheal lumen as a result of the suture. The orotracheal tube is reinserted and two more Vicryl sutures are placed in the tracheal incision to

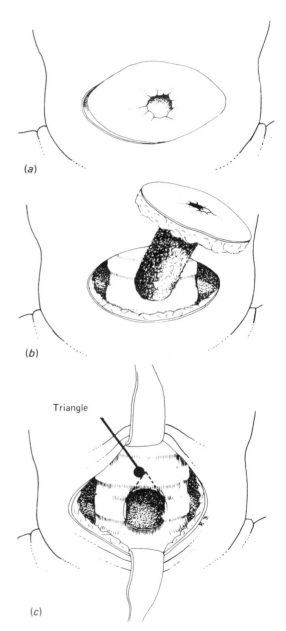

Figure 26.8 Surgical closure of the stoma: (*a*) the elliptical skin incision; (*b*) ellipse of skin with fibrous track around the stoma is freed by cutting diathermy; (*c*) a suprastomal triangle of anterior tracheal wall is excised

prevent the leakage of air into the neck tissues. After achieving haemostasis, the strap muscles, the subcutaneous tissues and skin are closed in layers. The child is sedated and taken back to the intensive care unit with the endotracheal tube still in place. Adequate humidification is maintained and the tube is now left in place for at least 24–48 hours. This is done to allow postoperative oedema to subside and a return to the otolaryngological ward is nearly always possible after 48 hours. Humidification is continued as required and the child is observed for a further 5 days before the skin sutures are removed. The child can then return home if the domestic arrangements are suitable.

There are several advantages in this approach which has been employed by the author for a period of 15 years:

1 It allows direct access to the tracheal stoma and permits the removal of any possible obstruction under direct vision
2 The suturing of the tracheal stoma reconstitutes the cylindrical wall of the trachea and, therefore, increases the strength of the trachea at this weakened point. In practice the closure does not produce narrowing of the lumen, which is prevented in any case by the presence of the endotracheal tube
3 The removal of the tough fibrous track hastens the healing in the soft tissues and the horizontal elliptical incision produces a better cosmetic result
4 It is well recognized that there is a high incidence of persistent tracheocutaneous fistulae following simple decannulation by tube removal. This is particularly so after long-term cannulation (as in subglottic stenosis) when the incidence may be 50% (Ochi, Bailey and Evans, 1992). The fistulous track will then need to be excised at a later date. By carrying out surgical decannulation such fistulae are avoided.

An obvious disadvantage of surgical decannulation is that an operation is required, but other disadvantages encountered have been relatively infrequent. In the author's experience, re-opening of the tracheostomy was necessary on two occasions within 3 days of the closure. In one there was a residual granuloma and the other developed marked surgical emphysema following inadequate suturing of the trachea. This resolved spontaneously.

This surgical method of decannulation was originally employed by the author to decannulate three children who had resisted all other attempts at decannulation (Rogers, 1980). It was so successful that the technique was initially used for all decannulations but is now reserved for the more difficult cases with large suprastomal granulations and suprastomal collapse. It is certainly a most useful addition to the available methods of treatment and the benefits have been confirmed by others (Joseph *et al.*, 1991; Al–Saati *et al.*, 1993).

Summary and conclusion

Tracheostomy in children is no longer the fearsome operation of the last century. There are still occasions when it is the primary treatment of choice, but its position has been largely usurped by intubation, particularly in inflammatory disease. The operation has become much safer by treating it as an elective procedure and emphasizing basic principles of surgical technique and aftercare. The mortality as a result of the tracheostomy itself is still around 5% even in the best hands and the main cause of death is obstruction of the tube at home. Decannulation is no longer a significant problem except in the worst cases of acquired subglottic stenosis and the scar on the neck is often unnoticeable by adulthood.

In the future the aim should be to eliminate the need for tracheostomy but, with the advances in neonatal medicine, cranial and thoracic surgery and the increase in the numbers and speed of motor vehicles, this is unlikely. There will gradually be changes in the types of tubes and their attachments and the operation itself may change as the age-old cricothyroidotomy and its successor, the minitracheostomy, are assessed more thoroughly.

References

AL-SAATI, MORRISON, G. A. J., CLARY, R. A. and BAILEY, C. M. (1993) Surgical decannulation of children with tracheostomy. *Journal of Laryngology and Otology*, **107**, 217–221

AZIZKHAN, R. G., LACEY, S. R. and WOOD, R. E. (1993) Anterior cricoid suspension and tracheal stomal closure for children with cricoid collapse and peristomal tracheomalacia following tracheostomy. *Journal of Paediatric Surgery*, **28**, 169–171

BENJAMIN, B. and CURLEY, J. W. A. (1990) Infant tracheostomy – endoscopy and decannulation. *International Journal of Pediatric Otorhinolaryngology*, **20**, 113–121

BLACK, R. J., BALDWIN, D. C. and JOHNS, A. N. (1984) 'Decannulation panic' in children: fact or fiction? *Journal of Laryngology and Otology*, **98**, 297–304

BLACK, T. L., FERNANDES, E. T. and CARR, M. G. (1988) Preventing accidental decannulations following tracheostomy. *Journal of Pediatric Surgery*, **23**, 143

BROCKHURST, P. J. and FELTOE, C. K. (1991) Corrosion and fracture of a silver tracheostomy tube. *Journal of Laryngology and Otology*, **105**, 48–49

CARTER, P. and BENJAMIN, B. (1983) Ten year review of pediatric tracheotomy. *Annals of Otology, Rhinology and Laryngology*, **92**, 398–400

COHEN, S. R., DESMOND, M. S., EAVEY, R. D. and MAY, B. C. (1977) Endoscopy and tracheostomy in the neonatal period. A 10-year review. *Annals of Otology, Rhinology and Laryngology*, **86**, 577–583

CRYSDALE, W. S. and SENDI, K. (1988) Evolution in the management of acute epiglottitis: a 10 year experience with 242 children. *International Anaesthesiology Clinics*, **26**, 32–38

FEARON, B. and COTTON, R. (1974) Surgical correction of subglottic stenosis of the larynx in infants and children. A progress report. *Annals of Otology, Rhinology and Laryngology*, **83**, 428–431

FROST, E. A. M. (1976) Tracing the tracheostomy. *Annals of Otology, Rhinology and Laryngology*, **85**, 618–624

FRY, T. L., FISCHER, N. D., JONES, R. D. and PILLSBURY, H. C. (1985) Comparisons of tracheostomy incisions in a pediatric model. *Annals of Otology, Rhinology and Laryngology*, **94**, 450–453

GERSON, C. R. and TUCKER, G. F. (1982) Infant tracheotomy. *Annals of Otology, Rhinology and Laryngology*, **91**, 413–416

GOODALL, E. W. (1934) The story of tracheostomy. *British Journal of Childhood Diseases*, **31**, 167–176

HOME, F. (1765) *An Enquiry into the Natural Causes and Cure of Croup*. Edinburgh: Kincaid and Bell

IRVING, R. M., JONES, N. S., BAILEY, C. M. and MELVILLE, J. (1991) A guide to the selection of paediatric tracheostomy tubes. *Journal of Laryngology and Otology*, **105**, 1046–1051

JOSEPH, H. T., JANI, P., PREECE, J. M., BAILEY, C. M. and EVANS, J. N. G. (1991) Paediatric tracheostomy: persistent tracheo-cutaneous fistula following decannulation. *International Journal of Pediatric Otorhinolaryngology*, **22**, 231–236

LINE, W. S., HAWKINS, D. B., KAHLSTROM, E. J., MACLAUGHLIN, E. F. and ENSLEY, J. C. (1986) Tracheotomy in infants and young children: the changing perspective, 1970–1985. *Laryngoscope*, **96**, 510–515

MADDERN, B. R., WERKHAVEN, J. and STOOL, S. E. (1989) Post-tracheotomy granulation tissue managed by carbon dioxide laser excision. *Annals of Otology, Rhinology and Laryngology*, **98**, 828–830

MALLORY, G. B., REILLY, J. S., MOTOYAMA, E. K., MUTICH, R., KENNA, M. A. and STOOL, S. E. (1985) Tidal flow measurement in the decision to decannulate the pediatric patient. *Annals of Otology, Rhinology and Laryngology*, **94**, 454–457

MUKHERJEE, D. K. (1979) The changing concepts of tracheostomy. *Journal of Laryngology and Otology*, **93**, 899–907

NELSON, T. G. (1958) *Tracheostomy: a Clinical and Experimental Study*. Baltimore: Williams and Wilkins

OCHI, J. W., BAILEY, C. M. and EVANS, J. N. (1992) Decannulation and suprastomal collapse. *Annals of Otology, Rhinology and Laryngology*, **101**, 656–658

OKAFOR, B. D. (1983) Tracheostomy in the management of paediatric airway problems. *Ear, Nose and Throat Journal*, **62**, 50–55

PRACY, R. (1976) Tracheostomy tubes. In: *Scientific Foundations of Otolaryngology*, edited by R. Hinchcliffe and D. Harrison. London: William Heinemann Medical Books. pp. 766–772

PRACY, R. (1979) Intubation of the larynx, laryngotomy and tracheostomy. In: *Scott-Brown's Diseases of the Ear, Nose and Throat*, 4th edn, edited by J. Ballantyne and J. Groves. London: Butterworths. pp. 567–586

PRESCOTT, C. A. and VANLIERDE, M. J. (1989) Tracheostomy in children – the Red Cross War Memorial Children's Hospital experience. *International Journal of Pediatric Otorhinolaryngology*, **17**, 97–107

PRESCOTT, C. A. J. (1992) Peristomal complications of paediatric tracheostomy. *International Journal of Pediatric Otorhinolaryngology*, **23**, 141–49

QUINEY, R. E., SPENCER, M. G., BAILEY, C. M., EVANS, J. N. G. and GRAHAM, J. M. (1986) Management of sub-glottic stenosis: experience from two centres. *Archives of Disease in Childhood*, **61**, 686–690

RAO, A. J., AIYER, C. R., KOMATSU, T., SHIMADA, Y., YANAGITA, N. and HATTORI, S. (1989) Model of a new generation of tracheostomy and endotracheal tubes. *Annals of Otology, Rhinology and Laryngology*, **98**, 157–159

REILLY, J. S. and MYER, C. M. (1985) Excision of suprastomal granulation tissue. *Laryngoscope*, **95**, 1545–1546

RODGERS, B. M., BROOKS, J. J. and TALBERT, J. L. (1979) Pediatric tracheostomy: long term evaluation. *Journal of Pediatric Surgery*, **14**, 258–263

ROGERS, J. H. (1980) Decannulation by external exploration of the tracheostomy in children. *Journal of Laryngology and Otology*, **94**, 454–457

SALMON, L. F. W. (1957) Tracheostomy: the evolution of an operation. *Guy's Hospital Gazette*, **71**, 233–242

SASAKI, C. T., FUKUDA, H. and KIRCHNER, J. A. (1973) Laryngeal abductor activity in response to varying ventilatory resistance. *Transactions of the American Academy of Ophthalmology and Otolaryngology*, **77**, 403–410

SONI, N. K., CHATTERJI, P. and THIND, S. S. (1984) Tracheostomy in children. *Indian Journal of Paediatrics*, **51**, 45–47

SWIFT, A. C. and ROGERS, J. H. (1987) The changing indications for tracheostomy in children. *Journal of Laryngology and Otology*, **101**, 1258–1262

TEPAS, J. J., HERDY, J. H., SHERMETA, D. W. and HALLER, J. A. (1981) Tracheostomy in neonates and small infants: problems and pitfalls. *Surgery*, **89**, 635–639

TOM, L. W. C., MILLER, L., WETMORE, R. F., HANDLER, S. D. and POTSIC, W. P. (1993) Endoscopic assessment in children with tracheotomies. *Archives of Otolaryngology and Head and Neck Surgery*, **119**, 321–324

TUCKER, J. A. and TUCKER, G. F. (1979) A clinical perspective on the development and anatomical aspects of the infant larynx and trachea. In: *Laryngo–Tracheal Problems in the Pediatric Patient*, edited by G. B. Healy and T. J. I. McGill Springfield, Illinois: Charles C. Thomas. pp. 3–8

WETMORE, R. F., HANDLER, S. D. and POTSIC, W. P. (1982) Pediatric tracheostomy experience during the past decade. *Annals of Otology, Rhinology and Laryngology*, **91**, 628–632

YUNG, M. W. and SNOWDON, S. L. (1984) Respiratory resistance of tracheostomy tubes. *Archives of Otolaryngology*, **110**, 591–595

27

Home care of the tracheostomied child

Rosalind Wilson

Tracheostomy is an essential part of many life-saving procedures in paediatric laryngology. The majority of children return to the community with the tracheostomy in place and with few exceptions they will be cared for at home by their parents. Tracheostomy care is a daunting undertaking for any family and the responsibility for training the care givers lies with the nursing staff on the ward, with the assistance of the liaison health visitor, the social worker and the clinical psychologist. As soon as it is known that a child is to have a tracheostomy, preparation of the care givers and liaison with the community must begin.

A tracheostomy is a frightening prospect for anyone and needs to be handled sensitively by experienced nursing staff. Most parents have little or no knowledge of basic anatomy, so clear explanations with the aid of diagrams are essential to clarify what the tracheostomy is and its purpose in respiration. In the discussion of the anatomy it is important to include how the child's ability to speak may be affected, and the need for humidification, as the normal airway is bypassed by the tracheostomy.

Time spent talking with the parents at this stage is valuable and a clearly defined plan should be made. It is essential that there is an agreed policy of teaching on the ward, to ensure consistency of information from all members of staff to avoid confusion and to promote confidence.

The new tracheostomy

Seeing their child with a tracheostomy for the first time is undoubtedly a very distressing sight for the parents, though the fact that the child no longer needs intensive care and is not struggling for breath but breathing easily and begining to feed normally helps significantly in the process of acceptance. Nursing staff must be aware of the parent's anxieties and give them time to adjust.

Parents often wrestle with mixed feelings of fear, guilt, inability to cope and sometimes even revulsion. Gradually after a few days of watching the child improving and observing the care given by the nurses, they feel able to start learning tracheostomy management themselves. All parents, however apprehensive, want to be able to care for their child at home. It is important that they know that the child will not be discharged until they are confident in the care required and the nursing and medical staff are confident that the child will be safely looked after.

Initially the child will be cared for by an experienced nurse, who will begin to show the parents what she is doing and why and which elements of the care will need to be continued at home. Two or 3 days after the formation of the tracheostomy, parents are usually willing to start learning to suction their child, observing the nurse's demonstration and then doing it themselves under supervision. They will become more familiar with the sounds the child makes, but learning to assess the child's need for suction takes time and the nurse will need to continue to advise them.

Suction of the tracheostomy

The aim of suction is to clear the tracheostomy tube and the secretions gathered at the tube tip, but not to suction the chest. When demonstrating the nurse must show the parents another tube so that they can get an idea of its length and how far to pass the catheter. The catheter should be passed no more than 1 cm beyond the tube tip to avoid damaging the trachea.

A new suction catheter must be used every time and the suction power applied only on the outward journey. It is safe to rotate the catheter while suctioning but only once one is sure that the tip of the catheter is in the tracheostomy tube not the trachea.

A child's need for suction must always be decided individually. It is dangerous to prescribe a routine.

As soon as the tracheostomy is formed the parents should be helped to understand the meaning of what they are hearing. Parents soon become tuned in to their child's needs and know exactly when to suction.

Concerns are often voiced about frequent suction provoking excess secretions. This will not happen if the suction is done properly. It is more dangerous to leave the child at risk of a blocked tube.

Becoming aware of the signs of increased respiratory effort is an essential part of caring for a child with any type of artificial airway. The carer must be able to identify deviations from the normal, to know what to do and when to seek assistance. During the first week postoperatively it is hoped that the parents will become familiar with suction and changing the tapes and will begin to take over responsibility for the child's daily care, hygiene, nutrition and general well-being. At this stage, although increasingly involving the parents, the stoma care should still be carried out by the nurse, as the stitches are still *in situ* and the wound may need attention.

The first tube change is not done until 7 days after the formation of the stoma to allow adequate epithelialization. It is done by, or under the supervision of the medical staff. The child is now breathing easily and the stoma healing so the remaining time in hospital is used to teach the parents how to change the tracheostomy tube and to begin to take on the complete care of their child, sleeping next to the child's bed to become accustomed to their suction needs at night, learning how to use the equipment and most importantly gaining confidence.

Changing the tracheostomy tube

The tracheostomy tube should be changed weekly unless the child has a chest infection, in which case it may be necessary to change the tube every 2–3 days due to the tenacity of the secretions and possible blockage. The tube changing procedure must become a routine part of the child's life, not a trauma. It is important that the child is gently encouraged to cooperate, a baby will find the experience distressing at first but if she is not frightened by restraint but held gently and soothed she will soon become used to the procedure. These children become cooperative at a surprisingly early age when they trust the carer and know what to expect.

For a routine tube change there should be two carers involved, one to carry out the tube change,

the other to assist. The major role of the assistant is to hold the tube in place following the instructions of the changer.

The tube change must be done with the suction pump to hand as it is likely to be needed during the procedure.

The new tube and tapes should be prepared; some people prefer to tie one side of the tapes to the tube before they start, a lubricant jelly spread thinly on the sides of the tube eases insertion.

1 The assistant holds the tube in place, one finger on each flange (Figure 27.1*a*)
2 The changer cuts and removes the tapes
3 The changer takes the new tube in one hand, removes the old tube with the other and quickly inserts the new tube through the stoma in a curved action that has been described as 'pouring a cup of tea' (Figure 27.1*b*)
4 The assistant holds the new tube in place (suction is often needed at this point)
5 The child is reassured and praised
6 The changer ties the tapes with at least three knots on the first side and a bow on the second side
7 Tape tension is tested with the assistant still holding the tube in place, the child is helped into a sitting position, one finger should fit between the tapes and the back of the neck (Figure 27.1*c*)
8 Once satisfied with the tension, the bow is converted into a knot by pulling the loops and adding more knots
9 When the tapes are firmly knotted on both sides the assistant can release the grip.

Changing the tapes

Tape changing should be done daily. Babies particularly need frequent tape changes as the tapes are likely to lie in a skin crease which can become red, excoriated and painful. The neck is cleaned and dried and new tapes are applied, one-quarter inch (0.6 cm) cotton tape is preferred as it will not slip. Cream is not recommended but a non-gauze dressing tucked under the flanges may be of use. The area must be kept clean and dry. The procedure itself is a modified version of the tube change and is best performed after the child's bath.

Sleeping and supervision

At home, the baby with a new tracheostomy should sleep near to the parents in order to familiarize them with the sound she makes and to become accustomed to the frequency of suction required.

Before leaving hospital it is essential that the primary carer has the opportunity to sleep close to the baby, to reassure herself and the staff that she will

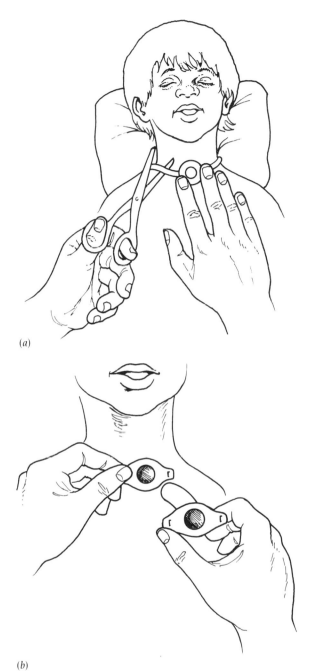

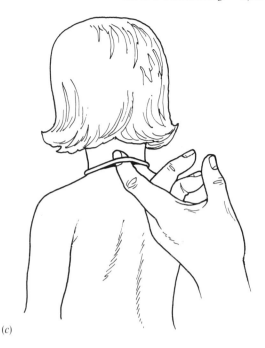

(a)

(c)

(b)

Figure 27.1   Changing the tracheostomy tube. (*a*) The assistant holds the tube in place; (*b*) removing and replacing the tubes; (*c*) tape tension is tested

wake up when the child needs suction. A few noisy toys in the cot are useful to alert the parent to a restless child. Very soon parents become acutely aware of any change in the child's condition. After a

few months the baby may be moved to a separate room, when a listening device can be used allowing the parent to move freely about the house and garden.

Bathing

As swimming is forbidden, parents may worry about the safety of bathing. Bathtime is not a problem if care is taken. All children must be supervised while in the bath and some splashing will not cause any harm. Hairwashing is best done with the child sitting up in the bath using a shower attachment or a jug so that the water flows down the child's back.

School

A child with a tracheostomy should go to a mainstream school. This often requires negotiation; teaching staff are frequently alarmed by the prospect of having such a child in their classroom. The opportunity to meet the child is extremely valuable to see that the child has a problem but is not unwell and is able to take part in all the activities of the classroom (Figure 27.2). A 'Statement of Educational Needs' is required to certify the child's suitability for mainstream school.

Letters from the otolaryngological surgeon may also be required to stress the need for a welfare assistant who must be employed to attend school with the child to take responsibility for all the tracheostomy care.

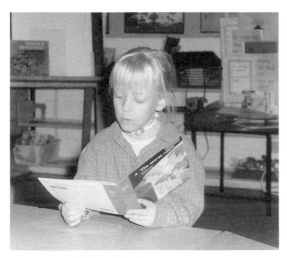

Figure 27.2   Child in school

Undoubtedly there will be some children with additional problems who need to be educated in special environments, but a tracheostomy alone should not preclude them from mainstream education alongside their peers.

Discipline

It is very important to react to the child's behaviour as one would to any other child. The tracheostomy may be part of the child's life for many years, so treating her as an invalid is not doing her any favours. A spoilt, indulged child is not a happy child.

The child should be encouraged to take part in all the activities of their peer group, with the exception of swimming. Many children with tracheostomies do gymnastics, ride horses and take part in many other energetic sports (Figure 27.3). A fine scarf or a purpose-made filter may be of use in dusty atmospheres, though the filters are not recommended for routine use as they tend to mask the need for suction.

Speech and language development

The presence of a tracheostomy is frequently believed to be a reason for a child's lack of speech and slow language development. So long as there is sufficient air leak around the tracheostomy tube to allow vocalization, the child should be encouraged to speak, just as any other infant of similar age.

Some babies may not be able to vocalize, due to the comparatively large size of the tube in the airway so they should be encouraged to copy oro-motor movements and to develop natural gesture and then

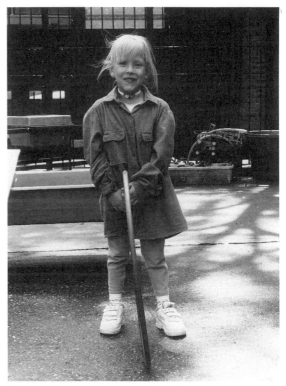

Figure 27.3   Child at activity in a park

signing. The Makaton signing system, which has been designed specially for children with communication disorders, is ideal for such children and does not stop them developing normal speech when they later acquire the ability to produce some sound.

Every tracheostomized child must be assessed by a speech and language therapist who can advise the parents and make recommendations to the local speech therapist. The child may be suitable for a speaking valve which, for the majority of children, improves the volume and clarity of the voice, a major factor in the child's development, integration into society and ability to cope in school.

Travel

Wherever the child goes the suction pump must go. The carer must also bring sufficient supplies for the time away: spare tracheostomy tubes, tapes, suction catheters, scissors, syringes and saline.

For car travel it is possible to get a recharging adaptor for the portable pump which is used in the dashboard cigarette lighter socket. Airlines will carry suction units by prior arrangement with the airport medical officer. Cabin air pressure does not have any adverse effects on the tracheostomized child. An adaptor may be required for differing electrical voltages abroad.

Equipment

Tracheostomy tubes

There are many types of tube available, silver and plastic, cheap and expensive. Simple one piece plastic tubes are often preferred by parents of babies and small children, while silver tubes with multiple parts are better suited to older children who can become independent in the care of their tracheostomies.

Commonly used tracheostomy tubes

Plastic tubes

1 *Great Ormond Street pattern* (Figure 27.4)
   Unobtrusive and parents prefer them visually
   Bevelled, making insertion easier
   Available with extensions to prevent occlusion
   Disposable after each use and relatively inexpensive.
2 *Portex paediatric tracheostomy tubes* (Figure 27.5)
   Often the most readily available
   Compatible with 'Rusch' speaking valves
   Blunt ended without an introducer
   Disposable single use items.
3 *Shiley paediatric tracheostomy tubes* (Figure 27.6)
   Blunt ended with an introducer
   Compatible with 'Rusch' speaking valves
   Available in shorter lengths for neonates
   Disposable single use items.

All plastic tracheostomy tubes are made from plastic that becomes softer at body temperature reducing the risk of trauma to the trachea and granulation formation. They are uncomplicated one piece tubes that are commonly preferred by parents.

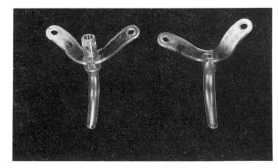

Figure 27.4 Great Ormond Street (GOS) tube. Left, extended; right, flat

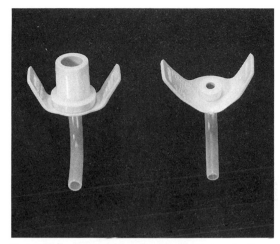

Figure 27.5 Portex tube. Left, with 15 mm termination; right, without termination

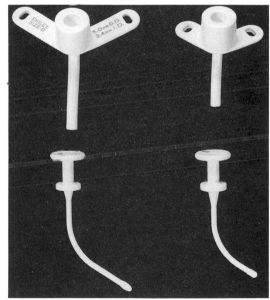

Figure 27.6 Shiley tube. Left, paediatric; right, neonatal, with introducers

Silver tracheostomy tubes (Figure 27.7)

Silver tubes are expensive but may be used for many years. There is a variety of designs most of which have five parts:

1 The main or outer tube
2 The inner, plain or sleeping tube
3 The speaking tube with valve and fenestration (suction must never be done through this tube)
4 The introducer
5 The blocker.

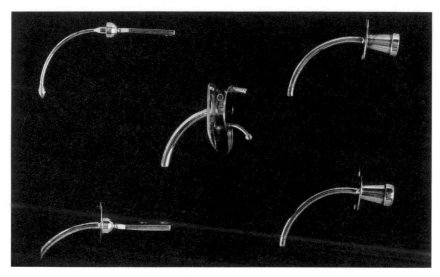

Figure 27.7 Silver tube. Clockwise from top left, introducer, plain or sleeping tube, speaking tube, blocker and in the centre, the tube itself

Silver tubes may irritate some children and they are believed to cause granulations to form in the trachea but they do allow the older child or teenager a far greater degree of freedom as the inner tube can be removed and cleaned by the young person when it becomes blocked. A plastic tube would need to be completely changed.

Suction catheters

All the suction catheters now available are plastic and are single use disposable items, under no circumstances should they be cleaned and reused.

Some have the advantage of a hole in the hub which enables the user to control the suction power without having to kink the catheter.

Suction pumps

A child with a tracheostomy needs three suction pumps. To the uninitiated this will seem excessive but their need soon becomes apparent because whenever the child goes suction must be available.

1 A powerful electric pump such as the Sam 12 is the most important, it must be placed permanently in a position where it is most useful, usually beside the child's bed (Figure 27.8a).
2 A portable pump, Laerdal or Vacu-Aide is essential to enable the mother and child to leave the house and return to their normal routines. These pumps are rechargeable and must be plugged into the mains when at home. They are not intended to be

used 24 hours a day, so at home the SAM 12 should be used (Figure 27.8b).
3 A portable foot pump, e.g. Ambu is vital in the event of a power cut or pump failure as it relies only on human effort, some parents find it useful to keep it in the boot of the car (Figure 27.8c).

All these pumps must be cleaned regularly with hot soapy water and a sterilizing solution. They need regular servicing and the filters are changed according to the manufacturer's instructions. Some hospitals are able to organize a loan of equipment but their provision is the responsibility of the local health authority.

Discharge planning

Discharge planning should start as soon as it is known that the child is to have a tracheostomy formed. It is the local health visitor's responsibility to provide the equipment and supplies, so it is important that she is given time to plan and, if possible, invited to meet the child and family prior to discharge.

The parents will have been taught all the direct care in the hospital but often value the advice and moral support of a local health professional that they can get to know well.

The hospital social worker can inform the parents about benefits they are entitled to and can liaise locally if further help is required.

Some local authorities are able to offer added bonuses such as providing a nurse overnight on a regular basis or giving the family a designated parking space outside the house.

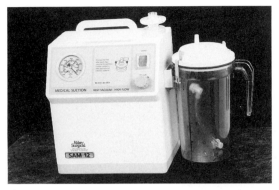

(a)

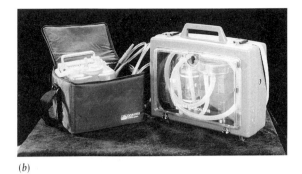

(b)

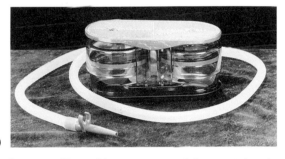

(c)

Figure 27.8 (a) Sam 12 suction pump; (b) portable suction pumps; left, Vacu-Aide, right, Laerdal; (c) Ambu foot pump

A child with a tracheostomy requiring admission for a chest infection or perhaps an unrelated condition does not necessarily need to go to the specialist hospital. It is important to forge links with the local hospital, so that they can get to know the child's needs and be able to offer respite care on occasion.

Dangers may arise with children's tracheostomies in hospitals not familiar with their care. Staff may not be aware of the need for constant supervision and isolate the child in a cubicle. If individual supervision is not available children are much better cared for in an open ward where staff are constantly at hand.

28

Neonatal pulmonary disorders

R. Dinwiddie

The establishment of breathing and the adaptation of the neonatal circulation to extrauterine life are two of the most important events which occur at the time of birth. These physiological changes are mediated by a number of factors acting both locally and systemically. The major control of these events is through the respiratory centres in the brain stem and it is therefore vital that these are present, intact and functioning normally if the adaptation to extrauterine life is to occur uneventfully. Most diseases seen in the neonatal period are a consequence of adverse effects on these natural physiological processes, including immaturity, infection, birth trauma or congenital malformation.

Onset of breathing

The onset of breathing is brought about by the responses to a number of complex reflexes which stimulate the respiratory centres. These include thermal stimulation such as cold, external tactile stimuli, and intrinsic reflexes within the rib cage which respond to the changes in chest wall shape as it passes through the birth canal and at the moment of birth itself. Chemical changes in the blood such as hypoxia and hypercarbia also have major stimulatory effects on the central nervous system as do acute cardiovascular pressure changes which occur after clamping of the umbilical cord. The inspiratory pressures required to open the lungs are relatively low, of the order of 10–20 cmH$_2$O; these are sufficient to overcome the resistive forces of the lungs, the residual fluid within them and the natural compliance of the chest wall.

The functional residual capacity is established within the first few breaths and a positive expiratory pressure is exerted during the latter part of these breaths in order to assist clearance of lung fluid. The normal functional residual capacity is approximately 30 ml/kg and is stabilized during the first 30–60 minutes of life.

The lungs of the functionally mature fetus are normally filled with surfactant-rich fluid which has the same volume as the subsequent functional residual capacity after birth. This liquid is emptied from the lungs during and after the birth process itself, partly by external compression of the chest as it passes through the vagina (or the uterine wall in cases delivered by caesarean section). This accounts for about one-third of the lung fluid, the remainder is absorbed directly across the pulmonary lymphatics or into the pulmonary capillaries during the first few minutes of life.

The changes in lung volume and compliance are matched by major circulatory adaptation which occurs at the same time. Before birth only about 10% of the cardiac output passes through the lungs because of the high pulmonary vascular resistance *in utero*. At birth the aeration of the lungs produces a rapid reduction in the pulmonary vascular resistance and this is accompanied by a rise in the P_aO_2 from intrauterine levels of 4 kPa (30 mmHg) to the postnatal levels of 8–12 kPa (50–90 mmHg). These changes stimulate the closure of the ductus arteriosus and the foramen ovale thus sealing off the large right to left intracardiac shunts which were present *in utero*. These fetal channels are however not irreversibly closed and can reopen during periods of stress or hypoxia.

Central control of breathing is vital to the maintenance of life, and the respiratory centres must remain intact during this period. They are particularly sensitive to hypoxic insult and respiratory and metabolic acidosis. They may be damaged by trauma or haemorrhage secondary to a particularly difficult or protracted delivery. They are also sensitive to the effect of drugs such as pethidine given to the mother for sedation or analgesia. Any interruption to the many complex natural processes occurring during birth can lead to asphyxial insult.

Birth asphyxia

Asphyxia during birth may be acute or chronic. Some babies suffer from acute hypoxia during the birth process, e.g. due to cord prolapse, while others have had chronic intrauterine asphyxia secondary to processes such as placental insufficiency which can occur for a number of reasons during pregnancy.

The major conditions leading to birth asphyxia can be divided into three categories: maternal, placental and fetal. Maternal predisposing factors include hypertension, diabetes, underlying cardiac or renal disease, abuse of drugs or alcohol, hypotension, or anaesthetic complications such as aspiration pneumonitis. Other causes include multiple births, abnormal presentation, cephalopelvic disproportion, and prolonged labour. Placental problems include abruption, placenta praevia, early separation and cord prolapse. Fetal conditions include pulmonary hypoplasia, anaemia secondary to rhesus disease, meconium aspiration and congenital malformations, particularly of the heart or lungs.

The events which occur during an asphyxial episode have been well described in the classical work of Dawes *et al.* (1963). The asphyxiated infant gasps initially and this is followed by a period of primary apnoea during which there is a decrease in heart rate, but maintenance of blood pressure and peripheral circulation. Hypoxaemia results in profound cyanosis. Resuscitation during this period will be effective using external stimulation and increasing the inspired oxygen to be inhaled during the next phase of breathing which begins within 1–2 minutes. This takes the form of gasping and lasts for a further 4–5 minutes following which terminal apnoea occurs. By this time there is profound hypoxia, hypercarbia, acidosis and circulatory collapse. After 7–8 minutes of significant hypoxia cerebral damage begins. Resuscitation at this stage requires positive pressure ventilation, usually following endotracheal intubation, using pressures of up to 20–30 cmH$_2$O with an initial breath of 3–5 seconds (Vyas *et al.*, 1981). Bag and mask ventilation can also be effective in the absence of personnel skilled in intubation. Circulatory support by external cardiac massage is essential in those with profound bradycardia or asystole. Intravenous drugs such as adrenalin (which can also be given topically via the endotracheal tube), glucose, sodium bicarbonate and calcium gluconate may also be required (Milner, 1991). Reversal of the effects of maternal sedative drugs such as pethidine, which prolongs the period of primary apnoea, can be achieved by the use of naloxone.

After acute resuscitation, such infants often require extensive support including ventilation, inotropic maintenance of heart rate and blood pressure, treatment of renal failure and correction of acid–base imbalance. Neurological outcome depends also on control of seizures and cerebral oedema in the neonatal period. The outcome is extremely variable, although a significant proportion of those who do survive the initial difficulties can turn out to be normal (Levene, 1993).

Respiratory distress syndrome

This condition, formerly called hyaline membrane disease, can arise in the newborn period for a number of reasons. The vast majority of cases, however, are due to surfactant deficiency in the preterm infant. It is the commonest cause of mortality and morbidity in this age group especially among those who weigh less than 1.5 kg at birth and whose gestation is less than 32 weeks. The illness is due to functional immaturity of the lungs resulting in a failure of adequate surfactant production by type II alveolar lining cells. Other predisposing factors include birth asphyxia, rhesus disease, maternal haemorrhage or diabetes, and multiple pregnancy.

The infant develops typical signs of respiratory difficulty within the first 2 hours after birth. These include indrawing of respiratory muscles, tachypnoea, sternal recession and expiratory grunting. The chest X-ray shows a typical ground glass appearance secondary to alveolar hypoventilation and an air bronchogram due to maintenance of large airway patency because of its cartilage. The differential diagnosis includes group B streptococcal pneumonia, persistent fetal circulation and underlying cardiac anomalies such as transposition of the great arteries.

Treatment

Treatment of respiratory distress syndrome is complex. Prevention of preterm delivery is desirable if possible. Antenatal steroids are helpful if given to the mother at least 24 hours and not more than 7 days before delivery (Crowley, Chalmers and Keirse, 1990). The administration of prenatal thyrotrophic hormone (TRH) is also useful. The use of surfactant in the past few years has made a significant difference to morbidity and mortality of this condition (Morley, 1991). These substances can be synthetic and consist mainly of phosphatidyl choline (PC) and phosphatidyl glycerol (PG) or they may be derived from natural sources such as bovine or pig lungs or human amniotic fluid. The surfactant can either be given prophylactically at birth to high-risk preterm babies or to those who have already developed symptoms of respiratory distress syndrome as 'rescue' therapy.

Mechanical ventilation is also used to support those infants who develop respiratory failure despite other supportive measures (Table 28.1).

Ventilation with positive end-expiratory pressure (PEEP) is indicated when there is recurrent apnoea or impending exhaustion. Inability to maintain P_aO_2 above 8 kPa (60 mmHg) in 60% oxygen or P_aCO_2 below 8 kPa (60 mmHg) would be indications for this level of support. A wide variety of machines and ventilatory techniques is now available for the treatment of this condition.

The aim is to keep the pressures applied to the lungs to the lowest level compatible with response so as to prevent acute complications such as pneumothorax or long-term problems such as chronic lung disease (Greenough, 1990). The use of rapid rate ventilation can also be helpful, particularly in the extremely small preterm infant. A few infants may benefit from paralysis, although this is not used regularly. High frequency ventilation is also used and can be successful.

Long-term risks include subglottic stenosis from long-term intubation but this should be avoidable with modern techniques of tube placement (Sherman and Nelson, 1989). A few such infants will still require surgery for this complication.

Other acute problems include secondary infection with Gram-positive or Gram-negative bacteria or fungi such as *Candida albicans*. Chronic lung disease/bronchopulmonary dysplasia remains a major complication in a small number of cases. Nowadays, with adequate support, 95% of infants with respiratory distress syndrome can expect to survive although the mortality rate remains higher in those weighing less than 1 kg at birth. Long-term outlook for lung function is good in the absence of chronic lung disease/bronchopulmonary dysplasia.

Transient tachypnoea of the newborn

This condition is seen in a number of infants who develop respiratory difficulties including tachypnoea, indrawing and cyanosis usually lasting for about 12–24 hours after birth. The chest X-ray shows bilateral haziness due to the presence of persistent interstitial lung fluid. The condition is more common in those born by caesarean section, probably because less fluid is squeezed from the lungs during the birth process itself. Treatment is supportive, including oxygen to maintain adequate blood gases. The need for ventilation is uncommon and most infants recover rapidly with no sequelae.

Patent ductus arteriosus

Persistent patency of the ductus arteriosus is rare in term infants. It is, however, extremely common in

Table 28.1 Treatment of respiratory distress syndrome

Surfactant
Neutral thermal environment
Oxygen P_aO_2 7–12 kPa (70–90 mmHg)
Correction of acid–base imbalance
Continuous positive airway pressure (CPAP)
Artificial ventilation
Paralysis – in selected cases
Pulmonary vasodilators
Antibiotics for other causes (group B streptococci)

infants with respiratory distress syndrome, reaching levels of 40% in those under 1 kg and 25% of those between 1.0 and 1.5 kg at birth. It is also more common in those with a higher fluid intake. Many preterm infants, especially those with respiratory distress syndrome, develop classical signs of patent ductus arteriosus towards the end of the first week of life. These include tachycardia, bounding peripheral pulses, a midclavicular murmur which becomes continuous, and a precordial thrill. At this stage the infant develops a left to right shunt through the ductus so flooding the lungs with extra blood flow. This results in pulmonary oedema, increased lung stiffness and a higher risk of acquiring secondary lung infection. The liver also enlarges indicating cardiac failure. Chest X-ray shows cardiomegaly and pulmonary plethora.

Management consists of fluid restriction to 60–70% of daily requirements, diuretics and increased end-expiratory pressure ventilation to reduce pulmonary oedema. If these measures fail then indomethacin, a prostaglandin synthetase inhibitor, is given in divided doses over 2–3 days, usually with a good response (Gersony *et al.*, 1983). Some ducts reopen after this treatment but by that stage there has usually been a sufficiently good response to allow weaning from the ventilator. If these measures fail then surgical ligation, preferably undertaken in the neonatal unit, is performed.

Persistent pulmonary hypertension (persistent fetal circulation)

Persistent fetal circulation occurs when the normal reduction in pulmonary vascular resistance fails to occur after birth. The normal stimuli for this process include the increased oxygen levels after breathing starts and the changes in circulatory pressures which occur with clamping of the cord. Increased tone of the pulmonary arterioles may be brought about by persistent hypoxia, especially in the presence of acidosis, and this results in an attempt to revert to the fetal circulatory pattern. This complication can occur in the baby with respiratory distress syndrome, but is more likely in those who have suffered from intrauterine asphyxia. It is also seen in those with meconium aspiration syndrome and where there is group B streptococcal pneumonia and septicaemia. Persistent fetal circulation can be difficult to distinguish from cyanotic congenital heart disease and echocardiography is required to exclude an underlying cardiac lesion.

Treatment consists of ventilatory support in an attempt to increase the pH to more than 7.48. At this level pulmonary vasodilation is more likely to occur. Hyperventilation to reduce P_aCO_2 level is useful if it can be achieved without significant barotrauma to the lungs. More recently, high frequency oscillation has been successful in maintaining oxygenation. Pulmonary vasodilators, such as tolazoline by continuous infusion, can be effective in some cases. Recently nitric oxide by continuous inhalation has also proved effective (Kinsella *et al.*, 1993). Where there is no response to these measures extracorporeal membrane oyxgenation can be used (Lancet, 1988).

Meconium aspiration syndrome

The passage of meconium before birth occurs in 8–15% of deliveries, however only a very small proportion, less than 1%, develop symptoms. The illness is usually seen in term or postmature babies and is rare in preterm infants. Meconium aspirated into the lower respiratory tract is extremely irritant to the lungs and it is this which results in the profound respiratory and circulatory changes which characterize the illness. This can occur *in utero* if there is fetal gasping which is a response to severe asphyxial insult. It is therefore possible for meconium to be aspirated into the trachea or even the peripheral parts of the lung before or during the birth itself. At birth large plugs in the trachea can cause acute airway obstruction and smaller plugs in the lower airways lead to partial airway obstruction and chemical pneumonitis which results in patchy lung collapse in some areas with overinflation and air trapping in others. The chest is classically barrel-shaped because of the overinflation in the lungs. Air leak is common and pneumothorax or pneumomediastinum occurs in as many as 40–50% of cases. The asphyxial and hypoxic insult often leads to an associated persistent pulmonary hypertension which can be severe.

The disease is preventable with proper antenatal care and the avoidance of fetal distress. At birth the airway, including the trachea, should be cleared by adequate suction if necessary. A chest X-ray should be taken in those who are symptomatic and will show patchy collapse in some areas with overinflation in others. Pneumothorax or pneumomediastinum may also be present.

Treatment is supportive and includes correction of acid–base imbalance, antibiotics for possible secondary bacterial infection and ventilation if necessary. Ventilation can be very difficult and some babies need to be paralysed, at least initially. Newer techniques of respiratory support including high frequency oscillation or extracorporeal membrane oxygenation (ECMO) have been used. Pulmonary vasodilators including tolazoline or nitric oxide may be required.

This condition carries a significant mortality in severe cases. A number of survivors have chronic neonatal lung disease and although the majority do make a complete recovery, a proportion have recurrent wheezy illness in the longer term (MacFarlane and Heaf, 1988).

Infections
Neonatal pneumonia

Pneumonia in the neonatal period is very common, especially in those who have other respiratory problems. It can be acquired before, during or after birth. The causative organisms can be bacterial, viral or fungal. The most serious bacterial pneumonia is due to the group B streptococcus. As many as 15% of mothers may harbour the organism in the birth canal and the baby will be in contact with this during the delivery. Despite this, less than 1% of such infants become clinically unwell. Their mortality however is extremely high. Predisposing factors include preterm delivery, prolonged rupture of the membranes and birth asphyxia. Presenting features are identical to classical respiratory distress syndrome. Chest X-ray shows the same appearance with bilateral ground glass shadowing. In the symptomatic infant the condition can be rapidly fatal unless early and appropriate antibiotics are given. Many are septicaemic at this stage and show evidence of shock and disseminated intravascular coagulation.

Treatment consists of circulatory support and antibiotics such as penicillin, gentamicin or a third generation cephalosporin. Maintenance of acid–base balance and ventilatory support are also vital. New forms of ventilation such as high frequency oscillation and other treatments such as ECMO have also been used successfully. Despite early and aggressive therapy the mortality for those with rapidly progressive disease remains high at about 60%.

A number of other bacteria can cause neonatal pneumonia including *Staphylococcus aureus*, *Staph. epidermidis*, *Pneumococcus* and *Listeria monocytogenes*. Gram-negative organisms such as *Escherichia coli*, *Klebsiella* and particularly *Pseudomonas aeruginosa* are also more common in infants who are ventilated for prolonged periods.

Chlamydia and fungi

Chlamydia trachomatis causes pneumonia in infants and should be looked for if there are persistent symptoms where conventional treatment is unsuccessful. It is usually associated with severe conjunctivitis as well. Fungi, including *Candida albicans* are pathogenic, especially in the debilitated neonate who has required several courses of antibacterial agents to control chronic chest infections. Extended treatment with antifungal agents is necessary.

Viral pneumonia

Viral pneumonia, caused by organisms such as cytomegalovirus, is well recognized in the neonatal period. As many as 0.3–1% of infants may be colonized with passively acquired cytomegalovirus at birth (Peckham *et al.*, 1983). A very small number develop persistent pneumonitis leading to recurrent wheezing and signs of respiratory infection. Sensorineural deafness is another well described complication. Ganciclovir, although toxic, can be used for treatment. The organism is readily cultured from the urine in such cases. Herpes simplex is another virus which can affect the neonate, infection with type I or II in the neonatal period can rarely lead to overwhelming infection with a high mortality and morbidity. Acyclovir is available for treatment.

Chronic lung disease
Bronchopulmonary dysplasia

A number of babies, especially those who are very low birthweight (< 1500 g at birth), develop chronic respiratory symptoms as a result of acute early neonatal lung disease. The incidence varies but is about 15–20% of babies in this weight range. The aetiology is multifactorial and includes impaired mucociliary clearance secondary to endotracheal intubation, barotrauma from ventilation, oxygen toxicity, chronic infection of the lower respiratory tract, and hypersecretion in the lungs. Other factors in some cases include patent ductus arteriosus and pulmonary oedema. Impaired vitamin intake and metabolism of vitamins A, D and E have also been implicated. Such infants remain oxygen dependent and have chronic lung changes evident both clinically and radiologically at 1 month of age.

Chest X-ray reveals two types of pathology, either bilateral haziness in lungs which are not overinflated (type I), or overinflated lung fields with cystic areas, especially in the lower zones (type II or classical bronchopulmonary dysplasia).

Treatment should consist of early weaning off ventilation if possible, adequate oxygenation, theophylline, diuretics and steroids (Greenough, 1990). Good nutrition is important but may be difficult if the infant is not tolerating feeds. Growth of the lungs is the key to recovery but this can take many months in the most severely ill. There is also a higher incidence of sudden

infant death in this group. Those with milder disease will gradually recover, although they are especially prone to lower respiratory tract infection in the first 2 years of life.

Recurrent apnoea

This is a common problem for preterm infants and is a variation of the normal pattern of periodic breathing seen at this age. Significant apnoea may be defined as episodes of cessation of breathing lasting for more than 20 seconds, or less than 20 seconds if accompanied by significant bradycardia. They may be central in origin due to immaturity or damage to the respiratory centres in the midbrain. They occur for a variety of other reasons including infections such as pneumonia, septicaemia or meningitis, metabolic acidosis, hypoglycaemia, seizures or as a complication of intracranial haemorrhage. Drugs such as phenobarbitone can suppress breathing. Apnoea also occurs as a consequence of respiratory or cardiac failure. Upper airway obstruction such as choanal atresia, micrognathia, for example in Pierre-Robin syndrome or cleft palate, can also precipitate attacks.

Those for whom no other underlying pathology can be found often respond to caffeine or theophylline. Attention should also be paid to the correction of any underlying severe anaemia, chronic hypoxia or acidosis. Those with severe episodes will require continuous positive airway pressure (CPAP) or ventilatory support until they are able to maintain an adequate respiratory drive spontaneously.

Congenital anomalies of the respiratory tract

These include abnormalities of the nose, palate, pharynx, trachea and major bronchi, lungs, rib cage and neuromuscular disorders. The range of anomalies is shown in Table 28.2.

Disease of the upper respiratory tract and larynx are considered elsewhere in this volume and will not be discussed further. Disorders of the lower respiratory tree, below the larynx are discussed in the following sections.

Trachea

Tracheal stenosis can be congenital or acquired. Affected infants present with biphasic stridor and respiratory difficulty, which may not necessarily be present at birth but which can first appear during an intercurrent respiratory tract infection. Wheezing is another common presenting feature due to retention of secretions below the level of the obstruction. Acquired tracheal stenosis is most commonly due to

Table 28.2 Congenital anomalies of the respiratory tract

Upper respiratory
Choanal atresia
Cleft lip and/or palate
Pierre Robin syndrome

Larynx
Laryngomalacia
Stenosis
Cleft
Web
Vocal cord paralysis
Atresia

Obstructive lesions of larynx
Haemangioma
Cysts
Papilloma

Tracheobronchial lesions
Tracheo-oesophageal fistula with or without oesophageal
   atresia
Tracheal pouch
Tracheomalacia
Tracheal stenosis
Tracheal agenesis
Bronchial stenosis
Bronchial agenesis

Extrinsic lesions
Vascular ring
Aberrant innominate artery
Bronchogenic cyst

Intrapulmonary lesions
Congenital lobar emphysema
Congenital lung cysts
Cystic adenomatoid malformation
Pulmonary sequestration
Pulmonary hypoplasia
Pulmonary agenesis

Diaphragm
Diaphragmatic hernia
Eventration of diaphragm
Paralysis of diaphragm

Rib cage
Asphyxiating thoracic dystrophy
Camptomelic dwarfism
Hypophosphatasia
Osteogenesis imperfecta

Neuromuscular disease
Congenital spinal muscular atrophy (Werdnig-Hoffman)
Neonatal myotonic dystrophy
Congenital myasthenia gravis

scarring secondary to prolonged endotracheal intubation. Direct tracheal surgery is possible and includes dilatation, stent insertion, primary resection and anastomosis or direct reconstruction using a cadaveric tracheal graft (Albert, 1995). Tracheal replacement can also be carried out as part of a transplantation procedure. Despite a number of advances in this field

all of these procedures remain high risk. If it is not possible to perform surgery then a tracheostomy may support the patient until natural growth occurs or surgical intervention can be undertaken.

Tracheal atresia is an extremely rare lesion and not usually compatible with life. It is commonly associated with malformation of the oesophagus since the two structures have a common embryological origin. Tracheomalacia is due to weakening of the tracheal wall, either spontaneously or in association with a compressive lesion such as an aberrant blood vessel or a vascular ring. It is also commonly found at the site of a tracheo-oesophageal fistula. Infants with significant tracheomalacia suffer from respiratory difficulties, particularly during intercurrent infection, and during expiration, when positive expiratory pressure in the lungs, which are hyperinflated, compresses the tracheal wall and causes dynamic collapse of the airway. If major apnoeic episodes are occurring as a consequence of this then an aortopexy may be necessary.

Extrinsic lesions

Lesions outside the trachea or major bronchi can produce respiratory obstruction by pressure on the airway. These include aberrant blood vessels, hyperdynamic arteries in association with a cardiac lesion causing a large left to right shunt, and bronchogenic cysts. Cystic hygroma can also produce tracheal compression if it lies in the upper mediastinum and particularly if there is a sudden haemorrhage into it which can occur occasionally. Vascular rings occur in various types and often produce pressure on the adjacent trachea and oesophagus. This can result in secondary tracheomalacia, which may persist postoperatively. Vascular anomalies take various forms including double aortic arch (54%), right aortic arch and left ligamentum arteriosum (16%), anomalous subclavian artery (12%), pulmonary artery sling (12%), and anomalous innominate artery (6%). Treatment is to re-route the aberrant vessels and to allow natural growth of the trachea and recovery of the tracheomalacia.

Lung abnormalities

Congenital lung cysts

Congenital lung cysts may be found incidentally on a chest X-ray when it is taken for other reasons, but they are more commonly noticed when they become infected. The main differential diagnosis is a postinfectious pneumatocoele, particularly following staphylococcal pneumonia. After the acute infection a lung cyst will not disappear, whereas a pneumatocoele will do so over a period of several months, providing the host is not immunodeficient. Lung cysts can also be seen in a sequestered lobe of lung which has become infected and this too must be excluded by subsequent investigation using a ventilation-perfusion lung scan. Treatment is by surgical removal since there is a high risk of recurrent infection in the future.

Cystic adenomatoid malformation

This anomaly is often found in the neonatal period when it may be associated with inability to establish normal breathing. A considerable number of cases are now diagnosed prenatally (Thorpe-Beeston and Nicholaides, 1994). It is also seen as a persistent shadow on the chest X-ray, either as an area of apparent non-aeration or with multicystic lesions present. It is more commonly seen on the left side (51%) than the right (35%) but can be bilateral in 14% of cases. Treatment is usually surgical, although about one in four will resolve without treatment. There is a significant prenatal and neonatal mortality for patients with this condition. The outlook for those who survive is however excellent.

Congenital lobar emphysema

This anomaly is thought to be due to an abnormality of the bronchial or mucosal lining in the associated airway. It is most frequently due to abnormal development of the cartilage in the airway, but may be secondary to extrinsic airway compression by a cyst, tumour or a blood vessel. The lobe progressively overinflates and presses on the surrounding lung. This will result in respiratory distress, wheezing and reduced air entry to the affected lobe. Most cases present in infancy but a few are found incidentally in later childhood and are relatively asymptomatic at this time. The lobes are affected in the following order: left upper, right middle, right upper, and rarely the lower lobes. A significant proportion (15%) of patients have associated cardiac anomalies and these should be excluded by echocardiography.

Treatment consists of lobectomy for those who have significant symptoms, particularly in the younger child. Those with few symptoms may be treated conservatively and the lung improves with natural growth and development (Kennedy *et al.*, 1991). The long-term lung function after surgery is good.

Lobar sequestration

These are areas of non-functioning lung tissue derived from abnormal embryonic development. They have aberrant connections to the tracheobronchial tree and an abnormal blood supply. They can be divided into two major groups – extralobar and intralobar. The extralobar type, which has its own separate pleura and an arterial blood supply, usually from the aorta, may communicate with the trachea or bronchus or occasionally with the gut. Intralobar sequestrations lie within the visceral pleura and are intimately associated with normal lung tissue. They may have tracheobronchial communication, but usually ventilate extremely poorly, they also have a systemic blood supply. Repeated infection in these lobes is not uncommon. On dynamic imaging they show extremely poor ventilation and no perfusion because they are not supplied from the pulmonary vascular bed. Treatment is by surgical removal since repeated infections commonly occur in these lesions.

Pulmonary agenesis and hypoplasia

Unilateral pulmonary agenesis may be asymptomatic and only found on incidental chest X-ray. There is, however, a significant incidence of related congenital malformations particularly affecting the vertebral column and the cardiovascular system. Chest X-rays show an opaque hemithorax with the heart shifted to the affected side. There is no specific treatment but the prognosis for lung function is good since the unaffected lung usually compensates to a very significant degree.

Bilateral pulmonary hypoplasia occurs in relation to a number of neonatal problems including renal agenesis (Potter's syndrome). It is also seen after prolonged amniotic fluid leak, intrauterine hydrops and skeletal abnormalities such as asphyxiating thoracic dystrophy. The outlook in this condition depends to a great extent on the degree of hypoplasia that is present. Severe cases are incompatible with life. Unilateral pulmonary hypoplasia can be found as an isolated finding, often without major functional effect unless it is associated with another malformation such as, for example, a diaphragmatic hernia.

Rib cage anomalies

Abnormalities of the rib cage occur in a number of neonatal syndromes, including asphyxiating thoracic dystrophy, camptomelic dwarfism, and osteogenesis imperfecta. Many of these are lethal in the neonatal period, although a number of patients have survived beyond this time with intensive respiratory support and surgery to enlarge the chest.

Neuromuscular disease

A number of infants are born with congenital neuromuscular disease which may be present at birth. Some babies have similar symptoms following severe birth asphyxia. The most common disease of this type is congenital spinal muscular atrophy (Werdnig-Hoffman disease), which presents with weakness, poor respiratory effort, feeding problems and often a history of reduced intrauterine fetal movements. Most infants die of respiratory failure secondary to associated swallowing difficulties and recurrent aspiration. Other conditions producing similar problems include neonatal myotonic dystrophy and congenital myasthenia gravis.

References

ALBERT, D. (1995) Mangement of suspected tracheobronchial stenosis in ventilated neonates. *Archives of Disease in Childhood*, **72**, F1–F2

CROWLEY, P., CHALMERS, I. and KEIRSE, M. J. N. C. (1990) The effects of corticosteroid administration before preterm, delivery: an overview of evidence from controlled trials. *British Journal of Obstetrics and Gynaecology*, **97**, 11–25

DAWES, G. S., JACOBSON, H. N., MOTT, J. C., SHELLEY, H. J. and STAFFORD, A. (1963) Treatment of asphyxia in newborn lambs and monkeys. *Journal of Physiology*, **169**, 167–184

GREENOUGH, A. (1990) Bronchopulmonary dysplasia: early diagnosis, prophylaxis, and treatment. *Archives of Disease in Childhood*, **65**, 1082–1088

GERSONY, W. M., PECKHAM, G. J., ELLISON, R. S., MIETTINEN, O. S. and NADAS, A. S. (1983) Effects of indomethacin in premature infants with patent ductus arteriosus: results of a national collaborative study. *Journal of Pediatrics*, **102**, 895–906

KENNEDY, C. D., HABIBI, H., MATTHEW, D. J. and GORDON, I. (1991) Lobar emphysema: long-term imaging follow-up. *Radiology*, **180**, 189–193

KINSELLA, J. P., NEISH, S. R., IVY, D. D., SHAFFER, E. and ABMAN, S. H. (1993) Clinical responses to prolonged treatment of persistent pulmonary hypertension of the newborn with low doses of inhaled nitric oxide. *Journal of Pediatrics*, **123**, 103–108

LANCET (1988) Persistent fetal circulation and extracorporeal membrane oxygenation. *Lancet*, ii, 1289–1291

LEVENE, M. I. (1993) Management of the asphyxiated full term infant. *Archives of Disease in Childhood*, **68**, 612–616

MACFARLANE, P. I. and HEAF, D. P. (1988) Pulmonary function in children after neonatal meconium aspiration syndrome. *Archives of Disease in Childhood*, **63**, 368–372

MILNER, A. D. (1991) Resuscitation of the newborn. *Archives of Disease in Childhood*, **66**, 66–69

MORLEY, C. J. (1991) Surfactant treatment for premature babies – a review of clinical trials. *Archives of Disease in Childhood*, **66**, 445–450

PECKHAM, C. S., CHIN, K. S., COLEMAN, J. C., HENDERSON, K., HURLEY, R. and PREECE, P. M. (1983) Cytomegalovirus infection in pregnancy: preliminary findings from a prospective study. *Lancet*, i, 1352–1355

SHERMAN, J. M. and NELSON, H. (1989) Decreased incidence of subglottic stenosis using an 'appropriate sized' endotracheal tube in neonates. *Pediatric Pulmonology*, **6**, 183–185

THORPE-BEESTON, J. G. and NICHOLAIDES, K. H. (1994) Cystic adenomatoid malformation of the lung: prenatal diagnosis and outcome. *Prenatal Diagnosis*, **14**, 677–688

VYAS, H., MILNER, A. D., HOPKIN, I. E. and BOON, A. W. (1981) Physiologic responses to prolonged and slow rise inflation in the resuscitation of the asphyxiated newborn infant. *Journal of Pediatrics*, **99**, 635–639

29

Diseases of the oesophagus

Lewis Spitz

Embryology

The oesophagus and trachea first become identifiable as separate structures when the embryo is 22–23 days old. The lung bud appears as a median ventral diverticulum in the developing foregut. Shortly thereafter the primitive stomach appears as a fusiform enlargement immediately caudal to the diverticulum. The oesophagus develops from the short area between the tracheal diverticulum and the stomach. As the trachea and oesophagus elongate ridges appear in the lateral walls. Fusion in the midline of these ridges separates the trachea from the oesophagus. The separation process commences caudally, proceeds cranially and is complete between days 34 and 36 of gestation. Elongation of the oesophagus relative to the rest of the developing fetus begins in the distal portion and is complete by 7 weeks. Kluth, Sterling and Seidl (1987) cast doubt on the lateral ridge theory of oesophagotracheal separation. They proposed a dorsal and lateral ridge theory.

The circular musculature of the oesophagus appears in the sixth week and by the end of that week innervation by the vagus nerve has commenced. During the seventh and eighth weeks, the epithelium of the oesophagus proliferates to such an extent that the lumen is virtually, but not completely, occluded. Initially the epithelium is ciliated but it is gradually replaced by stratified squamous epithelium.

Oesophageal atresia

This was a uniformly fatal congenital abnormality until 1939 when the first two survivors were reported independently by Levin (1941) and Ladd (1944). Both infants required multiple procedures – cervical oesophagostomy, feeding gastrostomy and subsequently oesophageal substitution. The first success with primary repair of the defect, which paved the way for future developments, was described by Haight in 1941 (Haight and Towsley, 1943). It is now rare for an infant with oesophageal atresia to succumb from the primary anomaly, unless it is associated with additional complex life-threatening anomalies or extreme prematurity (Rickham, Stauffer and Cheng, 1977; O'Neill, Holcomb and Neblett, 1982; Louhimo and Lindahl, 1983; Beasley and Myers, 1992).

Incidence

The incidence of abnormalities in oesophageal development is 1:3000–4000 live births (Myers, 1974). There does not appear to be any standard genetic pattern of inheritance, although the condition has been documented in siblings, in one and very occasionally in both twins and in two generations.

Embryology

The anomaly is thought to arise between the third and sixth weeks of intrauterine development. The precise cause and mechanism are unknown. Failure of complete separation of the foregut from the respiratory tract would appear to be the final common pathway for the development of the various types of defects. Oesophageal atresia may occur as an isolated anomaly but at least 40% of cases have additional malformations.

Types of anomaly

The variety and incidence of the different types of tracheo-oesophageal abnormalities are shown in Figure 29.1. These are as follows:

1 Oesophageal atresia with distal tracheo-oesophageal fistula – 87%

2 Oesophageal atresia without tracheo-oesophageal fistula – 6–7%

3 Oesophageal atresia with proximal tracheo-oesophageal fistula – 2%

4 Oesophageal atresia with proximal and distal tracheo-oesophageal fistula – <1%

5 Tracheo-oesophageal fistula without oesophageal atresia – 3–4%.

Associated anomalies

Additional congenital malformations are found in about one-half of infants with tracheo-oesophageal anomalies. The various systems affected are as follows with multiple defects occurring in many patients (Holder *et al.*, 1964; German, Mahour and Woolley, 1976; Chittmittrapap *et al.*, 1990):

1 Cardiovascular defects – 34%
2 Gastrointestinal (excluding anorectal) anomalies – 14%
3 Genitourinary anomalies – 12%
4 Anorectal malformations – 11%
5 Skeletal defects – 11%
6 Respiratory anomalies – 6%
7 Genetic/chromosomal defects – 2%
8 Miscellaneous anomalies – 10%.

The VATER complex of associated anomalies was described by Quan and Smith (1973). (The acronym stands for V = vertebral, A = anorectal, T–E = tracheo-oesophageal fistula and (o)esophageal atresia, R = radial and renal dysplasia.)

Ventricular septal defects are the single most common cardiac malformation (Greenwood and Rosenthal, 1976). Of the gastrointestinal anomalies, malrotation of the midgut occurs most frequently, followed by Meckel's diverticulum and duodenal atresia or stenosis. A variety of genitourinary anomalies occurs in association with oesophageal atresia, the most serious being bilateral renal agenesis (Potter's syndrome) which is incompatible with survival. The anorectal anomalies are equally divided between the supralevator (high) and translevator (low) defects.

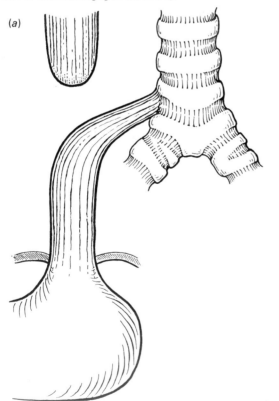
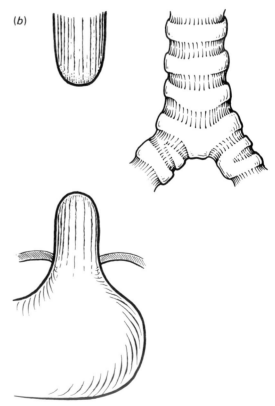

Figure 29.1 Types of oesophageal atresia. (*a*) Oesophageal atresia with distal tracheo-oesophageal fistula, 87%; (*b*) oesophageal atresia without tracheo-oesophageal fistula, 6–7%;

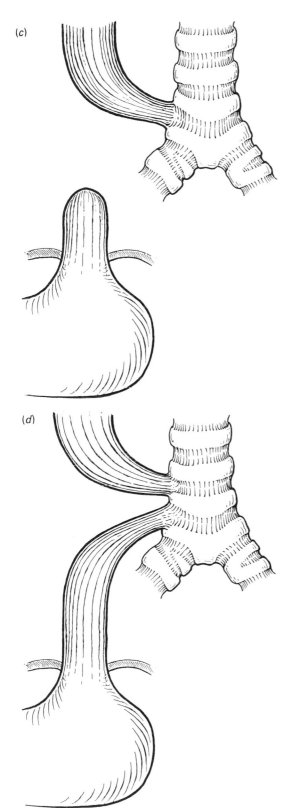

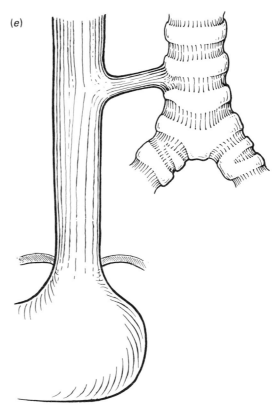

Figure 29.1 (*c*) oesophageal atresia with proximal tracheo-oesophageal fistula, 2%; (*d*) oesophageal atresia with proximal and distal tracheo-oesophageal fistula, <1%; (*e*) tracheo-oesophageal fistula without oesophageal atresia, 3–4%

Diagnosis

Polyhydramnios occurs in approximately 30% of mothers of infants with oesophageal atresia. Antenatal ultrasound scan may be diagnostic in oesophageal atresia without fistula because of failure to demonstrate the presence of intragastric fluid. The infant, at birth, is 'excessively mucusy' and requires repeated suction as it is unable to swallow saliva. Failure to recognize the anomaly at this stage will expose the infant to choking episodes and aspiration pneumonitis with the first feed. The diagnosis is confirmed by passing a large calibre (no. 10 French) firm catheter through the mouth and into the oesophagus. The position of arrest of the tube is confirmed on a chest X-ray (Figure 29.2). If the tube enters the stomach there is no oesophageal atresia. In the majority of cases with this condition the tube cannot be advanced more than 10 cm beyond the lower gum margin. It is important to include the abdomen on the original X-ray in order to assess the presence of intestinal gas

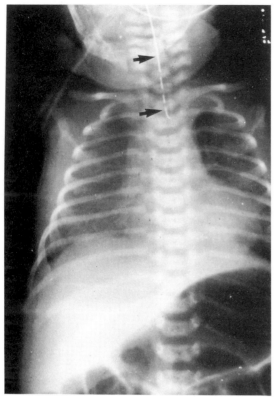

Figure 29.2 Plain X-ray of the chest and upper abdomen in an infant with oesophageal atresia. The radiopaque tube can be seen in the upper oesophagus. Gas in the intestines indicates the presence of a distal tracheo-oesophageal fistula

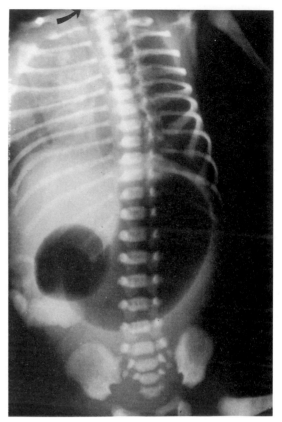

Figure 29.3 Plain X-ray of the chest and abdomen in an infant with oesophageal atresia – the tip of the catheter can be seen at the thoracic inlet. The gas pattern in the abdomen indicates the presence of a duodenal atresia ('double bubble')

shadows (Figure 29.3). Gas within the gastrointestinal tract implies the presence of a distal tracheo-oesophageal fistula while the distribution of the gas may indicate an additional intestinal anomaly, e.g. duodenal atresia or malrotation. The chest radiograph should be assessed for pulmonary pathology and the configuration of the heart shadow may be indicative of cardiac defects, e.g. Fallot's tetralogy.

Management

Treatment of infants with oesophageal atresia should be concentrated in centres where the surgical expertise, supportive services (anaesthesia, radiology, pathology) and specialized nursing care are available. Transfer to such centres should be effected promptly without exposing the infant to the risks of aspiration pneumonitis. The infant is transported in a portable incubator either in a lateral position or in the prone position in order to discourage reflux of gastric juice into the distal tracheo-oesophageal fistula, while continuous suction is applied to the upper pouch to prevent aspiration of saliva (Spitz, Wallis and Graves, 1984). Definitive repair may have to be postponed in the presence of aspiration pneumonitis which generally responds very rapidly to broad-spectrum antibiotics and vigorous chest physiotherapy (Koop, Schnaufer and Broennie, 1974; Randolph, Altman and Anderson, 1977; Grosfeld and Ballantine, 1978; Ito, Sugito and Nagaya, 1984). In the infant with severe respiratory distress requiring mechanical ventilatory support, consideration should be given to emergency ligation of the distal tracheo-oesophageal fistula to facilitate respiratory support and to prevent overdistension of the stomach and intestine (Jones *et al.*, 1980; Filstron *et al.*, 1982; Holmes, Kiely and Spitz, 1987; Malone *et al.*, 1990.)

The operative procedure is carried out under general endotracheal anaesthesia. Access is achieved via a right posterolateral extrapleural thoracotomy through the fourth or fifth intercostal space (deLorimier and Harrison, 1985). After dividing the azygos vein, the distal oesophagus is identified and traced proximally to its site of entry into the trachea.

Mobilization of the distal oesophagus should be kept to a minimum as its blood supply is derived segmentally direct from small aortic branches. Excessive mobilization may impair the blood supply to the anastomosis and lead to poor wound healing. The fistula is divided and the tracheal defect closed with fine interrupted non-absorbable sutures. The proximal blind end of the oesophagus is identified in the apex of the chest and mobilized sufficiently to effect an anastomosis with as little tension as possible. An end-to-end anastomosis is performed using a single layer of full thickness 5.0–7.0 polyglycolic acid or Prolene sutures (Figure 29.4).

An oesophagomyotomy (Livaditis, 1973), oesophagoplasty (Gough, 1980; Davenport and Bianchi, 1990) or the use of elective paralysis and mechanical ventilation for a few days postoperatively in an extremely tight anastomosis may be effective in reducing the incidence of anastomotic complications.

The passage of a fine silastic transanastomotic tube through the nose into the stomach will allow early enteral feeding postopeatively. A gastrostomy tube is no longer indicated in the routine repair of an oesophageal atresia. In fact, the fashioning of a gastrostomy exposes the infant to an increased incidence of gastro-oesophageal reflux which, in itself, predisposes the anastomosis to stricture formation (Kiely and Spitz, 1987; Chittmitrapap *et al.*, 1990).

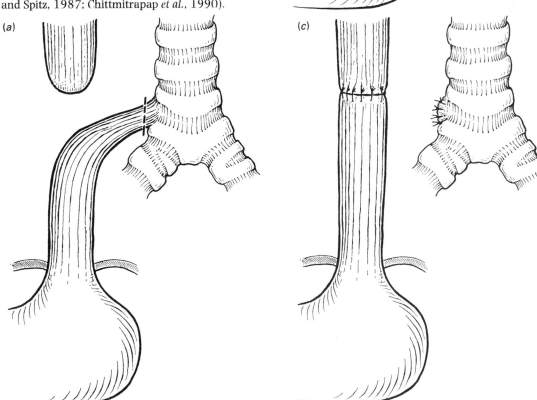

Figure 29.4 The technique of operative repair of oesophageal atresia with distal tracheo-oesophageal fistula. (*a*) Division of distal tracheo-oesophageal fistula. (*b*) Closure of tracheal defect with interrupted sutures. (*c*) End-to-end oesophago-oesophageal anastomosis with single layer of interrupted sutures

A contrast oesophagogram performed on the fifth postoperative day will determine the anastomotic integrity.

Patients with a long gap between the proximal and distal segment (particularly those with an isolated oesophageal atresia) require special attention. The alternative approaches available are to delay the repair pending differential growth of the oesophageal segments towards each other (3 months), or to perform a cervical oesophagostomy and carry out an oesophageal substitution (deLorimier and Harrison, 1986) at a later stage – colonic interposition (Waterston, 1969), gastric tube (Anderson and Randolph, 1978), or gastric transposition (Spitz 1984, 1992).

Results and prognosis

A total of 303 infants with tracheo-oesophageal anomalies were treated at The Hospital for Sick Children, London, in the period 1980–1989. The infants were allocated to risk groups according to the definitions of Waterston, Bonham-Carter and Aberdeen (1962, 1963) (Table 29.1). Group C infants were subdivided into those with associated anomalies compatible or incompatible with survival. The survival rates in this series are shown in Table 29.2.

Table 29.1 Risk groups for children with tracheo-oesophageal anomalies

Group	Birthweight (g)	Associated anomaly	Pneumonia
A	> 2500	None	None
B	1800–2500	None or moderate	±
C	< 1800	Severe and/or multiple	±

Table 29.2 Survival rates of 303 children with tracheo-oesophageal anomalies

Group	Number	Percentage	Percentage survival	
A	124	41	100	
B	65	22	91	86.5%
C1	101	33	79	
C2	13	4	0	

Complications

Complications of oesophageal atresia repair may be divided into early and late:

1 *Early complications* include anastomotic leak, strictures and recurrent tracheo-oesophageal fistula
2 *Late complications* comprise tracheomalacia, gastro-oesophageal reflux and disordered oesophageal peristalsis.

Anastomotic leaks

The incidence varies from 4 to 36% depending on the vigour with which the diagnosis is pursued. The majority of leaks are insignificant and are mainly detected on routine contrast studies. Minor leaks seal spontaneously but may lead to stricture formation. Major leaks present within 48–72 hours postoperatively and cause respiratory distress due to tension pneumothorax. They may be amendable to direct repair if promptly diagnosed, failing which cervical oesophagostomy and gastrostomy is the safest approach.

Anastomotic stricture

The stricture produces symptoms such as dysphagia or recurrent respiratory infections due to aspiration. The incidence varies from 10 to 50%. Strictures are caused by poor anastomotic technique, anastomotic leakage or gastro-oesophageal reflux. Most strictures respond to one or two dilatations but intractable strictures generally fail to respond to dilatations alone until the associated reflux is corrected (Chittmitrapap *et al.*, 1990).

Recurrent fistula

Recurrent fistulae develop in about 8% of patients (Ein *et al.*, 1983; Ghandour *et al.*, 1990). The diagnosis should be suspected in a child who develops respiratory symptoms during feeding or who suffers repeated respiratory infections. The investigation of choice is a tube oesophagogram with confirmation at endoscopy (bronchoscopy). Surgical division of the fistula is the only reliable method of treatment.

Tracheomalacia

This is due to a congenital weakness of the tracheal cartilage (Wailoo and Emery, 1979). It occurs in 10–20% of patients and is responsible for 'near miss' apnoeic and/or cyanotic attacks or recurrent respiratory infections. The condition affects the distal trachea and is diagnosed on bronchoscopic examination which reveals a slit-like aperture during expiration. Treatment is controversial. Many authors claim that the problem resolves spontaneously in time but the infant is at risk of sudden death. Operative correction consists of an aortopexy (Benjamin, Cohen and Glasson, 1976; Filler, Rosillo and Lebowitz, 1976; Kiely, Spitz and Brereton, 1987).

Gastro-oesophageal reflux

Careful investigation will reveal gastro-oesophageal reflux in up to 60% of children undergoing successful repair of oesophageal atresia. Various factors have been implicated in the pathogenesis of the reflux, particularly disordered oesophageal motility, displacement of the gastro-oesophageal junction and the use of a gastrostomy. The reflux causes recurrent vomiting which may lead to aspiration and respiratory infections or may produce a stricture at the anastomotic site. The diagnosis is established on barium oesophagogram and on pH monitoring. Medical treatment is successful in many cases but antireflux surgery may be necessary in selected cases (Ashcraft et al., 1977; Jolley et al., 1980; Chittmittrapap et al., 1990).

Disordered peristalsis

Swallowing difficulties may persist for many years as a result of the inherent oesophageal dysmotility affecting the distal segment in particular (Laks, Wilkinson and Schuster, 1972). The infant gradually learns to cope with this problem unless there is an associated anatomical defect (anastomotic stricture, gastro-oesophageal reflux or distal oesophageal stenosis). These infants are also prone to recurrent respiratory infections during the first few years of life (Martin and Alexander, 1985).

The mortality in oesophageal atresia is directly related to the severity of associated congenital anomalies particularly cardiac defects (Koop, Schnaufer and Broennie, 1974; Rickham, Stauffer and Cheng, 1977; Myers, 1979; Holder, 1986; Beasley and Myers, 1992; Spitz et al., 1993).

Achalasia

Achalasia is a motility disorder of the oesophagus characterized by an absence of peristalsis and failure of relaxation of the lower oesophageal sphincter (Henderson, 1966; Payne and King, 1983).

Incidence

Achalasia is rare in children (Azizkhan, Tapper and Eraklis, 1980). The incidence is one per 100 000 and approximately 5% of all patients with achalasia are symptomatic before the age of 15 years (Herman and

Moersch, 1929; Olsen et al., 1951). There are few reports of achalasia occurring in siblings (London et al., 1977; Stoddard and Johnson, 1982) and it has been reported in association with a number of syndromes, e.g. Riley-Day syndrome. Evidence for a familial incidence of the disease is lacking. Both sexes are equally affected.

Aetiology and pathogenesis

The aetiology of achalasia is unknown. Oesophageal dysmotility also occurs in Chaga's disease, scleroderma, oesophageal atresia, diabetes and secondary to gastro-oesophageal reflux, but the unique feature of achalasia is the constantly non-relaxing lower oesophageal sphincter.

Numerous theories exist regarding the pathogenesis of the condition, the primary defect being described variously as neurogenic, myogenic and hormonal. There is evidence suggesting that it is the result of an abnormality of parasympathetic innervation. Absence of ganglion cells in the myenteric plexus in the dilated portion of the oesophagus with normal ganglion cells in the distal non-dilated segment have been described (Gallone, Peri and Galliera, 1982). This, however, is not a constant feature and is reflected in the variable reports of the histopathology of some of the specimens of oesophageal muscle. These range from the total absence of ganglia, to the presence of normally ganglionated muscle or abnormal ganglion cell morphology. Histochemical staining for acetylcholinesterase may reveal the presence of ganglion cells and nerve trunks in the myenteric plexus, although their numbers are slightly reduced. Reports using electron microscopy (Friesen, Henderson and Hanna, 1983) and intestinal polypeptide hormonal assay support the theory that this is a neurogenic disorder (Aggestrup et al., 1983).

Diagnosis

Symptomatology

The principal symptoms of achalasia in childhood consist of vomiting, dysphagia, chest pain and weight loss. Dysphagia with the sensation of food sticking in the lower oesphagus and postprandial vomiting are the most frequent presenting symptoms. Retrosternal or epigastric pain occurs in one-third of the patients and in a few cases it is the primary presenting symptom. Weight loss of varying extent occurs in one-half of the patients. Nocturnal regurgitation may give rise to respiratory symptoms and recurrent respiratory infections may be experienced. A constant feature is the prolonged delay in establishing the precise diagnosis. The average duration of symptoms prior to diagnosis is 24 months and many children are treated for long periods for 'cyclic vomiting' or for 'anorexia nervosa' before achalasia is diagnosed.

Radiological features

The plain chest radiograph may show a dilated food-filled oesophagus with an air-fluid level in the distal third. In addition, there may be radiological signs of repeated aspiration pneumonitis. The chief characteristics on barium oesophagogram are a dilated oesophagus, the absence of a stripping wave, incoordinated oesophageal contractions and obstruction at the oesophagogastric junction with prolonged retention of barium in the oesophagus. Failure of relaxation of the lower oesophageal sphincter leads to classical rat-tail deformity of funnelling and narrowing of the distal oesophagus (Figure 29.5).

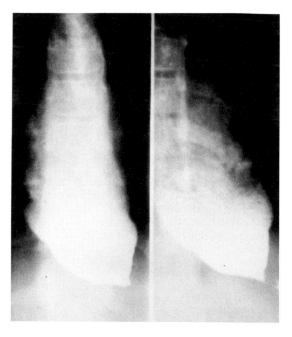

Figure 29.5 Barium swallow in a child with achalasia of the oesophagus with the classical 'rat-tail' deformity of the distal end

Endoscopy

Oesophagoscopy contributes little to the diagnosis, but retained food may be found within the dilated oesophagus. The main value of endoscopy is to exclude organic causes of obstruction in the oesophagus.

Oesophageal manometry

The diagnosis of achalasia is best confirmed by oesophageal motility studies using a constantly perfused catheter technique. The criteria for the diagnosis are:

1 A high pressure (> 30 mmHg) lower oesophageal spincter zone
2 Failure of the lower oesophageal sphincter to relax in response to swallowing
3 Absence of propulsive peristalsis
4 Incoordinated tertiary contractions in the body of the oesophagus (Figures 29.6 and 29.7).

Treatment

Three treatment options are available for the management of achalasia: pharmacological manipulation, forceful dilatation, and oesophageal myotomy with or without the addition of an antireflux procedure.

Pharmacological treatment

The manipulation of oesophageal motility disorders using pharmacological and dietary measures has been disappointing. Reports of the use of isosorbide dinitrate and nifedipine have been more encouraging (Blackwell, Holt and Heading, 1981; Gelfond, Rosen and Gilat, 1982). Nifedipine is a calcium entry blocker and since calcium ions are directly responsible for the activity of myofibrils and consequently the tension generated, their use in reducing the pressure in the lower oesophageal sphincter in achalasia, or for the vigorous oesophageal spasms, seems logical. Prostaglandin E2 has also been employed with some success. Its value in the long-term treatment of achalasia remains to be proven.

Forceful dilatation

Good palliation may be obtained by forceful dilatation. The most commonly used dilator consists of a single bag of fixed diameter which is inflated with water (Plummer) or air (Browne-McHardy, Rider-Moeller).

Forceful dilatation has been advocated as the treatment of choice in adults. Fellows, Ogilvie and Atkinson (1983) showed that, following pneumatic dilatation in adults, only 10% of patients subsequently required cardiomyotomy. In general, the results of pneumatic dilatation in children have been variable to poor (Vane *et al.*, 1988). Success rates, ranging from 40 to 60% have been reported in children (Payne, Ellis and Olsen, 1961; Berquist *et al.*, 1983). The aim of forceful dilatation is to disrupt the muscle fibres of the lower oesophageal sphincter. There is,

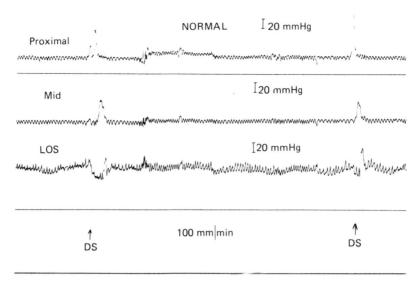

Figure 29.6 Oesophageal motility study in a normal child showing progression of the peristaltic waves through the oesophagus (DS = dry swallow)

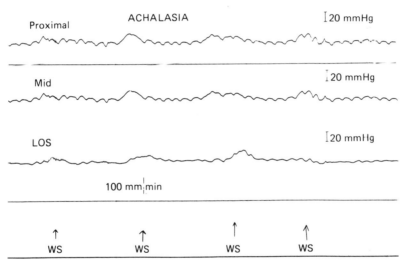

Figure 29.7 Oesophageal motility in a child with achalasia showing completely incoordinate oesophageal contractions (WS = wet swallow)

however, no evidence that the muscle fibres tear rather than stretch. Vantrappen and Janssens (1983) were unable to distinguish histologically between sphincter segments in dogs and monkeys subjected to forceful dilatations and those from normal controls. In general, older patients respond better to pneumatic dilatation (Azizkhan, Tapper and Eraklis, 1980). A report of 899 adult patients treated at the Mayo Clinic (Payne and King, 1983) concluded that myotomy was more successful and safer than dilatation, poor results being obtained twice as frequently following dilatation as after myotomy. The incidence of

perforation following pneumatic dilatation varies from 1 to 5% (Bennett and Hendrix, 1970; Vantrappen *et al.*, 1971; Fellows, Ogilvie and Atkinson, 1983).

Surgical procedure

Cardiomyotomy, as originally described by Heller in 1914, is the basis of all surgical procedures. The controversies concern the length of the oesophageal myotomy, the distance which the myotomy extends onto the stomach and the necessity for including an additional antireflux procedure (Jara *et al.*, 1979; Ballantine, Fitzgerald and Grosfeld, 1980; Buick and Spitz, 1985).

Myotomy may be performed either via an abdominal approach or by a left thoracotomy through the bed of the seventh or eighth rib. Taking care to protect the vagus nerves, a 5–7 cm incision is made through the muscle of the distal oeosphagus. The incision is deepened down through the muscle to the mucosa. Particular care must be taken to avoid opening the mucosa. The muscle wall is dissected laterally off the mucosa so that at least half the circumference of the oesophagus is exposed and the mucosa pouts freely through the incision. Ellis, Gibb and Crozier (1980) insist that to avoid reflux the incision should not extend for more than a few millimetres onto the stomach. If a longer incision is made onto the stomach wall, an antireflux procedure in the form of a short lax (floppy) Nissen fundoplication should be added to the procedure (Figure 29.8).

Oesophageal foreign bodies

Over 90% of ingested foreign bodies pass uneventfully through the gastrointestinal tract. If the foreign object fails to pass through, hold-up most commonly occurs in the oesophagus (Spitz, 1971).

Anatomy

There are four sites of anatomical narrowing in the oesophagus where foreign bodies are likely to impact. These are the postcricoid region, the level of the aortic arch, the level of the left main bronchus, and the level of the diaphragmatic hiatus (Slovis, Tyler-Werman and Solightly, 1982). Eighty per cent of impacted foreign bodies are held up at the level of the cricopharyngeus. Impaction may also occur at sites of pathological narrowing, e.g. strictures secondary to peptic oesophagitis, corrosive strictures, anastomotic strictures or congenital stenosis.

Clinical presentation

In the majority of cases there will be a clear history of ingestion of a foreign object. The child will present with acute symptoms of coughing, choking, excessive salivation, dysphagia or vomiting (Nandi and Ong, 1978; O'Neill, Holcomb and Neblett, 1983). If the foreign body remains impacted, adaptation may occur and the child will select foods which can be managed

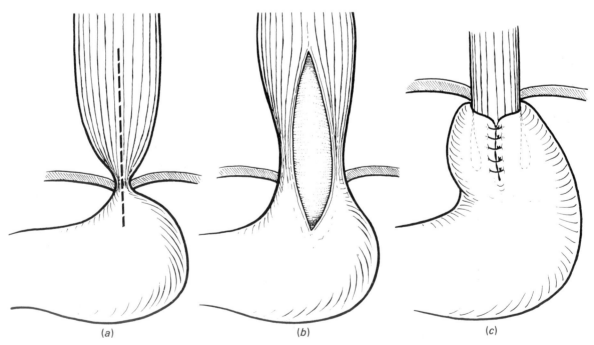

(a)   (b)   (c)

Figure 29.8 Operative procedure for achalasia – myotomy combined with a loose fundoplication. (*a*) Line of incision of myotomy from distal oesophagus through gastro-oesophageal junction onto body of stomach. (*b*) Myotomy completed. Mucosa bulging through defect in the muscle. The muscularis should be separated from the mucosa for half the circumference of the oesophagus. (*c*) Loose (floppy) fundoplication around distal 1.5–2.5 cm of oesophagus

without producing symptoms (Giordano *et al.*, 1981; O'Neill, Holcomb and Neblett, 1983). In other cases, there is no definite history or acute symptomatology and presentation occurs in an obscure fashion, e.g. chronic respiratory symptoms (stridor, wheezing, recurrent pneumonia) (Goldsher, Eliachar and Joachims, 1978), anorexia, haematemesis or pyrexia of unknown origin.

Diagnosis

The diagnosis will be confirmed on straight postero-anterior (PA) and lateral X-ray of the chest in those cases with a radiopaque foreign body ingestion. Further investigations are essential in patients in whom a foreign body is suspected but not evident on the plain X-ray. In these cases, a barium oesophagogram (Sharp, 1986), computerized tomography (Crenshaw, 1977) or endoscopy should be undertaken. In particular, it is the radiolucent foreign object which causes diagnostic difficulties. An aluminium can top can easily escape detection on plain X-ray (Figures 29.9 and 29.10) (Spitz and Hirsig, 1982).

Treatment

All foreign bodies lodged in the upper third of the oesophagus as well as sharp objects in the lower oesophagus should be removed using direct endoscopy. Rounded objects may be dislodged by means of a Foley balloon catheter. Rounded objects in the lower half of the oesophagus may be observed for 24–48 hours in anticipation of their spontaneous passage into the stomach following which passage through the rest of the gastrointestinal tract can be confidently predicted (Spitz, 1971). When the swallowed foreign body has been shown to be below the cardia, only patients who are symptomatic require further investigation. Searching of stools is both unpleasant and inaccurate (Stringer and Capps, 1991). Button batteries lodged in the oesophagus should be removed as soon as possible in order to avoid the danger of erosion through the wall of the oesophagus, e.g. the development of a tracheo-oesophageal fistula (Vaishnav and Spitz, 1989). Associated strictures of the oesophagus should be dilated and subsequently subjected to further investigation and definitive treatment.

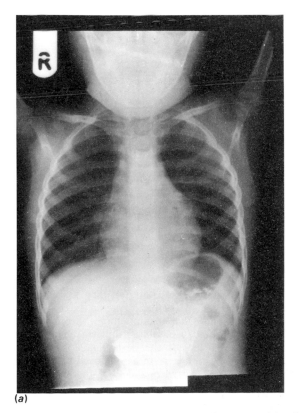

(a)

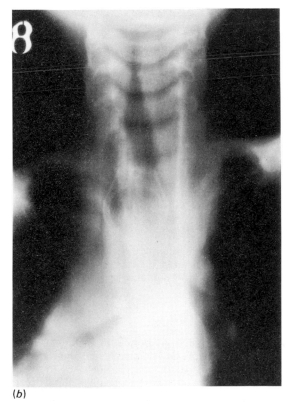

(b)

Figure 29.9 Radiolucent foreign body. (*a*) Plain X-ray of the chest in a child presenting with dysphagia. (*b*) Tomograph of same patient showing ring top lodged in upper oesophagus

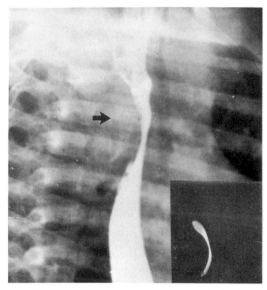

Figure 29.10 Barium swallow in an infant with dysphagia and respiratory symptoms. There is an indentation in the posterior wall of the upper oesophagus. This was caused by an abscess resulting from migration of a can tab (inset) through the oesophagus into the superior mediastinum

Complications

Problems usually arise in proportion to the duration of impaction (Clerf, 1975). Possible complications include ulceration, stricture formation, tracheo-oesophageal fistula, erosion through the wall of the oesophagus with mediastinal abscess or penetration into major blood vessels (Sharp, 1986). Perforation may also occur during attempts at endoscopic removal of a sharp object.

Corrosive injury to the oesophagus

Accidental ingestion of caustic substances has become relatively uncommon as a result of government legislation regulating their use in commercially available drain cleaners (Leape, 1986) and the introduction of child-proof containers.

Pathophysiology

Caustic soda (sodium hydroxide) ingestion can cause severe injury to the oropharynx, oesophagus or stomach. The strong alkali rapidly penetrates the body tissues producing an intense acute inflammatory reaction and oedema. If the concentration of the solution is high, transmural penetration occurs with resulting destruction of the musculature of the oesophagus,

penetration into the perioesophageal tissues with mediastinitis or frank perforation of the oesophagus. The acute phase is followed by sloughing of the necrotic tissue and replacement by granulation tissue. The final outcome varies from complete resolution in the mild case to extensive fibrosis of the entire oesophagus in the severely damaged cases. The extent and severity of the injury are directly related to the concentration of the lye ingested (liquid lye is more damaging than the granular form), the quantity ingested and the duration of contact (Ashcraft and Padula, 1974).

Clinical presentation

There is extensive oedema and swelling of the mouth and lips and the child is unable to swallow. Chest pain will occur if large quantities of lye reach the stomach. There may be haematemesis, dyspnoea, stridor and the other respiratory symptoms develop as a consequence of the resulting oedema or from direct laryngeal injury. Fibrosis of the lips and temporomandibular joint may develop as a result of severe oropharyngeal burns (Figure 29.11).

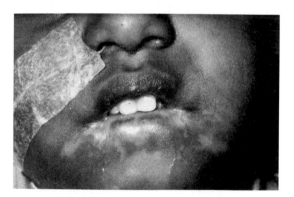

Figure 29.11 Fibrosis of the lips following severe oropharyngeal burns secondary to caustic soda ingestion

Diagnosis

It is important to ascertain whether the lye was actually ingested or whether it entered the oral cavity only. Early endoscopic examination, within 12–24 hours of the injury, should be undertaken to determine whether or not the oesophagus is affected. Assessment of the extent of oesophageal burn is not possible at this early stage and if the endoscopic examination is terminated once evidence of oesophageal injury is encountered, the risk of perforation is minimal (Leape, 1986).

An early contrast oesophagogram will reveal the

extent of the injury, determine the presence of a perforation and act as a baseline for evaluating future stricture formation (Figure 29.12).

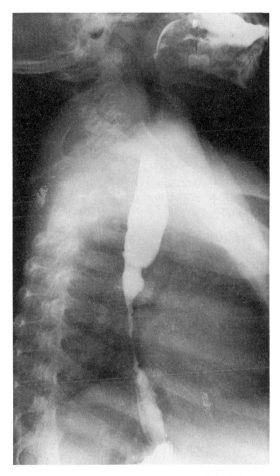

Figure 29.12 Barium oesophagogram in a child following ingestion of caustic soda. There is extensive stricture formation of the distal half of the oesophagus

Treatment

Emergency

Vomiting should not be induced. No neutralizing agents should be given as these produce heat when interacting with the corrosive substance and increase the severity of the injury. Admission to hospital of all suspected cases is imperative.

Continued management

Initial treatment should consist of broad-spectrum antibiotics and intravenous fluids. The use of steroids (prednisolone 2 mg/kg/day) as advocated by Haller and Bachman (1963), has recently been questioned and, in a prospective controlled trial, Anderson, Rouse and Randolph (1990) found systemic steroids to be of no benefit. If, on endoscopy, no oesophageal injury is found, treatment is stopped and the patient is discharged. If a burn is found, antibiotics are continued for 10 days and steroids for 3 weeks. Oral feeds are commenced as soon as the child is able to tolerate fluids. A gastrostomy for feeding purposes may be necessary in cases with severe burns. In these patients the opportunity should be taken to pass a string through the oesophagus to act as a guide for future dilatations.

A repeat oesophagogram is carried out 3 weeks after ingestion of the lye and oesophageal dilatations are commenced if a stricture is found. The dilatations are repeated at regular intervals until the stricture is eliminated. Ninety per cent of oesophageal strictures will respond to dilatation, the remaining cases will require oesophageal replacement.

Gastro-oesophageal reflux

Incompetence of the lower oesophageal sphincter is a common occurrence in newborn infants. In the vast majority of these infants maturation of the sphincter mechanism develops during the first year of life as the infant assumes the sitting and then the upright position (Carre, 1959).

Mechanisms of gastro-oesophageal reflux

Reflux of small amounts of gastric fluid may be regarded as physiological. It is only when the reflux is more frequent or prolonged that it becomes pathological. The normal mechanisms for the control of gastro-oesophageal reflux are:

1 Anatomical
   a lower oesophageal sphincter
   b intra-abdominal segment of oesophagus
   c angle of His
   d mucosal rosette in the lower oesophagus
   e phreno-oesophageal membrane
   f pinch-cock effect of the diaphragmatic crura
2 Physiological
   a effective peristaltic clearance of content from the distal oesophagus
   b prompt gastric emptying.

Pathophysiology

Gastro-oesophageal reflux may or may not be associated with an anatomical hiatus hernia. A sliding hiatus hernia is generally associated with reflux while a rolling hernia (paraoesophageal) causes symptoms by virtue of its intrathoracic volume or secondary to complications such as haemorrhage or perforation as a consequence of peptic ulceration or volvulus of the stomach. A paraoesophageal hernia always requires surgical correction (Ellis, Crozier and Shea, 1986) (Figure 29.13).

Acid-pepsin reflux into the lower oesophagus results in a chemical inflammation of the squamous mucosa which is ill equipped to resist the digestive enzymes. In the early stages there is an inflammatory cell infiltration with erythema of the mucosa. With continuing reflux the mucosa becomes friable and bleeds on contact. Later, ulceration develops which may proceed to stricture formation as fibrous tissue is laid down as a consequence of transmural damage.

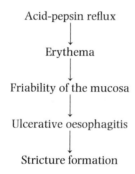

Acid-pepsin reflux

↓

Erythema

↓

Friability of the mucosa

↓

Ulcerative oesophagitis

↓

Stricture formation

Clinical presentation (Ramenofsky, 1986)

Early infancy

The infant presents with recurrent vomiting which may be projectile and may even mimic pyloric stenosis. The vomitus generally contains ingested milk only, but haematemesis in the form of fresh blood or of 'coffee-grounds' may occur as a result of ulcerative oesophagitis. With repeated vomiting the infant fails to gain weight at the expected rate and develops severe constipation. Presentation with recurrent respiratory infections or apnoeic attacks will be discussed under aspiration syndromes.

Later childhood

Persistent vomiting is still the major symptom in older children, but the problem may only occur in the form of night vomiting of mucus which is noted on the pillow in the morning. Heartburn caused by oesophagitis and dysphagia from ulcerative oesophagitis or stricture formation assume more prominence at this age. Hypochromic microcytic anaemia may develop as a consequence of constant slow blood loss from ulcerative oesophagitis. Asthma or recurrent respiratory infections may develop from recurrent aspiration of gastric contents.

Associated anatomical defects

Gastro-oesophageal reflux is more common in patients with corrected oesophageal atresia, diaphrag-

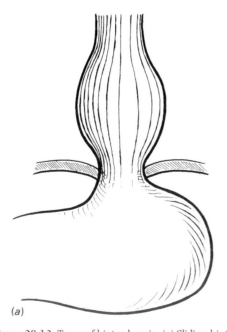

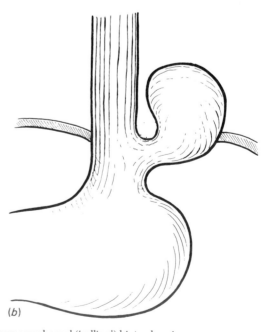

(a)   (b)

Figure 29.13 Types of hiatus hernia. (*a*) Sliding hiatus hernia; (*b*) paraoesophageal ('rolling') hiatus hernia

matic hernia or defects of the anterior abdominal wall, e.g. exomphalos. Precipitating causes are malrotation of the midgut and other causes of gastric outlet obstruction, e.g. pyloric stenosis or antral dysmotility.

Neurological abnormalities

The association between gastro-oesophageal reflux and severe mental retardation and other neurological abnormalities has only recently been appreciated. An estimated 10% of retarded children in institutional care manifest vomiting as a major problem. The tendency is to ascribe the vomiting to psychological causes and this has led to prolonged delay in diagnosis exposing the child to the development of complications from the reflux. Severe failure to thrive, iron deficiency anaemia, recurrent bouts of pneumonia and strictures frequently occur in these children (Abrahams and Burkitt, 1970; Sondheimer and Morris, 1979; Spitz, 1982).

Aspiration syndromes

Recurrent episodes of pneumonia (Ashcraft, Holder and Amoury, 1981; Jolley *et al.*, 1981), attacks of asthma and apnoeic episodes resulting in near-miss sudden infant death syndrome have been ascribed to aspiration of gastric contents (Beckwith, 1973; Leape *et al.*, 1977; Herbst, Books and Bray, 1978; Fontan *et al.*, 1984). Near-miss sudden infant death syndrome results from either laryngospasm (Downing and Lee, 1975) or reflex bradycardia (Kenigsberg *et al.*, 1983).

Unusual presentation

Abnormal head and neck contortions in association with ulcerative oesophagitis were first described by Sandifer in 1964 (Kinsbourne, 1964). The range of symptoms has been extended to torticollis, tics, dystonia and irritability. Protein-losing enteropathy may occur as a result of ulcerative oesophagitis.

Diagnosis

A range of investigations has been applied to establish the presence and severity of gastro-oesophageal reflux (Darling, 1975; McCauley, Darling and Leonidas, 1979).

Barium oesophagogram

The patient should be kept warm and comfortable during the examination. No attempt should be made to induce reflux by means of abdominal compression or other provocative manoeuvres. The patient is screened in the lateral, supine and prone positions.

Particular attention is paid to the following details:

1 Anatomy of the oesophagus and the presence of strictures (Figure 29.14), ulcerative oesophagitis (Figure 29.15), abnormal narrowing or displacement should be noted

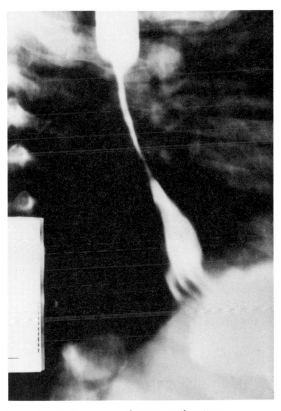

Figure 29.14 Barium oesophagogram showing an extensive stricture in the distal oesophagus and an associated sliding hiatus hernia

2 Peristaltic activity: primary contractions of the oesophagus occur during deglutition, secondary waves clear any residual content and may be normal, while tertiary waves are feeble attempts at contraction which are generally incoordinated and are always abnormal

3 Hiatus hernia: the presence of a sliding or paraoesophageal hernia will become evident during the examination

4 The degree of gastro-oesophageal reflux is graded according to the highest level of the refluxed barium content:
   grade 1 – distal oesophagus
   grade 2 – proximal/thoracic oesophagus
   grade 3 – cervical oesophagus
   grade 4 – continuous gastro-oesophageal reflux

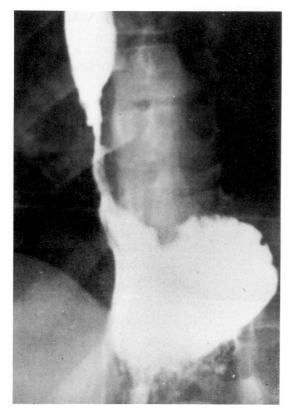

Figure 29.15 Barium oesophagogram showing extensive narrowing and ulcerative oesophagitis in the distal oesophagus with an associated sliding hiatus hernia

grade 5 – aspiration of barium into the tracheobronchial tree
grade 6 – delayed reflux on the 30 minute X-ray film
The rate of clearance of refluxed barium should also be noted
5 Evidence of gastric outlet obstruction or duodenal malrotation.

Oesophageal pH monitoring

Measurement of the pH in the distal oesophagus by means of an intraluminal pH probe is currently the most accurate method of documenting reflux (Jolley *et al.*, 1978, 1979; Boix-Ochoa, Lafuente and Gil-Vernet, 1980; Sondheimer, 1980; Ramenofsky and Leape, 1981). The recordings are monitored continuously over a 24-hour period. pH levels below 4 are regarded as significant and during the 24-hour recording the following parameters are examined:

1 Number of episodes when pH falls below 4
2 Duration of each reflux episode
3 Number of reflux episodes lasting more than 5 minutes

4 Total duration of reflux expressed as a percentage of recording time.

Oesophageal manometry

This is best measured by continuous infusion open-tipped catheters. A high pressure zone is normally present at the lower oesophageal sphincter. There is good correlation between reflux and decreased lower oesophageal pressure in adults, but measurements of the sphincter pressure in children is much more variable. Euler and Ament (1977) suggested that lower oesophageal pressure values may be useful in predicting those cases which would eventually require surgical treatment.

Endoscopy and oesophageal biopsy

Endoscopic examination of the oesophageal mucosa is required to document the degree of oesophagitis and should be supplemented by endoscopic biopsy to provide histopathological grading of inflammatory cell infiltration. Four grades of oesophagitis may be found at endoscopy:

grade I – erythema of the mucosa
grade II – friability of the mucosa
grade III – ulcerative oesophagitis
grade IV – stricture formation.

Scintiscanning

Technetium (^{99}Tc) sulphur colloid scans have been used in an attempt to define the presence of gastro-oesophageal reflux over a longer period than during the barium examination (Christie and Rudd, 1978; Jona, Sty and Glickich, 1981). They also provide evidence of pulmonary aspiration in delayed scans taken 24 hours later. Aspiration may also be confirmed by the presence of lipid-laden macrophages in tracheal aspirates.

Management
Medical treatment

Feeds

Small frequent feeds thickened with cornflour or Nestargel should be given to infants with reflux (Herbst, 1986).

Position

The 60° upright position used to be recommended but it was found that the infant slumps foward in this position, thus increasing the intra-abdominal pressure. The position most frequently adopted now is the 30° head elevated prone position (Orenstein and Whittington, 1983).

Antacids

Simple antacids such as magnesium or aluminium hydroxide are more effective in the liquid form. Antacids combined with alginic acid (Gaviscon) form a foam level in the fundus of the stomach which discourages reflux (Cucchiara *et al.*, 1984).

Hydrogen receptor antagonists (*cimetidine, ranitidine*)

These agents are particularly useful in the presence of severe oesophagitis in promoting healing and in achieving symptomatic relief of heartburn (Cucchiara *et al.*, 1984).

Other drugs

Drugs which increase the lower oesophageal pressure, e.g. metoclopramide, bethanechol, domperidone, cisapride, also stimulate gastric emptying (McCallum *et al.*, 1983).

Surgical treatment

The *indications* for a surgical approach are (Spitz and Kirtane, 1985):

1 Established oesophageal stricture
2 Failure of conservative medical measures
   a in the presence of an anatomical anomaly, e.g. oesophageal atresia, malrotation, exomphalos, etc.
   b in the presence of associated neurological damage. The response to medical treatment is notoriously poor and the additional nursing burden imposed by repeated vomiting adds significantly to the social stress of the family
   c apnoeic episodes and repeated respiratory infections which do not respond promptly
   d failure to thrive in spite of adequate treatment.

With the exception of near-miss sudden infant death syndrome, failure of medical treatment should not be considered until the treatment has been attempted for at least 3 weeks in hospital or 6–12 weeks at home.

The most widely adopted surgical procedure for the correction of reflux is Nissen fundoplication. This involves wrapping the fundus of the stomach around the distal 2–4 cm of oesophagus. The wrap should be lax and short to allow free passage of food through the oesophagus and to permit the patient to eructate, while at the same time preventing reflux (Figure 29.16). Postoperative complications are more frequent in patients with established strictures and in

debilitated children with severe retardation. Referral for surgery is invariably delayed in those children and earlier surgery may avoid many of the postoperative problems (Spitz, 1982).

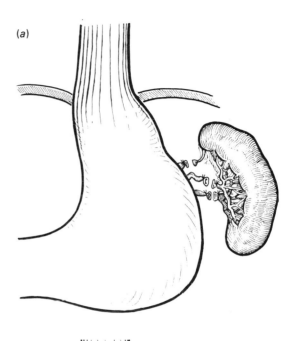
(a)

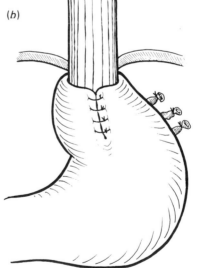
(b)

Figure 29.16 The operative technique for Nissen fundoplication. (*a*) The oesophagus is exposed at the hiatus and mobilized for a short distance into the posterior mediastinum. The short gastric vessels are ligated and divided. The hiatus is narrowed to prevent recurrence of the hernia. (*b*) The fundus of the stomach is wrapped around the distal 2–3 cm of oesophagus and sutured in position with interrupted non-absorbable sutures including the suture in the anterior (extramucosal) wall of the oesophagus

Complications

Early complications most commonly comprise those related to the respiratory system with atelectasis and pneumonia predominating.

Later complications include wrap disruption causing recurrent reflux, wrap dysfunction leading to dysphagia, gasbloat or 'abdominal meteorism' in 10–50% of cases and intestinal obstruction due to adhesions in around 5% of patients. Prolapse of the fundoplication into the posterior mediastinum or the development of a paraoesophageal hernia leads to recurrent symptoms and almost invariably necessitates revision surgery (Spitz and Hitchcock, 1990).

Congenital oesophageal stenosis

Stenosis of the oesophagus most commonly arises from acquired lesions, e.g. reflux oesophagitis, corrosive ingestion, foreign body impaction or secondary to surgical resection and anastomosis. Congenital stenosis is a rare anomaly which may be caused either by a membranous web or diaphragm, or may arise as a result of intramural deposits of tracheobronchial cartilaginous tissue. The latter pathology has been most frequently reported in association with oesophageal atresia and/or tracheo-oesophageal fistula (Nishina, Tsuchida and Saito, 1981; Yeung *et al.*, 1992).

Clinical features

In the presence of a complete web, presentation is similar to that of oesophageal atresia with symptoms occurring on the first day of life. In other cases, symptoms may develop at any stage of life through to adulthood but generally arise in early infancy. The symptoms include dysphagia, vomiting with food ingestion, failure to thrive, recurrent respiratory infections and foreign body impaction.

Diagnosis

Gastro-oesophageal reflux as a cause of the stenosis should always be excluded. The barium oesophagogram will identify the site of the lesion. Congenital webs are most commonly located in the middle third of the oesophagus and appear as shelf-like projections within the oesophageal lumen. Tracheobronchial remnants are generally located in the lower third of the oesophagus or at the gastro-oesophageal junction and they cause sharp narrowing at this point. The precise nature and anatomical location of the lesion should be confirmed by endoscopic examination.

Treatment

Dilatation alone may be sufficient for many oesophageal webs. Surgical resection of tracheobronchial cartilaginous tissue is generally recommended (Scherer and Grosfeld, 1986).

References

ABRAHAMS, P. and BURKITT, B. F. E. (1970) Hiatus hernia and gastro-oesophageal reflux in children and adolescents with cerebral palsy. *Australian Paediatric Journal,* **6,** 41–46

AGGESTRUP, S., UDDMAN, R., SUNDLER, F., FAHRENKRUG, J., HAKANSON, R., SØRENSON, H. R. *et al.* (1983) Lack of vasoactive intestinal polypeptide nerves in esophageal achalasia. *Gastroenterology,* **84,** 924–927

ANDERSON, K. D. and RANDOLPH, J. G. (1978) Gastric tube interposition. A satisfactory alternative to the colon for esophageal replacement in children. *Annals of Thoracic Surgery,* **25,** 521–525

ANDERSON, K. D., ROUSE, T. M. and RANDOLPH, J. G. (1990) A controlled trial of corticosteroids in children with corrosive injury of the oesophagus. *New England Journal of Medicine,* **323,** 637–640

ASHCRAFT, K. W. and PADULA, R. T. (1974) The effect of dilute corrosives on the esophagus. *Pediatrics,* **53,** 226–232

ASHCRAFT, K. W., GOODWIN, C. D., AMOURY, R. A. and HOLDER, T. M. (1977) Early recognition and aggressive treatment of gastroesophageal reflux following repair of esophageal atresia. *Journal of Pediatric Surgery,* **12,** 317–321

ASHCRAFT, K. W., HOLDER, T. M. and AMOURY, R. A. (1981) Treatment of gastroesophageal reflux in children by Thal fundoplication. *Journal of Thoracic Cardiovascular Surgery,* **82,** 706–712

AZIZKHAN, R. G., TAPPER, D. and ERAKLIS, A. (1980) Achalasia in childhood: a 20-year experience. *Journal of Pediatric Surgery,* **15,** 457–461

BALLANTINE, T. V. N., FITZGERALD, I. F. and GROSFELD, J. L. (1980) Transabdominal esophagomyotomy for achalasia in children. *Journal of Pediatric Surgery,* **15,** 457–461

BEASLEY, S. W. and MYERS, N. A. (1992) Trends in mortality in oesophageal atresia. *Pediatric Surgery International,* **7,** 86–89

BECKWITH, J. B. (1973) The sudden infant death syndrome. *Current Problems in Pediatrics,* **3,** 3–37

BENJAMIN, R., COHEN. and GLASSON, M. (1976) Tracheomalacia in association with congenital tracheoesophageal fistula. *Surgery,* **79,** 504–508

BENNETT, J. R. and HENDRIX, T. R. (1970) Treatment of achalasia with pneumatic dilatation. *Modern Treatment,* **7,** 1217–1228

BERQUIST, W. E., BYRNE, W. J., AMENT, M. E., FONKALSRUD, E. W. and EULER, A. R. (1983) Achalasia: diagnosis, management and clinical course in 16 children. *Pediatrics,* **71,** 798–805

BLACKWELL, J. N., HOLT, S. and HEADING, R. C. (1981) Effect of nifedipine on oesophageal motility and gastric emptying. *Digestion,* **21,** 50–56

BOIX-OCHOA, J., LAFUENTE, J. M. and GIL-VERNET, J. M. (1980) Twenty-four hour pH monitoring in gastroesophageal reflux. *Journal of Pediatric Surgery,* **15,** 74–78

BUICK, R. G. and SPITZ, L. (1985) Achalasia of the cardia in children. *British Journal of Surgery*, **72**, 341–343

CARRE, I. (1959) The natural history of the partial thoracic stomach (hiatus hernia) in children. *Archives of Disease in Childhood*, **34**, 344–353

CHITTMITTRAPAP, S., SPITZ, L., BRERETON, R. J. and KIELY, E. M. (1990) Anastomotic stricture following repair of esophageal atresia. *Journal of Pediatric Surgery*, **25**, 508–511

CHRISTIE, D. and RUDD, T. G. (1978) Radionuclide test for gastroesophageal reflux in children. *Pediatric Research*, **12**, 432

CLERF, L. H. (1975) Historical aspects of foreign bodies in the air and food passages. *Southern Medical Journal*, **68**, 1449–1454

CRENSHAW, R. T. (1977) 'Pop Top' ingestion: a technique for localization. *Journal of the American Medical Association*, **237**, 1928–1929

CUCCHIARA, S., STAIANO, A., ROMANIELLO, G., CAPOBIANCO, S. and AURICCHIO, S. (1984) Antacids and cimetidine treatment for gastro oesophageal reflux and peptic oesophagitis. *Archives of Disease in Childhood*, **59**, 842–847

DARLING, D. B. (1975) Hiatal hernia and gastroesophageal reflux in infancy and childhood: analysis of the radiologic findings. *American Journal of Roentgenology, Radium and Therapeutic Nuclear Medicine*, **123**, 724–736

DAVENPORT, M. and BIANCHI, A. (1990) Early experience with oesophageal flap repair for oesophageal atresia. *Pediatric Surgery International*, **26**, 89 91

DELORIMIER, A. A. and HARRISON, M. R. (1985) Esophageal atresia: embryogenetics and management. *World Journal of Surgery*, **9**, 250–257

DELORIMIER, A. A. and HARRISON, M. R. (1986) Esophageal replacement. In: *Pediatric Esophageal Surgery*, edited by K. W. Ashcraft and T. M. Holder. Orlando: Grune and Stratton pp. 89–136

DOWNING, S. E. and LEE, J. C. (1975) Laryngeal chemosensitivity: a possible mechanism for sudden infant death. *Pediatrics*, **55**, 640–649

EIN, S. H., STRINGER, D. A., STEPHENS, C. A., SHANDLING, B., SIMPSON, J. and FILLER, R. M. (1983) Recurrent tracheosophageal fistula: seventeen year review. *Journal of Pediatric Surgery*, **18**, 436–441

ELLIS, F. H., CROZIER, R. E. and SHEA, J. A. (1986) Paraesophageal hiatus hernia. *Archives of Surgery*, **121**, 416–420

ELLIS, F. H., GIBB, S. P. and CROZIER, R. E. (1980) Esophagomyotomy for achalasia of the esophagus. *Annals of Surgery*, **192**, 157–161

EULER, A. R. and AMENT, M. E. (1977) Value of esophageal manometric studies in the gastroesophageal reflux in infancy. *Pediatrics*, **59**, 58–61

FELLOWS, I. W., OGILVIE, A. L. and ATKINSON, M. P. (1983) Pneumatic dilation in achalasia. *Gut*, **24**, 1020–1023

FILLER, R. M. ROSILLO, P. J. and LEBOWITZ, R. L. (1976) Life threatening anoxic spells caused by tracheal compression after repair of oesophageal atresia: correction by surgery. *Journal of Pediatric Surgery*, **11**, 739–748

FILSTON, H. C., CHITWOOD, W. R., SCHKOLNE, B. and BLACKMAN, L. R. (1982) The Fogarty balloon catheter as an aid to management of the infant with esophageal atresia and tracheosophageal fistula complicated by severe RDS or pneumonia. *Journal of Pediatric Surgery*, **17**, 149–151

FONTAN, J. P., HELDT, G. P., HEYMAN, M. B., MARIN, M. S. and TOOLEY, W. H. (1984) Esophageal spasm associated with apnea and bradycardia in an infant. *Pediatrics*, **73**, 52–55

FRIESEN, D. L., HENDERSON, R. D. and HANNA, W. (1983) Ultrastructure of the esophageal muscle in achalsia and diffuse esophageal spasm. *American Journal of Clinical Pathology*, **79**, 319–325

GALLONE, L., PERI, G. and GALLIERA, M. (1982) Proximal gastric vagotomy and anterior fundoplication as complementary procedures to Heller's operation for achalasia. *Surgery, Gynecology and Obstetrics*, **155**, 337–341

GELFOND, M., ROSEN, P. and GILAT, T. (1982) Isosorbide dinitrate and nifedipine treatment of achalasia: a clinical, manometric and radionuclide evaluation. *Gastroenterology*, **83**, 963–969

GERMAN, J. C. MAHOUR, G. H. and WOOLLEY, M. M. (1976) Esophageal atresia and associated anomalies. *Journal of Pediatric Surgery*, **11**, 299–306

GHANDOUR, K. E., SPITZ, L., BRERETON, R. J. and KIELY, E. M. (1990) Recurrent tracheo-oesophageal fistula: experience with 24 patients. *Journal of Paediatric Child Health*, **26**, 89–91

GIORDANO, A., ADAMS, G., BORIES, L. and MEYERHOFF, W. (1981) Current management of esophageal foreign bodies. *Archives of Otolaryngology*, **107**, 249–251

GOLDSHER, M., ELIACHAR, I. and JOACHIMS, H. Z. (1978) Paradoxical presentation in children of foreign bodies in trachea and oesophagus. *Practitioner*, **220**, 631–632

GOUGH, M. H. (1980) Esophageal atresia – use of an anterior flap in the difficult anastomosis. *Journal of Pediatric Surgery*, **15**, 310–311

GREENWOOD, R. D. and ROSENTHAL, A. (1976) Cardiovascular malformation associated with tracheoesophageal fistula and esophageal atresia, *Pediatrics*, **57**, 87–91

GROSFELD, J. L. and BALLANTINE, T. V. (1978) Esophageal atresia and tracheoesophageal fistula: effect of delayed thoracotomy on survival. *Surgery*, **84**, 394–402

HAIGHT, C. and TOWSLEY, H. A. (1943) Congenital atresia of the esophagus with tracheoesophageal fistula and end-to-end anastomosis of esophageal segments. *Surgery, Gynecology and Obstetrics*, **76**, 672–688

HALLER, J. A. and BACHMAN, K. (1963) The comparative effect of current therapy of experimental caustic burns of the esophagus. *Journal of the American Medical Association*, **186**, 262

HELLER, E. (1914) Extramukose Cardiaplastik beim chronische Cardiospasm mit Dilatation de Oesophagus. *Mitteilungen Grenzgebiete Medizinische Chirurgie*, **27**, 141

HENDERSON, R. D. (166) *The Esophagus: Reflux and Primary Motor Disorders*. Baltimore/London: Williams & Wilkins. pp. 149–179

HERBST, J. J. (1986) Medical treatment of gastroesophageal reflux. In: *Pediatric Surgery*, edited by K. W. Ashcraft and T. M. Holder. Orlando: Grune and Stratton. pp. 181–191

HERBST, J. J., BOOKS, L. S. and BRAY, P. F. (1978) Gastroesophageal reflux in the 'near miss' sudden infant death syndrome. *Journal of Pediatrics*, **92**, 73–75

HERMAN, J. and MOERSCH, M. D. (1929) Cardiospasm in infancy and in childhood. *American Journal of Diseases of Children*, **38**, 294–298

HOLDER, T. M. (1986) Esophageal atresia and tracheosophageal fistula. In: *Pediatric Esophageal Surgery*, edited by K. W. Ashcraft and T. M. Holder, Orlando: Grune and Stratton. pp. 29–52

HOLDER, T. M., CLOUD, D. T., LEWIS, J. E. and PILLING, C. P. (1964) Esophageal atresia and tracheoesophageal fistula. A survey of its members by the surgical section of the American Academy of Pediatrics. *Pediatrics*, **34**, 542–549

HOLMES, S. J. K., KIELY, E. M. and SPITZ, L. (1987) Tracheo-oesophageal fistula and the respiratory distress syndrome. *Pediatric Surgery International*, **2**, 16–18

ITO, T., SUGITO, T. and NAGAYA, M. (1984) Delayed primary anastomosis in poor-risk patients with esophageal atresia associated with tracheoesophageal fistula. *Journal of Pediatric Surgery*, **19**, 243–247

JARA, F. M., TOLEDO-PEREYRA, L. H., LEWIS, J. W. and MAGILLIGAN, D. J., JR (1979) Long-term results of esophagomyotomy for achalasia of the esophagus. *Archives of Surgery*, **114**, 935–936

JOLLEY, S. G., HERBST, J. J., JOHNSON, D. G., BOOK, L. S., MATLAK, M. E. and CANDON, V. R. (1979) Patterns of postcibal gastroesophageal reflux in symptomatic infants. *American Journal of Surgery*, **138**, 946–950

JOLLEY, S. G., JOHNSON, D. G., HERBST, J. J., PENA, A. R. and GARNIER, R. C. (1978) An assessment of gastroesophageal reflux in children by extended pH monitoring of the distal esophagus. *Surgery*, **84**, 16–24

JOLLEY, S. G., JOHNSON, D. G., HERBST, J. J. and MATLAK, M. E. (1981) The significance of gastroesophageal reflux patterns in children. *Journal of Pediatric Surgery*, **16**, 859–865

JOLLEY, S. G., JOHNSON, D. G., ROBERTS, C. C., HERBST, J. J., MATLAK, M. E., MCCOMBS, A. *et al.* (1980) Patterns of gastroesophageal reflux in children following repair of esophageal atresia and distal tracheoesophageal fistula. *Journal of Pediatric Surgery*, **15**, 857–862

JONA, J. Z., STY, J. R. and GLICKICH, M. (1981) Simplified radioisotope technique for assessing gastroesophageal reflux in children. *Journal of Pediatric Surgery*, **16**, 114–117

JONES, T. B., KIRCHNER, S. G., LEE, F. A. and HELLER, R. M. (1980) Stomach rupture associated with esophageal atresia, tracheoesophageal fistula and ventilatory assistance. *American Journal of Roentology*, **134**, 675–677

KENIGSBERG, K., GRISWOLD, P. G., BUCKLEY, B. J., GOOTMAN, N. and GOOTMAN, P. M. (1983) Cardiac effects of esophageal stimulation: possible relationship between gastroesophageal reflux (GER) and sudden infant death syndrome (SIDS). *Journal of Pediatric Surgery*, **18**, 542–545

KIELY, E. and SPITZ, L. (1987) Is routine gastrostomy necessary in the management of oesophageal atresia. *Pediatric Surgery International*, **2**, 6–9

KIELY, E. M., SPITZ, L. and BRERETON, R. (1987) Management of tracheomalacia by aortopexy. *Pediatric Surgery International*, **2**, 13–15

KINSBOURNE, M. (1964) Hiatus hernia with contortions of the neck. *Lancet*, **i**, 1058–1061

KLUTH, D., STERLING, G. and SEIDL, W. (1987) The embryology of foregut malformations. *Journal of Pediatric Surgery*, **22**, 389–393

KOOP, C. E., SCHNAUFER, L. and BROENNIE, A. M. (1974) Esophageal atresia and tracheoesphageal fistula: supportive measures that affect survival. *Pediatrics*, **54**, 558–564

LADD, W. E. (1944) The surgical treatment of esophageal atresia and tracheoesophageal fistula. *New England Journal of Medicine*, **230**, 625–637

LAKS, B. H., WILKINSON, R. H. and SCHUSTER, S. R. (1972) Long-term results following correction of esophageal atresia and tracheoesophageal fistula. A clinical and cinefluorographic study. *Journal of Pediatric Surgery*, **7**, 591–597

LEAPE, L. L. (1986) Chemical injury of the esophagus. In:

Pediatric Esophageal Surgery, edited by K. W. Ashcraft and T. M. Holder. Orlando: Grune and Stratton. pp. 73–88

LEAPE, L. L., HOLDER, T. M., FRANKLIN, J. D., AMOURY, R. A. and ASHCRAFT, K. W. (1977) Respiratory arrest in infants secondary to gastroesophageal reflux. *Pediatrics*, **60**, 924–928

LEVIN, N. L. (1941) Congenital atresia of the esophagus with tracheoesophageal fistula: report of successful extrapleural ligation of fistulous communication and cervical and esophagostomy. *Journal of Thoracic Surgery*, **10**, 648–657

LIVADITIS, A. (1973) Esophageal atresia: a method of overbridging large segmental gaps. *Zeit Kinderchirugie*, **13**, 298–306

LONDON, F. A., RAAB, D. E., FULLER, J. and OLSEN, A. M. (1977) Achalasia in three siblings: a rare occurrence. *Mayo Clinical Proceedings*, **52**, 97–100

LOUHIMO, I. and LINDAHL, H. (1983) Esophageal atresia: primary result of 500 consecutively treated patients. *Journal of Pediatric Surgery*, **18**, 127–229

MCCALLUM, R. W., FINK, S. M., LERNER, E. and BARKOWITZ, D. M. (1983) Effects of metroclopramide and bethanecol on delayed gastric emptying present in gastroesophageal reflux patients. *Gastroenterology*, **84**, 1573–1577

MCCAULEY, R. G., DARLING, D. B. and LEONIDAS, J. C. (1979) Gastroesophageal reflux in infants and children: a useful classification and reliable physiologic technique for its demonstration. *American Journal of Roentology*, **130**, 47–50

MALONE, P. S., KIELY, E. M., BRAIN, A. J., SPITZ, L. and BRERETON, R. J. (1990) Tracheo-oesophageal fistula and preoperative mechanical ventilation: a dangerous combination. *Australian and New Zealand Journal of Surgery*, **60**, 525–527

MARTIN, L. W. and ALEXANDER, F. (1985) Esophageal atresia. *Surgical Clinics of North America*, **65**, 1099–1113

MYERS, N. A. (1974) Oesophageal atresia: the epitome of modern surgery. *Annals of the Royal College of Surgeons, England*, **54**, 277–287

MYERS, N. A. (1979) Oesophageal atresia and/or tracheo-oesophageal fistula. A study of mortality. *Progress in Paediatric Surgery*, **13**, 141–165

NANDI, P. and ONG, G. B. (1978) Foreign body in the oesophagus: review of 2394 cases. *British Journal of Surgery*, **65**, 5–9

NISHINA, T., TSUCHIDA, Y. and SAITO, S. (1981) Congenital esophageal stenosis due to tracheobronchical remnants and its associated anomalies. *Journal of Pediatric Surgery*, **16**, 190–193

OLSEN, A. M., HARRINGTON, S. W., MOERSCH, H. J. and ANDERSEN, H. A. (1951) The treatment of cardiospasm: analysis of a twelve year experience. *Journal of Thoracic Surgery*, **22**, 164–187

O'NEILL, J. A., HOLCOMB, G. W. and NEBLETT, W. W. (1982) Recent experience with esophageal atresia. *Annals of Surgery*, **195**, 739–745

O'NEILL, J. A., HOLCOMB, G. W. and NEBLETT, W. W. (1983) Management of tracheobronchial and esophageal foreign bodies in childhood. *Journal of Pediatric Surgery*, **18**, 475–479

ORENSTEIN, S. R. and WHITTINGTON, P. E. (1983) Positioning for prevention of infant gastroesophageal reflux. *Journal of Pediatrics*, **103**, 534–537

PAYNE, W. S. and KING, R. M. (1983) Treatment of achalasia of the esophagus. *Surgical Clinics of North America*, **63**, 963–970

PAYNE, W. S., ELLIS, F. H., JR and OLSEN, A. M. (1961) Treatment of cardiospasm (achalasia of the esophagus) in children. *Surgery*, **50**, 731–735

QUAN, L. and SMITH, D. W. (1973) The VATER association. *Journal of Pediatrics*, **82**, 104–107

RAMENOFSKY, M. L. (1986) Gastroesophageal reflux. Clinical manifestations and diagnosis. In: *Pediatric Esophageal Surgery*, edited by K. W. Ashcraft, and T. M. Holder. Orlando: Grune and Stratton. pp. 151–179

RAMENOFSKY, M. L. and LEAPE, L. L. (1981) Continuous upper esophageal pH monitoring in infants and children with gastroesophageal reflux, pneumonia, and apnoeic spells. *Journal of Pediatric Surgery*, **16**, 374–378

RANDOLPH, J. G., ALTMAN, R. P. and ANDERSON, K. D. (1977) Selective surgical management based upon clinical status in infants with esophageal atresia. *Journal of Thoracic and Cardiovascular Surgery*, **74**, 335–342

RICKHAM, P. P., STAUFFER, U. G. and CHENG, S. K. (1977) Oesophageal atresia: triumph or tragedy. *Australian and New Zealand Journal of Surgery*, **47**, 138–143

SCHERER, L. R. and GROSFELD, J. L. (1986) Congenital esophageal stenosis, esophageal duplication, mesenteric cyst and esophageal diverticulum. In: *Pediatric Esophageal Surgery*, edited by K. W. Ashcraft and T. M. Holder. Orlando: Grune and Stratton. pp. 53–71

SHARP, R. J. (1986) Esophageal foreign bodies. In: *Pediatric Esophageal Surgery*, edited by K. W. Ashcraft and T. M. Holder. Orlando: Grune and Stratton. pp. 137–149

SLOVIS, C. M., TYLER-WERMAN, R. and SOLIGHTLY, D. P. (1982) Massive foreign object ingestion. *Annals of Emergency Medicine*, **11**, 433–435

SONDHEIMER, J. M. (1980) Continuous monitoring of distal esophageal pH: a diagnostic test for gastroesophageal reflux in infants. *Journal of Pediatrics*, **96**, 804–807

SONDHEIMER, J. M. and MORRIS, B. A. (1979) Gastroesophageal reflux among severely retarded children. *Journal of Pediatrics*, **94**, 710–714

SPITZ, L. (1971) Management of ingested foreign bodies in childhood. *British Medical Journal*, **4**, 469–472

SPITZ, L. (1982) Surgical treatment of gastroesophageal reflux in severely mentally retarded children. *Journal of the Royal Society of Medicine*, **75**, 525–529

SPITZ, L. (1984) Gastric transposition via the mediastinal route for infants with long-gap esophageal atresia. *Journal of Pediatric Surgery*, **19**, 149–154

SPITZ, L. (1992) Gastric transposition for esophageal substitution in children. *Journal of Pediatric Surgery*, **27**, 252–259

SPITZ, L. and HIRSIG, J. (1982) Prolonged foreign body impac-

tion in the oesophagus. *Archives of Disease in Childhood*, **57**, 551–553

SPITZ, L. and HITCHCOCK, R. J. I. (1990) Gastro-oesophageal reflux in infants and children. *Current Practice in Surgery*, **2**, 51–56

SPITZ, L. and KIRTANE, J. (1985) Results and complications of surgery gastro-oesophageal reflux. *Archives of Disease in Childhood*, **60**, 743–747

SPITZ, L., WALLIS, M. and GRAVES, H. F. (1984) Transport of the surgical neonate. *Archives of Disease in Childhood*, **59**, 284–288

SPITZ, L., KIELY, E., BRERETON, R. J. and DRAKE, D. (1993) Management of esophageal atresia. *World Journal of Surgery*, **17**, 296–300

STODDARD, C. J. and JOHNSON, A. G. (1982) Achalasia in siblings. *British Journal of Surgery*, **69**, 84–85

STRINGER, M. D., and CAPPS, S. N. J. (1991) Rationalising the management of swallowed coins in children. *British Medical Journal*, **302**, 1321–1322

VAISHNAV, A. and SPITZ, L. (1989) Alkaline battery-induced tracheo-oesophageal fistula. *British Journal of Surgery*, **76**, 1045

VANE, D. W., COSBY, K., WEST, K. and GROSFELD, J. L. (1988) Late results following esophagomyotomy in children with achalasia. *Journal of Pediatric Surgery*, **23**, 515–519

VANTRAPPEN, G. and JANSSENS, J. (1983) To dilate or operate? That is the question. *Gut*, **24**, 1013–1019

VANTRAPPEN, G., HELLEMANS, J., DILOOF, W., VALEMBOIS, P. and VANDENBROUCKE, J. (1971) Treatment of achalasia with pneumatic dilatations. *Gut*, **12**, 268–275

WAILOO, M. P. and EMERY, J. L. (1979) The trachea in children with tracheoesophageal fistula. *Histopathology*, **3**, 329–338

WATERSTON, D. J. (1969) Reconstruction of the esophagus. In: *Pediatric Surgery*, edited by W. T. Mustard, M. M. Ravitch and W. H. Snyder. Chicago: Year Book Medical. p. 400

WATERSTON, D. J., BONHAM-CARTER, R. E. and ABERDEEN, E. (1962) Oesophageal atresia: tracheo-oesophageal fistula. A study of survival in 218 infants. *Lancet*, i, 819–822

WATERSTON, D. J., BONHAM-CARTER, R. E. and ABERDEEN, E. (1963) Congenital tracheo-oesophageal fistula in association with oesophageal atresia. *Lancet*, ii, 55–57

YEUNG, C. K., SPITZ, L., BRERETON, R. J., KIELY, E. M. and LEAKE, J. (1992) Congenital esophageal stenosis due to tracheobronchial remnants: a rare but important association with esophageal atresia. *Journal of Paediatric Surgery*, **27**, 852–855

30

Branchial cleft anomalies, thyroglossal cysts and fistulae

P. D. M. Ellis

Branchial cleft anomalies and thyroglossal cysts and fistulae are the end result of defects in development in the neck area of the embryo. In this chapter an attempt is made to show how such defects occur and the mechanisms by which various well recognized clinical conditions are created. It should be remembered that the development of the neck is complex and that our knowledge of the rapidly changing anatomical relationships between the various structures is incomplete. Nonetheless, when embryological knowledge is combined with a study of established clinical conditions, some degree of certainty and logic can emerge.

Branchial cleft anomalies

Embryology

In the early embryo, the foregut develops between the brain above and the primitive heart below (Hamilton, Boyd and Mossman, 1972). The mouth is separated from the pharynx by the buccopharyngeal membrane which disappears around the end of the third week when a series of bars appears in the walls of the pharynx. These bars are formed by mesodermal condensations and are known as the branchial arches. The arches fuse ventrally, thus forming U-shaped structures which support the pharynx. Initially there are six of these arches, but the fifth is vestigial and rapidly disappears.

Figure 30.1 shows how four branchial pouches internally, and four branchial grooves externally, separate the remaining five branchial arches. Each branchial pouch is lined by endoderm and each branchial groove by ectoderm, and these pouches and grooves are separated by a thin layer of mesoderm. In fish this endoderm–mesoderm–ectoderm layer breaks down so that a branchial cleft or gill-slit is formed. This does not normally occur in man but, should it do so, a branchial fistula may result.

A central core of cartilage develops in each arch and muscles differentiate from the surrounding mesoderm. Each arch is supplied by a cranial nerve and by an artery (aortic arch artery) which connects the ventral aortic sac to the dorsal aorta. Our knowledge of the exact derivatives of the arches is detailed in the more cranial arches, but becomes progressively less so in the caudal arches.

The first branchial arch gives rise to the maxilla, incus, malleus, anterior ligament of malleus, spheno-mandibular ligament and mandible. The muscles are the muscles of mastication and the nerve is the mandibular branch of the trigeminal nerve. The artery is the first aortic arch artery from which is formed the maxillary artery.

The second arch forms the stapes, styloid process, stylohyoid ligament and the lesser cornu and upper part of the body of the hyoid bone. Its muscles are the muscles of facial expression which are supplied by the facial nerve. The artery is the second aortic

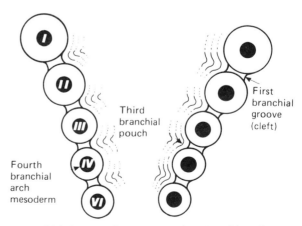

Figure 30.1 Diagram showing coronal section of 4-week-old embryo

arch artery which, rarely, may persist as the stapedial artery.

The third arch gives rise to the greater cornu and lower part of the body of the hyoid bone. Its nerve is the glossopharyngeal nerve and its artery is the third aortic arch artery which persists as part of the internal carotid artery.

The fourth and sixth arches form the laryngeal cartilages and the muscles of the pharynx and larynx which are supplied by the superior laryngeal (fourth arch) and recurrent laryngeal (sixth arch) branches of the vagus nerve. The fourth aortic arch artery forms the adult aorta on the left and the subclavian artery on the right while the sixth arch artery becomes the pulmonary trunk.

Between the branchial arches are the branchial pouches internally and the branchial grooves externally.

First branchial pouch and groove

The first pouch grows laterally to form the eustachian tube and middle ear while the groove deepens to form the external auditory meatus. The pouch and groove meet at the tympanic membrane where they are separated by a thin layer of mesoderm. This mesoderm persists as the middle fibrous layer of the tympanic membrane. Note that only the dorsal part of the first groove takes part in forming the external auditory meatus. The remainder of the groove normally disappears but may persist as a preauricular sinus or a collaural fistula. The pinna is formed from a number of tubercles which appear at the dorsal ends of the first and second branchial arches. These tubercles surround the dorsal end of the first groove which is to form the external auditory meatus (Figure 30.2).

Second, third and fourth branchial pouches and grooves

The dorsal part of the second pouch contributes to the middle ear while the ventral part forms the supratonsillar fossa. The dorsal part of the third pouch forms the inferior parathyroid gland while the ventral part forms the thymic duct. The dorsal part of the fourth pouch forms the superior parathyroid gland while the ventral part probably contributes to the thyroid gland. Externally, the second branchial arch grows caudally and covers over the third, fourth and sixth arches, thus creating a deep pit or sinus lined by ectoderm (Figure 30.3). The opening to this cervical sinus is normally closed by fusion of its lips so that an ectoderm-lined cystic space is produced; later the cyst is resorbed and disappears.

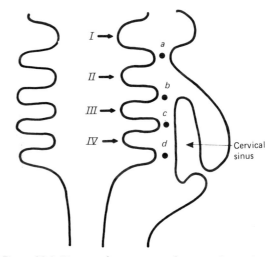

Figure 30.3 Diagram showing coronal section of 5-week-old embryo, a, b, c, d = sites of possible breakdown leading to a first, second, third or fourth branchial cleft fistula

Pathogenesis and pathology

Abnormal development of the branchial pouches and grooves may result in cysts, sinuses or fistulae.

A *cyst* is defined as a collection of fluid in an epithelium-lined sac. It may occur when part of a branchial groove or pouch becomes separated from the surface and fails to resorb. A cyst derived from a branchial groove will be lined by squamous epithelium; one derived from a branchial pouch will be lined by respiratory epithelium which may undergo squamous metaplasia after recurrent infections.

A *sinus* is a blind-ended track leading from an epithelial surface into deeper tissues. Such a sinus will occur when a branchial groove or pouch fails to resorb and remains open onto its epithelial surface.

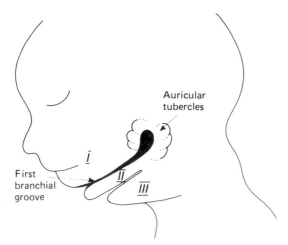

Figure 30.2 Diagram showing first, second and third branchial arches at about 7 weeks. (Modified from Frazer, J. E., 1926, *Journal of Anatomy*, **61**, by courtesy of Cambridge University Press)

A *fistula* is an abnormal communication between two epithelial surfaces. A branchial fistula is the human equivalent of the gill-slit in fish and passes from the skin externally to the pharynx or larynx internally.

It is important to note that inclusion dermoids can closely mimic cysts derived from branchial grooves. In both cases the cyst will be lined by squamous epithelium and may contain skin adnexae. Only if cartilage is present can the cyst be certainly ascribed to a branchial groove origin. Inclusion dermoids occur especially in relation to the tubercles which appear at the cranial ends of the first and second arches and form the pinna. Here it is often impossible to be certain whether a cyst or sinus is an inclusion dermoid or a true branchial groove abnormality.

Anomalies of the first branchial cleft

Abnormal development may result in periauricular sinuses, cysts and collaural fistulae. Accessory tragi are also conveniently considered here although they develop from branchial arch tissue rather than the branchial cleft itself.

Accessory tragi

Accessory tragi, or auricles, are the result of anomalous growth of the tubercles of the first or second branchial arches and are therefore not true *cleft anomalies*. They are usually found in the preauricular region but may also occur anywhere along a line passing down to the sternoclavicular joint. They often contain cartilage and may be associated with other first and second arch abnormalities such as cleft palate and mandibular hypoplasia. If they do not contain cartilage they may be indistinguishable from a simple skin tag. Unsightly accessory tragi should be removed.

Periauricular sinuses and cysts

It is difficult to decide whether these sinuses and cysts are inclusion dermoids resulting from epithelium trapped between the developing auricular tubercles or whether they are remnants of first branchial groove epithelium which has failed to resorb. Attempts have been made by Work (1972) and Batsakis (1980) to support one or other pathogenesis but the present author remains unconvinced, especially as there may be no pathological differences between the two. Perhaps one should simply state that superficial lesions may be a consequence of either, while the deeper lesions and especially those passing to the

nasopharynx are more certainly branchial cleft in origin.

The sinus or cyst is usually preauricular in site, although inferior and posterior lesions do occur. The commonest lesion is the preauricular sinus with its opening just in front of the ascending limb of the helix (Figure 30.4). Preauricular cysts are less common and, unless large, may only present when they become infected. An infected cyst may rupture or be drained onto the surface and thus be converted into a sinus. Both sinuses and cysts are lined by squamous epithelium and may contain skin adnexae in their walls. Many preauricular sinuses cause no trouble or may be kept quiescent by regular expression of any sebaceous material that collects. Others, however, become infected and cause recurrent pain, swelling and offensive discharge. Similarly, preauricular cysts often cause no symptoms and simply appear as an incidental finding on routine otolaryngological examination. If symptoms are sufficiently troublesome, excision of the cyst or sinus with its track must be considered. The difficulty, of course, is that an apparently simple cyst or sinus may have extensive and deep branching ramifications which pass close to the facial nerve (Ford *et al.*, 1992). The patient or parent must fully understand the risk of facial nerve

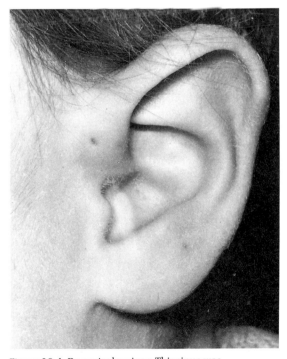

Figure 30.4 Preauricular sinus. This sinus was asymptomatic and required no treatment

damage before agreeing to operation. They must be sure that the severity of symptoms justifies the risk of surgically-induced facial paralysis.

At operation, in the case of a cyst, a vertical incision is made over the cyst just anterior to the pinna. In the case of a sinus a similar incision is made but it should be split to include the opening of the sinus (Figure 30.5). Injection of the sinus with methylene blue may be of help, but care should be taken as any extravasation of dye outside the track will make dissection more difficult. The vertical incision can be extended into a standard parotidectomy incision if necessary. Dissection should now proceed medially until the whole cyst or sinus has been excised. Usually the track peters out above the level of the bony tympanic plate but, if it passes deeply into the parotid gland, it is best to carry out a superficial parotidectomy, displaying the facial nerve and its branches. It will now be possible to excise the track completely while preserving the facial nerve.

Collaural fistula

A collaural fistula is the least common of the first branchial cleft anomalies. It runs from the external auditory meatus or tragal notch down into the neck where it opens at a point between the angle of the mandible and the sternomastoid muscle. The fistula is caused by a failure of resorption of the ventral part of the first branchial groove (Figure 30.6). The fistulous track runs through the parotid gland and may pass medial to, lateral to, or through the facial nerve (Belenky and Medina, 1980).

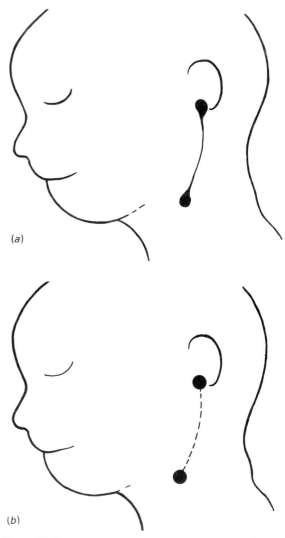

(a)

(b)

Figure 30.6 Formation of a collaural fistula; (a) showing the first branchial groove; (b) showing how the lips of the groove have fused causing a fistula which opens dorsally into the external auditory meatus and ventrally into the neck

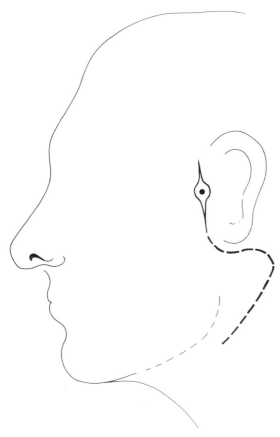

Figure 30.5 Incision for preauricular cyst and sinus. Note that it can be extended into a standard parotid incision if necessary

A fistula causing symptoms should be excised. A modified parotidectomy incision is made which should include both ends of the fistulous track. After the facial nerve has been displayed by a superficial parotidectomy, the track can be dissected and excised. It must be remembered, however, that recurrent infections and previous attempts at removal often cause extensive scarring and cystic masses. The facial nerve may be embedded in such tissue rendering it likely to damage. Patients *must* be warned of a possible facial paralysis.

Lastly, it should be noted that it is possible for the endoderm–mesoderm–ectoderm layer between the first branchial groove and first branchial pouch to disappear so that the two become continuous as a branchial fistula (see Figure 30.3). Should such a fistula persist there will be an internal opening in the region of the eustachian tube orifice and the fistula will pass to the surface between the internal and external carotid arteries. The author has no personal experience of such a case, but suggests that the medial extent of the fistula could be explored in the same way as other lesions in the parapharyngeal space.

Anomalies of the second branchial cleft

Anomalous development of the second branchial cleft can result in fistulae, sinuses or cysts. A fistula occurs when the cervical sinus persists and the layer of endoderm–mesoderm–ectoderm between the second branchial pouch and groove breaks down (see Figure 30.3). If the fistulous tract is incomplete an internal or external sinus is formed. Rarely, a true branchial cyst is caused by incomplete resorption of the cervical sinus after closure of its lips. Most so-called 'branchial cysts', however, are probably due to epithelial inclusions in lymph nodes. This controversy, and 'branchial cysts' in general, are further discussed in Volume 5, Chapter 16.

A second branchial cleft fistula opens externally into the lower third of the neck just anterior to the sternomastoid muscle (Figure 30.7). This external opening will have been present from birth unless it has been produced by incision and drainage of an abscess. Other members of the patient's family may be affected and the lesion is occasionally bilateral. Recurrent infection with abscess formation may occur in the fistulous tract or there may be an intermittent clear mucoid discharge through the external opening onto the skin of the neck. Pathologically, the fistula consists of a muscular tube lined by respiratory or squamous epithelium, the latter being more common after recurrent infection. There are often cystic dilatations along the course of the fistula and the submucosa may contain glandular elements as well as nerves and lymphoid tissue.

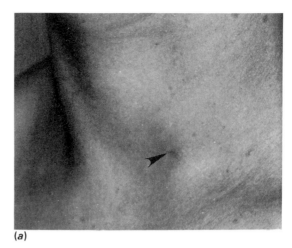
(a)

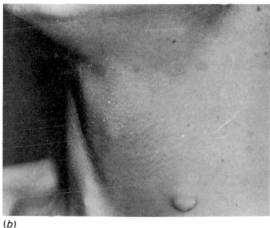
(b)

Figure 30.7 External appearances of second branchial cleft anomaly. (*a*) Fistulous opening; (*b*) skin tag

Fistulae which are the site of recurrent infection or discharge should be excised, but other fistulae can be left unless the external opening is cosmetically unacceptable. The extent of the tract can be assessed preoperatively by injection of a radiopaque dye. A complete fistula is uncommon and most sinuses end well before the pharynx is reached. At operation (Figure 30.8), a horizontal skin crease incision is made to include the external opening. Dissection follows the tract as it pierces the investing layer of deep cervical fascia and ascends along the carotid sheath. After recurrent infection the tract may be firmly adherent to the internal jugular vein or carotid artery so it is best to define these structures carefully as dissection proceeds. In long necks, and especially in complete fistulae, a further horizontal incision will be needed higher in the neck. The tract is delivered into the upper incision and can be followed as it passes to the pharyn-

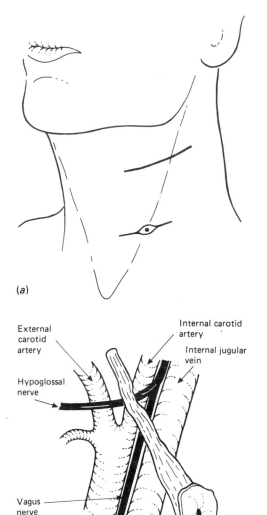

(a)

(b)

External
carotid
artery

Internal carotid
artery

Internal jugular
vein

Hypoglossal
nerve

Vagus
nerve

Figure 30.8 Operation for second branchial cleft fistula (*a*) showing two horizontal incisions, the lower one to include the fistulous opening; (*b*) the fistula is seen crossing the hypoglossal nerve to pass between the internal and external carotid arteries

geal wall. Figure 30.9 shows how the tract must pass between the internal and external carotid arteries and how it will be cranial or anterior to the glossopharyngeal and vagus nerves which are the nerves of the third and fourth arches. To ensure that symptoms will not recur, the whole tract should be excised up to and including its opening into the pharynx.

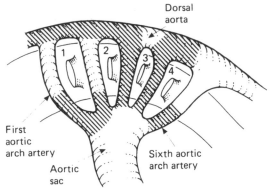

Dorsal
aorta

First
aortic
arch artery

Aortic
sac

Sixth aortic
arch artery

Figure 30.9 Diagram showing the relationship of branchial clefts to the developing aortic arch arteries. The branchial clefts are numbered 1, 2, 3, 4. The common carotid artery is formed from the aortic sac; the external carotid artery is formed from the roots of the first and second aortic arch arteries; the internal carotid artery is formed from the third aortic arch artery, then the dorsal aorta, then the cranial prolongation of the dorsal aorta. The fourth aortic arch artery forms the arch of the aorta on the left and the subclavian artery on the right. Note that derivatives of the first and second clefts will pass between the internal and external carotid arteries; derivatives of the third cleft will pass caudal, that is posterior to the internal carotid artery; derivatives of the fourth cleft will pass caudal, that is inferior to the arch of the aorta on the left and the subclavian artery on the right

Anomalies of the third and fourth branchial clefts

Third and fourth branchial cleft fistulae are rare and only a handful has been reported in the literature (Godin *et al.*, 1990; Takimoto *et al.*, 1990; Ford *et al.*, 1992). The author has treated one patient with a third cleft fistula and the case history will serve as a description.

The patient was a 12-year-old girl who had had 13 operations for drainage of recurrent neck abscesses. She presented to the author with a discharging opening in the neck just anterior to the sternomastoid muscle. At operation a fistulous tract was found which passed between the common carotid artery and the vagus nerve and ended in the pyriform fossa. The tract was completely excised and histological examination showed it to be lined by stratified squamous epithelium (Figure 30.10).

A fistula of the fourth cleft would have to pass caudal to the arch of the aorta or right subclavian artery and end in the upper oesophagus or pyriform fossa. Takimoto *et al.* (1990) described a case of a complete fistula but, more usually, only isolated branchial cleft remnants have been described along this anatomical pathway (Downey and Ward, 1969; Tucker and Skolnick, 1973).

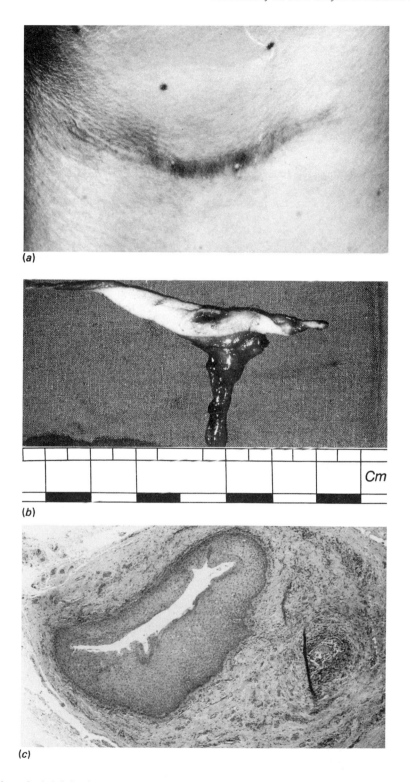

Figure 30.10 Third branchial cleft fistula. (*a*) Cosmetic deformity resulting from previous attempts at removal; (*b*) surgical specimen including ellipse of skin and fistulous track; (*c*) transverse section of fistula showing stratified squamous epithelium and surrounding scar tissue

Thyroglossal cysts and fistulae
Embryology

Towards the end of the third week of embryonic life a thickening of endoderm appears at the site of the tuberculum impar in the floor of the primitive pharynx. This endodermal thickening soon becomes evaginated to form the thyroglossal duct which descends into the neck between the first and second branchial arches so that it comes to lie in close relationship to the primitive aorta. Later the duct solidifies and is then known as the thyroglossal tract (Figure 30.11). When the thyroglossal tract reaches the front of the trachea it becomes bilobed to form the two thyroid lobes which are connected by the isthmus. Each thyroid lobe may also receive a contribution from the ventral part of the fourth pharyngeal pouch. Normally the rest of the tract disappears leaving the foramen caecum at the base of the tongue as the only adult indication of its place of origin.

Any part of the thyroglossal tract may persist into adult life. The commonest finding is persistence of the lowest part of the tract as the pyramidal lobe of the thyroid gland. Less frequently, the tract may fail to descend into the neck from the base of the tongue so that it persists as a lingual thyroid. Because of the early relationship of the tract to the aortic arch, islands of thyroid tissue have also been found in the superior mediastinum. The most common clinical condition resulting from persisting tract remnants is the thyroglossal cyst. A knowledge of the embryology of the thyroglossal tract is fundamental to an understanding of surgical treatment and so will be described in detail.

As mentioned previously the tract descends into the neck between the first and second branchial arches. This means that it must descend between the developing mandible (first arch) cranially and the hyoid bone (second and third arches) caudally. Figure 30.12 confirms that the tract passes into the neck cranial or anterior to the hyoid bone and laryngeal cartilage.

Frazer in 1940 discussed the intimate relationship between the tract and the hyoid bone. He noted that the hyoid bone changes from an ovoid shape in the embryo (see Figure 30.12) to a crescentic shape in the adult (Figure 30.13). He suggested that this

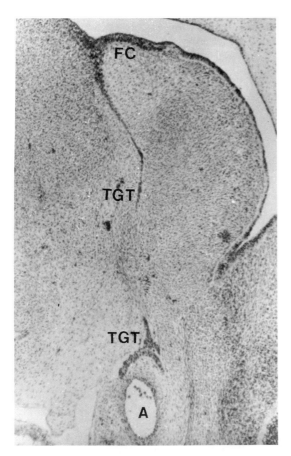

Figure 30.11 Three-week-old embryo showing the thyroglossal tract passing down through the tongue to the aorta. (TGT) thyroglossal tract, (FC) foramen caecum, (A) arch of aorta. (From Ellis, P. D. M. and van Nostrand, A. W. P., 1977, *The Laryngoscope*, **87**, by courtesy of the authors and publisher)

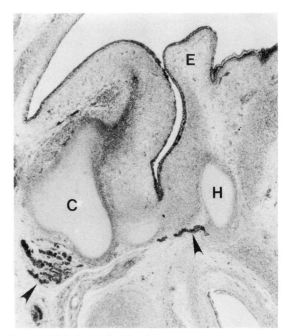

Figure 30.12 Six-week-old embryo. Sagittal section in which the thyroglossal tract (arrowed) is shown to remain anterior to the developing hyoid bone. (E) epiglottis, (H) hyoid bone precursor, (C) cricoid cartilage. (From Ellis, P. D. M. and van Nostrand, A. W. P., 1977, *The Laryngoscope*, **87**, by courtesy of the authors and publisher)

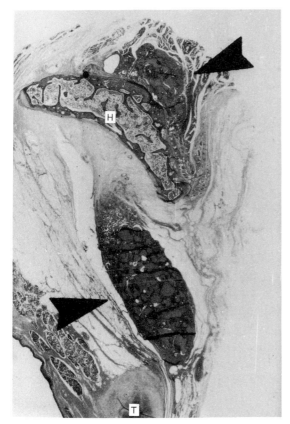

Figure 30.13 Sagittal section of adult larynx. Thyroglossal tract remnants are arrowed. (H) hyoid bone, (T) thyroid cartilage. Note: (1) crescentic shape of the hyoid bone; (2) intimate relationship of tract remnants to the hyoid bone; (3) the tract hooks around the inferior border of the hyoid bone to lie posterior to it before descending to the isthmus. (From Ellis, P. D. M. and van Nostrand, A. W. P., 1977, *The Laryngoscope*, **87**, by courtesy of the authors and publisher)

change of shape was a result of the downward pull of the strap muscles producing a downward projection of the body of the hyoid bone which thus indented the tract. In the adult, therefore, a persisting thyroglossal tract will pass down in front of the hyoid bone and then hook up around its inferior border to lie posterior to the bone before finally descending to the isthmus. Several authors (Ward, Hendrick and Chambers, 1949; Lawson and Fallis, 1969; Podoshin *et al.*, 1989) have stated that the tract may descend posterior to or even through the hyoid bone. They do not, however, supply convincing pathological evidence nor do they refute the embryological studies of Frazer (1940) and Hamilton, Boyd and Mossman (1972) which show conclusively that the tract descends cranial or anterior to the second and third branchial arches in which the bone develops. Ellis and van Nostrand (1977) studied 30 embryos at varying states of development, 200 adult larynges and 20 thyroglossal cyst specimens. In no instance did the tract pass down posterior to or through the hyoid bone. They suggested that reports of the tract passing through the hyoid bone could be due to misinterpretation of pathological specimens (Figure 30.14). All are agreed, however, that the tract is intimately related to the bone and that attempts to dissect the tract from its surface are likely to fail. The best way to remove all tract remnants and thus avoid recurrence is to excise the central part of the hyoid bone as recommended by Sistrunk in 1920 (see below).

Clinical features and management of thyroglossal tract remnants

Lingual thyroid

The thyroglossal tract may fail to descend into the neck so that the adult thyroid gland comes to lie at any point from the foramen caecum to the front of

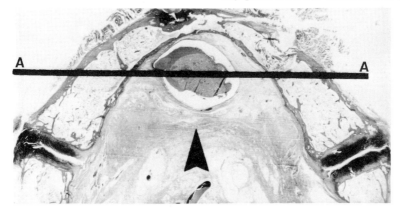

Figure 30.14 Horizontal section of an adult larynx at the level of the hyoid bone. The thyroglossal tract remnant is arrowed. As a result of the concavity of the posterior surface of the bone a section taken at (AA) may show thyroid tissue in a ring of bone. Note also the unusual finding of a jointed hyoid bone. (From Ellis, P. D. M. and van Nostrand, A. W. P., 1977, *The Laryngoscope*, **87**, by courtesy of the authors and publisher)

the trachea. The most common clinical condition is the so-called lingual thyroid. These patients usually present in childhood when a symptomless lump is noticed on the base of the tongue (Figure 30.15). Obstructive symptoms such as dysphagia or dysarthria are rare and usually occur only when the lump enlarges as a result of pregnancy, thyrotoxicosis or neoplasia. A thyroid scan must be performed if surgical excision is contemplated as the lingual thyroid may be the only functioning thyroid tissue present. Usually, however, no treatment is required and patients can be confidently reassured.

Thyroglossal cysts

Thyroglossal cysts occur equally in men and women and are usually noted in childhood, although they may present at any age. The cyst can occur at any point along the path of the tract from the base of the tongue to the thyroid isthmus, the commonest site being just above or just below the hyoid bone (Figure 30.16). Most cysts are midline, but those at the level

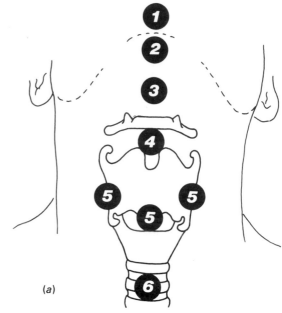

(a)

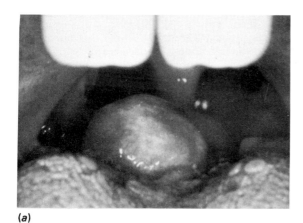

(a)

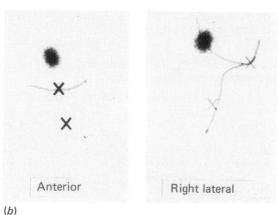

(b)

Figure 30.15 (a) A 10-year-old girl with a lingual thyroid. (b) The thyroid scan shows this to be her only functioning thyroid tissue

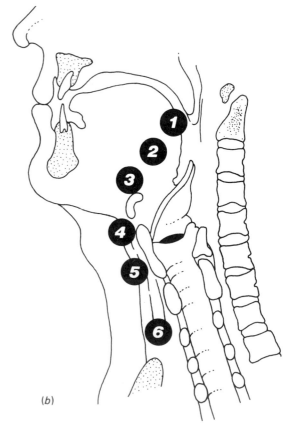

(b)

Figure 30.16 Possible sites of thyroglossal cysts. 1, base of tongue; 2, intralingual; 3, suprahyoid; 4, infrahyoid; 5, prethyroid; 6, pretracheal

of the thyroid cartilage may be pushed to one or other side, usually the left.

Most patients present with a symptomless lump in the midline of the neck. Examination will show that it is freely mobile from side to side and that it may transilluminate. The lump will rise on swallowing (on account of its attachment to the hyoid bone via the thyroglossal tract) and will also rise on protrusion of the tongue (because of its attachment to the base of the tongue via the thyroglossal tract) (Figure 30.17).

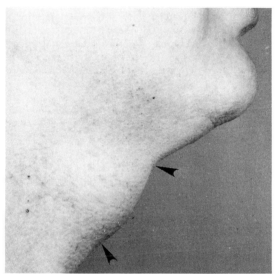

(a)

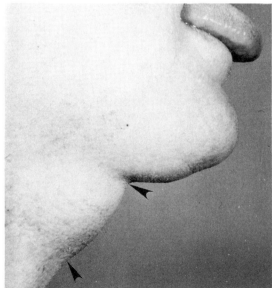

(b)

Figure 30.17 Large thyroglossal cyst (arrowed). Note that the cyst has risen on tongue protrusion (*b*). This physical sign is best demonstrated by palpating the cyst while the patient protrudes his tongue

No other midline neck lump rises on tongue protrusion, so this physical sign is virtually pathognomonic. Some patients present with acute infection and abscess formation (Figure 30.18) which may result in a sinus or fistula with intermittent discharge of a clear glairy mucus. Such a sinus or fistula is always acquired and may also follow inadequate surgical excision.

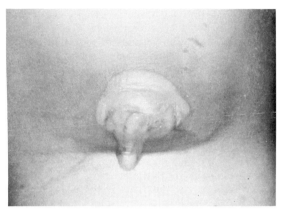

Figure 30.18 Infected thyroglossal cyst with spontaneous rupture and discharge

If the cyst is cosmetically unacceptable or is the site of recurrent infection and fistula formation it should be excised. Gross and Connerley (1940) have argued that small symptomless cysts may be left *in situ*. However, many cysts do eventually become the site of a recurrent inflammation and, very occasionally, a carcinoma may develop within the cyst. In most cases, therefore, surgical excision is the treatment of choice. A preoperative thyroid scan should be performed and this will usually show a normal thyroid gland in the normal position. Perhaps surprisingly, it is uncommon to find functioning thyroid tissue in relation to the cyst.

Sistrunk's operation for the removal of thyroglossal cysts

In 1920, Sistrunk described his technique for the removal of thyroglossal cysts. He had found that simple excision of the cyst was often followed by further cyst formation or a chronically discharging sinus at the operative site. He argued that these recurrences could be avoided only by removing the whole of the thyroglossal tract. To do this he advised excision of the central part of the body of the hyoid bone and a core of tongue muscle up to the foramen caecum. Using this technique on 270 patients at the Mayo Clinic, Brown and Judd (1961) were able to reduce the previously high recurrence rate to only 4%.

A horizontal skin crease incision is made at the level of the cyst including, if necessary, the external opening of any sinus or fistula. The cyst is easily defined lying anterior to the larynx and it will usually be possible to find a well-defined fibrous cord passing to the body of the hyoid bone (Figure 30.19). Using bone-cutting forceps, the body of the hyoid bone is transected on either side of the midline, thus freeing a central portion 1–2 cm in length. Patients seem to suffer no disadvantage through losing most of the body of the hyoid bone and there is no need to attempt to suture the cut ends of bone together. It may be possible to follow the fibrous cord superiorly through the tongue musculature to the base of the tongue but, more usually, the cord peters out above the hyoid bone. In all cases, however, a core of tongue tissue comprising parts of geniohyoid and genioglossus should be excised, thus ensuring that all tract remnants including accessory tracts are removed (Howard and Lund, 1986; Hoffman and Schuster, 1988). A useful manoeuvre at this stage is to place the index finger of the left hand in the mouth on the foramen caecum. This removes any uncertainty about which part of the tongue should be excised and allows dissection right up to the foramen caecum. Ideally dissection should stop just short of the mucosa at the foramen caecum. If the mucosa should be breached, a catgut purse string suture will produce satisfactory closure. During closure, great care should be taken to halt any bleeding and to drain the wound. A postoperative haematoma may cause respiratory obstruction and be life threatening. Close supervision is essential in the early postoperative period and stitch scissors and sinus forceps should be kept at the bedside so that any necessary drainage can be carried out.

Pathological examination of the cyst will show it to be lined by columnar epithelium, squamous epithelium or, occasionally, no epithelium at all. When the epithelium is columnar it is usually pseudostratified, ciliated and associated with mucous glands in the submucosa; the cyst itself contains mucus. When the epithelium is squamous it keratinizes so that the cyst contains keratin. After recurrent infections, epithelium is often absent and the cyst contains inflammatory exudate. Lymphoid tissue is not normally found in the cyst wall (contrast 'branchial cysts'), so that the infection of the cyst is probably either blood-borne or spreads down a patent thyroglossal duct from the foramen caecum. The cyst may be in continuity with a tubular or solid thyroglossal tract and the tract may be duplicated or branching, emphasizing again the importance of excising a wide core of tongue tissue with the specimen.

Thyroid carcinomas are occasionally found in thyroglossal cysts. Page *et al.* (1974) reviewed the literature and found 656 such cases, all of which were papillary carcinomas. Most had presented as simple cysts and were diagnosed only on pathological examination. Treatment is adequate surgical excision followed by suppressive doses of thyroid hormones.

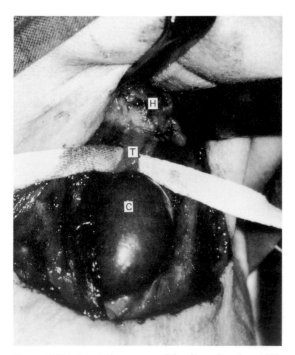

Figure 30.19 Surgical exposure of the thyroglossal cyst (C), tract (T) and hyoid bone (H)

References

BATSAKIS, J. G. (1980) *Tumours of the Head and Neck*, 2nd edn. Baltimore: Williams and Wilkins. pp. 514–520

BELENKY, W. M. and MEDINA, J. E. (1980) First branchial cleft anomalies. *Laryngoscope*, **90**, 28–39

BROWN, B. M. and JUDD, E. S. (1961) Thyroglossal duct cysts and sinuses. *American Journal of Surgery*, **102**, 494–501

DOWNEY, W. L. and WARD, P. H. (1969) Branchial cleft cysts in the mediastinum. *Archives of Otolaryngology*, **89**, 762–765

ELLIS, P. D. M. and VAN NOSTRAND, A. W. P. (1977) The applied anatomy of thyroglossal tract remnants. *Laryngoscope*, **87**, 765–770

FORD, G. R., BALAKRISHNAN, A., EVANS, J. N. G. and BAILEY, C. M. (1992) Branchial cleft and pouch abnormalities. *Journal of Laryngology and Otology*, **106**, 137–143

FRAZER, S. E. (1926) The disappearance of the precervical sinus. *Journal of Anatomy*, **61**, 139

FRAZER, S. E. (1940) *A Manual of Embryology*, 2nd edn. London: Balliere, Tindall and Cox. pp. 236–238

GODIN, M. S., KEARNS, D. B., PRANSKY, S. M., SEID, A. B. and WILSON, D. B. (1990) Fourth branchial pouch sinus: principles of diagnosis and management. *Laryngoscope*, **100**, 174–178

GROSS, R. E. and CONNERLEY, M. L. (1940) Thyroglossal cysts and sinuses: a study and report of 198 cases. *New England Journal of Medicine*, **223**, 616–624

HAMILTON, W. J., BOYD, J. D. and MOSSMAN, H. W. (1972) *Human Embryology*, 4th edn. Cambridge: W. Heffer. pp. 151–192

HOFFMAN, M. A. and SCHUSTER, S. R. (1988) Thyroglossal duct remnants in infants and children: reevaluation histopathology and methods for resection. *Annals of Otolaryngology, Rhinology, Laryngology*, **97**, 483–486

HOWARD, D. J. and LUND, V. J. (1986) Thyroglossal ducts, cysts and sinuses: a recurrent problem. *Annals of the Royal College of Surgeons of England*, **68**, 137–138

LAWSON, V. G. and FALLIS, J. C. (1969) Surgical treatment of thyroglossal tract remnants. *Canadian Medical Association Journal*, **100**, 855–858

PAGE, C. P., KEMMERER, W. T., HAFF, R. C. and MAZZAFEVRI, E. L. (1974) Thyroid carcinomas arising in thyroglossal ducts. *Annals of Surgery*, **180**, 799–803

PODOSHIN, L., FRADIS, M., GOLDSTEIN, J., MISSELEVITCH, I. and

BOSS, J. H. (1989) Intrahyoid thyroglossal cyst. *Journal of Laryngology and Otology*, **103**, 539–542

SISTRUNK, W. E. (1920) The surgical treatment of cysts of the thyroglossal tract. *Annals of Surgery*, **71**, 121–122

TAKIMOTO, T., YOSHIZAKI, T., OHOKA, H. and SAKASHITA, H. (1990) Fourth branchial pouch anomaly. *Journal of Laryngology and Otology*, **104**, 905–907

TUCKER, H. M. and SKOLNICK, M. L. (1973) Fourth branchial cleft (pharyngeal pouch) remnant. *Transactions of the American Academy of Ophthalmology and Otolaryngology*, **77**, 368–371

WARD, G. E., HENDRICK, J. W. and CHAMBERS, R. G. (1949) Thyroglossal tract abnormalities. *Surgery, Gynecology and Obstetrics*, **89**, 727–734

WORK, W. P. (1972) Newer concepts of first branchial cleft defects. *Laryngoscope*, **82**, 1581–1593

31

Tumours of the head and neck

R. Corbett, J. Pritchard and P. N. Plowman

Malignancy is relatively rare in childhood; only 120–140 out of every million children less than 15 years of age are diagnosed with cancer each year. However, cancer is the third most common cause of death in the paediatric population of the industrialized world. Those occurring most often are the acute lymphoblastic and myeloid leukaemias (30%), brain tumours (20%), Hodgkin's and non-Hodgkin's lymphomas (12%), neuroblastomas (7%), soft tissue sarcomas (6%), Wilms' tumour (6%) and bone tumours (5%).

Most head and neck masses which occur in childhood are benign. Of those that are biopsied, congenital lesions such as branchial cleft, thyroglossal duct and dermoid cysts are found most frequently (55%), followed by inflammatory lymphadenopathy (30%), malignant (10%) and benign (5%) neoplasms (Torsiglieri et al., 1988). The head and neck region is the primary site for about 5% of cancers; more than half occur in the neck and a painless mass is the most common clinical finding. The remainder are found, in descending order of frequency, in the nasopharynx and middle ear/mastoid, hypopharynx, nasal cavity, paranasal sinuses and oral cavity (Rapidis et al., 1988). Tumours occurring at these sites may initially present with seemingly 'innocent' problems such as serous otitis media, ear discharge or nasal obstruction before persistence of symptoms or a neurological deficit point towards a more serious diagnosis. In one study of nasopharyngeal malignancies in children, the median interval between onset of symptoms and diagnosis was 13 weeks (Tom et al., 1992). A thorough examination of the ear, nose and throat is warranted if a child presents with an unusual pattern of symptoms. In 10–20% of cases, a mass in the neck is not the 'primary' lesion but rather a secondary deposit from a nasopharyngeal cancer (Jaffe, 1973).

Lymphomas are the commonest type of paediatric head and neck cancer (50%), followed by rhabdo-myosarcoma (20%), nasopharyngeal carcinoma and neuroblastoma (6% each), thyroid carcinoma (4%) and a miscellany of other tumours such as sarcomas other than rhabdomyosarcoma, primitive neuroectodermal tumours (PNET) and carcinoma of the salivary glands (Rapidis et al., 1988). In contrast with adults, carcinomas are very rare in children, though almost half of childhood carcinomas occur in the head and neck region (thyroid gland and nasopharynx). The relative incidence of paediatric head and neck malignancies varies with age – rhabdomyosarcoma and neuroblastoma are commonest in the first 2 years of life. Thereafter, lymphoma is most frequently diagnosed (Robinson et al., 1988).

The length of the discussion apportioned to the various tumours in this chapter will not necessarily correspond with their rank order of incidence as this would be inappropriate for an otorhinolaryngological textbook. For example, children with lymphoma may initially present to the otolaryngology clinic but they are not subsequently managed there; therefore, lymphoma will be only broadly outlined in this chapter. Conversely, although salivary gland tumours and nasopharyngeal carcinomas are rare in childhood, these have been reviewed more extensively. Fibromatosis and Langerhans cell histiocytosis, both non-malignant conditions, are included in this chapter because they require multidisciplinary management, including input from the otorhinolaryngological team. Angiofibroma and laryngeal papilloma are primarily 'surgical' diseases and are discussed in Chapter 15.

Major advances in management over the last 25–30 years mean that 60% of children with cancer can now be completely cured. As a consequence, physicians and surgeons bear a great responsibility to minimize the late side effects of treatment while striving to achieve a cure. Unlike adult cancer most paediatric malignancies respond to chemotherapy.

For tumours located in and around complex and sensitive anatomical structures, shrinkage with chemotherapy prior to surgery is usually preferable to initial radical surgical excision and its inevitable morbidity. These days there is general agreement that children with *suspected* malignancies should be referred to regional paediatric oncology centres where multidisciplinary management can be coordinated. Here patients can benefit from the medical, nursing and psychosocial expertise that naturally develops when relatively large numbers of children are seen and treated. There is now *no* case for the 'occasional' child to be managed in an adult unit. For the convenience of the patient, some aspects of care, e.g. management of infections and follow up, may be shared with the local hospital and community paediatric team (Orton, 1994). It is quite possible that otolaryngological surgeons in local hospitals will be involved in the 'shared care' of children with head and neck malignancies.

Lymphoma of the head and neck

Overall, non-Hodgkin's lymphoma accounts for two-thirds of cases of childhood lymphoma and Hodgkin's disease for one-third. In the head and neck region, however, Hodgkin's and non-Hodgkin's lymphoma occur with equal frequency (Rapidis *et al.*, 1988). Boys are twice as commonly affected as girls. Enlarged *upper cervical* lymph nodes are usually due to a non-malignant process but lymphoma is diagnosed in one-third of cases with *supraclavicular* lymphadenopathy (Torsiglieri *et al.*, 1988).

Non-Hodgkin's lymphoma

Histologically paediatric non-Hodgkin's lymphoma (NHL) is almost always 'high-grade' and conveniently divided into three main subtypes. Terminology has been muddled by attempts to use the adult classification system for childhood non-Hodgkin's lymphoma. The European approach is to classify according to the normal cell counterpart based on immunophenotyping. About 80% of non-Hodgkin's lymphomas in children are 'small cell' tumours, subdivided into those of either T-lymphoblastic or B-lymphoblastic origin. The remaining 20% are 'large cell' non-Hodgkin's lymphomas, the major constituent of this group being the recently-described Ki-1 positive anaplastic large cell lymphoma (Reiter *et al.*, 1994). This classification system is of great practical importance because the clinical presentation, treatment and prognosis of the three non-Hodgkin's lymphoma subtypes are different.

The conventional distinction between lymphoblastic lymphoma and leukaemia based on the number of blasts in the bone marrow (< > 25%) is arbitrary and of little practical relevance. Childhood lymphoblastic lymphoma and leukaemia are considered as part of a spectrum of the same disease. 'Small cell' lymphomas can grow extremely rapidly so that symptoms may develop and progress over a surprisingly short period of time. 'Large cell' lymphomas tend to have a slower natural history, during which symptoms and signs may fluctuate. The non-Hodgkin's lymphomas are staged using the St Judes staging system (Table 31.1) (Murphy, 1980).

Table 31.1 St Jude staging system for non-Hodgkin's lymphoma

Stage	Definition
I	Single tumour (extranodal) or single anatomical area (nodal), excluding mediastinum or abdomen
II	Single tumour (extranodal) with regional node involvement; on same side of diaphragm: a Two or more nodal areas b Two single (extranodal) tumours with or without regional node involvement Primary gastrointestinal tract tumour (usually ileocaecal) with or without associated mesenteric node involvement, grossly completely resected
III	On both sides of the diaphragm: a Two single tumours (extranodal) b Two or more nodal areas; All primary intrathoracic tumours (mediastinal, pleural, thymic); All extensive primary intra-abdominal disease; unresectable All primary paraspinal or epidural tumours regardless of other sites
IV	Any of the above with initial CNS or bone marrow involvement (< 25%)

T-lymphoblastic non-Hodgkin's lymphoma

Most T-lymphoblastic non-Hodgkin's lymphomas occur in boys aged 5–15 years. These tumours usually arise in the mediastinum, probably in the thymus, as a large anterior mediastinal mass with or without a pleural effusion. Many, but not all, of these patients have palpable lymphadenopathy in the supraclavicular, upper cervical or axillary regions. Rapid enlargement may cause airway compression producing stridor and orthopnoea, or obstruction to the superior vena cava leading to facial swelling, congestion, and prominence of the veins in the head, neck and arms (Figure 31.1). Generalized lymphadenopathy and hepatosplenomegaly are more often associated with bone marrow infiltration which may lead to a typical 'leukaemic' presentation. Rarely, the meninges may be involved at diagnosis.

The diagnosis of T-cell non-Hodgkin's lymphoma

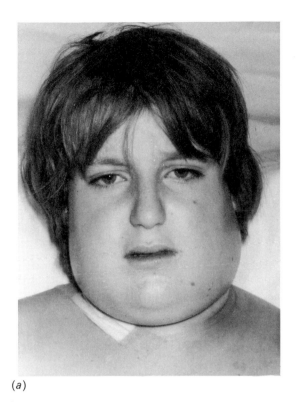

(*a*)

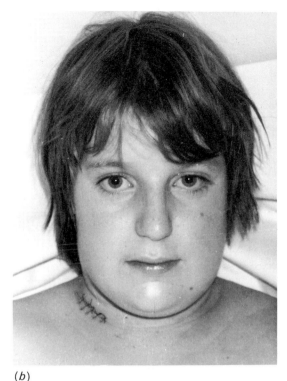

(*b*)

Figure 31.1 Twelve-year-old boy with nasopharyngeal non-Hodgkin's lymphoma (*a*) presenting with massive cervical lymph node enlargement, (*b*) 3 days after commencing chemotherapy. Note node biopsy scar

may be made from biopsy specimens of bone marrow, mediastinal mass or lymph node, or on pleural fluid aspirate. However, the child with a massive mediastinal tumour presents a major anaesthetic risk. Tumour compresses the intrathoracic airway, sometimes to a diameter of only a few millimetres, so that tracheostomy is not helpful. Under these circumstances treatment with vincristine and steroids may be indicated prior to making a tissue diagnosis. Tumours often shrink very rapidly and the diagnostic procedure (e.g. limited thoracotomy or biopsy via transbronchial mediastinoscopy) should be undertaken within a few days to ensure a tissue diagnosis. Hodgkin's disease and malignant germ cell tumours are the most important differential diagnoses.

The principle of treatment is based on studies undertaken by the Children's Cancer Study Group in America which showed that T-cell non-Hodgkin's lymphoma responds to treatment used for childhood acute lymphoblastic leukaemia (Anderson *et al.*, 1983). In the UK, pulsed treatment gave poor results. In contrast, sustained multiagent chemotherapy given over 2 years has improved the outlook for children with T-lymphoblastic non-Hodgkin's lymphoma with about 80% cured (Eden *et al.*, 1992). Therapy directed towards the central nervous system

is mandatory. Two randomized studies have shown that local radiotherapy to sites of initial bulky disease (e.g. the anterior mediastinum) does not improve disease-free survival (Murphy and Hustu, 1980; Mott, Eden and Palmer, 1984). This finding is not surprising because most relapses occur outside the original site of bulky disease.

B-lymphoblastic lymphoma

This disease, also referred to as Burkitt's lymphoma, occurs in two forms which are indistinguishable by immunophenotyping or histology. The endemic variety occurs in equatorial Africa. It is invariably associated with Epstein-Barr virus infection and often presents as a jaw mass. In contrast, the sporadic (or Western) variety is associated with Epstein-Barr virus infection in only 20% of cases and most often arises in the abdomen or Waldeyer's ring. Remarkable progress has been made in understanding the molecular genetics of these tumours since the observation that they are associated with chromosomal translocations involving chromosome 8. The breakpoint on this chromosome involves the *c-myc* oncogene which is translocated to the immunoglobulin heavy chain locus on chromosome 14 [t(8;14)] in most cases. The translocation of the *c-myc* oncogene close to a transcriptionally active immunoglobulin gene in the B cell leads to overproduction of *c-myc* protein which maintains the cell in a proliferative state (Brada, 1991). A small number of B-lymphoblastic lymphomas are associated with inherited and acquired immunodeficiency states including the acquired immune deficiency syndrome (Nadal *et al.*, 1994).

Overall, the jaw is the most common primary site in endemic Burkitt's lymphoma, particularly in children under 5 years of age (Burkitt, 1970). In contrast, only 20% of sporadic Burkitt's lymphoma occur in the head and neck; however, the jaw is the commonest site in this region followed by the tonsil/nasopharynx, skull, maxillary sinus, orbit and nose (Anavi *et al.*, 1990). The presenting features may include a jaw mass, toothache, sore throat, nasal stuffiness and cranial nerve palsies. Symptoms and signs often progress rapidly. Nasopharyngeal tumours are not easily detected at an early stage – they spread along contiguous planes and erode bone without necessarily producing a significant mass. Rapid onset of cranial nerve palsies should alert the clinician to the diagnosis. Speedy referral, diagnosis and treatment are of the essence. At the time of biopsy of the primary lesion or lymph node, bone marrow and CSF should be sampled. On occasions, 'lumpy' intracranial disease may produce signs in the absence of malignant cells in the CSF.

In contrast with T-cell non-Hodgkin's lymphoma, patients with B-cell disease benefit from intensive, pulsed chemotherapy (Anderson *et al.*, 1983). Substantial progress has been made in the treatment of this disease with regimens based on cyclophosphamide, vincristine, prednisolone, doxorubicin, high-dose methotrexate, cytarabine and etoposide. There is little role for surgery or radiotherapy; systemic treatment is combined with intrathecal chemotherapy and administered in pulses over about 6 months. The intensity of treatment and choice of drugs depends on the stage of disease. More than 90% of patients with stage I/II disease are cured compared with 80% for stage III. With more intensive treatment, 75% of patients who presented with bone marrow or central nervous system disease survive (Patte, Leverger and Perel, 1990; Patte *et al.*, 1991).

Anaplastic large cell lymphoma

Anaplastic large cell lymphoma is a recently described disease entity. In the past, most cases were labelled as 'histiocytic lymphoma'. It is now recognized that true histiocytic lymphoma is rare (Bucsky *et al.*, 1994). Anaplastic large cell lymphoma is recognized by the histological appearance; most cases express the Ki-1 antigen (CD 30) and are called Ki-1 positive anaplastic large cell lymphoma. The clinical course is usually characterized by protracted ill-health (lethargy, anorexia, weight loss and unexplained fever) and lymphadenopathy, most often in the cervical

region and mediastinum, which may wax and wane. In contrast with other types of non-Hodgkin's lymphoma and Hodgkin's disease, the adenopathy is often painful and may mimic an inflammatory process. Lung and skin disease are common, but bone marrow and CNS involvement are rare (Rubie *et al.*, 1994). The differential diagnosis includes infection (e.g. tuberculosis), immunodeficiency and Hodgkin's disease. In general treatment is based on regimens designed for B-lymphoblastic lymphoma, though CNS-directed treatment need not be so intensive. The outlook is at least as good as that for B-cell disease with 5-year survival around 80% (Reiter *et al.*, 1994).

Hodgkin's disease

There is a definite bimodal peak in the age incidence of Hodgkin's disease. The earlier peak occurs in the third decade in the 'industrialized' world, but before adolescence in the 'developing' world. Hodgkin's disease is rare before 5 years of age. There is a male predominance, most striking in the younger child. Viruses, in particular Epstein-Barr virus, may be implicated in the aetiology of Hodgkin's disease (Wolf and Diehl, 1994). The usual clinical presentation is that of painless supraclavicular or cervical lymphadenopathy; the glands often feel firmer than 'inflammatory' nodes and may occasionally be tender if they enlarge rapidly (Figure 31.2). Two-thirds of patients have mediastinal lymphadenopathy. As in T-lymphoblastic lymphoma, masses may obstruct the superior vena cava and trachea. About one-third of patients have non-specific symptoms such as unexplained fever, weight loss or drenching night sweats (so-called 'B' symptoms). The diagnosis is made by histological examination of a lymph node biopsy which reveals the presence of large, multinucleate cells called Reed-Sternberg cells, now thought to be the malignant clone in Hodgkin's disease. Reed-Sternberg cells are associated with variable degrees of sclerosis and infiltration with pleomorphic cells. Using these features, the disease is divided into four histological subtypes: nodular sclerosis is diagnosed in about 60% of children with Hodgkin's disease followed by mixed cellularity, lymphocyte predominant and lymphocyte depleted subtypes (Donaldson and Link, 1987).

The Ann Arbor staging system is still in common use (Table 31.2) (Carbone, Kaplan and Musshoff, 1971). In Europe, the disease is staged using imaging techniques alone, most often with CT scanning of the chest and abdomen after ingestion of oral contrast medium. Lymphangiography is not performed because of technical difficulties in carrying out and interpreting the test in children. Few institutions now use 'staging laparotomies' (splenectomy, liver and abdominal lymph node biopsy). Surgical

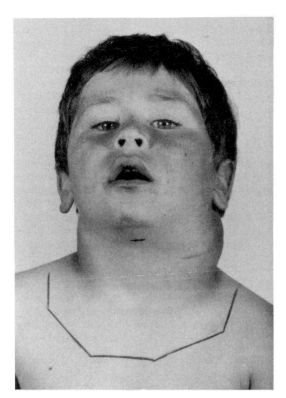

Figure 31.2 Cervical lymphadenopathy due to Hodgkin's disease

ences in staging techniques (Donaldson *et al.*, 1990).

Treatment for Hodgkin's disease involves radiotherapy and/or chemotherapy. Hodgkin's disease is extremely radiosensitive and conventionally-fractionated treatment to a total dose of 35–40 Gy is usually prescribed. The disease is also extremely chemosensitive. The prototype 'MOPP' regimen (mustine, vincristine, procarbazine and prednisolone) is very emetogenic and is associated with a 5–7% risk of second malignancy, notably acute non-lymphocytic leukaemia (Coleman, 1986). In children, 'ABVD' (adriamycin, bleomycin, vinblastine and dacarbazine) or 'ChlVPP' (chlorambucil, vinblastine, procarbazine and prednisolone) are preferred in many centres. 'ABVD' can cause cardiac and pulmonary toxicity, while 'ChlVPP' causes infertility in males. Conventional treatment for stage I and IIA disease involves either radiotherapy alone, or radiotherapy and a short course of chemotherapy. Longer courses of chemotherapy with or without radiotherapy are used for stage III and IV disease. There are, however, variations on this theme. For instance, children in the UK with stage I disease are treated with radiotherapy alone. With this approach, there is a higher rate of relapse outside the radiation field but most relapses are 'salvaged' with chemotherapy. Thus, survival rates are similar but with diminished long-term morbidity in the group overall (Barrett *et al.*, 1990). Actuarial 5-year survival is 97% for stage I, 94% for stage II, 92% for stage III and 74% for stage IV (Manley *et al.*, 1993; Radford *et al.*, 1993). Outcome for stage IV disease may be better if radiotherapy is given in addition to multiagent chemotherapy (Schellong *et al.*, 1987). With such excellent survival rates for stages I–III disease, the challenge for the future is to develop strategies which further reduce morbidity without compromising efficacy. Factors identifying patients with high-risk disease should be defined so that more intensive treatment is given to this group.

pathological staging is undoubtedly more accurate but it is generally felt that the morbidity associated with laparotomy/splenectomy in childhood (severe infections, adhesive intestinal obstruction, and possibly an increased incidence of second malignancies) is not justifiable because the outcome for patients with stage I or II disease is similar despite differ-

Table 31.2 Ann Arbor staging classification (Carbone, Kaplan and Musshoff (1971) with the permission of the editor of *Cancer Research (Baltimore)*)

Stage I:	Involvement of a single lymph node region (I) or a single extralymphatic organ or site (I_E)
Stage II:	Involvement of two or more lymph node regions on the same side of the diaphragm (II) or solitary involvement of an extralymphatic organ or site and of one or more lymph node regions on the same side of the diaphragm (II_E)
Stage III:	Involvement of lymph nodes regions on both sides of the diaphragm (III) which may be accompanied by localized involvement of extralymphatic organ or site (III_E) or by involvement of the spleen (III_S) or both (III_{SE})
Stage IV:	Diffuse or disseminated involvement of one or more extralymphatic organs or tissues with or without associated lymph node enlargement

Rosai-Dorfman disease

Sinus histiocytosis with massive lymphadenopathy (also known as Rosai–Dorfman disease) is a non-malignant disease, usually seen in the first decade of life. It is characterized by massive, painless, bilateral cervical lymphadenopathy. Histology shows intrasinusoidal histiocytosis featuring multinucleate phagocytes containing engulfed blood cells (Rosai and Dorfman, 1972). Other nodal groups may be involved. The lymph nodes are usually mobile and discrete at the outset, but become fixed and matted as the disease progresses. Extranodal involvement of tissues such as the eyelid, orbit and salivary gland may occur. The cause of the disease is unknown; it usually resolves without treatment within 3–9 months but very occasionally patients die of the disease (Foucar, Rosai and Dorfman, 1984). Corticosteroids are sometimes effective.

Sarcomas of the head and neck

Rhabdomyosarcoma

A sarcoma is a malignancy originating from primitive mesenchymal cells which, under normal circumstances, develop into supportive tissues such as muscle and bone. Most sarcomas show some evidence of differentiation into a particular supportive tissue but maturation is incomplete. The most common 'normal tissue' counterpart for childhood sarcomas is skeletal muscle, and tumours showing features of skeletal muscle differentiation are called rhabdomyosarcomas. Rhabdomyosarcomas account for 5–8% of childhood tumours. A small subset of children, mostly with genitourinary rhabdomyosarcomas, belong to families in which multiple cancers such as breast, lung and brain tumours, adrenocortical carcinoma and leukaemia also develop. Constitutional mutations in the p53 'tumour suppressor' gene, located on the long arm of chromosome 17, characterize this 'cancer predisposition syndrome' – the Li-Fraumeni syndrome.

Rhabdomyosarcomas arise from mesenchymal tissue. The head and neck region is the most common site of origin (40%), followed by the genitourinary tract (20%), extremities (20%) and trunk (10%). One-quarter of head and neck malignancies in childhood are rhabdomyosarcomas and the median age at diagnosis is 6 years (Rapidis *et al.*, 1988). Age-incidence studies reveal that rhabdomyosarcoma is the most common type of head and neck cancer in the first 24 months of life, but thereafter is second to lymphoma until at least the twelfth year (Robinson *et al.*, 1988). Fifty per cent of head and neck tumours arise in the orbit and nasopharynx (Anderson *et al.*, 1990). However, in terms of presentation and prognosis, it is convenient to subdivide head and neck rhabdomyosarcomas into those arising from the orbit

(25%), non-orbital parameningeal sites (nasopharynx, paranasal sinuses, middle ear/mastoid, pterygoid-infratemporal fossa, 50%) and non-orbital, non-parameningeal sites (e.g. mouth, neck, face, scalp, larynx, 25%). Tumours of the orbit usually present with proptosis and occasionally ophthalmoplegia, and are usually diagnosed when still relatively small; parameningeal extension is very unusual. Tumours of non-orbital, non-parameningeal sites usually present as localized, painless masses (Figure 31.3), but laryngeal tumours produce symptoms of upper airways obstruction (Kato *et al.*, 1991). Parameningeal tumours often initially masquerade as common childhood problems by producing obstruction to the nose, middle ear or paranasal sinuses (Figure 31.4). Persistent pain, sanguineous discharge or cranial nerve paralysis eventually point to a serious cause for the symptomatology, and the tumour is often large at diagnosis. When the tumour arises below a mucus-secreting epithelium, it may give rise to a 'botryoid' appearance that is almost diagnostic of rhabdomyosarcoma (Figure 31.5).

Once a tumour is suspected, it is important to delineate the extent of the local disease – the contrast resolution of MRI is superior to other techniques. For parameningeal tumours, MRI most precisely demonstrates the relationship of the tumour to normal anatomy at the base of the skull and identifies any intracranial extension. However, bony erosion at the base of the skull, characteristic of parameningeal spread, is best seen on CT scans set at bone windows. This investigation is mandatory if there is no other evidence of parameningeal infiltration such as cranial nerve palsy, CSF leak, malignant cells in the CSF or evidence of intracranial spread on MRI. Using these criteria, about 50% of these tumours will show evidence of parameningeal infiltration.

The next stage in management is to consider whether excision or biopsy is the optimum procedure. Anderson *et al.* (1990) reported that complete microscopic excision of 60 primary head and neck tumours was achieved in only four patients prior to chemotherapy. Unless there is a good chance of achieving clear surgical margins with minimal morbidity, it is best to err on the side of caution and aim only to biopsy the primary tumour at diagnosis. Histopathological diagnosis is straightforward if the tumour cells are spindle-shaped with eosinophilic cytoplasm, or if cross-striations are seen. More commonly, the appearance is that of an undifferentiated 'small, round, blue-cell' tumour of childhood with a differential diagnosis that includes neuroblastoma, the Ewing's sarcoma/primitive neuroectodermal tumour family of tumours and non-Hodgkin's lymphoma. Monoclonal antibodies directed against 'tumour-related' antigens such as desmin (rhabdomyosarcoma), leucocyte common antigen (lymphoma) and neuron-specific enolase (neuroblastoma and primitive neuroectodermal tumours) are helpful in establishing the

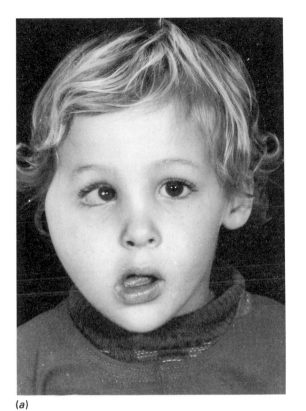

(a)

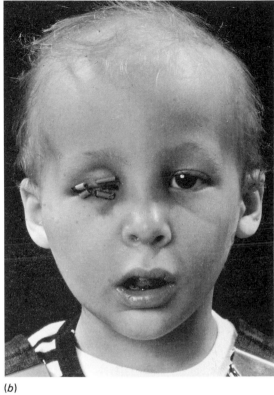

(b)

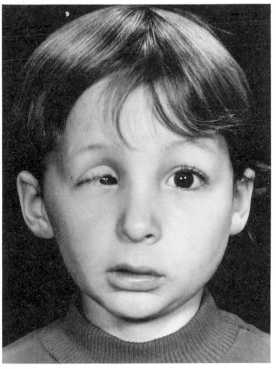

(c)

Figure 31.3 Massive facial rhabdomyosarcoma (initially misdiagnosed as unilateral mumps). (*a*) At diagnosis, age 5 years; (*b*) during therapy (note tarsorrhaphy, needed because of chemotherapy, and radiation-induced corneal ulceration); (*c*) 5 years after diagnosis showing maxillary hypoplasia due to radiation

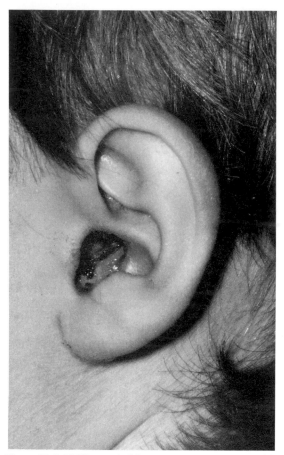

Figure 31.4 Middle ear rhabdomyosarcoma in a 5-year-old boy presenting with a botryoid (grape-like) mass at the external auditory meatus

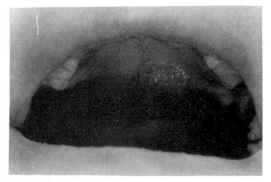

Figure 31.5 Palatal rhabdomyosarcoma: note botryoid appearance

diagnosis. There are three pathological subtypes of childhood rhabdomyosarcoma: embryonal, alveolar and pleomorphic. The pleomorphic variant, while the most common subtype in adults, is rare in children.

The botryoid variant is really an embryonal tumour arising in a submucosal location giving a 'grape-like' appearance to the tumour. This classification carries prognostic significance so that the outcome for patients with embryonal tumours is relatively good, but, because the tumours are more aggressive and tend to metastasize early, relatively poor for alveolar histology. In addition to the architectural appearance under the light microscope, alveolar and embryonal rhabdomyosarcomas are characterized by chromosomal abnormalities. Alveolar rhabdomyosarcoma is associated with a translocation between chromosomes 2 and 13 [t(2;13)], and embryonal rhabdomyosarcoma with loss of heterozygosity of the short arm of chromosome 11. The 2;13 translocation results in a fusion gene which brings together transcriptional regulators from each chromosome (Shapiro *et al.*, 1993). Fluorescent *in situ* hybridization (FISH) for t(2;13) provides an additional means of rapidly distinguishing alveolar from embryonal tumours.

Rhabdomyosarcoma may spread to regional lymph nodes (but this occurs in fewer than 5% of head and neck cases at diagnosis), lungs, liver, bone or bone marrow so that scans of the chest, abdomen, bones, and bone marrow aspirate and trephine biopsies, are performed in all patients. A lumbar puncture is indicated in all patients with parameningeal tumours. Distant spread is found in 8% of patients at diagnosis of head and neck rhabdomyosarcoma (Anderson *et al.*, 1990). Alveolar rhabdomyosarcomas metastasize more often compared with the embryonal type, but alveolar tumours are relatively rare in the head and neck region. Once this information is gathered, the patient is staged; most staging systems rely on surgical pathological data, e.g. the Clinical Grouping System used by the Intergroup Rhabdomyosarcoma Study group (Table 31.3).

Table 31.3 Intergroup Rhabdomyosarcoma Study clinical grouping system

Clinical group		Definition
I	A	Localized, completely resected, confined to site of origin
	B	Localized, completely resected, infiltrated beyond site of origin
II	A	Localized, grossly resected, microscopic residual
	B	Regional disease, involved lymph nodes, completely resected
	C	Regional disease, involved lymph nodes, grossly resected with microscopic residual
III	A	Local or regional grossly visible disease after biopsy only
	B	Grossly visible disease after ≥ 50% resection of primary tumour
IV		Distant metastases present at diagnosis

Treatment for rhabdomyosarcoma may involve chemotherapy, surgery and radiotherapy. Studies in the pre-chemotherapy era showed an actuarial 5-year survival rate of only 14% for children treated with surgery and/or radiotherapy (Kilman *et al.*, 1973). Most died of disease in the lungs or bone marrow indicating that 'micrometastatic' disease is present in the majority of patients at diagnosis and that 'systemic' therapy is essential. Fortunately, childhood rhabdomyosarcoma is a chemosensitive tumour. The most active agents are cyclophosphamide, ifosfamide, actinomycin D, vincristine, doxorubicin, etoposide, and platinum analogues (cisplatin and carboplatin). The intensity of treatment depends on a number of prognostic variables: first, the stage of disease, second, the site, and third, the histology (tumours of alveolar histology receive more intensive therapy). Patients with completely resected, non-alveolar disease are treated with vincristine and actinomycin D; other patients receive at least three drugs including cyclophosphamide or ifosfamide. For initially incompletely resected tumours and all those of alveolar histology, the Intergroup Rhabdomyosarcoma Study in the USA advocates radiotherapy plus chemotherapy, while the SIOP (International Society of Paediatric Oncology) group reserves radiotherapy for tumours which are incompletely resected after chemotherapy and all parameningeal tumours (Maurer *et al.*, 1992; Stevens *et al.*, 1993). The SIOP group approach results in more local recurrences, but many are salvaged with radiotherapy and second-line chemotherapy so that the long-term survival rate is very similar. The aim is to reduce the risk of late side effects caused by radiotherapy to the group overall. In some centres, surgery to residual masses is undertaken by expert head and neck cancer surgeons. It is believed that this offers the best chance of local clearance of tumour with least risk of functional and cosmetic morbidity.

Historically, children with regional nodal or metastatic disease have a poor outlook (around 20% survival) and are now treated intensively with most of the active drugs in rotation. Early results, however, suggest that this approach does not improve the prognosis.

The multidisciplinary approach to rhabdomyosarcoma, including multiagent chemotherapy, judicious surgery and radiotherapy to selected patients, has substantially improved the prognosis of patients with rhabdomyosarcoma of the head and neck. Survival at 5 years is 92% for tumours of the orbit, 81% for non-parameningeal, non-orbital head and neck sites and 69% for parameningeal disease (Maurer *et al.*, 1992). The challenge for paediatric oncologists is to develop chemotherapy strategies which more effectively eradicate residual disease after surgery.

Ewing's sarcoma/primitive neuroectodermal tumour family of tumours

This generic term embodies both Ewing's sarcoma and primitive neuroectodermal tumours (PNET), either of which may arise from bone or the soft tissues. These tumours share a specific chromosomal translocation [t(11q;22q)] and are thought to arise from post-ganglionic cholinergic neurons (Taylor *et al.*, 1993). The link between Ewing's sarcoma and primitive neuroectodermal tumours is supported by ultrastructural studies and *in vitro* cell cultures showing neurite outgrowth (Lancet, 1992). Ewing's sarcoma and primitive neuroectodermal tumours probably represent opposite ends of a spectrum of differentiation with the former the least differentiated and the latter showing some evidence of neuronal differentiation.

Until recently, primitive neuroectodermal tumour was usually mis-classified as either soft tissue Ewing's sarcoma or rhabdomyosarcoma so precise data on their behaviour are lacking. Most Ewing's sarcoma/primitive neuroectodermal tumours occur in the second decade of life and there is a slight male preponderance. However, primitive neuroectodermal tumour is commoner than Ewing's sarcoma in the first decade. These tumours are rare in blacks. Fewer than 10% arise in the head and neck region, most commonly the mandible, maxilla and nasopharynx (Mamede, Mello and Barbieri, 1990; Schmidt *et al.*, 1991). Paraspinal tumours may spread through intervertebral foraminae and cause spinal cord compression. Distant spread is to the lungs, bone and bone marrow and almost all patients have micrometastases at diagnosis. The usual management plan is initial biopsy followed by chemotherapy, with local treatment consisting of radiotherapy and/or surgery depending on the site and margins of resection. Drugs most effective against the Ewing's sarcoma/primitive neuroectodermal tumour family of tumours include cyclophosphamide, ifosfamide, doxorubicin, etoposide, vincristine and actinomycin D. Because of the site, local treatment to head and neck tumours usually consists of radiotherapy with 50–60 Gy delivered in 2 Gy fractions. However, mandibular tumours may be radically excised and the bone reconstructed (Langman, Kaplan and Matthay, 1989). With modern treatment, most recurrences occur at metastatic sites. The actuarial 5-year survival rate for all sites is 60–70% but, because of the high radiotherapy dose required, the cosmetic outcome may be poor.

Olfactory primitive neuroectodermal tumour (aesthesioneuroblastoma)

Because of the neuronal characteristics of the tumour, it is often labelled 'olfactory neuroblastoma' or 'aesthesioneuroblastoma'. However, it should not be confused with childhood neuroblastoma. Olfactory primitive neuroectodermal tumour is rare in children and the levels of urinary catecholamine metabolites in the urine (VMA/HVA) are normal. In contrast with neuroblastoma, the tumour spreads mainly by local invasion rather than distant metastases. Whang-Peng *et al.* (1987) reported the presence of the chromosomal translocation t(11;22) in so-called olfactory neuroblastomas – this cytogenetic abnormality is characteristic of the Ewing's sarcoma/primitive neuroectodermal tumour family of tumours. For these reasons, we prefer the label 'olfactory primitive neuroectodermal tumour' to distinguish this tumour from neuroblastoma.

There is a bimodal age incidence with the major peak in the fifth and sixth decades, and an earlier peak in the second decade; there is a slight male predominance (Elkon *et al.*, 1979). Olfactory primitive neuroectodermal tumours most often present with nasal stuffiness, discharge, epistaxis or pain (Mills and Frierson, 1985). Examination reveals a mass high in the nasal cavity in the region of the superior turbinate, cribriform plate and ethmoid sinus. The tumour grows relatively slowly but spreads to the other nasal cavity, paranasal sinuses and orbit leading to proptosis, and may erode the base of the skull leading to intracranial extension; occasionally, the course is aggressive. Spread to regional lymph nodes, bone, bone marrow, lung and spinal cord is described (Goldsweig and Sundaresan, 1990). The tumour may be staged according to the system of Kadish, Goodman and Wang (1976); group A, tumour confined to the nasal cavity; group B, tumour involving nasal cavity and paranasal sinuses; group C, tumour spreading beyond the nasal cavity and paranasal sinuses. Most tumours are stage B or C at presentation, but stage C disease is relatively commoner in younger patients (Kadish, Goodman and Wang, 1976; Mills and Frierson, 1985). Under the light microscope, the tumour may show evidence of neuronal differentiation (Homer-Wright rosettes, pseudorosettes, intercellular fibrillary background), or may appear as an undifferentiated small, round, blue-cell tumour. Electron microscopy usually reveals clear-cut neuronal differentiation with dense-core neurosecretory granules and neuritic processes (Taxy *et al.*, 1986). Nasal glioma, encephalocoele, extracranial meningioma and schwannoma may also occur at this site, but these are easily distinguished from olfactory primitive neuroectodermal tumour on histological grounds.

Conventional treatment for olfactory primitive neuroectodermal tumour includes surgery with or without conventionally-fractionated radiotherapy to a total dose of around 60 Gy. Extensive craniofacial resection is often required. Using this approach, the disease-free survival rate is dependent on the stage: 88% for stage A, 58% for stage B and 50% for stage C (follow up ranged from 4 to 8 years) (Dulguerov and Calcaterra, 1992). These figures should be viewed with caution as late recurrences occur. Recently, chemotherapy has produced responses in patients with extensive local or metastatic disease, or with recurrent tumour. Drug combinations include cyclophosphamide, actinomycin D, doxorubicin, vincristine and cisplatin (Goldsweig and Sundaresan, 1990). With the initial use of chemotherapy, the role of radiotherapy and extensive surgery must be redefined.

Osteosarcoma

This tumour arises from a primitive bone-forming mesenchymal cell. It is the commonest bone tumour in early life with its peak incidence in the second decade. Boys are more frequently affected than girls. Fewer than 10% occur in the head and neck. The commonest sites, in descending order of frequency, are the maxilla, mandible, skull and cervical spine (Dahlin, 1978). Osteosarcoma can be induced by therapeutic irradiation (so-called 'second tumours') and is commoner in patients with the hereditary form of retinoblastoma. The incidence of osteosarcoma is substantially increased when these risk factors are combined. Of 18 cases of osteosarcoma of the head and neck reported by Mark *et al.* (1991), three developed in patients with both these risk factors. Clinically osteosarcomas present as firm, fixed swellings with or without pain. Plain radiographs show areas of medullary destruction with osteosclerosis or osteolysis; 'sunray' spiculation radiating from the cortex into adjacent soft tissue may be a feature (Figure 31.6). Over 80% of patients have micrometastatic disease at the time of diagnosis, most commonly in the lungs.

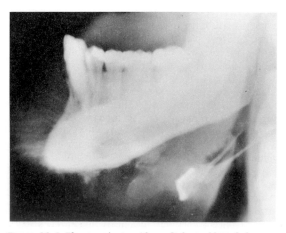

Figure 31.6 Plowman's sign (the radiological bearded chin), pathognomonic of mandibular osteogenic sarcoma

Chemotherapy definitely reduces the risk of meta-static recurrence (Link *et al.*, 1986). Active agents include doxorubicin, cisplatin, high-dose methotrexate, cyclophosphamide, ifosfamide and bleomycin. The modern management approach involves initial biopsy, then combination chemotherapy followed by surgical excision aiming to achieve clear surgical margins. Hemimandibulectomy or radical maxillectomy are undertaken in preference to radiotherapy because osteosarcoma is relatively radioresistant. 'Viable' tumour has been seen in amputation specimens which have been treated with 80 Gy or more (Lee and MacKenzie, 1964). The 5-year survival rate for osteosarcoma at all sites is 65–80% (Link *et al.*, 1986; Winkler *et al.*, 1990). Because the surgery is often difficult and, compared with limb osteosarcoma, the experience of individual surgeons is limited, osteosarcomas of the head and neck are associated with a higher risk of local failure compared with those of the extremities. Death from local failure is usually due to direct extension of tumour into the brain (Mark *et al.*, 1991).

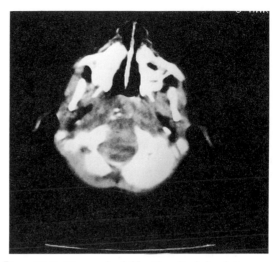

Figure 31.7 CT scan of a child with a clival chordoma. Destruction of bone at a level just rostral to the foramen magnum is clearly demonstrated

Chordoma

Chordomas are rare malignant tumours that develop from vestigial remnants of the notochord. These remnants are seen in about 2% of autopsies and correspond to the sites where chordomas typically occur – the sacrococcyx (50%), spheno-occiput (35%) and vertebrae (15%). Despite their embryonal origin, the peak age incidence for chordoma is in the fifth decade and it is rare before 30 years of age (Bianchi *et al.*, 1989). However, cranial cases usually occur at a younger age. Chordomas, which are commoner in men, grow slowly and tend to invade local structures. Metastases occur in only 10% of cases. Cranial chordomas, which usually involve the clivus, present with focal neurological deficits (due to posterior extension into the brain stem region) or obstruction to the nasopharynx due to anterior growth (Figure 31.7). These features are often preceded by a long history of headaches. Tomographic scans (either CT or MRI) delineate the tumour and extent of local spread. Radical resection is the optimum treatment but very difficult if there is intracranial extension. Chordoma responds to radiotherapy. O'Connell *et al.* (1994) used radiation doses of 65–75 Gy after surgery and reported survival rates of 50–60% at 8 years. Because clival chordomas abut the central nervous system meticulous radiation technique is required. Age appears to be an important prognostic factor; a recent analysis of 25 patients with spheno-occiput chordomas showed that all those under 40 years of age were alive after 5 years, whereas fewer than 40% of the older patients were alive ((Mitchell *et al.*, 1993). However, late recurrences are possible because the tumour often grows very slowly.

Ameloblastoma (adamantinoma)

The ameloblastoma is a rare tumour that arises, in descending order of frequency, in the mandible, maxilla and long bones (Kahn, 1989). The cell of origin is the enamel organ stem cell and tumours may be benign or malignant with solid and cystic components. Wide surgical excision is the treatment of choice; incomplete removal frequently leads to local recurrence (Sehdev *et al.*, 1974). Radiotherapy is reserved for those tumours where microscopic removal is incomplete. Local recurrence is more common for mandibular than maxillary lesions. Responsiveness to chemotherapy is unknown. Metastatic spread is exceedingly rare, but lung metastases have been reported many years after treatment for the primary tumour.

Neuroblastoma

Neuroblastoma is the most common extracranial solid tumour of childhood and accounts for 6–8% of malignancies in this age group. It is an embryonal tumour which develops from ventrally migrating neural crest cells destined to form the peripheral sympathetic nervous system. These sympathoblasts migrate to form the paravertebral sympathetic chain, adrenal medulla, paraganglion of Zuckerkandl, and the retroperitoneal sympathetic plexus. Almost all tumours arise from one of these structures and most head and neck neuroblastomas originate from the cervical sympathetic chain. Neuroblastoma is characterized by two remarkable biological features. First, the histological appearance of a tumour may change from a highly undifferentiated, malignant type to a completely differentiated and benign form. Second, tumours may spontaneously regress and disappear. Some infants present with widespread disease involving the liver, skin and bone marrow and an abdominal primary (occasionally it is cervical). This so-called 'stage 4S' disease usually resolves spontaneously. Recently, specific genetic changes in tumour cells such as amplification of the oncogene designated '*n-myc*' and deletion of the short arm of chromosome 1 (1p-) have been recognized and their presence associated with a poor outcome (Seeger *et al.*, 1985; Christiansen and Lampert, 1988). However, the relationship of these changes to the pathogenesis of the tumour is still unclear.

Most neuroblastomas arise in the abdomen (70%) and chest (20%). Head and neck manifestations of neuroblastoma are more likely to be due to secondary deposits from non-cervical primaries – left supraclavicular lymphadenopathy from primary intra-abdominal disease (Virchow-Troisier lymph node), bony swelling of the skull, maxilla or jaw, and periorbital bruising are typical of metastatic spread to this region. Only 5% of neuroblastomas originate in the head and neck. Overall, the median age at diagnosis is 2 years, but most primary cervical tumours present in the first year of life (Smith and Katz, 1990). Neuroblastoma is the second most common primary malignant head and neck tumour (after rhabdomyosarcoma) before the age of 2 years. The tumour usually presents as a painless, fixed, unilateral cervical mass. Local pressure may cause stridor, dysphagia or an ipsilateral Horner's syndrome due to interruption of the cervical sympathetic supply (Figure 31.8). Neurological signs and symptoms only predominate if the tumour grows through an intervertebral foramen and compresses the cervical spinal cord (a so-called 'dumb-bell' tumour) or if the child presents with opsoclonus-myoclonus (the so-called 'dancing eyes' syndrome). Well-differentiated tumours may secrete vasoactive intestinal polypeptide (VIP) resulting in diarrhoea and hypokalaemia. Manifestations of catecholamine hypersecretion such as hypertension and flushing are unusual compared with phaeochromocytoma. Primary cervical neuroblastomas rarely metastasize to distant sites.

The investigation, diagnosis and staging of suspected neuroblastoma are carried out in accordance with the recommendations of the International Neuroblastoma Staging System (INSS) (Brodeur *et al.*, 1993) (Table 31.4). The extent of the primary disease is assessed using tomographic scanning techniques. The elegant contrast resolution of MRI, in particular, precisely defines disease extent at the skull base, and the relationship to the great vessels and cervical spinal cord, making this modality preferable to CT scanning. Levels of homovanillic acid (HVA) and vanillylmandelic acid (VMA), metabolic byproducts

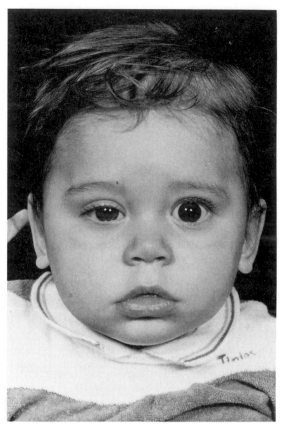

Figure 31.8 Infant with Horner's syndrome due to cervical primary neuroblastoma. The pupil was normally pigmented in this particular patient

of catecholamine breakdown, are raised in the urine of more than 90% of children with neuroblastoma. Neuroblastoma spreads to lymph nodes, bone, bone marrow and liver so that chest radiography, radioisotope bone scanning (more sensitive than skeletal survey), bilateral posterior iliac crest bone marrow aspirates and trephine biopsies, and abdominal ultrasound are important to evaluate distant metastatic spread. In addition, radiolabelled metaiodobenzylguanidine (mIBG), which is actively concentrated in neuroblastoma, may assist in making the diagnosis and defining distant metastases. Once the disease is 'staged', the primary tumour is either biopsied or excised. Histologically, there is a spectrum of appearances with completely differentiated tumour (ganglioneuroma) on the one hand and undifferentiated 'small, round, blue-cell' tumour on the other; partially differentiated ganglioneuroblastoma occupies the middle ground. Many head and neck primary tumours show features of differentiation such as intercellular neurofibrillary material and ganglion cells. However, the tumour may be difficult to distinguish from other 'small, round, blue-cell' tumours (see section on rhabdomyosarcoma).

In a study of 641 neuroblastomas, 84% of cervical neuroblastomas were stages 1 or 2, 16% were stage 3 and none was stage 4 or 4S (Berthold, 1990). Stages 1 and 2A disease is treated by surgical excision alone. Even if macroscopic residual disease is present after surgery in stage 2 patients, the prognosis is still very good, presumably because the disease regresses spontaneously (Matthay *et al.*, 1989). There is controversy over the optimal management of patients with ipsilateral lymph node involvement with some groups advocating chemotherapy in addition to surgery. For stages 3 and 4 disease, the tumour is biopsied in the first instance and chemotherapy given to try to eradicate metastases and render the primary tumour resectable. The agents most useful in neuroblastoma include cyclophosphamide, carboplatin and cisplatin, doxorubicin, etoposide and vincristine (Green, 1985). The European approach is to use OJEC (vincristine (Oncovin), carboplatin (JM8), etoposide and cyclophosphamide) or alternating courses of OJEC and

Table 31.4 International staging system for neuroblastoma

Stage 1
Localized tumour with complete gross excision, with or without microscopic residual disease; representative ipsilateral lymph nodes negative for tumour microscopically (nodes attached to and removed with the primary tumour may be positive)

Stage 2A
Localized tumour with incomplete gross excision; representative ipsilateral non-adherent lymph nodes negative for tumour microscopically

Stage 2B
Localized tumour with or without complete gross excision, with ipsilateral non-adherent lymph nodes positive for tumour. Enlarged contralateral lymph nodes must be negative microscopically

Stage 3
Unresected ipsilateral tumour infiltrating across the midline, with or without regional lymph node involvement; or localized unilateral tumour with contralateral regional lymph node involvement; or midline tumour with bilateral extension by infiltration (unresectable) or by lymph node involvement

Stage 4
Any primary tumour with dissemination to distant lymph nodes, bone, bone marrow, liver, skin and/or other organs (except as defined for stage 4S)

Stage 4S
Localized primary tumour (as defined for stage 1, 2A or 2B), with dissemination limited to skin, liver, and/or bone marrow* (limited to infants < 1 year of age)

OPEC (which are the same drugs as OJEC except with cisplatin substituting for carboplatin). In North America doxorubicin and higher doses of cyclophosphamide and cisplatin are often used. The actuarial survival at 6 years is related to stage: stage 1, 100% survival; stage 2, 94%; stage 3, 60–70%; and stage 4, 20–30%. Thus, the majority of patients with disease in the head and neck have an excellent outlook (Berthold, 1990).

At present the intensity of therapy is stratified according to the age of the patient and stage of the tumour. However, in future, treatment strategies will probably be influenced by an array of biological markers (such as serum ferritin, neuron-specific enolase, chromosome 1p deletion and n-myc amplification) which predict outcome more precisely.

Germ cell tumours

Germ cell tumours come from primordial germ cells which originate in the yolk sac endoderm in the embryo. These cells normally migrate to the gonadal ridge where they populate the developing testis or ovary. Occasionally, germ cells may inexplicably come to rest in an extragonadal location and multiply, producing a germ cell tumour. A germ cell tumour may be benign (in which case it is designated a teratoma) or malignant. As a group, these tumours most often occur in the sacrococcygeal region followed, in descending order of frequency, by the ovary or testis, mediastinum, brain and retroperitoneum. Only 4% of germ cell tumours are found in the head and neck, accounting for fewer than 1% of head and neck masses in children (Rapidis *et al.*, 1988). Jordan and Gauderer (1988) reviewed 212 cases of head and neck germ cell tumours (excluding intracranial sites); 90% occurred in the paediatric age group and 75% in neonates or stillborns. These tumours may occur in the midline or laterally, and are reported to involve the orbit, oral cavity, pharynx, face, neck or cervical spine. In the neonate they usually present as a well-defined, firm, mobile, multilobular, cystic swelling. Ultrasound usually reveals solid and cystic components, but calcification on plain radiographs is seen in only 16% of cases.

In adults, two-thirds of head and neck germ cell tumours are malignant, whereas probably less than 5% are malignant in childhood (Silberman and Mendelson, 1960). However, the importance of neonatal germ cell tumours lies in their often dramatic clinical presentation due to airway obstruction and the demand for urgent and skilful surgery.

Head and neck germ cell tumours have been categorized according to the age and clinical features at presentation (Jordan and Gauderer, 1988): group I, stillborn/moribund at birth (12%), group II, newborn with respiratory distress (46%), group III, newborn without respiratory distress (17%), group IV, children

1 month to 18 years (14%), and group V, adults (11%). The outcome was related to group so that whereas all patients in group I died, less than half of group II and very few in groups III and IV died.

Serum levels of alpha-fetoprotein (AFP) and beta-human chorionic gonadotrophin (beta HCG) levels should be measured *prior* to surgery in children with a suspected germ cell tumour. Raised levels indicate malignancy but it is important to compare with the age-related normal values. The upper limit of the normal range is high in the newborn, and declines to 'adult' levels by 21 weeks of age (Craft and Pritchard, 1994).

Nowadays, more than 80% of children with malignant germ cell tumours are cured with high-dose VAC (vincristine, actinomycin D and cyclophosphamide, with or without doxorubicin), BEP (bleomycin, etoposide and cisplatin) or JEB (bleomycin, etoposide and carboplatin) (Mann *et al.*, 1989). Conventional treatment involves 'second look' surgery for residual masses after chemotherapy. Radiotherapy is rarely needed. Marrow-ablative high-dose chemotherapy has a role in tumours resistant to conventional chemotherapy.

Carcinomas of the head and neck

Carcinomas are rare in children, accounting for no more than 1–2% of malignancies, but almost half occur in the head and neck region. The thyroid is the most common site (21% of carcinomas overall) followed by the nasopharynx (15%) and salivary glands (7%) with small numbers occurring in the mouth, orbit/periorbital region and maxillary antrum (McWhirter, Stiller and Lennox, 1989).

Thyroid carcinoma

The peak age range for the development of thyroid cancer is between 25 and 40 years; fewer than 10% of cases present in patients younger than 20 years of age (Mazzaferri, Young and Oertel, 1977). The sex distribution in children is similar to that for adults with three-quarters of thyroid cancers occurring in females. Radiation is an important aetiological factor, particularly in the USA and Israel. The practice of irradiating the head and neck in children suffering from thymic or tonsillar enlargement, acne, tinea capitis, eczema and cervical lymphadenopathy began in the USA in the 1920s and later spread to Israel. However, an association between this practice and thyroid malignancy was not noted until 1950 (Gorlin and Sallan, 1990). In its heyday, radiotherapy accounted for 75% of thyroid cancers in the young with boys and girls equally affected. Overall, about 7% of those irradiated developed thyroid malignancy

after a latency period of 5–40 years (Mehta, Goetowski and Kinsella, 1989). More recently, there has been a striking increase in the incidence of childhood thyroid carcinoma in regions neighbouring Chernobyl, due to the ingestion of radioiodines (Nikiforov and Gnepp, 1994). An increased risk of thyroid carcinoma is described in patients with familial adenomatous polyposis, Cowden's (multiple hamartoma) syndrome, familial non-medullary thyroid carcinoma and Hashimoto's thyroiditis.

Most children with thyroid cancer present with cervical lymphadenopathy indicating lymphatic spread at the time of diagnosis. A thyroid mass is often palpable, and sometimes visible (Figure 31.9). Adenomas account for one-third of thyroid nodules in children followed by carcinoma (22%), cyst (19%) and hyperplasia (13%). In contrast, only 1 in 200 thyroid nodules in adults are malignant (Fowler, Pokorny and Harberg, 1989). The most common histological subtype of thyroid carcinoma observed in children is papillary or mixed papillary-follicular, followed by follicular and very small numbers of medul-

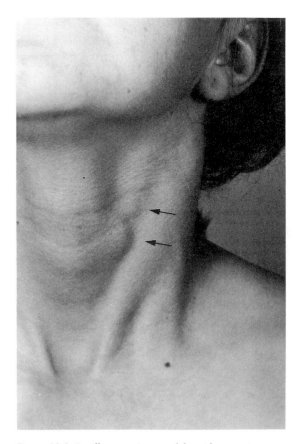

Figure 31.9 Papillary carcinoma of thyroid presenting as a discrete thyroid swelling in a teenage girl

lary, anaplastic and undifferentiated carcinomas. At the time of diagnosis of thyroid carcinoma in children over 50% have metastasized to cervical lymph nodes, and 10–20% to the lungs compared with 35% and 2% for nodes and lungs respectively in adults (Gorlin and Sallan, 1990). There is some relationship between histopathology and pattern of spread. Both papillary and follicular subtypes readily spread to lymph nodes, but the former has a predilection for the lungs and the latter for bones.

Histological diagnosis is made on a biopsy specimen of a cervical lymph node or thyroid nodule. Radical thyroidectomy – preserving the recurrent laryngeal nerves and at least one parathyroid gland – is the preferred therapeutic procedure. All involved lymph nodes must be excised from the deep cervical chain and, if shown on the CT scan, involved mediastinal nodes are also removed. Formal block dissection of the deep cervical chain is not routinely performed but is occasionally indicated. Following surgery, an ablation dose of iodine-131 is given to eradicate the normal thyroid remnant which is invariably present. If this iodine-avid tissue is not destroyed it will 'soak up' radioiodine during subsequent tracer studies and prevent visualization of metastases. Three months later a tracer iodine-123 or iodine-131 scan should reveal any lung, bone or residual nodal metastases which are treated with further 'ablative' doses of iodine-131 until scintigrams are clear of tumour.

There is good evidence that thyroid stimulating hormone (TSH) suppression with thyroid hormone after surgery reduces the risk of recurrence of well-differentiated thyroid carcinoma (Mazzaferri, Young and Oertel, 1977). Therefore, following radical thyroidectomy and radioiodine ablation of the thyroid remnant and metastases, patients are given T_4 in a dose titrated to reduce the TSH concentration to undetectable levels. Follow-up of the patient involves clinical examination (with meticulous examination of the neck), chest X-ray, tracer radioiodine scans and serum thyroglobulin estimation, the interval between assessments increasing with time. Our recommendations for serial radioiodine scans are based on the extensive studies of Pochin (1967) who found that more than 80% of well-differentiated thyroid cancers concentrated iodine. In addition, serum thyroglobulin is used as a marker of disease relapse, though levels may not always be raised in the presence of a positive radioiodine scan and circulating thyroglobulin autoantibodies may invalidate the assay (Grant *et al.*, 1984). Thus, while serum thyroglobulin estimations complement radioiodine scans in the follow up of patients with thyroid cancer, they do not provide a reliable substitute.

Thyroid cancer more often recurs in children than in adults. The cumulative risk of nodal relapse is 30% after 20 years compared with less than 10% in adults. Vigilance must be sustained because one-third of relapses occur 5 years after diagnosis and 15% are noted 15 or more years after diagnosis (Zimmerman *et al.*, 1988). The commonest site for relapse is in the cervical lymph nodes, followed by mediastinal nodes and the lungs. When a patient relapses with nodal disease, a tracer radioiodine scan must precede surgical resection of the involved nodes. Those with iodine-avid disease receive ablative doses of iodine-131 postoperatively. Relapse in the lung is treated with iodine-131, as long as the disease is iodine-avid.

Patients who are young at diagnosis and those without distant metastases fare better. The presence of cervical nodal metastases in children does not appear to have an adverse affect on outcome. Survival rates over 90% have been documented (Zimmerman *et al.*, 1988). In contrast to adults, distant metastases do not always confer a very poor prognosis. In one series, none of 19 children or young adults with pulmonary metastases from well-differentiated thyroid carcinoma treated with iodine-131 died of disease with a median follow up of 4.5 years (Vassilopoulou-Sellin *et al.*, 1992). Tubiana, Schlunberger and Rougier (1985) reviewed 38 children with thyroid cancer and noted an 88% survival at 15 years. Significantly, two deaths occurred after 20 or more years of follow up.

The treatment strategy for the small numbers of children with papillary or mixed disease limited to the thyroid gland is more contentious. The young patient with a localized intrathyroidal primary has an excellent prognosis. Is it necessary to perform radical thyroidectomy and radioiodine ablation, both of which are carry potential morbidity, in such a child? It may be argued that the best results in the Mazzaferri, Young and Oertel series (1977) were in the radically ablated patients, that papillary disease is often multifocal, and that modern thyroid surgery and radioiodine ablation are relatively safe. In addition, the late relapses and deaths in the less aggressively treated patients in the Tubiana, Schlunberger and Rouglier series (1985) has led our hospital to use conservative thyroidectomy followed by TSH-suppressive doses of T_4, while radioiodine therapy is withheld. Follow up consists of clinical examination and thyroglobulin assay, and may be supplemented with CT scanning to detect nodal or thyroid bed recurrence. If a recurrence is detected, ablation of the thyroid remnant precedes radioiodine treatment directed at disease. The treatment delay inherent in this approach is not a practical problem because of the slow pace of disease.

Nasopharyngeal carcinoma

Although nasopharyngeal carcinoma is a rare tumour representing less than 1% of childhood malignancies in the 'industrialized' world, it accounts for one-third of nasopharyngeal cancers in children. The most common nasopharyngeal cancer of childhood is rhabdomyosarcoma; lymphoma and nasopharyngeal carcinoma occur less often (Tom *et al.*, 1992). Fifteen per cent of all nasopharyngeal carcinomas occur in the paediatric population. In southern China nasopharyngeal carcinoma is endemic in adults though not in children. In contrast, nasopharyngeal carcinoma accounts for 10–20% of childhood malignancies in parts of northern Africa (Hidayatalla *et al.*, 1983). It is suggested that nasopharyngeal carcinoma is more common in black American children (Hawkins *et al.*, 1990). There is a striking association with Epstein-Barr virus infection. Epstein-Barr virus DNA is usually found in nasapharyngeal carcinoma tumour cells in children and antibody titres to viral antigens correlate with tumour bulk and disease activity (Naegele *et al.*, 1982). Presumably Epstein-Barr virus infection plays an integral part in the multi-step pathogenesis of nasopharyngeal carcinoma, entering epithelial cells of the nasopharynx after inhalation directly or delivery by Epstein-Barr virus-containing B lymphocytes.

Most nasopharyngeal carcinomas in childhood are characterized by a marked reactive lymphocytic infiltrate and were often labelled 'lymphoepitheliomas' in the past. In 1978 the World Health Organization (WHO) divided nasopharyngeal carcinoma into three subtypes (Shanmugaratnam and Sabin, 1978): type 1, squamous cell carcinoma with keratinization; type 2, non-keratinizing squamous cell carcinoma; type 3, undifferentiated carcinoma with no evidence of squamous cell differentiation. About two-thirds of childhood nasopharyngeal carcinoma are type 3 and one-third type 2, while type 1 is unusual in children. It is possible that the less differentiated tumours carry a better prognosis, probably because they are more responsive to chemo- and radiotherapy.

Over 80% of children with nasopharyngeal carcinoma present with asymptomatic cervical lymphadenopathy indicating spread to regional lymph nodes and usually this is the only presenting feature (Figure 31.10). There may, however, be local tumour infiltration causing nasal blockage and epistaxis, eustachian tube dysfunction with hearing loss and middle ear effusions, or sometimes extension to the base of the skull resulting in paralysis of cranial nerves. Metastases to lung, liver, mediastinum or bone are present in only a few children at diagnosis. Sometimes widespread disease may be associated with hypertrophic osteoarthropathy characterized by skeletal pain, joint swelling and clubbing. As cervical adenopathy is the most common presenting sign in nasopharyngeal carcinoma, the differential diagnosis includes inflammatory lymph node enlargement and Hodgkin's disease. Careful evaluation of the ear, nose, throat and thyroid gland is essential in children with persistent lymphadenopathy.

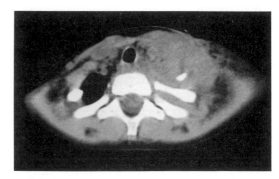

Figure 31.10 CT scan of neck demonstrating a large mass of lymph glands infiltrated by metastatic nasopharyngeal carcinoma. There was no discernible primary in the nasopharynx of this child

Once nasopharyngeal carcinoma is confirmed or suspected evaluation includes detailed examination of the cranial nerves and indirect nasopharyngoscopy by an otolaryngologist. MRI delineates the nasopharyngeal tumour more accurately than X-ray, but CT set at bone windows is important to determine whether there is erosion at the base of the skull. A bone scan, CT of the chest and abdominal scanning (either CT or ultrasound) are needed to determine whether or not distant metastases are present. Once the extent of local infiltration and metastases is defined a disease stage can be allocated. Because the majority of children present with lymph node metastasis, a modification of the American Joint Committee on Cancer Tumour, Node, Metastasis (TNM) Classification is proposed for children (Table 31.5) (Ho, 1977). In a study of 57 patients aged between 4 and 21

Table 31.5 TNM staging classification of nasopharyngeal carcinoma (UICC)

Stage	Classification
T0	No evidence of primary tumour
T1	Tumour limited to one region
T2	Tumour extending into two regions
T3	Tumour extending beyond the nasopharynx without bone involvement
T4	Tumour extending beyond the nasopharynx with bone involvement, including the cartilaginous portion of the eustachian tube
N0	No palpable cervical nodes
N1	Mobile ipsilateral cervical lymphadenopathy
N2	Mobile bilateral cervical lymphadenopathy
N3	Fixed cervical lymphadenopathy
M0	No metastases
M1	Metastases

years, 14 had stage T0-T1, 22 stage T2 and 21 stage T3 disease. Thus, most young patients have locally advanced disease usually with regional nodal metastases, but distant metastases are rare (Ingersoll *et al.*, 1990).

Nasopharyngeal carcinoma is radiosensitive and the treatment of children has been largely extrapolated from adult practice. Although the world's largest experience and excellent survival rates were published by Ho's group (Ho, 1978), the radiation technique is not ideal. In particular, the dissimilarly canted nasopharyngeal and neck fields produce awkward field junctions in the region of Rouviere's node and the uppermost deep cervical nodes. The radiation technique employed at St Bartholomew's Hospital, London, commences with the child in an individually-made shell with a dental splint keeping the tongue downwards and the floor of the mouth low and outside the radiation portals. The orbito-meatal line (Reid's baseline) is vertical and all planning, including field junctions, is parallel or perpendicular to this plane. Planning and treatment then continue in a manner similar to previously published techniques (Lederman and Mould, 1968). The recommended tumour doses are 40–50 Gy to children less than 4 years, increasing to 60 Gy for children older than 12 years. The total dose is conventionally divided into 175–190 cGy fractions. There is no evidence that higher doses are more effective in children and young adults (Jenkin *et al.*, 1981). By using a three-field boost to the nasopharynx the incidence of treatment-induced trismus is low. Even if clinically uninvolved, the neck nodes down to the clavicles receive a conventionally fractionated dose of 50 Gy. A good, reproducible radiation technique for nasopharyngeal carcinoma is a technically demanding exercise.

Ingersoll *et al.* (1990) reported 57 children and young adults (median age 18 years at diagnosis) with nasopharyngeal carcinoma. All received radiotherapy (median dose 64.5 Gy), but only 14 received chemotherapy. Twenty-seven patients relapsed, 20 at distant sites only (bone, lung, liver or mediastinal lymph nodes), six at both locoregional and distant sites, and one had a locoregional recurrence only. This study, and that of Pao *et al.* (1989), indicated that the majority of children fail at distant sites and that failure is more likely in higher T stage disease, independent of nodal status. These data indicate that patients with advanced local disease have micrometastatic deposits outside the proposed radiation field at diagnosis. Most children with nasopharyngeal carcinoma have Ho stage T2 or T3 so that systemic therapy is desirable in these patients. Nasopharyngeal carcinoma in adults is responsive to doxorubicin, platinum, bleomycin, vincristine, methotrexate and fluorouracil, and paediatric studies have used combinations of these agents together with radiotherapy. No prospective, randomized study has tested the utility of

chemotherapy in nasopharyngeal carcinoma and single-agent data are lacking in children. However, nasopharyngeal carcinoma is chemosensitive; 40 of 41 adolescents and adults had a major clinical response to three courses of epirubicin, bleomycin and cisplatin prior to radiotherapy, and all assessable patients had a complete response following radiotherapy (Bachouchi *et al.*, 1990). A pragmatic approach is taken at the Great Ormond Street Hospital for Children where six courses of alternating VAC (vincristine, actinomycin D and cyclophosphamide) and JEB (carboplatin – JM8, etoposide and bleomycin) precede radiotherapy as described above.

The outcome in children with nasopharyngeal carcinoma is mainly influenced by the extent of local disease. Adjusting staging to that of the Ho classification, survival for T1 disease is in excess of 80% at 16 years compared with 35% for T2 and T3 disease over the equivalent period of time (Pao *et al.*, 1989). The presence of metastases or cranial nerve palsies at diagnosis carries grave prognostic significance. There are two words of caution about interpreting results on nasopharyngeal carcinoma; first, it is suggested that the outlook for undifferentiated nasopharyngeal carcinoma is better than the more differentiated forms so that results of adult studies should be extrapolated to children with circumspection. Secondly, childhood nasopharyngeal carcinoma is so uncommon that studies reporting this condition have reviewed patients over a number of decades. Imaging techniques, chemotherapy and radiotherapy protocols, and supportive care have changed over the review period so that survival results from these studies should be seen as part of a continuum. Because most patients who relapse do so at distant sites, there is now a case to explore a cautious reduction in the total radiation dose, especially in young children, in order to reduce the considerable 'late-effects' of 'high-dose' radiotherapy, especially damage of the hypothalamic–pituitary axis. The major challenge now is to develop multiagent chemotherapy regimens with proven efficacy in children in order to eradicate micrometastatic disease.

Salivary gland tumours

In childhood, most salivary gland masses are not neoplastic and most neoplasms are not malignant. Even when salivary swellings are removed, 60% are non-neoplastic; two-thirds of these are mucocoeles and the remainder mainly sialadenitis, either non-specific or due to tuberculosis or sarcoidosis (Krolls, Trodahl and Boyers, 1972). Mucocoeles occur only in the minor oral salivary glands, most commonly in the lower lip. They tend to occur during 'teething' (either primary or secondary dentition) and probably result from injury to the secretory duct of the gland. The clinical picture is of a small, smooth, painless, unilocular swelling.

An analysis of 9823 salivary gland neoplasms showed that only 3% occurred in patients less than 16 years of age (Luna, Batsakis and El-Naggar, 1991). Two-thirds are benign and one-third malignant. Benign mesenchymal lesions, such as haemangiomas and lymphangiomas, are commoner than benign epithelial masses such as adenomas (Figure 31.11). Pleomorphic adenomas and haemangiomas together account for 80% of the total of benign masses. Other benign lesions, in descending order of frequency, include lymphangiomas, neural tumours, embryomas, lipomas, Warthin's tumour, cystadenoma and lymphoepithelial lesions. Malignant mesenchymal lesions such as rhabdomyosarcoma are rare; most malignant masses are of epithelial origin and half of the salivary gland cancers are mucoepidermoid carcinomas. Tomographic scans (either CT or MRI) are useful to determine whether a mass is intrinsic or extrinsic to the salivary gland and, if in the parotid region, to define the relationship to the facial nerve. CT with sialography is no longer recommended. The biopsy, examination of frozen section and the definitive surgical procedure are usually carried out in one session. Enucleation increases the risk of recurrence of pleomorphic adenomas and mucoepidermoid carcinomas and second-look parotid surgery

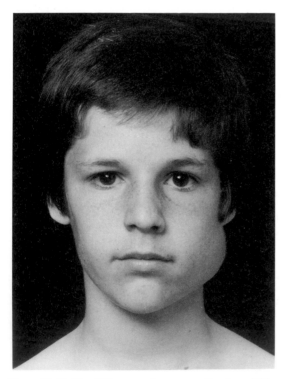

Figure 31.11 Parotid haemangioma presenting in a child with a long history of swelling. (Photograph by courtesy of Professor L. Spitz)

increases the risk of damage to the facial nerve; therefore, masses should be treated by wide excision in the first instance. Fine needle aspiration may be helpful in distinguishing the causes of salivary gland enlargement and assist in planning the extent of surgery (Callender *et al.*, 1992). However, expertise in cytology is often lacking in children's hospitals.

Pleomorphic adenoma accounts for one-quarter of neoplasms of the salivary glands in childhood (Luna, Batsakis and El-Naggar, 1991). In contrast with adults, monomorphic adenomas are exceedingly rare in children (Seifert, Okabe and Caselitz, 1986). Pleomorphic adenomas most commonly arise in the parotid gland, followed by the minor salivary and submandibular glands. The mass is usually painless and slow-growing and facial nerve palsy does not occur (Callender *et al.*, 1992). These slow-growing neoplasms are surrounded by an imperfect pseudocapsule that is crossed by 'fingers' of tumour so that simple enucleation results in a high risk of recurrence. Therefore, the treatment of choice for pleomorphic adenoma in the parotid is parotidectomy with preservation of the facial nerve. Tumours lateral to the facial nerve or in the tail of the gland may be removed by superficial parotidectomy whereas the rarer deep tumour is treated by nerve-sparing total parotidectomy. Treated this way, tumour recurrence is very unusual (Malone and Baker, 1984). These authors emphasized that the surgical treatment of recurrence after local excision or enucleation of the tumour may necessitate removal of the VIIth nerve so that initial local excision with or without radiotherapy is suboptimal management. Radiotherapy is reserved for the rare instance where radical surgery leaves residual disease. In these circumstances, postoperative radiotherapy is delivered with an appositional, lateral megavoltage electron source to a total dose of 60 Gy over 6 weeks. With this technique chronic dry mouth can be avoided, but late temporomandibular joint dysfunction and mandibular ramus hypoplasia may result. Pleomorphic adenomas of the submandibular and minor salivary glands are managed by complete excision. As with parotid lesions, incisional biopsy and enucleation should be avoided.

Malignancies of the salivary glands in childhood comprise mucoepidermoid carcinoma (50%), acinic cell carcinoma and adenocarcinoma (10% each), and small numbers of sarcoma, adenoid cystic carcinoma, carcinoma ex-pleomorphic adenoma and squamous cell carcinoma (Luna, Batsakis and El-Naggar, 1991). Half of the childhood mucoepidermoid carcinomas occur in patients younger than 10 years, usually in the parotid gland. The clinical presentation is a painless swelling although discomfort and facial nerve paralysis may be encountered. A histological grading system is prognostically useful; most tumours in children are low-grade (grade I histology). They are usually well-circumscribed, although there is little or no capsule. Tumours sometimes incite surrounding inflammatory changes which may explain the benign lymphadenopathy sometimes observed (Callender *et al.*, 1992). In principle, treatment of low-grade tumours is as for adenomas. The type of operation depends on the extent of the tumour. A subtotal, nerve-sparing parotidectomy is optimal if it complies with the principle of complete tumour excision with clear margins. Sacrifice of the facial nerve may be necessary if there is perineural invasion or if the intact nerve limits resection and is preferable to limited surgery followed by postoperative radiotherapy. Facial nerve grafting can restore deficits after nerve resection (Callender *et al.*, 1992). Low-grade tumours with unclear margins and high-grade tumours are treated with postoperative radiotherapy which improves the rate of local control. Mucoepidermoid carcinoma of the submandibular or sublingual glands is treated by radical resection of the gland and surrounding lymph nodes. Tumour may occasionally spread by local infiltration or to regional lymph nodes. Block dissection of the cervical lymph nodes is indicated if clinically involved at diagnosis or at relapse. There are few published data on the efficacy of chemotherapy in children. Combinations of 5-fluorouracil, doxorubicin, cisplatin and cyclophosphamide have produced responses in adults with recurrent or metastatic salivary gland tumours (Venook *et al.*, 1987). The prognosis for mucoepidermoid carcinoma is better in children and the survival rate is almost 95%.

The management of acinic cell carcinoma (a low-grade malignancy), adenocarcinoma and adenoid cystic carcinoma (both high-grade cancers) is similar to that described for mucoepidermoid carcinoma but the outcome is less favourable.

Fibroblastic proliferations of infancy and childhood

This heterogeneous collection of rare disorders is characterized by uncontrolled proliferation of fibrous tissue with a tendency to local recurrence after incomplete resection. Almost one-third occur in the head and neck region (Hayashi *et al.*, 1989). Conditions such as digital fibromatosis and fibromatosis colli ('sternocleidomastoid tumour') may be defined according to their anatomical location. The most important disorders from an oncologist's point of view are infantile 'aggressive' fibromatosis, infantile myofibromatosis and congenital infantile fibrosarcoma. Infantile myofibromatosis usually presents as single or multiple cutaneous or subcutaneous deposits – if multiple, the skeleton and internal organs (e.g. lung, myocardium and gastrointestinal tract) may be involved. Occasionally, infantile fibromatosis affects the upper respiratory tract or tongue (Wiswell *et al.*, 1988). Under the microscope, the condition is distinguished from the other fibrous proliferations of infancy on the basis of

myoblastic features as well as the fibroblastic component. Although excised lesions tend to recur, infantile myofibromatosis is a benign, self-limiting condition. Occasionally, extensive multifocal disease leads to death from organ failure.

Infantile 'aggressive' fibromatosis usually presents in the first 2 years of life and may be present at birth. It most often originates in the head and neck, upper torso and legs. In the head and neck region, the tongue, mandible, mastoid process and maxillary sinus or nasopharynx are most frequently involved. The condition presents as a firm, fixed, painless mass which may ulcerate overlying skin or mucosa (Figure 31.12). Bone erosion is often present and vital structures may be threatened. Congenital infantile fibrosarcoma is usually detected in the first year of life; over two-thirds of lesions arise in the extremities. Blocker, Koenig and Ternberg (1987) reported five of 52 infantile fibrosarcomas occurring in the head and neck region.

The outlook is good for both infantile fibromatosis and fibrosarcoma. The conventional treatment is wide local excision, but even extensive surgery in the head and neck region often fails to remove the tumour completely while placing the young child at risk of substantial morbidity (e.g. jaw hypoplasia

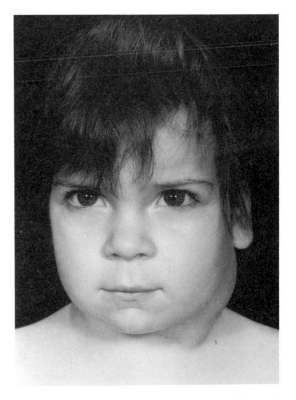

Figure 31.12 Cervical fibromatosis in a 4-year-old boy. There was slow spontaneous resolution over 2 years

requiring reconstruction). For these reasons, the efficacy of chemotherapy has been tested in both infantile fibromatosis and fibrosarcoma. Regimens based on vincristine, actinomycin D and cyclophosphamide/ifosfamide have produced impressive responses in both conditions (Raney *et al.*, 1987; Kynaston *et al.*, 1993). It is now reasonable to use chemotherapy as a first-line treatment for tumours whose position or size preclude adequate excision without morbidity. In view of the late unwanted effects of cyclophosphamide and ifosfamide, the vincristine/actinomycin D regimen is most often used. Patience is required because the response to chemotherapy is often slow. The initial objective is 'stabilization' of disease over a 2–3 month period.

Despite apparent histological differences, infantile fibromatosis and congenital infantile fibrosarcoma behave very similarly. This has led some authors to question whether congenital infantile 'fibrosarcoma' really is a malignancy. In addition, the rate of metastasis is very low, and the outlook excellent compared with other childhood sarcomas (Coffin *et al.*, 1994). However, occasional tumours do metastasize. Nonrandom chromosomal trisomies have been described in the infantile form of fibrosarcoma and may be useful in distinguishing fibrosarcomas with metastatic potential from those without (Schofield *et al.*, 1994).

Langerhans cell histiocytosis

The term Langerhans cell histiocytosis embraces the conditions known as histiocytosis X, eosinophilic granuloma, Hand-Schüller-Christian disease and Letter-Siwe disease. Whatever organ is involved the light microscopic appearances of Langerhans cell histiocytosis are characterized by the presence of Langerhans histiocytes accompanied by 'small round cells' and eosinophils. Langerhans cells, antigen-presenting cells of the monocyte-macrophage series, are normally only found in the skin. Their presence in other organs (where they are called 'LCH cells') is virtually pathognomonic of Langerhans cell histiocytosis. It had been thought that this is not a neoplastic disease and that the cellular infiltrate is due to an uncontrolled reaction of the antigen-presenting cell, possibly secondary to a defect in regulation of the immune system. However, recent experiments have shown that the LCH cells (but not the lymphoid cells) in Langerhans cell histiocytosis are 'clonal', indicating an intense proliferative stimulus (Willman *et al.*, 1994). It seems likely that the underlying abnormality is one of faulty communication between lymphocytes and Langerhans cells, perhaps because of abnormal production of cytokines (Kannourakis and Abbas, 1994).

The precise incidence of Langerhans cell histiocytosis is unknown; approximately 50 new cases are diagnosed in the UK per annum, but this is almost certainly an underestimate as mild cases may readily be misdiagnosed as seborrhoeic eczema. Also, oral/gut or lung involvement may be asymptomatic. The disease may occur in the newborn and the elderly, but the peak incidence is between 2 and 4 years of age. Boys are affected more frequently than girls (male: female is 1.5–2.0:1), but there is no difference in the degree of severity between the sexes. The sites of disease at presentation vary enormously and, as a result, symptoms are protean (Table 31.6). In over 50% of diagnosed cases, more than one organ is involved at presentation (multisystem disease). In the

Table 31.6 Presenting symptoms of 30 children with Langerhans cell histiocytosis

Symptom	Number of children*
Skin rash	15
Recurrent aural discharge	8
Bone pain	5
Scalp lump(s)	5
Proptosis	4
Failure to thrive	3
Breathlessness	3
Lymphadenopathy	2
Hepatosplenomegaly	1
Spinal cord compression	1

* Numbers add up to more than 30 as some children had multiple symptoms.

remainder only one organ or organ system is involved (single-system disease) though detailed investigation may reveal occult disease at other sites. The head and neck region is frequently involved. The yellow, scaly, 'seborrhoeic' rash often involves the scalp (particularly behind the ears) and intertriginous areas (Figure 31.13). A chronic, often smelly, aural discharge, is a common presenting feature. This is due to cutaneous infiltration of the external auditory canal, or polyps of histiocytic tissue projecting into the canal from the middle ear and mastoid (Irving, Broadbent and Jones, 1994). Secondary infection is common. A discharging ear in association with a 'seborrhoeic' rash should alert the clinician to the possibility of Langerhans cell histiocytosis. One or more bones are involved in 80% of patients. Lesions are solitary or multiple, and the skull is most frequently involved (Figure 31.14). Defects in the calvarium can often be palpated and there is sometimes an overlying soft tissue swelling. Radiologically, the lesions appear 'punched out'. Cervical lymphadenopathy is common and sometimes massive, producing symptoms of obstruction. Occasionally, the skin overlying a lymph node or bony lesion breaks down resulting in a chronically discharging sinus (Figure 31.15). Tracheal involvement has been described (Brickman, Nogrady and Wiglesworth, 1973). Early

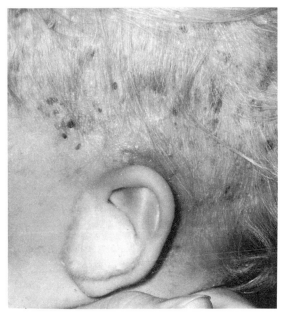

Figure 31.13 Langerhans cell histiocytosis – typical 'seborrhoeic' eczematous rash behind ear. This 2-year-old girl also had chronic aural discharge

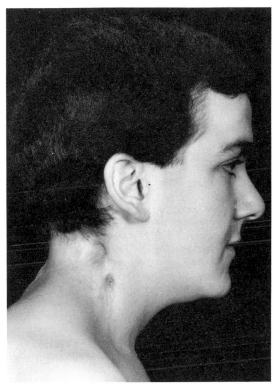

Figure 31.15 Langerhans cell histiocytosis: chronic dermal sinuses, the result of chronic underlying lymph node involvement

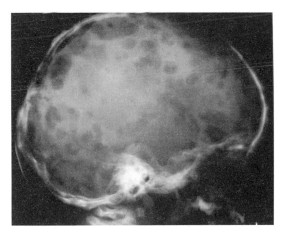

Figure 31.14 Lateral skull X-ray of a child with extensive skull involvement by Langerhans cell histiocytosis

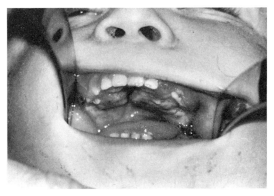

Figure 31.16 Langerhans cell histiocytosis: palatal fistula – a rare complication of oral involvement

manifestations in the mouth include granularity or thickening of the gingival mucosa (Betts and McNeish, 1972). More extensive involvement may be painful and, exceptionally, a palatal fistula may develop (Figure 31.16). Dental involvement may be due to underlying disease in the mandible or maxilla, or as a result of direct infiltration from the oral mucosa. In severe cases erosion of dental alveoli and gum retraction may cause premature eruption or loosening of the teeth. In these patients, loss of the dental lamina dura is an important radiological sign. Proptosis may be due to a retro-orbital deposit or bony lesion. Infiltration of the posterior pituitary gland or infundibulum, best shown by MRI, produces diabetes insipidus in 30–40% of cases (Greenberger *et al.*, 1981). The anterior pituitary gland may sometimes be involved causing growth hormone deficiency. Other organs that may be involved include the liver and spleen, bone marrow, lungs and gastrointestinal tract.

The diagnosis is made by histological examination of a biopsy of an involved organ, usually bone, skin or lymph node, but special techniques are required to confirm the diagnosis. Presence of the CD1a antigen is crucial and electron microscopy may reveal 'hand mirror'-shaped inclusion granules known as Birbeck granules (Nezelof, 1979). The Writing Group of the Histiocyte Society has published criteria for the diagnosis of Langerhans cell histiocytosis (Chu *et al.*, 1987). Because the precise underlying defect is unknown there is no scientifically rational approach to treatment. When Langerhans cell histiocytosis is limited to one system (most often the skeleton) spontaneous resolution usually occurs and a period of observation is appropriate. If intervention is needed because of persisting symptoms, intralesional corticosteroids are useful. Systemic treatment is required for patients with multisystem involvement. Langerhans cell histiocytosis is responsive to corticosteroids and chemotherapy, the two most active agents being a vinca alkaloid (vinblastine or vincristine) and etoposide. A world-wide study into the treatment of multisystem Langerhans cell histiocytosis is presently being conducted – the 'LCH 1' trial of the International Histiocyte Society started in 1992. All patients receive an initial high dose of steroids, and are then randomized to receive either vinblastine or etoposide. If patients fail on the initial treatment, they are 'crossed over' to the other regimen. The results of 'LCH 1' trial should be available in 1996 or 1997. Other measures may be helpful. Mustine HCl, applied topically, can be very effective for skin disease, and for otitis externa. Gingival infiltration is treated with surgical curettage and diabetes insipidus with DDAVP (a synthetic form of antidiuretic hormone).

The prognosis for patients with single system Langerhans cell histiocytosis is uniformly excellent and progression to multisystem disease is rare, but a few patients develop chronic problems. There is also a tendency for multisystem disease to 'burn out' over 1–5 years but, overall, patients fare less well. Some 10% die acutely (usually from liver or bone marrow failure), 40–50% achieve sustained complete remission and the remaining 40–50% enter a chronic, 'waxing and waning' phase of the disease. Chronic ear discharge, sometimes with conductive hearing loss, occurs in some of these survivors (Smith and Evans, 1984).

Unwanted effects of treatment

The unwanted effects of chemotherapy may be short-lived or may persist and can be grouped into those that are non-specific and the inevitable result of the cytotoxic action of the individual drugs, and those that are specific to one drug or group of drugs. Acute non-specific toxicity usually affects tissues whose component cells replicate rapidly, such as haemopoietic, mucosal and hair follicle cells. Acute bone marrow and immune suppression follows the administration of most types of chemotherapy, and places the patient at risk of bacterial, fungal and viral infections which require aggressive, broad-spectrum antimicrobial therapy. The duration and severity of bone marrow suppression depends on the combination of drugs used and the individual doses. Myelosuppression is usually the dose-limiting factor and has led to the convention of 'pulses' of chemotherapy being administered every 3 weeks. Drugs such as doxorubicin, actinomycin D, etoposide and carboplatin cause damage to the mucosa of the gastrointestinal tract, in particular the mouth and pharynx. Sometimes, pain from mucosal erosion is referred to the ear. Oral toilet is necessary to reduce the risk of superimposed infections.

There are relatively few otolaryngology-related drug-specific side effects. The mixed motor and sensory 'glove and stocking' peripheral neuropathy of vincristine and vinblastine is almost always transient and is usually less severe in children than in adults. Mononeuropathy can sometimes occur producing facial, phrenic or recurrent laryngeal nerve palsies. Jaw pain, sometimes referred to the ear, is another relatively common idiosyncratic side effect of the vinca alkaloids, especially in older children. The onset is usually within 24 hours of administration and the pain may be so severe as to warrant the use of narcotic analgesics. Cisplatin in conventional doses does not produce myelosuppression or mucositis but is associated with dose-dependent nephro- and ototoxicity. Hearing loss is unusual at cumulative doses of less than 300 mg/m^2 and tends to affect high frequencies initially, but extends to lower frequencies with increasing cumulative total dose (Brock *et al.*, 1991). Therefore, regular audiometry and assessment of the glomerular filtration rate is mandatory for patients receiving cisplatin. Carboplatin is much less oto- and nephrotoxic. The alkylating agents (e.g. cyclophosphamide and ifosfamide) produce a dose-dependent reduction in male fertility. Doxorubicin and daunorubicin may cause a dose-dependent cardiomyopathy.

Radiotherapy inevitably causes short-term hair loss in irradiated areas and may induce transient skin inflammation and mucosal erosion. Otitis externa is a common complication requiring treatment with steroid and antibacterial ear drops. In the long term, damage to the salivary glands, thyroid gland or hypothalamic–pituitary axis may produce, respectively, a sicca syndrome, hypothyroidism and varying degrees of hypopituitarism. Chronic otitis media, delayed or arrested tooth development and nasal voice changes may complicate radiotherapy to the head and neck (Jaffe *et al.*, 1984). In addition, radiotherapy causes hypoplasia of the facial bones and surrounding soft tissues, sometimes resulting in distressing facial malformation.

Radiotherapy and cytotoxic drugs can be mutagenic and 'second cancers' have been documented in patients treated with these modalities. Survivors of childhood cancer have a relative risk of developing a second cancer which is six times greater than the expected incidence 25 years after developing the initial cancer (Hawkins, Draper and Kingston, 1987). The commonest chemotherapy-induced second malignancy is acute myeloid leukaemia, and the alkylating agents (e.g. procarbazine and chlorambucil) and etoposide are particularly associated with this complication. The commonest radiation-induced second malignancies are sarcomas, particularly osteosarcomas. Radiotherapy involving the thyroid gland increases the risk of carcinoma arising in that organ. Clearly, the indication for using these therapies should be carefully considered but changes in treatment should not be undertaken should the chance of cure be compromised.

Future prospects

There has been a remarkable improvement in prognosis for children with cancer in the last three decades because of more accurate diagnosis and the use of multiagent chemotherapy in addition to radiotherapy and surgery. Most children with cancer in the 'industrialized' world are treated according to protocols devised by Children's Cancer Study Groups so that the efficacy and toxicity of combinations of treatment can be carefully assessed. It is this attention to detail which has led to major advances in treatment planning. An important thrust in paediatric oncology is to 'stratify' treatment so that more rigorous, and potentially more toxic treatment is only given to children whose cancers show adverse prognostic markers. In this way, alkylating agents with their leukaemogenic potential and risk of infertility in boys may be safely omitted in patients with 'good prognosis' cancer. The current objective of paediatric oncology teams is to achieve 'cure at least cost' rather than 'cure at any cost'. An important reason for the failure of therapy is the acquisition of drug resistance by the tumour. A particular type of multidrug resistance may be reversed by specific agents such as verapamil or cyclosporin (Ozols *et al.*, 1987). Another means of attack against drug resistance is to intensify treatment by giving the treatment over a shorter period of time (Skipper, 1990). In general, there is a tendency towards 'short, sharp' courses rather than protracted maintenance programmes. To this end, the recent use of cytokines such as granulocyte colony stimulating factor (G-CSF) and haemopoietic stem cell rescue to expedite marrow recovery allows greater doses of drugs to be given over shorter periods of time. Such measures may improve response rates in cancers with a high risk of recurrence.

References

ANAVI, Y., KAPLINSKY, C., CALDERON, S. and ZAIZOV, R. (1990) Head, neck and maxillofacial childhood Burkitt's lymphoma. A retrospective analysis of 31 patients. *Journal of Oral and Maxillofacial Surgery*, **48**, 708–713

ANDERSON, G. J., TOM, L. W. C., WOMER, R. B., HANDLER, S. D., WETMORE, R. F. and POTSIC, W. P. (1990) Rhabdomyosarcoma of the head and neck in children. *Archives of Otolaryngology – Head and Neck Surgery*, **116**, 428–431

ANDERSON, J. R., WILSON, F. J., JENKIN, D. T., MEADOWS, A. T., KERSEY, J., CHILCOTE, R. R. et al. (1983) Childhood non-Hodgkin's lymphoma. The results of a randomized therapeutic trial comparing a 4-drug regimen (COMP) with a 10-drug regimen (LSA$_2$-L$_2$). *New England Journal of Medicine*, **308**, 559–565

BACHOUCHI, M., CVIKOVIC, E., AZLI, N., GASMI, J., CORTES–FUNES, H. and BOUSSEN, H. (1990) High complete response in advanced nasopharyngeal carcinoma with bleomycin, epirubicin and cisplatin before radiotherapy. *Journal of the National Cancer Institute*, **82**, 616–620

BARRETT, A., CRENNAN, E., BARNES, J., MARTIN, J. and RADFORD, M. (1990) Treatment of clinical stage I Hodgkin's disease by local radiation therapy alone. A United Kingdom Children Cancer Study Group Study. *Cancer*, **66**, 670–674

BERTHOLD, F. (1990) Overview: biology of neuroblastoma. In: *Neuroblastoma: Tumour Biology and Therapy*, edited by L. Potchedly. Boca Raton, CRC. pp. 1–30

BETTS, P. R. and MCNEISH, A. S. (1972) Oral manifestations of Letter-Siwe disease. *Archives of Disease in Childhood*, **47**, 463–464

BIANCHI, P. M., MARSELLA, P., MASI, R., ANDRIANI, G., TUCCI, F. M., PARTIPILO, P. et al. (1989) Cervical chordoma in childhood: clinical statistical contribution. *International Journal of Pediatric Otorhinolaryngology*, **18**, 39–45

BLOCKER, S., KOENIG, J. and TERNBERG, J. (1987) Congenital fibrosarcoma. *Journal of Paediatric Surgery*, **22**, 665–670

BRADA, M. (1991) Impact of molecular biology on our understanding of non-Hodgkin lymphoma. *European Journal of Cancer*, **28**, 315–320

BRICKMAN, H. F., NOGRADY, M. B. and WIGLESWORTH, F. W. (1973) Scrofula and tracheal obstruction. *American Journal of Respiratory Disease*, **108**, 1208–1211

BROCK, P., BELLMAN, S. C., YEOMANS, E. C., PINKERTON, C. R. and PRICHARD, J. (1991) Cisplatin ototoxicity in children: a practical grading system. *Medical and Pediatric Oncology*, **19**, 295–300

BRODEUR, G. M., PRITCHARD, J., BERTHOLD, F., CARLSEN, N. L., CASTELBERRY, R. P., DEBERNARDI, B. et al. (1993) Revisions of the international criteria for neuroblastoma diagnosis, staging and response to treatment. *Journal of Clinical Oncology*, **11**, 1466–1477

BUCSKY, P., FAVARA, B., FELLER, A. C., NEZELOF, C., RADZUN, H.-J., SCHLEGELBERGER, B. et al. (1994) Malignant histiocytosis and large cell anaplastic (Ki-1) lymphoma in childhood, guidelines for differential diagnosis. *Report of the Histiocyte Society, Medical and Pediatric Oncology*, **2**, 200–203

BURKITT, D. P. (1970) General features of facial tumours. In: *Burkitt's Lymphoma*, edited by D. P. Burkitt and D. H. Wright. Edinburgh: Livingstone. pp. 6–15

CALLENDER, D. L., FRANKENTHALER, R. A., LUNA, M. A., LEE, S. S. and GOEPFERT, H. (1992) Salivary gland neoplasms in children. *Archives of Otolaryngology – Head and Neck Surgery*, **118**, 472–476

CARBONE, P. P., KAPLAN, H. S. and MUSSHOFF, K. (1971) Report of The Committee on Hodgkin's Disease Staging. *Cancer Research*, **31**, 1860–1861

CHRISTIANSEN, H. and LAMPERT, F. (1988), Tumour karyotype discriminates between good and bad prognostic outcome in neuroblastoma. *Cancer*, **57**, 121–126

CHU, T., D'ANGIO, G. J., FAVARA, B., LADISCH, S., NESBIT, M. and PRICHARD, J. (1987) Histiocytosis syndromes in children (letter). *Lancet*, i, 4142

COFFIN, C. M., JASZCZ, W., O'SHEA, P. A. and DEHNER, L. P. (1994) So called congenital-infantile fibrosarcoma: does it exist and what is it? *Paediatric Pathology*, **14**, 133–150

COLEMAN, C. N. (1986) Secondary malignancy after treatment of Hodgkin's disease. An evolving picture. *Journal of Clinical Oncology*, **4**, 821–824

CRAFT, A. and PRITCHARD, J. (1994) Malignant disease. In: *Clinical Biochemistry and the Sick Child*, 2nd edn, edited by B. E. Clayton and J. M. Round. Oxford: Blackwell Scientific Publiciations pp. 425–460

DAHLIN, D. C. (1978) Osteosarcoma of bone and a consideration of prognostic variables. *Cancer Treatment Reports*, **62**, 189–192

DONALDSON, S. S. and LINK, M. P. (1987) Combined modality treatment with low dose radiation and MOPP chemotherapy for children with Hodgkin's disease. *Journal of Clinical Oncology*, **5**, 742–749

DONALDSON, S. S., WHITAKER, S. J., PLOWMAN, N., LINK, M. P. and MALPAS, J. S. (1990) Stage I–II pediatric Hodgkin's disease: long-term follow-up demonstrates equivalent survival rates following different management schemes. *Journal of Clinical Oncology*, **8**, 1128–1137

DULGUEROV, P. and CALCATERRA, T. (1992) Esthesioneuroblastoma: the UCLA experience 1970–1990. *Laryngoscope*, **102**, 843–849

EDEN, O. B., HANN, I., IMESON, H. J., COTTERILL, S., GERRARD, M. and PINKERTON, C. R. (1992) Treatment of advanced stage T cell lymphoblastic lymphoma: results of the United Kingdom Children's Cancer Study Group (UKCCSG) Protocol 8503. *British Journal of Haematology*, **82**, 310–316

ELKON, D., HIGHTOWER, S. J., LIM, M. L., CANTRELL, R. W. and CONSTABLE, W. C. (1979) Esthesioneuroblastoma. *Cancer*, **44**, 1087–1094

FOUCAR, E., ROSAI, J. and DORFMAN, R. F. (1984) Sinus histiocytosis with massive lymphadenopathy. *Cancer*, **54**, 1834–1840

FOWLER, C. L., POKORNY, W. J. and HARBERG, E. J. (1989) Thyroid nodules in children: current profile of a changing disease. *Southern Medical Journal*, **82**, 1472–1478

GOLDSWEIG, H. G. and SUNDARESAN, N. (1990) Chemotherapy of recurrent esthesioneuroblastoma. *American Journal of Clinical Oncology*, **13**, 139–143

GORLIN, J. B. and SALLAN, S. E. (1990) Thyroid cancer in childhood. *Endocrinology and Metabolism Clinics of North America*, **19**, 649–653

GRANT, S., LUTTRELL, B., REEVE, T., WISEMAN, J., WILMHURST, E., STIEL, J. *et al.* (1984) Thyroglobulin may be undetectable in the serum of patients with metastatic disease secondary to differentiated thyroid carcinoma. *Cancer*, **54**, 1625–1628

GREEN, D. M. (1985), *Diagnosis and Management of Malignant Solid Tumours in Children.* Boston: Martinus Nijhoff Publishing. p. 217

GREENBERGER, J. S., CROCKER, A. C., VAWTER, G., JAFFE, N. and CASSIDY, J. R. (1981) Results of treatment of 127 patients with systemic histiocytosis (Letter-Siwe syndrome, Schuller-Christian syndrome and multifocal eosinophilic granuloma). *Medicine*, **60**, 311–338

HAWKINS, E. P., KRISCHER, J. P., SMITH, B. E., HAWKINS, H. K. and FINEGOLD, M. J. (1990) Nasopharyngeal carcinoma in children – a retrospective review and demonstration of Epstein-Barr viral genomes in tumor cell cytoplasm: a report of the Pediatric Oncology Group. *Human Pathology*, **21**, 805–810

HAWKINS, M. M., DRAPER, G. J. and KINGSTON, J. E. (1987) Incidence of second primary tumours amongst childhood cancer survivors *British Journal of Cancer*, **56**, 339–347

HAYASHI, Y., SPITZ, L., KIELY, E., PRICHARD, J. and PINCOTT, J. R. (1989) Fibrous tissue tumours. *Progress in Paediatric Surgery*, **22**, 121–132

HIDAYATALLA, A., MALIK, M. O. A., EL HADI, A. E., OSMAN, A. A. and YUTT, M. S. (1983) Studies on nasopharyngeal carcinoma in the Sudan, I. Epidemiology and aetiology. *European Journal of Cancer and Clinical Oncology*, **19**, 705–710

HO, J. H. C. (1977) Stage classification of nasopharyngeal carcinoma: a review. In *Nasopharyngeal Carcinoma: Etiology and Control*, edited by T. De The and Y. Ito. Lyon: Lyon International Agency for Research in Cancer. pp. 99–113

HO, J. H. C. (1978) An epidemiologic and clinical study of nasopharyngeal carcinoma. *International Journal of Radiation Oncology, Biology and Physics*, **4**, 183–198

INGERSOLL, L., WOO, S. Y., DONALDSON, S., GIESLER, J., MAOR, M. H., GOFFINET, D. *et al.* (1990) Nasopharyngeal carcinoma in the young: A combined M. D. Anderson and Stanford Experience. *International Journal of Radiation Oncology, Biology Physics*, **19**, 881–887

IRVING, R. M., BROADBENT, V. and JONES, N. S. (1994) Langerhans cell histiocytosis of childhood, management of head and neck manifestations. *Laryngoscope*, **104**, 64–70

JAFFE, B. F. (1973) Pediatric head and neck tumours. A study of 178 cases. *Laryngoscope*, **83**, 1644–1651

JAFFE, N., TOTH, B. B., HOAR, R. E., RIED, H. L., SULLIVAN, M. P., MCNEESE, M. D. *et al.* (1984) Dental and maxillofacial abnormalities in longterm survivors of childhood cancer: effects of treatment with chemotherapy and radiation of the head and neck. *Pediatrics*, **73**, 816–823

JENKIN, R. D. T., ANDERSON, J. R., JEREB, B., THOMPSON, J. C., PYESMANY, A., WARA, W. M. *et al.* (1981) Nasopharyngeal carcinoma – a retrospective review of patients less than thirty years of age. *Cancer*, **47**, 360–366

JORDAN, R. B. and GAUDERER, M. W. L. (1988) Cervical teratomas: an analysis. Literature review and proposed classification. *Journal of Pediatric Surgery*, **23**, 583–591

KADISH, S., GOODMAN, M. and WANG, C. C. (1976) Olfactory neuroblastoma, a clinical analysis of 17 cases. *Cancer*, **37**, 1571–1576

KAHN, M. A. (1989) Ameloblastoma in young persons: a clinicopathologic analysis and etiologic investigation. *Oral Surgery, Oral Medicine and Oral Pathology*, **67**, 706–715

KANNOURAKIS, G. and ABBAS, A. (1994) The role of cytokines in the pathogenesis of Langerhans cell histiocytosis. *British Journal of Cancer*, **70**, 337–340

KATO, M. A. D. P., FLAMANT, F., TERRIER-LACOMBE, M. J., HABRAND, J. L., SCHWAAB, G., LUBOINSKI, B. *et al.* (1991) Rhabdomyosarcoma of the larynx in children: a series of five patients treated in the Institut Gustave Roussy (Villejuif, France). *Medical and Pediatric Oncology*, **19**, 110–114

KILMAN, J. W., CLATWORTHY, H. W., NEWTON, W. A. and GROSFELD, J. W. (1973) Reasonable surgery for rhabdomyosarcoma: a study of 67 cases. *Annals of Surgery*, **178**, 346–351

KROLLS, S. O., TRODAHL, J. N. and BOYERS, R. C. (1972) Salivary gland lesions in children. *Cancer*, **30**, 459–469

KYNASTON, J. A., MALCOLM, A. J., CRAFT, A. W., DAVIES, S. M., JONES, P. H., KING, D. J. *et al.* (1993) Chemotherapy in the management of infantile fibrosarcoma. *Medical and Pediatric Oncology*, **21**, 488–493

LANCET (1992) Editorial: Ewing's sarcoma and its congeners: an interim appraisal. ii, 99–100

LANGMAN, A. W., KAPLAN, M. J. and MATTHAY, K. (1989) Ewing's sarcoma of the mandible. *Otolaryngology, Head and Neck Surgery*, **100**, 74–77

LEDERMAN, M. and MOULD, R. F. (1968) Radiation treatment of cancer of the pharynx: with special reference to telecobalt therapy. *British Journal of Radiology*, **41**, 251–274

LEE, S. and MACKENZIE, D. (1964) Osteosarcoma: a study of the value of preoperative megavoltage radiotherapy, *British Journal of Surgery*, **51**, 252–274

LINK, M. P., GOORIN, A. M., MISER, A. W., GREEN, A. A., PRATT, C. B., BELLASCO, J. B. *et al.* (1986) The effect of adjuvant chemotherapy on relapse-free survival in patients with osteosarcoma of the extremity. *New England Journal Medicine*, **314**, 1600–1606

LUNA, M. A., BATSAKIS, J. G. and EL-NAGGAR, A. K. (1991) Pathology consultation: salivary gland tumours in children. *Annals of Otology, Rhinology and Laryngology*, **100**, 869–871

MCWHIRTER, W. R., STILLER, C. A. and LENNOX, E. L. (1989) Carcinomas in childhood, a registry-based study of incidence and survival. *Cancer*, **63**, 2242–2246

MALONE, B. and BAKER, S. R. (1984) Benign pleomorphic adenomas in children. *Annals of Otology, Rhinology and Laryngology*, **93**, 210–214

MAMEDE, R. M., MELLO, F. V. and BARBIERI, J. (1990) Prognosis of Ewing's sarcoma of the head and neck. *Otolaryngology, Head and Neck Surgery*, **109**, 650–653

MANLEY, S. M., BARRETT, A., MARTIN, J. and RADFORD, M. (1993) Hodgkin's disease stage IV: results from UK Multicentre Study. *Medical and Paediatric Oncology*, **21**, 546 (abstract)

MANN, J. R., PEARSON, D., BARRETT, A., RAAFAT, R., BARNES, J. M. and WALLENDSZUS, K. R. (1989) Results of the United Kingdom Children's Cancer Study Group's malignant germ cell tumour studies. *Cancer*, **63**, 1657–1667

MARK, R. J., SERCARZ, J. A., TRAN, L., DODD, L. G., SELCH, M. and CALCATERRA, T. C. (1991) Osteogenic sarcoma of the head and neck, *Archives of Otolaryngology – Head and Neck Surgery*, **117**, 761–766

MATTHAY, K. K., SATHER, H. N., SEEGER, R. C., HAASE, G. M. and HAMMOND, G. D. (1989) Excellent outcome of stage II neuroblastoma is independent of residual disease and radiation therapy. *Journal of Clinical Oncology*, **7**, 236–244

MAURER, H. M., GEHAN, E. A., BELTANGADY, M., CRIST, W., DICKMAN, P. S., DONALDSON, S. S. *et al.* (1992) The Intergroup Rhabdomyosarcoma Study-II. *Cancer*, **71**, 1904–1922

MAZZAFERRI, E. L., YOUNG, R. L. and OERTEL, J. E. (1977) Papillary thyroid carcinoma: the impact of therapy in 576 patients. *Medicine (Baltimore)*, **56**, 171–196

MEHTA, M. P., GOETOWSKI, P. G. and KINSELLA, T. J. (1989)

Radiation induced thyroid neoplasms 1920 to 1987: a vanishing problem? *Journal of Radiation Oncology, Biology and Physics* **16**, 1471–1475

MILLS, S. E. and FRIERSON, H. F. (1985) Olfactory neuroblastoma: a clinicopathologic study of 21 cases. *American Journal of Surgical Pathology*, **9**, 317–327

MITCHELL, A., SCHEITHAUER, B. W., UNNI, K. K., FORSYTH, P. J., WOLD, L. E. and MCGIVNEY, D. J. (1993) Chordoma and chondroid neoplasms of the spheno-occiput; an immunohistochemical study of 41 cases with prognostic and nosologic implications. *Cancer*, **72**, 2943–2949

MOTT, M. G., EDEN, O. B. and PALMER, M. K. (1984) Adjuvant low dose radiation in childhood non-Hodgkin's lymphoma (Report from UK CCSG). *British Journal of Cancer*, **50**, 463–469

MURPHY, S. B. (1980) Classification, staging and end results of treatment of childhood non-Hodgkin's lymphoma: dissimilarities from lymphomas in adults. *Seminars in Oncology*, **7**, 332–339

MURPHY, S. B. and HUSTU, H. O. (1980) A randomised trial of combined modality therapy of childhood non-Hodgkins lymphoma. *Cancer*, **45**, 630–637

NADAL, D., CADUFF, R., FREY, E., HASSAM, S., ZIMMERMANN, E. R., SEIGNEURIN, J.-M. *et al.* (1994) Non-Hodgkin's lymphoma in four children infected with the human immunodeficiency virus: association with Epstein-Barr virus and treatment. *Cancer*, **73**, 224–230

NAEGELE, R. F., CHAMPION, J., MURPHY, S., HENLE, G. and HENLE, W. (1982) Nasopharyngeal carcinoma in American children, Epstein-Barr virus specific antibody titers and prognosis. *International Journal of Cancer*, **29**, 209–212

NEZELOF, C. (1979) Histiocytosis X: a histological and histogenetic study. *Pediatric Pathology*, **5**, 153–157

NIKIFOROV, Y. and GNEPP, D. R. (1994) Pediatric thyroid cancer after the Chernobyl disaster. Pathomorphologic study of 84 cases (1991–1992) from the Republic of Belarus. *Cancer*, **74**, 748–766

O'CONNELL, J. X., RENARD, L. G., LIEBSCH, N. J., EFIRD, T., MUNZENRIDER, J. E. and ROSENBERG, A. E. (1994) Base of skull chordoma: a correlative study of histologic and clinical features of 62 cases. *Cancer*, **74**, 2261–2267

ORTON, P. (1994) Shared care. *Lancet*, ii, 1413–1415

OZOLS, R. F., CUNNION, R. E., KLECKER, R. W., HAMILTON, T. C., OSTCHEGA, Y., PARRILLO, J. E. *et al.* (1987) Verapamil and Adriamycin in the treatment of drug-resistant ovarian cancer patients. *Journal of Clinical Oncology*, **5**, 641–647

PAO, W. J., HUSTU, H. O., DOUGLAS, E. C., BECKFORD, N. S. and KUN, L. E. (1989) Pediatric nasopharyngeal carcinoma: long-term follow-up of 29 patients. *International Journal of Radiation Oncology, Biology and Physics*, **17**, 299–305

PATTE, W. J., LEVERGER, G. and PEREL, Y. (1990) Updated results of the LMB86 protocol for the French Paediatric Oncology Society (SFOP) for B-cell non-Hodgkin's lymphoma (B-MHL) with CNS involvement (CNS +) and B-ALL. *Medical and Pediatric Oncology*, **18**, 397–403

PATTE, C., PHILIP, T., RODARY, C., ZUCKER, J.-M., BEHRENDT, H., GENTEL, J.-C. *et al.* (1991) High survival rate in advanced-stage B-cell lymphomas and leukemias without CNS involvement with a short intensive polychemotherapy: results from the French Pediatric Oncology Society of a randomized trial of 216 children. *Journal of Clinical Oncology*, **9**, 123–132

POCHIN, E. E. (1967) Prospects for the treatment of thyroid

carcinoma with radio-iodine. *Clinical Radiology*, **18**, 113–135

RADFORD, M., MARTIN, J., BARRETT, M. A., COTTERILL, S. and IMESON, J. (1993) Treatment of stage I Hodgkin's disease in children: report for the United Kingdom Children's Cancer Study Group. *Medical and Paediatric Oncology*, **21**, 543 (abstract)

RANEY, B., EVANS, A., GRANOWEITER, L., SCHAUFFER, L., URI, A. and LITTMAN, P. (1987) Nonsurgical management of children with recurrent unresectable fibromatosis. *Pediatrics*, **79**, 394–398

RAPIDIS, A. D., ECONOMIDIS, J., GOUMAS, P.D., LANGDON, J.D., SKORDALAKIS, A., TZORTZATOU, F. *et al.* (1988) Tumours of the head and neck in children: a clinico-pathological analysis of 1007 cases. *Journal of Cranio-Maxillo-Facial Surgery*, **16**, 279–286

REITER, A., SCHRAPPE, M., TIEMANN, M., PARWARESCH R., ZIMMERMANN, M., YAKISON, E. *et al.* (1994) Successful treatment strategy for Ki-1 anaplastic large-cell lymphoma of childhood: a prospective analysis of 62 patients enrolled in three consecutive Berlin-Frankfurt-Munster Group studies. *Journal of Clinical Oncology*, **12**, 899–908

ROBINSON, L. D., SMITH, R. J. H., RIGHTMIRE, J., TORPHY, J. M. and FERNBACH, D. J. (1988) Head and neck malignancies in children: an age-incidence study. *Laryngoscope*, **98**, 11–13

ROSAI, J. and DORFMAN, R. F. (1972) Sinus histiocytosis with massive lymphadenopathy: a pseudolymphomatous benign disorder. *Cancer*, **30**, 1174–1188

RUBIE, H., GLADIEFF, L., ROBERT, A., GAUBERT, I., HUGUET, F., ROCHAIX, P. *et al.* (1994) Childhood anaplastic large cell lymphoma Ki-1/CD30: clinicopathologic features of 19 cases. *Medical and Paediatric Oncology*, **22**, 155–161

SCHELLONG, G., HORNIG, I., BRAMSWIG, J. H., SCHWARZE, E. W. and WANNEMACHER, M. (1987) Favourable outcome of childhood stage IV Hodgkin's disease with Oppa/Copp chemotherapy and additional radiotherapy. *Medical and Paediatric Oncology*, **15**, 325 (abstract)

SCHMIDT, D., HERRMANN, C., JURGENS, H and HARMS, D. (1991) Malignant peripheral neuroectodermal tumor and its necessary distinction from Ewing's sarcoma: a report from the Kiel Pediatric Tumor Registry. *Cancer*, **68**, 2251–2259

SCHOFIELD, D. E., FLETCHER, J. A., GRIER, H.E. and YUNIS, E. J. (1994) Fibrosarcoma in children and infants. Application of new techniques. *American Journal of Surgical Pathology*, **18**, 14–24

SEEGER, R. C., BRODEUR, G. M., SATHER, H., DALTON, A., SIEGEL, S. E., WONG, K. Y. *et al.* (1985) Association of multiple copies of the N-myc oncogene with rapid progression of neuroblastomas. *New England Journal of Medicine*, **313**, 1111–1116

SEHDEV, M. K., HUVOS, A. G., STRONG, E. W., GEROLD, F. P. and WILLIS, G. W. (1974) Ameloblastoma of maxilla and mandible. *Cancer*, **33**, 324–333

SEIFERT, G., OKABE, H. and CASELITZ, J. (1986) Epithelial salivary gland tumors in children and adolescents: analysis of 80 cases (Salivary Gland Register 1965–1984). *ORL*, **48**, 137–149

SHANMUGARATNAM, K. and SABIN, L. (1978) *Histological Typing of Upper Respiratory Tract Tumours*. Geneva: World Health Organization, **19**, 32–33

SHAPIRO, D. N., SUBLETT, J. E., LI, B., DOWNING, J. R. and NAEVE, C. W. (1993) Fusion of PAX3 to a member of the forkhead family of transcription factors in human alveolar rhabdomyosarcoma. *Cancer Research*, **53**, 5108–5112

SILBERMAN, R. and MENDELSON, I. R. (1960) Teratomas of the neck. *Archives of Disease of Childhood*, **35**, 159–170

SKIPPER, H. E. (1990) Dose intensity versus total dose of chemotherapy: an experimental basis. In: *Important Advances in Oncology 1990*, edited by V. T. DeVita, S. Hellman and S. A. Rosenberg. Philadelphia: J. B. Lippincott. pp. 43–64

SMITH, R. J. H. and EVANS, J. N. G. (1984) Head and neck manifestations of histiocytosis X. *Laryngoscope*, **94**, 395–399

SMITH, R. J. H. and KATZ, C. D. (1990) Neuroblastoma of the head and neck. In: *Neuroblastoma: Tumour Biology and Therapy*, edited by C. Pochedly. Boca Raton: CRC Press. pp. 245–276

STEVENS, M., OBERLIN, O., FLAMANT, F., REY, A. and PRAQUIN, M.-T. (1993) SIOP MMT 89 protocol for non-metastatic rhabdomyosarcoma – an update. *Medical and Paediatric Oncology*, **21**, 554 (abstract)

TAXY, J. B., BHARANI, N. K., MILLS, S. E., FRIERSON, H. F. and GOULD, V. E. (1986) The specturm of olfactory neural tumors: a light-microscopic immunohistochemical and ultrastructural analysis. *American Journal of Surgical Pathology*, **10**, 687–695

TAYLOR, C., PATEL, K., JONES, T., KIELY, F., DE STAVOLA, B. L. and SHEER, D. (1993) Diagnosis of Ewing's sarcoma and peripheral neuroectodermal tumour based on the detection of t(11;22) using fluorescence in situ hybridisation. *British Journal of Cancer*, **67**, 128–133

TOM, L. W. C., ANDERSON, G. J., WOMER, R. B., WETMORE, R. E., HANDLER, S. D., POTSIC, W. P. *et al.* (1992) Nasopharyngeal malignancies in children. *Laryngoscope*, **102**, 509–514

TORSIGLIERI, A. J., TOM, L. W. C., ROSS, A. J. III, WETMORE, R. F., HANDLER, S. D. and POTSIC, W. P. (1988) Pediatric neck masses: guidelines for evaluation. *International Journal of Pediatric Otorhinolaryngology*, **16**, 199–210

TUBIANA, M., SCHLUNBERGER, M. and ROUGIER, P. (1985) Long-term results and prognostic factors in patients with differentiated thyroid carcinoma. *Cancer*, **55**, 794–804

VASSILOPOULOU-SELLIN, R., KLEIN, M. J., SMITH, T. H., SAMAAN, N. A., FRANKENTHALER, R. A., GOEPFERT, H. *et al.* (1993) Pulmonary metastases in children and young adults with differentiated thyroid cancer. *Cancer*, **71**, 1348–1352

VENOOK, A. P., TSENG, A. JR, MEYERS, F. J., SILVERBER, I., BOLES, R., FU, K. K. *et al.* (1987) Cisplatin, doxorubicin, and 5-fluorouracil chemotherapy for salivary gland malignancies: a pilot study of the Northern California Oncology Group. *Journal of Clinical Oncology*, **5**, 951–955

WHANG-PENG, J., FRETER, C. E., KNUTSEN, T., NANFRO, J. J. and GAZDAR, A. (1987) Translocation t(11;22) in esthesioneuroblastoma. *Cancer Genetics and Cytogenetics*, **29**, 155–157

WILLMAN, C. L., BUSQUE, L., GRIFFITH, B. G., FAVARA, B. E., MCCLAIN, K. L., DUNCAN, M. H. *et al.* (1994) Langerhans cell histiocytosis (histiocytosis X) – a clonal proliferative disease. *New England Journal of Medicine*, **331**, 154–160

WINKLER, K., BIELACK, S., DELLING, G., SALZER-KUNTSCHIK, M., KOTZ, R., GREENSHAW, C. *et al.* (1990) Effect of intraarterial versus intravenous cisplatin in addition to systemic doxorubicin, high-dose methotrexate, and ifosfamide on histologic tumor response in osteosarcoma, (Study COSS-86). *Cancer*, **66**, 1703–1710

WISWELL, T. E., DAVIS, J., CUNNINGHAM, B. E., SOLENBERGER, R. and THOMAS, P. J. (1988) Infantile neurofibromatosis: the most common fibrous tumour or infancy. *Journal of Paediatric Surgery*, **23**, 315–318

WOLF, J. and DIEHL, V. (1994) Is Hodgkin's disease an infectious disease? *Annals of Oncology*, **5**, 105–111

ZIMMERMAN, D., HAY, I. D., GOUGH, I. R., GOELLNER, J. R.,

RYAN, J. J., GRANT, C. S. *et al.* (1988) Papillary thyroid carcinoma in children and adults: long-term follow-up of 1039 patients conservatively treated at one institution during three decades. *Surgery*, **104**, 1157–1166

32

Salivary gland disorders in children

P. J. Bradley

Embryology

Both the major (parotid and submandibular) and minor salivary glands are derivatives of ectoderm. During their development they pierce the surrounding mesenchyme and arborize, before terminating as multiple acini. The proximal portion of the original primordium becomes the gland's main duct. The surrounding mesenchyme divides each gland into lobules and envelops it to form a capsule. The minor salivary glands are distributed over the entire oral cavity except on the alveolus of the jaws and the rosteromedial portion of the hard palate. Between the fourth to the sixth week (or the 10 mm stage) of embryonic life, the parotid is the first major salivary gland to develop as an epithelial ingrowth near the angle of the mouth on the inner surface of the cheek. As it grows rapidly backwards towards the ramus of the mandible it becomes a hollowed tube and, at this level, branches extensively into primordial ducts and acinar cells.

Although the parotid anlage is the first to appear, the mesenchyme surrounding the submandibular and sublingual glands condenses first, allowing them to become organized into solid and encapsulated organs. Condensation of the mesenchyme occurs later in embryonic life and, as a result, lymph nodes may become entrapped in the parotid gland. On the other hand, salivary gland tissue has also been found in lymph nodes in the submandibular triangle. These glandular elements have been known to undergo neoplastic change, with salivary gland tumours arising in a lymph node. Sebaceous gland elements are also found in the parotid gland, and are believed to originate from blind ending intercalated and striated ducts. The formation of the acinar epithelia is not considered the final stage of differentiation, as replacement and regeneration of acinar cells may occur from pre-existing acini and other cells of ductal origin. The origin of the myoepithelial cells is still not known.

The submandibular gland begins its development late in the sixth week as paired primordia arising near the midline under the tongue. They grow back along the floor of the mouth towards the angle of the mandible, turning inferiorly and superficially posterior and lateral to the mylohyoid muscle. Here the primordia begin to branch freely to form the body of the gland.

The sublingual glands arise in the eighth week of development as an independent row of small glands with individual ducts. The secretory portions of the gland are confluent with each other in a common connective tissue capsule. They originate as 10–20 primordia from the floor of the mouth under the tongue, but are arranged laterally along the course of the submandibular primordia (Johns, 1977).

Anatomy

The knowledge of the detailed anatomy of the major salivary glands is essential for the physician to understand the modes of presentation of salivary gland disease and also to be able to perform surgical procedures when indicated. The cranial nerves, facial nerve and its branches, lingual and hypoglossal nerves, are intimately related to these glands in a similar fashion to that found in the adult, and if damaged will produce considerable disability, both cosmetic and functional. However, the facial nerve needs to be considered in more detail when parotid gland surgery is contemplated in the young child. At birth the mastoid process is absent and the tympanic ring is narrow. In the newborn the facial nerve lies just under the skin as it exits the temporal bone and is therefore vulnerable to injury. The nerve assumes a deeper and more protected position between 2 and 4 years of age as the tympanic ring enlarges and the mastoid process forms (May, 1986).

Evaluation

Evaluation of salivary gland disorders in children should begin with a thorough history and physical examination. Specific points that need to be elicited include the onset and duration of symptoms, their periodicity, the presence or absence of swellings, and the character of the salivary secretions. The presence of systemic disease should be thoroughly investigated. The spectrum of salivary pathology, especially in the parotid gland, is similar to that encountered in the adult. In childhood inflammatory processes predominate and within this group those with a non-obstructive aetiology are more prevalent. Additionally, systemic disease may initially present as parotid gland enlargement and this should always be remembered.

Physical examination

Bimanual examination, as well as examination of any masses or swellings located in the anatomical area, is useful in the evaluation of salivary gland diseases in children. This procedure should consist of simultaneous palpation of the salivary structures intraorally and extraorally. It may be difficult to differentiate between a salivary gland enlargement and cervical adenopathy. The normal parotid gland cannot be demarcated by palpation, and therefore a localized swelling is usually of clinical importance. Cervical adenopathy is frequently preceded by a history of

fever, upper respiratory tract infection or dental treatment. In general, discrete, but multiple, lymph nodes in both sides of the neck may be involved. Massage of the normal parotid gland often produces a clear saliva flow from the opening of Stensen's duct. Any variation from the normal, e.g. a swollen puncta, particulate, mucoid or purulent secretions, should be noted and recorded. Abnormal salivary secretions should be further evaluated, both microscopically and also by culture and sensitivity testing. The disease process may be of a chronic nature and the patient may need to be re-examined frequently to ascertain the natural history of the disease process.

Three distinct observations need to be made when undertaking a physical examination of the parotid or submandibular glands:

1 Is the entire gland enlarged or just part of it?
2 If a part, is the mass in or adjacent to the gland?
3 If in the gland, is the mass solid or cystic in nature?

In addition one needs to note the associated signs of tenderness, facial nerve weakness, skin involvement, or fixity of the mass to surrounding structures.

Algorithms aid in the differentiation and management of salivary gland disorders in children. The pathological conditions encountered in the parotid gland can be divided into unilateral discrete, unilateral diffuse and bilateral diffuse conditions and separated into neoplastic and non-neoplastic disorders (Figures 32.1, 32.2 and 32.3).

Examination of the saliva

Three examinations can be performed – culture, cytology and sialochemistry. The validity of the culture

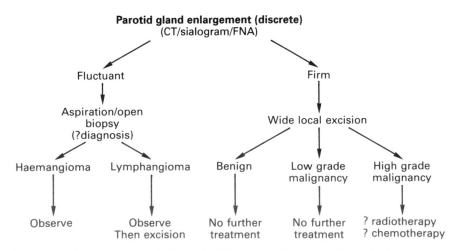

Figure 32.1 Algorithm for the management of salivary gland disorders – discrete parotid gland enlargement – in children

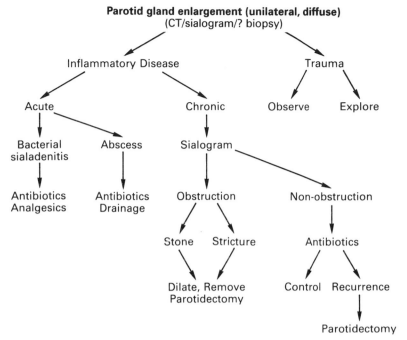

Figure 32.2 Algorithm for the management of salivary gland disorders – unilateral, diffuse parotid gland enlargement – in children

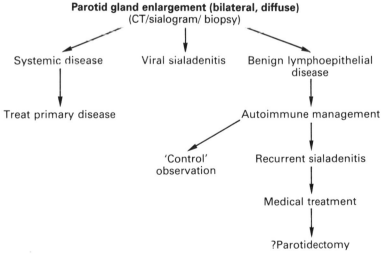

Figure 32.3 Algorithm for the management of salivary gland disorders – bilateral, diffuse parotid gland enlargement – in children

data is greatest when the specimen is carefully obtained. Ideally needle aspiration for culture (after careful skin preparation) or intraductal aspiration via a catheter should be attempted. Cultures obtained by simple swabbing of the duct opening usually grow mixed flora and result in misleading information. Cytology may be performed on saliva expressed or collected. Cells may also be obtained by fine needle aspiration. Sialochemistry is of little use in the evaluation of paediatric salivary gland disorders.

Radiological examination: diagnostic imaging

A variety of diagnostic imaging techniques is available for the investigation of salivary gland disorders. In the main these techniques are used to investigate the parotid and submandibular glands. Sialography of the sublingual glands can be performed but is usually unhelpful. Plain X-ray views are usually unhelpful unless the disorder is dental in origin or to detect a radiopaque calculus (see later). Sialography may be used to evaluate the presence of calculi, obstructive disease, inflammatory lesions, assessment of salivary (parotid) gland trauma and discrete swellings. This procedure may be carried out in the youngest of patients with minimal sedation if gently performed. Discomfort is generally slight and post-injection swelling short lived. The emptying time of the ductal system should be recorded. Sialography is best considered for studying the ductal system and glandular pattern.

Ultrasound is often able to distinguish intrinsic from extrinsic masses. This investigation is also helpful when inflammatory lesions are suspected. Ultrasound may also be useful to guide needle drainage of an abscess or in retrieving cells for cytology.

Computerized tomography (CT scan) is the study of choice currently for evaluating intrinsic and extrinsic parotid masses. CT scans, however, are not a substitute for histological diagnosis. The general appearance of the mass often gives considerable insight into its histological type – benign lesions are generally sharply circumscribed, whereas inflammatory and malignant lesions are often irregular, and infiltrative.

Magnetic resonance imaging (MRI scan) gives excellent soft tissue definition and is currently the imaging technique of choice in the evaluation of salivary gland swellings and lumps. Advantages of this technique include its ability to provide coronal, axial and sagittal views, as well as avoiding radiation exposure.

Acute suppurative parotitis

Acute suppurative parotitis may originate from a septic focus in the oral cavity, such as chronic tonsillitis or dental infection, which may suppress salivary secretions. The mode of transmission of the organism into the parotid gland may be due to a combination of factors, usually following decreased secretory function associated with dehydration and sepsis. Another possible mode of spread of organisms is through a transitory bacteraemia. Reduced salivary flow may also allow the ascent of any indigenous bacterial flora up Stensen's duct thereby triggering acute suppurative parotitis.

Staphylococcus aureus is the most common pathogen associated with acute parotitis, however streptococci (including *Streptococcus pneumoniae*) and Gram-negative bacilli (including *Escherichia coli*) have also been reported. The true incidence of anaerobic bacteria in suppurative parotitis has not been determined because most studies did not employ proper techniques to obtain culture material nor were the bacteria, when identified, considered to be pathogenic (Brook, 1992).

Parotitis is typically characterized by swelling of the gland, mainly at the angle of the jaw. Acute suppurative parotitis develops suddenly with induration and a warm erythematous swelling of the cheek. Bacterial parotitis is usually unilateral, the gland becomes swollen and extremely tender and the patient is frequently toxic, with marked fever. The mouth of the parotid duct is red and pouting, and pus may be seen exuding or may be expressed by gentle pressure on the parotid gland and duct. Because of the dense fibrous capsule of the gland, pus rarely points extraorally in the early stage of suppuration. The infection may extend locally, by rupture of the abscess, into the surrounding tissues, possibly causing septic arthritis of the temporomandibular joint or osteomyelitis of the mandible (Figure 32.4) or into the face or ear, or even down the fascial plane to the mediastinum. Examination of the pus from the parotid gland and the performance of Gram staining may support the diagnosis of suppurative infection. Specimens for anaerobic culture should not be obtained from around Stensen's duct because oropharyngeal contamination is certain. Needle aspiration of the parotid gland may allow better recovery of the causative organism. However, if no pus is obtained, introduction of sterile saline solution by needle and subsequent aspiration may yield the causative organism. Ultrasonography examination may help to localize areas where pus has accumulated. If no pus is obtained repeated aspiration may need to be performed at a later stage. The aspirated material should be cultured for aerobic as well anaerobic bacteria, fungi and mycobacteria. Surgical exploration and drainage may be indicated for diagnosis as well as for therapeutic reasons (Figure 32.5). If infection is not found, a search should be made for non-infective causes of parotid swellings.

Maintenance of adequate hydration and the administration of parenteral antimicrobial therapy are essential elements in the management of suppurative parotitis. The specific choice of antibiotic depends on the causal agent. A penicillinase-resistant penicillin or a cephalosporin is generally adequate. However, the presence of methicillin-resistant staphylococci (MRSA), mainly found in patients who have been in hospital for a long time, may mandate the use of vancomycin hydrochloride. Clindamycin hydrochloride, cefoxitin sodium, a combination of metronidazole and the macrolide imipenem, or a penicillin plus β-lactamase inhibitor will provide adequate coverage

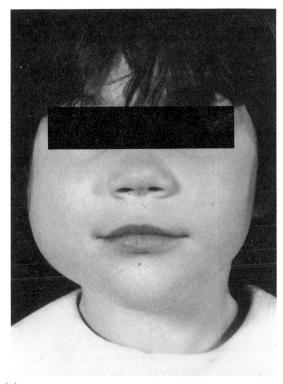

(a)

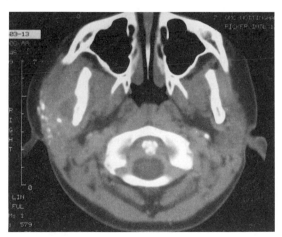

(b)

Figure 32.4 (*a*) Child with osteomyelitis of the mandible. (*b*) CT/sialogram of osteomyelitis of the right mandible with abscess

for anaerobic as well as aerobic bacteria. Empiric antimicrobial therapy before identification of organisms may be required. Following isolation of the causative organism and performance of antibiotic sensitivity testing, therapy may be adjusted accordingly (Brook, 1992).

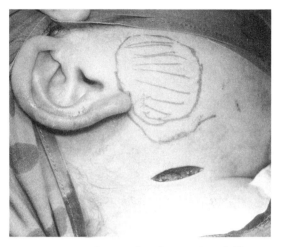

Figure 32.5 Surgical approach to drainage in a child

Non-tuberculous mycobacterial infections

Infection with non-tuberculous mycobacteria such as *Mycobacterium avium*, *Mycobacterium intracellulare*, *Mycobacterium scrofulaceum* and related organisms (MAIS complex) usually presents with cervical lymphadenitis in childhood. The diagnosis is established either by culture of the mycobacterium responsible from the affected lymph node or, where the culture is negative, by typical histological features and a positive intradermal skin test using non-tuberculous mycobacterial antigens in children, in whom skin testing with tuberculin PPD was negative.

This infection is most commonly seen in children between the ages of 2 and 5 years (Figure 32.6). The

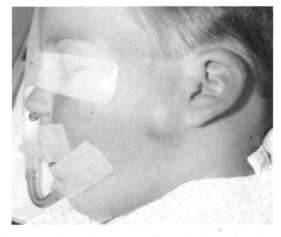

Figure 32.6 Parotid mass caused by atypical mycobacteria

fact that the lymph nodes involved are virtually all in the head and neck region supports the theory that the mouth or pharynx is the portal of entry (Pransky *et al.*, 1990).

Surgical excision of the involved lymph nodes is indicated and is necessary to eradicate the disease. Technical difficulties may arise in two situations. A discharging sinus forms when the disease has reached an advanced clinical stage with liquefaction and caseation in the infected lymph nodes. Complete excision in the presence of a discharging sinus is often impossible, but the alternative of curettage is associated with a higher rate of recurrence. The second difficulty arises when a lymph node involves the parotid area, where meticulous dissection, using a nerve stimulator, may be necessary to avoid damage to the facial nerve.

The term 'recurrence' lacks an accepted definition because of the difficulties in distinguishing true recurrence from reinfection. The overall recurrence rate is approximately 8% in children followed up for 6 months or more after excision biopsy.

This infective process is a clinically recognizable disorder in a population in which tuberculous lymph node infection is rare. Other organ involvement in non-tuberculous mycobacteria is extremely rare in otherwise healthy individuals, though it has been reported in immune compromised children. Delay in diagnosis, and therefore treatment, leads to recurrence of disease and undesirable scarring. Early diagnosis and adequate surgical resection is necessary to prevent long-term morbidity (Joshi *et al.*, 1989).

Acute non-suppurative parotitis

The most common cause of parotid swelling in childhood is epidemic mumps caused by paramyxovirus. Since the introduction of mumps vaccination the frequency of viral mumps has significantly decreased in the immunized population. Other viral agents associated with parotid infection are the enteroviruses such as coxsackie A, Epstein-Barr, influenza A, lymphocytic choriomeningitis and parainfluenza A. The viral agents may account for the occurrence of sporadic cases of viral parotitis and may explain the occurrence of multiple attacks of parotitis in the same individual.

Viral parotitis may involve the other salivary glands and the soft tissues, leading to facial swelling that can extend to the chest walls. Viral parotitis should be differentiated from acute suppurative parotitis because it is endemic and produces no pus. It should also be diagnosed and recognized as separate from other causes of parotid swellings. Mumps, as well as the other viral infections, can be diagnosed generally by a rising titre during serological examination. The serum amylase level is said to be elevated in up to 90% of patients with mumps, and may be useful in distinguishing parotitis from cervical adenitis or other masses in the neck. However, elevation of the serum amylase level is not specific for viral parotitis.

Specific viral parotitis (mumps)

Mumps is an acute, contagious illness that usually causes fever and painful non-purulent inflammation of the parotid glands. In many cases other organ systems involvement occurs such as meningoencephalitis, orchitis, pancreatitis or deafness. The cause is usually the mumps virus (paramyxovirus), however viruses such echovirus, coxsackie A and others have been implicated occasionally (Zollar and Mufson, 1970).

There is an 18–21 day incubation period and a 1–3 day prodromal period of malaise, fever and discomfort over the angle of one or both jaws prior to the development of parotitis. During the next 24–48 hours one or both parotid glands becomes tender and swollen, often with surrounding jelly-like neck oedema. The ear lobe may be displaced laterally and the smooth line of the jaw is lost. The parotid duct orifice is inflamed, but if pus exudes from it the diagnosis of septic parotitis and not mumps should be made. The acute infection subsides in 72 hours though the salivary gland swelling may persist for 7–10 days. In some cases the parotitis may be absent, in others all four major salivary glands may become acutely enlarged and rarely only one submandibular gland may be affected. This clinical picture has changed significantly since the introduction of the mumps vaccine. The peak incidence of mumps occurs in the 4–6-year-old age group. The diagnosis is made by demonstrating antibodies to the mumps S and V antigen and to the haemagglutination antigen. Studies have shown that more than 95% of adults have neutralizing antibodies. The diagnosis may also be made by isolating the virus from urine, this can be performed up to 6 days before and 13 days after the salivary gland symptoms appear. Approximately 40% of attacks are subclinical. Mumps meningitis is common, but carries a good prognosis. Cerebrospinal fluid (CSF) lymphocytosis occurs in approximately 65% of affected patients but many do not show any symptoms. Management of mumps consists of good oral hygiene. If the infection is associated with a history of fits, the temperature should be lowered by tepid sponging and antipyretics such as paracetamol (but not aspirin).

Mumps is spread by aerosol droplets from the saliva and nasopharyngeal secretions of an infected individual and spreads easily in highly populated urban areas. In unvaccinated communities, epidemics occur approximately every 3–4 years. Apart from isolation of an index case, little can be done to prevent the spread of a mumps outbreak. Neither normal human immunoglobulin nor high titre mumps immunoglobulin is recommended. One attack confirms lifelong immunity. Mumps during pregnancy occasionally causes fetal endocardial fibroelastosis, or if contracted in the first trimester, abortion may occur. Termination of pregnancy is not usually recommended. Protective amounts of antibody cross the placenta so that an infant whose mother has already had mumps is unlikely to develop the disease in the first 6–9 months of life.

In the USA the incidence of mumps has fallen by 90% following the introduction of a live attenuated vaccine in 1967. In the UK measles, mumps and rubella (MMR) vaccine has had an uptake of 88% since its introduction in 1988, resulting in the interruption of the 3-year epidemic cycle and has resulted in significant lowering of the incidence of mumps (Jones, White and Begg, 1991).

Juvenile recurrent parotitis

Recurrent parotitis in children is rare, but next to specific viral parotitis (mumps) it is the most common inflammatory salivary gland disease of childhood. The condition is characterized by periodic acute or subacute swellings of the parotid gland, usually associated with pain as well as fever and malaise. The exacerbations are predominantly unilateral, and when bilateral the symptoms are more prominent on one side. Between attacks the child is free from symptoms.

The disease usually presents in children between the ages of 5–7 years but children presenting earlier or later are well recognized. Exacerbations may occur over many years with attacks occurring every 3–4 months, but the clinical course may vary considerably between children. After puberty the symptoms usually subside and the clinical disease may resolve completely. However continued recurrent swelling may persist into adult life.

Histological examination of the affected glands in juvenile recurrent parotitis reveals areas with massive infiltration by lymphocytes with lymph follicle formation. There are cystically dilated interglandular ducts which, on the sialographic image, correspond to small spherical collections of contrast medium called salectases. Among aetiological factors to have been considered in the development of juvenile recurrent parotitis are congenital malformation of the parotid ducts, hereditary, primary or secondary infections, allergy, and local manifestation of systemic immunological disease (Konno and Ito, 1978).

Regrettably, no preventative therapy for this disease is available. During recurrences it is important to treat the acute inflammation of the glands to prevent further damage to the glandular parenchyma. In most cases penicillin V is effective. Clini-

cally there is no obvious reason to change from penicillin when recurrent attacks present. Staphylococcal bacteria generally do not form a major part of the oral flora of otherwise healthy children. Other effective antibiotics include cloxacillin and flucloxacillin in debilitated patients or in those with purulent discharge.

In the majority of cases there is decrease in frequency of symptoms at puberty and the disease clinically disappears in adult life. However, the sialographic changes remain almost unaltered into adult life (Geterud, Lindvell and Nyten, 1988) (Figure 32.7). Currently evidence suggests that the clinical disease is related to congenital ectasia of portions of salivary ducts and the infection is considered to ascend from the oral cavity (Ericson, Zetterlund and Öhman, 1991).

Sialolithiasis in children

Sialolithiasis is a condition common in adults, most frequently affecting the submandibular gland. This condition is considered to be related to the viscosity of the saliva and the length and tortuosity of Wharton's duct. Cases of sialolithiasis have occasionally been reported in children.

The average age of the children affected by salivary calculi is 10 years. There is a preponderance of boys to girls (2:1) with no apparent explanation for this sex difference. Sialolithiasis has frequently been present for many years asymptomatically or there may be long symptomless periods between episodes of pain or swelling. The symptoms vary considerably from a single localized tenderness in the floor of the mouth to acute swelling of the gland accompanied by high temperature, requiring admission to hospital and administration of intravenous antibiotics. The main complaint is usually submandibular swelling accompanied by pain that increases close to meal time, with a gradual decrease of pain and swelling afterwards. The pain usually occurs immediately before meals because discharge of saliva is stimulated and the gland swells because of the blocked duct. In younger patients, under 10 years of age, the glands are usually located intraorally but in those over 10 years, the gland is located both intraorally and extraorally. The location of the stone may also account for the differences in clinical symptoms and signs. Most of the stones found in the older age group are located posteriorly.

True occlusal radiographs show a stone in the anterior two-thirds of the duct. A stone in the posterior third of the duct, close to the gland or actually in the gland can be seen only by distal oblique occlusal radiographs (Figure 32.8). It is important to perform both views as the same patient, not infrequently, may have several stones. When stones do not appear

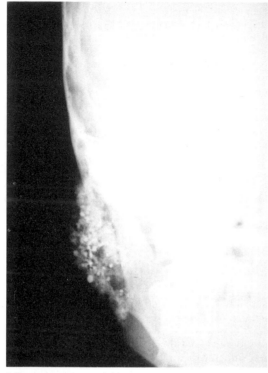

(a)

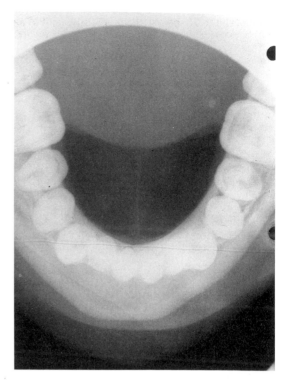

Figure 32.8 Occlusal view of floor of mouth showing a stone in the right floor of mouth and in the left submandibular duct

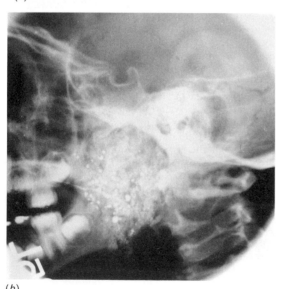

(b)

Figure 32.7 Radiograph of sialectasis: (a) anteroposterior, (b) lateral

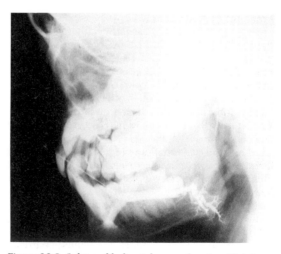

Figure 32.9 Submandibular sialogram showing dilated ductal system

on the radiograph then the possibility of a radiolucent stone should be considered; a sialogram may then be necessary (Figure 32.9).

Treatment is by sialodochotomy if the stone is located in the anterior two-thirds of the duct. The removal of the gland should be considered if the stone is located posteriorly or within the gland substance. Occasionally the stone will become impacted in the duct, leading to atrophy of the gland. In this situation no treatment is recommended. Sialolithiasis in the parotid gland of children has been reported only on two occasions to date (Kaufman, 1968).

Trauma

Injury to a major salivary gland is seldom an isolated incident and, more often, is associated with multiple trauma. In the evaluation of the trauma to the parotid gland the major concern is the facial nerve or its branches and the parotid duct. If a laceration extends anteriorly to a line dropped from the lateral canthus of the eye, the facial nerve does not need to be explored. It is said that satisfactory re-innervation will occur through cross branches. When a laceration is posterior to this line, the wound must be explored, the cut ends of the nerve identified and reapproximated. It is recommended that exploration should be performed within 72 hours.

The parotid duct is most likely to be injured if a laceration cuts through the masseter muscle. Pooling of saliva in the wound is frequently seen. Several options are available to treat parotid duct injury:

1 Ligation of the duct with glandular atrophy
2 The shortened duct may be moved and a new intraoral opening created
3 The duct can be repaired with 6/0 nylon over a polyethylene tube stent. This stent should left in place for 10–14 days before removal.

If for any reason the repair is delayed, the resulting inflammatory process will predispose to a salivary sinus.

Cysts and congenital salivary gland lesions

The parotid glands are affected more frequently by cysts and congenital lesions than any other of the salivary glands (Work and Hecht, 1968; Work, 1981). Ranulas affect the sublingual gland ducts and the lesser salivary glands are sites for the development of retention cysts which present on the tongue and the palate.

Cysts of the parotid gland are important since they account for 2–5% of all parotid gland lesions. A cystic lesion can occur in any portion of the parotid gland and can cause difficulties in diagnosis, particularly if the anatomical location is retromandibular and deep to the facial nerve. Many cystic lesions occur as a unilocular lesion in a single parotid gland. Multilocular cysts involving both glands are rare.

Cysts may also be acquired secondary to obstructive disease, neoplastic conditions, calculi, associated benign lymphoepithelial disease, trauma or parasites. Congenital cystic lesions mainly occur in the parotid gland and can be divided into dermoid cysts,

branchial cleft cysts (type I and type II, see Chapter 30), branchial pouch cysts and congenital ductal cysts.

A dermoid cyst can occur within the parotid gland as an isolated mass. Diagnosis may be made by CT scan or ultrasound, needle aspiration of fluid for cytology is helpful. Treatment is by complete surgical removal, otherwise recurrence is frequent. Care should be taken to preserve the facial nerve.

Congenital ductal cysts can occur in infancy and are manifest by enlargement of the parotid glands. These lesions can be demonstrated by sialography and are considered to be true congenital retention cysts. No treatment is indicated unless associated with repeated episodes of infection. Parotidectomy with preservation of the facial nerve is curative but should be delayed until the patient is older or adult.

Ranulas

Ranulas are benign space occupying lesions arising in the sublingual gland. An intraoral ranula is usually a readily recognizable lesion with a characteristic localization and appearance. A bluish, translucent and fluctuant swelling of the floor of the mouth, sometimes with a history of spontaneous rupture and expulsion of viscous fluid is nearly always pathognomonic (Batsakis and McClatchey, 1988). Infrequently it may present as a soft tissue mass with or without an intraoral component – known as the plunging ranula. The cervical ranula reaches to the neck either posteriorly (and may displace the submandibular gland) or through a discontinuous mylohyoid muscle.

Treatment in the past included marsupialization, radiation and excision. It has been established that the sublingual gland is the origin of cervical ranulas and the theory of extrasalivary origin is not proven. The majority of ranulas are pseudocysts without an epithelial lining. Marsupialization will inevitably lead to recurrence in the non-epithelial lined pseudocysts. An average of three operations was considered necessary before cure could be established (Van den Akker, Bays and Becker, 1978). The essential component of treatment of cervical ranulas must include removal of the sublingual gland from which the mucous secretions are arising (Black and Croft, 1982).

Granulomatous lesions

Granulomatous lesions as in other sites, produce a chronic inflammatory response in the salivary glands. Most frequently it involves the parotid glands but occasionally it is seen in the submandibular gland. Patients present with a localized nodule within the gland which is similar to the presentation of a neoplasm. The lesion frequently presents in isolation making the diagnosis difficult. However, suspicion is aroused when accompanied with signs and symptoms of systemic disease. The mass is usually painless, slowly progressive in size and often without surrounding inflammatory reaction. Salivary secretions are normal in amount and in colour. Sialography demonstrates extrinsic pressure on the ductal system, CT scan reveals a solid mass. Fine needle aspiration may not be helpful though should be performed. The possible causes include sarcoidosis, tuberculosis, atypical mycobacteria infection, actinomycosis and cat-scratch disease. Excision biopsy is frequently required to obtain tissue for analysis and culture. Subsequent treatment depends on the histopathological diagnosis. Bilateral cystic enlargement of the parotid glands has been reported and observed in HIV infected children, usually in combination with lymphocytic interstitial pneumonitis (De Vries *et al.*, 1988). Salivary gland involvement may be the initial manifestation of HIV with the parotid gland being the most frequently affected site (Falloon *et al.*, 1989).

Chronic diffuse parotid enlargement

It is not uncommon for the salivary glands to become enlarged in children due to metabolic or endocrine abnormalities. The parotid glands are frequently involved in a slow but progressive painless enlargement. This is not usually associated with inflammation but the glands may fluctuate in size during the early stages. Thyroid, diabetes mellitus and pituitary-adrenal hormone diseases are the most commonly associated entities. Parotid gland enlargement associated with hypothyroidism is not related to the magnitude of the deficiency but rather is thought to represent a true hypertrophy. Diabetes mellitus should be excluded in all children who present with bilateral parotid gland hypertrophy. Cushing's disease is associated with fatty infiltration of the parotids. The above endocrine disorders do not have any specific identifying histopathological features. There is fibrous atrophy followed by atrophy of the glandular elements with time. Because of this progressive atrophy, there may be an associated reduction of salivary volume. The ductal elements remain normal on sialography. *Cystic fibrosis* is also associated with salivary gland enlargement. More frequently the submandibular glands are enlarged and this disease can also affect the parotids. When children under the age of 2 years present with enlarged parotids without any associated inflammation, cystic fibrosis needs to be excluded by a sweat test.

Necrotizing sialometaplasia

This is a benign, self-limiting ulcerative disease of the minor salivary glands, usually seen in the oral cavity.

Histologically and clinically the disease may simulate the clinical presentations of squamous cell carcinoma or mucoepidermoid carcinoma. Necrotizing sialometaplasia was first reported in 1973 by Abrams, Melrose and Howell in a patient who presented with a lesion on the hard palate. It has been documented and reported in nearly all areas of the head and neck region where mucous secreting glands exist. The aetiology of the lesions appears due to ductal proliferation in response to trauma. All lesions are treated by incisional biopsy to confirm the diagnosis. Making the correct diagnosis may be difficult but it is essential for the clinician and the pathologist to be aware of this disease's existence to prevent mutilating surgery and to prevent the possibility of radiotherapy being given in addition. Necrotizing sialometaplasia is a benign condition that heals spontaneously in 6–12 weeks, although total excision of the lesion may be performed, more definitive therapy is unnecessary (Grillon and Lally, 1981).

Plexiform neurofibroma

Plexiform neurofibroma is an unusual tumour but has been reported and is said to represent 0.6% of all major salivary gland tumours in children (Castro *et al.*, 1972). All reported cases of neurofibroma in children are of the plexiform type. Cases have been reported arising in the submandibular and the sublingual glands (Weitzner, 1980). Plexiform neurofibroma is indicative of neurofibromatosis even though it may be the only clinical manifestation. The possibility of any given mass of the salivary gland in a child being a neurofibroma is remote but, in the presence of café-au-lait spots or other stigmata of von Recklinghausen's disease, a plexiform neurofibroma should be considered. Excision is the treatment of choice.

Salivary haemangioma

Salivary haemangioma affects girls in 80% of reported cases, most being present at birth; 90% have presented and are diagnosed within the first year of life. Eighty per cent of haemangiomas occur in the parotid gland, 18% in the submandibular gland and 1.1% in the minor salivary glands. Haemangiomas are encountered in the sublingual glands and have also been reported in the papilla of the submandibular ducts.

Haemangiomas may have attained a considerable size when diagnosed. The diagnosis is usually easy to make and is based on the colour, consistency and site of the tumour. Haemangiomas are classified according to their histological architecture into capillary, cavernous, mixed and hypertrophic categories. The classification loses its effectiveness because there is considerable overlap, especially in the capillary and cavernous components. It is believed that the hypertrophic form represents an immature capillary haemangioma and that the cavernous lesion is an end product of a maturing capillary haemangioma, thus classifying the various types along the continuum of histological maturation.

The tumour mass itself is most frequently confined to the intracapsular portion of the gland. The overlying subcutaneous tissue and skin are only occasionally involved. The histological appearances show that the lobular architecture of the salivary gland is maintained but the parenchyma is replaced by endothelial proliferation with vascular differentiation, which surrounds the glandular acini and ducts.

Treatment is more difficult. Surgery, if contemplated, should be postponed for as long as possible, because about 50% of these tumours resolve spontaneously within the first 3–4 years of life. A haemangioma spreads diffusely within the entire parotid gland and may on occasions penetrate the masseter muscle. It is obvious that dissection of the facial nerve can be difficult in such cases.

Any procedure that reduces the bulk of the haemangioma and thus postpones the necessity for surgery should be tried first. The following methods have been described:

1 Injection of sclerosing fatty acids prepared from cod's liver, quinine and hypertonic solutions. Complications of this technique have included facial nerve injury, bleeding and abscess formation.
2 Electrocautery of the haemangioma. Difficult and potentially traumatic.
3 Ionizing radiation should only used as a last resort, if at all, because of damage to the growth of bone and because of the associated danger of malignant transformation.
4 Injection of glucocorticosteroids especially for the rapidly growing haemangioma has been described as very effective in the capillary haemangioma type (Conley, 1975).

Lymphangioma and cystic hygroma

Lymphangioma and cystic hygroma are usually present at birth, but may only become clinically evident by the second year of life. The commonest site is the parotid gland area. An increase in size later in life is usually associated with infection or following trauma. The characteristics of the lymphangioma vary widely. The size may remain constant, increase suddenly or decrease slowly, but complete remission does not occur.

The lesion presents as a soft, non-tender swelling of the cheek which demonstrates ballotement because of its fluid content. As the tumour grows, the skin over it becomes thin and blue in colour. The danger of an excessive increase in size of the lymphangioma

is damage to bone by pressure absorption and vascular compression. The facial nerve is very resistant, however, and is almost never damaged. Aspiration and cytology biopsies may be required to make the diagnosis. Lymphangiomas should be removed because they do not undergo spontaneous regression and often increase in size. The timing of the operation is crucial, the optimum time being the fourth or fifth year of life. Dissection of the facial nerve fibres in very small children can be difficult since the nerves are surrounded by the cysts and can only be preserved by fine dissection (Conley, 1975). Sometimes a series of operations is preferable to avoid cosmetic disfigurement, reducing radicality and minimizing the possibility of facial nerve paralysis. These lesions are classified as lymphangiomas simplex (containing capillary-sized lymphatic channels), cavernous lymphangioma (with dilated lymphatic spaces) and cystic hygroma (composed of cysts of varying sizes) and are generally believed to be malformations rather than a true neoplasm. The salivary gland parenchyma is not replaced by lymphangiomatous tissue as is seen in the haemangioma condition but rather coexists as islands of normal glandular tissue surrounded by thin walled, lymph-containing spaces.

Salivary gland tumours

No more than 5% of all salivary gland neoplasms occur in children (Luna, Batsakis and El Nagger, 1991) and 3.3% of the neoplasms, benign or malignant, present in patients 16 years of age or younger. Salivary gland neoplasms in children account for 8% of all paediatric neck tumours. They are the fourth most frequent paediatric head and neck tumour after tumours of the nasopharynx, skin and thyroid in that order (Shikhani and Johns, 1988; Callander *et al.*, 1992).

Several features distinguish neoplasms in this age group from those in adults:

1 There is a much greater frequency of non-epithelial tumours
2 There is a higher proportion of malignant neoplasms when non-epithelial tumours are excluded
3 There is a preponderance of parotid gland involvement, e.g. 7:1 ratio with the submandibular gland.

Benign and malignant neoplasms of the salivary glands in children usually present as a painless, enlarging mass with no evidence suggesting inflammation or infection. The masses are typically slow growing, though they may enlarge rapidly. Pain and cranial nerve defects are usually absent, although they suggest malignancy when present. Regional lymphadenopathy may also be present, though its presence at the time of diagnosis has rarely been reported. In a review (Shikhani and Johns, 1988) there was a sex predilection in favour of females for all paediatric salivary gland neoplasms (female:male ratio 1:42). For the benign neoplasms, the ratio is even higher (1:57) and for the malignant tumours (1:28). Most of these tumours develop during the teens with very few tumours reported below the age of 8 years. Almost all the histological varieties of salivary gland tumours reported in adults have also been found in children (Table 32.1). There were no clinical features that differentiated between benign and malignant lesions with any degree of certainty.

Table 32.1 Benign salivary gland neoplasms

Histology	Number	%
Pleomorphic adenoma	214	87.7
Plexiform neurofibroma	8	3.2
Warthin's tumour	5	2
Cystadenoma	5	2
Lymphoepithelial lesion	3	1.2
Neurilemmoma	3	1.2
Embryoma	3	1.2
Xanthama	2	0.8
Adenoma	1	0.4
Total	244	100

The first principle in the management of salivary gland tumours is to establish a histological diagnosis. Incisional biopsy is to be condemned because the risk of damage to the facial nerve outweighs any clinical or management benefit. Fine needle aspiration is safer and should yield a correct diagnosis in more than 75% of cases with a negligible risk of 'seeding'. The greatest reliability of fine needle aspiration has been shown to occur with pleomorphic adenomas. The operative technique for removal of a parotid or submandibular gland in a child is not much different from that of the adult. It should be remembered that the facial nerve is more superficially placed in the very young child because the mastoid air cells have not fully developed. Thus, the facial nerve lies just medial or below the tip of the mastoid. The therapeutic plan is complete removal of the neoplasm without tumour spill or damage to the facial nerve. Frozen section support may be helpful for proper intraoperative decision.

A review of results has been reported when initial surgery was one of the three following surgical procedures: superficial parotidectomy, total parotidectomy or simple excision with emphasis on the recurrence rate and the final ultimate prognosis. The recurrence rate after enucleation of a parotid pleomorphic adenoma was high (39.3%) and hence must be condemned in children as it is in adults. The recurrence after superficial parotidectomy was 19.5%, a much higher rate than for the same procedure in adults.

This might be due to the increased risk of violation of the tumour 'capsule' and the resultant seeding, because of the small size of the facial nerve and associated structures of the child. The least recurrence risk (7.1%) occurred when a total parotidectomy was performed as part of the initial surgical management. The prognosis associated with pleomorphic adenoma surgery was good and a large majority of patients remained tumour free over a long period of follow up.

The mucoepidermoid carcinoma type is the most common salivary gland malignancy seen in childhood and made up 49.6% of all salivary gland cancers seen in a review (Luna, Batsakis and El-Nagger, 1991) (Table 32.2). The recurrence after superficial parotidectomy was 30.7% and after simple enucleation was 48.3%. There was no recurrence after a total parotidectomy or reported in the few cases where radiotherapy was added to the initial excision procedure. Lymph node metastases, when encountered, should be treated by selective neck dissection. Radiotherapy should only be considered if the tumour is very large, and when microscopic disease would appear to have remained despite aggressive surgical management. Acinic cell carcinoma, when present, should be treated similarly to mucoepidermoid carcinoma by total parotidectomy. Adenoid cystic carcinoma, when present in childhood, demonstrates a high recurrence rate and is associated with a relatively poor survival. This is because the disease is generally more extensive at the time of presentation and the failure to recognize microperineural extensions. The other malignant tumours of salivary type, when encountered in childhood, are associated with a poor prognosis. These other histological types, when diagnosed, are best managed by complete surgical removal of the tumour by total parotidectomy. Currently the role of postoperative radiotherapy is not clear, although it may be considered to be cura-

Table 32.2 Malignant salivary gland neoplasms

Histology	Number	%
Mucoepidermoid carcinoma	122	49.6
Acinic cell carcinoma	30	12.2
Undifferentiated carcinoma	22	8.9
Adenocarcinoma	19	7.7
Adenoid cystic carcinoma	16	6.5
Malignant mixed tumour	10	4.1
Rhabdomyosarcoma	6	2.4
Undifferentiated sarcoma	5	2.0
Mesenchymal sarcoma	5	2.0
Unclassified carcinoma	4	1.6
Squamous cell carcinoma	3	1.2
Lymphoma	3	1.2
Ganglioneuroblastoma	1	0.4
Total	246	100

tive, it may have devastating long-term sequelae when given to the young. Some authors have suggested that radiotherapy should only be given more for palliative rather than curative reasons (Baker and Malone, 1985).

Embryoma

This is a recognized epithelial salivary gland tumour unique to children (Batsakis *et al.*, 1988). To date this tumour has been recognized only in the newborn or during the first year of life. Embryomas are morphologically similar to stages of development of the embryonic anlage of the minor salivary glands. Less than 25% of the reported embryomas have shown histological and/or biological signs of malignancy. The majority have responded to surgical excision with a benign clinical course.

Minor gland tumours

There are only a few reports of epithelial neoplasms of the minor salivary glands in children. The neoplasms, when reported, have been almost exclusively located in the oral cavity. In a review of children with epithelial tumours of the intraoral minor salivary glands, only one child was below the age of 9 years (Waldron, El-Mefty and Gnepp, 1988). Two histological types dominate in series, the pleomorphic adenoma and the mucoepidermoid carcinoma (Gustafsson *et al.*, 1987). Complete surgical excision is the treatment of choice. Single cases have been reported of cystadenoma and adenocarcinoma lesions located in the oral cavity (Budnik, 1982). Surgical excision has been curative.

References

ABRAMS, A. M., MELROSE, R. J. and HOWELL, F. V. (1973) Necrolizing sialometaplasia: a disease simulating malignancy. *Cancer*, **32**, 130–135

BAKER, S. R. and MALONE, B. (1985) Salivary gland malignancies in children. *Cancer*, **55**, 1730–1736

BATSAKIS, J. G. and MCCLATCHEY, K. D. (1988) Cervical ranula. *Annals of Otology, Rhinology and Laryngology*, **97**, 561–562

BATSAKIS, J. G., MACKAY, B., RYKE, A. F. and SEIFERT, R. W. (1988) Perinatal salivary gland tumours (embryomas). *Journal of Laryngology and Otology*, **102**, 1007–1011

BLACK, R. J. and CROFT, C. B. (1982) Ranula: pathogenesis and management. *Clinicial Otolaryngology*, **7**, 299–303

BROOK, I. (1992) Diagnosis and management of parotitis. *Archives of Otolaryngology – Head and Neck Surgery*, **118**, 469–471

BUDNICK, S. D. (1982) Minor salivary gland tumours in children. *Journal of Dentistry for Children*, **49**, 44–47

CALLANDER, D. L., FRANKENTHALER, R. A., LUNA, M. A., LEE, S. B. and GOEPFERT, H. (1992) Salivary gland neoplasms in children. *Archives of Otolaryngology – Head and Neck Surgery*, **118**, 472–476

CASTRO, E. B., HUVOS, A. G., STRONG, E. W. and FOOTE, F. W. (1972) Tumours of the major salivary glands in children. *Cancer*, **29**, 312–317

CONLEY, J. (1975) *Salivary Glands and the Facial Nerve*. Stuttgart: Thieme

DE VRIES, E. J., KAPADIA, S. B., JOHNSON, J. T. and BONTEMPO, F. A. (1988) Salivary gland lymphoproliferation disease in acquired immune disease. *Otolaryngology, Head and Neck Surgery*, **99**, 59–62

ERICSON, S., ZETTERLUND, B. and ÖHMAN, J. (1991) Recurrent parotitis and sialectesis in childhood. *Annals of Otology, Rhinology and Laryngology*, **100**, 527–535

FALLOON, J., EDDY, J., WIENER, L. and PIZZO, P. A. (1989) Human immunodeficiency virus infection in children. *Journal of Paediatrics*, **114**, 1 30

GETERUD, A., LINDVALL, A. M. and NYTEN, O. (1988) Follow up study of recurrent parotitis in children. *Annals of Otology, Rhinology and Laryngology*, **97**, 341–346

GRILLON, G. L. and LALLY, E. T. (1981) Necrotizing sialometaplasia. *Oral Surgery*, **39**, 747–753

GUSTAFSSON, H., DAHLQVIST, A., ANNIKO, M. and CARLSÖÖ, B. (1987) Mucoepidermoid carcinoma in a minor salivary gland in childhood. *Journal of Laryngology and Otology*, **101**, 1320–1323

JOHNS, M. (1977) The salivary glands: anatomy and embryology. *Otolaryngologic Clinics of North America*, **10**, 261–271

JONES, A. G. H., WHITE, J. M. and BEGG, N. T. (1991) The impact of MMR vaccine on mumps infection in England and Wales. *Communicable Disease Report*, **1**, R 94–96

JOSHI, E., DAVIDSON, P. M., JONES, P. G., CAMPBELL, P. E. and ROBERTSON, D. M. (1989) Non-tuberculous mycobacterial lymphadenitis in children. *European Journal of Paediatrics*, **148**, 751–754

KAUFMAN, S. (1968) Parotid sialolithiasis in a child. *American Journal of Diseases of Children*, **115**, 623–624

KONNO, A. and ITO, E. (1978) A study on the pathogenesis of recurrent parotitis in childhood. *Annals of Otology, Rhinology and Laryngology*, **88**, 1–20

LUNA, M. A., BATSAKIS, J. G. and EL NAGGER, A. E. (1991) Salivary gland tumours in children. *Annals of Otology, Rhinology and Laryngology*, **100**, 869–871

MAY, M. (1986) *The Facial Nerve*. Stuttgart: Theme Inc

PRANSKY, S. M., REISMAN, B. K., KEARNS, D. B., SEID, A. B., COLLINS, D. and KROUS, N. F. (1990) Cervicofacial mycobacterial adenitis in children endemic to San Diego. *Laryngoscope*, **100**, 920–925

SHIKHANI, A. H. and JOHNS, M. E. (1988) Tumours of the major salivary glands in children. *Head and Neck Surgery*, **10**, 257–263

VAN DEN AKKER, H. P., BAYS, R. A. and BECKER, A. K. (1978) Plunging or cervical ranula. *Journal of Maxillofacial Surgery*, **6**, 293–301

WALDRON, C. A., EL-MEFTY, S. K. and GNEPP, D. R. (1988) Tumours of the intraoral minor salivary glands: a demographic and histologic study of 426 cases. *Oral Surgery, Oral Medicine and Oral Pathology*, **66**, 323–333

WEITZNER, S. (1980) Plexiform neurofibroma of major salivary glands in children. *Oral Surgery*, **50**, 53–57

WORK, W. P. (1981) Non-neoplastic disorders of the parotid gland. *Journal of Otolaryngology*, **10**, 35–40

WORK, W. P. and HECHT, D. W. (1968) Non-neoplastic lesions of the parotid gland. *Annals of Otology, Rhinology and Laryngology*, **77**, 462–466

ZOLLAR, L. M. and MUFSON, M. A. (1970) Acute parotitis associated with para influenza 3 virus infection. *American Journal of Diseases of Children*, **119**, 147–148

33

The drooling child

Michael J. Cinnamond

Drooling or sialorrhoea is defined as the overflow of saliva from the mouth. It can be classified as physiological, acute or chronic (Table 33.1).

Table 33.1 Classification of drooling

Physiological drooling
  infancy
Acute drooling
  acute epiglottitis
  post-tonsillectomy
Chronic drooling
  'Andy Gump' deformity
  oesophageal obstruction
  mental disability
  muscular spasticity or incoordination

Classification

Physiological drooling

Most normal healthy infants drool as will be self-evident to anyone who has ever nursed a baby on their shoulder. This will generally decline as infancy progresses, though it may increase temporarily during teething. Physiological drooling will usually have ceased by the time the baby is 18 months to 2 years of age.

Acute drooling

Acute drooling occurs in many inflammatory and other diseases of the mouth and pharynx. The most obvious examples of this phenomenon are acute epiglottitis and following tonsillectomy. The drooling in these cases is due to pain on swallowing and will disappear as soon as the inflammatory reaction begins to settle.

Chronic drooling

The vast majority of patients with chronic drooling are either mentally disabled, often severely so, or are afflicted with one of the various forms of congenital or acquired muscle spasticity or incoordination. The natural assumption is that saliva is being over-produced, and in some instances this may be partially true. It has been suggested, for example, that the tranquillizers or anticonvulsants that many of these patients take might have a cholinergic effect, though the evidence for this is scanty and it seems unlikely that it could account for the whole problem.

Formation of saliva is a continuous process, at least during the waking hours. The measurement of salivary volume is fraught with difficulty but has been estimated in normal individuals during a 24-hour period to lie in the range 500–700 ml. In those few studies which have been done on patients with drooling similar results have been obtained (Ekedahl and Hallén, 1973). It would seem, therefore, that drooling is not related to increased salivation. Instead, the problem is one of inadequate disposal of normal volumes of saliva.

Aetiology

In a very few cases, drooling may be due to total or near-total oesophageal obstruction. In others, damage to the muscles of the tongue or floor of the mouth, as can occur following partial resection of the lower jaw ('Andy Gump' deformity), may make initiation of swallowing difficult or impossible.

In the majority, however, other factors are responsible (Table 33.2). Most of these patients have severe

Table 33.2 Causes of drooling

Over-production of saliva
   tranquillizers
   anticonvulsants
Inadequate disposal of saliva
   outflow obstruction
   failure to initiate swallowing
   faulty head and jaw posture
   muscular incoordination
   inappropriate muscle activity

postural problems affecting the head and neck, typically adopting a head hanging, open-mouthed attitude, often with a drooping, everted lower lip (Figure 33.1) Palpation often reveals increased muscle tone especially in the floor of the mouth and lower jaw and it is this, rather than weakness of the jaw closing muscles, which leads to the open-mouthed appearance. Barium screening or videofluoroscopy may show evidence of incoordinated activity of the pharynx and upper oesophagus with resultant failure to complete the second phase of swallowing. Finally, in some patients, there is inappropriate muscle activity such as tongue thrusting.

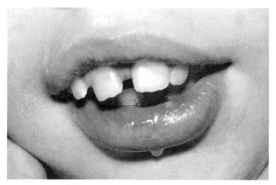

Figure 33.1 Typical appearance of the drooling child

The end product of these various factors is the inability to clear the mouth of saliva in the normal way, so that saliva tends to collect towards the front of the mouth in a pool which constantly overflows.

Clinical features

Most patients with drooling present because of social problems. Drooling is often seen as a sign of mental enfeeblement or slovenly behaviour and may result in withdrawal from social contact both on the part of the patient and the family. Children may be shunned by their peers, becoming objects of ridicule and insult. Others are frustrated because of constant soiling and damage to books or other household articles, such as the television remote control.

Most patients will require frequent changes of clothing, sometimes amounting to 10–15 changes per day. The need for constant laundering may put an intolerable burden on the mother, especially if there are other small children in the family and may also cause a serious drain on the family's financial resources. Excoriation of the skin over the chin and upper chest is common and is sometimes severe and extensive. In a very few cases, drooling may be so marked as to result in dehydration or electrolyte disturbance.

Management

Those responsible for the care of such patients, including their medical attendants, are often unaware of the possibility of treatment. Furthermore, there is a tendency to regard drooling as a problem of little or no consequence, especially in the presence of multiple handicaps. This is unfortunate as the quality of life in these patients can often be improved dramatically by relatively simple means.

The aim of treatment is either to improve swallowing or, if this proves impossible, to reduce the flow of saliva to the point where the patient's own defective clearance can cope. It is important to realize, however, that it is possible to be too successful in achieving a reduction in salivary flow. If the salivary gland output is reduced to less than 5% of normal, xerostomia will occur. Not only is this most unpleasant for the patient, much more so than the original drooling, but may have a disastrous effect on oral and dental hygiene. In addition, it must be borne in mind that drooling is not a serious or life-threatening condition. Treatment modalities which are likely to result in inadvertent damage to other structures should be avoided. In particular, impairment of facial nerve function, a serious and disfiguring injury in any patient, is likely to lead to an increase in drooling.

Despite these reservations, however, these patients can and should be helped. Many different modalities of treatment have been described, including both surgical and non-surgical methods (Table 33.3). Each of these can be considered under two main headings, improvement in swallowing and reduction of salivary flow.

Non-surgical methods
Improvement in swallowing
Physiotherapy

This form of treatment is usually designated as physiotherapy, but is actually carried out by speech and language therapists. Physiotherapy aims at improving the oral phase of deglutition by means of specific exercises for the muscles of the mandible, lips, tongue and palate (Ray, Bundy and Nelson, 1983; Waterman *et al.*, 1992). Thus jaw closure and stability are improved, mobility, positioning and coordination of

Table 33.3 Treatment of drooling

Non-surgical
  Improvement in swallowing
    physiotherapy
    biofeedback and behavioural modification
  Reduction of salivary flow
    drug therapy
    radiotherapy
Surgical
  Improvement in jaw posture
    mylohyoid myotomy
  Redistribution of salivary flow
    parotid duct relocation
    submandibular duct relocation
  Reduction of salivary flow
    excision of salivary glands
    ligation of salivary gland ducts
  Interruption of parasympathetic nerve supply
    division of auriculotemporal nerve
    extirpation of submandibular ganglion
    tympanic neurectomy (division of chorda tympani and
    excision of tympanic plexus)

the tongue and palate are enhanced, and better closure of the lips, especially during swallowing, is achieved. Such therapy probably works by substituting improved voluntary control for the normal, semi-automatic behaviour of the oral musculature during the first phase of swallowing. In those with severe mental disability or where drooling is excessive, little improvement can be expected, but in most patients physiotherapy enhances swallowing activity and may play an important role in management, especially in those in whom relocation of the salivary gland ducts is undertaken.

As Crysdale (1980) has pointed out, physiotherapy is unlikely to eliminate drooling entirely, but there are a few patients in whom a satisfactory result may be obtained with this method alone. For this reason a 6-month trial of physiotherapy is advocated prior to undertaking any surgical treatment.

Biofeedback and behavioural modification

Crysdale *et al.* (1985) reported a method of conditioning patients with drooling to respond to auditory stimuli. Electromyographic activity in the orbicularis oris and strap muscles is used to enhance awareness of swallowing activity. The achievement of proper motor responses triggers an auditory signal. After the training period, the patient is supplied with a timer which 'beeps' at pre-set intervals, thus supplying an auditory cue for swallowing to begin.

Reduction of salivary flow

Drug therapy

Anticholinergic drugs can produce a marked reduction in salivary gland output, witness the drying of the mouth induced by atropine and hyoscine. Unfortunately, however, at dosages sufficient to achieve control of drooling, these substances have unwanted and unpleasant side effects including constipation, urinary retention, restlessness or even xerostomia. In addition, such treatment would have to be continued more or less indefinitely. It seems unlikely, therefore, that these drugs offer a viable alternative to other methods of treatment.

Radiotherapy

Irradiation of the parotid, submandibular and sublingual glands has also been used as a method of reducing the flow of saliva. It is, however, extremely difficult to determine the radiation dosage required to cause cessation of drooling, while at the same time leaving sufficient flow to obviate against the development of xerostomia (Goode and Smith, 1970; Guerin, 1979). Furthermore, it is known that the serous elements of the salivary glands are more radiosensitive than the mucinous, so that the patient may be left with very thick, viscid saliva. The incidence of painful mucositis is high and there is at least a theoretical risk of inducing dysplastic or even neoplastic change in the salivary glands or thyroid. Radiotherapy is, therefore, too uncertain and too risky to be useful.

Surgical methods

Several different surgical approaches to the problem of drooling have been devised. Generally speaking these may be considered under two main headings: redistribution of flow and reduction of secretion. A third possibility is correction of the open-mouth posture by performing a mylohyoid myotomy. The basis for this operation is that poor jaw posture (see above) is related to hypertonicity of the muscles in the floor of the mouth, rather than weakness of the jaw muscles. The author has no personal experience of this procedure, but Crysdale (1980) considered it unacceptably aggressive.

Redistribution of salivary flow

In essence this means relocation of the submandibular or parotid ducts, from their normal position in the oral cavity to the tonsil fossa (Brody, 1977; Crysdale, 1982). The rationale for these operations is that saliva, when projected into the oropharynx, will stimulate the swallowing reflex. A successful outcome, however, obviously depends on the pharyngeal phase of swallowing being reasonably efficient. This is something that cannot be assumed in these patients, but is probably more likely to be true in those who have had preoperative physiotherapy.

Most authors on this subject have advocated removal of the tonsils as a separate procedure prior to relocating the ducts, and some have even commented on this as being a disadvantage of the procedure. Others, such as Crysdale (1989), now remove the tonsils only if these are filling the tonsil fossae. In the past, the author has tried transposing the submandibular duct onto the anterior pillar of the fauces, leaving the tonsil in position. This approach is not recommended, however, as it adds considerably to the difficulties of the operation and makes accurate placement of the duct orifice, which is a prerequisite to success, harder to achieve. There is also the concern that, should the patient subsequently require tonsillectomy, the relocated duct orifice will be jeopardized. There is, in any case, no necessity for the staged approach and the author routinely performs tonsillectomy as the initial step in the operation to relocate the ducts.

Parotid duct relocation

Transposition of the parotid ducts was first described by Wilkie (1967). The parotid duct, at the anterior border of the masseter, lies in close proximity to the upper and lower buccal branches of the facial nerve and to the buccal branch of the mandibular nerve. The operation is, therefore, not without significant risk. Moreover, complications such as duct stenosis, painful parotid swelling and septic parotitis have all been reported and may occur in as many as one-third of cases.

Submandibular duct relocation

Submandibular duct relocation, on the other hand, is a relatively simple and safe procedure. This procedure was first described in the English literature by Ekedahl (1974), though he mentioned Laage–Hellmann (1969) as having been the originator.

Routine tonsillectomy is first performed, paying particular attention to haemostasis. The ducts open on the summit of the sublingual papillae that lie on either side of the frenulum of the tongue. Following infiltration of the floor of the mouth with 1:80 000 adrenalin, a horizontally disposed elliptical incision is made to enclose both papillae. It is best not to separate the papillae at this stage. The ducts are, for the most part, easy to identify as thick white cords running backwards and laterally, but are often rather different in diameter. A combination of sharp and blunt dissection is used to separate the ducts from the surrounding sublingual tissues. The oval-shaped sublingual salivary gland is closely associated with the submandibular duct and, in part, drains into it. As damage to the sublingual glands is considered to be the main cause of ranula formation following this procedure, it is recommended that the sublingual sal-

ivary tissue is excised. Freeing of the ducts is carried backwards as far as possible, but at least beyond the midpoint of the distance between the frenulum and the tonsil fossa. In some cases the lingual and hypoglossal nerves will be seen, lying on either side of the duct, but it is unnecessary specifically to identify them. Provided that dissection is kept close to the duct, no harm should befall these structures.

A tunnel is then created sublingually on each side using long, straight artery forceps (Figure 33.2). With a finger in the tonsil fossa, the tip of the forceps is aimed to exit as low down in the fossa as possible. A thin red rubber catheter, introduced into the pharynx, is grasped by the forceps and drawn forwards through the tunnel. The ducts are separated from one another in the midline and each is sewn to the tip of its corresponding catheter (Figure 33.3), utilizing the surrounding cuff of mucosa to avoid damage to the duct itself. The catheters are drawn backwards avoiding twisting of the duct until the end of the duct appears in the tonsil fossa. It is essential that the duct should lie in its relocated position without tension. If this is not the case it will be necessary to free a little more of the duct and, in order to do this, it will be necessary to restore the duct to its normal position. The best way of achieving this is to leave a long tail on the suture fixing the duct to the catheter. When the duct has been relocated to the operator's satisfaction, the tonsil gag is re-inserted. The mucosal cuff on the end of the duct is sutured to the posterior aspect of the anterior faucial pillar and the catheter and retrieval suture are removed. Finally, the wound in the floor of the mouth is closed, either horizontally or vertically.

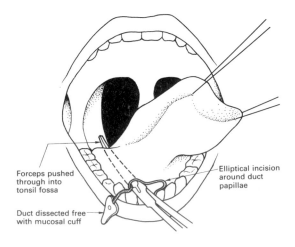

Forceps pushed through into tonsil fossa

Duct dissected free with mucosal cuff

Elliptical incision around duct papillae

Figure 33.2 Creating the sublingual tunnel

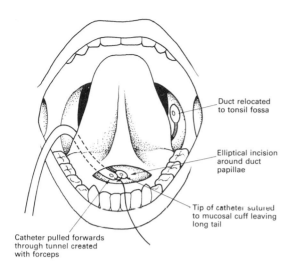

Duct relocated
to tonsil fossa

Elliptical incision
around duct
papillae

Tip of catheter sutured
to mucosal cuff leaving
long tail

Catheter pulled forwards
through tunnel created
with forceps

Figure 33.3 Relocating the submandibular ducts

A combination of a very small mouth, restricted jaw opening and a high arched palate may make it difficult or impossible to gain satisfactory access to the floor of the mouth. In these circumstances the best advice, gained from painful experience, is to abandon the procedure forthwith and consider tympanic neurectomy as an alternative.

Postoperatively, the patients seem to be no more uncomfortable than they would have been following tonsillectomy alone. In most, there is swelling of the floor of the mouth and a few also have some swelling of the submandibular glands. In both circumstances the swelling is transient and subsides within 24–48 hours. Ranulas are reported to occur in up to 10% of cases (Crysdale, 1989), and may on occasion prove difficult to treat. Excision of the sublingual gland at the time of duct relocation should, however, reduce the incidence of this complication. It has struck the author more than once that development of a submandibular duct calculus in a relocated duct could pose a rather tricky problem. So far, however, this complication has not been reported in the literature.

Reduction of secretion

There are three basic ways of doing this: excision of the glands, ligation of the ducts, or interruption of the parasympathetic nerve supply.

Excision of glands

Submandibular

Excision of the submandibular glands is a reasonably simple and safe operation and forms part of the surgical armamentarium of most otolaryngological

practitioners. There are, however, disadvantages; external scars are produced and there is some danger to the lingual and hypoglossal nerves and, in particular, to the cervical branch of the facial.

Parotid

While a reasonable case might be made for excision of the submandibular glands as a treatment for drooling there is no justification for parotidectomy, though this has been advocated. Total excision of both parotid glands is a formidable operation carrying an unacceptably high risk of permanent injury to the facial nerve even in expert hands. Its use in the management of chronic drooling is condemned unreservedly.

Ligation of the ducts

Ligation of both the parotid and submandibular ducts is a simple and relatively safe procedure (Glass, Nobel and Vecchione, 1978). There is, however, a significant postoperative morbidity with tender swelling of the glands, particularly the parotids, which in some cases is prolonged, lasting for weeks or even months.

Interruption of the parasympathetic nerve supply

Interruption of the parasympathetic secretomotor nerve fibres to the parotid, submandibular and sublingual glands would seem to be the ideal solution to the problem of drooling. There is a confluence of the fibres concerned in the middle ear, in the chorda tympani and the tympanic plexus. The approach to this area, via a postaural or endomeatal tympanotomy, is one in which all otolaryngologists should be well versed. Furthermore, the glands will continue to secrete at their basal or resting level, thus diminishing the risk of xerostomia and the saliva will be of normal composition. Although the middle ear operation has become the standard, two others should be mentioned if only for completeness. These are division of the auriculotemporal nerve and extirpation of the submandibular ganglion. Neither of these operations would seem to offer any advantage over the simpler and safer transtympanic approach.

Tympanic neurectomy and division of the chorda tympani

In 1946, Lempert described an operation for the relief of tinnitus aurium, which he called tympanosympathectomy. Sixteen years later, Golding–Wood (1962) revived the operation, which he renamed tympanic neurectomy, and described its use in the treatment of a variety of difficult otological problems including Frey's syndrome and chronic tympanic neuralgia.

In addition to fibres conveying taste sensation from the anterior two-thirds of the tongue, the chorda tympani carries parasympathetic, secretomotor fibres, taking origin from the superior salivary nucleus and ultimately being distributed to the submandibular and sublingual salivary glands.

In most instances the nerve is readily accessible, suspended in a mesentery of mucous membrane, lying first lateral to the long process of the incus and then medial to the handle of the malleus. Occasionally, however, it may be more difficult to find, being plastered onto the posterior wall of the middle ear just deep to the bony annulus or even within the facial recess. In very rare instances it may be absent.

The tympanic plexus is mostly derived from Jacobson's nerve, a branch of the glossopharyngeal, but receives sympathetic fibres from the internal carotid plexus via the caroticotympanic nerves. Occasionally, there is a small contribution from the facial nerve. The plexus supplies common sensation to the mucous membrane of the eustachian tube, middle ear cavity, mastoid antrum and mastoid air cells. In addition to the sympathetic fibres, it also carries parasympathetic fibres arising in the inferior salivary nucleus and distributed to the parotid gland and the mucous membrane of the mouth. These fibres reach their destination via the lesser superficial petrosal nerve and the otic ganglion.

The classical description of the plexus is of a single trunk running upwards in an oblique fashion over the promontory just anterior to the round window niche. As it ascends, often lying in a groove in the promontory, numerous fine branches are given off. Two surgically important variations on this theme

have been described. The main trunk of the plexus may lie within the substance of the bone of the promontory, sometimes deeply so. Second, Ross (1970) and Porto, Whicker and Proud (1978) showed that in 50% of ears there is an anterior or hypotympanic branch – this correlates well with the findings at operation (Figure 33.4). This branch leaves the main trunk low in the hypotympanum and may itself be covered by bone. It curves forwards around the base of the promontory in the direction of the eustachian tube orifice. There is very little symmetry in the pattern of the tympanic plexus.

As with all middle ear surgery, good visualization is important. It is, therefore, recommended that this operation is carried out under hypotensive anaesthesia. The approach to the middle ear is best done via a standard endomeatal tympanotomy though the flap should be positioned more inferiorly than normal, to improve access to the hypotympanum. With a small external auditory meatus, however, it may be necessary to employ the postaural route. This adds a little to the operation but has the advantage of allowing better access to the hypotympanum.

In dealing with the chorda tympani it is best to free the nerve from its mucosal fold with a Rosen's needle, to sever it at its point of exit from the posterior wall with microscissors and then to avulse the remainder of the nerve with fine crocodile forceps. This method protects the facial nerve and, at the same time, ensures that a long segment is removed.

The tympanic plexus is approached by elevating the mucous membrane from the promontory after first dividing it around the anterior rim of the round window niche. As much as possible of the mucosa

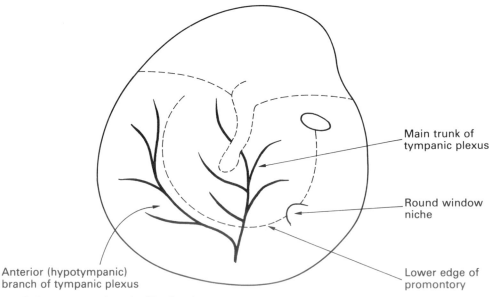

Main trunk of
tympanic plexus

Round window
niche

Anterior (hypotympanic)
branch of tympanic plexus

Lower edge of
promontory

Figure 33.4 The hypotympanic branch of Jacobson's nerve

covering the promontory and hypotympanum should be excised. In most instances this will reveal the main trunk of the nerve lying in a shallow groove on the promontory from which it can be easily elevated and a long segment avulsed. Side branches may already have been removed with the mucous membrane or may be seen running obliquely upwards across the promontory. Where the main trunk is not readily identifiable it will often be found in a small canaliculus covered by a thin plate of bone which may readily be breached with a sharp pick or needle. If, however, the trunk is more deeply placed within the substance of the promontory it can be uncovered by gentle drilling with a small diamond paste burr, bearing in mind the proximity of the basal turn of the cochlea.

It seems likely that the most common cause of an unsuccessful result in this operation is failure to identify and excise the hypotympanic branch. Unfortunately, the nerve tends to lie below the curve of the promontory in the hypotympanum and this area is not only difficult to visualize properly but, because the surface of the bone is often broken up by air cells, the overlying mucosa may be impossible to elevate and the nerve may remain hidden. The anterior branch may, itself, occupy a bony canal in which case it can be very difficult indeed to find. It is imperative, however, to make a thorough search for this branch in every case utilizing higher magnification. The anterior and inferior aspect of the promontory should be cleaned with a small House curette or by careful drilling with a diamond paste burr (Crysdale, 1980).

All middle ear operations involve risk to hearing; Smyth (1976) reported a significant hearing loss occurring in 1% of straightforward myringoplasties. It is, therefore, essential to carry out some form of audiological assessment before surgery and at least 6 weeks should be allowed to elapse before operating on the second ear. Ideally, the hearing should be tested using pure tone audiometry but, unfortunately, in the mentally handicapped patient, this is often not possible. In this situation consideration should be given to evoked response audiometry if this is available. Where the patient has only one hearing ear, it is probably wisest not to proceed with tympanic neurectomy and to consider some other method of treatment instead.

Concern has been expressed in the past about loss of the sense of taste consequent upon dividing both chordae tympani. To preserve the nerve on one side, however, undoubtedly compromises the chances of a worthwhile outcome. Furthermore, it has been the author's experience and that of others that in those patients capable of doing so, there is no complaint resulting from the loss of this faculty and in the rest there is no evidence of loss of appetite. The most likely explanation for this apparent anomaly is that olfaction, the taste buds on the posterior third of the tongue and the texture of food all contribute to the remaining sense of taste.

Results of surgical management

Of necessity, the assessment of the results of these procedures must be rather crude and anecdotal. It has been possible, however, to produce a rough guide based on direct observation of the patients by parents and nursing staff, coupled with an estimation of the decrease in the number of bib or clothing changes required. The criteria used in the assessment are expressed in Table 33.4.

Table 33.4 Criteria for assessment

Result	Meaning
Unchanged	
Improved	A noticeable improvement but drooling still a problem
Good	A noticeable improvement and drooling no longer a problem
Excellent	Drooling has ceased altogether

Surgical management of drooling results in about 85% of patients showing a sustained, good or excellent response. Reported success rates for relocation of the submandibular duct vary from 80–100% (Ekedahl, 1974; Guerin, 1979; Cotton and Richardson, 1981; Bailey and Wadsworth, 1985; Crysdale, 1989; O'Dwyer, Timon and Walsh, 1989). For tympanic neurectomy a successful outcome has been reported in 50–80% of cases (Goode and Smith, 1970; Friedman and Kaplan, 1975; Michel, Johnston and Patterson, 1977; Crysdale, 1980). From the author's own series, the corresponding figures are 71% for relocation of the submandibular ducts and 90% for tympanic neurectomy. If there is no worthwhile reduction in drooling following relocation of the ducts, subsequent tympanic neurectomy can be performed.

Some authors have stated that good results obtained initially with tympanic neurectomy are followed later by return of the initial problem. Crysdale (1980) has suggested that this may be due to regrowth of preganglionic fibres, but the author considers that it is much more likely to be due to failure to find and excise the hypotympanic branch. In the author's series, no patient complained of worsening of drooling following an initial good response to tympanic neurectomy, the follow-up period ranging from 1 to 15 years.

Conclusions

All patients presenting with drooling should be considered for treatment. However, as the presenting problems are almost always social rather than medical, it is essential that a full and frank discussion takes place before decisions are made. No method of treatment carries a guarantee of success. If surgery is considered, more than one operation may be required, some discomfort at least, in the postoperative period must be expected and complications do occur. For these and for many other reasons it is important to ensure that parents, teachers and the patient, if capable of doing so, understand fully the nature of the problem and the methods of dealing with it.

In the small child it would seem sensible to postpone any decisions regarding treatment until he might be expected to have outgrown the phase of physiological drooling. In addition, the technical difficulties of surgery are likely to be considerably greater in the small child than at a later stage of development. It is, therefore, recommended that, in most cases, active intervention should be left until at least the age of 6 years.

If physiotherapy has not already been tried an intensive course, lasting at least 6 months, should be undertaken before surgery is considered. The choice of operation depends on the general physical and mental state of the patient. Where there is evidence of poor swallowing as determined from the history, from discussion with the speech therapist involved or from the results of barium screening or videofluoroscopy, it is unlikely that relocation of the submandibular ducts will succeed. In these cases tympanic neurectomy with division of both chordae tympani is the method of choice. Finally, long-term follow up with continuing counselling and advice is vitally important and should be undertaken in every case.

References

BAILEY, C. M. and WADSWORTH, P. V. (1985) Treatment of the drooling child by submandibular duct transposition. *Journal of Laryngology and Otology*, **99**, 1111–1117

BRODY, G. S. (1977) Control of drooling by translocation of the parotid duct and extirpation of mandibular gland. *Developmental Medicine and Child Neurology*, **19**, 514–517

COTTON, R. T. and RICHARDSON, M. A. (1981) The effect of submandibular duct rerouting in the treatment of sialorrhea in children. *Otolaryngology – Head and Neck Surgery*, **89**, 535–541

CRYSDALE, W. S. (1980) The drooling patient: evaluation and current surgical options. *Laryngoscope*, **90**, 775–783

CRYSDALE, W. S. (1982) Submandibular duct relocation for drooling – how to do it. *Journal of Otolaryngology*, **11**, 286–288

CRYSDALE, W. S. (1989) Submandibular duct relocation for drooling: a 10-year experience with 194 patients. *Otolaryngology – Head and Neck Surgery*, **101**, 87–92

CRYSDALE, W. S., GREENBERG, J., KOHEIL, R. and MORAN, R. (1985) The drooling patient: team evaluation and management. *International Journal of Pediatric Otorhinolaryngology*, **9**, 241–248

EKEDAHL, C. (1974) Surgical treatment of drooling. *Acta Otolaryngologica*, **77**, 215–220

EKEDAHL, C. and HALLÉN, O. (1973) Quantitative measurement of drooling. *Acta Otolaryngologica*, **75**, 464–469

FRIEDMAN, W. H. and KAPLAN, B. (1975) Tympanic neurectomy. Correction of drooling in cerebral palsy. *New York State Journal of Medicine*, **75**, 2419–2422

GLASS, L. W., NOBEL, G. L. and VECCHIONE, T. R. (1978) Treatment of uncontrolled drooling by bilateral excision of submaxillary glands and parotid duct ligations. *Plastic and Reconstructive Surgery*, **62**, 523–526

GOLDING-WOOD, P. H. (1962) Tympanic neurectomy. *Journal of Laryngology and Otology*, **76**, 683–693

GOODE, R. L. and SMITH, R. A. (1970) The surgical management of sialorrhea. *Laryngoscope*, **80**, 1078–1089

GUERIN, R. L. (1979) Surgical management of drooling. *Archives of Otolaryngology*, **105**, 535–537

LAAGE-HELLMANN, J. E. (1969) Retroposition augl submandibularis utforsgong som behandling vid drazling. *Nordisk Medicin*, **82**, 1522–1529

LEMPERT, J. (1946) Tympanosympathectomy. *Archives of Otolaryngology*, **43**, 199–207

MICHEL, R. G., JOHNSTON, K. A. and PATTERSON, C. N. (1977) Parasympathetic nerve section for control of sialorrhea. *Archives of Otolaryngology*, **103**, 94–97

O'DWYER, T. P., TIMON, C. and WALSH, M. A. (1989) Surgical management of drooling in the neurologically damaged child. *Journal of Laryngology and Otology*, **103**, 750–752

PORTO, A. F. JR, WHICKER, J. and PROUD, G. O. (1978) An anatomic study of the hypotympanic branch of Jacobson's nerve. *Laryngoscope*, **88**, 56–60

RAY, S. A., BUNDY, A. C. and NELSON, D. L. (1983) Decreasing drooling through techniques to facilitate mouth closure. *American Journal of Occupational Therapy*, **37**, 749–753

ROSS, J. A. T. (1970) The function of the tympanic plexus as related to Frey's syndrome. *Laryngoscope*, **80**, 1816–1833

SMYTH, G. D. L. (1976) Tympanic reconstruction: fifteen year report on tympanoplasty – Part II. *Journal of Laryngology and Otology*, **110**, 713–741

WATERMAN, E. T., KOLTAI, P. J., DOWNEY, J. C. and CACACE, A. T. (1992) Swallowing disorders in a population of children with cerebral palsy. *International Journal of Pediatric Otorhinolaryngology*, **24**, 63–71

WILKIE, T. F. (1967) The problem of drooling in cerebral palsy – a surgical approach. *Canadian Journal of Surgery*, **10**, 60–67

34

Recurrent respiratory papillomatosis

J. N. G. Evans

The first description of this condition is that of Mackenzie in 1880 when he described papillomas in the larynx of a child and he used the term juvenile laryngeal papillomas. The viral aetiology of this condition was first suggested by Ullman in 1928, who reported the experimental transmission of warts to the vagina of a dog and to his own arm using an extract of human laryngeal papilloma. Recurrent respiratory papillomatosis is a better description of the condition since papillomas are also seen in the adult population and the whole of the respiratory tract may be involved from lips to terminal bronchi.

Aetiology

The infecting agent causing recurrent respiratory papillomatosis is now known to be the human papilloma virus (Gissman et al., 1983), a small DNA virus 50 nm in diameter. The demonstration of viral particles within laryngeal papillomas has met with only limited success (Svoboda, Kirchner and Provd, 1963; Boyle et al., 1973; Stephens et al., 1979).

There are over 70 types of human papilloma virus. This is a group of viruses which is the subject of a great deal of study and research. The genus is typed depending on the homology of their DNA molecules, i.e. the similarity of the sequence of the nucleotide pairings in their DNA molecules (McCance and Gardner, 1990).

Human papilloma viruses 6 and 11 are thought to be the main causal agents in recurrent respiratory papillomatosis; these are the same viruses that cause warts on the penis, vulva, cervix and perianal areas.

There is considerable circumstantial evidence that, in some patients, the disease may be transmitted at the time of delivery. If a child contracts the disease before the age of 5 years there is a 60% probability that the mother had genital warts at the time of delivery (Strong et al., 1976). It is because of this association that mothers should be advised to have subsequent children by caesarian section.

After infection the virus may remain in the basal layer of the mucous membrane replicating by a process known as episomal maintenance, where the virus itself is undetectable and its presence can only be determined by DNA hybridization (Lock et al., 1980; Braun et al., 1982; Terry et al., 1987; Quiney et al., 1989).

As the cells of the basal layer differentiate, changes in the host cell allow the viral genes to be switched on (transcribed) and viral particles can be identified in the stratum granulosum and corneum (Figure 34.1).

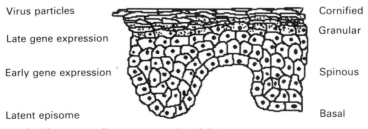

Figure 34.1 Replicative cycle of human papilloma virus in infected skin

Epidemiology

Recurrent respiratory papillomatosis has a worldwide distribution. The incidence in the USA was stated as 7 per million per year (Strong *et al.*, 1976) and in Denmark 3.84 per million per year (Lindeberg and Elbroend, 1990). These cases were distributed between children and adults; slightly more cases being diagnosed before the age of 16 years than after. Furthermore, recurrent respiratory papillomatosis is found in all socioeconomic groups and is not confined to the disadvantaged as was previously claimed. In children there is a female preponderance in contrast with the adult group where the reverse is true (Lindeberg *et al.*, 1986; Robb, 1987).

Presenting symptoms

The majority of children with recurrent respiratory papillomatosis present before the age of 4 years, although a not insignificant number may present during the first 6 months of life.

The initial symptom is hoarseness of voice or an abnormal cry. Increasing stridor and acute respiratory obstruction may occur but are usually late manifestations of the disease process. Papillomas form initially on the vocal cords themselves so interference with laryngeal function occurs early in the disease. Hoarseness in a child should not be dismissed as being the result of vocal abuse, an endoscopy must be performed to establish the diagnosis.

There is a tendency for papillomas to occur at the anterior aspect of the glottis and the anterior commisure itself is frequently involved. It is uncommon for the interarytenoid mucosa to be involved in early cases; perhaps the thickness of the mucus blanket and the more rapid rate of its movement exerts a protective role in this situation. When the larynx is extensively involved the normal flow of the mucus blanket is disrupted and the papillomas then invade the whole of the larynx with equal facility. The disruption of the tracheal mucus blanket that occurs after tracheostomy may also be a factor in the often explosive increase in tracheal papillomas that is seen after a tracheostomy has been performed. According to Batsakis, Raymond and Rice (1983), 2% of all affected patients will eventually develop bronchial involvement. It is for this reason that a tracheostomy should be avoided if it is possible to establish a normal airway by endoscopic removal of the papillomas.

Characteristics of the disease

The papillomas of recurrent respiratory papillomatosis are benign squamous papillomas that occur in clusters on the involved mucosa (Figure 34.2), the fronds of papilloma may be sessile and spread over a

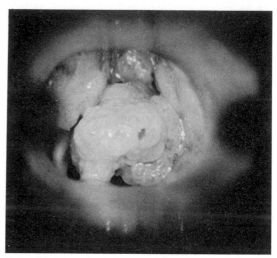

Figure 34.2 Fronds of papillomas filling the laryngeal lumen; the patient was tracheostomy dependent

wide area of mucosa or they may be pedunculated and localized (Figure 34.3).

It is characteristic that the lesions are multiple; occasionally at the onset of the disease or if the disease is about to become quiescent, only a single lesion may be manifest.

The lesions are notoriously recurrent even after the most radical extirpation. Recurrence may become an airway problem within 2 weeks or nothing may be visible for perhaps 5 or 20 years.

The presence of the viral episome in apparently normal cells accounts for the paradox of recurrence of papillomas after their complete removal.

On some occasions it appears that removal of the papillomas has an enhancing effect on the growth rate of the lesions, so that the recurrence may be larger than the original lesion.

Recurrent respiratory papillomatosis is a diffuse diathesis of the mucous membrane of the upper air and food passages; the papillomas may be encountered in the nostrils at the mucocutaneous junction, on the gingiva and lips (Figure 34.4), on both surfaces of the soft palate and the adjacent tonsillar pillars, in the larynx, in the tracheobronchial tree and occasionally in the pulmonary parenchyma and at the oesophageal inlet. The lesions have a predilection for points of airway constriction where there is increased air flow, drying, crusting and irritation; this is particularly evident around the tracheostomy site and at the tip of the tracheostomy tube. Most commonly the larynx is the site of greatest involvement and is often the only site (Strong *et al.*, 1976).

Remission

Remission of recurrent respiratory papillomatosis can take place at any age and at any time; whether

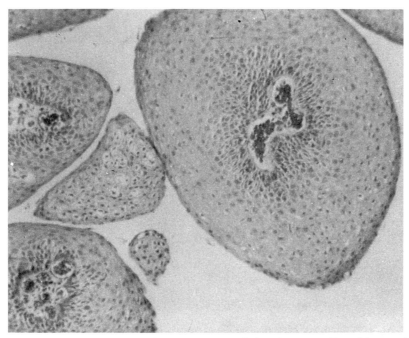

Figure 34.3 In each frond of papilloma the hyperplastic squamous epithelium is supported by a thin vascular core of connective tissue. Maturation takes place but ceases prior to keratinization unless the lesion is otherwise irritated or stimulated

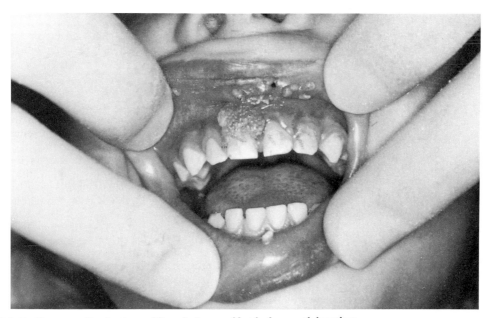

Figure 34.4 Papillomas on the gingiva and lips of a 5-year-old girl who mouth breathes

remission occurs or not appears to be unrelated to the thoroughness of the removal or to the method of removal of the disease. Table 34.1 shows that the chance of remission is greatest if the disease presents between the ages of 6 and 10 years ($P = 0.01$).

The overall chance of achieving remission in patients less than 16 years of age at the time of presentation is 46% if they are followed for 1 year and treated by appropriate endoscopy and laser destruction; this can be compared with a 26% chance of remission if

Table 34.1 Age of patients at time of remission

Age (years)	No. in remission (%)
1–5	15/46 (33)
6–10	16/23 (70)
11–13	6/12 (50)
Total	37/81 (46)

the disease becomes manifest at 16 years of age or later. Furthermore, the disease is more likely to undergo remission in the larynx (48%), than in the tracheobronchial tree (27%) or in the lungs (0%).

Duration of remission

The duration of remission varies from 2 years to life long. Relapses may occur at any time and for no apparent reason. Since a relapse may occur in any patient at any time, the best that can be hoped for at present is prolonged remission rather than cure (Strong, 1987).

Unfortunately, respiratory papillomatosis does have the potential to spread in a small number of cases from the larynx to involve the tracheobronchial tree. This is not uncommon and occurs in 11% of cases, with the lung parenchyma involved in 3% of cases (Strong, 1987).

In the lungs the disease produces cystic spaces which may be seen on X-ray. The cysts are lined with squamous epithelium and may be filled with fluid or air. The pulmonary spread is multicentric, relentlessly progressive and eventually fatal (Figure 34.5).

Malignant degeneration

The risk of malignant degeneration is extremely low unless radiotherapy had been used in an attempt to control the disease; thus radiotherapy is contraindicated in recurrent respiratory papillomatosis. In adults who smoke, malignant degeneration is not unusual; in Strong's series, reported in 1987, two cases of squamous cell carcinoma and three of verrucous carcinoma were encountered. A few other cases have been documented in the literature (Matsula *et al.*, 1985).

Management

The mainstay of treatment for juvenile respiratory papillomas is surgical extirpation. Vaporization with the CO_2 laser is the most acceptable mode of treatment as it carries the least risk of damage to the surrounding tissues. Nevertheless, scarring at the anterior commissure and posterior commissure is seen in a significant number of patients (Wetmore, Key and Swen, 1985; Crockett, McCabe and Shive, 1987; Saleh, 1992).

In order to reduce the scarring to a minimum great care should be taken by the endoscopist to try

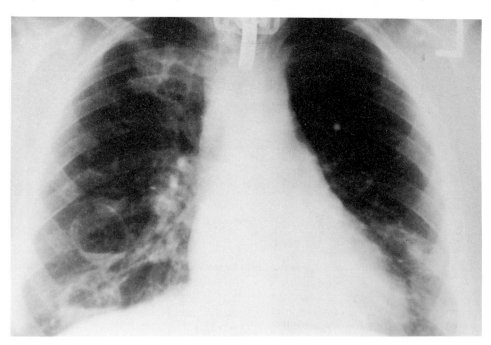

Figure 34.5 The multiple cysts in the right lung are lined with squamous epithelium, some contain air

to avoid damage to the underlying and adjacent mucous membranes with the avoidance of exposure of the vocalis muscle.

Papillomas at the anterior commissure are particularly prone to produce scarring so treatments should be separated by a month and only one cord treated at a time. Low power settings with the laser in intermittent mode or the newer microspot lasers also help to reduce scarring and web formation (Ossof, Wekhoven and Dere, 1991). Most of the papillomas can be removed around a metal or laser-proof tube introduced at the time of endoscopy (Figure 34.6). Those papillomas remaining at the posterior commissure can be dealt with after removal of the tube and with the patient breathing spontaneously or ventilation can be maintained with a ventive jet. Great care must be taken when using the laser to avoid accidental damage to the patient and to the theatre staff.

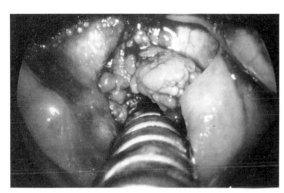

Figure 34.6 View of the larynx at microlaryngoscopy with metal laser-proof tube *in situ*

An additional hazard to theatre personnel may be the inhalation of smoke generated by the laser in which human papilloma viral DNA has been found (Ito, 1960; Ito and Evans, 1961; Kashima *et al.*, 1991).

The multifocal nature of the disease with dormant viral episomes present in the basal layer means that its definitive treatment must be medical. Patients with respiratory papillomatosis may demonstrate reduced immunocompetency (Perrick *et al.*, 1990) and both immunomodulating agents and antiviral agents have been employed. These include inosine pranobex (Patel, Gemmel and Carruth, 1987), adenine arabenoside (Hendrickse *et al.*, 1985), lysozyme chlorhydrate, (Altmar, 1990), acyclovir (Aguado *et al.*, 1991; Morrison and Evans, 1992) and ribavirin (Morrison, Kotecha and Evans, 1993). While some of these may have had a beneficial adjuvant effect, none has been established as having a major role in the treatment of respiratory papillomatosis.

The use of interferon, which acts by producing

enzymes to prevent viral replication and stimulate host defences by increasing lymphocytotoxic activity of killer lymphocytes, also enhances the activity of macrophages and increases antibody-dependent cell-mediated cytotoxicity. These activities have been extensively investigated by Lundquist *et al.* (1984), Healy *et al.* (1988), Benjamin *et al.* (1988), Leventhal *et al.* (1988), Mullooly *et al.* (1988) and Mattot *et al.* (1990). After initial enthusiasm for its use, substantial long-lasting remissions have not been seen in most centres including The Hospital for Sick Children, Great Ormond Street. A multicentre trial, which included our patients, showed that after the first 6 months of treatment the benefits were no longer significant (Healy *et al.*, 1988).

Conclusions

The treatment of recurrent respiratory papillomatosis has been bedevilled by false dawns of hope as each new treatment modality has been tried and success claimed. The treatment remains an enigma but careful removal of the papilloma using the CO_2 laser while awaiting a spontaneous remission seems to be the best available until we can stimulate the host response by adjuvant therapy to eradicate the causative viral episomes.

References

AGUADO, L. A., PINERO, B. P., BETANCOR, L., MENDEZ, A. and BANALES, E. C. (1991) Acyclovir in the treatment of laryngeal papillomatosis. *International Journal of Pediatric Otorhinolaryngology*, **21**, 269–274

ALTMAR, R. J. (1990) Lysozyme in the treatment of juvenile laryngeal papillomatosis. A new concept in its aetiopatheogenesis. *Anales Otorrinolaringologicos Ibero-Americanos*, **17**, 495–504

BATSAKIS, J. G., RAYMOND, A. K. and RICE, D. H. (1983) The pathology of head and neck tumors: papillomas of the upper aerodigestive tract. Part 18. *Head and Neck Surgery*, **5**, 322–344

BENJAMIN, B. N., GATENBY, P. A., KITCHEN, R., HARRISON, H., CAMERON, K. and BASTEN, A. (1988) Alpha-interferon (Wellferon) as an adjunct to standard surgical therapy in the management of recurrent respiratory papillomatosis. *Annals of Otology, Rhinology and Laryngology*, **94**, 376–380

BOYLE, W. F., RIGGS, J. L., OSHIRO, L. S., and LENNETT, E. E. H. (1973) Electron microscopic identification of papova virus in laryngeal papillomata. *Laryngoscope*, **83**, 1102–1108

BRAUN, L., KASHIMA, H., EGGLESTON, J. and SHAH, K. (1982) Demonstration of papillomavirus antigen in paraffin sections of laryngeal papillomas. *Laryngoscope*, **92**, 640–643

CROCKETT, M. D., MCCABE, F. B. and SHIVE, J. C. (1987) Complications of laser surgery for recurrent respiratory papillomatosis. *Annals of Otology, Rhinology and Laryngology*, **96**, 639–644

GISSMAN, L., WOLNICK, L., IKENBURG, H., KOLDOVSKY, U., SCHNURCH, H. G. and ZUR HAUSEN, H. (1983) Human papilloma virus types 6 and 11 DNA sequences in genital and laryngeal papillomas and in some cervical cancers. *Proceedings of the National Academy of Science USA*, **80**, 560–563

HEALY, G. B., GELBER, R. D., TROWBRIDGE, A. L., GRUNDFAST, K. M., RUBEN, R. J. and PRICE, K. N. (1988) Treatment of recurrent respiratory papillomatosis with human leucocyte interferon. Results of multi centre randomized clinical trial. *New England Journal of Medicine*, **319**, 401–407

HENDRICKSE, W. A., IRWIN, B. C., LEVINSKY, R. J., BAILEY, C. M., TYMM, G. and EVANS, J. N. G. (1985) Treatment of respiratory papillomatosis with adenosine arabinoside. *Archives of Diseases in Childhood*, **60**, 374–376

ITO, Y. (1960) A tumour producing factor extracted by phenol from papillomatous tissue of cottontail rabbits. *Virology*, **12**, 596–601

ITO, Y. and EVANS, C. A. (1961) Induction of tumours in domestic rabbits with nucleic acid preparations from partially purified shape papilloma virus and from extracts of the papillomas of domestic and cottontail rabbits. *Journal of Experimental Medicine*, **114**, 485–500

KASHIMA, H. G., KESSIS, T., MOUNTS, P. and SHAH, K. (1991) Polymerase chain reaction identification of human papilloma virus DNA in CO_2 laser plume from recurrent respiratory papillomatosis. *Otolaryngology – Head and Neck Surgery*, **104**, 191–195

LEVENTHAL, B. G., KASHIMA, H. K., WECK, P. W., MOUNTS, P., WHISNANT, J. K., CLARK, K. L. et al. (1988) Randomized surgical adjuvant trial of interferon alfa-nl in recurrent papillomatosis. *Archives of Otolaryngology – Head and Neck Surgery*, **114**, 1163–1169

LINDEBERG, H. and ELBROEND, O. (1990) Laryngeal papillomas: the epidemiology in a Danish sub-population 1965–84. *Clinical Otolaryngology*, **15**, 125–131

LINDEBERG, H., OSTER, S., OXLUND, I. and ELBROEND, O. (1986) Laryngeal papillomatosis; classification and course. *Clinical Otolaryngology*, **11**, 423–429

LOCK, E. E., JENSON, A. B., SMITH, H. G., HEALY, G. B., PASS, F. and VAWTER, G. F. (1980) Immunoperoxidase localization of human papillomavirus in laryngeal papillomas. *Intervirology*, **14**, 148–154

LUNDQUIST, P.-G., HAGLUND, S., CARLSOO, B., STRANDER, H. and LUNGREN, E. (1984) Interferon therapy in juvenile laryngeal papillomatosis. *Otolaryngology – Head and Neck Surgery*, **92**, 386–391

MCCANCE, D. J. and GARDNER, S. D. (1990) Papova viruses: papilloma viruses and polyoma viruses. In: *Principles and Practice of Clinical Virology*, 2nd edn, edited by A. J. Zuckerman, J. E. Banatvala and J. R. Pattison. Chichester: John Wiley and Sons. pp. 535–545

MACKENZIE, M. (1880) Diseases of the pharynx, larynx and trachea. *A Manual of Diseases of the Throat and Nose*. New-York. William Wood and Company. Vol. 1, p. 305.

MATSULA, H. M., THAWLEY, S. E., SPECTOR, G. J., MAUNCY, M. and PIKUL, F. J. (1985) Laryngeal epidermoid carcinoma associated with juvenile laryngeal papillomatosis. *Laryngoscope*, **95**, 1264–1271

MATTOT, M., NINANE, J., HAMOIR, M., MOULIN, D., MUSTIN, V., VERMYLEN, C. et al. (1990) Combined CO_2 laser and alfa

recombinant interferon treatment in five children with juvenile laryngeal papillomatosis. *Acta Clinica Belgica*, **45**, 158–163

MORRISON, G. A. J. and EVANS, J. N. G. (1993) Juvenile respiratory papillomatosis: acyclovir reassessed. *International Journal of Pediatric Otorhinolaryngology*, **26**, 193–197

MORRISON, G. A. J., KOTECHA, B. and EVANS, J. N. G. (1993) Ribavirin treatment for juvenile respiratory papillomatosis. *Journal of Laryngology and Otology*, **107**, 423–426

MULLOOLY, V. M., ABRAMSON, A. L., STEINBERG, B. M. and HOROWITZ, M. S. (1988) Clinical effects of alpha-interferon dose variation on laryngeal papillomatosis. *Laryngoscope*, **98**, 1324–1329

OSSOF, R. H., WEKHOVEN, J. A. and DERE, H. (1991) Soft tissue complications of laser surgery for recurrent laryngeal papillomatosis. *Laryngoscope*, **101**, 1162–1166

PATEL, P., GEMMELL, R. and CARRUTH, J. (1987) Inosine pranobex in recurrent laryngeal papillomatosis. *Journal of Laryngology and Otology*, **101**, 1306–1307

PERRICK, D., WRAY, B. B., LEFFEL, M. S., HARMON, J. D. and POROBSKY, E. S. (1990) Evaluation of immunocompetency in juvenile laryngeal papillomatosis. *Annals of Allergy*, **65**, 69–72

QUINEY, R. E., WELLS, M., LEWIS, F. A., TERRY, R. M., MICHAELS, L. and CROFT, C. B. (1989) Laryngeal papillomatosis: correlation between severity of disease and presence of H.P.V. 6 and 11 detected by in situ DNA hybridization. *Journal of Clinical Pathology*, **42**, 694–698

ROBB, P. J. (1987) The CO_2 laser and management of recurrent laryngeal papilloma: the Guy's experience. *Journal of Laryngology and Otology*, **101**, 369–75

SALEH, E. M. (1992) Complications of treatment of recurrent laryngeal papillomatosis with the carbon dioxide laser in children. *Journal of Laryngology and Otology*, **106**, 715–718

STEPHENS, C. B., ARNOLD, G. E., BUTCHKO, G. M. and HARDY, C. L. (1979) Autogenous vaccine treatment of juvenile laryngeal papillomatosis. *Laryngoscope*, **89**, 1689–1696

STRONG, M. S. (1987) Recurrent respiratory papillomatosis. In: *Scott Brown's Otolaryngology* 5th edn, edited by A. G. Kerr, vol. 6 *Paediatric Otolaryngology*, edited by J. N. G. Evans, London: Butterworth. pp. 466–470

STRONG, M., VAUGHAN, C. W., HEALY, B., COOPERBAND, S. and CLEMENTE, M. (1976) Recurrent respiratory papillomatosis. *Annals of Otology, Rhinology and Laryngology*, **85**, 508–516

SVOBODA, D. J., KIRCHNER, F. R. and PROVD, G. O. (1963) Electron microscopic study of human laryngeal papillomatosis. *Cancer Research*, **23**, 1084–1089

TERRY, R. M., LEWIS, F. A., GRIFFITHS, S., WELLS, M. and BIRD, C. C. (1987) Demonstration of hyman papillomavirus types 6 and 11 in juvenile laryngeal papillomatosis by in-situ hybridisation. *Journal of Pathology*, **153**, 245–248

ULLMAN, E. V. (1928) On the aetiology of laryngeal papilloma. *Acta Otolaryngologica*, **5**, 317–338

WETMORE, S. J., KEY, J. M. and SWEN, J. Y. (1985) Complications of laser surgery for laryngeal papillomatosis. *Laryngoscope*, **95**, 798–801

35

Paediatric anaesthesia

E. F. Battersby

There is no difference between adult and paediatric practice in the basic concepts of anaesthesia. There are, however, very important differences in the anatomy and physiology which have a significant impact on the conduct and safety of the anaesthetic. These differences are at their extreme in the neonatal period – the first 28 days of extrauterine life – but some remain of importance until 4–5 years of age (Table 35.1). Of equal importance is the infant's psychological development, particular problems being experienced at 2–3 years of age with the emergence of independence but the continuing need for security. Those who practise otolaryngological anaesthesia and surgery must appreciate the nature of the cardiorespiratory changes if the peri-anaesthetic period is to be conducted without morbidity, and optimum

conditions provided so that the correct diagnosis and treatment can be established. In no other branch of surgery is an understanding of each other's problems, cooperation and communication between surgeon and anaesthetist more important to the welfare of the patient.

Neonatal physiology

The respiratory system

Major changes occur in the respiratory system with the adaptation to extrauterine life and the gaseous expansion of the lungs during the first few breaths. Lung growth continues albeit at a reducing rate until about 5 years of age.

Table 35.1 Normal values in full-term infants compared with adults

	Infant	Adult
Weight (kg)	3.0	70
Surface area (m²)	0.19	1.8
Surface area/weight (m²/kg)	0.06	0.03
Respiratory frequency (breaths/minute)	30–40	12–16
Tidal volume (V_T) (ml/kg)	6–8	7
Dead space (V_D) (ml/kg)	2–2.5	2.2
V_D/V_T	0.3	0.3
Vital capacity (VC) (ml/kg)	35–40	50–60
Thoracic gas volume (TGV) (ml/kg)	35–40	30
Functional residual capacity (FRC) (ml/kg)	27–30	30
Lung compliance (C_L) (ml/cmH$_2$O)	5–6	200
Specific compliance (C_L/FRC) (ml/cmH$_2$O per ml)	0.04–0.06	0.04–0.07
Airways resistance (R_{aw}) (cmH$_2$O/l per s)	25–30	1.6
Work of breathing (g/cm per l)	2000–4000	2000–7000
Resting alveolar ventilation (V_A) (ml/kg per minute)	100–150	60
Resting oxygen consumption (V_{O_2}) (ml/kg per minute)	6.8	3.3

Anatomy of the airway

The neonate has a relatively large head and a short neck. The larynx lies opposite the lower border of the vertebral body of C4 and does not reach the adult position of C5–6 until 4 years of age. The epiglottis is inclined to the posterior pharyngeal wall at an angle of 45° and the glottis is in a more anterior position than in the adult. The tongue is relatively large. This combination of a high forward-looking larynx and a large tongue makes tracheal intubation difficult using a curved laryngoscope with the blade placed in the vallecula. A straight blade of the Magill type with the tip posterior to the epiglottis at the anterior commissure gives optimum conditions for tracheal intubation. The head should be in the neutral position (Creighton, 1994). By 1 year of age changes towards the adult position have occurred so that either method of intubation is satisfactory. Both straight and curved laryngoscopes should be available when anaesthetizing the small infant.

The narrowest part of the airway is the cricoid ring which is complete and may not accept a tracheal tube which has passed through the glottis. The cricoid is slightly elliptical in shape and, in a newborn infant weighing 2.5 kg, should have a sagittal diameter of 0.5 cm, a coronal diameter of 0.55 cm and a surface area of 0.25 cm². The variations in size and rate of growth of the cricoid cartilage are discussed by Too-Chung and Green (1974).

Minimal oedema at the cricoid ring may reduce the airway by up to 60% in the neonate. The trachea is about 4 cm in length. Unless measurement of tracheal tube length and fixation are carried out meticulously, accidental extubation or bronchus intubation may readily occur. Air entry to both lungs should always be checked after intubation in an infant.

The lung

Oxygen consumption in the normal newborn infant at neutral environmental temperature is 7 ml/kg per minute which is twice that of the adult on a weight basis. This requires a minute alveolar ventilation of 150 ml/kg per minute, twice that of the adult, which is achieved largely by an increased respiratory rate because of a relatively small inspiratory reserve volume in the neonate. There is a higher dead space ventilation per minute because of the higher rate of breathing. Falls in inspired oxygen concentration will rapidly affect arterial oxygen concentration. Airway resistance is high due to the small bore of the airways but an intrathoracic pressure change of only 5 cmH₂O is needed for normal tidal breathing. However, airway resistance forms a larger fraction of total resistance than in the adult, and infants are particularly at risk from the development of small airway obstruction.

Chest wall compliance in the neonate is about five times as great as lung compliance, whereas these are about equal in the adult. This more flexible chest wall means that relatively little work is required to move the chest cage in quiet breathing, but provides a rather unstable chest cage if the work of breathing is markedly increased due to airway obstruction or non-compliant lungs. The clinical assessment of increased work of breathing may be very difficult in the neonate as chest cage retraction and paradoxical breathing can leave the impression of good chest expansion in the presence of minimal alveolar ventilation. Increasing respiratory rates above 60 breaths per minute indicate the need for continuing close observation. Serial blood gas analysis is more helpful in the assessment of adequate alveolar ventilation in the neonate than it is in the older child.

The relatively low outward recoil force of the chest wall is probably the cause of the tendency of the newborn lung to stabilize with a relatively low functional residual capacity (FRC). This is also likely to be the cause of the tendency to peripheral airway closure with increased intrapulmonary shunting, hypoxia and peripheral gas trapping. These problems can be helped by the use of a continuous distending pressure applied to the airway (Figure 35.1). This forms an important aspect of the management of both respiratory failure and general anaesthesia in the newborn.

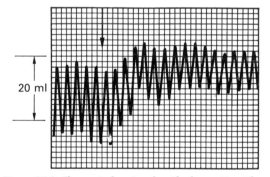

Figure 35.1 Change in functional residual capacity with continuous positive airway pressure (10 cmH₂O)

The healthy newborn infant uses about 1% of his energy expenditure in breathing, 75% of this to overcome elastic resistance and 25% flow resistance. A respiratory rate of 30–40 breaths per minute is the most efficient with regard to energy consumption. Increases in airway resistance or pulmonary stiffness will increase the work of breathing considerably so that it represents a very significant percentage of metabolic rate. Both these factors are likely to increase intrapulmonary shunting and consequently lower oxygen availability. Some reversal of this trend is achieved by the use of continuous positive airway pressure (CPAP) (Gregory *et al.*, 1971; Cogswell *et al.*, 1975).

The circulation

Major changes occur in the circulation at birth with the loss of the low resistance vascular bed of the placenta and the opening up of the high resistance pulmonary vascular bed. Pulmonary vascular resistance decreases dramatically after aeration of the lungs, but remains labile for some time until there is regression of the smooth muscle in the terminal arteriolar wall. A partial return to the circulation *in utero* may occur if the pulmonary vascular resistance rises and fetal anastomotic channels such as the ductus arteriosus and foramen ovale re-open. This is known as persistent pulmonary hypertension and up to 70–80% of the cardiac output may shunt right to left through these channels resulting in severe systemic desaturation. The pulmonary arteriolar smooth muscle constricts in response to hypoxaemia, hypercapnia and acidosis.

This damaging triad may be present in the neonate with severe airway obstruction and aggressive treatment is required if cerebral damage from hypoxia or venous congestion is to be prevented.

The neonate has a smaller percentage of myocardial contractile muscle mass than the adult, and severe hypoxaemia and acidosis may cause a 25% fall in cardiac output. Cardiac stroke volume remains relatively fixed in the neonatal period and cardiac output is closely related to cardiac rate, falling significantly at pulse rates below 100 per minute.

Several anaesthetic techniques which cause cardiac slowing will also cause a major fall in cardiac output.

The response to postural changes is less efficient so that hypovolaemia and head-up tilting are less well tolerated than in the older child. Normal pulse rate and blood pressure in childhood are shown in Tables 35.2 and 35.3).

Table 35.2 Normal heart rate (beats per minute)

Age	Average rate
Preterm	150 ± 20
Term	135 ± 20
1 month	160 ± 20
6 months	140 ± 20
1 year	120 ± 20
2 years	110 ± 20
5 years	90 ± 20
10 years	80 ± 20

Temperature control

The neonate is adversely affected by exposure to an environmental temperature just below normal body

Table 35.3 Normal blood pressure (mmHg)

Age	Blood pressure	Average range	
		Systolic	Diastolic
Neonate	80–50	80 ± 15	50 ± 15
6 months	90–60	90 ± 20	60 ± 10
1 year	95–65	95 ± 30	65 ± 20
2 years	100–65	100 ± 25	65 ± 25
5 years	95–55	95 ± 15	55 ± 10
10 years	110–60	110 ± 15	60 ± 10

temperature which is outside a very narrow range. The smaller the newborn the narrower is this neutral temperature range and the nearer it approaches normal body temperature.

There are several reasons for this; the newborn has a surface area relative to body mass nearly three times that of the adult and an insulating layer of subcutaneous tissue which at best is only half that of the adult and is frequently very much less. The normal mechanisms of cutaneous vasconstriction and dilatation do take place, but they can only compensate for very modest changes in environmental temperature.

About 70% of heat loss takes place by convection, radiation and conduction, and this can be greatly reduced by keeping the baby covered and nursed in a microclimate. This applies equally during transportation, resuscitation, induction of anaesthesia, application of monitoring equipment, surgery and recovery. Some exposure is necessary for adequate observation and the effects of this can be reduced by a warm draught-free operating theatre and the use of heating appliances such as an air mattress.

The principal mechanism for temperature maintenance in the neonate is increased heat production from the oxidation of triglycerides present in the brown fat deposits. The reaction is mediated via the sympathetic nervous system. Metabolism can increase threefold with a large increase in oxygen consumption, but this does not compensate for the large heat losses which occur in an unfavourable thermal environment. This metabolic response to cold is inhibited by hypoxia, which it may help to create and by hypoglycaemia, prematurity and general anaesthesia.

Day admission surgery

Day admission surgery is now well established and has many benefits in the paediatric field.

The requirements for safe and successful day case work are organization, careful case selection and a high standard of surgery and anaesthesia. The concept of 'inpatient for a day' expressed by Atkinson (1982) is important and haematological investigations and X-rays that are deemed necessary must be undertaken and the results seen before surgery commences. Case selection is important and reflects factors associated with the patient and with the operation. Patients should have a reasonable journey, adequate living conditions and be free of intercurrent infections. However, patients with long-term illnesses or malformations that have been fully investigated and are stable may be suitable for day-stay admission if the surgery and anaesthesia are unlikely to cause destabilization.

The type of surgery should preferably be less than 1 hour's duration, not enter body cavities, be unlikely to cause postoperative bleeding, and lead only to moderate pain that can be controlled by a local block or a mild oral analgesic. Operations suitable for day admission include minor nose operations such as diathermy to turbinates, antral washout, antrostomy and polypectomy. Minor surgery to the pinna, excision of accessory auricles, myringotomy, ventilation tube insertion and some patients for adenoidectomy are suitable, but the author's own policy does not include tonsillectomy because of the need for analgesic agents and the risk of haemorrhage during the first 24 hours. Laryngoscopy for minor stridor and some patients receiving laser treatment may be suitable for day discharge, but if doubt exists it is wise to warn parents that overnight admission may be necessary in the event of a more lengthy or major procedure being performed.

Anaesthesia has no particular restrictions but most children should not need premedication other than the use of Emla cream to aid the acceptance of venepuncture. Parental presence at induction of anaesthesia is now commonplace as the child is usually happier and more cooperative. This is not always the case and this complex issue has been studied by Bevan *et al.* (1990) and Vessey *et al.* (1994).

Premedication, intravenous and postoperative analgesics which are associated with nausea and vomiting should be avoided if at all possible, and if used, should be coupled with an antiemetic. Muscle relaxants are not contraindicated, but suxamethonium should be avoided in older children as its use is sometimes associated with postoperative muscle pains in ambulant patients. Tracheal intubation should not be withheld if the operation suggests its need, but it must be atraumatic with a loose-fitting tube. In most instances the laryngeal mask airway is a preferable alternative (Brain *et al.*, 1985; Mason and Bingham, 1990).

Patients should be kept under supervision for 2–4 hours after regaining consciousness and must be checked by a competent medical person before discharge. Parents should be advised about feeding, analgesics and possible significant postoperative complications before discharge.

Airway obstruction

Airway obstruction forms a major part of infant otolaryngology and ranges from the urgent diagnosis and relief of severe life-threatening obstruction to assessment of a variety of causes of stridor. The implication of some of the causes may mean a prolonged, difficult and disruptive period for both the parents and patient, often with a long-term tracheostomy and much surgery. Other diagnoses mean repeated inactivity and reassurance of the parents that significant and worrying stridor will eventually disappear. Nothing is more damaging to parental security and ability to manage than conflicting diagnoses and changing management regimens. Anaesthetists must be able to provide the surgeon with the operating conditions that allow the correct diagnosis to be made.

The newborn infant rarely presents with airway obstruction in the first days of life, but when this occurs it requires urgent and expert management. The older infant may present for the diagnosis and appropriate treatment of stridor. Over recent years small infants are seen who have been difficult to extubate or who have stridor appearing after satisfactory and successful care in a preterm neonatal intensive care unit where respiratory support has been required. Finally, older infants and young children who have been leading normal healthy lives may suddenly appear with an acute infective upper airway obstruction which is life-threatening. These will usually appear in non-specialist units and require prompt and correct management if damaging side effects or loss of life are to be avoided. Stridor in paediatric patients has been reviewed by Maze and Bloch (1979) and Hatch (1985).

The neonate

Airway obstruction is responsible for nearly all the otolaryngology admissions in the first 2 weeks of life and is the result of some form of developmental malformation. Infants with a lesser degree of congenital obstruction, or acquired lesions, will present later in infancy. Newborns presenting in the first 2 weeks of life will have serious problems which are likely to require urgent diagnosis and treatment, and the medical and anaesthetic management differs slightly from that in the older infant. The causes are shown in Table 35.4.

Airway obstruction that is severe or prolonged or has bouts of near total obstruction may be fatal or result in permanent neurological damage from cerebral hypoxia or intraventricular haemorrhage. Feeding is difficult, glycogen stores may be rapidly utilized and blood glucose may fall to a level which causes cerebral neuronal damage – below 1.7 mmol/l (30 mg%). Feeding by nasogastric tube is necessary but

Table 35.4 Causes of respiratory obstruction in the newborn

Nose
1 Bilateral postchoanal atresia
2 Absent nose

Pharynx
1 Maxillofacial deformities associated with mandibular hypoplasia such as Treacher Collins syndrome and Pierre Robin syndrome
2 Macroglossia
    Beckwith syndrome
    haemangioma
3 Lymphangioma
    cystic hygroma
4 Haemangioma

Supraglottis
1 Isolated cysts – vallecular or epiglottic
2 Multiple cysts – cystic hygroma

Glottis
1 Bilateral vocal cord palsy
    central nervous system and vagus nerve lesions
2 Laryngomalacia and atresia

Subglottis
1 Congenital stenosis or web
2 Haemangioma

Trachea
1 Tracheomalacia – unstable trachea
2 Microtrachea – small closed cartilage rings
3 Localized web or stenosis
4 Extrinsic compression
    vascular ring with localized tracheomalacia
    any intrathoracic tumour

may aggravate the airway obstruction as the newborn is an obligate nose breather. The neonatal trachea is soft and will collapse with respiratory effort in the presence of an obstructive lesion elsewhere in the airway, thus the differentiation from tracheomalacia may be difficult.

The classic signs of infant airway obstruction are stridor, intercostal indrawing, chest recession which is usually severe because of the compliant nature of the rib cage, and a respiratory rate increasing above 60 breaths per minute. The above may not be so obvious in the first days of life and the main signs may be non-specific, with an irregular breathing pattern, apnoeic attacks, intermittent cyanosis, bradycardia and peripheral circulatory failure. If doubt exists about the diagnosis because of atypical presentation, a rapid screen to distinguish from congenital heart disease, or primary pulmonary or intrathoracic pathology must take place, remembering that congenital malformations are often multiple.

Clinical examination must include a check for

facial, mouth and neck malformations, and patency of the posterior choana and oesophagus using a nasogastric tube. Assessment of cardiac and liver size and the presence of femoral pulses is an essential preliminary cardiovascular screen. A plain X-ray of neck, chest and abdomen is necessary to rule out pneumothorax, diaphragmatic hernia and other intrathoracic and thoracic inlet pathology. If doubt about heart disease exists then an electrocardiograph (ECG) and two-dimensional echocardiogram should be performed. X-ray contrast studies of the oesophagus to define a vascular ring may be omitted at this stage because of the danger of aspiration. Blood gas estimation is neither diagnostic of any one pathology nor the degree of obstruction, but an indication of the well-being of the neonate. Normal values of blood gases at 24 hours of age are shown in Table 35.5. Serial blood gases are only marginally helpful in making a decision to proceed to a surgical assessment of the obstruction which should, if possible, be carried out before these values deteriorate.

Table 35.5 Normal blood gases at age 24 hours

pH	7.35	7.35
P_aCO_2	4.5 kPa	34 mmHg
P_aO_2	10.6 kPa	80 mmHg
Base excess	– 4 mmol/l	– 4 mmol/l

Diagnostic laryngoscopy should be undertaken in an operating theatre with full surgical and theatre teams present. Premedication with atropine 0.1 mg intramuscularly helps to dry secretions, stabilize a more rapid pulse rate and maintains cardiac output. A precordial stethoscope, ECG, intravenous cannula and warm draught-free theatre are essential. Preoxygenation using a tight-fitting mask, end-expiratory pressure and assisted ventilation allows some further assessment of the degree of obstruction prior to attempted awake laryngoscopy and tracheal intubation. Problems with visualization of the glottis due to facial or pharyngeal malformations will already have been noted, and unexpected solitary supraglottic cysts are always anterior to the glottic opening. The passage of a laryngoscope will improve the airway in supraglottic pathology.

A problem with insertion of a tracheal tube through a normal-looking glottis is always due to a subglottic stenosis or web, which is not easily recognizable at first laryngoscopy. If a rigid preformed neonatal Cole pattern tracheal tube (internal diameter 1.5 mm, external diameter 3.0 mm) cannot be inserted, then a tracheostomy will almost certainly be necessary. This will require oxygen and halothane to be administered with assisted ventilation holding the tube impacted through the glottis, onto the stenosis, and local infiltration of the neck with 0.5 or 1% lignocaine. If the larynx appears easy to intubate at the preliminary inspection it may be preferable to use an inhalation induction and short-acting muscle relaxant for intubation.

Once intubated, anaesthesia should commence with oxygen and halothane 2%. The larynx should be sprayed with 10 mg of lignocaine and any additional monitoring applied. When settled, laryngoscopy and bronchoscopy can be carried out on a spontaneously breathing patient, so that a full assessment of the dynamic status of the trachea and larynx is possible. During any hypoventilation or breath holding, assisted or controlled ventilation is carried out via the ventilating Storz–Hopkins bronchoscope. The 2.5 mm bronchoscope is difficult to use as a ventilating bronchoscope with the telescope inserted as a consequence of the high gas flow resistance. Laryngoscopy is performed during emergence using 100% oxygen and spontaneous breathing so that vocal cord movement may be assessed. If continuing temporary airway assistance is required then a nasotracheal or nasopharyngeal tube can be inserted and the neonate allowed to breathe humidified air and oxygen via a breathing system allowing controlled continuous positive airway pressure.

The infant

The older neonate, infant or young child may present with upper airway obstruction from congenital or acquired causes (Table 35.6). The diagnosis is based on the presence of stridor. Stridor that is positional and only inspiratory suggests a functional supraglottic cause, while unremitting inspiratory and expiratory stridor – often referred to as two-way stridor –

Table 35.6 Acquired airway obstruction in infants (congenital causes see Table 35.4)

Infective stridor
  croup
  epiglottitis
  diphtheria
  retropharyngeal and tonsillar abscess
  cellulitis – floor of mouth and neck

Trauma
  foreign body
  external trauma
  chemical and thermal burns
  intubation and instrumentation – subglottic oedema
  long-term intubation
    granuloma
    web
    cricoarytenoid fixation
  recurrent laryngeal nerve damage – cord palsy

Neoplasia
  laryngeal papillomatosis
  tumours – thoracic inlet or chest

indicates anatomical subglottic or tracheal obstruction. The degree of obstruction is largely a clinical assessment based on the work required to achieve adequate alveolar ventilation. The more effort required, the greater the use of accessory muscles, and the more compliant the chest cage, the more indrawing and chest cage retraction is present. Blood gases are well maintained unless there is a concomitant pulmonary problem as is frequently seen in laryngotracheobronchitis. As obstruction increases, more respiratory effort is required but eventually fatigue occurs. Serious hypoventilation with less stridor, less chest retraction and rapidly deteriorating blood gases supervenes. Urgent relief is required as hypoxia, apnoea, cerebral damage and cardiac arrest rapidly follow. Obstruction must never be allowed to progress to this state. Indicators of deterioration include reluctance to drink, a respiratory rate rising above 60 breaths per minute, a rising pulse rate, sweating, pallor and a poor peripheral circulation. Factors contributing to deterioration include dehydration and secretion retention.

Most infants presenting to the anaesthetist have mild to moderate airway obstruction and are referred for diagnosis by microlaryngoscopy, bronchoscopy, and treatment if appropriate. The surgical requirements are a still, oxygenated spontaneously breathing patient who can be maintained almost awake, and without laryngospasm, so that a careful assessment of tracheal collapse and of cord and cricoarytenoid movement can be made. The basic technique requires good topical anaesthesia of the larynx and a light inhalational anaesthetic. Premedication consists of intramuscular atropine. Good drying of pharyngeal secretions is essential, so that topical anaesthesia is effective, thus making adequate preoperative starvation mandatory. Sedation should be avoided. Induction with halothane/oxygen is satisfactory and once consciousness is lost the use of a tight-fitting mask and semi-occlusion of the *T*-piece bag achieves considerable raised airway pressure. Functional stridor will reduce or disappear, but stridor caused by a fixed obstructive lesion such as a subglottic stenosis will only improve minimally.

Basic monitoring which does not disturb the infant should be applied at induction and while anaesthesia deepens using up to 4% halothane/oxygen, additional monitoring and an intravenous infusion are established and a decision made whether to intubate using deep anaesthesia or muscle relaxant. If mask ventilation is difficult a muscle relaxant must not be used and if any doubt exists preliminary inspection of the larynx will indicate the safety of muscle paralysis. The larynx is sprayed using a metered dose 10% lignocaine spray with a maximum dose of 4–5 mg/kg. Pelton *et al.* (1970) reported on the safety of lignocaine in a dose up to 3 mg/kg, but over many years others have used the larger maximum dose with no clinically definable problems and excellent clinical conditions (Eyres *et al.*, 1978). Care with maximum dosage is more important in those under 1 year of age (Whittet, Hayward and Battersby, 1988).

A modest-sized plastic nasotracheal tube is inserted through the glottis which allows a crude estimate of subglottic size and maintains anaesthesia during transport, the setting up of the suspension laryngoscope, and preliminary assessment. On the return of spontaneous breathing, the tube is withdrawn to the nasopharynx, oxygen/halothane insufflated for any minor surgery and the patient allowed to wake up with the laryngoscope tip positioned in the vallecula while vocal cord and cricoarytenoid movements are assessed. The use of an injector attachment to the laryngoscope is unsatisfactory in children aged under 5 years of age, as the gas jet causes distortion to the glottis, ventilation is usually inadequate and a functional assessment is impossible. Bronchoscopy is carried out first if the primary lesion is likely to be tracheal and is only performed at the end if the laryngoscopy is negative. Bronchoscopy is contraindicated in the presence of a significant subglottic stenosis, as postoperative oedema may precipitate an acute respiratory obstructive episode. Prophylactic intravenous dexamethasone (0.25–0.5 mg/kg) is given and is helpful, although it has not proved valuable in chronic subglottic oedema. Nebulized racemic adrenalin (0.05 ml/kg of 2.25% solution) has been widely used but a standard dilution of adrenalin 1:1000 is also effective.

Diagnostic bronchoscopy is performed with the Storz–Hopkins ventilating bronchoscope as its optical and lighting system provides excellent clarity of view. The system can be readily sealed and used as a ventilating bronchoscope but, in the sizes below 5 mm, the antifog sheath must not be used as the gas flow resistance for both spontaneous breathing and intermittent positive pressure ventilation is too high. The sheath is replaced by a spacing block which prevents the telescope from projecting beyond the end of the bronchoscope. The 2.5 mm bronchoscope

has a high gas flow resistance with the telescope in position and its use in this mode is accompanied by considerable airway obstruction. This situation is only partially remedied using the newer slim line telescopes. Intermittent removal of the telescope and occlusion of the proximal end of the bronchoscope allows ventilation to take place.

An alternative is to use the telescope on its own, with spontaneous breathing, which is necessary anyway to establish a diagnosis of generalized or localized tracheomalacia. Much of the visual quality is lost if this bronchoscope is used without the telescope, with proximal lighting and a magnification lens, but it is sealed and can be used in a ventilation mode. Table 35.7 demonstrates the airway resistance measured in the smaller bronchoscopes. The tip of the larger size paediatric bronchoscopes is slightly elliptical, but as it must pass the cricoid ring which is almost circular in infancy and the narrowest structure in the normal airway, the larger diameter is the most relevant. Table 35.8 shows bronchoscope tip sizes and the appropriate size instruments for normal patients in the lower age group.

The alternative Negus bronchoscope cannot be sealed and is therefore used with spontaneous breathing or with the Venturi injector in a paralysed or deeply anaesthetized patient (Sanders, 1967). Magnification can be provided by the use of a small telescope which is mounted on a moveable arm. The view for diagnostic assessment is much inferior to that provided by the Storz–Hopkins bronchoscope, and it is now rarely used. The Negus bronchoscope is tapered with a wide bore proximal opening thus allowing the use of a high pressure injector jet and gas entrainment to ventilate the lungs. There is a need to restrict either driving pressure or jet size in smaller patients to prevent barotrauma to the lungs. In addition, overventilation with CO_2 washout and removal of inhalational anaesthetic agent can occur very rapidly. Bethune *et al.* (1972) recommended appropriate jet sizes for different bronchoscopes using a standard

Table 35.7 Storz-Hopkins bronchoscopes

Bronchoscope size (mm)	Gas flow resistance (cmH$_2$O/l per s)			
	Measured at 5 l flow		*Measured at 10 l flow*	
	Bronchoscope only	Bronchoscope and telescope	Bronchoscope only	Bronchoscope and telescope
2.5	42	1512	80	2700
3.0	21	40	30	65
3.5 (short)	12	16	15	26
3.5 (long)	12	34	19	39
4.0	8	20	15	25
5.0	6	12	12	18

Battersby and Ridley (unpublished data).

Table 35.8 Storz-Hopkins bronchoscopes

Bronchoscope size (nominal) (mm)	Internal diameter (mm)	Maximum external diameter (mm)	Age normal airway
2.5	3.0	4.0	Neonate
3.0	4.0	5.0	Neonate–6 months
3.5	4.6	5.6	6–18 months
4.0	6.0	7.0	18 months–3 years
5.0	6.8	8.0	3–8 years

pipeline driving pressure. Miyasaka, Sloan and Froese (1980) reported the use of jet injectors in both tapered and tubular bronchoscopes, and confirmed the safety of a 19-gauge jet in the smaller size Negus bronchoscopes.

The ability to change from spontaneous breathing to intermittent positive pressure ventilation and back again during bronchoscopy allows a full assessment of organic and functional pathology to be carried out quickly and safely. Neither anaesthetic technique is always entirely adequate on its own, but muscle paralysis prevents functional assessment and should never be induced until there is certainty that ventilation will be achieved.

Monitoring is all important and requires close continuous clinical observation, a precordial stethoscope, ECG, pulse oximetry and blood pressure measurement as a minimum.

Acute infective obstruction

Acute epiglottitis and croup are the principal acute infective causes of airway obstruction in childhood. They are of special importance because of their widespread occurrence and potential danger to life. The clinical course and management of both conditions is very different and is dealt with fully in Chapter 24, but there are important implications for anaesthesia.

Acute epiglottitis

Acute epiglottitis is less common than croup and is usually caused by infection with *Haemophilus influenzae* type B. The time course is acute and death from airway obstruction as a result of the hugely swollen and inflamed epiglottis may occur within a few hours of the onset of symptoms. Breathing is easier in the sitting position, but swallowing is difficult and painful so that the characteristic picture is of a child with rapid onset stridor, sitting forward and dribbling. Attempted diagnosis by awake pharyngoscopy is dangerous as it may precipitate respiratory arrest. Lateral X-ray of the neck is contraindicated in the acutely ill child. It may at times be helpful in the clinically stable child with a questionable diagnosis, but must

be undertaken in the intensive care unit or operating theatre where full facilities and personnel for airway rescue are present (Butt *et al.*, 1988). The clinical picture is so characteristic and may change so rapidly that urgent direct laryngoscopy under general anaesthesia and tracheal intubation are indicated in all patients once the clinical diagnosis is suspected. Any preliminary disturbing episode that may precipitate acute airway obstruction should be avoided.

Anaesthesia is induced in the sitting position with oxygen (100%) and halothane, as recommended by Hannallah and Rosales (1978). As consciousness is lost the patient is placed flat and positive end-expiratory pressure and ventilatory assistance are applied via a tight-fitting mask while an assistant applies monitoring equipment and sets up an intravenous infusion. Muscle relaxants must not be given. Tracheal intubation is carried out orally with a smaller than usual size tube of adequate length and rigid enough to manipulate through the oedematous supraglottis. The essentials are reliable and duplicate equipment, a range of tracheal tube sizes already checked and competent assistance. Otolaryngological, nursing staff and functioning bronchoscopes must be available as, although it is usually feasible to insert a tracheal tube, it is sometimes extremely difficult. Surgical opinion and possible bronchoscopy may be required if the diagnosis is found to be incorrect.

Oedema begins to resolve rapidly and within 10 minutes is frequently lessening or has been displaced so that the change from an oral to a long-term nasotracheal tube is always easier. The nasotracheal tube should be small enough to insert easily, the tip should lie at midtrachea and fixation must be satisfactory. The method described by Reid and Tunstall (1966) has proved reliable over many years. Sedation will be required initially and the most satisfactory drugs to use are nasogastric chloral hydrate or intravenous morphine, midazolam or diazepam. The dose ranges are shown in Table 35.9.

Most patients with long-term nasotracheal tubes who breathe spontaneously are attached to a continuous flow, humidified, oxygen-enriched circuit where a continuous positive end-expiratory pressure of a few centimetres of water can be maintained, otherwise significant pulmonary atelectasis will occur. If

Table 35.9 Sedating agents in intensive care units

Chloral hydrate	20–30 mg/kg	Oral nasogastric tube
Morphine		
infusion	0.5 mg/kg in 50 ml at 2 ml/hour	5% dextrose
bolus	0.1–0.2 mg/kg	Intravenously
Diazepam	0.1–0.2 mg/kg	Intravenously
Midazolam	0.1–0.2 mg/kg	Intravenously

secretions are minimal the management may be easier with a condenser–humidifier on the tracheal tube. Minimal sedation is required, the child is mobile and, if necessary, arm splints may be used to prevent self-extubation. Systemic dehydration must be avoided. Because of the rapid response to antibiotics and airway relief, oedema resolves rapidly and extubation is usually possible within 24–36 hours, so that there is no place for tracheostomy in the management of this condition.

Acute laryngotracheobronchitis

Acute laryngotracheobronchitis, or croup, is a viral infection of the entire airway, but its initial clinical presentation is stridor, with slowly increasing upper airway obstruction. The condition has a prolonged course and only a small proportion of patients need airway relief. Excessive airway secretions may be extremely difficult to remove by coughing because of their viscosity, dyspnoea and subglottic oedema. The increased viscosity reflects dehydration which occurs because of the rapid respiratory rate and unwillingness to drink. Early and adequate intravenous fluid replacement is an integral part of the treatment of this condition. If lower airway infection and secretions are significant then hypoxaemia may occur.

Indications for airway relief are clinical and are based on continuous close observation of the patient, assessing the respiratory work used to achieve alveolar ventilation. Increasing chest cage retraction, inability to cough, agitation, restlessness and fatigue are indicators that relief is required. Blood gas deterioration is a late feature so serial blood gases are usually of little help, although a falling arterial Po_2 due to peripheral lung secretions may indicate the need for earlier relief.

In severe cases, oral tracheal intubation under general anaesthesia relieves the obstruction caused by subglottic oedema and allows aspiration of retained airway secretions. A small dose of intravenous diazepam 0.1–0.2 mg/kg may be given at the commencement of anaesthesia if the infant is agitated. Oxygen/halothane is a suitable induction agent and assisted ventilation quickly allows a level of anaesthesia where laryngoscopy is well tolerated. Visualization of the larynx is easy as supraglottic oedema is insignificant, but the subglottis may cause considerable resist-

ance to the passage of even a very small bore tube. It is essential that a variety of tube sizes of adequate length is available and that the tubes can be made stiffer by the use of a semi-rigid tube introducer.

The use of a short-acting muscle relaxant is contraindicated. The principle of not giving short-acting muscle relaxants to patients with airway obstruction until it is known with absolute certainty that the airway can be secured, must be followed at all times. There is no exception. After initial clearance of airway secretions the oral tube is changed to a nasotracheal tube of correct size and length which is fixed in position. The nasotracheal tube must be several sizes smaller than would be used for routine anaesthesia and preferably should allow a small air leak when positive pressure is applied. Resolution of laryngotracheobronchitis is slow so that intubation is likely to be necessary for several days. Antibiotics may be required for lower airway infection. Sedation, physiotherapy and good hydration are essential and the nursing management of the intubated patient must be of a high standard. A small percentage of patients will eventually require a tracheostomy because of significant intubation trauma or the development of severe subglottic narrowing (McEniery *et al.*, 1991).

Microlaryngeal surgery

The suspension laryngoscope allows a number of surgical procedures to be carried out on the larynx, usually without a preliminary tracheostomy. Anaesthesia must take place with the patient's airway shared and the anaesthetic airway not obtrusive in the glottis. This is difficult in the small child where the glottic diameter may only be 5–8 mm. A number of techniques has proved satisfactory, although none is devoid of problems.

Tracheal anaesthesia and insufflation

Spontaneous breathing with deep inhalational anaesthesia, using halothane or isoflurane is combined with topical anaesthesia of the larynx. A small-sized tracheal tube is positioned either anteriorly or posteriorly in the glottis, while the major part of the surgical procedure is carried out, and is then withdrawn to the pharynx for the final part of the operation. The disadvantages are some obstruction to the surgical field initially and no control of ventilation latterly, but in practice the technique is very satisfactory for relatively short procedures on the glottis even in very small infants. No special equipment is required.

High pressure jet ventilation

This is a derivative of the Sanders bronchoscopic jet ventilation, but as there is no tapered tube there is no Venturi effect and so little gas entrainment. The jet is pressurized at 30–60 psi (207–413 kPa) and a near normal ventilatory rate is used. The injector jet system has been shown to maintain satisfactory blood gases (Spoerel and Greenway, 1973) and can be used for a relatively long period of time. Deep anaesthesia is necessary initially with topical anaesthesia to the larynx and complete muscle paralysis throughout the procedure. Anaesthesia may need to be maintained by intravenous supplementation with propofol. The jet can be sited on the laryngoscope blade 1–2 cm above the larynx, but this is not always satisfactory in the lower age groups. It is difficult to maintain alignment with the trachea as glottic distortion occurs, surgery may interfere with ventilation or blood and debris may be blown into the trachea. The jet may also be sited in the midtrachea as described by Benjamin and Gronow (1979). The 'Ben-jet' has four small soft side flanges near the tip so that the jet is maintained in the midtracheal diameter thus avoiding damage to the tracheal mucosa and recoil as the jet is pressurized. The paediatric tube is 16G and measured at 5 cm. It has been found satisfactory in infants over 3 years of age, but its flammability makes it unsuitable for use with the laser. This size of jet requires a driving pressure well below standard compressed gas pipeline pressure and there is a number of devices available which allow adjustment of the driving pressure. A fine bore intratracheal metal jet can be used with the laser, but it requires careful placement and fixation to avoid damage to the tracheal mucosa. It is essential that the peak jet pressure is not too high and that the expiratory phase, which takes place through the glottis, is not obstructed at any time.

Muscle relaxation must be fully maintained during the procedure to avoid the danger of sudden unexpected glottic closure, and the operative procedure must not occlude the glottis at any time. Failure to observe these provisos has resulted in serious barotrauma to the lungs with bilateral pneumothoraces and mediastinal emphysema. This technique should only be used by an experienced team because of the potential for serious complications.

High frequency jet ventilation

The use of high frequency positive pressure (jet) ventilation has been reviewed by Sjöstrand (1980).

The technique has been used for laryngoscopy and bronchoscopy (Eriksson and Sjöstrand, 1977) and has been administered by a transglottic insufflation catheter (Borg, Eriksson and Sjöstrand, 1980) and via a percutaneous transtracheal catheter (Klain and Smith, 1977), thus avoiding any glottic tube.

The advantages of high frequency positive pressure ventilation are the reduced risk of barotrauma as the peak inspiratory pressure is usually below that required for conventional positive pressure ventilation, improved intrapulmonary gas distribution, and, as there is no entrainment, the delivered gas mixture can be precisely controlled. However, as expiration is continuous and takes place around the catheter or endoscope an open glottis is essential and full muscle paralysis must be maintained at all times. Obstructive pulmonary disease is probably a contraindication to its use because of the risk of serious gas trapping. Borg, Eriksson and Sjöstrand (1980) recommended a frequency of 60 breaths per minute with a fixed inspiratory time of 22%. Much higher frequencies have been used, although there seems little advantage in their use during laryngeal surgery. Carbon dioxide elimination is influenced mainly by the absolute tidal volume rather than the frequency or inspiratory/expiratory (I/E) ratio (Rouby et al., 1985). However, intrapulmonary gas trapping or positive end-expiratory pressure increases with an increase in inspiratory/expiratory ratio, driving pressure and frequency. End-expiratory pressure may be measured and correlates with increasing pulmonary volume (Bourgain et al., 1990). Avoidance of excessive gas trapping at very high frequencies is likely to result in CO_2 retention as the absolute tidal volume will be reduced. This technique requires the use of a specially designed high frequency jet ventilator and most now incorporate an airway pressure measurement facility which automatically stops the fresh gas flow if the airway pressure rises due to obstructed expiration. If the high frequency jet ventilator is used for any length of time there is a potential for major changes in $P_{a}CO_2$. As chest movement, the traditional clinical method of assessment of ventilation is not present, both $P_{a}CO_2$ and oxygen saturation should be measured.

Lindahl, Yates and Hatch (1987) have demonstrated a close relationship between arterial ($P_{a}CO_2$) and end-tidal CO_2 ($P_{ET}CO_2$) in normal infants and children. Measurement of end-tidal CO_2 during high frequency jet ventilation is achieved by intermittent disruption of ventilation so that an end-tidal sample is obtained. This technique requires a sampling port within the lower trachea. Dhara and Butler (1992) achieved this by the use of a triple lumen vascular access catheter placed in the trachea as the high frequency jet, with pressure and CO_2 measurement ports.

High frequency jet ventilation in children is an area where transcutaneous CO_2 measurement may be a more satisfactory means of assessing adequacy of ventilation than end-tidal sampling and as an alternative to direct arterial sampling.

Specific conditions

Choanal atresia

Bilateral choanal atresia may be membranous or bony, but in either case, nasal breathing is completely obstructed.

The neonate alternates between normal crying and rest which results in cyanosis and apnoea as breathing becomes obstructed. Temporary relief is obtained by insertion of a small plastic airway which can be strapped in position until surgical relief is obtained. During this period orogastric tube feeding is necessary as the baby cannot feed and breathe.

Anaesthesia consists of awake intubation in the neonate if there is likely to be difficulty in the procedure because of associated anomalies such as the Charge association. A kink-proof tube under a tongue blade is used as the approach is similar to that for a tonsillectomy. Maintenance with nitrous oxide and oxygen and a muscle relaxant such as atracurium or vecuronium with intermittent positive pressure ventilation using a *T*-piece and bag is satisfactory. Monitoring and temperature maintenance are necessary. The approach is usually to drill from the nose through the posterior choanae using a shielded dental drill, until an adequate-sized dilator can be passed into the pharynx. More rarely a transpalatal approach is used and this may involve blood loss of a magnitude that requires replacement. Splints made from a plastic nasal tracheal tube are inserted into each nostril and fixed in position with a heavy nylon tie around the nasal septum. They are left in position for about 6 weeks. These provide a patent nasal airway so that termination of anaesthesia should be trouble-free. Dilatation of the posterior choanae may be required after the splints have been removed.

Supraglottic cysts

These are rare and are usually single but may be multiple in association with cystic hygroma. Single cysts are always anterior and may present with episodes of airway obstruction in between periods of apparent normality, but they can nearly always be seen on a good quality lateral X-ray of the neck. The surgical treatment is to deroof the cyst and marsupialize the base which is frequently wide and usually in the vallecula. This is undertaken using the suspension laryngoscope and tracheal anaesthesia. Inhalational anaesthesia with oxygen 100% and halothane should be used and orotracheal intubation performed as soon as possible. This may be difficult with large cysts but the glottic opening is always found posteri-orly. In extreme difficulty the cyst may be partially aspirated with a needle attached to a suction unit. Once the larynx is intubated the area should be sprayed with topical lignocaine and, if practical, the tube changed to a nasotracheal tube as this sits in a better position when using the suspension laryngoscope. Anaesthesia may be continued with nitrous oxide, oxygen and halothane, but preferably with the use of a muscle relaxant and intermittent positive pressure ventilation as rapid complete awakening is required. Awake extubation is usually trouble-free and as tissue damage is minimal, postoperative oedema is unlikely.

Multiple cysts associated with cystic hygroma are unpredictable and range from small pedunculated cysts on the epiglottis and aryepiglottic folds to cystic tissue in the pyriform fossa, pharyngeal wall and tongue. Anaesthesia is managed as for a solitary cyst, but the surgical interference should be minimal and only to relieve obstructive symptoms. The more severe forms of cystic hygroma cannot be excised totally and some postoperative obstruction may persist so that rapid and complete awakening is required. Occasionally adequate relief is impossible and tracheostomy is required, but this will usually be associated with a major resection of cystic hygroma from the neck.

Laryngeal cleft

Patients with posterior laryngeal cleft are unable to achieve competent glottic closure during swallowing and so have frequent episodes of aspiration. The more extreme forms, extending to the upper trachea and oesophagus, develop severe aspiration pneumonias from very early in life. They are initially managed with a low tracheostomy and gastrostomy feeding and later have a direct repair via an anterior laryngofissure approach or a lateral pharyngotomy. The minor forms are usually not diagnosed until later because the recurrent bouts of chestiness are not initially attributed to aspiration. Direct laryngoscopy can easily overlook the defect as the superficial appearance of the glottis may be normal but a probe will readily reveal the deficiency of interarytenoid tissue. The minor forms that are associated with aspiration are closed by direct suture using the suspension laryngoscope and an anteriorly placed kink-proof tracheal tube under the laryngoscope blade.

Laryngeal papillomatosis

Laryngeal papillomatosis is caused by a viral infection, probably with a DNA virus of the papova group. Management depends on the extent of the infection and the degree of airway obstruction, and is based on the destruction of individual papillomas by burning.

In the upper airway this is most easily and atraumatically accomplished by the use of the CO_2 laser and in the lower airway by laser bronchoscopy or the use of a fibreoptic bronchoscope with an argon laser (Bailey *et al.*, 1992). Some of the more severe and intractable clinical states require a long-term tracheostomy for safe and adequate management.

The carbon dioxide laser is used with an operating microscope, the invisible CO_2 laser beam being marked by a visible helium neon tracer. The beam can be directed very accurately and the depth of tissue destruction controlled by a combination of power and exposure time. There should be minimal damage to the surrounding tissue so that there is little pain and oedema with good healing and minimal scarring (McGill, Friedman and Healy, 1983). Excessive use of the laser damages tissue beyond the papilloma and may result in permanent scarring and damage to the larynx. The use of the laser poses some anaesthetic problems, the principal difficulty being the ignition of rubber and plastic tracheal tubes, combustion being supported by both oxygen and nitrous oxide. The laser beam passes through gas mixtures which will only ignite, explode or decompose if a non-metallic solid object first absorbs the beam and produces heat. The beam is deflected and the energy scattered by metallic objects. The essential protective requirements are that all tracheal and tracheostomy tubes and injectors should be metal (Norton and de Vos, 1978), metal foil wrapped or made of laser-proof material. Reflecting impregnated plastic wrap is unsatisfactory (Sosis, 1989). All theatre personnel must wear protective glasses to avoid accidental corneal burns. The patient's eyes, mouth and exposed areas which could be accidentally burned must be protected by moist gauze swabs.

Anaesthesia can be maintained with one of several techniques but all require good topical anaesthesia of the glottis. A simple technique is spontaneous breathing with oxygen, air and halothane or isoflurane via a metal tracheal tube. The tube is withdrawn to the pharynx for the final part of the laser procedure to allow the posterior commissure to be treated. This is a safe and simple technique which works well in smaller patients. Alternatively, a muscle relaxant technique with ventilation using either a laser-proof intratracheal jet or a supraglottic laryngoscopic jet may be used, although the latter becomes increasingly unsatisfactory with smaller patients. High frequency jet ventilation using a foil wrapped multilumen tube has been described (Dhara and Butler, 1992). Lower tracheal laser is easily managed using a muscle relaxant technique and a ventilating laser bronchoscope.

Laryngotracheoplasty

Laryngotracheoplasty is the operative correction of a subglottic or upper tracheal stenosis. The patient will usually have a low tracheostomy which should not have been allowed to stenose and the chest must be as clear of secretions as can be achieved immediately prior to operation.

The surgical approach is through a small collar incision immediately above the tracheostome. The cricoid ring is enlarged or, if too abnormal or if the upper tracheal ring is stenosed, a costal cartilage graft is inserted. The trachea and cricoid are closed over a rolled silastic splint which is left in place for 6 weeks.

Anaesthesia consists of any technique using muscle paralysis and intermittent positive pressure ventilation. The glottis is sprayed with lignocaine and the chest cleared of any viscid secretions by the use of normal saline and suction. The most stable airway conditions are achieved by the use of a cuffed armoured tube inserted into the trachea via the tracheostome and taken through 180° to connect with the anaesthetic breathing system over the thorax. It is essential that the cuff is entirely within the trachea, otherwise the tube is likely to extrude during the operation. The tube tip must be clear of the carina so that both lungs are ventilated. If the baby is too small to allow the use of a flexible cuffed tube, a shortened preformed plastic tube provides a stable airway, but allows an air leak into the operation site and may allow tracheal aspiration of blood. The shoulders are placed over a sandbag and the neck extended. Extensive monitoring is required and should include a precordial stethoscope, an airway pressure gauge and ventilator disconnection alarm. Close continuous monitoring of the ventilatory state is essential. Electrocardiograph, blood pressure, pulse oximetry and end-tidal CO_2 monitoring should be routine.

Intravenous fluids must be continued postoperatively as the silastic splint, if too long, may sometimes result in aspiration. Chest physiotherapy is important as there is nearly always a short-term deterioration in the chest status with an increase in secretions. If a rib graft has been taken, a postoperative chest X-ray to exclude a pneumothorax must be carried out.

Cricoid split

Small infants who cannot be extubated due to laryngeal oedema and damage following prolonged intermittent positive pressure ventilation may have a single stage repair without a prior tracheostomy. Poor pulmonary function must not be the cause of extubation failure. The repair may be either an anterior split of the cricoid ring or the insertion of a small anterior rib cartilage graft.

The patient will already be intubated with a small size nasotracheal tube and anaesthesia is carried out with an anaesthetic gas mixture, muscle relaxant and intermittent positive pressure ventilation. Extensive monitoring is essential.

Once the cricoid ring is divided there will be an air leak from the operation site and ventilation may need adjusting. The tracheal tube will require changing to one of a larger diameter as this forms the postoperative splintage for the repair. It is essential that the tube is the correct length so that it is inserted well beyond the cartilage graft but is also well clear of the carina. Experienced nursing care is required postoperatively to prevent tube blockage or extubation and steroid cover prior to extubation is helpful in the prevention of oedema. The tube is maintained for about 5 days so that there is a continuing need for intensive therapy unit care.

Aryepiglottoplasty

Some 10% of infants with laryngomalacia have stridor of sufficient severity to benefit from surgical excision of redundant mucosa over the arytenoid cartilages and the aryepiglottic folds (Jani *et al.*, 1991). There is a reduction in night-time desaturation and a return to normal oral feeding.

Anaesthesia requires a spontaneously breathing patient with good topical anaesthesia of the larynx so that microlaryngoscopy can confirm the diagnosis and identify the major area of mucosal prolapse. The tracheal tube is re inserted and the mucosa excised endoscopically using microlaryngeal scissors. It is important that the posterior laryngeal commissure is not damaged so that adhesions or web formation are avoided. Extubation at the end of the procedure is usually uneventful with an immediate reduction in the degree of stridor.

Tracheostomy

The principal indication for tracheostomy in the infant is for the long-term bypass of congenital or acquired upper airway obstructive lesions while growth and corrective surgery take place. Most airway maintenance for respiratory support is managed by long-term nasotracheal intubation, but this may be changed to a tracheostomy in some patients with intractable cardiorespiratory or neurological disease where the duration of intermittent positive pressure ventilation is likely to be many months. Tracheostomy should be performed under tracheal general anaesthesia on a still, non-congested and oxygenated patient.

Oxygen/halothane or intravenous induction are suitable but a short-acting muscle relaxant such as suxamethonium should be avoided in difficult obstructive lesions, or if there is recent demyelination from neurological disease. If the subglottis is very narrow in the neonate, intubation may be possible using the rather stiff Cole pattern neonatal resuscitation tube (internal diameter 1.5 mm, external diameter 3.0 mm). Maintenance of anaesthesia can be managed by any method, but muscle paralysis and intermittent positive pressure ventilation ensures oxygenation and prevents venous congestion due to coughing.

The neck is fully extended over a sandbag in the small infant, but only moderately extended in the child as there is the risk of making the tracheostomy in the thoracic trachea. The tracheal incision should be vertical through the third and fourth rings without excision of cartilage. The tracheal incision can be opened by the use of plastic surgical skin hooks, so that insertion of the tracheostomy tube under direct vision is easy once the tracheal tube is withdrawn to just above the opening. The tracheostomy tube is tied firmly in place before the tracheal tube is finally removed. Nylon stay sutures on the tracheal wall either side of the incision help to open the trachea in the event of early accidental decannulation, although the risk of making a false passage into the anterior mediastinum is still considerable.

Conventional tracheostomy dilators are no help in this emergency situation in the small infant. The operation must be followed by a chest X-ray to check the position of the tube tip but, more importantly, to exclude a pneumothorax. The tracheostomy is initially most easily managed using a plastic tube, but after 1 week the tube may be changed to another type if more appropriate.

Foreign body

Inhaled foreign body is commonest in the 1–3-year-old age group and although a wide range of small objects has been incriminated, the most universal is a peanut fragment. There is frequently a history suggestive of inhalation and X-ray signs of obstructive emphysema or collapse. Bronchoscopic removal under general anaesthesia is performed in nearly all instances and involves identifying the nature and location of the foreign body, its removal with the appropriate type of forceps, and a check bronchoscopy to ensure that removal is complete. Adequate preoperative starvation and an intramuscular atropine premedication are essential prerequisites, induction of anaesthesia being by inhalation oxygen/halothane or a small dose of intravenous thiopentone. A short-acting muscle relaxant such as suxamethonium allows the application of good topical anaesthesia to the trachea and glottis prior to orotracheal intubation. Anaesthesia is deepened with oxygen/halothane up to 4% during spontaneous breathing, while the final monitoring is applied. Supplementation with isoflurane is satisfactory if preferred.

In theatre, the tracheal tube is exchanged for a bronchoscope and the foreign body is located. It is preferable at this stage to allow spontaneous breathing to continue with 100% oxygen and the appropriate amount of halothane to maintain a deep level of anaesthesia, but if necessary, ventilatory assistance can be carried out by ventilation through the Storz-Hopkins bronchoscope or use of the Venturi injector on the Negus bronchoscope. It is not unusual for several attempts to be necessary to grasp the foreign body and remove it up the trachea and it is usually necessary to remove the bronchoscope and foreign body together through the glottis. The bronchoscope must be reinserted to check that removal is complete. The combination of a stable base of deep inhalational anaesthesia and the ability to carry out intermittent positive pressure ventilation via the bronchoscope provides the anaesthetist with good control and allows the surgeon considerable flexibility in approach.

The exercise may be prolonged due to inexperience of the operator or difficulty in manipulating the available forceps to grasp the object. If the foreign body has not been removed within 45 minutes the procedure should be abandoned and rescheduled with a more experienced operator or different equipment. Bronchoscopy must be followed by efficient physiotherapy and usually a short course of an antibiotic. As several insertions of the bronchoscope may be necessary a possible sequel is the development of subglottic oedema and a single prophylactic dose of dexamethasone should be given and repeated if stridor becomes apparent. The intravenous infusion line should be kept for 10 hours to maintain hydration until a complete and uneventful recovery has occurred.

Vascular ring

Malformations of the aortic arch may cause compression of the trachea and oesophagus, although the malformation may not always be a complete ring. The most common type of defect is some form of double aortic arch. The degree of compression is determined partly by the type of vascular malformation present and by its severity. Symptoms are stridor, feeding difficulty and aspiration, and these are present at birth in 50% of patients, but nearly all have presented by 6 months of age. Diagnosis is by history, chest X-ray, echocardiogram and contrast oesophagogram, which should be performed in all patients, but great care is needed in the severely obstructed neonate in the first days of life where there is the danger of serious aspiration. Bronchoscopy is unlikely to alter the surgical management and, as it may increase oedema at the obstruction site, it is best avoided just before surgery. If a complex cardiac defect exists full cardiac assessment is necessary.

The operation involves division and sometimes reimplantation of the aberrant vessel or abnormal arch. Complete dissection of the oesophagus and trachea from surrounding fibrous tissue is necessary to achieve satisfactory relief. The more severe forms are associated with a localized tracheal malformation or tracheomalacia at the site of the compression and this results in some residual stridor which occurs in under 10% of patients. Incomplete surgical correction should be considered in cases of continued stridor. Bronchoscopy is essential to determine the extent of any tracheomalacia. Anaesthesia is managed with topical anaesthesia, oxygen/halothane and spontaneous breathing, so that segmental tracheal collapse can be readily identified, but as chest aspiration may have been severe, coughing and breath holding may require intermittent positive pressure ventilation to maintain satisfactory oxygenation. Occasionally, an undiagnosed vascular ring may present to the otolaryngology department for assessment of stridor in infancy.

Adenotonsillectomy and otitis media

The last decade has seen several changes in the surgical management of otitis media and pharyngeal lymphoid tissue hypertrophy. The apparent increased incidence of otitis media with effusion has led to surgical middle ear drainage by myringotomy, ventilation tube insertion and adenoidectomy at the earlier age of 1–2 years. The effective treatment of acute bacterial tonsillitis with antibiotics has resulted in a more conservative approach to tonsillectomy and a reduction in the number of older children requiring tonsillectomy for recurrent tonsillitis.

The 2–3-year-old child is at one of the most difficult ages in terms of the psychological impact of hospitalization and operation. The most satisfactory means of coping with this is a good rapport between medical and nursing staff and the parents, with as much ward involvement for the parents as is possible.

This requires effort, understanding, tact and patience in informing the more aggressive and insecure parents and encouraging the timid or apparently disinterested parent. Education should commence at the first outpatient consultation with information about hospitalization and operations in children. Several books are available to help parents discuss this with their own children and many hospitals produce their own advisory pamphlets. These should be available at the first outpatient visit, and an opportunity made for parents to ask questions relating to the operation and hospitalization. From the child's point of view the essentials are kindness, honesty and an attitude of calmness and security from all the strangers in whose care the child is placed. Hospital admission should be for the shortest time practical, with unrestricted visiting if a parent is unable to be resident in hospital with the child. A parent should be with the child soon after consciousness has returned after the operation, and there are certainly no medical grounds for restricting parental access after tonsillectomy. In contrast, the family needs to keep a sense of proportion and to realize that tonsillectomy is a significant operation, the patient will not feel well afterwards and is not helped by a large family gathering at the bedside on operation day. With a sympathetic and informative attitude on the part of all hospital staff there are few problems.

Many younger children requiring simple procedures such as myringotomy and adenotonsillectomy have signs and symptoms of acute upper respiratory tract infection on admission. Although there have been conflicting views on the safety of anaesthesia in the presence of upper respiratory tract infection, there is good evidence that a recent viral infection increases the risk of anaesthesia. Arterial haemoglobin oxygen desaturation is common both intraoperatively and postoperatively. There is increased risk of laryngospasm and particularly if intubation is required, a hyperresponsiveness of the lower airway resulting in bronchospasm (DeSoto *et al.*, 1988; Dueck, Prutow and Richman, 1991). Anaesthesia for elective surgery is contraindicated. A mild running nose of long-term duration due to vasomotor rhinitis, probably carries little risk. A careful history and clinical examination is essential in order to establish the cause of a running nose, if doubt exists the operation should be postponed.

The anaesthetic management for adenotonsillectomy is frequently difficult and requires an experienced anaesthetist if disasters are to be avoided. The requirements are:

1 A reasonable but safe level of analgesia and sedation
2 Quiet, non-depressed breathing with complete absence of airway obstruction during the surgery so that bleeding due to a raised venous pressure is avoided
3 The prevention of aspiration of blood both during surgery and afterwards by rapid awakening and the return of an active cough reflex
4 An adequate fluid intake must be maintained during the day without stimulating vomiting.

Myringotomy and ventilation tube insertion

These procedures are well suited to day admission. Premedication is not usually necessary although Emla cream reduces the discomfort of venepuncture. A mild non-emetic analgesic such as codeine phosphate or DF 118 may be given intramuscularly during the anaesthetic. Induction by inhalational nitrous oxide, oxygen, halothane or intravenous thiopentone or propofol, is suitable with maintenance by nitrous oxide, oxygen and halothane administered using a *T*-piece circuit. Airway maintenance using a laryngeal mask has proved entirely satisfactory.

Adenotonsillectomy

Adenoids are removed because they cause obstruction to the eustachian tubes and the nasopharyngeal airway. Tonsils are removed because of recurrent bouts of acute tonsillitis, peritonsillar abscess, or oropharyngeal airway obstruction. Serious degrees of upper airway obstruction are not uncommon. This may be aggravated by the presence of congenital maxillofacial and mandibular malformations such as occur in Treacher Collins and Pierre Robin syndromes. Disproportion may be present in other congenital disorders such as Down's syndrome and the mucopolysaccharidoses where there is also the risk of instability of the upper cervical spine (Skeletal Dysplasia Group, 1989). In some of these patients the upper airway obstruction may be associated with considerable anaesthetic difficulties in airway maintenance and tracheal intubation. Immediate postoperative improvement may be minimal.

Chronic upper airway obstruction may cause the development of the sleep apnoea syndrome with disordered central control of respiration and incoordination of the oropharyngeal musculature which may take some time to correct after removal of the obstruction (Guilleminault, Tilkian and Dement, 1976; Brouillette, Fernbach and Hunt, 1982; Bradley and Phillipson, 1985; Thach, 1985). Hypoxaemia and hypercapnia may cause pulmonary vasoconstriction with right heart failure (Macartney, Panday and Scott, 1969). In those rare patients where pulmonary hypertension has developed, tonsillectomy represents a significant risk. The preoperative status may be improved by airway support at night using a continuous positive airway pressure mask. Klein and Reynolds (1986) reported the use of continuous insufflation of the pharynx as a means of helping to improve the preoperative status of children suffering from the sleep apnoea syndrome. Catley *et al.* (1985) have shown that, in adults, postoperative disturbances of respiration and sleep are associated with the use of opiate analgesia and result in episodes of hypoxaemia. Oxygen therapy corrects the hypoxaemia, but not the respiratory disturbances (Jones *et al.*, 1985). There is every reason to believe that a similar state of affairs is present after adenotonsillectomy in children who have exhibited obstructive sleep apnoea and episodes of hypoxaemia may continue in the immediate postoperative period. It may be that failure to appreciate this has been the cause of some of the perioperative fatalities associated with adenotonsillectomy.

Preoperative assessment of the patient must include a history relating to airway obstruction and disturbed sleep patterns and this may indicate the need for night-time sleep desaturation studies. Patients with episodes of severe nocturnal desaturation should be examined for evidence of pulmonary hypertension. Bleeding tendencies in the patient or a near relative should be noted. Recent ingestion of non-steroidal anti-inflammatory drugs may cause a prolongation of the bleeding time due to platelet dysfunction. A minor degree of increased bleeding time which has little effect on an operation may be disastrous in an adenotonsillectomy and the operation should be postponed until the haematological status is fully assessed.

In no other operation is it so important to adjust the type and dose of premedication to suit both the preoperative status of the patient and the intended anaesthetic technique. Premedication should be regarded as an integral part of the overall anaesthetic management. Patients who have severe upper airway obstruction from adenoidal hypertrophy and a history of a disturbed sleep pattern should receive atropine only. The same applies to patients with less severe obstruction but coexisting maxillofacial deformities as these will not be relieved by surgery. Many children require no premedication. If children under 5 years of age require sedative premedication, trimeprazine and atropine provide reasonable sedation, are given orally and have a significant antiemetic effect. Emla cream allows pain free venepuncture and reduces the need for sedative premedication in older children. Adenoidal curettage may cause bradycardia and it is wise to give intravenous glycopyrrolate or atropine at induction if a vagal blocking agent has not been given.

Anaesthesia for adenotonsillectomy was traditionally carried out using ether insufflation and a Boyle Davis gag. The newer inhalational agents are unsatisfactory and have an inadequate safety margin for this technique. The introduction of the Doughty (1957) split tongue blade and compression-proof tracheal tube connectors has allowed orotracheal intubation to provide safe access for both surgeon and anaesthetist. Modern preformed plastic tubes are not always satisfactory as they may compress under the tongue blade if the tube is small or the gag requires excessive opening or traction in a patient with difficult oral access. In addition, they are frequently long and may predispose to bronchial intubation. An alternative airway may be provided using a reinforced laryngeal mask airway (Williams and Bailey, 1993). Once positioned it does not usually obstruct the surgical field, provides good protection against aspiration of blood, and may be left in position until recovery of reflexes. Maintenance with nitrous oxide, oxygen and halothane with spontaneous breathing is satisfactory in most patients, but it is a difficult technique if opiates have been used for premedication as irregular breathing and hypoventilation occur. Deep anaesthesia with palatal relaxation is then difficult to achieve and is followed by delayed awakening. This can be avoided by the use of a medium-duration muscle relaxant, such as atracurium or vecuronium, and positive pressure ventilation. Both spontaneous breathing and controlled ventilation have their advocates, both are satisfactory provided that the other aspects of the anaesthetic are adjusted appropriately.

Termination of the anaesthetic is the most critical time and one is faced with a choice of awake extubation usually preceded by coughing, straining and increased bleeding, or deep extubation with the possibility of aspiration, laryngospasm and hypoxia during emergence. In practice, children given only trimeprazine and halothane can usually be extubated deeply, regain consciousness very quickly and rarely exhibit laryngospasm. Patients given opiate premedication, thiopentone and halothane have a high incidence of serious laryngospasm if extubated deeply and may take a considerable time to wake up. They should always be extubated awake and this is more easily achieved with the use of muscle relaxants and minimal or no halothane. If there has been pre-existing serious airway obstruction or anatomical difficulty in intubation, extubation must only take place when fully awake.

Bleeding must be controlled, and the mouth, pharynx and postnasal space cleared of blood clot prior to extubation. This should be in the 'tonsil position' on the side and head down, so that any residual blood can drain out through the mouth and nose. Close competent supervision of the patient must be maintained in the theatre until emergence from anaesthesia is complete, with no bleeding, a good cough reflex and a purposeful response to spoken commands.

Traditionally pain relief following tonsillectomy has been by the use of intramuscular opiates given either before or during the operation. Some anaesthetists have used only oral analgesia such as paracetamol. This has frequently resulted in over sedation or inadequate pain relief.

Diclofenac given before the operation has been reported as a satisfactory analgesic for tonsillectomy (Watters *et al.*, 1988) and to produce a calmer and more wakeful child in comparison to those given papaveretum (Bone and Fell, 1988). This however has not been a universal finding and was not substantiated by Thiagarajan *et al.* (1993) who assessed the risk of perioperative haemorrhage as a result of diclofenac-induced platelet dysfunction. There is no convincing evidence that bleeding is increased in those patients given diclofenac.

The present position is that rectal diclofenac is a very useful addition to the drugs available for pain management in children undergoing tonsillectomy. It is particularly useful in those patients with a compromised airway where opiate-based drugs are contraindicated. Other non-steroidal anti-inflammatory drugs may be shown to be more effective in the future.

Restlessness during emergence from anaesthesia is not uncommon after tonsillectomy and is caused by pain which should be treated. Codeine phosphate intramuscularly is satisfactory, supplemented by a non-steroidal anti-inflammatory agent such as diclofenac which may be given rectally after induction of anaesthesia. Paracetamol is helpful when swallowing is manageable. However, continuing restlessness later in the day is much more likely to be the result of a combination of bleeding, airway obstruction or aspiration and should not be treated with analgesics. A careful clinical examination of the operation site and the patient's cardiorespiratory status is required. Blood volume should be restored, if indicated and consideration given to reoperation for bleeding.

The in-theatre blood loss associated with adenotonsillectomy has been variously reported as ranging from 5 to 10% of the circulating blood volume (75–80 ml/kg) with an occasional patient losing up to 20%. This means that, although few patients require blood, many come close to a volume loss which needs replacement. Continuing postoperative loss can be extremely difficult to estimate as much of the blood is swallowed. An intravenous cannula is an integral part of this operation and should remain *in situ* until recovery is clearly satisfactory. Crystalloid fluid should always be given to patients under 13 kg body weight. Older children manage very well without intravenous fluids, but the fluid balance status should be noted until there is no doubt about the adequacy of oral intake. Fluid should be given if minor bleeding continues, there is vomiting, excessive insensible loss in hot weather, or there are additional medical problems where fluid and calorie restriction is contraindicated.

The bleeding tonsil

The bleeding tonsil or adenoid bed presents one of the more high risk situations in anaesthesia. Most patients who require reoperation have never really stopped bleeding and a little more patience at the original operation would have averted the situation. The common error is to underestimate the blood loss which is difficult to assess as much of it is swallowed. The danger signs are restlessness, pallor, tachycardia, poor peripheral circulation and swallowing. A fall in blood pressure is a relatively late indicator of hypovolaemia in children. Vomiting blood clot usually means that a significant loss has occurred. Bleeding that has continued for 2 hours does not usually stop until clot has been cleared from the bleeding site and a decision to reoperate should be made before the patient's condition deteriorates. Blood should be cross-matched early and blood volume restored before operation with volume boluses of 20 ml/kg until the peripheral circulation is satisfactory.

The most important factors in theatre are usually technical as most mortality and morbidity occur through loss of control of the airway with aspiration, obstruction and hypoxaemia. Induction of anaesthesia should take place with the patient on the side with the head down, so that clot vomited in early induction is not aspirated. Because of residual seda-

tion and anaesthesia, loss of consciousness is readily achieved with halothane and oxygen. Intubation, which may require a smaller size tube than that used during the initial procedure, can be carried out using suxamethonium and cricoid pressure, after first visualizing the pharynx so that any obstructive clot can be cleared. Rapid sequence thiopentone and suxamethonium have been advocated, but thiopentone is contraindicated if hypovolaemia exists and there is little time to remove obstructive clot from the pharynx before hypoxaemia occurs. Ventilation via a face mask may precipitate massive regurgitation of clot from the stomach.

Important factors are the use of a technique which is familiar, to have adequate competent assistance and correctly functioning equipment with duplicate tracheal tube, laryngoscope and high level wide bore suction. Once the airway is secured and the lungs ventilated with oxygen the tracheal tube should be aspirated to remove any blood and a wide bore stomach tube used to clear the stomach. However, it is virtually impossible to empty the stomach completely of clot, and vomiting always occurs during emergence, so that extubation must be delayed until consciousness has returned. Postoperatively little analgesia is required and is contraindicated in the presence of a postnasal pack. Maintenance intravenous fluid should always be given until the following day. Continuing oozing demands that a full coagulation screen and bleeding studies are performed without delay if this has not been undertaken already, and fresh frozen plasma or platelets given as indicated.

The ear

Major ear surgery in the very young is confined to exploration of congenital middle ear atresia with reconstruction of an external auditory canal so that a hearing aid may be used. Older children may require a myringoplasty if infection has damaged the tympanic membrane, sometimes exploration of the ossicles, and more rarely exploration of the mastoid air cells to remove chronic infection or cholesteatoma and allow adequate drainage. Cochlear implantation is increasingly carried out in the young child as is the provision of osseo-integrated hearing aids.

The anaesthetic requirements are a stationary bloodless field so that an operating microscope can be used, preservation of the facial nerve, if necessary, by monitoring its function, prevention of tympanic membrane graft displacement by nitrous-oxide induced pressure changes in the middle ear, and prevention of postoperative vomiting.

Congenital defects of the ear

Defects in the development of the first and second branchial arches give rise to a condition known as hemifacial microsomia. Asymmetric hypoplasia of the malar, maxilla and mandible occurs and there is deformity or absence of the pinna, external auditory canal and middle ear. A further progression of this deformity known as Goldenhar's syndrome involves the cervical spine and the heart, the usual defects being a ventriculoseptal defect or tetralogy of Fallot. Treacher Collins syndrome is an autosomal dominant mandibulofacial dysostosis which includes mandibular hypoplasia, often severe, and malformation of the pinna and external auditory canal. Conductive deafness occurs in 40% of patients.

Exploration of the middle ear, followed by the formation of an epithelial lined external auditory canal allows a hearing aid to be used to maximize residual hearing. The use of osseo-integrated implanted hearing aids has increased. Some cosmetic reconstruction of the pinna is usually necessary and the surgery is likely to be staged. Although the anaesthetic requirements are simple, considerable difficulty may be experienced in airway maintenance on induction and awakening, and in tracheal intubation. This is because the oropharyngeal airway is narrow as a result of micrognathia and relative macroglossia due to posterior displacement of the tongue. Maxillary and palatal abnormalities may narrow the nasopharyngeal airway. The larynx is high as a consequence of the mandibular hypoplasia and mouth opening may be restricted.

Anaesthetic management requires careful assessment of any upper airway obstruction and avoidance of longer-acting sedating agents if any obstruction is present. Assessment includes the measurement of mouth opening which should be greater than 2 cm, and the prominence of the upper dentition and its occlusal relationship to the lower teeth. Plain X-rays of the head and neck may show cervical vertebral abnormalities such as fusion or hemivertebrae. Nichol and Zuck (1983) have shown that, if the distance between the posterior arch of the atlas vertebra and the occiput is narrow, extension of the head will cause anterior bowing of the cervical spine, which may lift the larynx out of view. Delegue *et al.* (1980) have stressed the importance of the maxillopharyngeal angle which is created by the intersection of a line along the upper teeth and one along the posterior pharyngeal wall. Angles below 90° are associated with inability to visualize the glottis by direct laryngoscopy, while angles greater than 100° are associated with easy visualization provided that the mouth opens.

A simple bedside assessment has been suggested by Frerk (1991) using a modified Mallampati test (Mallampati *et al.*, 1985; Samsoon and Young, 1987) and measurement of the thyromental distance. Patients in whom the posterior pharyngeal wall could not be visualized below the soft palate and who had a short thyroid cartilage-to-bony chin distance were likely to be very difficult to intubate.

In practice, it is nearly always possible to intubate orotracheally those patients in the younger age group, although a small percentage may present difficulties. Rarely, older children with these syndromes may be impossible to intubate by conventional means, but they can usually be identified by careful preoperative assessment, so that a decision can be made to use a different technique such as a laryngeal mask airway, a fibreoptic scope or a technique using awake intubation under local anaesthesia.

An inhalational induction technique with halothane is satisfactory and spontaneous breathing with a face mask is usually trouble free once an appropriate-sized oropharyngeal airway can be used. The use of continuous distending pressure will relieve minor degrees of airway obstruction. The laryngeal mask airway has been a major advance in airway maintenance in these difficult patients, either as the definitive intraoperative airway or prior to tracheal intubation.

Intubation requires a precise and careful technique with a range of tube sizes and laryngoscopes available. Visualization of the larynx is aided by a firm posterior push on the larynx provided this does not cause distortion, lateral displacement or glottic closure. The use of a semi-rigid gum elastic bougie is helpful in directing a tube into an anteriorly placed larynx. The head should be in a neutral position (Creighton, 1994). Elevation of the shoulders converts a difficult intubation into one which is impossible. The use of a short-acting muscle relaxant makes laryngoscopy neither easier nor more difficult. It does, however, place a finite time limit on the procedure before hypoxia ensues. Careful documentation of the technique used and degree of difficulty encountered must be kept as this may allow the use of a different technique on a subsequent occasion and help future anaesthetists when repeated surgery is required.

Once intubation is accomplished in the more difficult patients, anaesthesia should be maintained with a muscle relaxant, intermittent positive pressure ventilation and minimal supplement, so that extubation can be carried out with the return of full consciousness at the end of the operation and thus avoid postoperative airway obstructive problems.

Myringoplasty and cochlear implantation

Graft procedures on the tympanic membrane or operations on the ossicular chain are always carried out using the microscope and the requirements are a stationary and bloodless field.

Bleeding may be arterial or venous in origin and the poorest fields are most likely to be associated with venous bleeding. This will occur if the pressure in the internal jugular vein or superior vena cava is raised

(Figures 35.2 and 35.3), and the causes usually relate to poor anaesthetic technique such as partial airway obstruction in a spontaneously breathing patient, a high mean airway pressure in a ventilated patient, or abdominal compression. Careful positioning on the theatre table is essential to prevent venous obstruction from causes such as tight clothing, drapes or cables lying across the neck. There should be enough head-up tilt, 15°–20°, to lower the venous filling level in the external jugular vein well below the angle of the jaw.

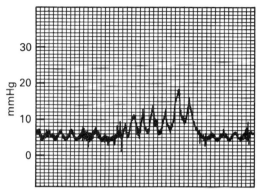

Figure 35.2 Venous pressure in the superior vena cava. Effect of moderate bag inflation of lungs in a 5-year old child

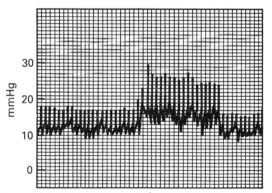

Figure 35.3 Venous pressure in the superior vena cava. Effect of operator's arm resting across the upper abdomen of a 15-month-old infant

Arterial bleeding has only a loose relationship with peak systolic pressure, although bleeding will increase with high arterial pressure and be less at pressures below 85 mmHg. Cardiac output increases with cardiac rate in children, until severe tachycardia occurs, and bleeding is always more significant if the rate is elevated. The damaging effects of a stormy induction with crying, coughing and straining, last up to half an hour or more due to increased catecholamine secretion, with a higher cardiac rate, arterial pressure and venous congestion. Heavy sedating premedication may be indicated if the patient is unwilling and apprehensive.

Anaesthetic techniques which provide an impeccable airway, no increase in mean airway pressure, a modest reduction in $P_a\text{CO}_2$, some peripheral vascular dilatation and a normal or reduced cardiac rate, will always provide satisfactory operating conditions if the patient is positioned correctly on the operating table. For the majority of patients there is little difference between a technique employing spontaneous breathing with any of the currently used inhalational agents, or muscle paralysis with *d*-tubocurarine and modest hyperventilation. Hypoventilation and obesity are better managed using a mechanical ventilation technique, as are operations expected to take much longer than 1 hour.

Any well-managed anaesthetic will probably produce a peak arterial pressure of about 85 mmHg measured in the arm at the level of the heart. This represents a lower cerebral arterial pressure depending on the degree of head-up tilt. The mean arterial pressure in the brain should be maintained above 50 mmHg.

Local vasoconstriction by the use of topically applied adrenalin 1:1000 is effective and there is little evidence of significant systemic absorption – this may be all that is required to produce good conditions.

Reduction of peak arterial pressure below 80 mmHg will usually require the use of a specific hypotensive agent. The choice currently rests between three such drugs.

Labetalol (Trandate)

This is the most satisfactory agent from the practical point of view and probably the only agent that should be used for ear surgery. It induces hypotension by blocking alpha-adrenoreceptors in the peripheral arterioles. There is also some concurrent beta-blockade so that compensatory tachycardia is avoided. Modest reductions in both pulse rate and systemic pressure occur readily and there is a synergistic action with halothane. Administration is by incremental intravenous boluses commencing with a dose of about 0.2 mg/kg repeated at 5-minute intervals until the desired effect is achieved. This will always be at a dose below the maximum of 1 mg/kg. As the mean duration of effect is about 1 hour there is no sudden rebound hypertension. However, postural hypotension may occur for some hours after the operation. Labetalol should be avoided in asthmatics as bronchospasm may be induced. Excessive bradycardia is responsive to atropine in increased dosage.

Sodium nitroprusside (Nipride)

This is a powerful direct-acting peripheral vascular dilator which produces a profound hypotension rapidly, but fairly transiently, as there is rapid conversion to cyanide and later thiocyanate which are inactive.

Its administration requires precision as it is a very potent drug and it should be given by a slow infusion syringe pump in a solution of 1.5 mg/kg in 5% glucose in a 50 ml syringe, starting at a rate of 0.2–0.4 ml/hour which gives a dose of 0.1–0.2 μg/kg per minute. Satisfactory control of the blood pressure should be achieved with a dose below 1–3 μg/kg per minute, and if this is arrived at by a very slow increase in dose, tachycardia and tachyphylaxis may be avoided. Doses above 8 μg/kg per minute lead to excessive levels of cyanide in the blood which inhibit cellular oxidative metabolism and lead to a profound metabolic acidosis. Cyanide and thiocyanate interfere with the metabolism of vitamin B_{12} (cyanocobalamin) so that sodium nitroprusside is contraindicated in vitamin B_{12} deficiency, poor liver function and Leber's optic atrophy. Blood pressure measurement must be carried out accurately and frequently because of the profound and labile nature of the hypotension. Direct invasive percutaneous arterial pressure monitoring is necessary.

Nitroglycerine (Tridil)

Nitroglycerine is a direct-acting peripheral vascular dilator which probably affects the venous system more than the arterial system. The main use is in adults as a coronary artery dilator. It is a safe, easy to use agent causing modest hypotension with few side effects at a dose of 1–3 μg/kg per minute and in children it is used as a peripheral dilator during cardiac surgery. Direct arterial pressure monitoring is advisable.

These three agents do not currently hold a product licence for use in children in the UK, although they have been used widely for many years in paediatric practice.

The indications for specific hypotensive drugs in ear surgery are minimal and their use must be carefully equated with the small but definite increased risk to the patient. Hypotensive drugs should never be used in an attempt to compensate for a poorly given general anaesthetic. If required, which will be more to reduce heart rate than blood pressure, labetalol is the most satisfactory agent to use.

Graft displacement

Tympanic membrane graft displacement is a theoretical and at times a practical problem if nitrous oxide is used for the anaesthetic. There is a 35-fold difference in the blood:gas partition coefficients between nitrous oxide (0.46) and nitrogen (0.013). After commencement of anaesthesia there is rapid diffusion of nitrous oxide into air-containing body cavities, reaching a peak in about 30 minutes. The body cavity either undergoes distension, or if non-distensile is subject to a significant increase in pressure. The middle ear will intermittently lower this pressure a little by discharge through the eustachian tube if it is patent. When nitrous oxide is withdrawn middle ear pressure will become negative once the cavity is closed and this may cause displacement of an underlay graft. To avoid this, nitrous oxide should be withdrawn 20 minutes before the middle ear is closed, and anaesthesia continued with oxygen or oxygen/air, and an increased dose of an inhalational agent, so that consciousness does not return. There should be a firm agreement between surgeon and anaesthetist about the use of nitrous oxide before the operation commences, so that the anaesthetic can be planned in a rational manner.

Fluid and electrolyte balance

Infants and small children have a high metabolic rate and therefore a high calorie and water turnover so that prolonged periods of fluid deprivation are not well tolerated. There is evidence that the postoperative well-being of patients is better if fluid depletion is avoided. All patients coming to theatre suffer some withholding of food and fluid because of the danger of vomiting or regurgitating and aspirating gastric contents during general anaesthesia. This is particularly important in otolaryngological surgery because of the site of the operation and the frequent application of topical anaesthesia to the larynx. No food is given for 6 hours before anaesthesia, but clear fluids may be given up to 3–4 hours before the operation (Welborn *et al.*, 1993). These times will sometimes be longer because of variations in the operating schedule, but should not be shorter.

Following tonsillectomy, fluid intake may be delayed because of pain on swallowing, and after ear surgery, there is a high incidence of vestibular disturbance resulting in nausea or vomiting. Antiemetic drugs induce drowsiness and this may cause delay in adequate oral intake. Infants with serious airway obstruction are always likely to have a significant fluid deficit particularly if nasogastric tube feeding has not been commenced. Many infants and young children are likely to suffer significant fluid depletion during the first 12 hours postoperatively and benefit from intravenous fluid replacement. Serious electrolyte disturbances are unlikely so that the principal concern is a satisfactory fluid maintenance regimen.

Normal daily requirements of fluid and electrolytes

Many methods have been used for calculating daily water requirements based on either body weight or surface area. For practical purposes the information must be simple and prescribed in terms such that nursing staff can readily relate it to the moment-to-moment management of an intravenous burette infusion. For this reason prescriptions should be in millilitres per hour derived from basic data in millilitres per kilogram per hour, although calculations dealing with major fluid and electrolyte imbalances should be based on 24-hour estimations. Basic water requirements for healthy non-surgical infants are shown in Table 35.10.

Table 35.10 Normal daily water requirements

Days of age	ml/kg per hour	ml/kg per day
Neonate		
1	2	50
5	4	100
10	6	150
15	6–7.5	150–180
Infants and children		
Body weight (kg)		
2	7.5	180
5	6	150
10	5	120
15	4	100
20	3	75
25	2.5	60
40	2	50

Carbohydrate

The infant metabolic rate is nearly twice that of the adult and the glucose requirement is about 5 g/kg per day. This can be supplied if all the daily maintenance fluid contains 5% glucose. Underweight neonates with little carbohydrate reserves tend to become hypoglycaemic with glucose levels below 1.7 mmol/l (30 mg%). If levels below this are maintained for several hours in full-term neonates, severe cortical neuronal damage is likely and non-specific symptoms such as fits, twitching and apnoea may occur. If oral or nasogastric feeding cannot be instituted glucose 10% should be given until blood glucose levels are satisfactory, although excessive amounts may cause an osmotic diuresis especially in the preterm baby. Routine 6-hourly blood glucose estimations are required in the at-risk group.

Early reports of hypoglycaemia associated with preoperative starvation have not been substantiated (Nilsson *et al.*, 1984; Redfern, Addison and Meakin, 1986). It seems that infants will not become hypoglycaemic provided preoperative starvation is not excessive and oral intake commences within 4 hours of surgery. Prolonged withholding of food due to swallowing difficulties, vomiting, increased demand as a result of pyrexia, glycogen storage disorders or diabetes, require that an appropriate intravenous fluid containing glucose is given.

Sodium

The daily requirement of sodium in the neonate is about 1–2 mmol/kg per day, and this requirement will be met if daily maintenance fluid contains one-fifth normal saline. Surgery in the adult increases aldosterone secretion and thus some sodium retention. Studies in children show no increase in aldosterone secretion for moderate surgery which will include most otolaryngological surgery, although increased aldosterone secretion is seen after major abdominal surgery. Gastric secretion in infancy has a higher sodium content than in the adult and gastrointestinal fluid loss must be replaced with normal saline.

Insensible fluid loss from the skin has a sodium content equivalent to one-third normal saline, but fluid lost through the respiratory tract is only water.

Potassium

The daily requirement of potassium is about 0.5–1 mmol/kg per day. Ninety-eight per cent of total body potassium is intracellular and serum potassium more often reflects pH than total body potassium content. There is an obligatory daily renal loss of potassium and additional loss in gastric aspirate or diarrhoea. Respiratory alkalosis will depress serum potassium and this may be important for cardiac rhythm if operative or postoperative hyperventilation occurs in a dehydrated infant. Routine postoperative fluid comprising one-fifth normal Hartman's solution and 5% glucose contains 1 mmol/l of potassium, but if intravenous fluid is required beyond 24 hours this will need to be increased by the addition of 0.5 g KCl to 500 ml of intravenous fluid (13.4 mmol KCl/l). Quantities greatly in excess of this will be needed if there is a large potassium loss, which is unlikely to occur in otolaryngological practice. If serum potassium remains persistently below 3 mmol/l additional KCl at the rate of 0.5–1 mmol per hourly fluid volume may be safely given until the serum level reaches 3.5 mmol/l, provided that there is ECG monitoring, adequate urine output and careful control of the intravenous infusion rate.

Calcium

Hypocalcaemia may occur in the first days of life probably as a result of immaturity of the parathyroid glands. Slightly later hypocalcaemia may occur in babies fed on cows' milk which has a high phosphate content and so precipitates insoluble calcium phosphates in the gut. Hypocalcaemia may present with non-specific neurological irritability and fits such as are seen in hypoglycaemia. Treatment with calcium gluconate (1 mg/kg of 20% calcium gluconate as bolus) is required if there are symptoms or a serum ionized calcium level below 0.7 mmol/l. A calcium level above 0.3 mmol/l is adequate for blood clotting and above 0.5 mmol/l for efficient myocardial contractility. Problems with calcium are unlikely to occur in otolaryngological practice outside the neonatal age group.

Intraoperative fluids

Intraoperative fluid may be given as intravascular volume replacement in the form of blood, plasma or other colloid, or as extracellular fluid replacement in the form of water containing electrolytes. Both may be necessary.

Intravascular replacement

Intraoperative blood loss of 10% or less of the calculated circulating blood volume (Table 35.11) does not require blood replacement unless the haemoglobin is below 1.24 mmol/l (8 g/dl) or considerable postoperative loss is anticipated. Losses of 20% or over should be replaced with whole blood or equivalent with an additional allowance of 5 ml/kg. Further volume will be required if postoperative loss continues. With a loss between 10 and 20% blood replacement will only be indicated if the haemoglobin is below 1.71 mmol/l (11 g/dl), significant postoperative loss is anticipated, or further staged surgery is to follow shortly. Otherwise appropriate volume replacement should be carried out using a colloid substitute or plasma. High haematocrit blood products must be used with great care so that high haemoglobin levels are avoided.

Table 35.11 **Average blood volume**

Age	Blood volume (ml/kg)
Newborn	80–85
6 weeks–2 years	75–80
2 years–15 years	70–75

Crystalloid replacement

The fluid maintenance requirement under anaesthesia has been estimated at 3–4 ml/kg per hour. An additional factor which adds to this amount is the use of dry gas which requires humidification in the patient's upper airway. An additional water content of about 2.5 ml/l of minute ventilation per hour is required to saturate gas in a non-rebreathing system.

Translocation of extracellular fluid into areas where it is removed from effective circulation occurs in the first few hours of surgery. The quantities are extremely variable depending on the site of surgery and the degree of manipulation and trauma involved, but range from 1 ml/kg per hour in minor surgery which will include most otolaryngological procedures, to 10 ml/kg per hour in upper abdominal surgery.

Incompletely corrected preoperative loss is likely to be minimal in otolaryngology except in the case of emergency relief of airway obstruction where pre-existing fluid deficits may be considerable.

Usually in otolaryngology, if maintenance fluid is given, then little more than basic requirements are necessary and a one-fifth normal saline solution in 5% glucose is satisfactory.

Postoperative fluid

The minimum fluid requirements for the first 24–48 hours postoperatively are a similar volume to the intraoperative requirements, namely 3–4 ml/kg per hour. This quantity requires to be increased depending on environmental factors such as temperature, humidity, pyrexia, airway obstruction and the use of infrared heaters, which all affect the insensible loss, sometimes considerably. Additional volumes of the appropriate electrolyte content are required to make up gastrointestinal loss. Maintenance fluid should be given as 5% glucose in one-fifth Ringer's lactate solution or a similar solution. In the presence of continuing pyrexia, sweating and acidosis, two-fifths of the volume should be Ringer's lactate solution. If hydration is satisfactorily maintained then an average urine output of 0.3–0.5 ml/kg per hour in the neonate and 0.5–1 ml/kg per hour in the infant should be achieved readily without recourse to diuretics. Early return to oral feeding should be possible after most otolaryngological surgery.

References

ATKINSON, R. S. (1982) Anaesthesia for day-case surgery. In: *Recent Advances in Anaesthesia and Analgesia*, edited by R. S. Atkinson and C. Langton–Hewer. Edinburgh: Churchill Livingstone. vol. 14, pp. 81–88

BAILEY, A. G., VALLEY, R. D., AZIZKHAN, R. G. and WOOD, R. E. (1992) Anaesthetic management of infants requiring endobronchial argon laser surgery. *Canadian Journal of Anaesthesia*, **39**, 590–593

BENJAMIN, B. and GRONOW, D. (1979) A new tube for microlaryngeal surgery. *Anaesthesia and Intensive Care*, **7**, 258–263

BETHUNE, D. W., COLLIS, J. M., BURBRIDGE, N. J. and FORSTER, D. M. (1972) Bronchoscope injectors. A design for use with pipeline oxygen supplies. *Anaesthesia*, **27**, 81–83

BEVAN, J. C., JOHNSTON, C., HAIG, M. J., TOUSIGNANT, G., LUCY, S., KIRNON, V. et al. (1990) Preoperative parental anxiety predicts behavioural and emotional responses to induction of anaesthesia in children. *Canadian Journal of Anaesthesia*, **37**, 177–182

BONE, M. and FELL, D. (1988) A comparison of rectal diclofenac with intramuscular papaveretum or placebo for pain relief following tonsillectomy. *Anaesthesia*, **43**, 277–280

BORG, U., ERIKSSON, I. and SJÖSTRAND, U. (1980) High-frequency positive-pressure ventilation (HFPPV). A review based upon its use during bronchoscopy and for laryngoscopy and microlaryngeal surgery under general anaesthesia. *Anesthesia and Analgesia*, **59**, 594–603

BOURGAIN, J. L., DESRUENNES, E., COSSET, M. F., MAMELLE, G., BELAICHE, S. and TRUFFA–BACHI, J. (1990) Measurement of end-expiratory pressure during transtracheal high frequency jet ventilation for laryngoscopy. *British Journal of Anaesthesia*, **65**, 737–743

BRADLEY, T. D. and PHILLIPSON, E. A. (1985) Pathogenesis and pathophysiology of the obstructive sleep apnoea syndrome. *Medical Clinics of North America*, **69**, 1169–1185

BRAIN, A. I., MCGHEE, T. D., MCATEER, E. J., THOMAS, A., ABU-SAAD, M. A. and BUSHMAN, J. A. (1985) The laryngeal mask airway. Development and preliminary trials of a new type of airway. *Anaesthesia*, **40**, 356–361

BROUILLETTE, R. T., FERNBACH, S. K. and HUNT, C. E. (1982) Obstructive sleep apnoea in infants and children. *Journal of Paediatrics*, **100**, 31–40

BUTT, W., SHANN, F., WALKER, C., DUNCAN, A. and PHELAN, P. (1988) Acute epiglottitis: a different approach to management. *Critical Care Medicine*, **16**, 43–47

CATLEY, D. M., THORNTON, C., JORDAN, C., LEHANE, J. R., ROYSTON, D. and JONES, J. G. (1985) Pronounced episodic oxygen desaturation in the postoperative period. Its association with ventilatory pattern and analgesic regimen. *Anesthesiology*, **63**, 20–28

COGSWELL, J. J., HATCH, D. J., KERR, A. R. and TAYLOR, B. (1975) Effects of continuous positive airway pressure on lung mechanics of babies after operation for congenital heart disease. *Archives of Disease in Childhood*, **50**, 799–804

CREIGHTON, R. E. (1994) The infant airway. *Canadian Journal of Anaesthesia*, **41**, 174–176

DELEGUE, L., ROSENBERG–REINER, S., GHNASSIA, M.D., MANLOT, G. and GUILBERT, M. (1980) L'intubation tracheale chez les enfants atteints de dysmorphie cranio-faciales congenitales. *Anesthesia Analgesia Reanimation*, **37**, 133–138

DESOTO, H., PATEL, R. I., SOLIMAN, I. E. and HANNALLAH, R.S. (1988) Changes in oxygen saturation following general anesthesia in children with upper respiratory infection signs and symptoms undergoing otolaryngological procedures. *Anesthesiology*, **68**, 276–279

DHARA, S. S. and BUTLER, P. J. (1992) High frequency jet ventilation for microlaryngeal laser surgery. An improved technique. *Anaesthesia*, **47**, 421–424

DOUGHTY, A. G. (1957) A modification of the tongue blade of a Boyle Davis gag. *Lancet*, i, 1047

DUECK, R., PRUTOW, R. and RICHMAN, D. (1991) Effect of parainfluenza infection on gas exchange and FRC response to anesthesia in sheep. *Anesthesiology*, **74**, 1044–1051

ERIKSSON, I. and SJÖSTRAND, U. (1977) A clinical evaluation of high frequency positive pressure ventilation (HFPPV) in laryngoscopy under general anaesthesia. *Acta Anaesthesiologica Scandinavica Supplementum*, **64**, 101–110

EYRES, R. L., KIDD, J., OPPENHEIM, R. and BROWN, T.C.K. (1978) Local anaesthetic plasma levels in children. *Anaesthesia and Intensive Care*, **6**, 243–247

FRERK, C. M. (1991) Predicting difficult intubation. *Anaesthesia*, **46**, 1005–1008

GREGORY, G. A., KITTERMAN, J. A., PHIBBS, R. H., TOOLEY, W. H. and HAMILTON, W. K. (1971) Treatment of idiopathic respiratory distress syndrome with continuous positive airway pressure. *New England Journal of Medicine*, **284**, 1333–1340

GUILLEMINAULT, C., TILKIAN, A. and DEMENT, W. C. (1976) The sleep apnoea syndromes. *Annual Review Medicine*, **27**, 465–484

HANNALLAH, R. and ROSALES, J. K. (1978) Acute epiglottitis: current management and review. *Canadian Anaesthetists' Society Journal*, **25**, 84–91

HATCH, D. J. (1985) Acute upper airway obstruction in children. In: *Recent Advances in Anaesthesia and Analgesia*, edited by R. S. Atkinson and A. P. Adams. Edinburgh: Churchill Livingstone. pp. 133–153

JANI, P., KOLTAI, P., OCHI, J. W. and BAILEY, C. M. (1991) Surgical treatment of laryngomalacia. *Journal of Laryngology and Otology*, **105**, 1040–1045

JONES, J.G., JORDAN, C., SCUDDER, C., ROCI, E. D. A. and BARROWCLIFFE, M. (1985) Episodic postoperative oxygen desaturation: the value of added oxygen. *Journal of the Royal Society of Medicine*, **78**, 1019–1022

KLAIN, M. and SMITH, R. B. (1977) High-frequency percutaneous transtracheal jet ventilation. *Critical Care Medicine*, **5**, 280–287

KLEIN, M. and REYNOLDS, L. G. (1986) Relief of sleep related oropharyngeal airway obstruction by continuous insufflation of the pharynx. *Lancet*, i, 935–939

LINDAHL, S. G. E., YATES, A. P. and HATCH, D. J. (1987) Relationship between invasive and non-invasive measurements of gas exchange in anaesthetised infants and children. *Anesthesiology*, **66**, 168–175

MACARTNEY, F. J., PANDAY, J. and SCOTT, O. (1969) Cor pulmonale as a result of chronic nasopharyngeal obstruction due to hypertrophied tonsils and adenoids. *Archives of Disease in Childhood*, **44**, 585–592

MCENIERY, J., GILLIS, J., KILHAM, H. and BENJAMIN, B. (1991) Review of intubation in severe laryngotracheobronchitis. *Pediatrics*, **87**, 847–853

MCGILL, T., FRIEDMAN, E. M. and HEALY, G. B. (1983) Laser surgery in the pediatric airway. *Otolaryngologic Clinics of North America*, **16**, 865–870

MALLAMPATI, S. R., GATT S. P., GUGINO, L. D., DESAI, S. P., WARAKSA, B., FREIBERGER, B. *et al.* (1985) A clinical sign to predict difficult tracheal intubation: a prospective study. *Canadian Anaesthetists' Society Journal*, **32**, 429–434

MASON, D. G. and BINGHAM, R. M. (1990) The laryngeal mask airway in children. *Anaesthesia*, **45**, 760–763

MAZE, A. and BLOCH, E. (1979) Stridor in pediatric patients. *Anesthesiology*, **50**, 132–145

MIYASAKA, K., SLOAN, I. A. and FROESE, A. B. (1980) An evaluation of the jet injector (Sanders) technique for bronchoscopy in paediatric patients. *Canadian Anaesthetists' Society Journal*, **27**, 117–124

NICHOL, H. C. and ZUCK, D. (1983) Difficult laryngoscopy – the 'anterior' larynx and the atlanto-occipital gap. *British Journal of Anaesthesia*, **55**, 141–144

NILSSON, K., LARSSON, L. E., ANDRÉASSON, S. and EKSTRÖM–JODAL, B. (1984) Blood glucose concentrations during anaesthesia in children. *British Journal of Anaesthesia*, **56**, 375–378

NORTON, M. L. and DE VOS, P. (1978) New endotracheal tube for laser surgery of the larynx. *Annals of Otology, Rhinology and Laryngology*, **87**, 554–557

PELTON, D. A., DALY, M., COOPER, P. D. and CONN, A. W. (1970)

Plasma lidocaine concentrations following topical aerosol application to the trachea and bronchi. *Canadian Anaesthetists' Society Journal*, 17, 250–255

REDFERN, N., ADDISON, G. M. and MEAKIN, G. (1986) Blood glucose in anaesthetised children. *Anaesthesia*, 41, 272–275

REID, D. H. S. and TUNSTALL, M. E. (1966) The respiratory distress syndrome in the newborn. A method of treatment using prolonged nasotracheal intubation and intermittent positive pressure ventilation. *Anaesthesia*, 21, 72–80

ROUBY, J. J., SIMONNEAU, G., BENHAMOU, D., SARTENE, R., SARDNAL, F., DERIAZ, H. *et al.* (1985) Factors influencing pulmonary volumes and CO_2 elimination during high frequency jet ventilation. *Anesthesiology*, 63, 473–482

SAMSOON, G. L. T. and YOUNG, J. R. B. (1987) Difficult tracheal intubation: a retrospectve study. *Anaesthesia*, 42, 487–490

SANDERS, R. D. (1967) Two ventilating attachments for bronchoscopes. *Delaware Medical Journal*, 39, 170–175

SJÖSTRAND, U. (1980) High-frequency positive pressure ventilation (HFPPV): a review. *Critical Care Medicine*, 8, 345–364

SKELETAL DYSPLASIA GROUP (1989) Instability of the upper cervical spine. *Archives of Disease in Childhood*, 64, 283–288

SOSIS, M. B. (1989) Evaluation of five metallic tapes for protection of endotracheal tubes during CO_2 laser surgery. *Anesthesia and Analgesia*, 68, 392–393

SPOEREL, W. E. and GREENWAY, R. E. (1973) Technique of ventilation during endolaryngeal surgery under general anaesthesia. *Canadian Anaesthetists' Society Journal*, 20, 369–377

THACH, B. T. (1985) Sleep apnoea in infancy and childhood. *Medical Clinics of North America*, 69, 1289–1315

THIAGARAJAN, J, BATES, S., HITCHCOCK, M. and MORGAN-HUGHES, J. (1993) Blood loss following tonsillectomy in children. A blind comparison of diclofenac and papaveretum. *Anaesthesia*, 47, 132–135

TOO-CHUNG, M. A. and GREEN, J. R. (1974) The rate of growth of the cricoid cartilage. *Journal of Laryngology and Otology*, 88, 65–70

VESSEY, J. A., BOGETZ, M. S., CASERZA, C. L., LIU, K. R. and CASSIDY, M. D. (1994) Parental upset associated with participation in induction of anaesthesia in children. *Canadian Journal of Anaesthesia*, 41, 276–280

WATTERS, C. H., PATTERSON, C. C., MATHEWS, H. M. L. and CAMPBELL, W. (1988) Diclofenac sodium for post tonsillectomy pain in children. *Anaesthesia*, 43, 641–643

WELBORN, L. G., NORDEN, J. M., SEIDEN, N., HANNALAH, R. S., PATEL, R. I., BROADMAN, L. *et al.* (1993) Effect of minimizing preoperative fasting on perioperative blood glucose homeostasis in children. *Paediatric Anaesthesia*, 3, 167–171

WHITTET, H. B., HAYWARD, A. W. and BATTERSBY, E. F. (1988) Plasma lignocaine levels during paediatric endoscopy of the upper respiratory tract. Relationship with mucosal moistness. *Anaesthesia*, 43, 439–442

WILLIAMS, P. J. and BAILEY, P. M. (1993) Comparison of the reinforced laryngeal mask airway and tracheal intubation for tonsillectomy. *British Journal of Anaesthesia*, 70, 30–33

Volume index

Cumulative index

This index is intended as a general guide only of the main heading entries covered in the six volumes of *Scott-Brown's Otolaryngology*, and is not comprehensive. For more detailed treatment of a subject refer to the individual volume indexes.

Entries are indexed by volume, chapter and page number. Volume numbers are indicated in **bold** type.